Principles and Practice of PEDIATRICS

SECOND EDITION

J.N. SHARMA
Retired Professor of Pediatrics
Gauhati Medical College, Guwahati, Assam
NEIGRIHMS, Shillong, Meghalaya

Peepee Publishers and Distributors (P) Ltd.®

Principles and Practice of Pediatrics

Published by
Pawaninder P. Vij and Anupam Vij

Peepee Publishers and Distributors (P) Ltd.
Head Office: 160, Shakti Vihar, Pitam Pura
Delhi-110034 (India)

Correspondence Address:
7/31, First Floor, Ansari Road, Daryaganj
New Delhi-110002 (India)
Ph: 41512412, 23246245, 9811156083
e-mail: peepee160@yahoo.co.in
e-mail: peepee160@rediffmail.com
e-mail: peepee160@gmail.com
www.peepeepub.com

First Edition: **2014**
Second Edition: 2018

ISBN : 978-81-8445-246-4

PREFACE TO THE SECOND EDITION

In view of the rapid advances in medical science, all textbooks need to be revised and updated to include the latest information and recommendations. It is primarily to inform and serve the needs of the students as well as practitioners.

Besides a thorough revision and remodelling of all chapters, this edition of the book provides up-to-date information about the neonatal advance life support and some diseases in the newborn, respiratory diseases, viz., Pneumonia and Asthma, recent recommendations of treatment of infectious diseases like Malaria, Dengue, Tuberculosis and AIDS.

To complete any such work, you need the good wish and all round help of well-wishers. I must mention that my most important driving force is the students. Their appreciation and good words about the book was the sole inspiration for this revised edition.

I take this opportunity to express my heartfelt thanks and gratitude to Dr. Santanu Deb, Senior Pediatrician, Nazareth Hospital, Shillong, Dr. Anupama Deka, Professor and HOD, Pediatrics, Silchar Medical College, Dr. Gautam Medhi, Associate Professor, FAAMC, Barpeta for going through the newly written as well as the revised and modified chapters and good suggestions. My heartfelt thanks also to Dr. Ripon Debbarma, Assistant Professor of Pediatrics, Agartala Government Medical College, Tripura, for the photograph of the child in the cover.

Last but not the least I am grateful to Mr. Pawaninder Pal Vij, Director, Peepee Publishers and Distributors (P) Ltd. for taking the task of publishing the second edition of this book.

J.N. Sharma

PREFACE TO THE FIRST EDITION

Pediatrics as an independent subject was ultimately started and the first batch of undergraduate students of the Medical Colleges of Assam appeared for the final professional Part II examination with a full paper in Pediatrics including Neonatology in 2003.

A syllabus was suggested by MCI indicating the theoretical as well as the practical part. It was felt from the beginning that there should be a book available for the undergraduate students, on the basis of the syllabus. The books available are too extensive and faculty as well as the students of Gauhati Medical College expressed the need for a concise textbook for the undergraduate students.

The idea of such a book first came to the mind of the author when once in Kolkata for conducting postgraduate examination a request came from one of the senior professors of Kolkata Dr (Mrs.) Madhurima Lahiri to write a textbook on Pediatrics. The initiation was by preparing notes for the undergraduate students for theory classes as well as tutorial classes. The notes became popular among students as well as faculties and a request came for publishing the notes as a book.

This book is written primarily for undergraduate students and pediatric practitioners as well as for the postgraduate students who may use it as a revision book before examinations. While compiling the book, the author has followed the recommendations by the MCI and the education cell of IAP. However, besides the syllabus cited by the MCI, a few chapters as well as topics have been added with a view to give an idea about the status of these diseases in children. Inclusion of these topics may help the general practitioners to screen the children and refer at an early date to the appropriate facility. Students may ignore these chapters for examination purpose.

With the belief that illustrations are more helpful than only text, descriptions in the book has been supported by figures, photographs and X-rays as much as possible. Detailed chapters on pediatric oncology, common surgical problems and rheumatic diseases have been included specially to help graduate doctors and practising pediatricians to help in early diagnosis and referral.

Pediatrics is still a developing subject with ever changing concepts. Moreover, the diseases which are prevalent in our country are different than those in western countries. There is definitely a need for books which gives stress on the diseases and disease pattern prevalent in our country. The books written by western authors are definitely of high standard but befitting their country.

I am indebted to all the well wishers who encouraged me for writing this book especially my undergraduate and postgraduate students. Hope the book shall be of help to them. I take this opportunity to offer my heartfelt thanks to Dr. Shaumendu and Dr. Pradipta for being all along with me in the preparation of this book. I would like to offer my thanks and gratitude to Dr. N.C. Bhattacharyya, presently Professor and Head, Pediatric Surgery who went through the chapter of 'Common Pediatric Surgical Problems' and advised me for corrections. I am indebted to the faculty members Dr. Pranita Kalita, Dr. Nripen Pathak, Dr. M.N. Baruah, Dr. Ranjit Agarwalla, Dr. Chandrajyoti Bora, Dr. Rakesh, Dr. Pubali Deka, Dr. Vivek Choudhury and PGT Dr. Sujib, who went through the proof for correction.

Last but not the least I am grateful to Mr. Pawaninder Pal Vij, Director, Peepee Publishers (P) Ltd for taking the task of publishing this book.

J.N. Sharma

CONTENTS

1

Childhood and Maternal and Child Health Services

OUTLINES

What is Childhood?

The Government of India has decided to include children upto 18 years in the pediatric age group. Children upto 12 years constitute 40% and below 18 years around 60% of the population. India has therefore a huge number of prospective and productive populations to be reared with scientific methods to build them up into useful citizens. The child is never a miniature adult. Then how do children differ from adults?

Differences Between an Adult and a Child

1. Anatomy and physiology of children are different from adult. Childhood is a period of growth and development, both physical and mental, upto adolescence. The child is in a state of increase in size of body and organs and maturation of physiological functions.
2. The disease rate in children is two times that of adult. In the preschool period, the child in the developing countries, suffer atleast 3 – 4 times from acute respiratory infection and 3 – 4 times acute diarrhoea resulting in protein energy malnutrition leading to high morbidity and mortality.
3. Disease pattern is different in different age groups. The child suffers from a peculiar set of disease which is not seen in an adult viz. vaccine preventable infectious diseases. In addition, most of the inborn errors of metabolism as well as congenital malformations present during early childhood.
4. Disease presentation and therapy are different. Moreover, the same disease can present with different manifestation in different age group.
5. Drug doses in children should be calculated on the basis of per kg body weight or per square metre body surface.
6. Organs are immature and developing. The child therefore needs rational treatment to avoid side effects and damage to organs.
7. Special attention should be given to growth monitoring and nutritional needs and prevention of diseases. Nutritional disorders and recurrent infectious diseases, during childhood can cause gross physical and mental handicap.

Periods of Childhood

The childhood is divided into the following periods:

Newborn	:	0 to 28 days
Infant	:	0 to 1 year
Preschool child	:	1year to 5 years
School child	:	Above 5 years to 10 years (girls)
		Above 5 years to 12 years (boys)
Adolescent child	:	Girls 10 years to 18 years
		Boys 12 years to 20 years

Vital Statistics

Why Important?

Workers all over the world agree that the most important public health step would be institution of a proper statistical system. This applies to most tropical regions in the world. Without an adequate knowledge of disease incidence, suitable preventive and curative measures cannot be put into practice while there is no yardstick by which one can measure improvement or deterioration of the child health situation.

Ideally vital statistics should include stillbirth, neonatal, infant and maternal mortality rates as well as the incidence of low birth weight together with the mortality and morbidity within these groups. The most important of these are the infant mortality rate which is discussed in details.

Current Health Indicators in Infants and Children

Accepted definitions to express perinatal mortality and morbidity are essential to compare with other national and international studies. The definitions described below are those duly approved and adapted by the task force of National Neonatology Forum, India.

Early Childhood (1-4 years) Mortality Rate: It is defined as the number of deaths at ages 1-4 years in a given year, per 1000 children in that age group at the midpoint of the year concerned. It excludes the infant mortality.

Under 5 Proportionate Mortality Rate: It is the proportion of total deaths occurring in the under 5 age group. This rate can be used to reflect both infant and child mortality rates.

Gestational age: Gestational age is calculated from the first day of the last menstrual period till the date of birth and is expressed in completed weeks, e.g., 37 weeks + 6 days are considered as 37 weeks only. On the basis of the gestational age, a newborn is classified as follows:

Term: Babies with gestational age between 37 and 41 weeks.

Preterm: Babies with gestational age less than 37 completed weeks.

Post term: Babies with gestational age of 42 weeks or more.

Live birth: Live birth is defined as complete expulsion or extraction from the mother, of the product of conception (irrespective of the duration of pregnancy) and which after such separation, breathes or shows any other evidence of life such as beating of the heart, pulsation of the umbilical cord or definite movements of the voluntary muscles irrespective of the attachment of placenta and/ cord.

It needs mention that infants weighing less than 500 grams at birth should show signs of life for at least one hour before they are designated as live born.

Still birth: Intermediate and late fetal death are designated as still birth. Death at gestational age between 22 and 27 weeks or a fetus weighing between 500 grams and 999 grams or with crown heel length between 25 cm and less than 35 cm is called *intermediate fetal death*. Death at a gestational age of 28 weeks or more or a fetus weighing 1000 grams or more and crown heel length of at least 35 cm is called *late fetal death.*

Birth weight: It is the first weight of a live or still born infant which should be preferably taken within first hour of life or during first day of life before any significant postnatal weight loss has occurred. On the basis of birth weight neonates are classified as follows:

- *Low birth weight*: Birth weight less than 2500 grams irrespective of gestation.
- *Very low birth weight*: Birth weight less than 1500 grams.
- *Extremely low birth weight*: Birth weight less than 1000 grams.

Perinatal Period: Perinatal period extends from the 28th week of gestation to the 7th day of life.

Extended Perinatal Period: This period extends from the 22nd week of gestation (or > 500 grams) to 7th day of life.

In view of the increasing survival of the infants weighing less than 1000 grams as a result of improvement in the perinatal care, the concept of extended perinatal period has been introduced.

Perinatal Mortality Rate: It is defined as late fetal and early neonatal (first week) death of infants weighing more than 1000 grams (or 28 weeks of gestation or more) at birth per thousand total births weighing 1000 grams.

Neonatal Period: It is the period extending from birth up to 28 days. An infant up to 28 days is called a neonate. The first 7 days after birth is referred to as early neonatal period and the period between 7 days and 28 days is referred to as late neonatal period.

Neonatal Mortality Rate: The neonatal mortality rate is defined as the number of death per thousand live births in the first 28 days after birth.

Early Neonatal Mortality Rate: It is defined as neonatal deaths of infants weighing over 1000 grams during the first 7 days after birth per 1000 live births.

Late Neonatal Mortality Rate: It is defined as neonatal deaths of infants weighing over 1000 grams during 28 days of life per 1000 live births.

Extended Neonatal Mortality Rate: The extended neonatal mortality rate can be calculated by including infants weighing up to 500 gram.

Infant Mortality Rate

Definition

Infant mortality rate is the ratio of deaths under 1 year of age in a given year to the total number of live births in the same year; usually expressed as a rate per 1000 live birth.

Difficulties in Collecting Data

It is agreed upon worldwide that infant mortality rates quoted from the underdeveloped and developing countries must be accepted with considerable reserve, as they are often unreliable and incomplete owing to difficulty of ensuring the accurate collection of data.

Criteria for Accurate Collection of Data

Compulsory birth and death registration with well-organized health staff is the most important criteria for accurate collection of data, which is not available in most developing countries. Estimates of infant mortality in technically underdeveloped countries are, therefore, very approximate and often represent an underestimate.

Causes of Infant Mortality

Demographers describe the infant mortality rate as the most sensitive index of health and level of living of people of a country. It is given a separate treatment because:

1. Infant mortality is the largest single age category of mortality.
2. Deaths at this age are due to a peculiar set of diseases.
3. Infant mortality is affected rather quickly and directly by specific health programmes and therefore may change more rapidly than the death rate.

Infant mortality rate includes the neonatal mortality and the post neonatal mortality. Neonatal mortality rate has been further described as the early, late and extended neonatal mortality rates.

Causes

50% of infant death occurs during the first 7 days after birth out of which 60% occurs within first 24 hours.

Infant mortality which occurs within first 4 weeks is called neonatal mortality; that which occurs between 28 days and 1 year is called post neonatal death.

Table 1.1: Showing the causes of infant mortality

Causes of neonatal death	*Causes of post neonatal death*
1. LBW – Immaturity*	1. Diarrheal diseases
2. Birth asphyxia	2. Acute respiratory infection
3. Infection	3. Other communicable diseases
4. Congenital malformation	4. Protein energy malnutrition
	5. Congenital malformation
	6. Accidents

*Immaturity: Birth weight < 750 grams, hyaline membrane disease and intraventricular hemorrhage.

Factors Leading to High Infant Mortality

Socioeconomic Factors

The interrelationship between poor socioeconomic condition and high infant mortality is well-known. The mortality rate is higher in the lower socioeconomic group of the population as well as in the underdeveloped countries compared to developed countries.

Prenatal Factors

A significant proportion of the high infant mortality in tropical countries can be traced to maternal malnutrition and ill health during pregnancy which for practical purposes can be considered to produce three ill-effects:

(i) **Fetal malnutrition:** A woman with a pre-pregnancy weight of < 40 kg and height of < 145 cm, which indicates chronic protein energy malnutrition in the first 5 years of life and through adolescence, is at high risk of delivering low birth weight babies.

Fetal storage of minerals like iron and calcium and vitamins viz. vitamin A occurs during last trimester of pregnancy. If there are inadequate depots as a result of maternal deficiency, the store will be depleted early resulting in deficiency states in the child in the later part of infancy. Pre-existing malnutrition may be exaggerated, in the mother during pregnancy, by restriction of high protein diet as a food taboo or in the hope of producing a smaller baby in order to have an easy delivery.

(ii) **Preterm birth:** Prematurity along with all the functional disadvantages, is one of the most important causes of neonatal mortality. Complications during pregnancy, e.g., PET; APH etc. may lead to preterm delivery. Further, any severe acute illness during pregnancy may result in preterm delivery.

(iii) **Fetal infection:** Maternal TORCHS infections may be communicated to the fetus and may be responsible for death in infancy. Placental malaria, with no clinical consequences for the mother, can result in low birth weight neonates.

Natal and Neonatal Factors

A large number of deliveries still occur at home in our country as well as other developing countries. Unskilled and unclean obstetrical practices by untrained birth attendants are responsible in part for a high natal and neonatal mortality from dystocia, birth trauma and infections (umbilical infection, septicemia, neonatal tetanus). The dangers of labour are further increased by customary absence of antenatal care.

Post Neonatal Factors

Diarrhea often heads the list among the post neonatal causes. It is usually of infective origin associated with dirt, flies, contaminated water supply and faulty excreta disposal. The traditional tendency to treat such cases with prolonged semi starvation often leads to malnutrition or aggravates pre-existing malnutrition to severe forms of protein energy malnutrition and eventually death.

Acute respiratory tract infection (viz. pneumonia) is another post neonatal cause related to ill ventilated, smoky, housing and cross infection as a result of overcrowding. *Whooping cough* may attack young infants and prove fatal. *Tuberculosis*, spread by droplet infection, may lead to serious disease viz. miliary tuberculosis and disseminated tuberculosis during infancy. *Severe malaria* is an important cause of mortality in the latter half of infancy, in hyper endemic areas. *Neonatal septicemia, tuberculosis without meningitis, neonatal tetanus* are still important causes of infant mortality in many developing countries. *Congenital syphilis*, an important cause of infant mortality in many tropical countries is not so in India.

Protein energy malnutrition does not play a dominant role as a cause of mortality in the first year of life largely because most babies are breast fed in the first 6 months of life and they thrive well. However, in the latter half of infancy breast milk supply decreases, complementary feeding is inadequate; the child's demand is more and hence fails to thrive. The severe form of protein energy malnutrition viz. marasmus however, can occur in early infancy in the event of unsuccessful breastfeeding. This is more prevalent in the urban areas and urban slums especially under the influence of subtle suggestion of advertisements of infant foods. Another serious form of malnutrition of tropics (not in India at present) which can be a major contributor to infant death is *infantile beriberi*. This condition is still seen in rice eating countries of South East Asia and classically kills infants rapidly with convulsions and acute heart failure. Infantile beriberi is unique in that it is caused exclusively by maternal malnutrition, being due to low thiamine diet during pregnancy and lactation.

Measures to Bring Down Infant Mortality Rate

Under ideal condition of social welfare, no baby should die, except possibly the few who are born with serious handicaps such as congenital abnormalities or disorders originating in the intrauterine life. It is notable that only a multi-pronged attack will reduce infant mortality. To achieve a reduction of the infant mortality rate one has to concentrate attention on the following interventions:

1. Care of the girl child during the first 5 years, adolescence, and care of the women during

pregnancy and lactation to provide optimal health care, nutrition and health education. The girl child should have a normal weight and height for age during the first five years of age and during adolescence. This will help in adequate development of the various organs including the reproductive system during the adolescent period. Every parent should be advised a target of 40 kg weight and a height of 145 cm for their girl child at 18 years of age.

2. All pregnant women should have the requisite number of antenatal check-ups and proper screening for complications and prompt referral. All deliveries should be conducted by skilled birth attendants.
3. Promotion of exclusive breastfeeding and timely introduction of complementary feeding.
4. Universal immunization of child and mother.
5. Encourage family planning.
6. Efficient maternal and child health services.
7. Improvement of economic condition and standard of living.
8. Promotion of female literacy.
9. Health education, family life education and training on mother craft skills.

Maternal and Child Health Services

From time to time since independence, the government has come up with different maternal and child development programmes with the help of international agencies like WHO, UNICEF etc. The following programmes need mention:

1. Integrated child development services scheme (ICDS).
2. Child survival and safe motherhood (CSSM).
3. Reproductive child health (RCH).
4. Integrated management of neonatal and childhood illness (IMNCI).

Integrated Management of Neonatal and Childhood Illness (IMNCI)

The IMNCI (Integrated management of neonatal and childhood illness) is the ongoing programme in our country. Over the last three decades the annual number of deaths among children less than 5 years of age has decreased by almost a third. However, this reduction has not been evenly distributed throughout the world. At present, every year more than 10 million children die in developing countries before they reach their fifth birthday. Seven in ten of these deaths are due to acute respiratory infection (mostly pneumonia), diarrhoea, measles, malaria or malnutrition – and often to a combination of these illnesses.

Many prevention and treatment strategies included in different earlier programmes viz. ICDS, CSSM, RCH have already proven effective for saving young lives. UIP has successfully reduced death due to measles. Oral rehydration therapy has contributed largely to reduction of diarrhoeal deaths. Effective antibiotic therapy has saved millions of children with pneumonia. Prompt treatment of malaria has allowed more children to recover. A modest improvement in practice of exclusive breastfeeding has reduced childhood mortality.

While each of these interventions has been successful, accumulating evidence suggests that an integrated approach is needed to manage sick children to achieve better outcome. Child health programmes need to move beyond single diseases to addressing the overall health and wellbeing of the child. Because many children present with overlapping signs and symptoms of diseases, a single diagnosis can be difficult and may not be feasible or appropriate. This is especially true for the first level health facilities where examinations involve few instruments, negligible laboratory tests and no radiology.

During the mid-1990s, the World Health Organization, in collaboration with UNICEF and many other agencies, institutions and individuals, responded to this challenge by developing a strategy known as the Integrated Management of Childhood Illness (IMCI). Although the main reason for developing the IMCI strategy stemmed from the needs of curative care, the strategy also addresses aspects of nutrition, immunization, and other important elements of disease prevention and health promotion. The objectives of the strategy are to reduce death and the frequency and severity of illness and disability and to contribute to improved growth and development. This strategy has been expanded in India to include the neonates and hence renamed as Integrated Management of Neonatal and Childhood Illness (IMNCI).

Target Population and Clinical Guidelines

The IMNCI clinical guidelines target children less than 5 years old. This is the age group that bears the highest burden of deaths from common childhood diseases. The guidelines represent an evidence based, syndromic approach to case management that includes rational, effective and affordable use of drugs and diagnostic tools.

Components of the Integrated Approach

The IMNCI strategy includes both preventive and curative interventions that aim to improve practices in health facilities, the health system and at home. The core of the strategy is integrated case management of the most common causes of neonatal and childhood problems with a focus on the common cause of death viz. ARI, diarrhoea, malaria and measles.

The strategy includes three main components:

1. Improvement of case management skills of health staff through provision of locally adapted guidelines on Integrated Management of Neonatal and Childhood Illness and activities to promote their use.
2. Improvements in the overall health system required for effective management of neonatal and childhood illness.
3. Improvements in family and community health care practices.

The Principles of Integrated Care

Depending on the child's age, various clinical signs and symptoms differ in their degrees of reliability and diagnostic value and importance. Therefore, the IMNCI guidelines recommend case management procedures based on two age categories:

1. Young infants age up to 2 months.
2. Children aged 2 months up to 5 years.

The IMNCI guidelines are based on the following principles:

1. All sick young infants up to 2 months age must be assessed of "possible bacterial infection / jaundice". They must be routinely assessed for major symptom "diarrhoea".
2. All sick children aged 2 months up to 5 years must be examined for "general danger signs" which indicate the need for immediate referral or admission to hospital. They must then be routinely assessed for major symptoms: cough or difficulty in breathing, diarrhoea, fever and ear problems.
3. All sick young infants and children aged 2 months up to 5 years must also be routinely assessed for nutritional and immunization status, feeding problems, and other potential problems.
4. Only a limited number of carefully selected clinical signs are used, based on evidence of their sensitivity and specificity to detect disease. These signs were selected considering the conditions and realities of the first level health facilities.
5. A combination of individual signs leads to an infant's or a child's classification(s) rather than a diagnosis. Classifications indicate the severity of the condition(s). They call for specific actions based on whether the infant or child (a) should be urgently referred to a higher level of care, (b) require specific treatment (such as antibiotics, antimalarial), or (c) may be safely managed at home. The classifications are colour coded: "pink" suggests hospital referral or admission, "yellow" indicates initiation of specific treatment and "green" calls for home management.
6. The IMNCI guidelines address most, but not all, of the major reasons a sick infant or child is brought to the clinic. An infant or child with chronic problems or less common problems may require special care. The guidelines do not describe the management of trauma or other acute emergencies due to accidents or injuries. They also do not cover care at birth.
7. IMNCI management procedures use a limited number of essential drugs and encourage active participation of caretakers in the treatment of infants and children.

Parents, if correctly informed and counselled, can play an important role in improving the health status of their children by following the advice given by a health care provider, by applying appropriate feeding practices and by bringing sick children to a health facility as soon as symptoms arise. Hence an essential component of the IMNCI guidelines is the counselling of the caretakers about home care, including counselling about feeding, fluids and when to return to a health facility.

National Health Mission (NHM)

The Government of India launched the NRHM (National Rural Health Mission) programme in 2005, now renamed as National Health Mission (NHM) with an aim to improve the quality of life of its citizens for a period of 7 years. It is operational in the whole country with special focus on 18 states viz. 8 empowered action group states (Bihar, Jharkhand, Madhya Pradesh, Chhattisgarh, Uttar Pradesh, Uttaranchal, Orissa and Rajasthan), 8 north eastern states (Assam, Arunachal Pradesh, Meghalaya, Mizoram, Nagaland, Manipur, Tripura and Sikkim), Himachal Pradesh and Jammu and Kashmir. The mission adopts a synergic approach by relating health to determinants of good health viz. nutrition, sanitation, hygiene and safe drinking water by making necessary changes in the basic health care delivery system. It also brings the Indian system of medicine (AYUSH) to the mainstream of health care.

The programmes integrated in the NRHM are the following existing programmes of health and family welfare including RCH II, national vector borne disease control programmes (against malaria, filaria, kala azar, dengue fever/dengue hemorrhagic fever, Japanese encephalitis), national leprosy eradication programme, revised national tuberculosis control programme, national programme for control of blindness, iodine deficiency disorder control programme and integrated disease surveillance project. The principle aim of NRHM is to provide accessible, affordable, accountable, effective and reliable primary health care, and bridging the gap in rural health care through creation of a cadre of accredited social health activist (ASHA). ASHA will be a health activist in the community who will create awareness on health. The Anganwadi worker will guide ASHA in performing her duty.

(*For further reading about the programmes, students can refer to a standard book of Community Medicine*).

Suggested Reading

1. Textbook of Preventive and Social Medicine edited by JE Park and K Park, 20th edition, 2009.
2. Students' Handbook IMNCI, Ministry of Health and Family Welfare, Government of India.
3. National Neonatology Forum, National Neonatal—Perinatal data base: Report for the year 1995, New Delhi, 1996.

2

Disorders of Fluid, Electrolyte and Acid-base Balance

OUTLINES

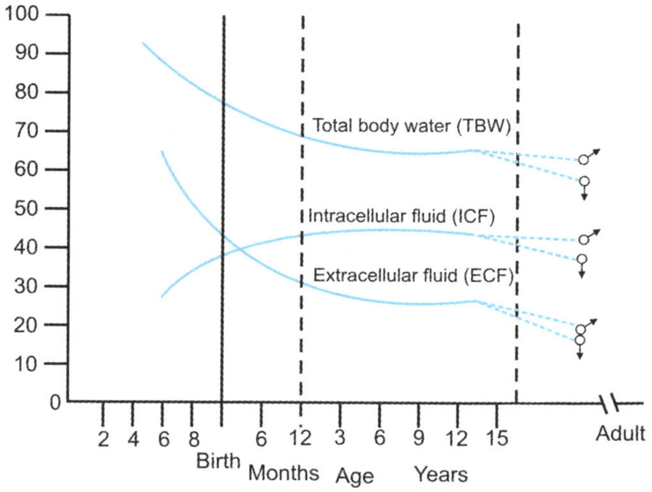

Fig. 2.1: Total body water, intracellular fluid, and extracellular fluid as a percentage of body weight (From The body fluids in pediatrics. Editor Winters R W. Little Brown and Company 1973, Boston)

Composition of Body Fluids

The components of human body include water, protein, minerals, fat and a small amount of carbohydrate. Water is the most plentiful constituent.

Total Body Water

The total body water (TBW) as a percentage of body weight varies with age (Fig. 2.1) The high fetal TBW gradually decreases to 75% of the body weight in a term infant. Preterm babies, therefore has a higher TBW than term infants. After birth during the first year of life, the TBW decreases to about 60% of body weight and remains at this level until puberty. By the end of puberty, TBW in boys remains at 60% whereas the TBW in girls decreases to about 50%. This is because at puberty, the fat content of girls increases and the boys have an increase in muscle mass and fat has a very low water content whereas muscle has a high water content.

Fluid Compartments

The TBW is divided into two main compartments: intracellur fluid (ICF) and extracellular fluid (ECF). In the fetus and newborn, the ECF volume is larger than the ICF volume. The postnatal diuresis causes an immediate decrease in the ECF volume. The ICF volume continuously expands from the postnatal period as a result of cellular growth and by one year age the ratio of ICF volume to ECF volume approaches adult levels.

The ECF volume is about 20–25% of body weight and ICF volume is about 30–40% of the body weight. Post pubertal boys have a higher ICF volume as a result of increase muscle mass. There is no significant difference in the ECF volume between post pubertal boys and girls.

The ECF volume is further divided into the plasma water and the interstitial fluid constituting 5% and 15% of body weight respectively. Plasma along with the blood cells constitutes the blood volume. The blood volume given a hematocrit of 40% is usually 8% of body weight. It is, however, higher in neonates and young infants. In preterm neonates it is around 10% of body, weight. The reduction of interstitial fluid manifests as dehydration and increase results in edema.

The Normal Equilibrium Between the Intravascular and Interstitial Fluid

Normally a delicate equilibrium is maintained between the intravascular fluid and the interstitial fluid. The intravascular volume, which is crucial for proper tissue perfusion, is regulated by the balance between the oncotic and hydrostatic forces.

The intravascular fluid has a higher concentration of albumin than the interstitial fluid and the consequent oncotic force draws water into the intravascular space. Maintenance of this gradient depends on the limited permeability of albumin across the capillaries. On the other hand, the hydrostatic pressure of the intravascular space, which is due to the pumping action of the heart, drives fluid out of the intravascular space.

In the capillaries, these forces favour movement of fluid into the interstitial space at the arterial end of the capillaries. Dilutional increase in albumin concentration resulting in decrease hydrostatic forces and increased oncotic forces causes movement of fluid into the capillaries at the venous end of the capillaries. Overall there is a net movement of fluid out of the intravascular space but this fluid is returned to the circulation via the lymphatics.

Electrolyte Composition

The composition of the solutes in the ECF and ICF are different (Fig. 2.2). Sodium and chloride are the dominant cations and anions respectively in the ECF whereas potassium is the most abundant cation in the ICF. The concentration of potassium within the cells is approximately 30 times higher than in the ECF. The anions in the ICF include predominantly proteins and phosphate in abundance.

The dissimilarity in the anions between the ECF and ICF is largely determined by the presence of intracellular molecules that do not cross the cell membrane, i.e., the barrier between the ECF and ICF. The difference in the distribution of cations viz sodium and potassium, on the other hand is due to the activity of the Na^+ K^+ ATPase which uses cellular energy to extrude sodium from cells and move potassium into the cells.

The chemical gradient between the intracellular and the extracellular potassium concentration creates the electrical gradient across the cell membrane. The concentration dependent movement of potassium out of the cell makes the intracellular space negative relative to the extracellular space.

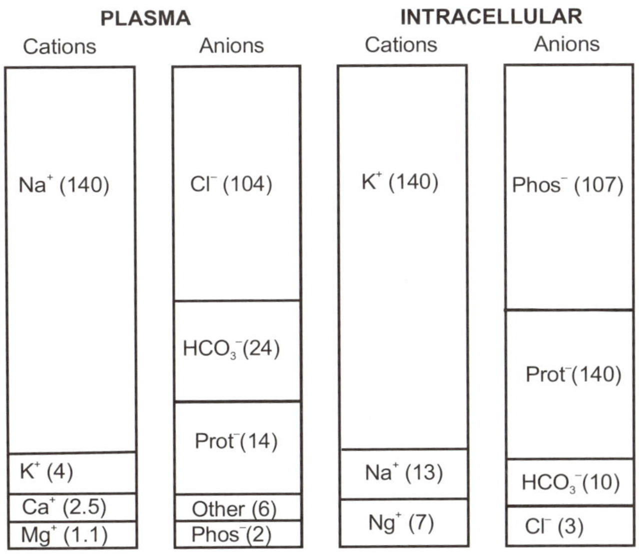

Fig. 2.2: Concentrations of the major cations and anions in the intracellular space, plasma, expressed in mEq/L

Osmolality

Osmolality refers to the number of mols in a kilogram of solvent. Osmolarity refers to the number of mols in a litre of solution. For clinical purposes, osmolarity which is expressed as mols/litre is a close approximation to osmolality. The osmolality, expressed as mols/kg determines the movement of water across a semi-permeable membrane.

The cell membrane is freely permeable to water. Hence the ICF and ECF are in osmotic equilibrium. If the osmolality of one compartment change, then movement of water leads to rapid equalization of the osmolality. Proper functioning of the cells requires close regulation of plasma osmolality and intravascular volume. The plasma osmolality is normally 285 – 295 mOsm / kg. It is measured by the degree of freezing point depression. It can also be calculated based on the following formula:

$$\text{Osmolality} = 2 \times (\text{Na}) + (\text{Glucose}) / 18 + (\text{BUN}) / 2.8$$

Glucose and BUN are measured in mg/dL. Division by 18 and 2.8 converts the units into mmol /L. Multiplication of sodium by 2 accounts for its accompanying anions chloride and bicarbonate. The calculated osmolality is usually slightly lower than the measured osmolality.

Regulation of Osmolality

Regulation of plasma osmolality to maintain it between 285 and 295 mOsm/kg is necessary for proper functioning of cells. Two factors which maintain normal plasma osmolality are modification of water intake and excretion by kidneys (Fig. 2.3).

An elevated effective osmolality leads to secretion of ADH by neurons in the supraoptic and paraventricular nuclei in the hypothalamus, the axons of which terminate in the posterior pituitary. The circulating ADH binds to its V_2 receptors in the collecting duct cells of the kidney and generates cAMP thereby causes insertion of water channels (aquaporin - 2) into the renal collecting tubes. This produces increased permeability to water, permitting reabsorption of water into the hypertonic renal medulla resulting in increased concentration of urine and decrease ion water excretion. Urinary water losses cannot be totally eliminated because there is obligatory excretion of urinary solutes viz. urea and sodium. The regulation of ADH secretion is linked to plasma osmolality, with responses detectable with a 1% change in the osmolality. ADH secretion virtually disappears when the plasma osmolality is low, and this allows excretion of maximally dilute urine.

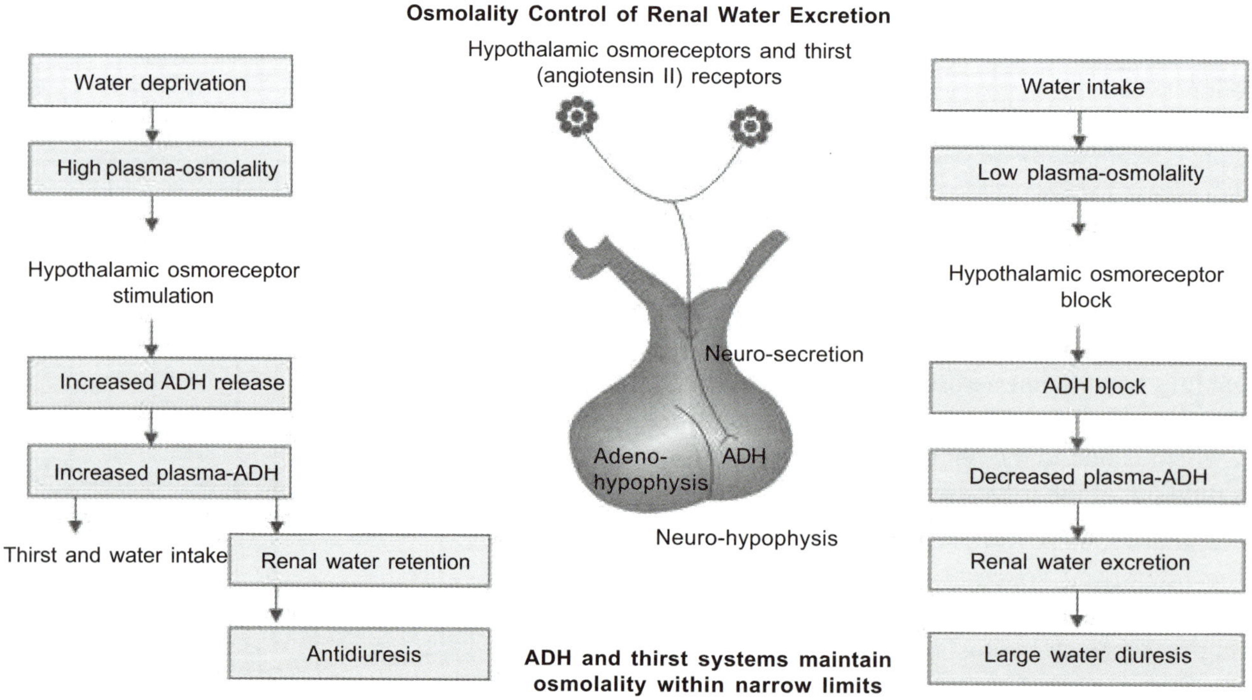

Fig. 2.3: Figure showing control of osmolality

The consequent loss of free water (i.e. water without sodium) corrects the plasma osmolality.

Water intake is regulated by several mechanisms. Osmoreceptors in the hypothalamus which are different from the osmoreceptors that determine ADH secretion regulate water intake. These osmoreceptors stimulate thirst when the serum osmolality increases, by linking to the cerebral cortex. Volume depletion can stimulate both thirst and ADH secretion regardless of plasma osmolality. The sensation of thirst requires moderate volume depletion, but only 1 – 2% change of plasma osmolality. Angiotensin II, which is increased during volume depletion, is also known to stimulate thirst. Baroreceptors when sensing volume depletion may also stimulate thirst.

Regulation of Sodium and Water Balance

Maintenance of an appropriate intravascular volume is critical for survival. Sodium and chloride, the principal extracellular cation and anion restricted to the ECF are necessary for maintenance of intravascular volume. For simplicity sodium balance is considered the main regulator of volume status because body content of sodium and chloride usually changes proportionately. However, chloride depletion is considered the dominant derangement causing volume depletion in metabolic alkalosis. Sodium depletion may exceed chloride depletion in metabolic acidosis with volume depletion.

The kidney is the organ which determines the sodium balance. The interplay of factors regulating body water and sodium in shown in Fig. 2.4.

The renin angiotensin system is an important regulator of renal sodium excretion. The juxtaglomerular apparatus produces renin in response to decreased effective intravascular volume. Renin, a proteolytic enzyme cleaves angiotensin; producing angiotensin I. Angiotensin converting enzyme (ACE) converts angiotensin I to angiotensin II which stimulates the proximal tubule to increase sodium reabsorption and stimulates the adrenal gland to increase aldosterone secretion. Aldosterone, through its action in the distal convoluted tubule and the collecting duct increases sodium absorption. Along with increasing urinary sodium loss, angiotensin II is a vasoconstrictor, which helps to maintain an adequate blood pressure in the presence of volume depletion.

Volume overload occurs when sodium intake exceeds output. Volume expansion stimulates synthesis of atrial natriuretic peptide (ANP), a hormone which is produced by the atria of the heart in response to distension. The ANP increases the GFR, inhibits sodium reabsorption in the medullary portion of the collecting duct thereby facilitating an increase in urinary sodium excretion.

Regulation of Potassium Balance

Potassium is primarily an intracellular electrolyte. The highest amount is contained in the muscles. As the muscle mass increases there is an increase in body potassium.

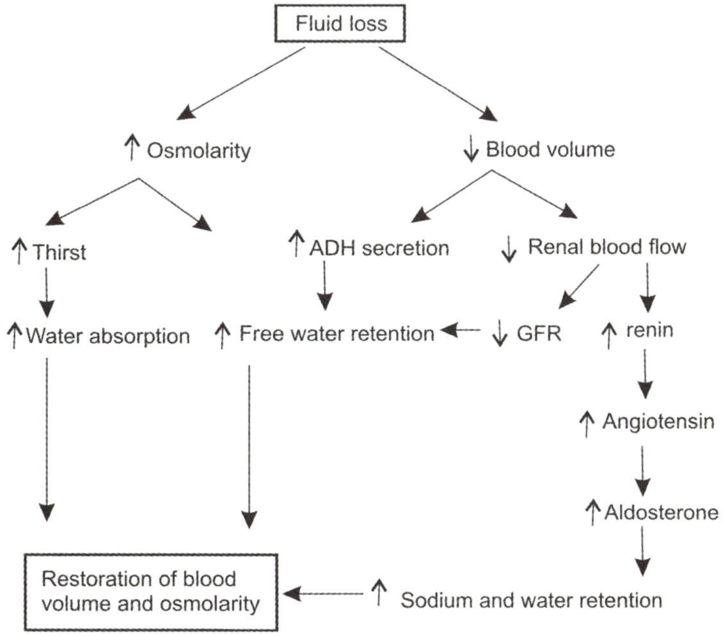

Fig. 2.4: Regulation of water and sodium balance in the body

Therefore, there is an increase in body potassium during puberty which is more significant in boys. The majority of extracellular potassium is in the bone; less than 1% of total body potassium is in plasma. The $Na^+ K^+$-ATPase maintains the high intracellular potassium concentration by pumping sodium out of the cell and potassium into the cell.

The kidneys are the principal regulator of chronic potassium balance. Potassium is freely filtered at the glomerulus, but 90% is reabsorbed. The distal tubule and the collecting duct have ability to absorb as well as secrete potassium. The amount of tubular secretion regulates the amount of potassium that appears in the urine. The plasma potassium concentration directly influences the secretion in the distal nephron, i.e., as potassium concentration increases, secretion increases.

The principal hormone regulating potassium secretion is aldosterone. It is released by the adrenal cortex in response to increase plasma potassium. Its main site of action is the cortical collecting duct, where aldosterone stimulates sodium movement from the tubule into the cells. This creates a negative charge in the tubular lumen, facilitating potassium excretion. In addition, the increased intracellular sodium stimulates the $Na^+ K^+$-ATPase, causing more potassium to move into the cells lining the cortical collecting duct.

Principles of Fluid and Electrolyte Therapy

Maintenance and Replacement Therapy

A normal child has large variations in daily intake of water and electrolytes. The calculated water and electrolyte needs which form the basis of maintenance therapy are not absolute requirements. These calculations actually provide reasonable guidelines for intravenous therapy. Maintenance intravenous fluids are used in children who cannot be fed enterally due to some pathological process. Children should not be placed on intravenous fluids simply because their intake is being monitored in hospital and they do not take maintenance fluid orally. Maintenance fluids are most commonly necessary in preoperative and postoperative patients.

Maintenance Fluid

The components of maintenance water include urine 60%, insensible losses 35% (skin and lungs) and stool 5%. Maintenance fluids are generally composed of a solution of water, 5% glucose, sodium and potassium. The maintenance fluid should provide sodium (2–3 mEq/kg/day) and potassium (1–2 mEq / kg/day). Such a solution usually achieves the goals of maintenance fluids which include prevention of dehydration, electrolyte imbalance, starvation ketoacidosis and protein degradation. Patients on maintenance fluid receives inadequate calories and loose 0.5–1% body weight/24 hours. Hence patients should not remain on maintenance fluid indefinitely. Total parenteral nutrition should be started in patients who cannot be started on enteral feeds for more than a few days.

Table 2.1 : Calculation of maintenance fluid volumes

Weight	*Fluid volume*	*Fluid rate*
0 – 10 kg	100 ml / kg	4 ml /kg /hour
11 – 20 kg	1000 ml + 50 ml/kg for each kg > 10 kg	40 ml/ hr + 2 ml/kg/hr × (wt – 10 kg)
Above 20 kg	1500 ml + 20 ml/kg for each kg > 10 kg*	60 ml/hr + 1 ml/kg/hr × (wt – 20 kg) **

* The maximum total fluid / day is normally 2400 ml.
** The maximum fluid rate is normally 100 ml/hour.

The children on maintenance fluid may require replacement fluids if they have excessive losses, e.g., from nasogastric suction, high urine output, and ongoing losses (due to loose motions and vomiting) during acute watery diarrhoea.

Intravenous Solutions

Half normal saline and one fourth normal saline in 5% dextrose are the fluids used for maintenance therapy in children. They may contain potassium 20 mEq/L, 10 mEq/L or no potassium. Normal saline and Ringer lactate are isotonic solutions which have approximately the same tonicity as plasma. These fluids are generally used for correction of intravascular volume correction.

Table 2.2 : Composition of intravenous solution

Fluid	*Na^+*	*Cl^-*	*K^+*	*Ca^{++}*	*lactate-*
Normal saline (0.9 % NaCl)	154	154	–	–	–
½ normal saline (0.45% NaCl)	77	77	–	–	–
¼ normal saline (0.225% NaCl)	38.5	38.5	–	–	–
Ringer lactate	130	109	4	3	28

The normal plasma osmolality is 285–295 mOsm/ kg. Intravenous fluids are generally designed to have an osmolality that is either close to or moderately more than plasma. Infusing fluids of low osmolality peripherally can cause water to move into RBCs and cause hemolysis. Therefore one fourth saline and half normal saline which are solutions with very low osmolality, should be administered mixed with 5% dextrose which increases the osmolality to 355 (one fourth saline) and 472 (half normal saline).

Selection of Maintenance Fluid

The first step is to calculate the requirement of water and electrolyte needs. Children weighing less than 20–25 kg have a high water need/kg. Hence the best maintenance fluid for them is one fourth saline in 5% dextrose + potassium, 20 mEq/L. In larger children the ideal maintenance fluid is half normal saline in 5% dextrose + potassium 20 mEq/L. It should be noted that these solutions are for children with normal homeostatic mechanism. Disease process will require adjustment e.g. low potassium in renal failure.

Replacement Fluids

Replacement fluids are required for correction of current losses in next 24 hours. It is difficult to predict current loss. Therefore it should be replaced when it happens. Replacement fluids should be advised in addition to maintenance fluid. The most frequent source is gastrointestinal loss in the form of loss of fluid and electrolytes in diarrhoea and gastric juice in vomiting. Diarrhoea usually leads to loss of potassium and bicarbonate resulting in hypokalemia and metabolic acidosis whereas vomiting/nasogastric aspiration can cause alkalosis. Urine output is the other cause of water loss. However, urine output may decrease or increase depending on a disease process. Accordingly the fluid has to be adjusted.

Ideally, for replacement of current losses, the exact amount of fluid loss should be measured, its electrolyte content estimated and then replaced in a specific time period with a fluid with same electrolyte composition.

Adjustment of Replacement Fluid Therapy

1. *Diarrhoea*: The average electrolyte content of diarrhoea stools is sodium: 55 mEq/L, potassium 25 mEq/L and bicarbonate: 15 mEq/L. The replacement can be done either by WHO oral rehydration solution or with the intravenous solution ¼ normal saline in 5% dextrose + 15 mEq/L bicarbonate + potassium 25 mEq/L. In case of IV solution infusion, the loss is replaced every 1–6 hours depending on the rate of loss. In case of ORS, an average amount of 15-20 ml/kg should be given after every loose motion.
2. *Vomiting or nasogastric losses*: The average electrolyte composition of gastric fluid is sodium: 60 mEq/L, potassium: 10 mEq/L and chloride: 90 mEq/L. The replacement of ongoing loss can be done by the intravenous solution ¼ normal saline in 5% dextrose + 10 mEq/L potassium chloride. The loss is replaced every 1–6 hours. For example if 200 ml is lost, it should be replaced as 50 ml/ hour in 4 hours.
3. *Oliguria/anuria*: In cases with anuria and oliguria, the replacement requirements include insensible water loss (one third maintenance) + urine output. The urine output should be replaced mL/mL with half normal saline.
4. *Polyuria*: In case of polyuria, the replacement requirements are insensible loss (one third maintenance) + urine output. As the urine output is excessive, it is important to measure urinary sodium and potassium concentration to help in formulating the replacement fluid.
5. *Chest tube drains and third space loss:* These losses are to be replaced when it is significant. They can be measured and replaced. The third space loss which is due to shift of fluid from the intravascular space to the interstitial space is difficult to measure. Hence replacement is empirical and should be anticipated in patients who are at risk. The third space loss and chest tube drains are isotonic. So it can be replaced with normal saline or Ringer lactate. Protein losses from chest tube drainage can be significant requiring replacement with 5% albumin solution.

Deficit Therapy

Deficit therapy is necessary when a child develops dehydration. The fluid and electrolyte deficit in mild to moderate dehydration can be treated with oral rehydration therapy whereas severe dehydration needs intravenous fluids for correction.

Calculation of Deficits

The calculation of deficits will depend on the type of dehydration, i.e., isonatremic, hyponatremic or hypernatremic.

Majority of patients have **isonatremic/isotonic dehydration** where the serum sodium levels are normal. The water deficit is calculated on the basis of degree of dehydration, i.e., percent dehydration × weight. The sodium and potassium deficit is calculated from the water deficit as water deficit × 80 mEq/L and water deficit × 30 mEq/L respectively. The entire fluid deficit is corrected by 24 hours.

Mild and moderate dehydration are treated with oral rehydration fluid (WHO) unless enteral therapy is not possible. *Severe dehydration* requires intravenous fluid therapy. To restore intravascular volume in severe dehydration with shock, fluid boluses of normal saline/Ringer lactate 20 ml/kg over 20–30 minutes is used until intravascular volume is restored. The half of the calculated deficit fluid should be given in the first 8 hours after subtracting the bolus fluid. The rest of the fluid should be infused in the next 16 hours.

Hyponatremic dehydration is seen in 10–15% of patients with diarrhoea. It occurs when large amount of electrolytes especially sodium, are lost in stool out of proportion to loss of fluid. It occurs more frequently with dysentery and cholera. Hyponatremia may develop or worsen if during diarrhoea there is an increased oral intake of low electrolyte or electrolyte free fluids.

Mild to moderate hyponatremic dehydration can be treated with oral rehydration solution (WHO). In *severe dehydration*, the goal of treating hyponatremia is correction of intravascular volume depletion with an isotonic solution (Normal saline/Ringer lactate). Hyponatremic dehydration requires correction of sodium and water losses. The sodium deficit can be calculated by the formula: sodium deficit = 0.6 × Wt. × $[(Na^+)_d - (Na^+)_I]$ where $(Na^+)_d$ = desired sodium concentration and $(Na^+)_I$ = initial sodium concentration and Wt = weight in kilograms. In general it is not necessary to increase sodium concentration beyond 135 mEq /L. It is important to avoid increasing sodium by more than 12 mEq/L each 24 hours.

Despite the increased sodium deficit in comparison to isotonic dehydration, ¼ saline in 5% dextrose with 20 mEq/L of potassium (if not contraindicated) is usually effective. Half of the total calculated fluid is administered in 8 hours and rest in next 16 hours. Hyponatremia with neurological symptoms (seizures) needs treatment with 3% sodium chloride to rapidly increase the serum sodium concentration. Each ml/kg of 3% sodium chloride increases the serum sodium by approximately 1 mEq/L. An infusion of 4–6 ml/kg often results in resolution of the symptoms.

Hypernatremic dehydration results from disproportionately large net losses of water compared with losses of electrolytes. It is seen in 10–20% of patients with diarrhoea. It may occur when oral home-made electrolyte solutions with high concentration of salt are administered or when infants are fed boiled skimmed milk during the course of diarrhoea. Feeding boiled skimmed milk produces a high renal solute load and increased urinary water loss. The other causes of hypernatremia may be presence of fever, high environmental temperature, which causes evaporative loss of water; hyperventilation, and decreased water intake. Hypernatremia can cause complications like cerebral hemorrhage and thrombosis. This results from movement of water from the brain cells into the hypertonic extracellular fluid causing brain cell shrinkage and tearing of blood vessels within the brain. The movement of water from the intracellular space to extracellular space protects the intravascular space. The children therefore look less ill and urine output is preserved longer than in isotonic dehydration.

Children with hypernatremic dehydration are lethargic but irritable when touched. Hypernatremia can cause fever, increased tone, and hyperreflexia. Cerebral edema can be a complication during treatment which is characterized by seizures, brain herniation and death.

Mild to moderate hypernatremic dehydration can be treated with oral rehydration solution (WHO). The initial management of *severe dehydration* requires restoration of intravascular volume with normal saline as in other types of dehydration. Ringer lactate should not be used because it is more hypotonic than normal saline and may cause too rapid a decrease in the serum sodium concentration, especially if multiple fluid boluses are necessary. The fluid deficit is corrected slowly in order to prevent cerebral edema. Therefore fluid is not run at a faster rate during the first 8 hours. The rate of correction of hypernatremia depends on the initial sodium concentration as follows:

Serum sodium	Time
145 – 157 mEq/L:	24 hours
158 – 170 mEq/L:	48 hours
171 – 183 mEq/L:	72 hours
184 – 196 mEq /L:	84 hours

A child with dehydration and only water loss (diabetes insipidus) usually needs a more hypotonic solution than a child with fluid and electrolytes loss as in cases of diarrhoea. It should be noted that a vigilant monitoring of sodium concentration and adjustment of the therapy is more important than choice of a fluid. In general, the appropriate starting fluid for the neonate is ¼ saline in 5% dextrose whereas for older children ½ normal saline in 5% dextrose. Both fluid should contain 20mEq/L potassium, if not contraindicated. If the serum sodium concentration decreases too rapidly, sodium concentration of IV fluid should be increased or rate of administration decreased. If serum sodium decreases too slowly, the sodium concentration of IV fluid should be decreased or the rate of administration of IV fluid increased. The amount of maintenance fluid should be between 1.25–1.5 times the normal.

Cerebral edema can occur as a result of rapid decrease of serum sodium concentration during correction of hypernatremic dehydration and manifest with seizures. It can be reversed by acute correction of sodium concentration with 3% sodium chloride.

Oral fluids if allowed during rehydration of hypernatremic dehydration should be adjusted in the intravenous fluid. It should be in the form of oral rehydration solution (WHO). Infant formula which has a low sodium content should not be given because it may cause rapid decrease of serum sodium concentration.

Hypokalemia

Hypokalemia is defined as serum potassium less than 3.5 mEq/L. There are four basic mechanism of hypokalemia. They are low intake, nonrenal losses, and renal losses all of which are associated with total body potassium depletion. Acute gastroenteritis is the most common cause of hypokalemia in children.

Common Causes

Non-renal losses : Acute diarrhoea, laxative abuse, nasogastric suction, vomiting, drugs (beta adrenergic agonist, theophylline, barium). Hypokalemic periodic paralysis.

Renal losses : Diabetes ketoacidosis, proximal renal tubular acidosis, diuretic phase of acute tubular necrosis, post obstructive diuresis, interstitial nephritis, drugs (loop and thiazide diuretics, aminoglycosides, cisplatin, amphotericin).

Decreased intake: Low chloride formula.

Clinical Features

The consequences of hypokalemia are mainly observed in skeletal muscles and heart. The clinical consequences in skeletal muscles include muscle weakness and cramps. Muscle paralysis can occur at serum potassium levels of less than 2.5 mEq/L. Paralysis usually starts in the legs followed by the arms and even respiratory paralysis. Hypokalemia also causes slowing of gastrointestinal motility which may manifest as constipation or paralytic ileus when the serum potassium is less than 2.5 mEq/L. Hypokalemia impairs bladder function and cause urinary retention.

The consequences of involvement of heart muscles are shown in ECG changes which include a flattened T wave, depressed ST segment and appearance of a U wave, which is located between the T wave, if visible and P wave. In presence of underlying heart disease, ventricular fibrillation may occur.

Hypokalemia may worsen existing hepatic encephalopathy by stimulating renal ammonia production. Chronic hypokalemia may cause interstitial nephritis, renal cysts and failure to thrive.

Diagnosis

Hypokalemia is a clinical diagnosis with the help of a good history. The serum potassium will be low. Sometimes a differentiation between renal and non-renal loss may be required which may be established by estimation of urinary potassium loss.

Treatment

Therapy for hypokalemia depends on factors like potassium level, clinical symptoms, renal function, presence of intracellular shift, and ongoing losses. With decreased renal function one should be more cautious in correcting hypokalemia. It should be noted that the plasma potassium level does not always provide an accurate estimation of the total body potassium deficit. This is because there may be shifts of potassium from the intracellular space to plasma. With correction of the precipitating causes there may be movement of potassium into the intracellular space resulting in more need for potassium supplementation. However, patients with ongoing losses need correction of potassium deficit and replacement of ongoing losses.

Transient, asymptomatic, or mild hypokalemia may resolve spontaneously or may be treated with oral potassium supplement (2–3 mEq / kg /day in 3 divided doses. Severe hypokalemia require intravenous potassium at a dose of 0.5–1 mEq/kg (maximum dose 40 mEq) usually given at the rate of maximum 10 mEq/1 hour.

Hyperkalemia

Hyperkalemia is defined as a serum potassium level greater than 6 mEq/L. measured in non-hemolysed serum. Hyperkalemia is of concern when serum potassium levels exceed 6.5 mEq/L or if ECG changes have developed.

Common Causes

Increased Intake

Oral or intravenous, blood transfusion.

Non-renal Causes

Tumour lysis syndrome, digitalis toxicity, flouride toxicity, hemolysis, hematomas and bleeding, insulin deficiency, malignant hyperthermia, exercise, tissue necrosis, hyperkalemic periodic paralysis.

Renal Causes

Renal failure, primary adrenal disease (e.g. 21 hydroxylase deficiency), lupus nephritis, sickle cell disease, urinary tract obstruction, kidney transplant, medications like ace inhibitors, angiotensin II blockers, potassium sparing diuretics, cyclosporin, NSAIDs, trimethoprim.

Spurious Hyperkalemia

Hemolysis, tissue ischemia during blood drawing, thrombocytosis, leucocytosis.

Clinical Features

Spurious hyperkalemia is very common in children. A repeat serum potassium is often appropriate. If there is leucocytosis or thrombocytosis, then the repeat estimation should be from plasma.

Cardiac toxicity usually precedes clinical symptoms like paresthesia, weakness and tingling. An ECG should be done when the serum potassium level is high. The ECG changes are peaked T waves to start with progressing to widened QRS complexes, bradycardia, tachycardia, supraventricular tachycardia, ventricular tachycardia, ventricular fibrillation and asystole.

Treatment

The child with oliguria/anuria should not receive any potassium containing food, fluid or medicine until adequate renal function is reestablished. Washed RBCs should be used for packed cell transfusion. If the potassium level is greater than 6.0–6.5 mEq/L an ECG should be ordered.

Serum potassium level should be measured every 12–24 hours and an ECG obtained if necessary. If serum potassium level rise upto 5.5 mEq/litre, measures to deplete body potassium should be initiated with sodium polystyrene sulphonate resin, 1 gm/kg orally suspended in 2 ml /kg 70% sorbitol. It can also be given per rectally suspended in 20% sorbitol 10 ml/kg. Resin therapy is repeated 2 hourly. One gram resin/kg body weight reduces serum potassium by 1 mEq/L.

If the serum potassium rises above 7 mEq/litre, the following emergency measures are to be started, awaiting dialysis, in addition to resins and given sequentially:

(i) 10% calcium gluconate 0.5 ml/kg IV over 10 minutes.

(ii) 7.5% sodium bicarbonate 3 mEq/kg IV slowly.

(iii) 50% glucose (1gm/kg) with regular insulin (1 unit/5 gm glucose) IV over 1 hour.

(iv) Salbutamol 5–8 microgram/kg IV or by inhalation.

It should be noted that the duration of action of these measures is only a few hours. Persistent hyperkelemia, especially in patients requiring emergency measures should be treated with dialysis.

Management of chronic hyperkalemia includes reduction of intake by dietary changes and eliminating and reducing medications that cause hyperkalemia. Some patients may require drugs to increase excretion of body potassium like polystyrene sulphonate and thiazide diuretics. Some infants with chronic renal failure may require dialysis. It is rarely necessary in older children.

Acid Base Equilibrium

An acid is a substance that releases a hydrogen ion (H^+). A base is a substance that accepts a hydrogen ion.

The pH is the negative log of the hydrogen ion concentration. There is an inverse relationship between the pH and the hydrogen ion concentration. When the hydrogen ion concentration decreases, the pH increases and when the hydrogen ion concentration increases, the pH decreases. The normal pH is 7.35–7.45. Maintaining a normal pH is necessary because hydrogen ions are highly reactive and are especially likely to combine with proteins altering their function.

Normal Acid Base Balance

Close regulation of pH is necessary for cellular enzymes and other metabolic processes that function optimally at a normal pH. Chronic mild derangements in acid base status may interfere with normal growth and development, whereas acute severe changes in pH can be fatal. The body attempts to maintain arterial pH, PCO_2 and bicarbonate (HCO_3) within narrow physiological parameters.

Control of acid base balance depends on the buffer system, the lungs and kidney. The buffer system is the first to come into play when there is an imbalance of the acid-base in the body followed by the lungs and the kidney.

Buffer System

Buffers are substances that attenuate the change in pH that occurs when acids or bases are added to the body. There are a variety of physiologic buffers that protect the body against major changes in pH. They are divided into bicarbonate and non-bicarbonate buffers.

The *bicarbonate buffer system* is based on the relationship between carbon dioxide and bicarbonate. Bicarbonate acts as a conjugate base for the H^+ and accepts it when released after carbon dioxide combines with water ($CO_2 + H_2O = H^+ + HCO_3$). The bicarbonate buffer system is very effective because of two reasons (1) The body bicarbonate concentration is very high (24 mEq/L); and (2) It is an open system. It is an open system because the lungs increase the carbon dioxide excretion when the blood carbon dioxide concentration is increased. In a close system, the carbondioxide would increase. The bicarbonate buffer system is routinely monitored clinically.

The *non-bicarbonate buffers* include proteins, phosphate, and bone. *Protein* buffers consist of extracellular proteins, mostly albumin and intracellular proteins including hemoglobin. Proteins are effective buffers largely due to the presence of the amino acid histidine, which has a side chain that can bind or release hydrogen ion. Hemoglobin and albumin have 34 and 16 histidine molecules respectively. *Phosphate* can bind upto three hydrogen molecules. The concentration of phosphate in the extracellular space is relatively low, which limits the overall buffer capacity of phosphate. Hence it is less important than albumin. In the intracellular space it is bound to organic molecules like ATP. Still phosphate is an effective buffer. However, phosphate is at a much higher concentration in the urine, where it is an important buffer. *Bone* is composed of sodium bicarbonate and calcium bicarbonate. Dissolution of bone releases base. This can buffer an acid load, although at the expense of bone density if this occurs over an extended period of time. In contrast, bone formation by consuming base helps to buffer base excess. The bone is an important buffer.

Clinically the extracellular pH is measured. Intracellular pH need not be measured because changes are parallel.

The Lungs

The normal acid base balance is maintained by the lungs and kidney. The lungs prevent an increase in the partial pressure of CO_2 (PCO_2) in the blood by excreting the CO_2 produced by the body. The pulmonary response to changes in CO_2 occurs via central sensing of the PCO_2 and a subsequent increase or decrease in ventilation to maintain a normal PCO_2 (35–45 mmHg). An increase in ventilation decreases the PCO_2 and a decrease in ventilation increases the PCO_2.

While the lungs excrete CO_2, the kidneys must deal with the endogenous production of acid.

The Renal Mechanism

The reabsorption of filtered bicarbonate is the necessary first step in renal regulation of acid base balance. The proximal tubule reclaims about 85% of the filtered bicarbonate. The rest 15% is reclaimed mostly in the ascending loop of Henle.

In the Proximal Tubule

1. The $Na^+ K^+$ -ATPase excretes sodium across the basolateral membrane to maintain low intracellular sodium.
2. The low intracellular sodium concentration provides energy for the Na^+, H^+ antiporter which exchanges sodium from the tubular lumen for intracellular hydrogen ions.
3. The hydrogen ions that are secreted into the tubular lumen then combine with filtered bicarbonate to generate carbonic acid. Carbon dioxide and water

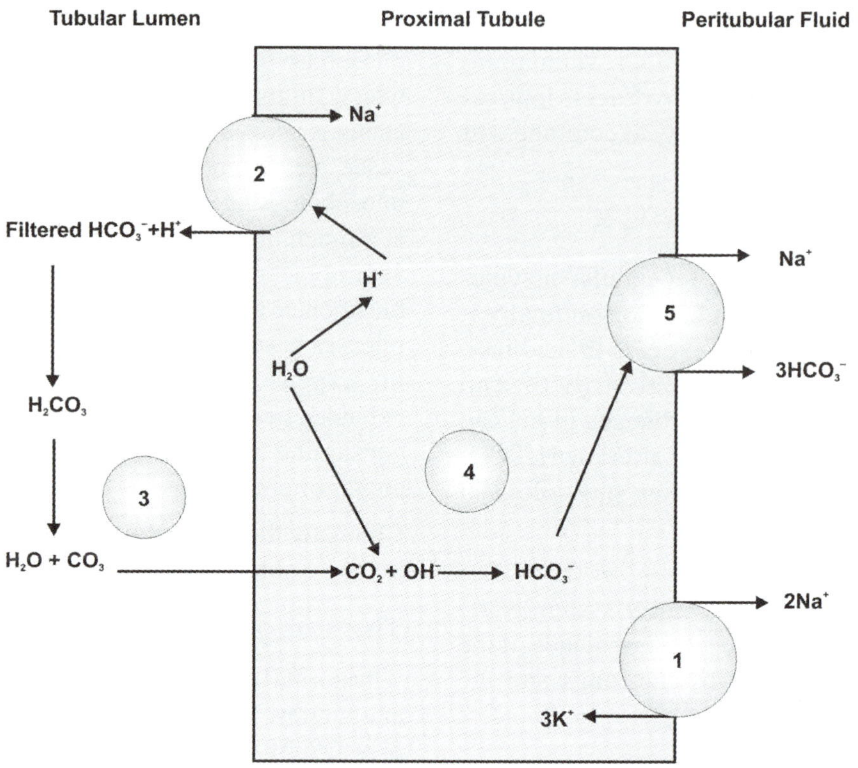

Fig. 2.5: Renal mechanism in the proximal tubule

are produced from carbonic acid. This reaction is catalyzed by luminal carbonic anhydrase.

4. Carbon dioxide diffuses into the cell and combines with OH^- ions to generate bicarbonate. This reaction is catalyzed by an intracellular carbonic anhydrase.
5. The dissociation of water generates an OH^- ion and an H^+ ion. The Na^+, H^+ antiporter secretes the hydrogen ions. The bicarbonate ions cross the basolateral membrane and enter the blood via the $3HCO_3^-$ / 1 Na + co-transporter. The energy for this co-transporter comes from the negatively charged cell interior, which makes it electrically favourable to transport a net negative charge (i.e. 3 bicarbonates and only one sodium).

The second step in renal acid base handling consists of excretion of the endogenous acid production. The excretion of acid occurs mostly in the collecting duct and a small part in the distal tubule.

Adequate excretion of endogenous acid requires the presence of urinary buffers because secretion of hydrogen ions by the tubular cells alone cannot lower the urine pH below 4.5. The hydrogen ion concentration at pH 4.5 is less than 0.04 mEq/L which would require more than 25 litres of water at a pH 4.5 to excrete 1 mEq of hydrogen ion. This necessitates the presence of urinary buffers. Presence of buffers in urine can attenuate the decrease in pH. The two principal urinary buffers are phosphate and ammonia. Phosphate and ammonia buffer the hydrogen ions secreted by the collecting tubules.

In the Collecting Tubule

1. The dissociation of water generates an OH^- ion and an H^+ ion. The H^+ ATPase secretes hydrogen ions into the tubular lumen.
2. Bicarbonate is formed when OH^- ion combines with carbon dioxide in a reaction mediated by carbonic anhydrase.
3. The bicarbonate ions cross the basolateral membrane and enter the blood via the HCO_3^- / Cl^- exchanger. The hydrogen ions in the tubular lumen are buffered by phosphate and ammonia. Ammonia (NH_3) can diffuse from the peritubular lumen, but ammonium (NH_4) cannot pass through the cells of the collecting duct.

The phosphate is an effective buffer but its buffering capacity is limited by its concentration. Urinary phosphate is proportional to dietary intake. There is no mechanism for increasing urinary phosphate excretion in response to changes in acid base status.

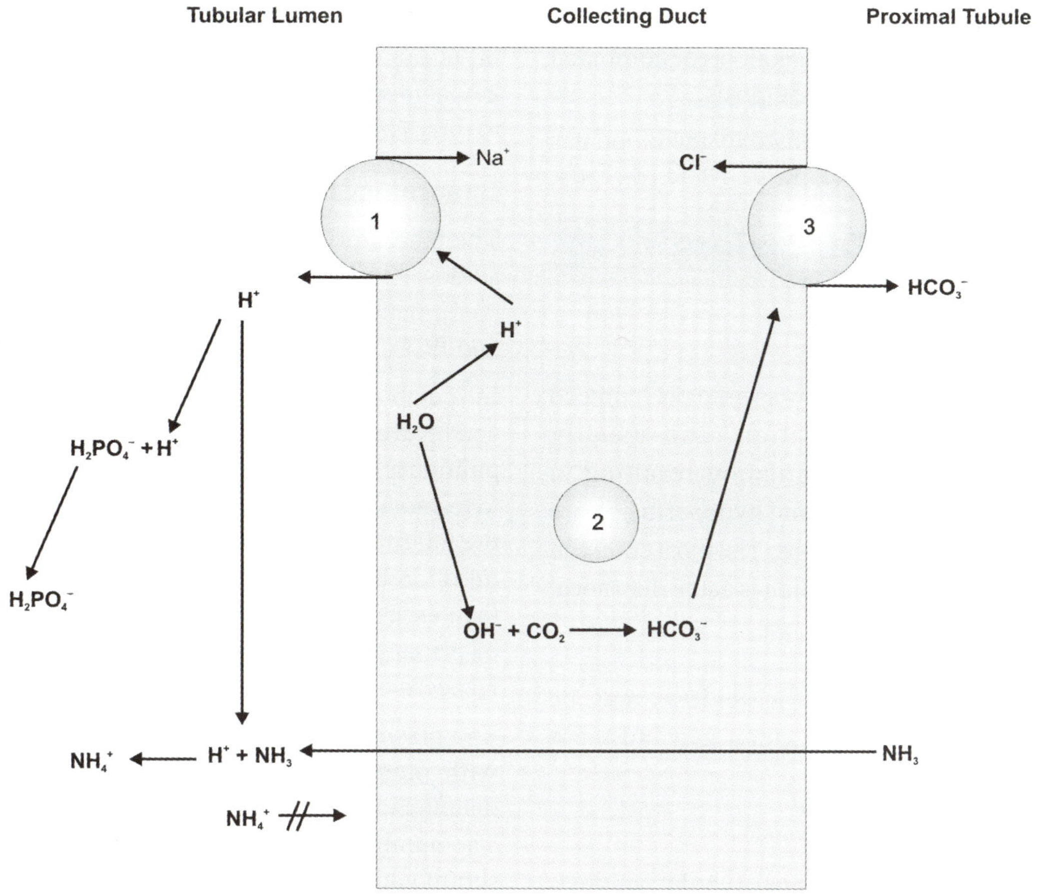

Fig. 2.6: Mechanism in collecting tubule

The buffering capacity of ammonia is based on the reaction of ammonia with hydrogen ions to form ammonium ($NH_3 + H^+ = NH_4$).

Ammonia is excreted from the cells of the proximal tubules mostly through metabolism of glutamine. The ammonia excreted is reabsorbed by cells of the ascending limb of loop of Henle resulting in a high medullary interstitial concentration of ammonia with low concentration of ammonium ions in the tubular fluid entering the collecting tubules.

The cells of the collecting tubule secrete hydrogen ions and regenerate bicarbonate, which is returned into the blood stream. This bicarbonate neutralizes the endogenous acid production. Phosphate and ammonia buffer the hydrogen ions secreted by the collecting tubules.

Ammonia is an effective buffer because of the high concentrations in the medullary interstitium and because the cells of the collecting duct are permeable to ammonia but not to ammonium. Because the luminal pH is lower than the pH in the medullary interstitium, there is a higher concentration of ammonia within the medullary interstitium than in the medullary lumen. This favours movement of ammonia into the tubular lumen. The cells of the collecting duct are impermeable to ammonium preventing back diffusion of ammonium out of the tubular lumen even though the concentration of ammonium is higher in the tubular lumen than in the interstitium.

Clinical Assessment of Acid Base Disorders

The normal pH is 7.35 to 7.45. *Acidemia* is a pH below 7.35 and *alkalemia* is a pH above 7.45. *Acidosis* is a pathological process that causes an increase in the hydrogen ion concentration and *alkalosis* is a pathological process that causes a decrease in the hydrogen ion concentration. Acidemia and alkalemia indicate a pH abnormality whereas acidosis and alkalosis indicate the pathologic process that is taking place.

A *simple acid base disorder* is a single primary disturbance, e.g., metabolic acidosis and alkalosis, respiratory acidosis and alkalosis. A *mixed acid base disorder* is said to be present when there is more than one primary acid base disturbance e.g. combination of respiratory acidosis and metabolic alkalosis or combined metabolic acidosis and respiratory acidosis.

The acid base status can be determined by the blood gas analyzer which will show the pH, pCO_2, HCO_3, directly.

Acid Base Disorders

Metabolic Acidosis

It is a condition characterized by low arterial pH, reduced plasma bicarbonate concentration, and usually compensatory alveolar hyperventilation resulting in decreased PCO_2. Acute diarrhoea and hypoperfusion are common causes of metabolic acidosis. The most common cause of metabolic acidosis in children is acute diarrhoea.

Etiology

The important causes of metabolic acidosis may be classified as those with a normal anion gap and those with an increased anion gap.

Common Causes

Normal anion gap: Diarrhoea, renal tubular acidosis (proximal, distal and hyperkalemic), urinary tract diversions.

Increased anion gap: Lactic acidosis, ketoacidosis, renal failure, poisoning (salicylate, methanol, ethylene glycol), inborn errors of metabolism (aminoacidopathies, organic acidemias).

Clinical Features

The signs and symptoms of mild and moderate acidosis are usually obscured by the clinical features of the underlying disorder. Mild acidosis may present with lassitude, nausea and vomiting.

The characteristic finding in severe metabolic acidosis is increased ventilation which occurs as a part of respiratory compensation. Initially there is increase depth of breathing. Later there is deep and rapid pursed lip breathing (Kussmaul breathing). Severe acidosis with pH levels less than 7.2, may cause circulatory shock due to impaired myocardial contractility and decrease response to catecholamines. In presence of an underlying heart disease or other predisposing electrolyte disorders there is an increased risk of arrhythmias.

There may be signs of ECF volume depletion especially in patients with gastrointestinal volume loss or with diabetic ketoacidosis. Chronic metabolic acidosis causes failure to thrive in children.

Laboratory Findings

The laboratory tests include tests to confirm metabolic acidosis and those to diagnose the cause. The tests for confirmation include arterial pH, plasma bicarbonate level, and PCO_2 and plasma anion gap.

In metabolic acidosis, the arterial pH is less than 7.35 and bicarbonate is less than 21 mEq/L. In the absence of pulmonary disease, the PCO_2 is less than 40 mm Hg due to respiratory compensation. In simple metabolic acidosis, the fall in PCO_2 may be about 11–13 mmHg for each 10 mEq/L reduction in plasma bicarbonate. A greater or less than expected fall in the PCO_2 suggests the coexistence of primary respiratory alkalosis or respiratory acidosis respectively.

The plasma anion gap is useful for evaluating patients with metabolic acidosis and divides them into two diagnostic groups *viz.* normal or increased anion gap. The number of serum anions must equal the number of serum cations in order to maintain electrical neutrality. The anion gap is the difference between the measured cations (sodium) and the measured anions (chloride + bicarbonate). The anion gap is also the difference between the unmeasured cations (potassium, magnesium and calcium) and the unmeasured anions (albumin, urate, phosphate, sulphate). An increased anion gap occurs when there is an increase in unmeasured anions. A normal anion gap metabolic acidosis occurs when there is a decrease in the bicarbonate concentration without increase in unmeasured anions. A normal anion gap is 8–16. The anion gap can be determined by the following formula: Anion gap = $(Na^+)-[(Cl^-) + (HCO_3^-)]$.

The laboratory tests for etiological diagnosis include BUN, creatinine, serum glucose, and urine analysis and electrolytes estimation.

For example in presence of metabolic acidosis, an elevated BUN and creatinine indicates renal insufficiency, an elevated BUN /creatinine ratio supports a diagnosis of pre-renal azotemia. Hyperglycemia, glycosuria and ketonuria and metabolic acidosis indicate diabetic ketoacidosis as the diagnosis. Presence of metabolic acidosis with glycosuria and normoglycemia occur in children when type II renal tubular acidosis is a part of

Fanconi syndrome. The serum potassium level may be normal or abnormal with metabolic acidosis; being low when associated with acute GI loss or elevated when associated with renal insufficiency.

Treatment

Treatment of cause is the most effective approach in patients with metabolic acidosis. Correction of the basic disorder results in normalization of the acid base status. Bicarbonate therapy as a short term measure is indicated in acute renal failure until the kidney functions returns to normal, and poisonings (salicylate, methanol, ethylene glycol). Long-term therapy is required in cases where the underlying disorder is irreparable e.g. renal tubular acidosis and chronic renal failure.

Oral or intravenous bicarbonate therapy can be used. Intravenous therapy is generally used when a rapid response is necessary. In emergency situations, 7.5 %/ 8.4% sodium bicarbonate 1 mEq / kg / dose diluted in equal volume of distilled water is given slowly (1 mEq / minute). A more gentle approach is to add the total requirement to the patient's intravenous fluids remembering to remove an equal amount of sodium chloride from the solution to avoid giving an excessive sodium load. Careful monitoring is mandatory to appropriately titrate the dose of sodium bicarbonate.

Metabolic acidosis associated with renal insufficiency may require peritoneal dialysis. Hemodialysis is indicated in patients with renal insufficiency with significant uremia and hyperkalemia, treatment of poisonings.

Metabolic Alkalosis

It is a condition characterized by elevated pH, increased plasma bicarbonate concentration, and usually compensatory alveolar hypoventilation resulting in increased PCO_2. Metabolic alkalosis in children is most commonly secondary to vomiting or diuretic use.

Etiology

The causes of metabolic alkalosis are divided into two categories on the basis of urinary chloride. Causes with low urinary chloride are also called chloride responsive because alkalosis is maintained in these cases by volume depletion and is corrected by volume repletion. Causes with high urinary chloride do not respond to volume repletion and they are called chloride resistant.

Common Causes

Low urinary chloride (< 15 mEq / L) / chloride responsive

Gastric losses viz. vomiting, nasogastric suction, diuretics (loop, thiazide), chloride loosing diarrhoea, cystic fibrosis.

High urinary chloride (> 20 mEq/L) / chloride resistant

Renovascular disease, renin secreting tumour, Cushing's syndrome, adrenal adenoma and hyperplasia, hyperaldosteronism, base administration.

Clinical Features

Children with causes of metabolic alkalosis with low urinary chloride often present with symptoms of volume depletion. In contrast, children with high urinary chloride have symptoms related to hypertension.

The symptoms of metabolic alkalosis include carpopedal spasm (tetany) and seizure as a result of low ionized calcium during alkalemia as a result of increased binding of calcium to albumin. Arrhythmias are a potential complication with increased risk when there is concomitant hypokalemia. Hypoventilation in patients with severe metabolic alkalosis can cause hypoxia in patients with normal lungs.

Laboratory Findings

The laboratory tests include tests to confirm metabolic alkalosis and those to diagnose the cause. The tests for confirmation include arterial pH, plasma bicarbonate level and PCO_2.

The arterial pH is > 7.45 and HCO_3 > 40 mEq/L. In simple metabolic alkalosis, the PCO_2 may be expected to rise about 6–7 mmHg for each 10 mEq/L increment in plasma bicarbonate. A greater or less than expected increase in the PCO_2 suggests the coexistence of respiratory acidosis or respiratory alkalosis respectively. There may be an increase in PCO_2 levels as high as 50– 60 mmHg in patients with mild renal insufficiency.

The laboratory tests for etiological diagnosis include urinary chloride level, renin and aldosterone levels, 24 hours urinary cortisol level, electrolytes, sweat chloride test etc. Urinary chloride estimation helps to classify the causes with low and high levels. The cases with high levels are further classified into those with hypertension and without. For example elevated renin and aldosterone levels are characteristic of renin vascular disease and renin secreting tumours. They are low in children with Cushing's syndrome. Aldosterone is high and renin low in patients with adrenal adenomas, or hyperplasia and hyperaldosteronism. An elevated 24-hour urinary cortisol level with metabolic alkalosis is diagnostic of Cushing's syndrome.

Treatment

Children with mild metabolic alkalosis (HCO_3< 32 mEq/L) does not require any intervention. However, a worsening mild metabolic alkalosis due to nasogastric suction will need treatment.

Intervention is usually necessary with moderate and severe metabolic alkalosis. The most effective approach is to treat the underlying cause. Most children have one of the chloride responsive causes with fluid losses, in whom metabolic alkalosis responds to administration of sodium chloride and potassium chloride to correct volume deficit and potassium deficit. In case of volume depletion due to diuretics, the diuretic may be stopped; the doses reduced or use potassium sparing diuretics. In cases of alkalosis resulting from nasogastric suction it may be decreased or discontinued. Alternatively, a gastric proton pump inhibitor can be added to reduce gastric secretion and losses of hydrochloric acid. With adequate intravascular volume, and a normal serum potassium concentration, the kidney is able to excrete the excess bicarbonate in a few days.

In children with chloride resistant causes, ideal treatment is elimination of excess aldosterone effect. Volume repletion is contraindicated because it will not correct metabolic alkalosis and may cause exaggeration of hypertension.

Respiratory Acidosis

It is a condition characterized by low arterial pH, hypoventilation resulting in an elevated PCO_2, and usually compensatory increase in plasma HCO_3 concentration.

Etiology

The causes of respiratory acidosis may be pulmonary or non-pulmonary.

Common Causes

Pulmonary (lower airway)

Pneumonia, bronchiolitis, asthma, pneumothorax, pulmonary edema and hemorrhage, neonatal and adult respiratory distress syndrome, meconium aspiration syndrome, bronchopulmonary dysplasia, hypoplastic lungs.

Pulmonary (upper airway)

Aspiration, laryngospasm, angioedema, obstructive sleep apnea, tonsillar hypertrophy, vocal cord paralysis.

Disorders of CNS

Encephalitis, head trauma, brain tumour, stroke, hypoxic brain damage, increased intracranial pressure, obesity-hypoventilation, medications (narcotics, barbiturates, benzodiazepines).

Disorders of spinal cord, peripheral nerves and neuromuscular junction

Diaphragmatic hernia, Guillain-Barré Syndrome, botulism, spinal cord injury, myasthenia gravis, medications (aminoglycosides, organophosphates and vecuronium).

Respiratory muscle weakness

Muscular dystrophy, hypokalemia, hypothyroidism, malnutrition, medications (corticosteroids, succinylcholine).

Miscellaneous

Decreased diaphragmatic movement due to ascites, kyphoscoliosis and cardiac arrest.

Pathophysiology

Hypoventilation can occur due to decrease activity of the respiratory centre, respiratory muscle failure and ventilation-perfusion imbalance. Disorders of CNS causes the depression of respiratory centre and reduces the ventilatory drive. Respiratory muscle failure can be secondary to depression of the respiratory centre, phrenic nerve paralysis, and defect in the neuromuscular junction. Pulmonary conditions cause reduction in alveolar surface area for gas exchange leading to ventilation-perfusion imbalance. Upper airway disease can decrease ventilation by impairing air entry into the lungs. Increased respiratory muscle work due to any cause also increases carbon dioxide production.

Clinical Features

The symptoms of respiratory acidosis depend on the PCO_2 level. It is more symptomatic when onset is acute. Symptoms are increased by concurrent hypoxia or metabolic acidosis.

The most characteristic change is a metabolic encephalopathy with presenting symptoms that includes headache, confusion, drowsiness progressing to stupor and coma. The onset is usually gradual with advancing respiratory failure. It may be abrupt when precipitated by drugs and pulmonary causes. There may be asterixis, myoclonus, hallucination, psychosis and seizures. Occasionally there may be papilledema as a result of increased intracranial pressure. The encephalopathy is reversible if hypoxic ischemic damage has not occurred. Respiratory acidosis increases the risk of cardiac arrhythmia especially in a child with underlying cardiac disease.

Laboratory Findings

In acute respiratory acidosis, the arterial pH is low with a high PCO_2. The HCO_3 level may be normal or slightly increased. An abrupt increase of PCO_2 is associated with a rise in plasma HCO_3 of no more than 3 – 4 mEq/L as a result of cellular buffering. A greater or lesser than expected increase in plasma HCO_3 indicates the coexistence of primary metabolic alkalosis or acidosis respectively.

Treatment

Treatment of cause is the most effective approach in patients with respiratory acidosis. In children with a chronic respiratory acidosis, there is no curative therapy, although an acute respiratory illness superimposed on the chronic respiratory condition is usually reversible.

All cases with respiratory acidosis are hypoxic. Therefore they need supplemental oxygen. Sedatives should be avoided except as necessary to facilitate mechanical ventilation. Children with significant respiratory acidosis due to a central nervous system disease usually require mechanical ventilation because these disorders usually take a long time to respond to therapy. In chronic respiratory acidosis, oxygen should be administered cautiously. Such patients have adapted to chronic hypercapnia so that their major respiratory stimulus is hypoxemia. Therefore the lowest oxygen concentration required to elevate the PaO_2 to acceptable level, i.e., greater than 50 mmHg should be given. Excessive use of oxygen can blunt the respiratory drive and increase the PCO_2. It is best to avoid mechanical ventilation in a patient with chronic respiratory acidosis. However it may be necessary in a superimposed acute illness. In such cases, the PCO_2 should be lowered to the patient's normal base line and it should be done gradually. These patients normally have elevated plasma HCO_3 as a result of metabolic compensation for the respiratory acidosis. A rapid lowering of PCO_2 can cause a severe metabolic alkalosis potentially leading to complications like cardiac arrhythmias, decreased cardiac output, and decreased cerebral blood flow. Further, prolonged ventilation at a normal PCO_2 causes the metabolic compensation to resolve. When the patient is subsequently extubated, the patient will no longer be benefited from metabolic compensation, causing a more severe acidemia due to respiratory acidosis.

Respiratory Alkalosis

It is a condition characterized by elevated arterial pH, hyperventilation resulting in a low PCO_2 and usually a compensatory decrease in plasma HCO_3 concentration. There is inappropriate reduction in PCO_2 usually due to hyperventilation. A respiratory alkalosis not due to hyperventilation may occur in children receiving extra-corporeal membrane oxygen (ECMO) or hemodialysis with carbon dioxide lost directly from the blood in the extracorporeal circuit.

Etiology

An increase in the ventilatory drive leading to alkalosis can result from hypoxemia/ tissue anoxia, stimulation of the lung receptors and central stimulation.

Common Causes

Hypoxemia/Tissue Anoxia

Pneumonia, asthma, severe anemia, high altitude, laryngospasm, carbon monoxide poisoning, laryngospasm.

Stimulation of Lung Receptors

Pneumonia, asthma, pneumothorax, hemothorax, pulmonary edema, neonatal and adult respiratory distress syndrome.

Central Stimulation

CNS diseases (meningitis, encephalitis, brain tumor, sub-arachnoid hemorrhage), fever, pain, anxiety, liver failure, medications (salicylate, theophylline, caffeine), mechanical ventilation and ECMO.

Pathophysiology

Arterial hypoxemia or tissue hypoxia stimulates the peripheral chemoreceptors which in turn stimulates the respiratory centre in the medulla to increase ventilation. The resultant increased respiratory effort increases the oxygen content of the blood but depresses the PCO_2. Acute hypoxia is a more potent stimulation than chronic hypoxia. Common causes of hypoxemia are primary lung disease, severe anemia and carbon dioxide poisoning.

The lung receptors respond to irritants and stretching, which in turn stimulates the respiratory centre to increase ventilation. Most of the causes that activate the receptors may also cause hypoxemia or tissue hypoxia and lead to hyperventilation by two mechanisms. Primary lung disease may initially have respiratory alkalosis but with respiratory failure in late stages go to respiratory acidosis.

Direct stimulation of respiratory centre occurs with primary CNS diseases like meningitis, trauma etc. A lesion near the respiratory centre in the midbrain is frequently fatal.

Liver diseases can cause respiratory alkalosis proportionate to the degree of liver failure. The exact mechanism is not known. Salicylates directly stimulate the respiratory centre to produce respiratory alkalosis. Pain, stress or anxiety can cause hyperventilation. Respiratory alkalosis is common in children on mechanical ventilation because ventilation is not under control of the respiratory centre. In addition, these children may have a decreased metabolic rate and hence less carbon dioxide production because of sedation and paralytic medications.

Clinical Features

The characteristic symptoms are produced by cerebral vasoconstriction and hypoxia as a result of rise in pH of both plasma and brain as the PCO_2 and the cerebral tissue PCO_2 falls.

When respiratory alkalosis is due to cerebral or metabolic causes the rate and depth of respiration increase markedly. In others the breathing pattern varies from frequent, deep, sighing respiration to sustained, obviously rapid breathing.

Acute respiratory alkalosis may cause chest tightness, lightheadedness, circumoral numbness and paresthesias of lower limbs. Less common manifestations are tetany, seizures, muscle cramps and syncope. Chronic respiratory alkalosis is usually asymptomatic since metabolic compensation decreases the magnitude of alkalemia.

However, it should be noted that the disease process that is causing the alkalosis is usually more concerning than the clinical manifestations of respiratory alkalosis.

Laboratory Findings

In acute respiratory alkalosis there is a rapid fall of PCO_2 to 20–25 torr and a drop of HCO_3 of no greater than 3–4 mEq/L and which usually does not go below 17 mEq/L. A greater or lesser than expected fall of HCO_3 suggest coexistent primary metabolic acidosis or alkalosis respectively.

Treatment

Specific treatment of respiratory alkalosis is rarely needed. Treatment focuses on the underlying cause.

Hyperventilation due to anxiety requires reassurance to the child as well as the parents. Benzodiazepines may be sometimes prescribed. During an acute episode of psychogenic hyperventilation, the patient is advised rebreathing into a paper bag which increases the patients PCO_2 and decreases the symptoms. Rebreathing should be advised only when other causes of hyperventilation are excluded. The rebreathing should be assessed with pulse oximetry.

Arterial Blood Gas (ABG) Analysis

ABG analysis measures the oxygen and carbon dioxide content, and acidity in arterial blood. ABG analysis is used to evaluate respiratory diseases and other conditions that affect the lungs. It is used to determine the effectiveness of oxygen therapy. The acid base component of the test gives information about kidney function.

Table 2.3 : Normal blood gas values at sea level

Parameters	*Arterial blood*
pH	7.35 – 7.45
PCO_2	35 – 45 mm Hg
PaO_2	75 – 100 mmHg*
HCO_3	22 – 26 mEq/L
Oxygen saturation (SaO_2)	94 – 100%

* At levels 3000 feet and above, the oxygen values are lower.

Collection of Blood Sample

The blood sample may be collected from the radial artery in the wrist, femoral artery in the groin or brachial artery in the arm using a fine needle. After the blood is drawn, pressure must be applied to the puncture site for atleast 5 minutes to completely stop bleeding. The sample should be analyzed immediately. The radial artery is the most common site for puncture.

How to Analyze the ABG

Study the pH whether it is low (acidosis) or high (alkalosis).

If it is low, look at the PCO_2.

1. If PCO_2 is high, it is respiratory acidosis. If PCO_2 is low, it is metabolic acidosis.

Table 2.4 : Blood gas findings in simple acid-base disturbances

Disorder	*Initial change*	*Compensatory Change*
Metabolic acidosis	Decrease HCO_3	$PCO_2 = 1.5x.[HCO_3] + 8+/-2$
Metabolic alkalosis	Increase HCO_3	PCO_2 increases by 7 mm Hg for each 10 mEq /L increase in serum HCO_3
Respiratory acidosis	Increase PCO_2	**Acute:** HCO_3 increases by 1 for each 1 mm Hg increase in PCO_2 **Chronic:** HCO_3 increases by 3.5 for each 10 mmHg increase in PCO_2
Respiratory alkalosis	Decrease PCO_2	**Acute:** HCO_3 falls by 2 for each 10 mm Hg decrease in PCO_2 **Chronic:** HCO_3 falls by 4 for each 10 mm Hg decrease in PCO_2

2. If PCO_2 is high and HCO_3 is high, it is compensated respiratory acidosis. If PCO_2 is low and HCO_3 is low, it is compensated metabolic acidosis.

If the pH is high, look at PCO_2.

1. If PCO_2 is low, it is respiratory alkalosis. If PCO_2 is normal or high, it is metabolic alkalosis.
2. If PCO_2 is high and HCO_3 is high, it is compensated metabolic alkalosis. If PCO_2 is low and HCO_3 is low, it is compensated respiratory alkalosis.

   NB: In a compensated process, PCO_2 and HCO_3 will be going the same direction. Both will be high or both will be low.

Shock

Shock is a complex clinical syndrome in which the cardiovascular system fails in its primary function of substrate delivery and metabolic removal, resulting in anaerobic metabolism and tissue anoxia.

Definition

The American college of critical care medicine guidelines defined shock, in pediatric patients, as tachycardia with signs of decreased organ or peripheral perfusion viz. decreased peripheral pulses compared with central pulses, altered alertness, capillary refill > 2 seconds, mottled or cool extremities, or decreased urine output.

Peculiarities in Children

1. Hypotension is a late sign of shock in children due to a high SVR and vasoactive capacity in infants and children. This is a survival mechanism designed to counter balance the limited cardiac reserve in children.
2. During states of shock, neonates, infants and children compensate by peripheral vasoconstriction to maintain adequate perfusion to the heart, brain, and kidney and hence hypotension is a poor prognostic sign.
3. Children often maintain their blood pressure until the late stages of shock. Therefore, as in adults, presence of systemic hypotension is not essential to make an early diagnosis of shock in children.

Clinical Stages of Shock

Shock is a progressive process. It is due to the continued presence of the initiating factor plus exaggerated and potentially harmful neuro humoral, inflammatory and cellular compensatory responses. Initially, shock may be compensated but then may progress to an uncompensated condition.

In *compensated* shock, homeostatic mechanisms maintain perfusion of the essential organs. Blood pressure, cardiac function and urine output is maintained. Hence the child appear to be normal.

Decompensated: The circulatory compensation fails leading to manifestations of abnormalities in all organ systems.

Irreversible: There is irreversible functional damage to essential organs and death is inevitable. The clinical and laboratory features of different stages of shock are shown in Table 2.5.

Table 2.5: Showing the features of different stages of shock

Organ system	*Compensated shock*	*Decompensated shock*	*Irreversible shock*
CNS	Agitation, anxiety, lethargy, somnolence	Altered mental status Encephalopathy HIE	HIE and cell necrosis
CVS	Tachycardia	Tachycardia, Bradycardia	Myocardial ischemia Cell necrosis
Lungs	Tachypnea Increased work of breathing	Acute respiratory failure	Acute respiratory failure
Kidneys	Oliguria Increased urinary osmolality Increased urinary sodium (FE_{Na} < 1)	Acute tubular necrosis Acute renal failure	Tubular necrosis
GIT	Ileus Feeding intolerance Stress gastritis	Pancreatitis Acalculus cholecystitis GI bleeding Gut translocation	GI bleeding Sloughing
Liver	Elevated transaminases	Shock liver	Hepatic failure
Blood	Platelet activation	DIC	DIC
Metabolic	Normal	Hypoglycemia	Hypoglycemia
Immune system	Immunoparalysis	Immunoparalysis	Immunoparalysis

Adapted from 'Shock: A Review' by Joseph A. Carcillo *et al.* in Pediatric Critical Care Medicine edited by Derreck S. Wheeler *et al.* 2007 published by Springer-Verleg, London Limited.

Categories of Shock

Shock is divided into three major categories with a degree of overlap into hypovolemic, cardiogenic and distributive. The end result, however, is failure to provide energy substrates to meet the metabolic demand of the tissues.

Hypovolemic shock is a result of inadequate circulating blood volume, owing to blood or fluid loss or insufficient fluid intake. This is the most common type of shock seen in children.

Cardiogenic shock occurs when cardiac compensatory mechanisms fail. It is usually seen in infants and young children and in patients with pre-existing myocardial disease or injury.

Distributive shock viz. septic and anaphylactic shock is associated with decreased venous return to the heart. It results from peripheral vasodilatation, arterial and capillary shunting past tissue beds with pooling of venous blood.

Pathophysiology

An initial insult triggers shock. This leads to inadequate oxygen delivery to organs and tissues.

Compensatory mechanisms like increasing cardiac output and systemic vascular resistance tries to maintain the blood pressure.

The body also attempts to optimize oxygen delivery to the tissues by increasing oxygen extraction and redistributing blood flow to the brain, heart and kidneys at the expense of skin and gastrointestinal tract. These responses lead to an initial state with maintenance of blood pressure.

If treatment is not initiated or is inadequate during this period, decompensation develops with hypotension, tissue damage and multisystem organ dysfunction and ultimately death.

A decrease in oxygen delivery to meet tissue oxygen requirement can be a result of any of the three basic abnormalities:

1. Hypovolemia.
2. Impairment of cardiac function.
3. Inappropriate distribution of cardiac output secondary to abnormal vasodilatation.

Hypovolemia may be true or relative. In true hypovolemia there is an actual sudden loss of circulating blood volume,

Table 2.6: Showing the causes of shock

Hypovolemic shock	*Cardiogenic shock*	*Distributive shock*
Fluid and electrolyte loss Diarrhoea, Vomiting, Excessive sweating, Diuretics, Heat stroke.	**Myocardial insufficiency** Myocarditis, Congestive cardiac failure, Cardiomyopathy.	Septic shock, Anaphylaxis, Drugs, Toxins, Neurogenic shock, Prolonged hypoxia or ischemia.
Blood loss External or Internal hemorrhage.	**Arrhythmias** Supraventricular tachycardia.	
Plasma loss Burns, Nephrotic syndrome, Sepsis, Intestinal obstruction, Peritonitis.	**Metabolic** Hypothermia, Hypoglycemia, drugs, toxins Acidosis, Hypoxia.	
Endocrine Diabetes mellitus, Diabetes insipidus, Adrenal insufficiency.	**Outflow obstruction** Cardiac tamponade Pneumopericardium Tension pneumothorax Pulmonary embolism Poor myocardial perfusion Kawasaki disease congenital coronary artery abnormality.	

as a consequence of loss of fluid and electrolytes (e.g., diarrhoea and vomiting) or acute blood loss (internal or external). Relative hypovolemia occurs secondary to peripheral pooling of blood volume and third space loss caused by a loss of vascular tone and increased capillary permeability. It is most often seen in septic shock.

The loss of circulatory blood volume is followed by a series of cardiac and peripheral homeostatic adjustments directed at restoration of systemic arterial blood pressure and perfusion of critical organs viz. heart and brain.

The extent and progression of hypovolemic shock hence depends on (1) the extent and rapidity with which hypovolemia occurs and (2) the child's pre-existing hemodynamic status which will determine whether the adjustments are adequate to maintain cardiovascular homeostasis.

Impairment of cardiac function is basically an event with inadequate stroke volume mostly as a result of decreased myocardial contractility (e.g., myocarditis) and infrequently due to mechanical obstruction to blood flow (e.g., cardiac tamponade).

Low cardiac output, decreased blood pressure and poor tissue perfusion produce inadequate oxygen delivery to tissues and microcirculatory failure. It may be best viewed as a pump failure. It needs to be mentioned that children rarely go through a compensated phase of cardiogenic shock.

Inappropriate distribution of cardiac output secondary to abnormal vasodilatation is a result of maldistribution of blood volume. The basic defect is massive injury to capillary endothelium resulting in loss of its integrity and leakage of fluid to the interstitial space or so called third space. Septic shock is a classic example.

Septic shock results when infectious agents or infection induced mediators in blood stream induce cardiovascular decompensation. In the early stages, there is a decrease in systemic vascular resistance and an increase in cardiac output (warm shock). Hemodynamically it is characterised by low cardiac filling pressure, increased cardiac output, tachycardia and decreased whole body oxygen consumption. The latter effect is due to impaired mitochondrial oxygen utilisation and deficient oxygen delivery to cells despite an increase in overall cardiac output (maldistribution of cardiac output). Later, there is decline in cardiac output and profound hypotension and hypoxia (cold shock).The end stage is often associated with multiple organ system failure with profound derangements in cardiovascular, pulmonary and renal systems.

Clinical Manifestation

It is not difficult to diagnose shock in a child with a full blown picture with *hypotension, lethargy, poor peripheral perfusion and cold extremities*. However, in such cases the likelihood of successful intervention would be limited. Hence it is important to recognise shock and initiate therapy before it causes irreversible vital organ damage.

Just as any other disease, shock is diagnosed by history and physical examination using laboratory investigations to further delineate the disease.

History

In case of an overt hemorrhage, the cause of shock is obvious. A detailed history in less obvious situations is important to make decisions regarding appropriate management.

For an early diagnosis, knowledge of predisposing conditions and comorbidities to shock is important. Children with fever, who have an identifiable source of infection or who are hypovolemic are at increased risk of developing shock.

In case of trauma, history regarding the mechanism of trauma, amount of blood loss and level of consciousness before arrival to hospital is important. A history of immunodeficiency, use of immunosuppressive agents, duration and height of fever, and associated features like lethargy, vomiting, diarrhoea, decreased oral intake, and decreased level of awareness or consciousness, may suggest infection and possibility of septic shock.

Physical Examination

A rapid cardiopulmonary assessment helps in early recognition of shock. The following examinations help:

Heart rate and pulse volume, core and peripheral temperature gap, capillary refill time, color of the skin, blood pressure, respiratory rate, liver span, urine output and level of consciousness.

Heart rate and pulse volume: *Tachycardia* is the earliest sign of shock though not a very sensitive sign. It is an attempt to maintain cardiac output. *Bradycardia* in a child in shock is an ominous sign. One should be aware of the normal heart rates at different age group for proper assessment.

Table 2.7: Showing normal heart rates at different age

Age	*Awake rate (per min)*	*Mean (per min)*	*Sleeping rate (per min)*
Birth to 3 months	85-205	140	80-160
3 months to 2 years	100-190	130	75-160
2 to 10 years	60-140	80	60-90
Above 10 years	60-100	75	50-90

The *pulse volume* should be palpated simultaneously over the femoral (central) and dorsalis pedis (peripheral) arteries. Absent or diminished distal pulse volume indicates decompensated shock. It is a result of vasoconstriction, a compensatory measure to preserve blood flow to vital organs. Absent central pulse is a pre-morbid sign indicating very rapid intervention. In early septic shock, on the other hand there is bounding distal pulse as a result of a high output state and low systemic vascular resistance.

Core-peripheral temperature gap: Should be assessed by comparing simultaneously the warmth of the skin over the trunk and that of the peripheries. A core toe temperature difference of more than 2 degrees centigrade is a sign of poor skin perfusion. This is a consequence of a falling cardiac output which results in cooling of the skin which begins in the periphery and extends proximally towards the trunk.

Skin temperature should be measured with the dorsal surface of the examiner's hands or fingers because these areas are most sensitive to temperature perception. Patients are considered to have cool extremities (a) if all examined extremities are cool to the examiner or (b) if only the lower extremities are cool, despite warm upper extremities in the absence of peripheral vascular disease.

Capillary refill time (CRT): Has become widely accepted as a reflection of intravascular volume in children. A value of < 2 seconds at normal ambient temperature is considered adequate. A prolonged CRT, in pediatric patients, has been found to be a good predictor of dehydration, reduced stroke volume, and increased blood lactate levels. Serial determination at frequent intervals is an excellent indicator of response to treatment. A gradual improvement in capillary refill is evident with response to treatment.

CRT is assessed by lifting the extremity slightly above the level of the heart and applying enough pressure to blanch the skin.

Decreased skin temperature and perfusion reflects a predominance of the sympathetic neuro hormonal response to hypovolemia. Studies have shown that monitoring of CRT and skin temperature are valuable in hemodynamic monitoring during circulatory shock and should be the first approach to assess any critically ill patient. However, less data are available regarding the clinical utility of these parameters once the patient is admitted to the ICU.

Color of the skin: Cold, pale, clammy, and mottled skin, and peripheral cyanosis associated with an increase in CRT are clinical signs of poor peripheral perfusion.

Blood pressure: The vasomotor tone can increase dramatically in children presenting with shock. Hence the blood pressure is often higher than normal for age in critically ill children in early shock. However, initially the pulse pressure is decreased, often because of some decrease in systolic blood pressure and increase in diastolic pressure. Later, both systolic and diastolic pressures fall indicating a major hemodynamic compromise. Hypotension is therefore a late sign. Hypovolemic shock in children may not occur until there is 30% volume loss. Therefore, hypotension cannot be overvalued as an overall indicator in assessment of shock.

Liver span: Increase in the liver span in a child with shock indicates myocardial dysfunction (cardiogenic shock). The measurement of liver span also indirectly helps evaluation of myocardial response to fluid management and inotropes therapy in absence of invasive hemodynamic monitoring.

Respiratory rate: A child with shock may present with tachypnea or hyperapnea.

Urine output: The child with shock may present with oliguria or anuria. Oliguria is a sign of vital organ hypoperfusion. Urine output of 1 – 2 ml/kg/hour is a reassuring sign of normal renal perfusion in children with shock.

Level of consciousness: Can assess the degree of vital organ hypoperfusion. The signs of brain hypoperfusion are an inconsolable cry, increasing drowsiness, a weak cry and hypotonia in young infants. Loss of eye contact (not focussing on mother's eyes) in an infant more than 2 months old is an early and ominous sign of cerebral hypoperfusion. Lethargy, agitation, confusion, often alternating with drowsiness are signs in older children. Presence of unequal pupil is the earliest sign of raised intracranial tension.

Table 2.8: Showing signs for early recognition of shock

Systems	*Symptoms and signs*
Cardiopulmonary	• Heart rate: Tachycardia • Pulse volume: Diminished distal pulse volume • Core and peripheral temperature gap > 2°C • Capillary refill time > 2 secs • Color of the skin: Cold, pale, clammy, and mottled skin, and peripheral cyanosis • Blood pressure: Higher than normal
Respiratory	• Respiratory rate: Tachypnea, hyperapnea
GIT	• Liver span: Increased
Kidney	• Urine output: Oliguria, Anuria
CNS	• Level of consciousness: See Table 2.9

Table 2.9: Showing signs of hypoperfusion of brain (level of consciousness)

Infants	*Older children*
(a) An inconsolable cry	(a) Lethargy, agitation, confusion, often alternating with drowsiness
(b) Increasing drowsiness	(b) Presence of unequal pupil is the earliest sign of raised intracranial tension
(c) A weak cry	
(d) Hypotonia	
(e) Loss of eye contact (not focussing on mother's eyes)	

Features of Prolonged Cerebral Hypoperfusion

Children with shock are usually hypotonic. However, intermittent flexor or extensor posturing may occur with extreme hypoxia and prolonged cerebral hypoperfusion. It needs emphasis that in presence of such abnormal movements in presence of shock, the child needs aggressive treatment of hypoxia and shock. Over enthusiastic anticonvulsive therapy in such cases can worsen the cardiopulmonary status. The signs of vital organ dysfunction include the following:

Cerebral : Hypotonia, intermittent flexor or extensor posturing

GIT : Erosive gastritis, ischemic pancreatitis

Liver : Ischemic hepatitis–elevation of transaminases and bilirubin

Hematologic: Coagulation abnormality, elevated PT, PTTK, severe DIC and Thrombocytopenia.

Septic Shock: Early Signs

The physical findings of early septic shock are different from other types of shock as the patient may have fever, chills. The peripheral tissues are initially well perfused and warm. Peripheral pulse rate and volume are increased. Pulse pressure is widened, precordium is hyperdynamic and diastolic blood pressure is low. Presence of acidosis is sign of early septic shock.

Table 2.10: Showing early physical signs in septic shock

(a) Fever with chills
(b) Warm peripheries
(c) Peripheral pulse rate increased
(d) Peripheral pulse volume high
(e) Low diastolic pressure and wide pulse pressure
(f) Precordium is hyperdynamic
(g) Presence of acidosis

However, once multiple organ failure sets in, the patient becomes cold, has decreased pulse volume, low blood pressure, and signs of decompensated shock. The society of critical medicine, USA has proposed a grading of severity of sepsis and septic shock applicable for all age as follows:

Table 2.11: Grading of sepsis and septic shock

Term	*Definition*
SIRS (Systemic inflammatory response syndrome)	Two or more of the following present: Tachycardia, Tachypnea Hyperthermia (>101°F / > 38°C) Hypothermia (< 96°F / 35.5°C) WBC > 12000/cumm / < 4000 /cumm Or, > 10% band cells
Sepsis	SIRS + Clinical Evidence of infection
Severe sepsis	Sepsis + Evidence of altered organ dysfunction, hypoperfusion or hypotension with 1 or more of the following: Acute change in mental status Low PaO_2 or FiO_2 Increased lactate Oliguria (urine output < 0.5 ml/kg for at least 1 hour)
Septic shock	Sepsis with hypotension or fall in mean arterial pressure by > 10 mm Hg from base line and perfusion abnormalities that is responsive to fluid resuscitation
Refractory or nonresponsive septic shock	Sepsis with hypotension that lasts for > 1 hour not responsive to IV fluid (20 ml/kg of normal saline over 30 minutes) or pharmacologic interventions (requiring vasopressor, e.g., dopamine > 10 mcg/kg/min)

Laboratory Markers of Shock

Serial blood gas and arterial lactate evaluation are the widely used markers to complement the clinical assessment of systemic perfusion and providing useful trends to titrate therapy.

It needs emphasis that normalization of blood pressure may not indicate reversal of the shock state in a patient who has ongoing metabolic acidosis and/or elevated arterial lactate. Recent studies have used central venous oxygen saturation ($ScvO_2$) to detect global oxygen deficiency. $ScvO_2$ can be monitored continuously with fiberoptic probes.

In clinical setting, a decrease in mixed venous O_2 saturation of 5% from its normal value (i.e., 65–77%) represents a significant fall in oxygen delivery (DO_2) and/or an increase in O_2 demand.

Laboratory Tests to Assess Severity and Etiology

Assessment of severity and etiology is greatly assisted by the following laboratory investigations:

1. Complete blood count.
2. Serum total protein and albumin.
3. Urea, serum creatinine, serum calcium (preferably ionised).
4. ABG, LFT, arterial blood lactate.
5. Coagulation profile.
6. X-ray chest.
7. Appropriate microbiological tests.

Arterial blood gas analysis is a very valuable aid in the management of shock. It helps in determining the adequacy of ventilatory functions. Determination of pH and base deficit aids in the quantification of tissue hypoperfusion, as the degree of metabolic acidosis correlates with severity of tissue perfusion. A simultaneous mixed venous oxygen tension can help quantifying the oxygen consumption.

Management

The approach to a patient who is potentially in shock requires that examination and resuscitation go hand in hand.

The Initial Resuscitation

The initial resuscitation involves securing a patent airway, administration of oxygen, establishment of intravenous excess and optimisation and stabilisation of cardiac output and systolic arterial blood pressure. These therapies are common to all forms of shock.

(a) A patent airway is to be maintained, if necessary, by using airway supports viz. nasopharyngeal airway, oral airway and endotracheal intubation.

(b) Oxygen should be administered initially to all patients in shock with an attempt to achieve an arterial oxygen saturation of 90% or higher. Continuous assessment of oxygenation can be guided by use of pulse oximetry. However, alteration in management must be based on direct assessment of arterial blood gas.

(c) A venous access must be obtained immediately. In children below 6 years, intraosseous route may be used for administration of fluids and drugs when I.V. access is not obtained within 1 to 2 minutes.

(d) Restoration of effective circulating volume by replacement of fluid is the key step. Almost all patients with hypovolemic and neurogenic shock and 20 to 30% with septic shock will respond well to fluid alone.

(e) If there is poor therapeutic response after two boluses (of 20 ml/kg normal saline/Ringers lactate IV in 30 minutes) or if there is evidence of cardiac or renal disease CVP measurement should be undertaken to evaluate the need and response to further fluid therapy.

Signs of Response to Fluid Bolus

1. Improvement in pulse volume.
2. Decrease capillary refill time.
3. Improvement of sensorium.
4. Decrease of tachycardia.
5. Elevation of initial decreased blood pressure.
6. Adequate urine output > 1 ml/kg/hr.

Administration of Vasoactive Drugs

Use of vasoactive drugs is a cornerstone because all shock states including hypovolemic have some form of impairment of myocardial function whether primary or secondary. It helps in optimisation of cardiac output.

In general, inotropic and vasodilator drugs should be used once volume resuscitation has been achieved. Even in cardiogenic shock, if there are no signs of CCF, Ringer's lactate in 5-10 ml/kg aliquots should be given while monitoring perfusion. However, in septic shock it is sometimes essential to start vasoactive drugs at the same time as the fluid infusion if the patient has profound hypotension or end organ failure.

Initial therapy should be undertaken with drugs with a mixed inotropic and vasopressor effect, e.g., dopamine, epinephrine, or norepinephrine. Addition of an inotropic agent, e.g., dobutamine may be considered if presence of myocardial dysfunction is suspected or confirmed. It is ideal to start with dopamine at a dose of 10 microgram/kg/min. Dobutamine can be added if response is inadequate.

In a patient who is in a low cardiac output state and where blood pressure appears adequate dobutamine may be the drug of first choice. In a patient who fails to respond to maximal increases in dopamine or dobutamine more potent agents viz. epinephrine, norepinephrine and isoproterenol must be considered. Adrenaline is useful in patients with left ventricular dysfunction that does not respond to dopamine and dobutamine. It is usually started at 0.1 microgram/kg/min and increased rapidly (max dose not to exceed 2-3 micrograms/kg/min. Norepinephrine is useful in septic shock when dopamine fails to reverse hypotension by improving arterial BP and urine flow.

Management of Neurogenic Shock

1. Trendelenburg position and compression leg wrap.
2. Ringer's lactate/Normal saline in 10-20 ml/kg aliquots.
3. Vasopressor drugs: Phenylephrine, 1-10 microgram/kg continuous infusion (1-10 microgram/kg/min in 5 to 10 minutes).

Specific Therapy of Hemorrhagic Shock

1.	Blood loss	< 15%	:	Ringer's lactate 20 ml/kg bolus
2.	Blood loss	15-30%	:	Ringer's lactate + whole blood (10-15 ml/kg)
3.	Blood loss	30-40%	:	Whole blood (10-15 ml/kg)

N.B.: 1. Replacement should be done as soon as possible.

2. Use of fresh blood (< 48 hours old) is preferable.

Management of Cardiogenic Shock

1. With no signs of CCF: Ringer's lactate 5-10 ml/kg aliquots should be given while monitoring perfusion. Fluid is stopped if there is no improvement.

2. If signs of CCF (viz. increased JVP, pulmonary edema, enlarged tender liver) develop/present vasoactive drugs are to be started.

Management of Septic Shock

1. Ringer's lactate/Normal saline rapidly in 20 ml/kg aliquots, if possible through two large bore peripheral IV catheters until perfusion, tachycardia and hypotension resolve. Successful outcome depend on the rapidity of infusion.

   If the administration of 60 ml/kg of crystalloid results in no improvement, myocardial dysfunction should be considered and vasoactive drugs (dopamine, epinephrine, norepinephrine, milrinone and vasopressin) needs to be started. The complex etiology of myocardial dysfunction often necessitates a combination of these agents.
2. Start vasoactive drugs initially if the patient has profound hypotension or end organ failure.
3. A broad spectrum antibiotic should be started after sending blood for culture. The choice of antibiotics depends on the specific predisposing risk factors.

Table 2.12: Showing the dosage schedule of vasoactive agents

Medications	*Dosage schedule*
Dopamine	10 mcg/kg/min IV continuous infusion increased slowly to a maximum of 30 mcg/kg/min
Dobutamine	5 – 20 mcg/kg/min IV continuous infusion
Epinephrine	0.1 ml/kg/dose of 1:10000 solution to be flushed with 5 ml of normal saline
Norepinephrine	0.05 – 0.1 mg/kg/min. Dose titrated to the desired effect (max dose 2 mg/kg/min)
Milrinone	50 – 75 mg/kg loading dose followed by 0.25 – 1.0 mg/kg/min continuous infusion
Vasopressin	0.3 – 2.0 units/kg/min

Adapted from Drug Dosages in Children by Meherban Singh and Asok Deorari, 8th edition, 2011.

Outcome

The effective treatment of shock requires a high index of suspicion and early diagnosis. Aggressive and early management is associated with intact survival. The mortality depends on the underlying etiology, being as high as 50% with septic shock. The bad prognostic factors are low body temperature (< 37°C), pulmonary disease, low cardiac index (<3.3l/min/m^2) and decreased oxygen utilisation.

Application of conventional goals of resuscitation, viz. ABC for airway, breathing and circulation, added by D for increasing the delivery of oxygen to level that meet the metabolic demands of all tissues in the body will help to prevent continued oxygen deficit and reduce the possibility of irreversible organ dysfunction and death.

Anaphylaxis

Anaphylaxis is a clinical condition in which there is a sudden release of potent biologically active mediators from mast cells and basophils leading to cutaneous, respiratory, cardiovascular and gastrointestinal symptoms.

Anaphylaxis represents the most severe allergic reaction in previously sensitized persons. It is a medical emergency and requires immediate medical attention because respiratory and cardiovascular collapse can occur within minutes after exposure to the allergic substance. Fatality is uncommon but may occur most commonly from airway obstruction and cardiovascular collapse.

Etiology

Potentially any substance is able to cause anaphylaxis. However, the common causes include drugs, intravenous immunoglobulin, latex, radio contrast dye, food, insect sting, exercise, exposure to cold, idiopathic.

Pathogenesis

Most cases of anaphylaxis are the result of activation of mast cells and basophils via cell bound allergen specific IgE molecules. As with any IgE mediated reaction, the patient must first be exposed to the responsible allergen to generate allergen specific antibodies. In many cases, the child and the parents are unaware of the initial exposure, which may be passage of food proteins in mother's milk. With re-exposure to the sensitizing allergen there is release of a variety of mediators (viz. histamine, tryptase) and cytokines by mast cells and basophils and possibly macrophages, which can produce allergic symptoms in any or all target organs.

Besides IgE mediated reactions, clinical anaphylaxis can also occur by direct release of mediators from mast cells by medications and physical factors (like exercise and exposure to cold), disturbance of leukotriene metabolism (Aspirin and NSAIDs), immune aggregates and probable complement activation (e.g., radio contrast dyes).

Table 2.13: Showing causative agents of anaphylaxis

Drugs	*Insects*	*Food*
Aspirin, NSAIDs, Penicillin, Cephalosporin, Chloroquine	Hornet, bee and wasp stings	Peanut, tree nuts, fish, sea food, milk, nut, eggs, mango, banana, soy, mustard and wheat.
Acetaminophen, morphine,	Honey bee stings are most dangerous.	
ACE inhibitor, IV contrast		

Clinical Manifestations

Symptoms and signs of anaphylaxis may be related to skin, respiratory, cardiovascular, gastrointestinal and neurologic system.

System	*Clinical features*
Cutaneous	Pruritus, urticaria, erythema, angioedema
Respiratory	Cough, sneezing, nasal congestion/itching, chest tightness, wheeze, stridor, laryngeal edema
Gastrointestinal	Nausea, vomiting, dysphagia, abdominal pain, fecal incontinence
Cardiovascular	Tachycardia, hypotension, syncope
Neurologic	Headache, change of mental status
General	Anxiety, sense of impending doom, pallor.

Respiratory features are result of swelling and edema of the respiratory mucosa and bronchospasm. Laryngeal edema may occur immediately after the exposure to an anaphylactic stimulus and result in upper airway obstruction and death if not treated. Shock due to peripheral vasodilatation can occur with or without respiratory symptoms.

Anaphylaxis can present with any combination of the above features. The onset of symptoms may vary depending on the cause of the reaction. The reaction from ingested allergens viz. food and medications are delayed in onset by minutes to 2 hours in comparison to those with injected allergens viz., stings and parenteral medications. The symptoms generally last for less than 24 hours. Majority of cases present with cutaneous features. Respiratory symptoms are the second in line followed by cardiovascular and gastrointestinal symptoms.

Treatment

Anaphylaxis is a medical emergency and may progress to shock and death if not treated immediately. There may be a biphasic reaction, which occurs around 4 hours after apparent resolution of symptoms, especially in patients in whom the symptoms at presentation were severe and treatment was started late. The cause is not known. It is characterized by recurrence of symptoms. Therefore, a child should be kept under observation for at least 4 hours after resolution of symptoms following treatment.

Steps of Treatment

Initial Management

1. Maintain ABC of resuscitation.
2. The approximate weight of the child should be calculated on the basis of the formula 2 × age + 9.
3. Stop administration of suspected medication, contrast medium, remove allergen from patient's mouth and scrap out bee sting.
4. Administration of oxygen by mask at 6–8 litres/minute.
5. Administration of Epinephrine (1:1000) IM in the dose of 0.01 ml/kg upto maximum of 0.03 ml/kg. Can be repeated every 5–15 minutes until anaphylaxis is controlled or signs of toxicity viz. palpitation, tremor and uncomfortable apprehension appear.
6. In patients with severe hypotensive shock Epinephrine (1:10000) should be given IV. If patient still remains in shock an intravenous infusion @ 0.25 micrograms/kg/minute should be started and titrated according to response.
7. When signs of laryngeal edema and upper airway obstruction are suspected, early intubation should be done as a life saving measure. The patient should be kept in trendelenburg position.
8. If there is severe laryngospasm, bronchospasm, shock or coma, intermittent positive pressure ventilation should be started.
9. When there is no response to initial epinephrine, patients with persistent hypotension should receive IV fluid challenge (20 ml/kg of normal saline/Ringers lactate).

Additional Measures in Initial Management

1. Slow IV doses of Promethazine (0.5–1 mg/kg) and Ranitidine (1 mg/kg).
2. Hydrocortisone 2–6 mg/kg or dexamethasone (0.1 – 0.4 mg/kg). It should be noted that corticosteroids do not reverse acute symptoms but may help prevent or minimize second phase reaction. Despite the controversy of corticosteroids in treatment of anaphylaxis, it is widely acceptable as a part of initial management.
3. Salbutamol nebulization for treatment of bronchospasm.
4. Nebulized epinephrine (1: 1000) for laryngeal edema may be tried but intubation should not be delayed.
5. To slow absorption of injected antigen (e.g., insect stings), a tourniquet may be placed proximal to the injection site. It should be released every 5 minutes. The total duration of tourniquet application should not exceed 30 minutes. Alternatively, aqueous epinephrine (1:1000) 0.1 – 0.2 ml may be injected into the site.

Supportive Treatment

1. Observe vital signs frequently. Monitor ECG and pulse oximetry.
2. All patients who have suffered from severe reaction should be admitted to hospital. Patients who remain unstable after initial management should be admitted to PICU.
3. For a less severe reaction, an asymptomatic patient may be discharged after 4–8 hours of observation. However, they should be cautioned about the second phase reaction which may occur even after 38 hours.

Suggested Reading

1. Steven M. Hollenberg, Joseph E. Parillo. Shock in Harrison's Principles of Internal Medicine, volume I, 14th edition, McGraw-Hill (Health Professions division) 1998; 214-222.
2. Menon PSN, Lodha R. Shock, in Medical Emergencies in Children Ed. Meherban Singh, Sagar Publications, 72, Janpath, Ved Mansion, New Delhi, 3rd edition, 2000; 176-192.
3. Crone RK. Acute Circulatory Failure in Children. Pediatr. Clin. North Am 1980; 27:525-538.
4. Gadeit Rainer, Maredante Karen. Recognition and Treatment of Shock in Children, IJPP 2000; 2:310-314.
5. Tobin JR, Wetzel RC. In Textbook of Pediatric Intensive Care. Ed. Rogers MC. Media, Pennsylvania. Williams and Wilkins 1996; 555-605.
6. Bergman KS, Harris BH. Arteriovenous pH difference–a new index of perfusion. J. Pediatr. Surg 1988;23:1190.
7. Wetzel RC, Rogers MC. Pediatric monitoring In Textbook of Critical Care. Ed. Shoemaker WC, Ayer S, Grevil A, Hollbrook PR, Thompson WL. Philadelphia. W B Saunders Co 1989; 215.
8. Saavedra JM, Harris GD, Finberg L. Capillary refilling in assessment of dehydration. Am. J. Dis. Child 1991;145:296.
9. Vega RM, Arner JR. A prospective study of usefulness of clinical and laboratory parameters for predicting percentage of dehydration in children. Pediatr. Emerg Care 1997;13:179.
10. Society of Critical Care Medicine. Consensus Conference. Definition for sepsis and organ failure and guidelines for the use of innovative therapy in sepsis.
11. Singhi Sunit. Management of Shock. Ind. Pediatr 1999;36:265-288.
12. Tobius JD. Shock in Children. The first 60 minutes. Pediatr. Ann 1996; 26(6):330-338.
13. Bengur AR, Meliones JR. Cardiogenic Shock. New horizon 1998; 6:139-140.

3

Breastfeeding and Lactation Management

OUTLINES

Breast milk is natural and normal food for the baby. Exclusive breast feeding during the first six months of life has been increasingly recognized to be of vital public health importance to all members of the society in the developing as well as the industrialized world. It has added advantage in terms of food security to the children of the developing world, where the incidence of malnutrition is very high. Exclusive breast feeding is advantageous for all–the baby, mother, family and the society. It is a perfect food even when the mother is ill, pregnant, menstruating or undernourished. Breastfeeding saves life. An exclusively breast fed infant is 14 times less likely to die from diarrhea, 4 times less likely to die from respiratory diseases and 3 times less likely to die from infections as compared to a bottle fed infant.

Advantages of Exclusive Breastfeeding

What is Exclusive Breastfeeding?

Exclusive breastfeeding means the infant receives only breast milk (from mother) and no other liquids, not even water or any complementary food with the exception of undiluted vitamin/mineral syrups and medicines.

Benefits to the Baby

1. Breast milk contains the right kind of proteins, fats, lactose, vitamins, minerals, enzymes and water in the amounts necessary for optimum growth and development of the infant during the first 6 months.
2. Breast milk is readily available, at the correct temperature and in required amounts. It does not require preparation, hence free from contamination.
3. It enhances the emotional bonding between the mother and the child.
4. It contains anti-infective factors including leucocytes, immunoglobulin and antibodies which protects the infant against infections like diarrhea, respiratory infections.
5. Exclusively breast fed babies have been shown to have a higher IQ and some studies have shown that breast fed babies develop better mathematical abilities than do infants that are not breast fed.

6. Breast fed babies are less prone to develop asthma and other allergic disorders. They have less chances of developing obesity and resultant diseases like diabetes, hypertension and coronary artery disease.

Benefits to the Mother

1. Breastfeeding soon after birth prevents postpartum haemorrhage; hence anemia and maternal death. Postpartum hemorrhage is the main cause of maternal death in our country at present.
2. It saves time and energy of the mother because she does not need time to prepare milk every 2 – 3 hours day and night.
3. It helps the mother regain her figure by utilizing the extra fat, laid down during the third trimester of pregnancy in production of breast milk. So obesity is less common in breastfeeding mothers.
4. Mothers who exclusively breastfeed their babies are better adjusted with their babies as far as rearing and behavioural adjustment is concerned.
5. Exclusive breastfeeding has a protective effect against breast and ovarian cancer and incidence of obesity.
6. Exclusive breastfeeding has contraceptive effect in the first 4 – 6 months.

Benefits for the Family and Society

1. Breastfeeding saves money, time and conserves energy. It saves money because breast milk does not need money to buy. A baby on exclusive breast-feeding suffers less from diseases; hence the family spends less on medicines and hospitalisation. Exclusive breastfeeding promotes family planning and thereby child survival.
2. Exclusive breastfeeding conserves energy because manufacture of artificial milk needs setting up of factories and spending of energy whereas breast milk production is at the expense of mother's energy. However, the mother requires an additional amount of only 600 calories extra for maintaining her health during lactation.

Disadvantages of Breast Milk Substitutes

The breast milk substitutes include animal milk (commonly cow, goat and buffalo) and commercially available dried powder milk in packets and tins. The disadvantages of breast milk substitutes include the following:

1. It is less nutritious and expensive. It does not contain nutrients in proper concentration suitable for the human baby. It has to be bought from the market and is costly.
2. Causes digestive problems as the composition is not suitable for human infants. It can cause malnutrition (undernutrition and obesity) if not fed in the recommended dilution of powder and milk.
3. Does not contain the anti-infective substances. Hence cannot protect child from infection.
4. Has to be prepared. Hence more chances of contamination.
5. Increase risk of allergic problems in baby as they are exposed to foreign protein present in cow's milk.
6. Does not protect mother from ovarian and breast cancer. It may result in early pregnancy.
7. Not suitable for proper brain development because cow's milk does not contain taurine and cystine.
8. Do not nurture bonding of mother and child.

Feeding Breast Milk Substitutes

The common indication is an orphan whose mother died during delivery. Even in such cases breast milk substitutes should be started only when a wet nurse is not available to breast feed the infant.

The commonly used and safer animal milk is cow's milk in our part of the country. Goat milk should not be advised as it contains very low amount of folic acid and if fed without supplementation for a prolonged period can cause megaloblastic anemia. Buffalo milk is very high in fat content which may not be tolerated by many infants. In a way dried powder milk is more hygienic than animal milk. This milk is supplemented with vitamins and minerals but still far inferior than breast milk.

Preparation

Cow's milk requires some humanization. It is done by boiling for 5–6 minutes and adding sugar. Boiling of cow's milk serves several purposes. It breaks down the complex proteins in cow's milk into simpler proteins so that the infant can digest. It also sterilizes the milk and makes it free of germs. The carbohydrate content of cow's milk is much less than human milk. Therefore for every 100 ml of cow's milk, 5 grams sugar should be added to increase the carbohydrate content and make it sweet. There is no need to dilute cow's milk but before boiling a small amount of water is to be added to prevent thickening of the milk. The added water evaporates during boiling.

All infants fed exclusively on cow's milk should receive supplements of vitamin B complex, Vitamin C and iron from the neonatal period. Vitamin C in cow's milk is destroyed during boiling and cow's milk iron is not absorbed adequately. So infants fed exclusively on cow's without supplements is at risk of suffering from scurvy and iron deficiency anemia.

When dried powder milk is used, a good and reliable brand should be selected. Every container of powdered milk contains a measure spoon. The proportion of milk powder and water (1 measure spoonful in 30 ml water) should be strictly adhered to so that the infant gets appropriate nutrition. Dilute milk causes malnutrition whereas concentrated milk causes intolerance and constipation.

Composition of Breast Milk

Breast milk is an ideal food because it contains all the nutrients that an infant needs for the first six months of life. The composition of breast milk is different at different stages of lactation. Hence it is referred to with different names like colostrum, transition milk, mature milk, and preterm milk.

Colostrum

Colostrum is the milk secreted in the first 7 days of life. It is thick, sticky, yellowish or clear. It is secreted in small amounts (30–100 ml).

Colostrum works as first defence against infections by providing 30–80 times higher concentration of white cells (mostly macrophages and some T and B lymphocytes) than mature milk, more antibodies and lysozymes. Hence it is called the first immunization. Antibodies and other immune factors probably work as modifying agents, preventing allergies in later life.

Composition of Colostrum (1–3 days)

Volume	2–20 ml per feed (30–100 ml/ 24 hours)
Colour	Lemon yellow
Specific gravity	1.040–1.060
Energy	67 kcal /10 ml
Protein total	2.3 gm/dl
Fat total	2.9 gm /dl
Lactose	5.5 gm /dl
Vitamin A	151 mg/dl
Vitamin E	1.5 mg/dl
Iron	0.5 – 0.8 mg/L
Cells	3–8 × 106 / ml

Colostrum works as a purgative and clears bilirubin from gut rapidly thereby preventing jaundice. Colostrum is rich in growth factors and some vitamins, e.g., vitamin A (3 times that of mature milk). Growth factors make intestinal surface villi grow and make intestine nonleaky. Vitamin A reduces the severity of infection. Cholesterol in colostrum helps in brain growth and growth of Bifidus flora in the gut. Colostrum contains antioxidants which trap neutrophil generated reactive oxygen metabolites. The yellow color of colostrum is due to beta carotene. Carotenoids are ten times and vitamin E is 2–3 times more than that in mature milk.

Although secreted in small amounts, it is sufficient to meet the calorie needs of a normal newborn infant in the first few days of life.

Transition Milk

It is the milk secreted in the following two weeks of life. The quantity of milk increases while IgG and protein content decrease and fat and sugar increases.

Mature Milk

It is the milk secreted after around two weeks of life. It contains all the nutrients needed for healthy physical and mental development of the infant. Mature milk changes even during the length of a single feed to exactly suit the needs of the infant. Mature milk has two parts viz. fore milk and hind milk.

a. **Fore Milk:** It comes at the start of a feed. It is watery and bluish in color. It has a low level of fat, and is high in lactose, protein, vitamins, minerals and water. It is produced in larger amounts than hind milk and it quenches the baby's thirst.

b. **Hind Milk:** It comes later in the feed. The consistency is thicker than fore milk and contains more fat. The fat content increases gradually from the beginning to the end of a feed. There is no sudden change from fore milk to hind milk. This extra fat makes it look whiter than fore milk. Hind milk supply energy and satisfy the baby's hunger.

It is important for the infant to have both fore milk and hind milk to get a complete meal and water that the infant needs and have an appropriate weight gain. Therefore it is important not to take infant of the breast until the infant is satisfied and the infant leaves the breast on its own.

Preterm Milk

Breast milk is not only species specific but also baby specific. Preterm milk is produced by a woman who delivers prematurely. The mother can produce milk suitable for the baby according to gestation. Preterm milk has a different composition from mature milk. It contains more protein, minerals, immunoglobulin and lactoferrin, more sodium, chloride and iron, less lactose than mature milk, which is essential and best suited for the growth and survival of the preterm baby. The increase amount of protein suit the fast growing needs of the preterm infant.

Breast Milk in the Second Year

Breast milk produced in the second year of life can provide 30% of child's energy requirement and protein needs, and 45% of Vitamin A requirement. Extended breastfeeding upto 2 years age can supply an ample amount of energy and protein to children of poor families who cannot afford to eat protein rich food.

Table 3.1 : Comparison between human milk and cow's milk

Component	*Human milk*	*Cow's milk*
1. Protein	0.9 g/100 g	3.3 g/100 g
2. Fat	3.8 g/100 g	3.8g/100 g
3. Enzyme lipase	Present	Absent
4. Lactose	7 g/100 g	4.8 g/100 g
5. Sodium	7 mEq/L	22 mEq/L
6. Chloride	11 mEq/L	19 mEq/L
7. Potassium	13 mEq/L	35 mEq/L
8. Calcium	34 mg%	117 mg%
9. Phosphorous	15 mg%	92 mg %
10. Iron	0.5 mg/L	0.5 mg/L
11. Zinc	4 mg/L	4 mg/L
12. Water	88%	88%
13. Protective substances	Present	Absent
14. Bacterial contamination	None	Likely

Superiority of Human Milk

1. Human milk has a high percentage of lactose and galactose which are an important component of galactocerebroside which is essential for brain growth as well as absorption of calcium. It contains amino acids like taurine and cystine which are important neurotransmitters.
2. The fats are mostly polyunsaturated fatty acids which are necessary for the myelination of the central nervous system.
3. It contains vitamins, minerals and electrolytes in the right proportion. The iron content is almost similar in amount in human and cow's milk but whereas absorption of iron from human milk is around 60%, cow's milk iron is only 10%.
4. The proteins of breast milk are mostly lactalbumin (> 60%). It forms soft curd which is easy to digest. The baby's intestine does not contain lipase. Breast milk contains lipase which helps in digestion of fat present in human milk.
5. Breast milk also contains hormones and epidermal growth factors which are necessary for maturation of intestinal tract.
6. Breast milk contains protective factors viz. secretory IgA, macrophages, lymphocytes, bifidus factor, unsaturated Lactoferrin, Lysozyme, complement and Interferon and Intestinal growth factor. These factors protect the respiratory tract and GI tract from invasion by harmful organisms.

Anatomy of Breast

Before learning the technique of breastfeeding one should be acquainted with the anatomy of breast, the parts of the breast which are related to breast milk production and the physiology of breast milk production and flow.

The human breast is an exocrine gland that produces milk. The shape and size of the breast varies from woman to woman just as the body build and the facial characteristics. It should be noted that production of milk has no relation to the size of breast.

The skin of the breast includes the nipple, the surrounding areola and the general skin. Bulk of the *nipple* is composed of smooth muscular tissue arranged in inner longitudinal and outer circular and

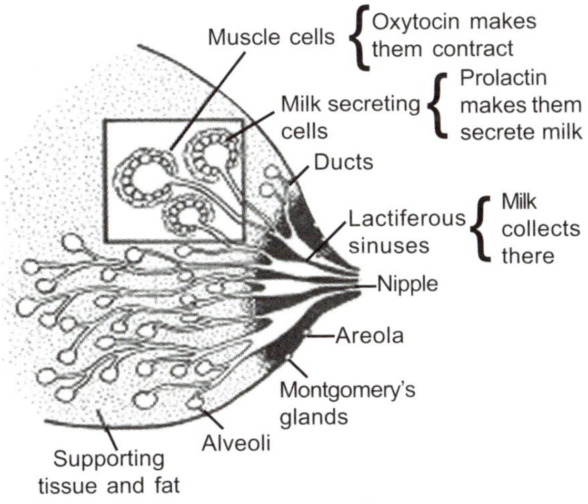

Fig. 3.1: Anatomy of the breast

radial fashion. Each nipple contains 20-25 lactiferous ducts surrounded by fibromuscular tissue. The nipple is richly innervated by unmyelinated sensory nerve endings. The nipple has not much role in breast-feeding. Breastfeeding can be successful in presence of a flat or inverted nipple.

The *areola* is the circular pigmented area surrounding the nipple. It is important to know that the lactiferous sinuses, the store of milk lies below the areola. For effective sucking and flow of milk the baby should suck the areola and not the nipple.

The *breast tissue* consists of two main parts, the parenchyma and the stroma. The *stroma* includes connective tissue, fat, blood vessels, nerves and lymphatics. The *parenchyma* is composed of alveoli lined with milk secreting cells, which secrete milk when hormone prolactin is released. Each lobulus of the breast contains 10 to 100 alveoli. The alveoli are connected by ducts which join to form lactiferous sinuses where milk collects before ejected out. The alveoli, the ducts and the lactiferous sinuses are wrapped by a net of myoepithelial cells. These cells contract and help to force out the milk into the lactiferous sinuses through the ducts and then eject the milk out of the breast when the hormone oxytocin is released.

The important anatomical part of the breast related to successful breast feeding therefore is the areola under which the lactiferous sinuses – the reservoir of milk is situated. The infant has to suck the areola in order to empty the breast and not the nipple.

Physiology of Lactation

Lactation is the physiologic completion of reproductive cycle. Throughout pregnancy the breast develops and soon after delivery of the infant, the breast responds to changes in the hormonal milieu and the suckling of the infant to produce and release milk.

Role of Hormones

Hormonal control of lactation can be divided into three stages: mammary growth, initiation of milk production and maintenance of established lactation.

Mammary Growth

Mammary growth starts in utero and ends in early pregnancy. The primary and secondary ducts of the breast develop in the fetus in utero and continue to grow after birth. In females before puberty, there is rapid expansion of these ducts under the influence of hormone estrogen. After puberty, there is extensive branching of the ducts with proliferation and canalization of the lobulo-alveolar units. In early pregnancy, there is marked increase in ductular sprouting, branching and lobular formation. This is evoked by the leutal and placental hormones. Irrespective of the size of the breast, the lobulo-alveolar units is same. For the same reason, there is no difference in the amount of milk production and the size of the breast.

Initiation of Milk Secretion

The initiation of milk secretion and maintenance of established lactation depends on the changes in the hormonal milieu of the mother and the reflexes in the infant. Full milk production may take 2–12 days post-partum, sometimes longer.

Colostrum production in small amount starts from the 16th week of pregnancy. Colostrum consists partly of fluid secretions and partly of whole and fragmented alveolar cells and some white blood cells. These cells produce antibodies which help protect both the breast itself and the intestine of the baby against infection. Prolactin secreted from the anterior pituitary and lactogen from placenta stimulates glandular production of colostrum. After delivery the placental inhibition of milk synthesis is removed and the woman's blood level of progesterone declines rapidly after the delivery of placenta. The breast fills with colostrum and the woman experiences breast fullness and engorgement described as 'milk coming in'.

Usually by 2–3 days postpartum, there is copious secretion of milk and changes in milk composition which continues until about 10 days when mature milk secretion is established. It has been observed that suckling of breast ad libitum commonly results in production of a large volume of milk by 24–48 hours after birth. This event marks the shift of lactation under endocrine control to lactation under autocrine control. Thus it is not the level of maternal hormones but the efficiency of infant suckling and/or emptying of milk from the breast which governs the volume produced in the breast. Both breasts are subject to same hormonal control but the volume each produces corresponds to that removed by the infant.

Maintenance of Established Lactation

Several breastfeeding reflexes have been described which are essential for maintenance of established milk secretion. These reflexes are the 'cornerstones of lactation'. One can often find the reason of a breast-feeding problem in the failure of one of them. The reflexes are as follows:

1. Reflexes in the mother
   a. Prolactin/milk production reflex
   b. Oxytocin/milk ejection reflex.
2. Reflexes in the infant
   a. Rooting
   b. Sucking
   c. Swallowing.

Reflexes in the Mother

The maternal reflexes viz. *prolactin/milk production reflex and oxytocin/ milk ejection reflex* involve the hormones prolactin and oxytocin respectively. Stimulation of the nerve endings in the nipple by suckling of the infant sends afferent impulses to the hypothalamus. This results in secretion of prolactin from anterior pituitary and oxytocin from the posterior pituitary. Prolactin helps in secretion of milk by directly acting on the milk secreting cells in the alveoli. It is present in the blood for about 30 minutes after the feed. It makes the breast produce milk for the next feed. So the more the baby sucks, the more prolactin is released and more milk is secreted. Hence the simplest way to increase milk production is to let the baby suckle more often. While the baby sucks, oxytocin contracts the myoepithelial cells forcing the milk out into the ducts giving the mother the feeling of milk let down as a warm and tingling sensation in the breast and transfer

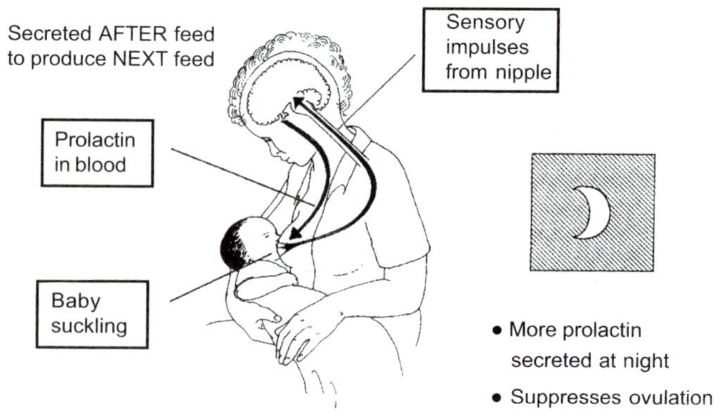

Fig. 3.2: Figure showing prolactin reflex

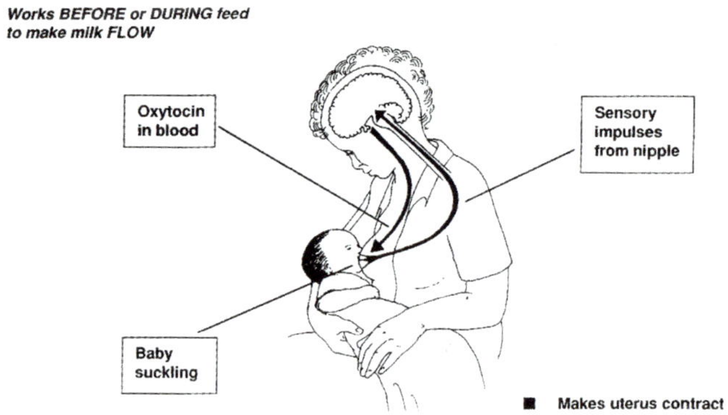

Fig. 3.3: Figure showing oxytocin reflex

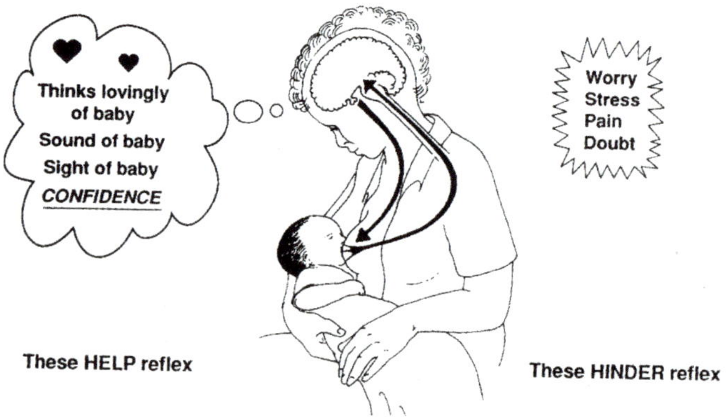

Fig. 3.4: Figure showing oxytocin reflex

of milk from the breast to the infant. Oxytocin is produced with the start of the suckling and sometimes even before that. It is produced for the feed.

Factors Affecting the Maternal Reflexes

The milk ejection reflex is influenced by the woman's psychological state. Thinking lovingly of the baby, sound and sight of the baby, and confidence in the mother help the reflex while worry, stress, pain and doubt in the mother's mind hinder the reflex. Same factors may be true for the milk production reflex. However, the milk production reflex depends on the amount of sucking. More the suckling more is the production. If the mother has twins breast milk production increases due to increased suckling. Prolactin secretion is more at night. Hence night feeds increases milk production on the following day. Increase prolactin secretion suppress ovulation and that is how exclusive breastfeeding helps in spacing of birth.

Reflexes in The Infant

The *rooting reflex* programmes the infant to search the nipple while gaping the mouth widely enough to take a mouthful of breast tissue. The *sucking reflex* is triggered when the nipple touches the palate. The swallowing reflex occurs when the infant's mouth fills with milk after 2–3 sucks.

All the three reflexes in the infant happen automatically without the baby having to learn to do that. For an appropriate feeding behaviour which mean emptying the breast efficiently and frequently, the mother should take the baby in the proper position so that the infant is attached properly to the breast.

Technique of Breastfeeding

- Baby placed in the correct position on the mother's lap.
- The mother touches the angle of the mouth of the baby with the nipple of the breast (Rooting reflex). The baby will open the mouth and protrude the tongue.
- The mother will then put the nipple and areola into mouth of the baby and see that there is proper latching.
- When there is proper latching, the baby will start feeding with a rhythm of 3–4 sucks followed by swallowing.
- One feeding time is 10–20 minutes. The time should not exceed 30 minutes. A feeding time of more than 30 minutes indicates inadequate breast milk production.

What is the Correct Position?

- A comfortable position for the mother and relaxed.
- Head, neck and body straight, baby's shoulders on the elbow of the mother.

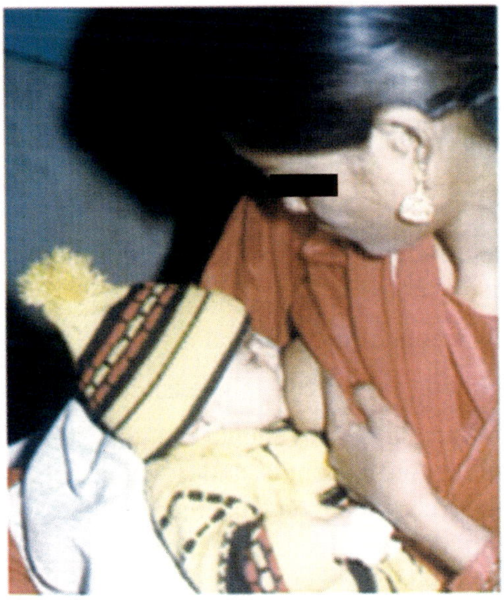

Fig. 3.5: Figure showing proper positioning

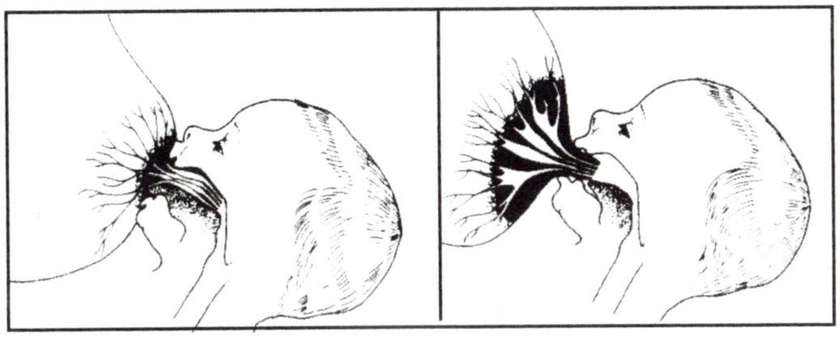

Fig. 3.6: Correct vs. incorrect latching

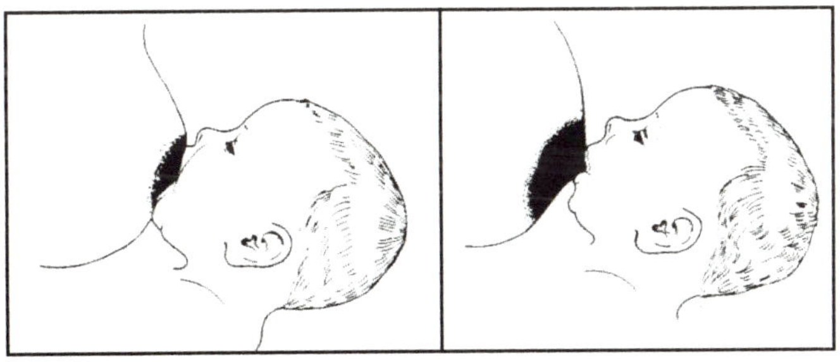

Fig. 3.7: Correct vs. incorrect latching

- Baby should face the mother's breast.
- Baby's abdomen touching the mother's abdomen.
- Mother's one hand on baby's buttock, the other free.

What is Good Attachment/Proper Latching?

- Baby's mouth will be wide open.
- Most of the areola will be inside the mouth. More areola will be seen above the upper lips less below the lower lips.
- Baby's lower lip will be curled outwards.

- Nose will be placed away from the breast and chin touching the breast.
- The baby will feed with slow and deep sucks. Mother does not feel pain during feeding.

Principles of Breastfeeding

1. When to start? Within 1 hour of birth irrespective of mode of delivery.
2. How frequently? On demand.
3. How long each feed? Till satisfied.
4. How long? The baby should continue exclusive breast feeding upto 6 months, and extended breast feeding upto 2 years or beyond together with age appropriate complementary feeding.

Why Breastfeeding Should be Started Early?

After the baby is born, the baby should be dried and immediately given to the mother in the first half an hour. The baby should be placed skin to skin with mother and offered breast milk within 1 hour after birth irrespective of mode of delivery. Starting breastfeeding early is important because:

1. Early initiation results in early production, more production, prolonged production of breast milk.
2. Both mother and the newborn are alert during first 30 – 60 minutes and the sucking reflex is most active in the baby during this time.
3. Early start ensures success of exclusive breast-feeding. Colostrum, which is the first secretion from the breast, is full of anti infective substances that protects the baby from infection like a vaccine. Hence feeding colostrum is considered as the first immunization in the child.
4. It reduces postpartum hemorrhage. Sucking stimulates secretion of hormone oxytocin which helps in early expulsion of placenta as well as involution of uterus.

Why Start Within 1 Hour?

Labour and delivery are stressful situations for both mother and baby. The stress leads to high levels of catecholamines in both mother and baby which keep them alert for first 30 minutes to 60 minutes. Moreover the sucking reflex in the baby is very active at birth. After this period both goes to sleep for few hours. Hence, if breastfeeding is not initiated during the first hour, it may be delayed to hours, only after the mother and the baby wakes up.

No prelacteal feeds should be given before initiating breastfeeding. Prelacteal feeds are a source of infection and they delay initiation of breastfeeding.

Why Breastfeeding is an Ideal Food Beyond 6 Months?

Breastfeeding should be continued beyond six months age together with age appropriate complementary food because of the following reasons:

1. Protective effects of breastfeeding continue beyond 6 months.
2. Breast milk remains a high quality, nutrient rich and energy rich food which is easy to digest. Sick babies often do not feel like eating food, but have appetite for breast milk.
3. Breast milk contains factors that help in absorption of nutrients.
4. It can provide 30% of child's energy and protein needs, 45% of Vitamin A requirement during the second year of life.

Adequacy of Breast Milk

Breastfeeding should be adequate for the baby for proper growth and development. Inadequate breast milk feeding is one of the common causes of nutritional marasmus during infancy. The mother should be made aware of the signs of adequacy of breast milk to avoid unnecessary tension of her thinking that she is not producing enough milk or not reporting early for actual inadequacy.

The signs of adequacy of breast milk include the following:

1. One feeding time of 10–20 minutes (a feeding time of more than 30 minutes indicates inadequacy of breast milk).
2. The baby sleeps or is quiet and content in between feeds.
3. The baby passes 6 or more times urine after the sixth day of life. In the initial period it may be 2–5 times.
4. The baby passes stools typical for a breast fed baby. The stool is golden yellow in color, contains stool matter, some mucous and water and smell sour.
5. The baby gains weight at the rate of 30 gms/day in the first 3 months, 20 gms/day in the next 3 months.

Lactation Management

Just because breastfeeding is natural (i.e. physiological), and nearly all mothers do it, it does not follow that they do so instinctively. Even normal feeding requires a technique that has to be learned, especially with the first baby. Suckling of the baby is learned rather than instinctive behaviour in many other mammals too. For example, when an elephant has her first calf, the experienced females surround her and guide her to feed. Dolphins behave in a similar way. If a woman has a problem with breastfeeding, as commonly happens, she has no inborn knowledge of what to do if her baby refuses to suck, if her nipples get hurt, or if her milk supply seems to be diminishing.

About one third of women in an industrialized society breast feed uneventfully and happily without any problem. In rural societies the proportion may be greater. There remain the other two thirds of the women who have all sorts of problems. These may vary from a minor problem like leaking or a more serious problem like a breast abscess. There are ways to overcome all these difficulties and it is essential for a health care provider to know how to deal with them.

Lactation is highly individual. It varies so much from one woman and one baby to another that it is difficult to formulate general rules.

In order to help mother breast feed successfully she should be counseled and prepared physically and mentally in the antenatal period itself.

Antenatal Counseling

The best time for counseling is the second trimester of pregnancy. During the first trimester, the mother is still not ready for the care of the baby. Moreover she may be sick with hyperemesis. During the third trimester, she is tense because the time of delivery is nearing. Hence second trimester is the best time to prepare the mother physically and mentally and counsel her regarding successful lactation. Many pregnant women arrive at the labour room. Some come early and some come late. This is also an opportune time to prime the mind of the mother if not already done. After the initial assessment, a staff nurse or a doctor should briefly explain the mother especially about early initiation, and the importance of colostrum.

Check List of Information to the Expectant Mother Include

1. Initiation of breastfeeding within an hour of birth irrespective of the mode of delivery.
2. Colostrum is good for the infant. Because of the high level of protective substances it is often referred to as the first immunization.
3. Sucking in the first few days is very essential for adequate production of milk.
4. The small amount of milk produced in the first few days is usually enough for the infant's needs. Supplementary feeds are rarely necessary.
5. Sucking prevents postpartum bleeding by helping involution of the uterus.
6. The ability to breast feed does not depend on the breast size. The size and condition of the nipple has little role in successful breastfeeding.
7. The quantity of breast milk is always good irrespective of nutritional status of mother. Overt vitamin deficiencies (viz. Vitamin A and D) in the mother may result in low levels in breast milk. These infants should receive vitamin supplementation in such situations.
8. Artificial feeding has many disadvantages and bottle feeding is dangerous as it can be a vehicle for organisms.

Physical and Mental Preparation

1. Examine the nipple for abnormalities and reassure the mother if the nipple is abnormal. The nipple has little role in successful breastfeeding.
2. Antenatal advice
   a. Talk about
      i. Advantages of EBF and dangers of artificial feeding, advantages of early initiation.
      ii. Dangers of prelacteal feeds. Prelacteal feeds include honey, water, animal milk etc which are customarily given to newborn before starting breastfeeding. They can act as a vehicle for infection. They delay initiation of breastfeeding.
      iii. Mechanism of breast milk production and technique of breastfeeding.
      iv. Dietary advice during pregnancy and lactation as regards additional calories and

protein. All mothers should be advised an additional 500 calories during lactation. This will replenish the additional calories required by the body for breast milk production and maintain mother's health. She should also be advised to continue iron and folic acid supplementation.

b. Advise mother to make one or two dresses open at front to facilitate breastfeeding.

c. Teach the signs of adequacy of breast milk.

Postnatal Informations

In the immediate postnatal period, the mother should be advised the following:

- No prelacteal feeds. They are harmful.
- Start breastfeeding within 1 hour.
- Bedding in of baby and frequent suckling.
- Mother should remain free from anxiety and tension.

A nutritious diet and iron folic acid supplementation to continue.

Problems During Breastfeeding

Problems may arise during breastfeeding. Helping mothers to solve these problems is one of the foremost responsibilities of health professionals. It is important to deal with the problems faced by the mothers because it may result in stoppage of breastfeeding, introduction of supplementary animal milk or commercial milk formula.

General Problems

1. **My milk has not started coming:** This is a very common problem. The mother complains when she finds that milk does not come out when the breast is squeezed in the first one to two days. Normally on the first and second day only small quantities of colostrum is secreted. Though small in quantity it is adequate for most babies. With frequent and demand feeding, lactation is well established by third or fourth post natal day.
2. **Too little milk:** Some mothers may have too little milk after delivery. Most of these mothers are able to produce enough milk and feed a baby normally after about two weeks. During this time, while the mother is waiting for the milk to increase, she needs support, encouragement, and supervision, so that she does not give up. If the infant loses weight to the extent of more than 10% of birth weight or shows signs of dehydration, expressed breast milk (EBM) can be given from another lactating mother. If EBM is not available, hygienically prepared supplementary milk can be given with cup after each breast feed.
3. **Too much milk too fast:** A mother may produce too much milk and it flows too fast out of the breast due to forceful ejection reflex. The milk fills the infant's mouth quickly and chokes it. In such a situation, the mother should express some milk before the infant start feeding.
4. **Leaking of milk:** In some mothers, leaking of milk can occur from the nipple during first few weeks of lactation. It is because of lack of tone of the sphincter muscles around the milk ducts. Leaking is strongest when the ejection reflex is active and occurs simultaneously from both breasts. So while feeding one breast, the milk leak from the other. Leaking considerably reduces after the first few weeks. Reassurance, frequent suckling and expressing of milk when at work can considerably give relief of leaking of milk.
5. **Blood in milk:** Some mothers may notice a little blood in milk, even in absence of a fissure. It is usually harmless and self limiting condition. The mother should be advised to continue breastfeeding.
6. **Too thin milk:** Some women may complain that their milk is very thin. They should be reassured that it is natural. Human milk is thinner than cow's or buffalo milk because of the lower fat content. Moreover, fore milk is thin and bluish in color whereas hind milk is whiter and thick because hind milk has a higher fat content.
7. **The baby cries too much:** The cry, in the infant, is the only way of communication to the world. Infants develop many kinds of cry. The hunger cry is only one of them. The infant may cry when the napkin is wet or soiled, when she/he feels cold or hot, for insect bites, for an uncomfortable bed or lap, if milk is insufficient, if there is a nose block. A shrill cry may indicate an intracranial infection. A few infants may be just criers or naturally angry babies expressing anger by crying. It should be noted that hunger is the most common discomfort experienced by an infant. The mother should be thus asked to put the baby on the breast whenever it cries. In 80% cases, the child stops crying. If the baby does not stop crying, other causes should be looked for.

8. **Breast refusal and late starters:** Some infants have a difficulty in attaching at the breast of the mother in spite of mother being motivated and frequently attempting to feed. This problem can occur in absence of any abnormality in the infant or the mother. Such infants may start late and have successful breast-feeding. In such infants, mother's milk may be expressed into a container and dropped slowly on her breast when the infant is assisted at the breast (drop and drip method).

Not Enough Milk

It is one of the most common reasons for introducing supplementary milk or early termination of breastfeeding.

The facts about production of enough breast milk are: (a) Almost all mothers can produce enough breast milk provided the baby suckles effectively and feeds on the breast as often as needed; (b) The amount of milk the breasts produce depends on the amount of milk the baby needs; (c) A malnourished woman can produce adequate amount of breast milk for good infant growth; (d) Even when the mother delivers twins or triplets, the mother can secrete enough milk for her babies.

A Practical Stepwise Approach

A practical stepwise approach to the problem of not enough milk involves the following three steps:

First step: To decide whether the infant is getting enough milk or not

To decide whether the infant is getting enough milk or not, one should look for the following reliable signs.

Signs of Getting Enough Milk

The signs of adequacy of breast milk include the following:

1. One feeding time is 10 – 20 minutes. A feeding time of more than 30 minutes indicates inadequacy of breast milk.
2. The baby sleeps or is quiet and content in between feeds.
3. The baby passes 6 or more times urine after the sixth day of life. In the initial period it may be 2 – 5 times.
4. The baby passes stools typical for a breast fed baby. The stool is golden yellow in color, contains stool matter, some mucous and water and smell sour.
5. The baby gains weight at the rate of 30 gms/day in the first 3 months, 20 gms/day in the next 3 months.

Signs of Not Getting Enough Milk

The following complaints by the mother should lead one to suspect inadequacy of breast milk. However, in such situations, one should check for the reliable signs to be certain whether or not baby is getting enough milk.

Complaints regarding the infant include:

- Not satisfied after a breast feed. Wants frequent breast feeds.
- Refuses to feed. Takes very long breast feeds (> 30 minutes).
- Have hard, dry or green stools.

Maternal complaints: A mother may complain that:

- Her breast did not enlarge during pregnancy.
- Breast milk did not "come in" after delivery.
- No milk comes out on expression.

The two reliable signs which indicate that the infant is not getting enough milk include:

1. Baby is below its birth weight after 2 weeks or gains less than 500 grams a month during the first 4 months, the baby is probably not getting enough milk. In order to establish that a baby is not getting enough milk, atleast two weight recordings at 2 weeks interval are needed. A baby should normally gain 250 grams or more in 2 weeks.
2. If the baby passes less than 6 times urine (after 5 days of birth) which is yellow and strong smelling, the milk is not enough.

Second step: If the baby is not getting enough breast milk decide why

To decide why the infant is not getting enough milk, a thorough history and observation of the infant feeding on the breast is necessary. Observing the infant feeding will give information about proper positioning and latching during the whole feed, and the length of feed.

Causes

In most situations, where an infant does not get enough breast milk, the cause is inadequate suckling or ineffective suckling by the infant. In extremely rare situations, poor glandular development of the breast or hormonal disturbances could be a cause.

Breastfeeding Factors

- Delayed start.
- Infrequent feeds, no night feeds, short feeds, and addition of any other fluid leads to less prolactin release.
- Poor attachment.

Maternal Psychological Factors

- Lack of confidence, worry, stress leads to poor oxytocin reflex.
- Dislike of breastfeeding, rejection of baby, tiredness in mother keeps the baby away from the mother.

Physical Conditions in the Mother and Baby

These are less common reasons for not enough milk. These may be considered when a possible solution could not be found after helping the mother.

Mother

- Use of contraceptive pills, diuretics.
- Pregnancy.
- Severe PEM, alcohol consumption, smoking.
- Poor breast development.

Baby

- Illness and abnormality.

Third step: Decide how to help the mother and baby

If the baby is *not getting enough milk* the following steps should be followed:

1. Reassurance to mother. The reason for which the baby is not getting enough milk should be explained to the mother. She should be reassured that she can produce as much milk as her baby needs.
2. The mother should be helped to improve the baby's attachment to the breast if necessary.
3. Frequent suckling (10–12 times/day) and for as long as it wishes should be advised. The baby should be allowed to suckle both breasts.
4. Mother should be helped to gradually reduce (30–60 ml/day) and stop supplementary milk if already started. She can reduce more if the infant is satisfied and gaining weight or less if weight gain is slow. She should use a cup to feed and advised to offer milk after the baby has breast fed for as long as it wants – not instead of a breast feed. The milk should be hygienically prepared and in proper dilution. The baby should be followed every day until baby starts gaining weight, then weekly until mother has gained confidence that her baby is gaining weight satisfactorily on exclusive breastfeeding.
5. If baby is above 4 months age and the above measures have failed, complementary feeding can be started. Animal milk in the form of cow's milk or formula is best avoided. If below 4 months, artificial feeding should be advised prepared in an hygienic way and in proper dilution.

If the baby is *getting enough milk*, which is confirmed by the presence of the reliable signs, the following steps should be followed:

1. The mother should be reassured. She should be explained the reasons for the signs that have made her doubt her milk production. She should be shown that her baby is gaining weight appropriately and that is a reliable sign of the baby getting enough milk.
2. The mother should be helped to improve the attachment of the baby to her breast.
3. The mother should be explained about the advantages of exclusive breastfeeding and dangers of supplements. She should be informed about the role of oxytocin reflex in getting milk down and that building up of confidence can help her come out of the problem.
4. The mother should be followed up every week until she has gained confidence.

Nipple Problems

Flat nipple, inverted nipple: The nipple is a guide to show where the baby has to take the breast. The length of the resting nipple is not important for breastfeeding. A protractility test (Fig. 3.8) helps to assess the working nipple. The woman tries to hold and pull out the nipple. If it can be pulled out it is protractile. Occasionally, a nipple does not protract and on attempting to pull out, the nipple goes deeper into the breast. This is an inverted nipple. In any case, the mother should be reassured that she will be able to breast feed. The inverted nipple should be treated in the post natal period. Nipple exercises and nipple shield

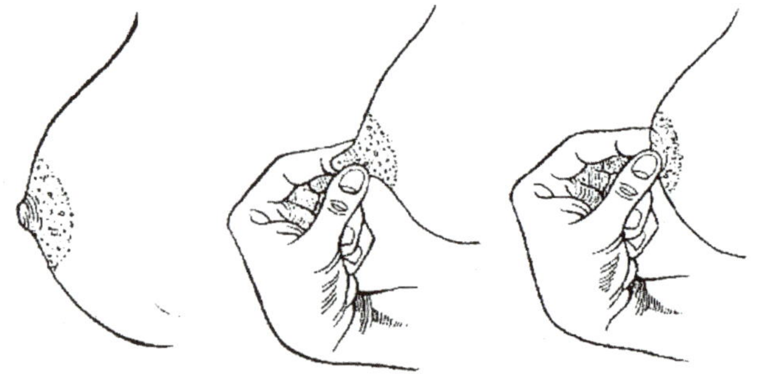

(a) A short nipple. Is it protractile or not?

(b) If you can pull it out like this, then it protracts well

(c) If it goes in like this when you try to pull it out, then it is not protractile

Fig. 3.8: Testing a nipple for protractility

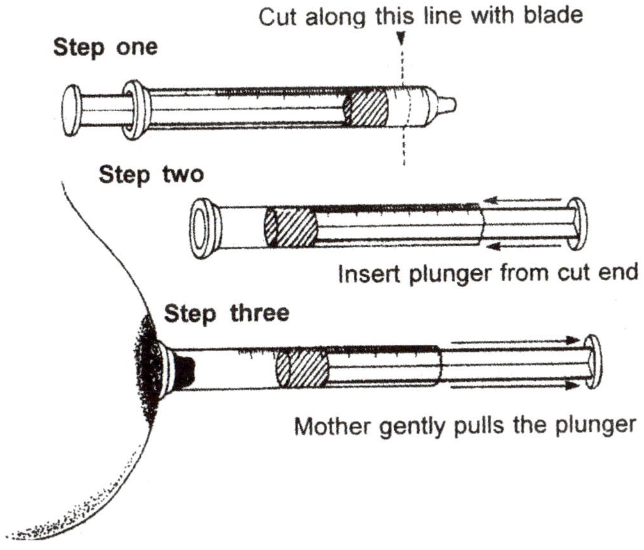

Fig. 3.9: The steps of treatment of inverted nipple

are of no value. The protractile flat nipple does not require any treatment.

The procedure for treatment of inverted nipple by using a disposable syringe is as follows:

- Cut the nozzle end of the syringe.
- Introduce the piston from the ragged cut end side.
- Ask the mother to apply the smooth side on the nipple and gently pull it out and let her wait for a minute.
- The nipple will protrude into the syringe. Ask the mother to slowly release the suction and put the baby to breast. It helps the nipple to erect out and the baby is able to suckle in proper position.
- The nipple then may retract back but doing the procedure each time over a period of days would help solve the problem.

Long nipple: With a long nipple, the baby may suck on the nipple alone and may not be able to take enough breast tissue into the mouth. The mother should be asked to bring the baby closer to the breast to enable it to take more breast tissue into the mouth. With time, the baby gets accustomed and breast feed even with the long nipple.

Sore nipple and cracked nipple: Sore nipple result from improper attachment of the baby's mouth to the breast in the early part of breastfeeding. If the baby continues to breast feed in this wrong position it may lead to cracked nipple, breast engorgement, mastitis and breast abscess. Oral thrush in the baby is another important cause. It usually develops after a few weeks of breastfeeding.

The treatment consists of exposure of the nipple to air and sun, correction of position and attachment. No ointment is necessary to treat the sore. Application of ointment may worsen the condition. The mother can put hind milk over the nipple after every feed. The sore heals in a few days. For oral thrush, 1% gentian violet or Cotrimazole should be applied over the nipple as well as inside the mouth of the baby. Systemic antifungal drugs may be needed for the mother if there is deep pain and itching.

Breast Problems

Breast engorgement: If enough milk is not removed from the breast, engorgement may result. The engorged breast feels tight, looks shinny and is painful. The milk may stop flowing. The baby cannot feed in correct position for tightness and the mother avoids feeding because of pain. This further aggravates the condition. Engorged breast may cause a mild fever (milk fever) in mother which subsides spontaneously. The common causes of breast engorgement are as follows:

- Prelacteal feeds.
- Delayed initiation of breastfeeding.
- Long intervals between feeds.
- Short feeds.
- Sore nipple.

Management includes frequent breastfeeding which relieves mild engorgement of breast. If pain and tightness of breast is severe, expression of breast milk can relieve pain and allow breastfeeding. If breast suckling is not possible, expressed breast milk can be given with cup and expression is continued till mother is comfortable.

Blocked duct, mastitis and breast abscess: A lactiferous duct may be blocked by thick milk if the baby does not suck well on a particular segment. This results in a painful hard swelling. If the blocked duct or engorged breast and sore nipple persist, infection may supervene. The sore is a good portal of entry and milk is a good nidus for bacterial growth. Breastfeeding should be continued in the normal breast and restarted in the other breast as early as possible.

Frequent breastfeeding on the affected breast in case of a blocked duct and massaging of the lump towards the nipple to promote emptying of breast should be advised.

With mastitis, the breast becomes hot, tender and swollen. If left untreated, an abscess may form as a hot, tender and fluctuant swelling, often associated with fever.

Treatment of mastitis consists of rest, frequent expression of breast milk, antibiotics and analgesic. Warm water fomentation may help to alleviate pain in mastitis. Antibiotics like Cloxacillin/Amoxicillin clavulinic acid should be started in case of mastitis and breast abscess. Paracetamol should be advised for pain. An abscess will need incision and drainage.

Breastfeeding should be started from the infected breast as soon as possible. Manual expression of breast milk in the affected breast should be advised till recovery to maintain lactation. The mother should be taught correct position and attachment during breastfeeding to prevent recurrence.

Expression of Breast Milk

All mothers should learn to express their breast milk. This can be taught during pregnancy and practised soon after birth. Expression of breast milk is useful in the following circumstances:

1. Feeding a low birth weight or sick neonate.
2. To relieve engorgement of breast.
3. Maintain milk supply when mother is sick and cannot feed the baby.
4. Relieve leaking breasts.
5. Leave milk for the baby when the mother goes out or to work.
6. Feed a baby when it learns to feed from an inverted nipple.

Method of Expression

Milk may be expressed by a pump (hand or mechanical) or by hand. Hand expression is the most useful method. A woman should express her own milk.

Steps of Expression

1. The mother should be psychologically prepared by building her confidence, reducing anxiety and pain and helping her to have good thoughts and feeling.
2. The mother should select a quiet place and ensure privacy. She should wash her hands and sit or stand comfortably holding a clean container near the breast.
3. The thumb and the index finger should be placed above and below the nipple opposite each other. The thumb and the finger should be pressed inwards towards the chest wall, and then the areola behind the nipple should be pressed between the finger and

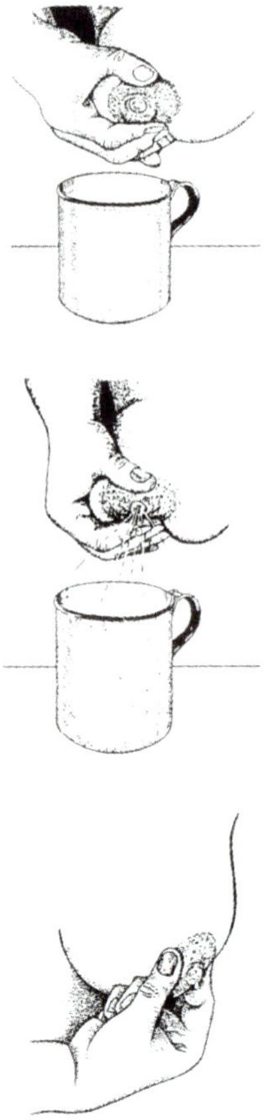

Fig. 3.10: Figure showing how to express milk

thumb so that the lactiferous sinuses beneath the areola are compressed.

4. Pressure should be alternatively given and released till the milk flow starts. Milk flow usually starts only after pressing for 4–5 times. If the procedure produces pain, the technique is wrong.
5. Pressure should be given on all sides to ensure expression from all segments of the breasts. Expression should be done alternately in both breasts for 3–5 minutes in each or till milk flow slows. To express milk adequately it takes about 20–30 minutes.

Special Situations

Working mothers: It is preferable that the working mothers practise exclusive breastfeeding for 6 months. It can be possible by adopting the following means:

- Exclusive breast feeding during the period of maternity leave. The total period of maternity leave can be taken after delivery. The leave can be further extended for the rest of the period with some other type of leave.

- If such leave is not possible after 4 months, the mother should give breastfeeding in the early morning and before going to work place. She can express milk before she leaves for work. This milk can be fed to the baby with a cup by the care giver. Breast milk can be stored at room temperature in a container with a cover for 6–8 hours and for 24 hours in the refrigerator. The mother can come from work in-between and feed the baby or express milk while at work and keep it for her baby. She should breast feed after return from work.
- After 4 months complementary feeding can be started but cereal based diet are not ideal, because infants under 6 months lack the enzyme pancreatic amylase necessary to digest starch.

At present many state governments have allowed 6 months maternity leave. Hope all government, public and private organisations follow suit.

Cleft lip and cleft palate: With only cleft lip there is no difficulty in breastfeeding. Some babies with partial cleft palate can be trained to breast feed in an upright position. Others may need cup, spoon or tube feeding.

Full term twins: Mothers have the capacity of producing milk for two babies. With two babies sucking, the breast milk production will increase. The mother should be explained these facts and shown the method to breast feed twins. Family support is very essential in such cases.

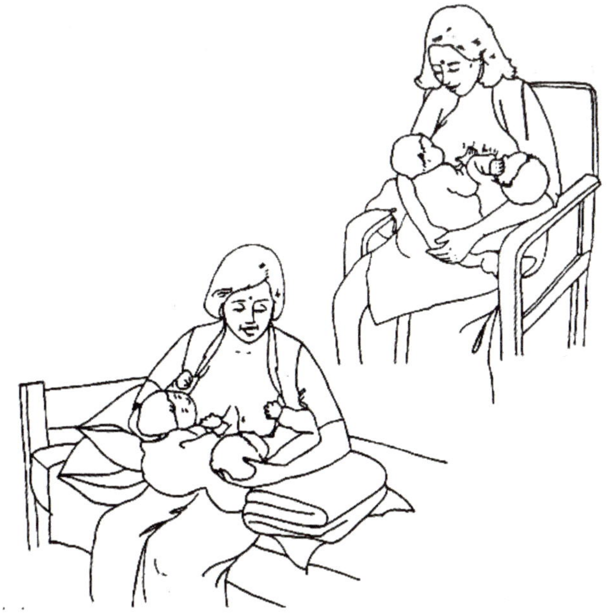

Fig. 3.11: Two ways of breast feeding twins

Maternal illness: Common maternal illness is not a contraindication of breastfeeding. During illness, the antibody produced in the mother is transferred to the baby through breast milk and protects the child (Fig. 3.12). Physically incapacitating systemic illness and psychosis may necessitate discontinuation.

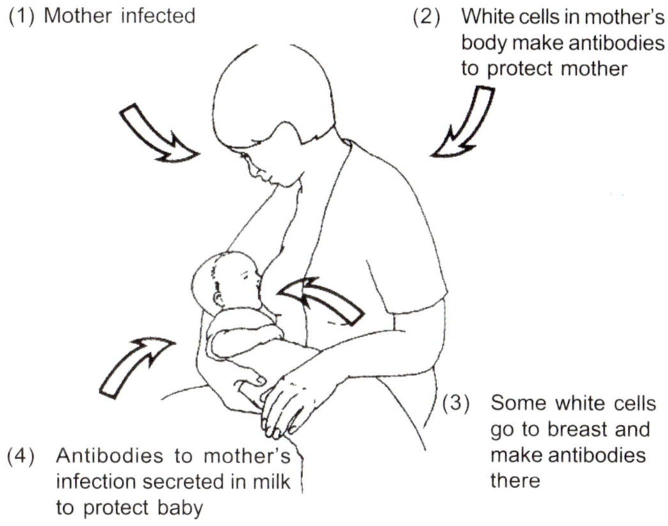

Fig. 3.12: Mechanism of protection of infant during common illness in mother

In HIV positive mothers, the WHO recommends that in under developed countries, the parents should be explained about the risk of transmission of virus in breast milk and allowed to take a decision on their own. In these countries, breastfeeding can protect the HIV infected child from other infections.

(See chapter on HIV/AIDS)

Malnutrition in mother: The quantity and quality of breast milk is maintained in a malnourished mother. Breastfeeding should be continued. The mother should be advised an adequate diet to improve her health.

Pregnancy: A mother can safely continue to breast feed the older child during a subsequent pregnancy. She should eat well to maintain her health.

Mother on drugs: Breastfeeding is contraindicated in a mother who is on anticancer drugs, radioactive substances, repeated doses of ergot (one dose postpartum is not harmful) and lithium. Most other drugs are safe. However, to be 100% safe, the lactating mother should be advised to take the drug doses immediately after a breast feed so that by the time the baby has the next feed, i.e., by 2–3 hours, the drug disappears from breast milk.

Sick baby: Breastfeeding should be continued in sick babies. The mother should be always hospitalized together with the baby. Breast milk is nutritious and easily digested, especially in babies suffering from diarrhea. It also supplies antibodies. The sick infant may refuse other food but usually accepts breast milk.

Low birth weight baby: Babies above 1800 gms should be encouraged breastfeeding. Babies weighing below that may need cup or nasogastric feeding. They should be fed expressed breast milk.

Complementary Feeding in Exclusively Breast-fed Infants

Complementary feeding is providing other foods or liquids along with breast milk. Breast milk is the ideal and appropriate food upto around 6 months age. After the age of 6 months, complementary feeding should be introduced to meet the nutritional needs of the growing child. Some infants may need complementary food after the age of 4 months if they are not growing adequately or appear hungry despite adequate breastfeeding. *However, no animal milk or formula milk should be fed after 4 months age in case of inadequate breast milk.* Again if need be, the infant should not be started on cereals between 4–6 months, as they cannot digest starch adequately because of lack of pancreatic amylase. Complementary food, at this age, can be started with fruits like ripe banana, papaya.

During the major part of the second half of first year the energy and nutrient contribution from breast milk is maintained at almost the same level as at 6 months of age. Complementary feeding is started with an education diet in very small amounts with an aim for new taste development. It is followed by transitional foods which are specifically prepared to meet the physiological and nutritional needs of the infants.

Therefore energy supplied by family foods during first year complements breast milk. It is only during the second year that the complementary feeding really replaces breast milk.

Physiological Development and Young Child Feeding

Rooting, sucking and swallowing reflexes, present at birth, facilitate breastfeeding. Sucking-swallowing coordination is present only from 34 weeks of gestation. Hence breastfeeding is possible only after 34 weeks of gestation. Below 34 weeks the infant should be fed expressed breast milk by gavage feeding to start with, followed by cup feeding and then breastfeeding. Presence of the gag reflex interferes with introduction of solids during the first 6 months of age. Pancreatic enzymes are suboptimal in the first 6 months. Hence cereals should not be started before 6 months age. The strength of voluntary sucking and swallowing is increased during 4–7 months.

By 7th month age, the locus of sensitivity to stimulation of gag reflex moves from the mid portion to the posterior third of tongue facilitating feeding of solid food. The pancreatic enzymes are adequate by this time.

Up and down movements of the mandible called munching or biting first become apparent by 5 months and helps in consumption of semi solid food.

Lateral movements of the tongue which move the food gruel to molar teeth develop by 12–18 months which help in handling of fibrous foods like raw vegetables and fibrous fruits.

The child actually learns to chew by 7–9 months age. Therefore, it is believed that if the stimulus for development of chewing is not applied at the appropriate age, the infant will always be a poor chewer and will be poor in eating solids.

Ideal Characteristics of Complementary Food

Complementary food should have the following characteristics: (1) Rich in energy and nutrients (2) Clean and safe (3) Easy to prepare from family food (4) Locally available and affordable (5) Culturally acceptable (6) developmentally appropriate (7) varied in taste, viscosity, flavour and taste.

Infant is Ready for Solid Food When They

- Hold tongue steady and sit without support.
- Can follow food with their eyes.
- Can open their mouth when they see food coming.
- Draw their lower lip as a spoon is removed from their mouth.
- And can move food from the front of their mouth to the back of their tongue to swallow.

Complementation Should not be Early Because

- Exclusive breastfeeding protects against infection in early life. Early complementation deprives baby of the unique nutritional benefits of breast milk as well.

- Early complementation has high risk of diarrhea and ARI.
- Digestive system and kidneys are immature to handle solids.
- Infant can develop food sensitivity and allergy with early exposure to solid food.
- Due to presence of strong extrusion and gag reflex and lack of muscle coordination for swallowing solids infants may choke on food they cannot swallow.

Ideal Diet Chart of the Child From Birth to 1 Year

Birth to 6 months: Only breast milk.

6 months to 9 months: Semisolids + breastfeeding.

9 months to 1 year: Solids + breastfeeding.

Above 1 year: Family food + breastfeeding upto 2 years or beyond.

Types of Complementary Food

- *Grain products:* Rice cereal (rice powder, rice flakes, puffed rice) wheat cereal (semolina, dalia, atta and maida).
- *Vegetables* viz. green leafy vegetables, potato, carrot, peas to start with.
- *Fruits:* Banana, papaya, mango citrous etc.
- Seeds and nuts.
- *Milk products:* Cheese, plain yogurt, butter.
- *Oils:* Ground nut oil and sunflower oil.
- Egg yolk, egg white, fish and meat.

Feeding Guidelines

At 6 Months Age

At 6 months age complementary feeding should be started preferably with a cereal. The preparation should be soft and flowing, thicker than breast milk and homogenous. When the infant has accepted soft food, different tastes should be gradually introduced while increasing the thickness. Small chopped pieces of food can be mixed by 7–9 months age to encourage chewing. Between 6–9 months one can also start pureed vegetables and tubers (green leafy, peas, carrot, potato etc.) and mashed fruit (banana, papaya, mango etc.), mashed rice and dal/khichri, bread crumbs in dal + oil, properly cooked green leafy vegetables.

At 9–12 Months Age

At 9–12 months age the infant can be started on unmashed rice, dal, roti, bread, vegetables, seasonal fruits, soft fish, egg yolk, curd, kheer, dalia.

From 1 Year Age

From one year age the child should be given food from the family pot except meat which should be given after 2 years age, because it is difficult to digest.

Fruit juices can be given from 6–9 months age. However, the amount should be restricted to 125 ml/ day. Larger amounts can cause distension of abdomen and osmotic diarrhoea due to the high content of glucose. Moreover, fruit juice does not contain many nutrients except water, glucose and Vitamin C. A large amount can fill the stomach and the child will refuse normal nutritious diet. Fleshy fruits like ripe banana (any kind), mango, papaya are better than fruit juices. They are whole some food and contains lot of nutrients especially vitamins and minerals.

Breastfeeding should be continued along with complementary food preferably upto 2 years age or beyond. Even if it is not possible, there is no need to supplement breast milk with animal milk or formula milk on the plea that breast milk is decreasing. Instead, solid food containing a mixed diet should be increased as the child grows. Animal milk or formula milk does not contain the nutrients of a balanced mixed diet. Supplementary milk may decrease the amount of age appropriate mixed diet to be taken by the infant; hence hamper growth. The biological availability of iron in cow's milk is only 10%. If children miss a mixed diet for cow's milk, they suffer from iron deficiency anemia. PEM and iron deficiency anemia causes loss of appetite and further reduce the amount of mixed diet.

Frequency of Complementary Food

At 6 months once a day and increase gradually

6–8 months	:	2–3 times/day
9–11 months	:	3–4 times/day
12–24 months	:	5–6 times/day
2–5 years	:	6 times/day

However, the ideal amount and frequency of complementary food is as much as the child desires and whenever the child is hungry.

Time for Feeding

Each feeding should not be for more than 15– 20 minutes.

Increase in Number of Food Items

- One item at 6 months, two mix by 8 months.
- Three mix by 9 months, four to five mix by 1 year.
- Five to six after 1 year.

While Increasing the Items of Food the Following is To Be Kept in Mind

1. Breastfeeding frequency maintained + night feeds.
2. Recipes, taste and flavors of food should be changed.
3. Baby's food should be prepared from family food to help develop taste.
4. The viscosity, texture of food should be gradually changed, i.e., to start as purees followed by gelatinous and then solids.

Preparation of the Meal

a. **Cereal meal:** The *rice cereal* (pithaguri/rice powder) should be cooked in oil and water and then mixed with breast milk or dal.

   The *wheat cereal* (semolina) should be prepared by frying in vegetable oil, cooked in water with sugar added.

b. **Rice and dal meal:** The rice and vegetables should be mashed and initially the proportion should be rice: dal (1: 3). Gradually by 9–12 months it should be 1:1. After 9 months the infant should be given unmashed rice.

Disadvantages of Commercially Available Complementary Foods

The commercially available complementary foods may seem convenient but they are disadvantageous for the infant because they are:

1. Expensive than home prepared food without any added nutritional value.
2. Usually of same taste. Monotonous food interferes with development of taste in the baby.
3. Usually of same texture which prevents development of chewing habit at proper age of the baby. The child starts to learn to chew at around 7 to 9 months of age. If they are not given food of proper texture, they do not learn to chew.

How to Feed the Child?

1. Children can usually feed themselves by one year of age but they need supervision and help.
2. The care giver should have patience and time and should show pleasure in feeding the child.
3. The children should be encouraged to feed by themselves with fingers or spoon by one year. They should be given food in a separate dish.
4. Food should be offered only when the child is hungry and interested in eating. If the child does not appear interested, it is better to play with him without forcing to eat. The care giver should avoid showing annoyance, but encourage the child to eat when hungry.

Care During Preparation of Food

1. Hands should be washed before preparing food or feeding the child.
2. Utensils should be washed with water and soap.
3. Clean water should be used to prepare the food.
4. Food should be kept covered and protected from flies and other insects.
5. Cooked food should be used within 3 hours. If necessary reheated and temperature checked before feeding.
6. Parents should themselves taste any food before feeding the child.

Suggested Reading

1. Breastfeeding in practice. A manual for health workers. Elisabet Helsing with Savage King, 1984, Oxford University Press, Delhi.
2. Infant feeding and complementary feeding, Editor Naval Kishore, published by Breast Feeding Network of India.
3. The science of infant feeding, Edited by R.K.Anand, N. B. Kumta, RP Kushwaha and Arun Gupta, Jaypee Brothers, Medical Publishers (P) Ltd., New Delhi.

4

Clinical Immunology and Immunization

OUTLINES

The Immune System

Immunity means the capability of the human body to resist organism and toxins that lead to damage of the tissues and organs. Immunity may be innate immunity, resulting in the body itself or may be acquired, which develop after the body is first attacked by an organism or a toxin. Acquired immunity often requires weeks or months to develop.

Innate Immunity

Innate immunity includes the following:

1. Phagocytosis of organisms by white blood cells and tissue macrophages.
2. Destruction of swallowed organisms by the acid secretions of the stomach and the digestive enzymes in the intestine.
3. Resistance of the skin to invasion by organisms.
4. Presence in the blood of certain chemical compounds that attack the foreign organisms or toxins and destroy them. These include lysozyme (a mucolytic polysaccharide that attacks bacteria and causes them to dissolute), basic polypeptides (which react with and inactivate certain types of gram positive bacteria), complement system (that can destroy bacteria) and natural killer lymphocytes (that can recognize and destroy foreign cells, tumor cells and even some infected cells).

Acquired Immunity

The ability of the human body to develop powerful specific immunity against individual invading agent viz. lethal bacteria, viruses, toxins and foreign tissues of other animals is called acquired immunity. Acquired immunity is caused by a special immune system that forms antibodies and /or activated lymphocytes that attack and destroy the specific invading organism or toxins. Acquired immunity can often bestow almost full protection and hence the importance of immunization in protection against diseases and toxins.

T lymphocytes

Acquired immunity is the product of the body's lymphocyte system. Two types of lymphocytes viz. T and B lymphocytes promote acquired immunity.

The T lymphocytes are preprocessed in the thymus gland. After their origination in the bone marrow, they migrate to the thymus gland. Here they divide rapidly and at the same time develop extreme diversity for reacting against specific antigens i.e. one of the T lymphocytes develops specific reactivity against one antigen. They are responsible for cell mediated immunity.

The T cells are of three major types viz. T helper cells, cytotoxic T cells and suppressor T cells with specific functions of their own.

The helper T cells constitute more than three fourth of the total T cells. They help in the functions of the immune system and virtually act as the major regulator of all immune functions. The helper T cells do so by forming a series of protein mediators called lymphokines (viz. interleukin 2, 3, 4, 5, 6, granulocyte-monocyte colony stimulating factor etc).

The specific regulatory functions of lymphokines are as follows:

1. Stimulation of growth and proliferation of cytotoxic T cells and suppressor T cells.
2. Stimulation of B cell growth and differentiation to form plasma cells and antibodies.
3. Activation of macrophage system.
4. Feedback stimulatory effect on helper T cells

Cytotoxic T cells/Natural Killer Cells

The cytotoxic T cell is a direct attack cell that is capable of killing micro-organisms and at times some of body's own cells; hence also called natural killer cells. The receptor proteins on the surfaces of the cytotoxic cells cause them to bind tightly to those organisms or cells that contain the appropriate binding specific antigen. Then they kill the attacked cells by secreting hole forming proteins, called perforins that literally punch large holes in the membrane of the attacked cells. Then fluid flows rapidly into the cell from the interstitial space. In addition, the cytotoxic T cells release cytotoxic substances directly into the attacked cell. The attacked cell almost immediately becomes greatly swollen dissolving thereafter. The cytotoxic T cells can also destroy cancer cells, heart transplant cells or other types of cells that are foreign to the body.

Suppressor T cells

Suppressor T cells are capable of suppressing the functions of both cytotoxic and helper T cells. It is believed that these suppressor functions serve the purpose of regulating the activities of the other cells, keeping them from causing immune reactions that might be damaging to the body's own tissues; hence they are also called regulatory T cells. They limit the ability of the immune system to attack the person's own body tissue. This is called immune tolerance.

B lymphocytes

The B lymphocytes are preprocessed in the liver during mid fetal life and in the bone marrow in late fetal life and after birth. They secrete antibodies and are responsible for humoral immunity. B lymphocytes are different from T lymphocytes in two ways: (1) like the T cells they do not develop reactivity against the antigen; instead they actively secrete antibodies that are reactive agents. These agents are large protein molecules that are capable of combining with and destroying the antigen. (2) The B lymphocytes have greater diversity than the T lymphocytes thus form many millions of types of B lymphocyte antibodies with different specific reactivities. These antibodies act mainly by two ways to protect the body from the invading agents:

1. By direct attack on the invader; and
2. By activation of the complement system.

There are five general classes of antibodies viz. IgM, IgG, IgA, IgD and IgE out of which three viz. IgG, IgE, IgM are of particular importance. Of these, IgG constitutes about 75% of the antibodies in the normal body. IgE constitute only a small percentage and is especially involved in allergy. The IgM is the class of antibodies which are formed during a primary response after exposure to an antigen.

The antibodies have a bivalent nature and most invading agents have multiple antigen sites. The antibodies can inactivate the invading agents in one of the several ways: (1) Agglutination (2) Precipitation (3) Neutralization (4) Lysis.

These are direct actions of the antibodies on the attacking antigens but they are often not strong enough to play a major role in protecting the body. Most of the protection comes through the amplifying effect of the complement system.

Complement System

Complement system is a collection of about 20 proteins out of which 11 are important. They are designated as C1 through C9, B and D. All these proteins are present normally among the plasma proteins in the blood as well as among the proteins that leak out of capillaries into the tissue spaces.

The classic pathway of the complement system is activated by an antigen antibody reaction setting into action a cascade of sequential reactions beginning with activation of proenzyme C1. The C1 enzymes that are formed then activate successively increasing quantities of enzymes in the later stages of the system, so that from a small beginning, an extremely large amplified reaction occurs. Multiple end products are formed during the reaction and several of these cause important effects that help to prevent damage of the body's tissues caused by the invading organism or toxin. The other effects of the complement cascade are the following:

1. *Phagocytosis and Opsonization:* The product C3b activates phagocytosis of bacteria to which antigen antibody complexes are attached by polymorphs and macrophages. This process is called opsonization.
2. *Lysis:* The product lytic complex which is a combination of multiple complement factors (C5b6789) has a direct effect of rupturing the cell membrane of the invading organism.
3. *Agglutination:* It is the effect of complement products leading to adherence of bacteria to one another.
4. *Neutralization of viruses:* The complement enzymes and other complement products can attack the structures of some viruses and thereby render them nonvirulent.
5. *Chemotaxis:* Chemotaxis of phagocytes (polymorphs and macrophages) is facilitated by complement fragment C5a. This helps in migration of these cells to the tissue area adjacent to the antigenic agent.
6. *Activation of mast cells and basophils:* The complement fragments C3a, C4a and C5a activate mast cells and basophils. These cells cause release of histamine, heparin and several other substances into the local fluids resulting in increased blood flow, increased leakage of fluid and plasma protein into the tissues and other tissue reactions that help inactivate and immobilize the invading organism.
7. *Inflammatory cells:* Besides the above mentioned cells, several other complement products contribute to local inflammation thus preventing the movement of the invading organism through the tissues.

Evaluation of Suspected Immunodeficiency

Recurrent infections usually presenting with fever is among the most common clinical problems in children. A major cause of recurrent infection among children is repeated exposure to common and usually benign infectious agents in early childhood. However, the number of children suspected of having a primary or secondary immunodeficiency far exceeds the number of actual cases, as most of the patients with recurrent infections do not have identifiable overt immunodeficiency disorders.

Primary immunodeficiency is usually not screened for at any time during life; and most affected do not have abnormal physical features. In addition, extensive use of antibiotics may mask the classic presentation of many primary immunodeficiency states. A high index of suspicion is therefore necessary for early diagnosis of an immunodeficiency disorder so that appropriate treatment can be instituted before irreversible damage develops.

Evaluation of immune function should be initiated in (a) Those rare infants or children who do have clinical manifestations of specific immune disorder; and (b) In all who have unusual, chronic, or recurrent infections such as:

1. One or more systemic bacterial infections (sepsis, meningitis).
2. Two or more serious respiratory or documented bacterial infections (cellulitis, abscesses, draining otitis media, pneumonia, lymphadenitis) within 1 year.
3. Serious infections occurring at unusual sites (liver and brain).
4. Infections with common childhood pathogens but of unusual severity.
5. Infections with unusual pathogens viz. Pneumocystis jiroveci, Aspergillus, Serratia marcescens, Nocardia, Burkholderia cepacia.

Additional clues to immunodeficiency include (i) Failure to thrive with or without chronic diarrhoea; (ii) Persistent infections after receiving live vaccines; and (iii) Chronic oral or cutaneous moniliasis.

It needs mention that children with defects in antibody production, phagocytosis or complement proteins have recurrent infections with encapsulated bacteria. They may grow and develop normally despite the recurrent infections unless they develop a complication like bronchiectasis from repeated lower respiratory tract bacterial infections or suffer from persistent enterovirus infections of the central nervous system.

In contrast, patients with deficiency of T-cell function usually develop opportunistic infections or serious illness from common viral agents in early life, and they fail to thrive. However, it should be noted that patients with repeated mild viral infections usually are not likely to have an immunodeficiency.

The evaluation of a suspected immunodeficiency disorder hence comprises history and a physical examination to start with, followed by investigations. A thorough family history can give a lot of clue to the diagnosis. It also needs mention that most immunological disorders can be excluded with proper choice of screening tests.

Table 4.1: Showing the cost effective screening tests
Complete blood count, differential count and ESR
• Absolute neutrophil count
• Absolute lymphocyte count
• Platelet count
• Howell-Jolly bodies
• ESR

The most cost effective screening tests are a complete blood count, a manual differential count and ESR. If an infant's neutrophil count is persistently elevated in the absence of any sign of infection, a leukocyte adhesion deficiency should be suspected.

If the ESR is normal, chronic bacterial or fungal infections are unlikely. If the absolute neutrophil count is normal, congenital and acquired neutropenia as well as leukocyte adhesion defects are excluded.

T cells normally constitute 70% of circulating lymphocytes and their absence will result in striking lymphopenia. If the absolute lymphocyte count is normal, a severe T cell defect is ruled out.

Absence of Howell-Jolly bodies or pitted erythrocytes in the peripheral smear rules out congenital asplenia. Normal platelet size or count excludes Wiskott-Aldrich syndrome. Lymphopenia observed by cord blood examination can detect severe combined immunodeficiency at birth. Early detection can facilitate life saving reconstitution to the affected infants shortly after birth.

Some of the above mentioned abnormalities may prove to be laboratory artifacts. Conversely, an apparently straight forward diagnosis may prove to be a much more complex disorder. Therefore children found to be having screening tests positive should be characterized fully before any type of immune therapy is begun, unless there is a life threatening illness.

In a child with recurrent or unusual bacterial infections, evaluation of T-cell and phagocytic cell functions is indicated even if the results of the initial screening tests (see Table 4.2) are normal.

B Cell Deficiency

Measurement of Serum IgA is a simple screening test for B cell defect. If IgA level is normal, selective IgA deficiency, which is the most common B cell defect, is excluded. In addition, permanent types of hypogammaglobulinemia are also excluded since IgA is very low or absent in these conditions.

If IgA is low, IgG and IgM should also be measured. Patients who are receiving corticosteroids or who have protein loosing states (e.g. nephrotic syndrome, protein loosing enteropathy) often have low serum IgG levels but produce antibodies normally. Therefore, in such cases, it is important that before starting intravenous immunoglobulin therapy it should be determined whether the levels are low because of inadequate synthesis or due to protein loss. This can be done by measuring antibody titres to specific antigens before institution of intravenous immunoglobulin therapy.

Another useful test for B cell function is to determine the presence and titre of isohemagglutinins or antibody titres to type A and B red blood cells polysaccharide antigens. This test measures predominantly IgM antibodies. It should be remembered that isohemagglutinins may be absent in the first 2 years of life and are always absent if the patient is blood type AB.

Antibody response to vaccine antigen is also a useful test. Most infants are immunized with diphtheria, tetanus and pertussis, conjugated hemophilus influenzae type B and in some countries pneumococcal conjugate vaccines. It is often informative to test for specific antibodies to these antigens. If the titres are low, measurement of antibodies to diphtheria or tetanus toxoid before and 2 weeks after DTaP or DT booster is helpful in assessing the capacity to form IgG to these antigens.

To evaluate a patient's ability to respond to polysaccharide antigens, antipneumococcal antibodies can be measured

Table 4.2: Table showing the laboratory tests in immunodeficiency

Screening tests	*Advanced tests*	*Special tests*
B cell deficiency IgG, IgM, IgA and IgE levels Isohemagglutinin titre Antibody response to vaccine antigens (tetanus, diphtheria, pneumococci, hemophilus influenzae)	B cell enumeration (CD19 or CD 20) Antibody response to boosters or to new vaccines	Advanced B cell phenotyping Biopsies (lymph nodes) Antibody response to special antigen (e.g. bacteriophage), mutation analysis
T cell deficiency Lymphocyte count Chest X-ray examination for thymus size Delayed skin tests (Candida skin test)	T cells subset enumeration (CD3, CD4, CD8) Proliferative responses to mitogens, antigens, allogenic cells HLA typing Chromosomal analysis	Advanced flow cytometry Enzyme assays (e.g. ADA, PNP) Thymic imaging Mutation analysis T cell activation studies Apoptosis studies, biopsy
Phagocyte deficiency WBC count, morphology Respiratory burst assay	Adhesion molecule assays (e.g. CD11B/CD 18, selectin ligandin Mutation analysis	Mutation analysis Enzyme assays (e.g. G6PD, NADPH oxidase, MPO)
Complement deficiency CH_{50} assay, C3, C4 level	AH 50 activity Component assays Activation assays (e.g. C3a, C4a, C4d, C5a)	

(ADA, adenosine deaminase, CH, hemolytic complement, G6PD, glucose 6 phosphatase dehydrogenase, MPO, myeloperoxidase, NADPH, nicotinamide adenine dinucleotide phosphate, PNP, purine nucleoside phosphorylase)

Adapted from Nelson Textbook of Pediatrics, 19th edition, 2011, Elsevier, Saunders

before and 3 weeks after immunization with pneumococcal polysaccharide vaccine, in patients more than 2 - 3 years old. Antibodies detected in these tests are of IgG isotype. In children below 2 years age with low antipneumococcal antibody titres, it is useful to first boost with 2 doses of conjugate pneumococcal vaccine 1 month apart. Then give a polysaccharide pneumococcal vaccine 1 month later and then measure antibody titres after 3 weeks. Patients with significant or permanent B cell defects do not produce either IgM or IgG antibodies normally.

If results from these tests are found to be normal and the immunoglobulins remain low, studies should be performed to evaluate the possible loss of immunoglobulin through the urinary or gastrointestinal tract.

IgG subclass measurements are seldom helpful in assessing immune function. It is occasionally helpful when profound antibody deficiencies are detected despite normal levels of immunoglobulins. It is believed that specific antibody measurements are far more cost effective than IgG subclass determinations.

Patients found to be having agammaglobulinemia should have their blood cells enumerated by flow cytometry using dye conjugated monoclonal antibodies to B cell specific CD antigens (usually CD19 or CD20).

Normally, approximately 8-10% of circulating lymphocytes are B cells. B cells are absent in X-linked agammaglobulinemia (XLA) and present in common variable immunodeficiency (CVID), IgA deficiency and hyper IgM syndromes.

Patients with XLA have a high susceptibility to persistent enteroviral infections, whereas those with CVID have more problems with autoimmune diseases and lymphoid hyperplasia. Specific molecular diagnostic tests for XLA are necessary in cases without a family history to aid genetic counselling. Other B cell defects also require molecular testing.

T Cells Deficiency

T cell and T cell subsets can also be enumerated by flow cytometry using dye conjugated monoclonal antibodies recognizing CD antigens present on T cells (CD2, CD3, CD4 and CD8). CD3+ T cells usually constitute 70% of peripheral lymphocytes. So it is an important test for any infant who is lymphopenic.

Infants with severe combined immunodeficiency (SCID) are unable to produce T cells. So they are lymphopenic at birth. It is a pediatric emergency and can be successfully treated by stem cell marrow transplantation. It needs an early diagnosis before serious untreatable infections develop. Normally, there are roughly twice as many CD4+ (helper) T cells as there are CD8+ T cells. There are examples of severe immunodeficiency in which phenotypically normal T cells are present. Hence tests for T cell function are more informative and cost effective then enumeration of T cell subpopulation by flow cytometry.

The Candida skin test is a cost effective test for T cell function. It can be done in children older than 6 years age. It is done by intradermal injection of 0.1 ml of a 1:1000 of a known potent Candida albicans extract. If the test result is negative, at 24 hours, 48 hours and 72 hours, a 1:100 dilution should be used. A positive test is defined as erythema and induration of 10 mm or more at 48 hours and if it is greater than that in 24 hours, all primary T cells defects are precluded. Such a situation obviates the need for tests like lymphocyte phenotyping or assessment of response to mitogens.

Natural Killer Cells (NK cells)

Natural killer cells can be enumerated by flow cytometry using monoclonal antibodies to NK specific CD antigens, CD 16 and CD 56.

Phagocytic Cell Deficiency

Killing defects of phagocytic cells should be suspected when there is history of recurrent staphylococcal abscesses or gram negative infections. The most reliable and useful test for this defect is a flow cytometric assessment of the respiratory burst using rhodamine dye. Leukocyte adhesion deficiencies can be diagnosed by flow cytometry assays of blood lymphocytes or polymorphs using monoclonal antibodies to CD18 or CD11. The phagocytic cell defect can be further defined according to their molecular cause.

Complement Deficiency

An effective screening test for complement defects is a CH50 assay. It is a bioassay that measures the intactness of the entire complement pathway. It yields abnormal results if the complement has been consumed from the specimen for any reason.

Genetic deficiencies in the complement system are usually characterized by extremely low levels of CH50. For an accurate result, the specimen should be quickly transported to the laboratory. It is important to identify which component is deficient because disease susceptibilities are different for different components. However, only C3 and C4 immunoassays are commercially available. Other component assays are available only in research laboratories. Identification of mode of inheritance is also important for genetic counselling. While properdin deficiency is sex linked other complement deficiencies are autosomal.

Historical Aspects: Immunization and Programmes

Dhanvantri, the father of Indian medicine, spoke of preventing infectious diseases through immunization. However, Edward Jenner, who used cowpox vaccination to protect against smallpox in human beings, developed the first successful vaccination in 1796. Around 100 years later in 1885, Louis Pasteur developed a very effective vaccine against Rabies.

An organized immunization programme, at global level, was first declared by World Health Organization in 1974 which was named as 'Expanded Programme of Immunization' (EPI). The EPI Programme focused on vaccination of children below 5 years age and pregnant women. The vaccines included were BCG, DPT, OPV, Measles and T. toxoid. Government of India adopted it in 1978.

When independent evaluation revealed very low coverage in many parts of the country through the EPI programme, the Universal Immunization Programme (UIP) was started in 1985. The primary objectives of the UIP programme were the following:

1. Universal immunization and reduction in infant mortality and morbidity due to vaccine preventable diseases.
2. Self-sufficiency in vaccine production, supply and training of medical and paramedical personnel.
3. Establishment of a functional cold chain system; and
4. Introduction of district level monitoring system.

The vaccines recommended were BCG, DPT, OPV and measles for infants and T.Toxoid for pregnant women. The age group was brought down to 1 year instead of 5 years. The Government of India, through UIP envisaged 100% coverage of pregnant women and 85% coverage for infants.

The UIP became an integral part of Child survival and safe motherhood programme (CSSM) in 1992 and subsequently a part of the Reproductive and child health programme (RCH) in 1997.

The Pulse polio programme (PPP) has been started in 1995. It includes supplementary immunization activities against poliomyelitis, as a part of the polio eradication programme.

BASIC IMMUNOLOGY

"Immune" is a Greek word which means, "to be protected". Protection can be obtained by acquired immunity offered by the introduction of various antigens and antibodies into the body. This process by which the body acquires immunity is called *immunization.*

There are two types of immunization: *active immunization* when specific antigens evoke the acquired immune response in the system and *passive immunization* when antibodies are supplied readymade in the form of immunoglobulins and sera. After immunization, there is a change from antibody negative state to antibody positive state. This is called *seroconversion.* The state of protection due to presence of humoral antibody (antibody detected in plasma / serum) is called *seroprotection.*

WHAT IS A VACCINE?

When an organism induces disease in the human body, the host immune system responds with immunity, first to ensure recovery and then to offer protection from the disease if the same pathogen were to be encountered again.

A vaccine is composed of one or more antigens of a pathogen, which will induce a protective immune response. Therefore, vaccines mimic infection with the respective pathogen, but without the risk of developing the disease.

Immune Response After Vaccination

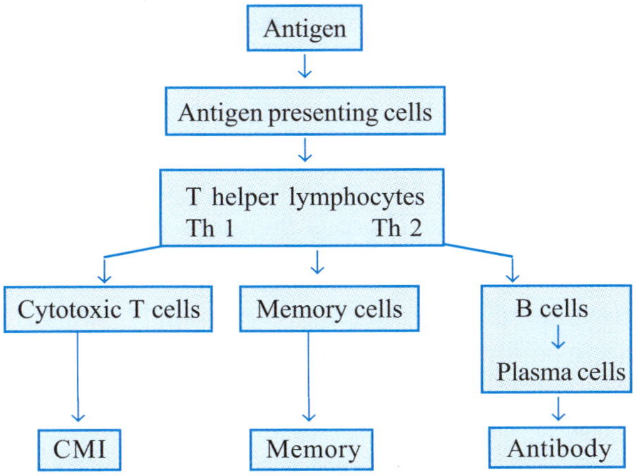

Fig. 4.1: Immune response after vaccination

After vaccination, the consequent immune response may be manifested through humoral (i.e. antibody) immunity or cell mediated immunity (CMI) or both. If the antigen preferentially stimulates Th 1 series of T helper lymphocytes, then a strong lymphocyte response is obtained. If Th 2 series is preferentially stimulated, the immunity is predominantly humoral. Carbohydrate vaccines are T cell independent. Therefore, they directly stimulate the B cells without T helper cell modulation. This results in a predominantly IgM response without IgG production or induction of immunological memory. Some vaccines like BCG elicit CMI without an easily demonstrable humoral component.

TIMING OF VACCINES

The timing of vaccines depends on the age at which the disease is anticipated, presence of maternally derived immunity as well as the feasibility of administering the vaccine at that time.

BCG, oral polio vaccine and Hepatitis B vaccine can be given soon after birth, as the maternally derived immunity apparently does not interfere with the vaccine "take". All the other vaccines should be given at the age according to the schedule. This is because of presence of detectable maternal antibody in the infant's circulation, which may inhibit the vaccines.

Most of the currently used childhood vaccines do not interfere with the vaccine "take" of other vaccine. Therefore, multiple vaccines can be given in combination or simultaneously. However, administration of Measles and Varicella may be associated with short lasting suppression of the immune system. Therefore, it may be advisable to keep an interval of 4 weeks between administration of these two vaccines and the other vaccines.

IMMUNIZATION SCHEDULE

The WHO declares an immunization schedule from time to time. The different countries adopt the schedule with some modifications depending on the prevalence of the diseases in the respective countries. Hence, the immunization schedule is different in different countries. Moreover, the schedule changes from time to time, with the change of prevalence of a disease. Starting with 3–4 vaccines in 1974, the number of vaccines has increased significantly in our country. Some of them are very costly not affordable by all sections of people. So when formulating a schedule for a particular child it should be effective as well as cost effective.

In India, the Indian Academy of Pediatrics, a body that works for welfare of the children has also formulated an immunization schedule. It includes all essential vaccines but not cost effective. Therefore, the responsibility lies on the provider to choose the most essential vaccines, which are, yet to be included in the national immunization schedule. The following is the present schedule of immunization in our country.

Table 4.3: National Immunization Schedule (2016)

Age	*Schedule*
Birth	BCG, OPV 0, Hepatitis B birth dose
6 weeks	OPV 1, RVV 1, f IPV 1, Pentavalent 1, PCV 1**
10 weeks	OPV 2, RVV 2, Pentavalent 2
14 weeks	OPV 3, RVV 3, f IPV 2, Pentavalent 3, PCV 2**
9 months	MCV 1, JE 1, PCV 3**, Vit A
16 – 24 months	DTwP- Booster 1, OPV- Booster, MCV 2, JE 2, Vit A
5 – 6 years	DTwP- Booster 2
10 years	TT
16 years	TT
Pregnant women	TT 1 and TT 2

RVV = Rota virus vaccine, Pentavalent: DPT + HIB + Hepatitis B, PCV = Pneumococcal vaccine, MCV = Measles containing vaccine, f IPV = fractional IPV.

** In selected states. Not in Assam.

It should be noted that many essential vaccines have been now included in the national schedule. However, some more vaccines viz. MMR, Typhoid, Hepatitis A, and Varicella needs to be included with future provision for the rest of the vaccines. Until then, the additional vaccines should be advised after one to one discussion with parents.

ABOUT THE VACCINES

BCG vaccine: The BCG vaccine first developed in1921 is derived from the bovine strain of mycobacterium tuberculosis. It continues to be the only effective vaccine against tuberculosis. However, it is more effective in prevention of hematogenous spread of Mycobacterium tuberculosis, which results in miliary tuberculosis and tubercular meningitis with a protective efficacy of 50 – 80% against these forms of tuberculosis. The protective efficacy against pulmonary tuberculosis is 50%.

The vaccine is heat and light sensitive and deteriorates on exposure to ultraviolet rays. The vaccine should be reconstituted with sterile normal saline. Once reconstituted, it should be used within 4 hours and the left over discarded. This is because the vaccine does not contain any antibacterial; hence contamination can occur with repeated use.

Dosage Schedule

The recommended dose is 0.1 ml irrespective of age and weight of the baby. It should be given intradermal, using a BCG syringe and a 26 gauge needle on the convex part of deltoid for easy visualization of the scar. The site of injection may be swabbed with normal saline.

The preferred time for BCG vaccination is soon after birth but there is no upper limit to BCG vaccination. However, to accrue the maximum benefit it should be given as early as possible within the age of 9 months. There is no need to repeat vaccination in a child who does not develop a scar.

Reaction

A successful intradermal injection is indicated by formation of a wheal of 5 mm. The wheal disappears within a short time. After 2 – 3 weeks, a papule develops which reaches a maximum size of 4 – 8 mm by the end of 5 – 6 weeks. There is repeated ulceration and healing until a scar is formed by 5 – 6 weeks.

Adverse Reactions

The adverse reactions include secondary infection at the site of vaccination, BCG lymphadenopathy and disseminated BCG infection.

Secondary infection at the injection site may require administration of antibiotics. It results from use of unsterile needle.

BCG lymphadenopathy may develop in the ipsilateral axillary / cervical lymph glands after a few weeks / months after vaccination. The nodes regress spontaneously after a few months. In some cases, the nodes may liquefy and result in an abscess. Surgical removal or repeated aspiration is the treatment of choice in such cases.

It should be noted that fine needle aspiration cytology of the gland may be positive for acid-fast bacilli but these are bovine strains and should not be misinterpreted as tubercular disease. There is therefore no place of anti-tubercular therapy in BCG lymphadenopathy.

Disseminated BCG infection is extremely rare but may occur in children with cellular immunodeficiency.

Storage

BCG vaccine can be stored at 2 – 8 °C upto 12 months without losing potency.

Polio Vaccine

The polio vaccine is of two types: oral polio vaccine (OPV) and inactivated polio vaccine (IPV).

Oral Polio Vaccine

The oral polio vaccine is a live attenuated vaccine containing a suspension of over 1 million particles of poliovirus type 1, 2 and 3 together. With polio eradication, approaching, trivalent OPV (tOPV) will no longer be available, having been replaced by bivalent OPV (bOPV) or monovalent OPV (mOPV). It is supplied with a stabilizing agent viz. magnesium chloride. Therefore, the potency is quite stable under refrigeration or freezing.

For reasons not clearly known, the "take rate" is relatively low. Therefore, multiple doses are necessary before 90 – 95% of children develop immune responses to all the 3 polioviruses.

Dosage Schedule

According to the National Immunization schedule, the oral polio vaccine should be started with the 0 dose within 14 days after birth followed by 3 primary doses at 6 weeks, 10 weeks and 14 weeks age and a booster dose at 16 – 24 months age.

If a substantial amount of the vaccine is vomited out or regurgitated within 5 – 10 minutes of administration, the dose should be repeated. If the repeat dose is also not retained, neither dose should be counted. The vaccine should be administered at a later visit. Breastfeeding can be allowed before and after vaccination and mild diarrhea is not a contraindication to OPV administration.

Storage

OPV should be stored at – 20°C at the district and state level and in the freezer compartment of the domestic refrigerator at the clinic level. The vaccine must be carried to outreach centres in a vaccine carrier at 2 – 8°C.

Adverse Reactions

OPV is a very safe vaccine and the best for eradication of polio. However, two major problems are faced with continued use of OPV. These are occurrence of Vaccine Associated Paralytic Poliomyelitis (VAPP) and emergence of circulating Vaccine Derived Polioviruses (cVDPVs).

At a time when the world is moving towards a polio free environment, the increasing incidence of VAPP has been a major concern. The risk would continue as long as OPV is used for prevention of poliomyelitis. Approximately 50% of VAPP cases are associated with poliovirus type 2.

Vaccine derived polioviruses (cVDPVs) are mutants of polio vaccine viruses that reacquire properties of wild virus. They have been associated with outbreaks of paralytic polio. It is usually seen in communities with low immunity especially when polio vaccine coverage rates decline but use of OPV continues. So in order to decrease the risk of emergence of cVDPVs very high immunization coverage is mandatory with OPV. Whereas VAPP occurs in individual cases, cVDPVs can result in large outbreaks.

To eliminate the risk of VAPP and emergence of cVDPVs it has been suggested that the mass OPV campaigns should be synchronized with the cessation of OPV use once eradication of wild poliovirus is achieved.

Inactivated Polio Vaccine (IPV)

Inactivated polio vaccine contains formaldehyde killed poliovirus types 1, 2 and 3. It is highly immunogenic. Seroconversion rate is 90 – 95% with 2 doses and 99% with 3 doses. It produces excellent humoral immunity as well as local pharyngeal and, possible intestinal immunity. IPV is the ideal vaccine for prevention of polio in immunocompromised children and symptomatic HIV infected child.

The ideal age to administer the first dose is 8 weeks. The interval between two doses should be 8 weeks. It can be used as a combined vaccine with DPT and Hib without compromising seroconversion and side effects. According to the National Immunization Schedule, the 1st dose of IPV should be given at 6 weeks and a 2nd dose at 14 weeks together with oral polio vaccine.

Three doses at 4 – 6 weeks interval is still considered the best option but 2 doses at 8 weeks interval can also be used if primary vaccination is started at 8 weeks age. IPV catch up schedule includes 2 doses at 2 months apart followed by a booster after 6 months.

Fractional Dose Inactivated Polio Vaccine (f IPV)

f IPV is a safe and reliable vaccine. It is a reduced dose (volume) IPV. It is found to be highly immunogenic. It is given intradermal. Dose is 0.1 ml.

It is a liquid vaccine. No reconstitution is required. It should be stored at 2 – 8 °C. An open vial can be used upto 28 days after opening

The advantages are three-fold viz. can stretch limited supplies and lower cost with high immunogenicity. Two doses at 6 weeks and 14 weeks are recommended. f IPV is also endorsed for outbreak response.

The 2 doses of f IPV, according to the national schedule, is accepted in view of shortage of IPV and the urgent need of providing immunity against type 2 polio virus. However, a full dose of IPV after 8 weeks of the second dose of f IPV has been recommended for better immunity.

DTwP Vaccine/Triple Antigen

It is one of the oldest combination vaccines. It is a combination of diphtheria toxoid, tetanus toxoid and whole cell killed pertussis vaccine; hence also called 'triple antigen'. The two toxoids are highly immunogenic (95–100%) whereas the pertussis vaccine, even after 3 doses has a protective efficacy of about 70–90% only.

Dosage Schedule

According to the National Immunization Schedule 3 primary doses should be administered at 6 weeks, 10 weeks and 14 weeks as in the combined Pentavalent vaccine followed by booster doses with DTwP at 16–24 months and 5–6 years age.

The vaccine should be injected deep intramuscularly on the anterolateral aspect of the thigh. Gluteal region should be avoided for two reasons. It may cause injury to the sciatic nerve. Secondly, as there is abundance of fat in this region, the vaccine may be deposited in the fat hampering absorption and decrease immune response.

Adverse Reactions

Local reactions include pain, swelling, redness at the injection site and inability to move the limb for about 24 hours. Systemic reaction includes moderate fever. All these reactions are thought to be almost entirely due to the pertussis component. *Convulsion* following DTwP vaccine is very rare and may be fever triggered. Studies have shown that there is no causal relationship between administration of DTwP vaccine and development of chronic neurologic disease.

Table 4.4: Showing adverse reactions after DTwP vaccination

Local	*Systemic*
Pain, swelling, redness, at the injection site Inability to move the limb for about 24 hours	Moderate to high fever Persistent inconsolable cry Seizures Severe allergic reaction Hypotonic hypo responsive episodes

Children who develop **high fever** (fever > 40 °C) within 48 hours, **persistent inconsolable cry** of > 3 hours duration, **seizures** (with or without fever within 72 hours), **severe allergic reaction and hypotonic-hypo responsive episodes** after the first dose of DTwP vaccine needs careful evaluation before the second dose. Administration of DTaP vaccine (i.e., containing acellular pertussis) may be considered under such circumstances.

Contraindications

DTwP vaccine is contraindicated in children with progressive neurological disorders. The vaccine should not be denied to children with seizure disorders and static neurological disorders like cerebral palsy and developmental delay.

DTaP Vaccine

This is a combined vaccine consisting of diphtheria and tetanus toxoid with acellular pertussis vaccines. It is not more efficacious than DTwP vaccine. Hence, the continued use of DTwP vaccine has been endorsed in UIP because of its low cost, proven efficacy and safety. The DTaP vaccine may be preferred in those children with history of severe adverse effects following DTwP vaccine. Like DTwP vaccine, DTaP vaccine should not be used in children above 7 years of age because of increased reactogenicity. The dosage schedule of DTaP is same as DTwP vaccine. The vaccine should be stored at 2–8°C.

Td Vaccine

This vaccine contains the usual dose of tetanus toxoid and only 2 units of diphtheria toxoid. The dose is 0.5 ml IM. It should be stored at 2–8°C. This vaccine is recommended to be used as replacement for DTwP/DTaP/DT for catch up vaccination on children aged above 7 years.

Tdap Vaccine

It contains Tetanus toxoid full dose with lesser dose of diphtheria toxoid and acellular pertussis. The minimum age for vaccination is 7 years. IAP advocates 1 dose to all adolescents aged 11 years through 12 years and one dose to pregnant women during every pregnancy (preferred during 27 through 36 weeks). The dose during pregnancy is believed to prevent pertussis in newborn.

Tetanus Toxoid

According to the National Immunization Schedule, Tetanus toxoid (TT) is given as boosters at 10 years and

16 years age. Thereafter it should be continued every 10 years. If a girl child takes 7 doses starting at 6 weeks with DPT vaccine / Pentavalent vaccine + 4 booster doses upto 16 years, there is no need for additional doses during pregnancy for next 10 years. Thereafter one single dose would be sufficient to extend immunity for another 10 years.

For pregnant women not being previously immunized, two doses of T. toxoid vaccine should be given 4 weeks apart, the second dose at least 2 weeks before delivery so that protective antibodies in adequate titre are transferred to the newborn for prevention of neonatal tetanus. For subsequent pregnancy within 5 years one dose of T. toxoid would suffice. Beyond 5 years 2 doses would be necessary again.

For previously unimmunized school children, primary immunization against tetanus consists of 2 primary doses given at 4 weeks apart, a third dose after 6 months to one year.

It is administered deep intramuscular over the shoulders in older children. It has no side effects. It is a cost effective vaccine.

Storage

The DTwP, DTaP, DT, Td, Tdap and TT vaccines should be stored at 2 – 8°C. These vaccines should never be frozen. Freezing will cause precipitation of the insoluble aluminum salts in which the toxoids are adsorbed and make it unusable.

Measles Vaccine

Measles vaccine is derived from live attenuated Edmonston Zagreb strain grown in human diploid cell culture. The virus strain is so named after the name of a child named Edmonston from whom the original virus strain was isolated. The vaccine is supplied freeze dried. The reconstituted vaccine should be kept in the refrigerator or a vaccine carrier. The reconstituted vaccine is heat labile and should be used within 4 hours and the unused vaccine discarded. Measles vaccine does not contain any anti-bacterial. Therefore strict asepsis should be maintained while aspirating contents from the multi dose vial.

At What Age?

The recommended age for measles vaccination is 9 months completed (270 days+) followed by a booster dose at 16 – 24 months. However, in case of an outbreak, the vaccine can be given as early as 6 months age, which should be followed by revaccination after 3 months or MMR vaccine at 15 months age. The measles vaccine should be injected subcutaneously over right upper arm. It can also be injected in the anterolateral aspect of the thigh.

Reaction

The response to vaccination may present as a short fever of 2 – 3 days starting from 5 – 10 days after immunization. Some 2 – 5% of children may have a few spots of rash visible over fair skin. The child should be examined for other causes if the fever persists for more than 3 days.

Adverse Reaction

Some cases of staphylococcal shock syndrome have been reported. This is believed to have occurred from bacterial contamination of the vaccine.

Storage

The vaccine should be stored at 2 – 8°C.

Toxic Shock Syndrome (TSS)

TSS is an acute multi system disease caused by TSST 1 producing strains of staphylococcus aureus.

Clinical Features

It is characterized by abrupt onset high fever, vomiting, diarrhea, accompanied by sore throat, headache and myalgia to start with. A diffuse erythematous macular rash (sunburn like or scarlatiniform) appears within 24 hours with subsequent desquamation on the hands and feet. It is accompanied with conjunctival and pharyngeal hyperemia. A strawberry tongue is commonly seen. Symptoms often include alteration of consciousness, oliguria, and hypotension, which in severe cases may progress to shock and DIC.

The *three major criteria* required for diagnosis includes abrupt onset fever; temperature > 38.8°C, hypotension (orthostatic or shock) and rash (erythematous with late desquamation).

Complications

The complications include adult respiratory distress syndrome, myocardial failure and renal failure depending on the degree of shock.

Laboratory Diagnosis

There is no specific laboratory test for diagnosis. Tests for multi organ system involvement may be positive. A positive culture for S. aureus from the focus helps but not mandatory for diagnosis.

Treatment

Treatment consists of parenteral administration of a beta lactamase-resistant anti-staphylococcal antibiotic (Vancomycin 40 mg/kg/day 6 hourly IV infusion) over 60 minutes 6 hourly. It should be ideally started after appropriate cultures are sent. The addition of clindamycin (20–40 mg/kg 6–8 hourly) in severe or unresponsive cases may terminate toxin production. Drainage of focal infected sites if any is important for successful treatment.

Supportive treatment includes fluid replacement, treatment of hypotension, renal failure and cardiovascular collapse. Inotropic agents may be required to treat shock. Corticosteroids and intravenous immunoglobin may be required for severe cases.

Outcome

Recovery occurs within 7–10 days and is associated with desquamation, particularly of palms and soles. Loss of hair and nails has also been observed after 1–2 months.

Prevention

TSS occurring after measles vaccination can be prevented by using mono dose vials of the vaccine, administration of the vaccine within 4 hours of reconstitution and use of auto disabled (AD) syringe.

Hepatitis B Vaccine

Hepatitis B vaccine is a highly purified recombinant DNA vaccine. The vaccine is highly immunogenic and seroconversion rates are greater than 95% after a 3 dose schedule.

The recommended pediatric dose is 0.5 ml corresponding to 10 microgram of the antigenic component. The adult dose is double the pediatric dose. The dose may be increased when vaccinating immunocompromised individuals, e.g., patients on chemotherapy for malignant diseases or those with chronic renal failure awaiting dialysis.

Dosage Schedule

The recommended dosage schedules are:

(a) For infants

Birth dose, then at 6, 10, 14 weeks.

(b) For older children, adolescents

Elected date, 1 month and 6 months.

The vaccine should be given intramuscularly over the anterolateral aspect of thigh in infants and over the deltoid muscles in older children. It forms a component of the Pentavalent vaccine in use now.

Storage

The vaccine should be stored at 2 – 8°C. The vaccine is adjuveneted with aluminum salts; hence should not be frozen. If frozen accidentally, the vaccine should be discarded.

Hib Conjugate Vaccine

Hemophilus influenzae type b (Hib) vaccine is a very effective and safe vaccine. The protective efficacy is 95%. This vaccine is at present included in the National Immunization Schedule. It is one of the components of the Pentavalent vaccine in use. This vaccine is also indicated prior to splenectomy and in patients with sickle cell disease.

Vaccine Schedule

According to the National Immunization Schedule, 3 doses should be given at 6 weeks, 10 weeks and 14 weeks age as one component of Pentavalent vaccine. IAP recommends a booster dose at 12 through 18 months age. The vaccine should be given intramuscular in the anterolateral aspect of thigh. The vaccine should be stored at 2 – 8°C.

Japanese Encephalitis (JE) Vaccine

Japanese encephalitis (JE) is one of the most important causes of viral encephalitis in Asia. The risk is highest in children aged 1-18 years, in rural areas and in the monsoon/post monsoon season. Japanese encephalitis has high mortality and morbidity. JE vaccination remains the single most important control measure.

No serious side effects have been reported with this vaccine. However, minor side effects that have been reported are mild fever, rash, tenderness at injection site and irritability. The vaccine should be stored at 2 – 8°C.

JE vaccine is recommended for individuals living in endemic areas till 18 years of age as well as those who travel to endemic areas. The National Immunization Schedule has recommended primary vaccination with two doses at 9 months and 16 – 24 months for routine immunization in all endemic areas. For catch up vaccination, all susceptible children upto 18 years should be vaccinated during disease outbreak / ahead of anticipated outbreak in campaigns.

Pneumococcal Conjugate Vaccines (PCVs)

Two vaccines are available: Pneumococcal polysaccharide vaccine (PPV 23) and Pneumococcal conjugate vaccine (PCV 10 and 13). Both the vaccines should be stored at 2–8°C.

The *polysaccharide vaccine* is poorly immunogenic in children below 2 years, has low immune memory, do not reduce nasopharyngeal carriage and does not provide herd immunity. It has at best 70% efficacy against prevention of invasive pneumococcal disease in the high-risk population but it is a safe vaccine with only occasional local side effects.

The *conjugate pneumococcal vaccine* was developed to increase immunogenicity in children below 2 years who are at the highest risk of developing pneumococcal disease. Two vaccines viz. PCV 10 and PCV 13 are licensed for children from 6 weeks to 5 years. In addition, PCV 13 is licensed for prevention of pneumococcal disease in adults.

Dosage Schedule

Pneumococcal conjugate vaccine (PCV): Primary schedule for both PCV 10 and 13 includes 3 doses of 0.5 ml at 6, 10, 14 weeks and 1 booster at 12 through 15 months.

Pneumococcal polysaccharide vaccine: Not recommended for routine vaccination in healthy children; recommended for vaccination of children with certain high risk factors. The high risk factors include sickle cell disease and other hemoglobinopathies, hyposplenia, asplenia, those on immunosuppressive therapy, congenital or acquired immunodeficiency, renal failure, CSF leak, cochlear implant, Nephrotic syndrome and HIV infection. Minimum age for vaccination is 2 years. For children with high risk factors 1 dose of PPSV should be given atleast 8 weeks after the last dose of PCV. An additional dose should be administered after 5 years in children with anatomic or functional asplenia or an immuno-compromising condition. PPSV should not be used alone for prevention of pneumococcal diseases amongst high risk individuals.

Rotavirus Vaccine (RVV)

Two types of vaccines are available in India: Rotarix TM and Rota Teq TM.

The Rotarix TM (Monovalent) Vaccine (RV1) is available as a lyophilized vaccine to be reconstituted with liquid diluent prior to administration. The vaccine and the diluent should be stored at 2 to 8°C and must not be frozen.

Dosage Schedule

The vaccine should be administered promptly after reconstitution. The dose is 1 ml orally, 2 doses at 4 weeks interval. The first dose can be administered at the age of 6 weeks and not later than 12 weeks age. If the infant spits or regurgitates the entire vaccine dose then the dose may be repeated at same visit.

Rota Teq TM Vaccine (Pentavalent) is available as a liquid vaccine mixed with buffer and no reconstitution is needed. It should be stored at 2–8 °C.

Dosage Schedule

It is administered orally in a three-dose schedule at 2, 4, 6 months age. The vaccination should not be initiated for infants more than 12 weeks old and all 3 doses should be administered before the age of 32 weeks.

The National Immunization Schedule includes 3 doses of RVV at 6, 10, 14 weeks. Vaccination should not be initiated for infants aged 15 weeks, 0 days or older. The maximum age for the final dose in the series is 8 months 0 days.

Vaccination should be strictly as per schedule as there is a potentially higher risk of intussusception if vaccines are given to older infants. In preterm, vaccination should be considered when they are clinically stable and atleast 6 weeks age. The infant can be allowed to take breast milk before or after vaccination.

MMR Vaccine

The MMR vaccine contains three vaccines viz. measles, mumps and rubella. It is supplied freeze dried. After reconstitution it should be used within 4 hours and the remaining vaccine discarded. It is an essential vaccine but yet to be included in the National Immunization schedule.

At What Age?

The minimum age is 9 months or 270 completed days. It is administered subcutaneously over the upper arm or anterolateral aspect of the thigh. The vaccine can be administered along with other vaccines viz. DPT, OPV and Hib.

IAP recommends 3 doses, the 1st dose at 9 months and a 2nd dose at 15 months and 3rd dose at 4 through 6 years age. IAP approves the 3rd dose as MMRV (MMR + Varicella) at 4 – 6 years age in place of only MMR.

Storage

For long-term storage it must be frozen. For clinic use it can be stored at 2 – 8 °C.

Typhoid Vaccine

Vaccination against typhoid is necessary in view of the high prevalence of the disease. At present there are two vaccines in use for prevention of typhoid: the Vi capsular polysaccharide (ViPS) vaccine and ViPS conjugate vaccine.

The Vi capsular polysaccharide vaccine (ViPS) has a reasonable efficacy and low reactogenicity. Protection begins within 2 weeks of vaccination. It provides modest and short lasting protection. It is not very effective below the age of 2 years because it is a polysaccharide vaccine. The ideal age for vaccination is 2 years plus and to be repeated every 3 years. The vaccine can be given intramuscularly / subcutaneously in the dose of 0.5 ml. Adverse effects are mild and include pain and swelling at the injection site. The vaccine should be stored at 2 – 8 °C. It should not be frozen.

Vi capsular polysaccharide conjugate vaccine (ViPS conjugate): Considering the epidemiology of typhoid in the country, there is definite need of protection against typhoid fever in children below 2 years of age; hence the need for typhoid conjugate vaccines. It is effective below 2 years of age also and capable of providing superior long-lasting protection.

Primary immunization: The ideal age is at 9-12 months of age. Only a single dose of the vaccine is recommended for primary series. An interval of at least 4 weeks with the measles/MMR vaccine should be maintained since the data on interference with the measles/MMR vaccine are not yet available.

Boosters: Those who received a dose of conjugate vaccine at 9-12 months can be prescribed booster of either Vi polysaccharide (Vi-PS) or the ViPS conjugate vaccine at 2 years of age. Those who have received booster of ViPS vaccine will need revaccination every 3 years till the intended duration of protection. The need of further boosters after ViPS conjugate vaccine is not yet determined since long term data are not yet available.

Catch-up schedule: Catch-up vaccination is recommended up to 18 years of age. Below 2 years, only conjugate vaccine is recommended while above 2 years of age any of the two can be employed.

Hepatitis A Vaccine

Hepatitis A vaccine can be used any time after 1 year of age because by then maternally derived antibody levels decline. The protective efficacy is 94 – 100%. Immunity is long lasting.

Dosage Schedule

Two vaccines are available. *Inactivated Hepatitis A vaccine* should be started at 12 through 23 months and second dose after 6 to 18 months. *Live attenuated H2 – strain Hepatitis A vaccine* is a single dose vaccine and can be started at 12 through 23 months of age. Either of the two vaccines can be used in catch up schedule beyond 2 years of age. Two doses of inactivated vaccine atleast 6 months apart should be administered to unvaccinated persons and only 1 dose of live attenuated H2 vaccine.

For catch up vaccination pre-vaccination screening for Hepatitis A antibody is recommended in children older than 10 years as at this age the estimated seropositive rates exceed 50%.

Adverse Reactions

These include local pain and induration.

Storage

The vaccine should be stored at 2 – 8 °C.

Varicella Vaccine

The varicella vaccine is highly effective, the protective immunity is humoral as well as cellular and develops in 95 – 99% individuals, and the immunity appears to be long lasting.

The vaccine can be administered to any healthy individual above the age of 12 months who has not suffered from varicella previously.

Dosage Schedule

Minimum age for vaccination is 12 months. The recommended schedule is to administer the first dose at age 15 through 18 months and a second dose at 4 through 6 years. The risk of breakthrough Varicella is lower if given 15 months onwards.

Adverse Reactions

Include fever, pain, swelling and redness at the vaccination site and rash.

Storage

The vaccine should be stored at 2 – 8 °C.

Routine Vaccination of Hepatitis A and Varicella Vaccines: Is It Necessary?

Both these vaccines are not included in the National Immunization Schedule. Hence the present recommendation is that it should be given on a one to one named child basis. Both vaccines are essential vaccine but costly. Ideally, it should be offered to all young children and adolescents who have not suffered from Hepatitis A and Varicella during childhood and are leaving home for studies in residential schools/colleges.

For High Risk Children

The *Hepatitis A vaccine* should also be administered in all cases of chronic liver disease. It may also be considered in children attending crèches and day care centres and in travellers from abroad visiting endemic areas. The *varicella vaccine* is also indicated in children with chronic lung/heart disease, humoral immunodeficiency, HIV infection (with CD 4 count above 25% of the age related norms), leukemia, and those on long-term salicylates and steroids.

Post Exposure Prophylaxis

Both these vaccines can be used for post exposure prophylaxis. The *Hepatitis A vaccine* should be given within 10 days of exposure. However, it may not be effective always like in case the contact has had the same source of infection as the index case. The *Varicella vaccine* should be given within 72 hours of exposure. The efficacy of post exposure prophylaxis is not very clear.

Yellow Fever Vaccine

Yellow fever vaccine is a live attenuated vaccine. It is available as a freeze dried preparation. The vaccine as well as the reconstituted vaccine should be stored at 2–8 °C and discarded within 1 hour of reconstitution. It can be safely given with all other childhood vaccines. Immunogenicity and efficacy are greater than 90%. Protective immunity is attained by 10th day and lasts for atleast 10 years. This is an important vaccine for travellers to South Africa and Sub Saharan Africa. A traveller should take the vaccine atleast 10 days before departure.

Dosage Schedule

The dose is 0.5 ml subcutaneously. Because serious side effects are common, the vaccine is contraindicated in infants below 6 months age, in those with history of thymus disease and HIV disease with CD4 count = /< 15% of age related cut off point and in those with history of serious egg allergy. The vaccine should be avoided in pregnant and lactating women and individuals = / > 65 years.

Side Effects

The incidence of serious adverse events is 1 per 400,000 doses. They include yellow fever associated neurologic disease (YEL-AND) viz. encephalitis, acute disseminated encephalomyelitis and Guillain-Barré Syndrome and yellow fever associated viseroptic disease (YEL-AVD) which mimics wild yellow fever and is often fatal.

Influenza Vaccine

The influenza vaccine is given before the peak influenza season. There are two types: Inactivated influenza vaccine (IIV) and live attenuated influenza vaccine (LAIV). Both vaccines should be stored at 2–8 °C. Best time to vaccinate is just before the onset of rainy season or just prior to onset of winter based on local epidemiology data.

II Vaccine: It is licensed to be used in children aged 6 months or older. It provides 70–90% efficacy against laboratory confirmed disease in healthy adults. The efficacy is around 50% in children under 5 years age. The vaccine is administered IM, the dose being 0.25 ml in children below 3 years age and 0.5 ml thereafter. *Side effects* include fever, rash and injection site reaction. Rarely serious side effects like GBS (1 case per million people) can occur. All the currently available IIVs contain the swine flu or A(H1N1) antigen; hence no need to vaccinate separately for swine flu.

LAI Vaccine: It has been approved by US FDA for use in individuals from 2–49 years. It is administered as a nasal spray. This vaccine has a superior efficacy than IIV in children below 5 years age.

It is not licensed to be used in children below 2 years, pregnant women and in presence of any chronic disease due to lack of efficacy and safety studies. This vaccine should also be avoided in children less than 5 years age with history of reactive airway disease, those with history of hypersensitivity to eggs and those with history of GBS in the past.

The *side effects* include mild fever, runny nose and sore throat.

The influenza vaccines are given before the peak influenza season in countries of high prevalence. IIV is recommended only for children with high-risk conditions. LAIV is recommended only in healthy children aged 2 through 18 years. For healthy children aged 2 through 18 years, either LAIV or IIV may be used.

The IAP recommends using the influenza vaccine in all children with risk factors as mentioned below and also wherein the vaccine is desired/requested by parents (discussing with them the benefits and limitations of the vaccine).

At risk children

- Congenital or acquired immunodeficiency
- Chronic cardiac, pulmonary, hematologic, renal, liver disease and diabetes mellitus
- Children on long term aspirin therapy
- Any neurologic disease that might cause respiratory compromise or impair ability to handle secretions
- Asthma requiring long term oral steroids

Dosage Schedule

IIV: First time vaccination: 6 months to below 9 years 2 doses 1 month apart; 9 years and above single dose. For annual vaccination single dose.

LAIV: First vaccination 2 – 9 years 1 or 2 doses as per annual recommendation. For 9 years and above single dose.

Meningococcal Vaccine

The available data on the background incidence of meningococcal disease in India are suggestive of low incidence of meningococcal disease and are less than that due to streptococcal pneumoniae and H influenzae type b. Hence routine childhood vaccination with meningococcal vaccine is not a priority presently.

A quadrivalent A, C, Y and W-135 conjugate vaccine has been licensed for use in individuals aged 11-55 years in USA (2-55 years in Canada). A single dose of 0.5 ml IM is recommended.

Human Papilloma Virus (HPV) Vaccine

It is a vaccine for protection of cervical cancer. The currently available vaccines are safe and efficacious but costly. The vaccine should be stored at 2–8°C, must not be frozen and protected from light.

Two vaccines are lincensed and available, HPV4 and HPV2. The minimum age for vaccination is 9 years. The dose is 0.5 ml IM in the deltoid and 2 doses at 0 and 6 months in girls between 9 and 14 years. At present no boosters are recommended. For girls 15 years and older and immunocompromised individuals 3 doses are recommended. In a 3 dose schedule, either HPV4 (0,2, 6 months) or HPV2 (0, 1, 6 months) is recommended.

For catch up vaccination, either HPV2 or HPV4 can be administered at the age of 13 years through 45 years if not previously vaccinated.

Immunization of Adolescents

Adolescence should be considered an appropriate age for catch up immunization as well as for administration of certain vaccines which may not have been available earlier.

Preferred Age

The preferred age for administration is at 10-12 years but catch up may be done till 18 years.

Routine Immunization

The recommended routine vaccines for adolescents are the following:

Vaccine	*Schedule*
Tdap/Td/TT*	10 years
HPV	10 to 12 years

* Recommended in the National Immunization Schedule.

Tetanus toxoid (TT), which is in use at present, is also an effective vaccine and is included in the National Immunization Schedule at 10 years and 16 years. HPV is recommended only for females, three doses at 0, 1 or 2 (depending on the vaccine used) and 6 months. The disadvantages of HPV vaccine are as follows:

- Available vaccines do not protect against serotype 35, the common serotype.
- Prevalent serotypes in West, Central and East India are not known.
- High cost; hence not affordable by all sections of people.
- Periodic screening for carcinoma cervix is found to be more cost effective.
- The present incidence of cervical carcinoma in India does not allow universal immunization.

Catch Up Immunization

It is important to catch up for missed vaccines in adolescents. It should be noted that a natural infection with varicella and Hepatitis A before adolescence, gives natural immunity and hence vaccination may not be required. Important vaccines for adolescents in our country are Hepatitis B, MMR, typhoid and TT/Tdap/Td vaccine and Hepatitis A and Varicella as indicated.

Catch Up Vaccination for Adolescents

Vaccine	*Schedule*
MMR	2 doses at 4 – 8 weeks interval
Hepatitis B	3 doses 0, 1 and 6 months
Hepatitis A*	2 doses at 0 and 6 months
ViPS Typhoid***	1 dose every 3 years
Varicella**	2 doses at 4 – 8 weeks interval

* For Hepatitis A prior check for Anti HAV IgG may be cost effective. Combination of Hep B and Hep A may be used in 0, 1, 6 schedule.

** Varicella 2 doses at 4-8 weeks interval, one dose if previously vaccinated with one dose.

*** A minimum interval of 3 years should be observed between 2 doses of typhoid vaccine.

Adolescent Immunization in Special Circumstances

At present JE, Pneumococcal and Rabies vaccine are important immunizations in our country.

Vaccine	*Age recommended*
Influenza	1 dose every year
JE*	Catch up upto 15 years
Pneumococcal	2 doses 5 years apart
Rabies**	0,3,7,14,28

* Only in endemic area as catch up. Maximum number of doses – Two.

** Rabies Vaccine: As soon as possible after exposure. Preventive vaccination in areas of high incidence of Rabies.

Vaccines for Adolescent Travellers (IAP)

All age appropriate vaccines should be completed before travel. In addition, those listed below should be administered depending on the travel area.

Vaccine	*Place of travel*	*Dose recommended*
Meningococcal*	USA/UK/endemic area, Saudi Arabia, Africa	2 doses 4–8 weeks apart
Yellow fever**	South Africa, Sub Saharan Africa	1dose 10 days before travel
Oral cholera	Endemic area or area with an outbreak	2 doses 1 week apart
JE	Endemic areas	Single dose
Rabies	For going on trekking	3 doses, 0, 7, 28 days

* Quadrivalent vaccine for those travelling to the US and Bivalent (A+C) or Quadrivalent for those travelling to the UK.

** Mandatory for all travellers to yellow fever endemic zones as per International Health Regulations.

Immunization in Special Circumstances

Immunization in preterm/Small for date infants: All vaccines are recommended to be administered as per schedule according to the chronological age irrespective of birth weight or period of gestation except Hepatitis B vaccine. If the weight is less than 2 kg, and the mother is HbsAg –ve, Hepatitis B vaccination is delayed for 1 month as immunogenicity is lower if administered earlier.

Since preterm and low birth weight infants have increased susceptibility to infections, the pneumococcal conjugate vaccine, Rota virus and influenza vaccines should be administered if resources permit.

Children receiving corticosteroids, other immunosuppressive therapy viz. chemotherapy and radiotherapy: Children receiving corticosteroids in high doses (Prednisolone 2 mg/ kg body weight) for 14 days or more should not receive live virus vaccines until steroid has been discontinued for 1 month. Killed vaccines are safe but may be less efficacious. Children on lesser doses of steroid, inhaled or topical steroid may be safely and effectively given the age appropriate vaccine.

Children on other immunosuppressive therapy should avoid live vaccines during therapy unless benefits outweigh risks. Children on chemotherapy and radiotherapy for malignancy should avoid all vaccines during therapy and for atleast 3 months after stopping therapy.

Lapsed immunization: A drop out from the immunization schedule does not require reinitiating the entire vaccine series. However, in case of uncertain or unknown immunization status, it is appropriate to start the schedule as in an unimmunized child. At present, there is no evidence to indicate that administration of vaccines to already immune recipients is harmful.

Immunization during illness: There is no contraindication to vaccination during minor illness viz. viral upper respiratory infections, mild diarrhea, and minor skin infections like boils, scabies. During a major illness (bed ridden or hospitalized), all immunization should be postponed till the child is well. In hospitalized children, immunization should be completed at the time of discharge.

Children with chronic diseases can be given safely all vaccines. However, the immunogenicity, efficacy, and duration of protection are lower than in healthy children. Hence, may require higher antigen content (e.g., Hepatitis B vaccine) and repeated boosters (e.g., Hepatitis A and Hepatitis B vaccines). In patients with planned splenectomy, vaccination should be initiated atleast 2 weeks prior to surgery with pneumococcal, Hib, and meningococcal vaccines.

Immunization in children with history of allergy: Children with history of egg allergy should not receive influenza and yellow fever vaccine. All other vaccines can be given safely. Children who have had a serious hypersensitivity reaction/anaphylaxis to a particular vaccine must never receive that vaccine again. A mild reaction, however, is not a contraindication. However, every child should be kept under observation for atleast 15 minutes after vaccination for allergic reaction.

Vaccination schedule for a child not immunized in time: In these children, the schedule has to be individualized. Any number of vaccines, live/inactivated, can be given on the same day maintaining a gap of 5 cm between the sites of injection. However, BCG and measles/MMR should not be given on the same day. If not given on the same day there should be a gap of 4 weeks between two live vaccines especially MMR and varicella.

HIV infected children: Vaccination of a baby born to a HIV positive mother but with indeterminate status should be done as per normal schedule.

The WHO recommended vaccines (viz. BCG, DPT, OPV, measles/MMR, hepatitis B vaccines) can be given to the HIV infected asymptomatic children. In HIV infected known symptomatic children BCG and OPV vaccine cannot be given. The other vaccines can be given safely to all HIV infected children. Hepatitis A vaccine and IPV can be given to all HIV infected infants. Varicella and MMR vaccines can be given to an infant with asymptomatic HIV infection and symptomatic infants with CD4 count > 15%.

An infant born to hepatitis B positive mother: If a mother is HBsAg positive (and specially HBeAg positive), the first dose of hepatitis B vaccine and HBIG (0.5 ml IM) should be given to the infant within 12 hours of birth. HBIG may be given upto 48 hours but efficacy after 48 hours is not known. Two more doses of hepatitis B vaccine should be given at 1 month and 6 months age. The closely spaced schedule should not be used.

If HBIG is not available or is unaffordable, hepatitis B vaccine may be given at 0, 1 and 2 months followed by an additional dose between 9–12 months. The efficacy of prophylaxis with both HBIG and hepatitis vaccine is 85–95%. With only hepatitis B vaccine it is 70–75%. All infants born to HBsAg positive mothers should be tested for HBsAg and anti HBsAg antibodies at the age of 9–15 months to identify carriers/non-responders.

In a preterm/small for date baby, if the mother is HbsAg + ve, then both Hepatitis B vaccine and Hepatitis B immunoglobulin is administered within 12 hours of birth followed by another 3 doses of the vaccine at 6 weeks, 14 weeks and 6–12 months. If Hepatitis B immunoglobulin is not available or affordable, only Hepatitis B vaccine should be given.

If the mother's HBsAg status is not known, it is important that Hepatitis B vaccination should begin within a few hours of birth so that perinatal transmission can be prevented. Any one of the following schedules may be used for this purpose; birth, 6 and 14 weeks or birth, 6 weeks and 6 months.

Tetanus prophylaxis in wound management: The type of prophylaxis will primarily depend on three factors: (1) Type of wound; (2) Previous immunization status; (3) Time of booster.

- A child with a clean, minor wound, unknown immunization status / with a history of < 3 doses of TT needs a full course of TT vaccination.
- A child with clean minor wound with history of 3 or more TT doses with a booster within 10 years needs only wound toilet. No TT vaccine. Beyond 10 years needs 1 booster.
- A child with other wounds, unknown immunization status/with a history of < 3 doses needs both Tetanus Immunoglobulin (250 IU, IM) and TT vaccine.
- A child with other wounds, with history of 3 or more TT doses with a booster within 5 years needs only wound toilet. Beyond 5 years needs 1 booster TT.
- For children below 7 years, DTwP/DTaP vaccine should be given. Above 7 years TT/Td.

Dog bite and rabies vaccine: All tissue culture vaccines (viz. human diploid cell vaccine, purified chick embryo cell vaccine, and vero cell vaccine) have almost equal efficacy and any one of them can be used. Rabies vaccine can be administered pre exposure or post exposure.

Pre exposure prophylaxis is necessary for the high-risk group. The high-risk group consists of young infants, veterinarians, wildlife staff, postal delivery staff and lab staff working with Rabies vaccine.

Irrespective of age, 1 ml vaccine is given intramuscularly over the deltoid region (anterolateral aspect of thigh in children below 2 years) on day 0, 7 and 28 days. A booster dose is given one year after the primary doses and every 5 years thereafter.

Post exposure prophylaxis is indicated following a significant contact with a warm blooded animal such as dog, cat, cow, buffalo, sheep, goat, pig, donkey, horse, camel, fox, jackal, monkey, mongoose, bear etc. Post exposure prophylaxis is not recommended, at present in case of rodent bites.

Infancy, pregnancy and lactation are not contraindications. A child presenting days/months/years after the bite should be managed in a similar manner as a child recently bitten as rabies has a long incubation period.

Classification of Rabies Exposure

WHO classifies rabies exposure into three categories as follows:

Category	*Description*	*Recommended treatment*
I	Licks on intact skin	None, if case history is reliable
II	Nibbling of uncovered skin, minor scratches, or abrasions without bleeding, licks on broken skin	Administer vaccine
III	Single or multiple trans-dermal bites, scratches. Contamination of mucous membrane with saliva (i.e., licks) or exposure to bats	Administer RIG and vaccine immediately

Post exposure prophylaxis of Rabies consists of (a) Cleaning of wound (b) Tetanus prophylaxis (c) Administration of Rabies immunoglobulin, and (d) Administration of Rabies vaccine.

Cleaning of wound: The first step in management is thorough cleaning of the wound with soap and then flushing under running water for 10 minutes. This should be followed by irrigation of wound with a virucidal agent such as 70% alcohol or providone iodine. Suturing of wound should be avoided. In case it is unavoidable for hemostasis, RIG infiltration should be done prior to it. Antibiotics should be given as indicated.

Administration of Rabies immunoglobulin: RIG (Human RIG 20 i.u./Kg or equine 40 i.u./kg) by infiltrating around the wound in case of category III bites. If RIG is not available, two doses of the vaccine can be given on day 0. It is, however, not a substitute of RIG.

Tetanus prophylaxis: As in wound management.

Vaccine Administration: The standard schedule is five doses on days 0, 3, 7, 14 and 30 with 0 being the day of commencement. A sixth dose on day 90 is optional and may be offered to patients with severe debility or those who are immunosuppressed. The dose of vaccine is same for children and adults.

For re-exposure, at any point of time, after a completed (and documented) pre or post exposure prophylaxis, two doses should be given on days 0 and 3 at any time after the full course.

Pet Animal Bite

In case of *bites of pet animals*, post exposure prophylaxis, may be deferred only if the pet at the origin of exposure is more than 1 year old and has a vaccination certificate indicating that it has received atleast two doses of a potent vaccine, the first not earlier than 3 months age and the second within 6 to 12 months of the first dose in the past one year.

The post exposure prophylaxis should be done as follows:

- Observe the animal for 10 days.
- Start vaccination 0, 3.
- If animal asymptomatic after 10 days, administer the day 7 dose at 28 days in case of unimmunized. If previously immunized stop after second dose.
- If the animal dies or gets lost: Complete 5 doses if unimmunized. Stop after second dose if previously immunized.
- In highly endemic area: Full vaccination as indicated. No observation.

Vaccination During Epidemics: There are two vaccines recommended during epidemics: Japanese B encephalitis and Meningococcal vaccine. The former vaccine is recommended for use in endemic areas during epidemic situation. The latter is indicated in persons at risk during epidemics.

Japanese B Encephalitis vaccine should be considered for all people travelling to countries where the disease is endemic. Along with infants, all susceptible children upto the age of 18 years should be administered catch up vaccination.

Meningococcal vaccines are recommended only in high-risk situations in children aged 2 years or more (3 months or more during outbreaks or with close household contacts). The polyvalent vaccine is preferred. A single dose of 0.5 ml SC/IM is recommended. In infants aged 3 months to 2 years, 2 doses 3 months apart are recommended. Revaccination with one more dose 2–5 years after the first dose may be preferred in children who remain at high risk or who have been vaccinated at an age younger than 4 years. Due to poor performance of the polysaccharide vaccine below 24 months of age, conjugate vaccines are now recommended for use in outbreak situations from 12-24 months.

Immunization in Travellers: A uniform vaccination schedule is not possible because the epidemiology of diseases differs in various geographical areas. The two steps in immunizing travellers are (a) to update routine immunization and (b) to provide travel specific immunizations. For fully immunized Indians travelling abroad, the recommended vaccine is yellow fever vaccine for those travelling to South Africa and Sub-Saharan Africa. Vaccines to be recommended for fully immunized children travelling from Western countries to India are BCG, typhoid, hepatitis A, hepatitis B, rabies and Japanese encephalitis (if visiting JE endemic areas in JE season). Further, children intending to go on Haj pilgrimage in Saudi Arabia should be advised meningococcal vaccine.

Immunization of Children with Bleeding Disorders: Subcutaneous route for vaccination can be used safely. Those vaccines which can be given only by intramuscular route should be scheduled after factor replacement therapy. Needle size of less than 23G should be used and firm and sustained pressure should be applied for atleast 5 minutes over the injection site.

Indian Academy of Pediatrics (IAP) Recommended Immunization Time Table

The IAP Coordination Committee of Immunization has formulated an immunization time table for the children of India. This is not yet totally accepted by the Government of India. Primarily following the government recommended vaccine schedule, the additional vaccines included over and above those vaccines in the IAP time table can be advised to parents on one to one named child basis.

Table 4.5: IAP immunization time table 2016

Age (completed weeks/months/years)	*Vaccines*
Birth	BCG, OPV_0, Hep – B 1
6 weeks	DTwP1, IPV1, Hep B 2, Hib 1, Rota virus 1, PCV1
10 weeks	DTwP 2, IPV 2, Hib 2, Rota virus 2, PCV 2
14 weeks	DTwP 3, IPV 3, Hib 3, Rota virus 3, PCV 3
6 months	OPV 1, Hep B 3
9 months	OPV 2, MMR1
9–12 months	Typhoid conjugate vaccine
12 months	Hep A 1
15 months	MMR 2, Varicella 1, PCV booster
16–18 months	DTwP booster 1/DTaP booster 1, IPV booster 1, Hib booster 1
18 months	Hep A 2
2 years	Typhoid conjugate booster
4–6 years	DTwP booster 2/DTaP booster 2, OPV 3, Varicella 2, MMR 3
10–12 years	Tdap/Td, HPV

IAP recommended vaccines for high-risk children:

1. Influenza vaccine.
2. Meningococcal vaccine.
3. Japanese encephalitis vaccine.
4. Cholera vaccine.
5. Rabies vaccine.
6. Yellow fever vaccine.
7. Pneumococcal vaccine (PPSV 23).

High-risk children include those with:

1. Chronic cardiac, pulmonary (including asthma if treated with prolonged high dose oral steroids), hematologic, renal (including Nephrotic syndrome), liver diseases.
2. Children on long term steroids, salicylates, immunosuppressive or radiation therapy.
3. Diabetes mellitus, CSF leak, Cochlear implant, malignancies.
4. Children with functional/anatomic asplenia/hyposplenia.
5. Disease outbreaks.
6. Laboratory personnel and health care workers.
7. Travellers.
8. Having pets at home.
9. Children with higher threat of being bitten by dogs viz. hostellers, risk of stray dog menace.

Adverse Events Following Immunization

Adverse events following immunization are rare. However, every doctor who is dealing with an immunization procedure should be prepared to manage these rare events when they occur. Hence it is mandatory for every immunization clinic to have an emergency set up ready to tackle such post immunization events.

Every vaccine passes through purity and sterility tests. Even then some reaction either inherent to the vaccine or as a sequel to its administration can rarely occur. The symptoms and management of the adverse events following immunization is shown below in a tabular form:

Adverse events	*Vaccine*	*Symptoms*	*Management*
Anaphylaxis	Any vaccine	Within minutes Circulatory collapse Hypovolemic shock Laryngospasm/ edema Acute respiratory distress	Adrenaline CPR Volume expanders Hydrocortisone Inotropes
Hypotensive-Hyporesponsive Episode	DPT	Within 12 hours acute paleness, transient decreased/ loss of consciousness, decreased/ loss of muscle tone	IV fluids Dexamethasone Oxygen
Incessant cry	DPT	Within 48–72 hours Excessive inconsolable crying	Sedation with trichlorophos (50 mg/kg/day) and paracetamol
Toxic shock syndrome	Contamination of measles vaccine with S. aureus	Within 30 minutes to few hours Mounting fever Vomiting, diarrhea Shock	IV fluids Cloxacillin 50-100 mg/kg/day Steroids, Supportive therapy
Bacterial abscess	Any vaccine	Within 72 hours Abscess with or without fever	Antibiotics Drainage
Sterile abscess	DPT, DT, TT typhoid and HB	Abscess formation by 72 hours	Drainage
Moderate to severe local	Any vaccine	Swelling and redness 3–10 cm size at injection site	Paracetamol
Febrile seizure	DPT, measles	Generalized seizure	Anticonvulscent Paracetamol

Cold Chain

The cold chain is a system of storing and transporting vaccines at recommended temperatures from the point of manufacture to the point of use.

The key elements of the cold chain are:

- *Personnel* to manage vaccine storage and distribution.
- *Equipment* to store and transport vaccine and to monitor temperature.
- *Procedures* to ensure that vaccines are stored and transported at appropriate temperatures.

Keeping vaccines at the right temperature is not an easy task, but the consequences of not doing so can be disastrous. Once vaccine potency is lost, it cannot be

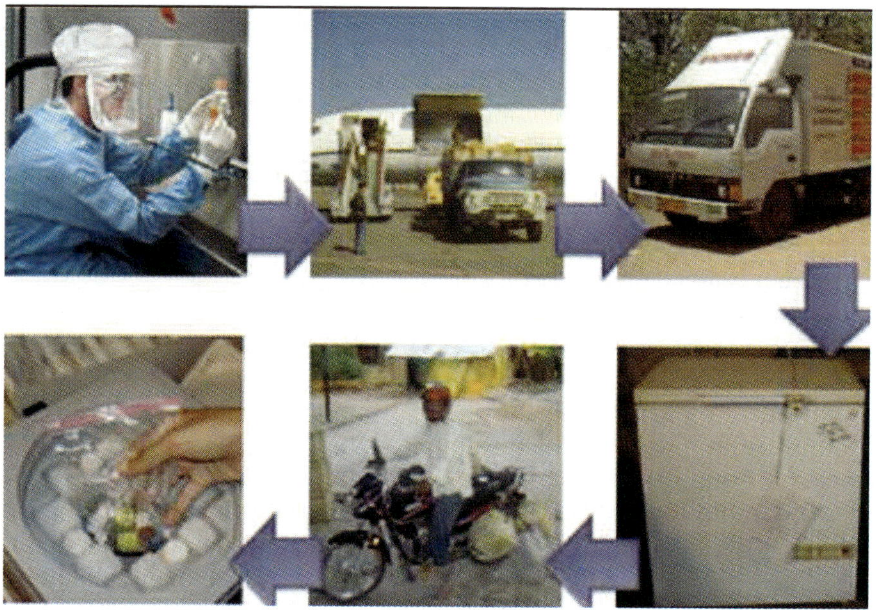

Fig. 4.2: Cold chain system from the manufacture to the point of use

regained. The damaged vaccines must be destroyed, leading to inadequate vaccine stocks and wastage of expensive vaccines. Moreover, children and women who receive a vaccine that is not potent are not protected. The Table 4.7 summarizes the sensitivity of vaccines to heat, light and freezing.

Table 4.7 : Summary of vaccine sensitivities

Vaccine	*Exposure to heat/Light, exposure to cold*	*Temperature at PHC*
Heat and light sensitive vaccines		
BCG	Relatively heat stable but sensitive to light. Not damaged by freezing	**+2°C to +8°C**
OPV	Sensitive to heat Not damaged by freezing	**+2°C to +8°C**
Measles	Sensitive to heat and light Not damaged by freezing	**+2°C to +8°C**
Freeze sensitive vaccines-C		
DPT vaccine	Relatively heat stable, Freezes at–3°C (Should not be frozen)	**+2°C to +8°C**
Hepatitis B	Relatively heat stable Freezes at - 0 .5°C (Should not be frozen)	**+2°C to +8°C**
DT	Relatively heat stable Freezes at–3°C (Should not be frozen)	**+2°C to +8°C**
TT	Relatively heat stable Freezes at–3°C (Should not be frozen)	**+2°C to +8°C**

At the PHC level, all vaccines are kept in the ILR for a period of one month at temperature of +2°C to +8°C.

Thermosensitivity of Vaccines

The vaccine most sensitive to heat is BCG (after reconstitution) followed by OPV, measles, DPT, BCG (before reconstitution), DT, TT, hepatitis B, Japanese encephalitis in descending order.

The vaccine most sensitive to freezing is hepatitis B vaccine followed by DPT, DT and TT in descending order.

The Safe Zone of Temperature for Vaccine Storage

To maintain the potency of the vaccine a safe zone of temperature is mandatory.

a. For short term (1 to 2 months): + 2 to + 8°C
b. For long term: - 20°C for BCG, OPV, measles and MMR only.

Multi-Dose Opened Vial Policy: Use After Reconstitution

Opened vials of measles, BCG and yellow fever vaccines, reconstituted vials of measles, BCG and yellow fever vaccines must be discarded at the end of each immunization session or at the end of six hours, whichever comes first.

Time limits for using vaccines after reconstitution:

- Varicella = 30 min (and protect from light).
- MMRV = 30 min (and protect from light).
- Yellow fever = 1 hour.

- Measles/MMR = 4 to 6 hours.
- Meningococcal Polysaccharide Vaccine single dose vial = 30 min.
- DTaP/Hib Combination = 30 min.

Vaccine Damage

The physical appearance of the vaccine may remain unchanged even after it is damaged. However, the loss of potency due to either exposure to heat or cold is permanent and cannot be regained.

Heat Damage

All vaccines are damaged by temperatures more than + 8°C, whether they are exposed to a lot of heat in a short time (e.g., as a result of keeping vaccine in a closed vehicle in the sun) or a small amount of heat over a long period (e.g. as a result of the frequent opening of lid of ILR). Reconstituted BCG, measles and JE vaccines are the most sensitive to heat and light. Since these live vaccines do not contain preservatives, there is risk of contamination with staphylococcus aureus leading to toxic shock syndrome and, therefore, they should not be used after 4 hours of reconstitution.

Checking for Heat Damage: The Vaccine Vial Monitor (VVM): A VVM is a label containing a heat-sensitive material which is placed on a vaccine vial to register cumulative heat exposure over time. The combined effects of time and temperature cause the inner square of the VVM to darken gradually and irreversibly. Before opening a vial, the status of the VVM should be always checked.

Does a VVM Measure Vaccine Potency?

No, the VVM does not directly measure vaccine potency but it gives information about the main factor that affects potency: heat exposure over a period of time. The VVM does not, however, measure exposure to freezing that contributes to the degradation of freeze-sensitive vaccines.

Reading the Stages of the VVM

1. The square is lighter than the circle. *If the expiry date has not been passed:* ***USE*** *the vaccine.*
2. The square is lighter than the circle. *If the expiry date has not been passed:* ***USE*** *the vaccine.*
3. The colour of the square matches that of the circle: ***DO NOT*** *use the vaccine.*
4. The colour of the square is darker than the circle: ***DO NOT*** *use the vaccine.*

Symbol	Explanation	Stage
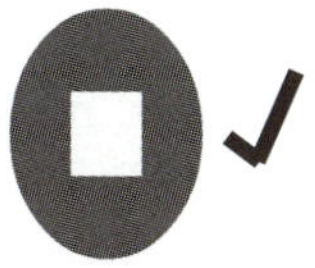	The inner square is lighter than the outer circle. If the expiry date has not passed, **USE** the vaccine.	I
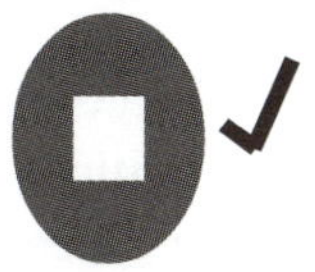	As time passes the inner square is still lighter than the outer circle. If the expiry date has not passed, **USE** the vaccine.	II
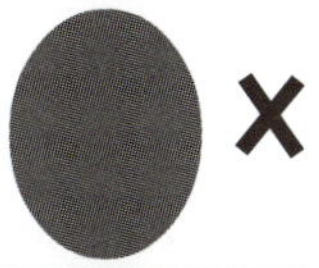	**Discard point:** The color of the inner square matches that of the outer circle. **DO NOT USE** the vaccine.	III
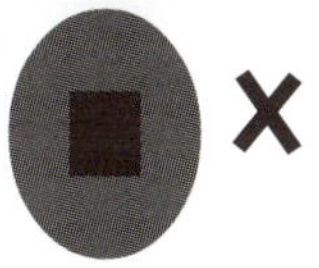	Beyond the discard point inner square is darker than the outer circle. **DO NOT** USE the vaccine.	IV

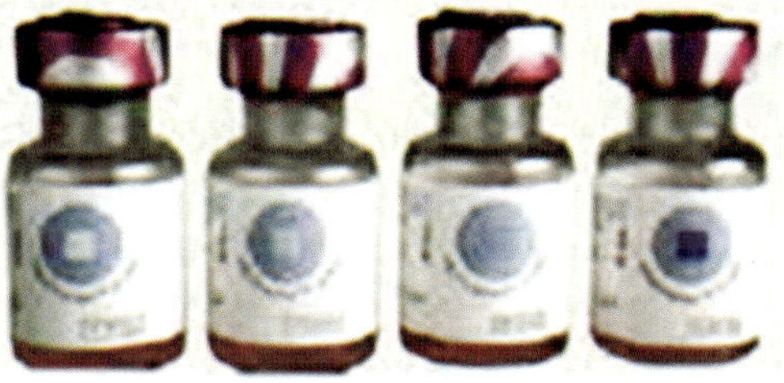

Source : WHO (www.who.int)

Fig. 4.3: Different stages of VVM

Correct Storage and Use of Diluents

Only the diluents supplied and packaged by the manufacturer with the vaccine should be used, since the diluent is specifically designed for the needs of that vaccine, with respect to volume, pH level and chemical properties.

The diluents should be stored between +2°C to +8°C in the ILR. If there are constraints of space, then diluents should be stored outside the cold chain. However, diluents should be cooled for at least 24 hours before use to ensure that vaccines and diluents are at +2°C to +8°C when being reconstituted. Otherwise, it can lead to thermal shock, i.e., the death of some or all the essential live organisms in the vaccine. The diluents and droppers should be stored with the vaccines in the vaccine carrier during transportation. Diluents should not come in direct contact with the ice pack.

Freeze Damage

Hepatitis B, DPT, DT and TT vaccines lose their potency if frozen. Freezing dissociates the antigen from the adjuvant alum thus interfering with the immunogenicity of the vaccine. Moreover, the risk of adverse events following immunization, such as sterile abscesses, may increase. Therefore, 'T-series' vaccines (DPT, DT, TT) and hepatitis B vaccine should be always stored between +2°C and +8°C.

If the vials are found to be frozen or contain floccules, the vials should be discarded. The shake test should be conducted if one suspects that vials could have been frozen.

The *shake test* is designed to determine whether adsorbed vaccines (DPT, DT, TT or hepatitis B) have been frozen at some point of time in the cold chain. Once the vaccine is frozen it tends to form flakes which gradually settle to the bottom after the vial is shaken. Sedimentation occurs faster in a vaccine vial which has been frozen as compared to a vaccine vial which has not been frozen.

Light Damage

BCG and measles vaccines are also light-sensitive, which is why they are supplied in amber-colored vials. Therefore, they need to be kept away from light.

Equipments for Storage

Cold chain equipment, both electrical and non-electrical, is used for storing vaccines and/or transporting them at appropriate temperatures. The cold chain equipments supplied under the UIP are as follows:

Deep freezers (DFs): Maintain a cabinet temperature between–20°C to–25°C; and store OPV and prepare ice packs at the district level. At the PHC level, deep freezers are used only for preparation of ice packs and are not to be used for storing UIP vaccines. About 20- 25 icepacks can be prepared by a 140 liter DF in 24 hours with at least 8 hours of continuous electricity supply.

Ice lined refrigerators (ILRs): Maintain a cabinet temperature between +2°C to +8°C; and are used to store all UIP vaccines at the PHC level. ILRs are lined with tubes or ice packs filled with water which freezes and keeps the internal temperature at a safe level despite electricity failure. ILRs can keep vaccine safe with as little as 8 hours continuous electricity supply in a 24-hour period. Since ILRs are top-opening, they can hold the cold air inside better than a front opening refrigerator. If baskets are not available, store vaccines (other than OPV and measles) over two rows of empty ice-packs kept on the platform of the ILR. Measles and OPV can be kept over two rows of empty ice packs on the floor of the ILR.

Domestic refrigerators: Also maintain a cabinet temperature between +2°C to +8°C with a holdover time of only 4 hours. Therefore, they are not recommended for common use in the UIP. However, they are used in urban dispensaries and by private practitioners in urban areas due to more assured power supply and non-availability of ILRs and DFs.

Cold boxes are insulated boxes used to collect and transport monthly supplies of vaccines from district stores to the health facility. They are also used to store vaccines when the ILR is out of order and when defrosting the freezer to keep frozen ice packs.

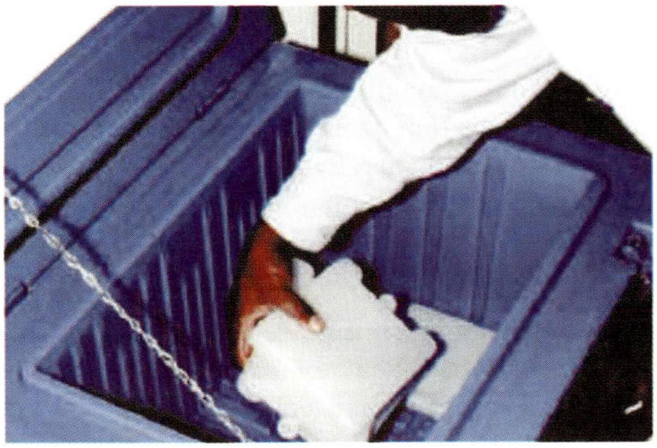

Fig. 4.4: Figure showing a cold box

Before the vaccines are placed in the cold box, fully frozen ice packs should be placed at the bottom and sides of the cold box. Thereafter, vaccines should be placed in cartons or polythene bags and placed in the cold box. The vaccines should be covered with a layer of fully frozen ice packs before the cold box is closed.

The vials of DPT, DT, TT and hepatitis B should not be placed in direct contact with the frozen ice packs. Note that vaccines should be transported or stored in cold boxes only with a sufficient number of hard frozen ice packs. In such a case, vaccines can be stored for 90 hours in a 5 litres cold box and for six days in a 20 litres cold box. The temperature of the cold box should be monitored by keeping a dial thermometer inside the cold box.

Vaccine vans: Are insulated vans used for transporting the vaccines in bulk. The vaccines should be transported to the last cold storage point only through vaccine vans.

Approximately 6 lakh to 10 lakh mixed antigen can be transported at a time. Vaccines should be transported only in cold boxes with the desired number of conditioned ice packs.

Vaccine carriers (with 4 conditioned ice packs): Maintain the inside temperature between +2°C to +8°C for 12 hours, if not opened frequently. They are used for carrying vaccines (16-20 vials) and diluents from PHCs to session sites. The return of unused vaccine vials from session sites to the PHC on the same day in the cold chain should be ensured. Unused vaccines that can be used in subsequent sessions should be kept. Vaccines that have been returned unopened more than thrice should be discarded. One should not keep any used vials in the cold chain. Day carriers which contain 2 ice packs or thermos flasks should never be used for routine immunization. Any screw driver or any other sharp shaft should not be used to open the lid of vaccine carrier.

Ice packs are plastic containers filled with water. These are frozen in the deep freezer and when placed in non-electrical cold chain equipment such as vaccine carriers and cold boxes, help increase the holdover time.

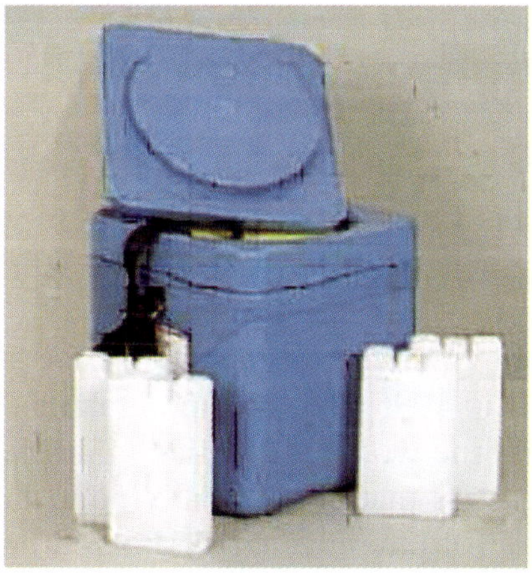

Fig. 4.5: Vaccine carrier with 4 ice packs

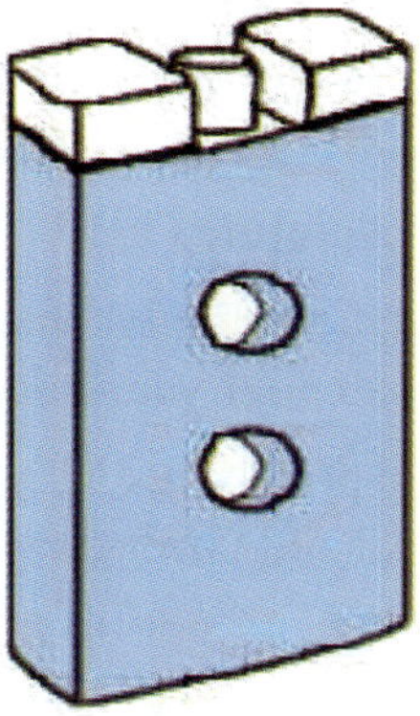

Fig. 4.6: Figure showing an ice pack

Conditioned ice packs: The most common cause of exposure to freezing temperatures is the failure to correctly condition ice packs prior to transport. Conditioning prevents freezing of freeze-sensitive vaccines. When ice packs are removed from a freezer, at say–25°C, they need to be kept at room temperature for long enough to allow the temperature of the ice at the core of the ice pack to rise to 0°C. This process is called conditioning. An ice pack is adequately conditioned as soon as beads of water cover its surface and the sound of water is heard on shaking it.

Thermometers: Whether, dial or stem (alcohol) are used to measure the temperature during storage of vaccines. Alcohol thermometers are more sensitive and accurate as they can record temperatures from–50°C to + 50°C and can be used for ILRs and deep freezers.

Correct Use of Thermometers

- Place a functional dial / stem thermometer in every cold chain equipment.
- Hang it vertically in the centre, away from direct contact with vaccine boxes and walls.
- Do not take it out of the equipment or hold for long. Read it where it is placed.
- Use it to monitor and record temperature every morning and evening.
- Take action to correct storage temperatures when the temperature record is outside recommended ranges.
- Replace the thermometer immediately if broken.

How to Store the Vaccines in the Different Storage Equipments

1. **Domestic refrigerators:** The OPV vaccine should be kept in the freezer compartment along with the ice packs. The rest of the vaccines in the non-freezing lower compartments with BCG and measles vaccines in the upper most shelf followed by DPT, DT, TT vaccines, hepatitis A and B and varicella in the middle shelf and diluents in the lower shelf. If the domestic refrigerator is used to store vaccines the following instructions should be followed:

   a. It should be used for storage of vaccines only. No food or drinks should be stored along with the vaccines. No vaccines should be stored in the baffle tray or the door shelves.

b. The refrigerator should be placed at least 10 cm away from the wall. It should be kept in a cool room away from direct sunlight.

c. The vaccines should be kept neatly with space between stacks for circulation of air. The refrigerator should be kept locked and opened only when necessary.

d. The refrigerator should be defrosted periodically. It should be on continuously.

e. A dial thermometer should be kept hanging on the top shelf for temperature monitoring.

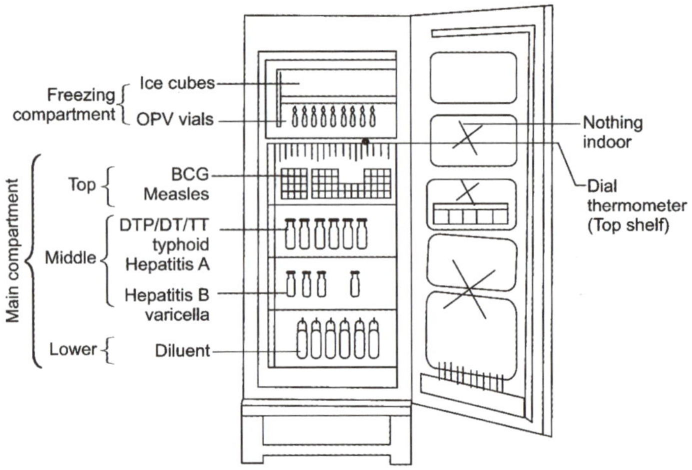

Fig. 4.7: Domestic refrigerator and vaccine storage

2. **Ice lined refrigerators:** While storing the vaccines in the ILR, the OPV should be kept in the bottom followed by BCG, measles and MMR. The DPT, DT, TT, hepatitis B, hepatitis A, varicella at the top.

3. **Vaccine carriers:** The oral polio should be kept at the bottom, followed by BCG, measles and MMR. The DPT, TT and TT should be kept at the top in a plastic bag to avoid direct contact with the ice packs.

Monitoring of Temperature

Dial thermometers are used to monitor temperature in ILR and domestic refrigerator. Alcohol thermometers are used to monitor temperature in the deep freezer. The temperature monitoring should be done 2 times a day.

Organization of the Immunization Clinic

Every hospital should have an immunization clinic and immunization should be carried out preferably every day. The immunization clinic should be adjacent to a well baby clinic. The objectives of the well baby clinic include assessment of growth and development, advice regarding exclusive breast feeding and complementary feeding, immunization and treatment of minor ailments. The immunization clinic should be run under the supervision of a doctor. Auto disabled syringe should be used for administration of all vaccines. The nurses and doctor on duty should be trained regarding the adverse reactions and their management.

The immunization clinic must be equipped for cold chain maintenance. It must be equipped for management of adverse reaction to vaccination particularly anaphylaxis. The vaccines can be stored in a domestic refrigerator or an ice lined refrigerator. A resuscitation tray should be available with drugs like adrenaline, hydrocortisone, dexamethasone, inotropes and intravenous fluids. Adrenaline should be pre-filled in a disposable syringe every day and discarded if not used. An oxygen cylinder, infusion sets should be available at hand. All health workers should also be trained in cardiopulmonary resuscitation.

Intensive Pulse Polio Immunization (IPPI)

In 1988, the 41st world health assembly launched a global initiative to eradicate polio by the end of the year 2000. This commitment was reaffirmed at the World Summit for Children in 1990. The Government of India started the Pulse Polio Immunization initiative for eradication of poliomyelitis in 1995. The IPPI programme is likely to continue until the world is certified to be eradicated of polio. Even areas that are currently polio free have to continue with IPPI to prevent risk of importing the wild virus into such areas.

Pulse polio immunization means administration of oral polio vaccine simultaneously to all susceptible children i.e. children below the age of 5 years.

Polio eradication is defined as:

1. No case of paralytic poliomyelitis caused by wild polio virus in last 3 calendar years along with.
2. Absence of wild polio virus in the community, where excellent clinical and virological surveillance exists; and
3. The coverage of pulse polio immunization is more than 80%.

Strategies for Eradication of Poliomyelitis

1. Routine immunization in infants.
2. Pulse polio immunization to all children below the age of 5 years regardless of whether they have been vaccinated before.
3. Effective disease surveillance (known as acute flaccid paralysis (AFP) surveillance) to detect all cases of acute flaccid paralysis, report them and investigate for poliovirus etiology. Confirmation of wild polio virus by genome analysis.
4. House to house mop up campaigns to ensure that every child is vaccinated and to break the final chains of transmissions.

Why Pulse Polio Immunization?

1. In developing countries where the incidence of poliomyelitis was high in the pre immunization era, only routine immunization of children with OPV vaccine could not eradicate poliomyelitis. In such countries, pulse polio vaccination is necessary to eradicate poliomyelitis.
2. With only routine immunization, there will be certain pockets of uncovered population, which may harbor wild polio virus, which will be transmitted to the newly born babies and other nonimmunized population. Thus there will remain a pool of non-immunized population in the community, which will continue to transmit the disease.
3. Children receiving doses additional to routine immunization will develop high immunity levels and children not receiving OPV previously will be immunized at the time of PPI.
4. The only way to protect children from polio is by stopping the circulation of wild polio virus from the environment. This is possible only if children less than 5 years of age simultaneously receive additional doses of OPV as is done in PPI. As all children are immunized simultaneously, the wild virus will be replaced in the intestine of the children as well as destroyed in the atmosphere. This will interrupt circulation of wild polio virus and thus eradicate polio.

Pulse Polio Immunization: Messages for the Community

1. Polio vaccine is one of the safest vaccines. Repeated doses will not do any harm to the child. The same OPV vaccine is used in all countries throughout the world.
2. The newborn baby should be given pulse polio immunization.
3. Even an ill child admitted in the hospital should receive OPV drops during PPI.
4. The child should be given PPI dose even if it falls one day after the routine OPV dose. However, if the routine immunization falls on the day of PPI, two doses are not required.
5. If the child is accidentally given more than 2 drops, it is still safe.

Acute Flaccid Paralysis (AFP) Surveillance

Acute flaccid paralysis means that paralysis is of acute onset (< 4 weeks) and the affected limb or limbs are flaccid, tone is diminished but sensation is not affected.

A case of AFP is defined as any child aged < 15 years who has acute onset of flaccid paralysis for which no obvious cause (such as trauma or electrolyte imbalance) is found.

AFP surveillance is carried out of all cases of AFP and not just for poliomyelitis. Therefore all cases of AFP should be reported regardless of the final diagnosis.

The Aim of AFP Surveillance

1. To detect polio virus transmission. In the initial stage, a good and sensitive surveillance helps in identifying the poliomyelitis cases and thus areas having wild polio virus transmission. In the later stage AFP surveillance is the only tool to establish the absence of wild virus transmission.
2. Surveillance should detect all cases of AFP, report them and investigate for polio virus etiology. When a polio virus is detected it should be examined by genome analysis to identify it as a wild virus, distinguish from vaccine virus and facilitate recording the incidence of vaccine associated paralytic poliomyelitis (VAPP).

AFP Case Investigation

1. **Reporting** to district immunization officer (DIO). The DIO should start investigation within 48 hours.
2. **Stool specimen collection:** It has been shown that for the purpose of eradication of wild polio virus, the

stool specimen culture is by far the best diagnostic test. Two specimens, at least 24 hours apart and within 14 days of onset of paralysis should be collected. Each specimen should be adequate volume (8–10 gms or size of a thumb). If cases are seen late (i.e. > 2 weeks after the onset of paralysis) stool specimen can still be collected upto 60 days after the onset of paralysis. Maximum chance of yielding a positive result is however within 2 weeks. Collection responsibility is on the DIO.

3. **Stool specimen transport:** Storage during transport should be in the freezer or any container that can maintain temperature below 8°C. A vaccine carrier can be used for the purpose.
4. **Polio virus isolation and typing** is done in the WHO accredited laboratories. For Assam the recommended laboratory is Institute of Serology, Calcutta.
5. **AFP surveillance good indicators:** The two most critical ways of assessing the quality of surveillance are:
   a. Rate of non-polio AFP: At least 1 case of non-polio AFP is to be reported per every 1 lakh children under the age of 15 years.
   b. Proportion of AFP cases with adequate stools within 2 weeks after onset of paralysis should be 80%.

Suggested Reading

1. Textbook of Medical Physiology by Guyton and Hall, 10th edition 2000, Saunders, Philadelphia.
2. Nelson Textbook of Pediatrics. Edited by Kliegman, Stanton, St. Geme, Schor and Behrman, 19th edition 2011, Saunders, Philadelphia.
3. IAP guide book on immunization. IAP Committee on Immunization 2005–2006.
4. IAP guide book on immunization. IAP Committee on Immunization 2007–2008.
5. Immunization handbook for health workers. Government of India, Ministry of Health and Family Welfare, New Delhi, 2006.
6. IAP guide book on immunization. IAP Committee on Immunization 2009–2011.

5

Growth and Development: Normal and Abnormal

OUTLINES

Growth and development are the most distinctive attributes of children which distinguishes them from adults. Growth and development constitute a continuous process from fertilization to maturity. Growth and development usually proceed concurrently, but may not always be interrelated. They are not interchangeable because they represent two different facets of the dynamics of change i.e. those of quantity and quality respectively.

Growth

Definition

It denotes an increase in the size of the body due to increase in the number and size of the cells resulting in an overall increase. It is attributed largely to hyperplasia, hypertrophy and differentiation of cells and tissues. Hyperplasia is evidenced by increase in DNA content of tissues and hypertrophy manifest as increase in protein to DNA ratio. Hypertrophy or increase cell size contributes to a lesser extent.

Laws of Growth

There are three laws of growth. They are as follows:

1. Growth and development in children is a continuous and orderly process. The sequence or pattern of growth in children is comparable but the rate is not always uniform.
2. Growth pattern of every individual is unique. The order of growth in human beings is cephalocaudal and distal to proximal. For example, growth of head occurs before that of neck and arms grow before legs. Distal parts of the body such as the hands grow before the upper arms.
3. Different tissues of the body grow at different rates:

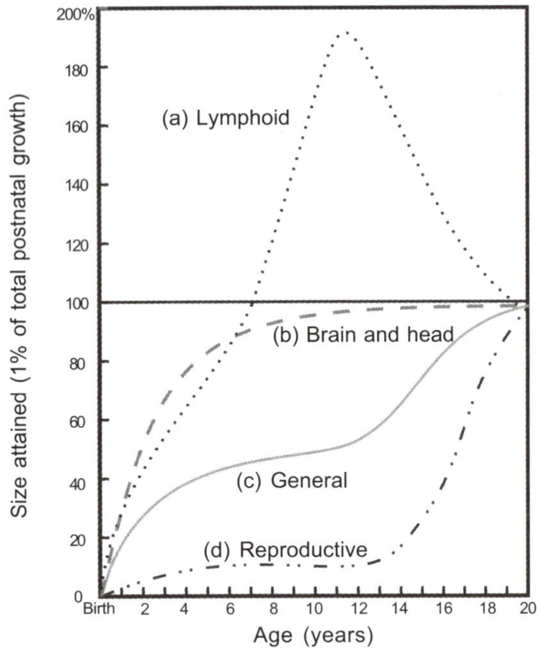

Fig. 5.1: Schematic growth curves of different tissues (From Tanner JM, Growth at Adolescence. Oxford, Blackwell Scientific Publications, 1955)

General body growth: General tissue includes whole body linear dimensions, respiratory and digestive organs, kidneys, aortic and pulmonary trunks, and musculature and blood volume. General body growth follows a sigma shaped curve. It is rapid during fetal period and first 1 to 2 years of post natal life, between 6–8 years age and during puberty. Growth is not uniform and hence the child's appetite which depends on the velocity of growth. It is more during the periods of rapid growth. So the child should be offered food whenever hungry and as much as he/she desires.

Brain and head growth: It includes brain and its parts, dura, spinal cord, optic system and cranial dimensions. Brain growth is very rapid during the 20–36 weeks of intrauterine life and during the first year of life, attaining around 67% at birth, 80% at 1 year and 90% at 5 years of adult size. Cerebellum reaches adult size by 15 months age. Brain myelination is complete by 7 years of age. Prevention of malnutrition during this period is important. Severe malnutrition can adversely affect brain development.

Growth of gonads: Reproductive tissues include testes, ovaries, epididymis, prostate, seminal vesicles, and fallopian tubes. Gonadal growth is dormant during childhood and becomes conspicuous during puberty. A normal nutritional status is an important factor influencing proper gonadal growth. Malnutrition during this period may result in underdeveloped reproductive organs.

Lymphoid growth: Lymphoid tissue includes thymus, lymph nodes, and intestinal lymph masses. Lymphoid growth attains peak during mid childhood (4–8 years), thereafter it declines. During this period, the child may normally have palpable glands. The school child is also vulnerable to enlargement of lymph glands due to various diseases. A child should be investigated for palpable lymph glands only when there is significant lymphadenopathy. Lymph gland size > 1.5 cm in cervical and axillary regions, > 2 cm in inguinal region and > 0.5 cm in epitrochlear region is called significant lymphadenopathy.

Periods of Growth

a. Prenatal period i.e. ovum 0–14 days, embryo 14 days to 9 weeks, fetus 9 weeks to birth.
b. Perinatal period i.e. growth from 28 weeks of gestation to 7 days after birth.
c. Post natal period includes newborn (birth to 4 weeks), infancy (first year of life), toddler (1–3 years), preschool child (3 to 6 years), school child (boys 6 to 12 years, girls 6–10 years) and adolescence.

Growth Spurts

Despite the continuous nature of growth from conception to maturity, the rate of growth is not the same at all time. There are periods of acceleration of growth. These periods of acceleration are known as growth spurts. In human there are three growth spurts:

a. Fetal and infantile growth spurt which is primarily a biophysical process.
b. Mid growth spurt is observed between the ages 6 – 8 years. It is of equal intensity and timing in both sexes but sometimes more pronounced in boys. This spurt is so small that it can be detected only on longitudinal assessment. The mid growth spurt coincides with differentiation of zona reticularis in adrenal cortex and secretion of adrenal androgens (adrenarche).
c. Adolescent growth spurt is a result of neuro humoral stimulation of the hypophysis by the hypothalamus.

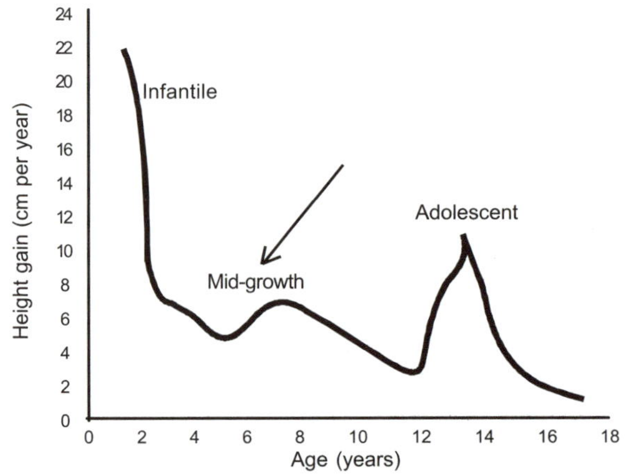

Fig. 5.2: Growth spurts in a longitudinal growth study

Endocrinology of Growth

The principal hormones affecting somatic and skeletal growth at different periods are as follows:

1. **Fetal period:** Insulin and thyroid (in later part).
2. **Infancy:** Growth hormone and thyroid hormone.
3. **Mid growth spurt:** Adrenal androgens.
4. **Adolescence:** Gonadal hormones.

Actions of the Different Hormones

Growth hormone plays a pivotal role in controlling post-natal growth. It is not an essential hormone for intrauterine fetal growth. The effects of growth hormone in vivo are mediated by somatomedins viz. Insulin like growth factors I and II (IGF-I and II). IGF- I is synthesized in the liver. It is the chief somatomedin involved in growth. IGF-II is a mitogen acting on bone cells but its exact function is not known.

The major actions of growth hormone are either direct or indirect. The direct actions are those on lipid and fat metabolism that are synergistic with cortisol and opposite to the actions of insulin and somatomedins. The indirect anabolic and growth promoting actions of growth hormone are mediated by somatomedins and include cell proliferation and protein synthesis in both skeletal and non-skeletal tissues. These actions are insulin like.

Thyroid hormone is secreted by the human fetus from 12th week of gestation. It plays an important role in post natal somatic growth. The crucial period of thyroxine dependent brain growth extends from the last part of gestation to several months post natally. The thyroid hormone promotes cartilage growth and maturation. It also influences synthesis and secretion of growth hormone. Hence thyroxine deficiency does not affect linear growth of fetus but it significantly retards skeletal maturation in the fetus.

Insulin is the chief hormone required for fetal growth. Insulin may bind to IGF- I receptor and promote growth. High insulin level may lower the levels of IGF binding proteins thereby increase free IGF and potentiate the action of IGFs. In mothers with overt or latent diabetes, the fetus is usually large with excessive birth weight.

Glucocorticoids inhibit growth by direct action on target tissues.

Androgens viz. testosterone and dihydrotestosterone accelerate linear growth and weight gain. They also appear to enhance secretion of growth hormone.

Peptide growth factors viz. EGF, TGF alpha, TGF beta, FGF, platelet derived growth factor etc. Their chief mode of action is paracrine or autocrine.

Growth in Low Birth Weight Infants

The low birth weight infants can be categorized into term or post term appropriate for date, preterm appropriate for date and small for date (preterm or term).

After birth, the small for date infants if fed early and adequately do not lose weight and start gaining weight within 2–3 days of life. In preterm babies, there is cumulative weight loss of upto 15% of birth weight in the first 3–4 days. The weight remains stationary for the next 4–5 days, then there is weight gain at the rate of 1–1.5% of body weight /day and birth weight is regained by the end of second week of life.

The small for date infants have a slightly faster growth rate in the first 3 months of life compared to preterm appropriate for dates. Thereafter growth slows down and by 18–24 months age, the small for dates are significantly lighter compared to the preterm. Preterm infants, on the other hand, catch up with the small for date babies by 6–9 months and overtake them.

The preterm appropriate for dates catch up and reach to the term appropriate for dates by 2–5 years age. If corrected for gestational age, the growth curve of the preterm runs parallel to the standard curves. The term small for date after an initial phase of rapid growth slows down and remain smaller. The preterm small for date infants are the worst sufferers.

Normal Postnatal Growth Pattern and Velocity of Growth

Growth During Infancy (Birth to 1 Year)

1. **Weight:** The normal average weight of a term neonate is 2800 grams (male) and 2750 grams (female). A term infant loose upto 10% of birth weight in the first week of life. This occurs as a result of excretion of extravascular fluid and possibly poor intake. Infants regain or exceed birth weight by 2 weeks of age and thereafter gain weight at the rate of approximately 30 grams / day during first 4 months, 20 grams/day during 5–8 months, 15 grams/day during 9 to 12 months age. Roughly, the infant doubles the birth weight by 5 months and triples by 1 year.
2. **Length:** The normal average length at birth is 50 cm. There is a gain of 3.5 cm/month in the first three months, 2 cm/ month in next 3 to 6 months, 1.5 cm/ month in next 6 to 9 months and 1.2 cm/month in 9 to 12 months age.
3. **Head circumference:** The normal average head circumference at birth is 32 to 35.5 cm. The head grows at the rate of 2 cm/month till 3 months age, 2 cm/ 3 months between 3months and 1 year.
4. **Chest circumference:** At birth, the chest circumference is about 3 cm less than head circumference. By 1 year age the two are almost equal. Thereafter the chest circumference should exceed head circumference.

Growth in Preschool Period (1 to 5 Years)

In the second year of life, the growth rate further slows down. Brain growth, however, continues with myelination throughout the second year. Between 1 and 3 years, weight gain is 3 kg/year, between 3 and 5 years it is 2 kg/ year. The gain in length in the second year is 2.5 cm, in the third year 7.5 to 10 cm, in 3–5 years 5–7.5 cm/ year. The growth in head circumference is 1 cm / year in 1 to 3 years age and 1 cm / year in 3 to 5 years age. The adult head size is achieved between 5 to 6 years age. The mid arm circumference is relatively constant between 16.5 to 17.5 cm between 1 to 5 years age. The upper segment to lower segment ratio is 1.7: 1 at birth. There is a gradual reduction in the ratio by 0.07–0.1 every year until ratio is around 1:1 at 10–12 years. In adults it is 1:1.1.

Growth in School Going Age (5 to 12 years)

The weight gain averages 3–3.5 kg and height gain 6 cm/year. The head grows only 2–3 cm. Myelination is complete by 7 years of age.

Table 5.1 : Velocity of growth

Weight		*Height*		*Head circumference*	
Age	*Rate*	*Age*	*Rate*	*Age*	*Rate*
0-4 mon	30 gm/day	birth	50 cm	birth	35 cm
5-8 mon	20 gm/day	1st year	25 cm	till 3 mon	2 cm/mon
9-12mon	10 gm/day	2nd year	12.5 cm	3-12 mon	2 cm/3 mon
1-2 yrs	3 kg/year	3rd year	7.5-10 cm	1-3 yrs	1cm/6 mon
3-12 yrs	2 kg/year	3-12 years	5- 7.5 cm	3-5 yrs	1 cm/year

Development

Definition

Development is defined as maturation of functions. It represents the qualitative aspect of the dynamics of change and indicates the acquisition of a variety of skills for optimal functioning of an individual. It usually proceeds concurrently with growth.

Principles

Development is a continuous process from conception to maturity. It begins in utero and birth is merely an event in the course of development. It is the most distinctive attribute of childhood. It is related to the maturation and myelination of the nervous system. The sequence of development is same in all children, but the rate varies from child to child. As in case of growth, development also proceeds in a cephalocaudal direction. Progress of development replaces mass activity by specific individual responses. Primitive reflexes have to be lost before voluntary movement is acquired. For example the walking and placing reflexes have to be lost before the child starts walking.

Important Developmental Milestones

Children accomplish maturation of different biological functions (level of development or milestones) at an anticipated age, with a margin of a few months on either side. The milestones may be divided into those pertaining to gross motor, fine motor adaptive, social and language development. Gross motor development involves control of child over his body.

Gross Motor Developmental Milestones

	Age	*Milestones*
1.	4 months	No head lag.
2.	6 months	Sits with support.
3.	8 months	Sits without support.
4.	9 months	Stands with support.
5.	10 months	Can pull itself to sitting position from supine.
6.	11 months	Walks with support.
7.	12 months	Stands without support. Walk few steps independently.
8.	13 months	Walks without support.
9.	15 months	Takes steps sideways. Can creep upstairs and kneel without support.
10.	18 months	Can get up and downstairs without help.
11.	24 months	Walks up and downstairs. Kicks a ball.
12.	30 months	Can walk tip toes, jump on both feet.
13.	36 months	Can go upstairs with one foot on each step. Can ride a tricycle.
14.	48 months	Can skip on one foot.
15.	60 months	Can skip on both feet.

Fine Motor, Adaptive Milestones

1.	1 month	Hands mostly closed due to grasp reflex.
2.	3 months	Hands mostly open. Plays with rattle when placed in hand.
3.	5 months	Grasp object with both hands, puts object into mouth.
4.	6 months	Drops one object when another is given.

Contd.

Contd.

5.	7 months	Approaches object with one hand, transfers from hand to hand. Retains one cube in hand while another is offered.
6.	9 months	Pincer grasp.
7.	12 months	Can put one object after another into basket.
8.	15 months	Feeds self from cup. Builds a tower of 2–3 cubes.
9.	18 months	Can self feed with a spoon. Makes a tower of 3–4 cubes.
10.	24 months	Puts in and takes of socks, shoes and pants. Can make a tower of 6–7 cubes.
11.	30 months	Can hold pencil in hand to scribble lines.
12.	36 months	Can draw a circle. Can make a tower of 9–10 cubes. Can dress and undress.

Social Development

1.	1 month	Regards mother.
2.	2 months	Social smile appears.
3.	3 months	Recognizes mother.
4.	6 months	Smiles at mirror image.
5.	7-8 months	Expresses anxiety on meeting strangers, imitates action and sound, responds to name.
6.	9 months	Waves good bye.
7.	12 months	Shakes head for 'No'.
8.	36 months	Knows gender, attends to toilet needs except for wiping.

Language Development

1.	1 month	Turns head to sound.
2.	3 months	Begins cooing.
3.	6 – 7 months	Speaks monosyllables.
4.	9 months	Speaks bisyllables.
5.	1 year	Speaks 2 – 3 words with meaning
6.	1½ years	Jargon speech, 6 – 20 words with meaning.
7.	2 years	Speak simple sentences.
8.	3 years	Vocabulary of about 250 words. Can tell a story.
9.	4 years	Can account experiences and events.

Delays in Development

It is very difficult to draw to a distinct dividing line between normal development and delayed development. Only the average level of development can be determined. Development delay should be suspected if a child is not able to perform the given task by the indicated ages. It is very importent to detect delayed miletone as early as possible so that early interventional measures can be started. For this purpose, the following four important milestones in the first year of life is shown to be very useful.

1. Social smile by 2 months.
2. Head holding by 4 months.
3. Sitting without support by 8 months.
4. Standing without support by 12 months.

Ideally, a mother should be made aware of these four milestones at the time of discharge from the hospital after delivery and advised to report immediately if there is a delay beyond the cutoff point because such infants require a thorough neurodevelopmental workup to exclude a developmental anomaly.

Factors Influencing Growth and Development

The factors affecting growth and development can be broadly classified into genetic factors and environmental factors.

Genetic Factors

1. *Parental inheritance* viz: Phenotype, intelligence and personality depend on inheritance from parents.
2. *Race*: Growth has a racial influence. The tribals are in general shorter people compared to the non-tribals.
3. *Sex*: There is no difference in the first year of life. Growth spurt during adolescence is earlier in girls; hence growth ceases earlier. On maturity, mean height and weight of girls is less than that of boys. Girls tend to walk, speak and acquire sphincter control earlier than boys.
4. *Biorhythm and maturation*: Daughters have similar age of menarche and similar length of menstrual cycle as their mothers.
5. *Genetic disorders:* Children with Down syndrome, Turner syndrome etc are short statured with variable degree of mental retardation.

6. Children of *multiple pregnancies*: Are seen to be associated with higher incidence of mental retardation, cerebral palsy etc. than single pregnancy.
7. *Birth order*: The first born tends to be more intelligent than subsequent children. However, there are exceptions.

Environmental Factors

Prenatal Factors

1. *Parental age*: Increased age of mothers is associated with chromosomal disorders like Down's syndrome. Increased paternal age is related to skeletal abnormalities like achondroplasia.
2. *Maternal height and weight, maternal nutritional status*: A weight < 40 kg and height < 145 cm in women indicates chronic protein energy malnutrition in the preschool years and adolescent period. Such women gives birth to low birth weight babies who in their turn become women with short stature.
3. *Personal factors*: A couple's desire to have a child of a particular gender may affect development. If the child is of the desired sex, overprotection and overindulgence may occur. If not, there may be rejection.
4. *Physical activity of mother*: Strenuous physical activity adversely affects the intrauterine growth. On the other hand, normal physical activity helps fetal growth.
5. *Parity:* Mean birth weight increases till 4th or 5th parity; thereafter the pattern is reversed.
6. *Placental dysfunction* as a result of PIH, PET, due to any cause, adversely affects fetal growth.
7. *Drugs used by mother*: Most of the drugs used by mother are transferred across the placenta. The drugs known to affect the fetus are many. The common ones include thalidomide, antiepileptics, Warfarin, antimitotics, antidepressants, antibiotics, antiemetics, lithium, magnesium sulphate etc. Smoking during pregnancy increases the risk of low birth weight, still birth, APH, mental and physical retardation, and later learning disabilities and overactivity. Alcohol excess in pregnancy causes fetal alcohol syndrome. Drug addiction may affect the father's sperm and cause damage to the fetus.
8. *Maternal infections,* the common ones that may damage the fetus include rubella, syphilis, toxoplasmosis, hepatitis B, CMV and HIV. Hereditary diseases include diabetes, hypothyroidism, phenylketonuria. Maternal diabetes is associated with fetal anomalies. The level of thyroid hormone in women with thyroid disease is a factor related to the motor competence of their children. High phenyl alanine levels during pregnancy can cause mental retardation in the child.
9. *Sex of the baby*: Male babies are heavier after 24 weeks of gestation under influence of testosterone.
10. *Exposure to irradiation in utero*: Accidental irradiation of the fetus in utero may cause severe brain damage. The defects (viz. mental subnormality, microcephaly and cataract) are more common in those exposed before 18 weeks of gestation. Exposure of males to irradiation may also cause fetal abnormalities.

Post Natal Factors

1. *Nutrition:* Balanced nutrition is required for adequate growth. Nutrition deficiency causes growth retardation and overnutrition causes obesity.
2. *Infections and infestations:* Persistent or recurrent acute respiratory infection, diarrhea or parasitic infestation causes growth retardation.
3. *Chemical agents:* Androgenic hormones increases growth but epiphyses of bones closes early and bone growth ceases early affecting the ultimate height.
4. *Trauma:* Fractures of bone ends may cause damage to the epiphysis and hamper skeletal growth.
5. *Social factors:* Children belonging to lower socio-economic background have inferior nutritional status and have growth retardation.
6. *Emotional factors:* viz. Broken homes, family problems, children in orphanage have a negative impact on the growth and development.
7. *Cultural factors:* viz. Child rearing practices and feeding habits have a great impact on the growth and development.
8. *Inappropriate stimulation during the sensitive period:* Sensitive period is a particular stage of development during which learning in response to appropriate stimuli is earlier than that at other times. For example if an infant is not given solid food which he can chew, usually at 6–7 months, it becomes increasingly difficult to get him to solids later on.

9. *Early learning:* During the first 5 years of life, children can learn early than at any other period of life. However, the child should not be stressed; rather child should be motivated to find pleasure in learning.

Assessment of Growth

Assessment of growth and development is an essential component of health surveillance in children and adolescence because any problem within the physiologic, interpersonal and social domains can adversely affect growth and development and thereby lower productivity in adult life.

Prerequisites for Assessment of Growth and Development

1. The child should be in good mood.
2. Child should not be hungry, sleepy or wet.
3. The mother should be present but should not help the child.
4. The developmental examination of young children should be always performed before the physical examination.

Methods of Assessment of Growth

1. Physical growth.
2. Skeletal growth.
3. Tissue growth.
4. Dental age.
5. Secondary sexual characters.

Assessment of Physical Growth

The assessment of physical growth is done by anthropometric measurements. The tools required for growth assessment are as follows:

1. Weighing scales viz. Electronic type, beam type and Salter spring balance for measuring weight. Electronic weighing scales should be preferred for their accuracy and convenience. Beam type weighing machines are preferred to spring balance because of their accuracy.
2. Infantometer, Wall scale or stadiometer for measurement of length/height.
3. Fibre glass measuring tape for measuring circumferences.
4. Herpenden's calipers for measuring skin-fold thickness.

The anthropometric measurements which are used in children may be age dependent or age independent. The age dependent anthropometric measurements include *weight for age, length/height for age, head circumference, and chest circumference.* The age independent criteria include *mid arm circumference, weight for height, quack sticks, Kanawati and Mclaren index, and Quetlet's index.* When the parents do not know the exact age of the child then the age independent anthropometric measurements are used.

The anthropometric measurements used for assessment of physical growth in adolescent children are *weight for age, height for age, weight for height, arm span, skin-fold thickness and body mass index.*

Technique of Measurement

Weight: Weight is a measure of total body mass and is sensitive to change in body fluid, fat, muscle mass, skeleton and body organs. Measurement of weight and rate of gain in weight are the best single parameters for assessment of physical growth. It cannot only detect malnutrition but can also detect the degree of malnutrition. The disadvantages of weight as a tool for assessment of nutrition are that it is an age dependent criteria and determination of the exact age is a prerequisite which is not always possible. It can measure only acute malnutrition and it is fallacious in presence of edema. Measurement of weight requires weighing machines which are difficult to carry in community surveys. It requires training of personnel.

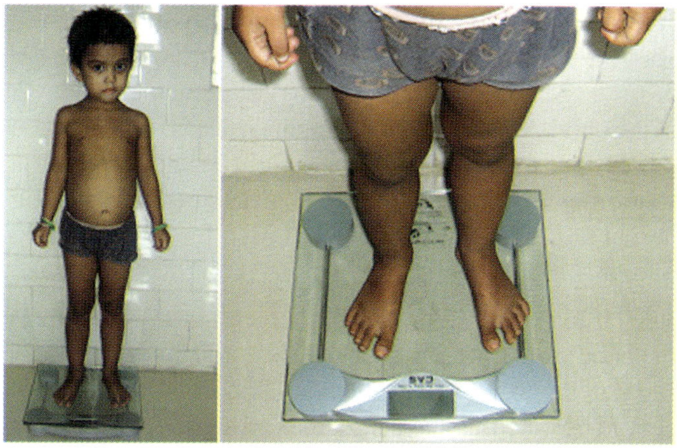

Fig. 5.3: Figure showing measurement of weight

A child should be nude or have bare minimum clothes (an under pant) and without shoes for weight measurement. The weight should be measured nearest to 25 grams accuracy. In a beam type or spring balance, the zero error in the machine should be corrected before use. In an electronic machine, one should wait till the '0' appears. The child is asked to stand straight on the machine, look forward and the weight is recorded.

Length: The measurement of length is the measurement of linear growth in children upto 2 years age. The child can stand properly only at 2 years of age. Moreover, upto 2 years age the child has a physiological lordosis which prevents accurate measurement of height. The length is taken on an infantometer.

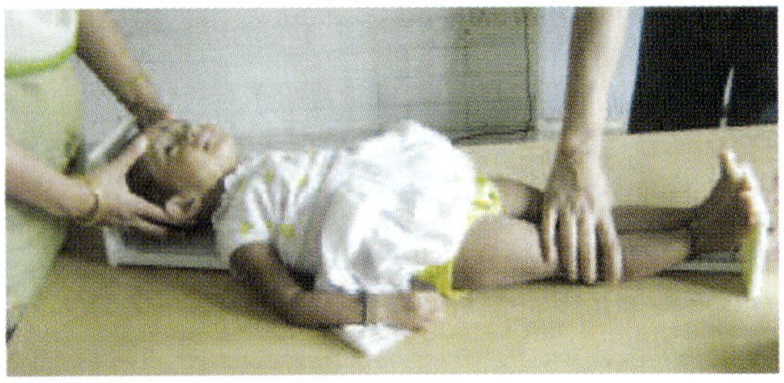

Fig. 5.4: Figure showing measurement of length

The child is placed supine on the infantometer and an assistant holds the head firmly with fixed head piece in such a way that the vertex looks upwards, the outer canthus of the eye is in the same vertical plane as the external auditory meatus and there is no gap between the head piece of the infantometer and the head. The knees of the child are pressed on the measuring board to keep the knee extended. Now the movable foot piece is glided along the measure board till it touches and flushes against the sole of the feet at right angle. The measurement is done nearest to 0.1 cm.

Height: Height is a measure of linear growth of children above 2 years age. Nutritional deprivation over a period of time (generally over 6 months) affects linear growth of the child. Measurement of height is helpful for detection of chronic malnutrition. The height is measured in a stadiometer. The sitting height is measured by the sitting height table. The sitting height is used for measurement of body proportion.

The child should stand with bare feet on the platform of the stadiometer with feet parallel and heels slightly separated. The heels, buttocks, shoulders and occiput should be touching the height measuring rod. The head is so positioned that the child looks directly forward with the Frankfurt plane (the line joining floor of the external auditory meatus to the lower margin of the orbit) and the biauricular plane being horizontal. The head piece is kept firmly over the vertex to compress the hair. The measurement of height is then recorded by exerting gentle traction on the mastoid process asking the child to be as straight as possible, take a deep breath, breathe out and relax.

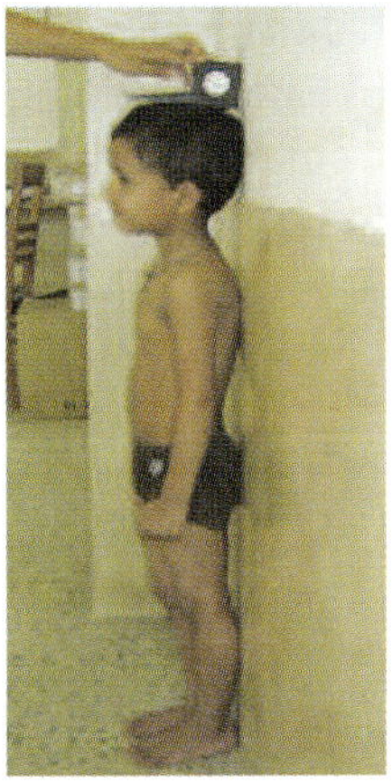

Fig. 5.5: Figure showing measurement of height

Head Circumference: The growth of head circumference gives an idea of the growth of brain. The head circumference at birth is an indicator of intrauterine brain growth. If the head growth exceeds 1 cm in 2 weeks during the first three months after birth, hydrocephalous should be suspected. Mental subnormality of early onset and late onset can be differentiated from the head circumference. The head is likely to be small if severe mental subnormality develops any time in the first year and remains normal when onset is after one year.

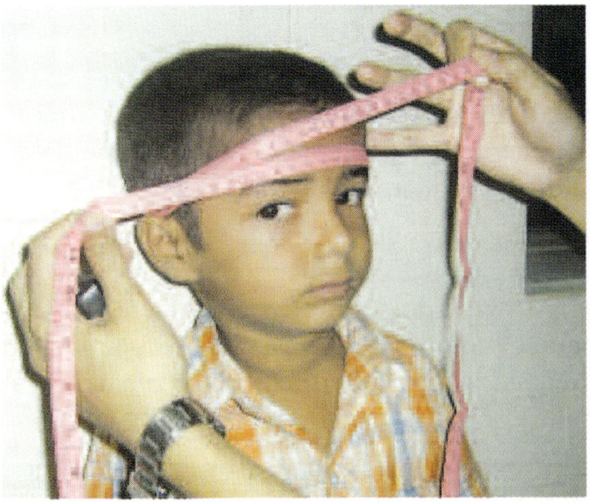

Fig. 5.6: The measurement of head circumference

A fibre glass tape is encircled over the most prominent part of the occiput and the supraorbital ridges in front and the reading is recorded. It is recorded nearest to 0.1 cm.

Head circumference measurement is important upto the age of 5 years.

Chest Circumference: At birth the head circumference is larger than chest circumference upto 3 cm. At birth the head circumference is larger by > 3 cm than chest circumference in preterm, small for dates and infants with hydrocephalous. At 6–9 months age, chest circumference may exceed head circumference in preterm babies. In malnourished babies, chest circumference may be significantly smaller than head circumference.

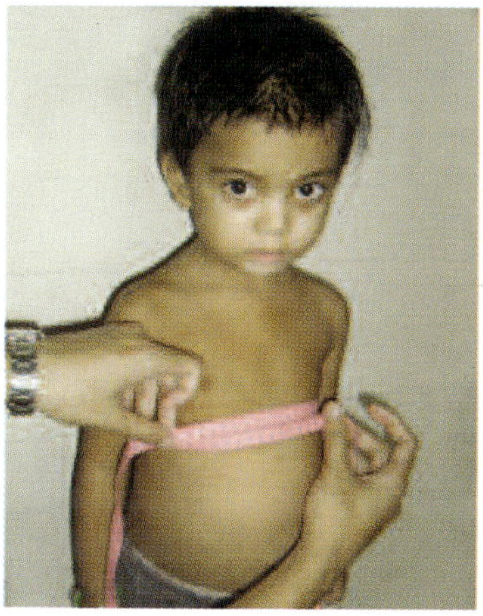

Fig. 5.7: Measurement of chest circumference

To measure the chest circumference, the fibre glass tape is passed through the xiphisternal junction to surround the chest in that plane. The measurement is recorded midway between inspiration and expiration nearest to 0.1 cm. The tape should not be passed through the nipple line as the position of the nipple may be variable.

Mid Upper Arm Circumference (MUAC): Mid arm circumference is an age independent anthropometric measurement. It is useful only in the age group of 1 year to 5 years. During this period the arm circumference remains reasonably static at 16.5 –17.5 cm among healthy children because the fat of early infancy is gradually replaced by muscles. It is a simple method and requires no sophisticated equipment for measurement. It requires minimal training and can be operated by workers at all levels: doctors to grass root workers. Measurement of MAC can assess malnutrition in presence of edema because in edematous protein energy malnutrition, the upper arm is spared. It cannot assess the degree of malnutrition.

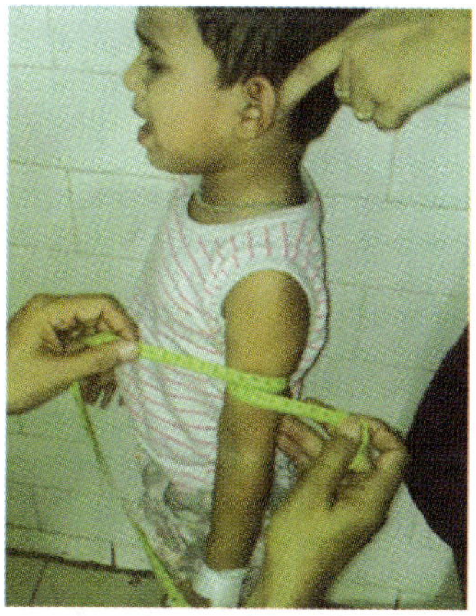

Fig. 5.8: Measurement of mid arm circumference

The mid upper arm circumference is measured at the mid point of left upper arm i.e. midway between the tip of acromion process of scapula and olecranon process of ulna. It is recorded nearest to 0.1 cm. The left arm is used as a universal standard. While measuring, the arm should be kept hanging by the side of the body to keep the muscles relaxed.

A MUAC < 12.5 cm indicates malnutrition. MUAC between 12.5 and 13.5 cm indicates impending malnutrition and MAC above 13.5 cm indicates normal nutrition.

Shakir Tape and Bangle Test: These are two methods based on the principle of MUAC. The Shakir tape is a fibre glass tape with three colour zones. The red zone indicates a MUAC < 12.5 cm, the yellow zone indicates MUAC between 12.5 cm and 13.5 cm and green zone indicates MUAC > 13.5 cm. The interpretation is same as in MUAC measurement.

The bangle test is used for quick assessment of arm circumference. A fibre glass bangle with internal diameter of 4 cm is slipped into the arm through the forearm. If the ring passes above the elbow, it indicates that the arm circumference is < 12.5 cm and the child is malnourished.

Quacstick: The quacstick is a meter rod where values of 80% MUAC for height are marked at corresponding height levels. If a child is found taller than his arm circumference on the stick he/she is considered to be malnourished.

Kanawati and Mclaren Index: It is the ratio of MUAC in cm and head circumference in cm. If the ratio is between 0.320–0.330 it is normal. A ratio between 0.280 – 0.320 indicates mild malnutrition, that between 0.250 – 0.279 indicates moderate malnutrition and that < 0.249 indicates severe malnutrition.

Quetlet's Index: It is a ratio between weight in kg by height in cm multiplied by 100. The normal value is 0.14–0.16.

Weight for Height: Weight for height below 5th percentile is the single best growth chart indicator of acute malnutrition.

Arm Span: It is the distance between the tips of the middle fingers of both arms outstretched at right angles to the body. The arm span is measured across the back of the child. In children less than 5 years age, the span is 1–2 cm less than the body length. In the 10–12 years age, the span is equal to height. An abnormally large span is seen in children with arachnodactyly, Klinefelter's syndrome, coarctation of aorta and eunuchoidism.

Body Mass Index (BMI): The body mass index can be calculated as weight/height^2 when weight is in kilograms and height is in metres. According to the CDC, a BMI over the 95th percentile indicates obesity, between 85th and 95th percentile is risk of overweight and below the 5th percentile is under weight.

Body Proportion: The upper segment lower segment ratio helps in diagnosis of the type of short stature, proportionate or disproportionate.

The upper segment is measured from the vertex to the upper edge of symphysis pubis and the lower segment from the upper edge of symphysis pubis to the heels. In the infants the upper segment can be measured with the help of an infantometer. The lower segment can be obtained by subtracting the upper segment from the length. The ratio of upper segment to lower segment (U/L) is approximately 1.7 at birth, 1.3 at 3 years and 1.0 after 7 years. Higher U/L ratios are characteristic of short limb short stature (e.g. achondroplasia) or bone disorders such rickets.

Assessment of Skeletal Growth

The skeletal growth is assessed by determination of bone age with the help of radiography. It is a useful tool for diagnostic evaluation of children with failure to thrive, short stature and disorders of sexual growth. The skeletal age should be estimated by the radiologist without considering the clinical profile of the case. Skeletal maturity is linked more closely to sexual maturity rating (SMR) than to chronological age. The bones to be evaluated at different age are as follows: (a) X-ray of foot and knee in the newborn, (b) X-ray of shoulder in the age group between 3 – 9 months, (c) X-ray wrist and hand in 10–13 years age group, and (d) X-ray elbow and hip at 14 years.

Assessment of Tissue Growth

Tissue growth can be assessed by radiography and measurement of skin-fold thickness.

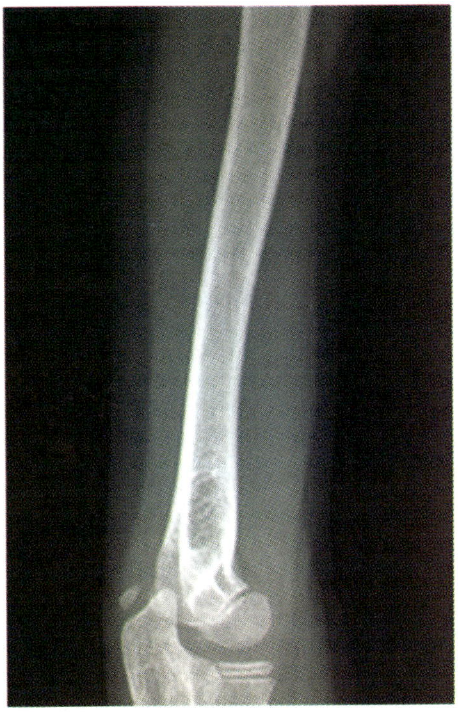

Fig. 5.9: AP view of arm showing bone, muscle and subcutaneous fat layers

An X-ray of the upper arm is taken and the different layers viz. the subcutaneous fat and the bone widths are measured. The muscle mass can be calculated as:

Muscle mass = total width of the arm – (bone width + subcutaneous fat).

Skin-Fold Thickness

The subcutaneous fat thickness can be measured at standard sites viz. biceps, triceps, intrascapular and supra-iliac regions. The subcutaneous fat thickness is 10 mm or more among healthy children between 1 and 6 years age. If it is less than 6 mm it indicates moderate to severe malnutrition. A skin-fold thickness > 85th percentile indicates obesity.

Measurement of skin-fold thickness (SFT) gives the estimate of body fat. Peripheral fat is measured by triceps and biceps SFT and central fat is measured by subscapular and suprailiac SFT. A Lange or Herpenden caliper is used for the purpose.

Method: The skin is picked up and the skin-fold held with one hand (*See* Fig. 5.10), while it is measured by the caliper held in the other hand. Three measurements should be taken at each site and the average noted.

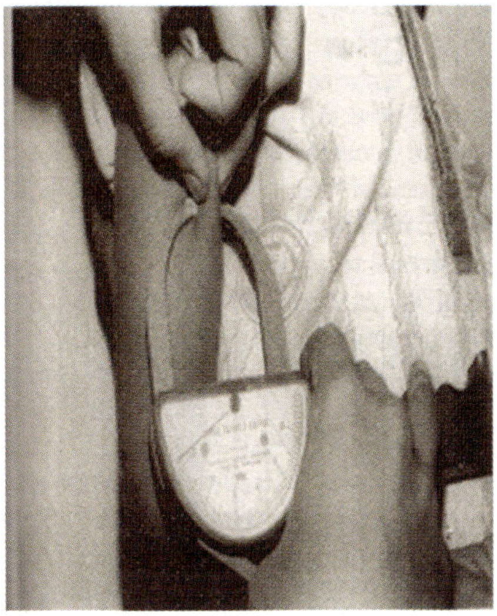

Fig. 5.10: Lange caliper for measurement of skin-fold thickness

Biceps SFT is measured at the mid point of the muscle belly, a point generally opposite the nipple. *Triceps SFT* is measured between the tip of the olecranon process of ulna and the acromian process of scapula. *Subscapular SFT* is measured below the inferior angle of scapula 45° to vertical. The skin-fold just under the shoulder is picked up following the natural fold of skin. The *suprailiac SFT* is measured above the iliac crest in the mid axillary line (approximately 2.5 cm above hip bone). Children having triceps and subscapular SFT > 85th percentile are considered obese, and < 5th percentile indicates thinness.

Assessment of Dental Development

It is done by counting the number of teeth erupted fully or partially. Delayed eruption is usual considered when there are no teeth by approximately 13–16 months.

Primary Teeth Eruption

The teeth in the upper jaw erupt earlier then those in the lower jaw, except for the lower central incisors. The primary teeth appear in the following order:

- Lower central incisors appear, usually, between the ages of 5 and 8 months.
- Upper central incisors appear 1 month later.
- Lateral incisors within next 3 months.
- The first molar usually appear around the age of 12–15 months.
- Canine between the ages of 18–21 months.
- Second molars at the age of 21–24 months.

Permanent Teeth Eruption

The permanent teeth appear in the following order:

- First molar: 6 years.
- Central and lateral incisors: 6–8 years.
- Canines and premolars: 9–12 years.
- Second molar 12 years.
- Third molar: 18 years or later.

Assessment of Secondary Sexual Characteristics

The stages of sexual maturation are assessed by the Sexual Maturity Rating (*See* Pages 91-92).

Assessment of Development

Developmental assessment of children is essential for detection of abnormal developmental delays. The infant's behavior should be studied and appraised in terms of the chronological age. In preterm infants, age correction should be done upto 2 years of age as follows: Correction of age = Chronological age–Number of weeks born prematurely.

Developmental assessment consist of (a) identification of developmental delay, (b) developmental diagnosis.

Identification of Developmental Delay can be done by (i) Assessment of milestones viz. gross motor, fine motor adaptive, social and language; (ii) By using developmental screening charts.

Developmental Diagnosis should be done when a child is identified to have a potential problem. It includes history, physical examination and laboratory investigations.

A thorough family history, antenatal, natal and post natal history is of particular importance. A *family history* may shed light on multigenerational diseases. A search for teratogenic exposures including drugs, radiation, addiction, infectious illness and trauma are important informations to be obtained in the *antenatal history*. The *natal history* should include birth weight, gestational age, Apgar score and any pregnancy induced complications. The *postnatal history* should include chronic respiratory or allergic diseases, otitis media, head trauma and sleep problems (signs of obstructive sleep apnea). *Physical examination* include (a) A complete evaluation of growth parameters, (b) Measurement of head circumference, (c) Examination for facial dysmorphism, signs of neurocutaneous disorders viz. café-au-lait spots, adenoma sebaceum, hypopigmented macules, (d) Test for vision and hearing.

Laboratory Examination should be picked up according to the clinical diagnosis for confirmation. The investigations may include:

1. Tests for inborn errors of metabolism viz. PKU, serum ammonia.
2. Tests for hypothyroidism viz. TSH, T3 and T4.
3. Tests for galactosemia e.g. presence of non-glucose reducing substances in urine and enzyme study.
4. Tests for iron deficiency and lead poisoning viz. serum lead levels, PBS etc.
5. Tests for mucopolysaccharidoses.
6. EEG and CT scan in cases with seizures or encephalopathy with microcephaly.
7. Chromosomal analysis.

Optimal Time for Developmental Assessment

For following up of large number of babies in the well baby clinic, it is ideal to assess them at 2, 4, 8 and 12 months of post natal life. However, contact points of primary immunization are also convenient and hence recommended. Development assessment is indicated:

1. As a part of follow-up of high risk neonates for early detection of cerebral palsy and mental retardation. The high risk neonates include ELBW, VLBW babies, and preterm babies, babies with neurological disorders like hypoxic ischemic encephalopathy, intraventricular hemorrhage, persistent seizure, hyperbilirubinemia, hypoglycemia, meningitis, infants with congenital malformations, congenital infection, babies with history of meconium aspiration syndrome and respiratory distress syndrome.
2. For complete evaluation of children with chromosomal disorders.
3. For complete evaluation of children with retardation in one field of development such as walking, speech or sphincter control.

Prerequisites for Developmental Assessment

1. It should be performed before physical examination or undertaking any painful procedures.
2. There should not be any distractions for the child.
3. The child should be in an amiable and cooperative mood.
4. Parents are allowed to be present at the time of examination, but they must not help the child.

Developmental Screening Tests

A number of sophisticated, contemporary developmental screening charts are available for use in children. The most commonly used ones are as follows:

1. Denver developmental screening tests (DDST): The original and DDST- II.
2. Bayley's scales of infant development.
3. Phatak's Baroda screening test.
4. Trivandrum development screening chart.
5. Amiel Tison method for neurological assessment.

Denver developmental screening test: This is the most widely used and researched test. It was first developed in 1967 and later revised in 1992 and presented as Denver II. It can be used in children from birth to 6 years. It contains 125 items and can assess in the 4 domains viz. gross motor, fine motor adaptive, social and language. The disadvantage of this chart is that it fails to identify children with subtle delay and its ability to predict cognitive delays at a later age (i.e. predictive validity) is modest.

Bayley's scales of infant development (BSID): It is an objective and sensitive scale, requires the services of a highly trained examiner and takes about 45 minutes to complete the test. There are 67 items in motor scale and 163 items in the mental scale.

Phatak's Baroda developmental screening test: It is a simplified version of Bayley's scales of infant development with 22 motor and 31 mental items.

Trivandrum developmental screening chart (TDSC): It is suitable for children below 2 years. It is a simple chart which can be operated even by paramedical health workers. It is a simplified version of Baroda developmental screening test. It is best suited to use in infants around 1 year of age because one year is an ideal age for formal developmental assessment in a community setting. Most of the items are concentrated around that age period. There are 17 test items in the chart. Another TDSC has been developed. There are 27 items in this chart and can be used in children 0 - 3 years (*see* appendix).

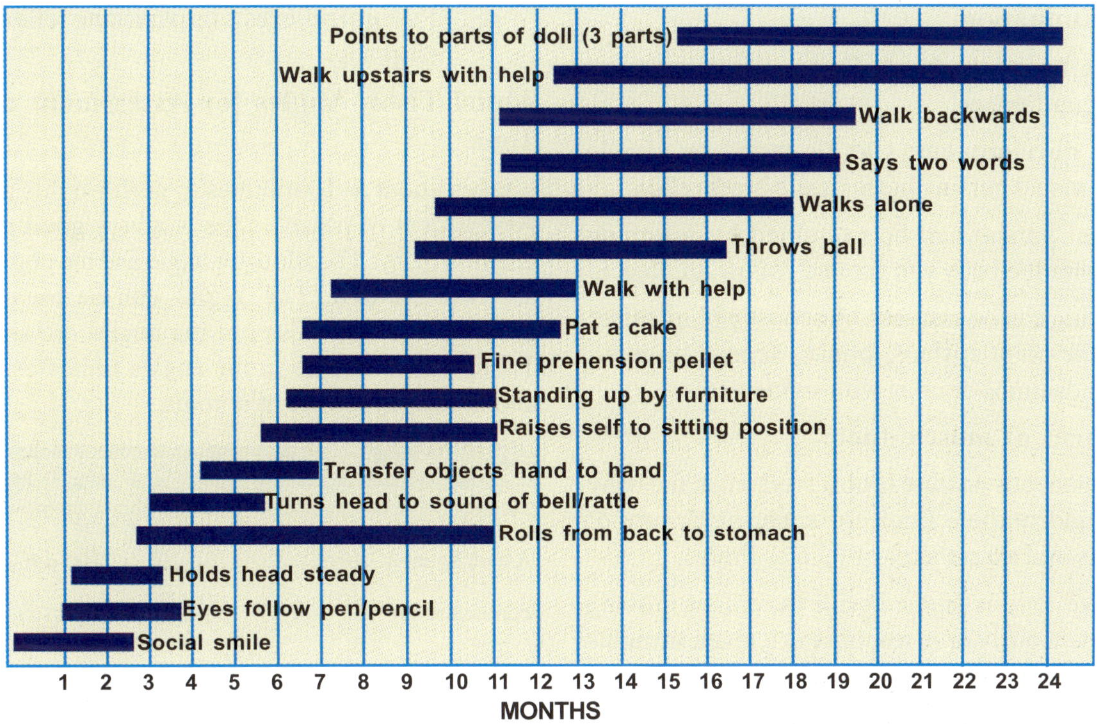

Fig. 5.11: Trivandrum development screening chart

The operation of the chart is easy. The milestones are represented by horizontal bars. The age is indicated by vertical lines. The left edge of each horizontal bar represents the age at which 3% of children passed the item and the right edge represents the age at which 97% of children passed the item. A pencil is kept vertically at the level of the chronological age of the child who is to be tested. If the child fails to pass any item that lies to the left of the age marker, the child is considered to have developmental delay. The test takes 5–7 minutes to perform.

It is a screening test. An infant who is suspected to have developmental delay by TDSC should be subjected to further neurodevelopmental assessment by standard developmental tests.

Amiel Tison Method of Neurological Assessment

This method of neurological assessment was described in France in the early part of this century. It was studied extensively by Claudine Amiel Tison and presented in a tabulated form. It is a simple test, easy to learn and does not need a kit. It is a strictly neurological test and does not take mental development into account and hence cannot replace standardized developmental tests. An infant, who is suspected to have abnormal tone by the assessment of Amiel Tison angles for assessment of passive tone, should be subjected to further neurological assessment.

This examination should be ideally done every month. For practical purpose, however, four testings at 3, 6, 9 and 12 months are enough. For preterm babies, corrected age or postconceptional age should be used rather than chronological age. Age correction should be done upto 2 years of age as follows:

Correction of age = Chronological age–Number of weeks born prematurely.

Method of Neurological Assessment by Amiel Tison Method

Evaluation of muscle tone is the fundamental part of Amiel Tison method of neurological assessment. Hence the evolution of muscle tone in the first year of life has to be clearly understood to interpret the results.

Evolution of Muscle Tone

From 28–40 weeks of gestation, acquisition of muscle tone and motor function spread from the lower extremities towards the head i.e. in a caudocephalic direction. After 40 weeks, the process is reversed, so that relaxation and motor control proceed downwards from head to the lower extremities in a cephalocaudal direction in the next 12–18 months.

Prerequisites for the Examination

The baby should be alert, wide awake, not crying and made to lie straight with the head in the mid line.

Steps of Examination

1. **Examination of the head:** Sutures, fontanelle and head circumference.
2. **Sensory development:** Can be tested by simple tests like visual pursuit and acoustic blink reflex.
   a. Visual pursuit can be examined by watching whether the baby can fix and follow an object.
   b. Hearing can be assessed by acoustic blink reflex i.e. the baby stiffens, blinks, screws up eyes, extends limbs or cries with sudden noise.
3. **Assessment of muscle tone:**
   a. Spontaneous posture is observed when the baby lies undisturbed. Look for constant closure of hands and asymmetry of face or limbs.
   b. Active tone is studied with the infant moving spontaneously or in response to a given stimulus e.g. pull to sit, pull to stand.
   c. Passive tone is studied by the maneuvers viz. adductor angle, heal to ear, popliteal angle, scarf sign and dorsiflexon at foot (Fig. 5.12).
   d. Primitive reflexes viz. stepping and placing reflexes, and tendon reflexes viz. knee jerk and ankle clonus are to be examined.
   e. Postural reflexes viz. parachute reflex and lateral dropping.

Amiel Tison Angles for Assessment of Passive Tone

It takes about 5–10 minutes to perform this assessment. Assessment of passive tone is a very good predictor of cerebral palsy. The adductor angle and the popliteal angles are best studied. The angles can be measured by a goniometer. The values of the angles are shown in the Table 5.2. Decrease in the angles indicates hypertonia and increase indicate hypotonia.

Table 5.2 : Value of the angles at different age

Months	*3 months*	*6 months*	*9 months*	*12 months*
Adductor angle	40–80°	70–110°	100–140°	130–150°
Popliteal angle	80–100°	90–120°	110–160°	150–170°

Method of Measurement of the Amiel Tison Angles

Adductor Angle: With the infant lying supine, the legs are extended and pulled apart as far as possible. The angle formed by the legs at this point is called the adductor angle. Any decrease or increase of the angle and asymmetry between the right and left legs is noted.

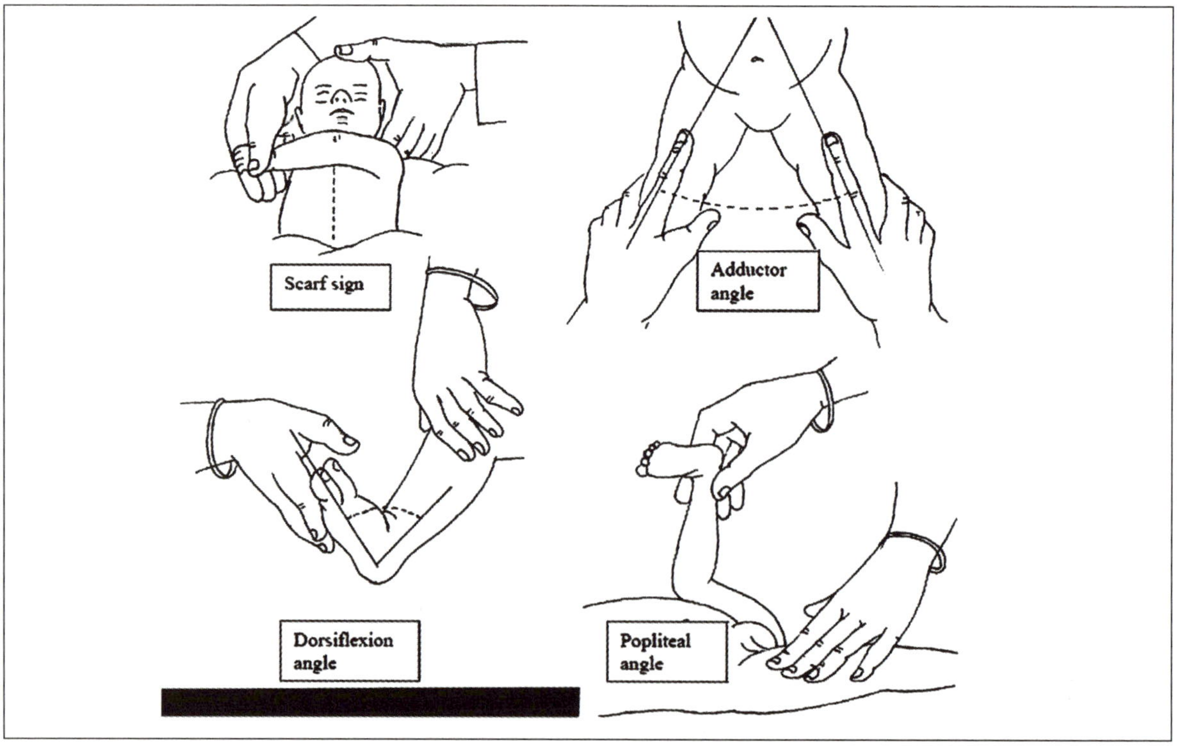

Fig. 5.12: Amiel Tison angles for assessment of passive tone

Popliteal Angle: The thighs are flexed laterally at the hip along both sides of the abdomen. While holding the infant in this position, the examiner presses the lower legs as far as possible towards the thigh. The popliteal angle is formed by the calf and the thigh. It is estimated in both the legs simultaneously.

Dorsiflexon of the Foot: The examiner holds the infant's legs straight and flexes the foot towards the leg. This is accomplished by applying pressure with the thumb to the sole of the foot. The dorsum of the foot and anterior aspect of the ankle form the angle.

Scarf Sign: The infant is held in a semi reclining position supported by the examiner's palm. The examiner takes the infant's hand and pulls the arm as far as possible across the chest towards the opposite shoulder. Four positions are possible in describing the position of the elbow in relation to the umbilicus. They are as follows:

a. The elbow does not reach the midline (normal).

b. The elbow crosses the midline.

c. The arm encircles the neck and the elbow reaches the axilla.

d. The arm encircles the neck like a scarf and the elbow is beyond the axilla.

The angles for assessment of passive tone can be taught to the mothers of infants at risk of cerebral palsy. They should be advised to report if there is a feeling of stiffness or looseness while performing the angles.

The passive angles can also be used for physiotherapy in the infants at risk of developing CP starting while in the NICU. Hence it will not only help in early detection of tone abnormalities in the infant but also provide early physiotherapy.

Assessment of Intelligence

Assessment of intelligence is done by intelligence tests. These tests attempt to measure a child's ability to learn. The results of these tests are expressed as mental age or intelligent quotient (IQ). Some commonly used tests are as follows:

1. Good enough draw a man test for children between 3 and 15 years age.
2. Bhatia's battery of performance tests of intelligence.
3. MISIC – Verbal (Malin's Intelligence Scale for Indian Children).
4. Stanford Binet test from 2 years to adult.
5. Wechsler test for children between 3 and 15 years age.

Good Enough Draw a Man Test

It is a simple test for assessment of IQ. It can be used for children aged 3–15 years of age. It is a paper and pencil test. The child is asked to draw a man. There is no time limit. The child receives 1 point for each of the item, which is present in the drawings. For each 4 points, one year is added to the basal age, which is 3 years. IQ can be calculated as mental age/chronological age × 100.

Assessment of Hearing Loss

An infant with hearing impairment from birth may develop developmental delay due to lack of orientation, mobility, and experiences. A child cannot talk unless he can hear. Hence if the problems of hearing are not detected early, it will cause problems with speech, language and cognitive development as well as impairment of receptive and expressive skills. It affects education, social, intellectual, cognitive and emotional development. Moreover, with late identification hearing is never at par with hearing peers.

Hearing develops from 24–25 weeks of gestation. Hence a hearing defect can be suspected in utero by USG examination. Normally on production of sound, there is startle with increase of heart rate. The earliest sign to suspect hearing defect after birth is absence of startle reflex (characterized by quieting or crying, blinking, momentary catch in respiration and change in heart rate after a sound) in the neonate. Absence of hearing can be suspected at 1 month age if the child does not turn head to sound.

The American Academy of Pediatrics endorses the goal of universal detection of hearing loss in infants before 3 months of age with appropriate intervention no later than 6 months of age. When universal screening is not possible, one can use the high risk criteria for assessment of hearing. The high risk factors include the following:

1. Admission to NICU 48 hours or more.
2. Family history of hereditary sensory neural hearing loss.
3. Intrauterine infection: TORCH.

4. Craniofacial anomalies.
5. Birth weight <1500 gms.
6. Hyperbilirubinemia requiring exchange.
7. Ototoxic medications (aminoglycoside for 7 days or more).
8. Bacterial meningitis.
9. Apgar score 0–4 at 1 min, 0–6 at 5 min.
10. Mechanical ventilation lasting 5 days or longer.

Screening Techniques

The recommended screening techniques for hearing are either auto acoustic emissions (OAE) testing or auditory brainstem evoked responses (ABER). The OAE tests are quick, easy to administer and inexpensive and provide a sensitive indication of the presence of hearing loss. The ABER test, an auditory evoked electrophysiological response correlates highly with hearing. It is useful for screening newborns as well as to identify the degree and type of hearing loss. Those children who fail OAEs should undergo ABER for more definitive evaluation.

Hearing Loss Beyond Neonatal Period

Many children become hearing impaired after the neonatal period and therefore are not identified by newborn screening programmes. Those who are congenitally deaf because of autosomal recessive inheritance or subclinical congenital infection are often not identified until 2–3 years of age. The following checklist may be helpful in early detection of hearing defect and aid early referral.

Hearing Checklist

A child with normal hearing should be able to achieve the following:

By 3 months: Startle or cry when there are loud noises, shows signs of waking up to loud sounds.

By 6 months: Stop playing when there is an interesting sound, enjoy toys that make noise.

By 9 months: Understands words like “no” and “bye”, show signs of responding to soft sounds, turn head to find source of interesting sounds.

By 12 months: Try to imitate the speech sounds you make, can point to familiar objects when asked.

By 15 months: Follow simple spoken instructions, speaks simple words.

Referral Criteria for Speech Delay

Children should be referred for audiological assessment if they fail to achieve the following:

By 12 months: No differentiated babbling or vocal imitation.

By 18 months: No use of single words.

By 24 months: Less than 10 single words.

By 30 months: Fewer than 100 words, no 2 word combinations and unintelligible speech.

By 36 months: Fewer than 200 words, no telegraphic sentences, clarity of speech less than 50%.

By 48 months: Fewer than 600 words, no use of simple sentences, and clarity of speech less than 80%.

Growth Monitoring

Growth monitoring means longitudinal follow-up of growth in a child. When the child’s weight is plotted on the growth chart against his /her age it gives the growth curve of the particular child over a period of time. This methodology is called growth charting or monitoring. Growth monitoring helps early detection of onset of growth failure.

Components of Growth Monitoring

The components of growth monitoring include the following:

a. Weighing the child.
b. Visualizing the weight by plotting on the growth chart.
c. Consultation with the mother.
d. Advice to the mother.

Tools for Growth Monitoring

The tools of growth monitoring are growth charts.

Who will Monitor?

At the hospital/clinics by doctors, at community level by Anganwadi workers, dais, mothers and school teachers.

When to Monitor and How Long to Monitor?

Monthly during the 1st year, every 2 months during the 2nd year and thereafter every 3 months upto 5 years.

Growth Charts

1. The WHO road to health chart.
2. Growth chart recommended by Government of India and used in ICDS projects.
3. Growth chart adopted by Indian Academy of Pediatrics.
4. WHO Growth charts (*See* appendix).

WHO Road to Health Chart

It can be used for both sexes. The upper curve represents the median (50th percentile) for boys and the lower curve represents the 3rd percentile for girls. The space between the two lines is the road to health. This will include the zone of normality for 95% children population upto 5 years.

It is helpful for detection of early growth faltering when a child is longitudinally followed up. There is also pictorial directives regarding starting of complementary food. The disadvantage of this growth chart is that it cannot grade protein energy malnutrition. This chart is kept with the mother and she should be instructed to bring the chart at every visit to the Anganwadi centre.

Interpretation

a. If the child is growing normally, its growth curve will be above 3rd percentile and will run parallel to the road to health curves. It is the direction of the growth that is more important than position of the dots in the line.

b. Faltering or falling of the child's weight curve signals growth failure which is the earliest sign of PEM and may precede clinical signs by weeks or even months. Such a child needs special care.

c. The objective of child care is to keep the child above the 3rd percentile.

ICDS Growth Chart

It contains three reference curves in addition to the standard (50th percentile representing 80%). They are 70%, 60% and 50%. It helps to determine the degree of malnutrition. This is kept in the Anganwadi centers.

Operation and Interpretation

The weight of the child should be plotted on the chart corresponding to the age and observed. The child is

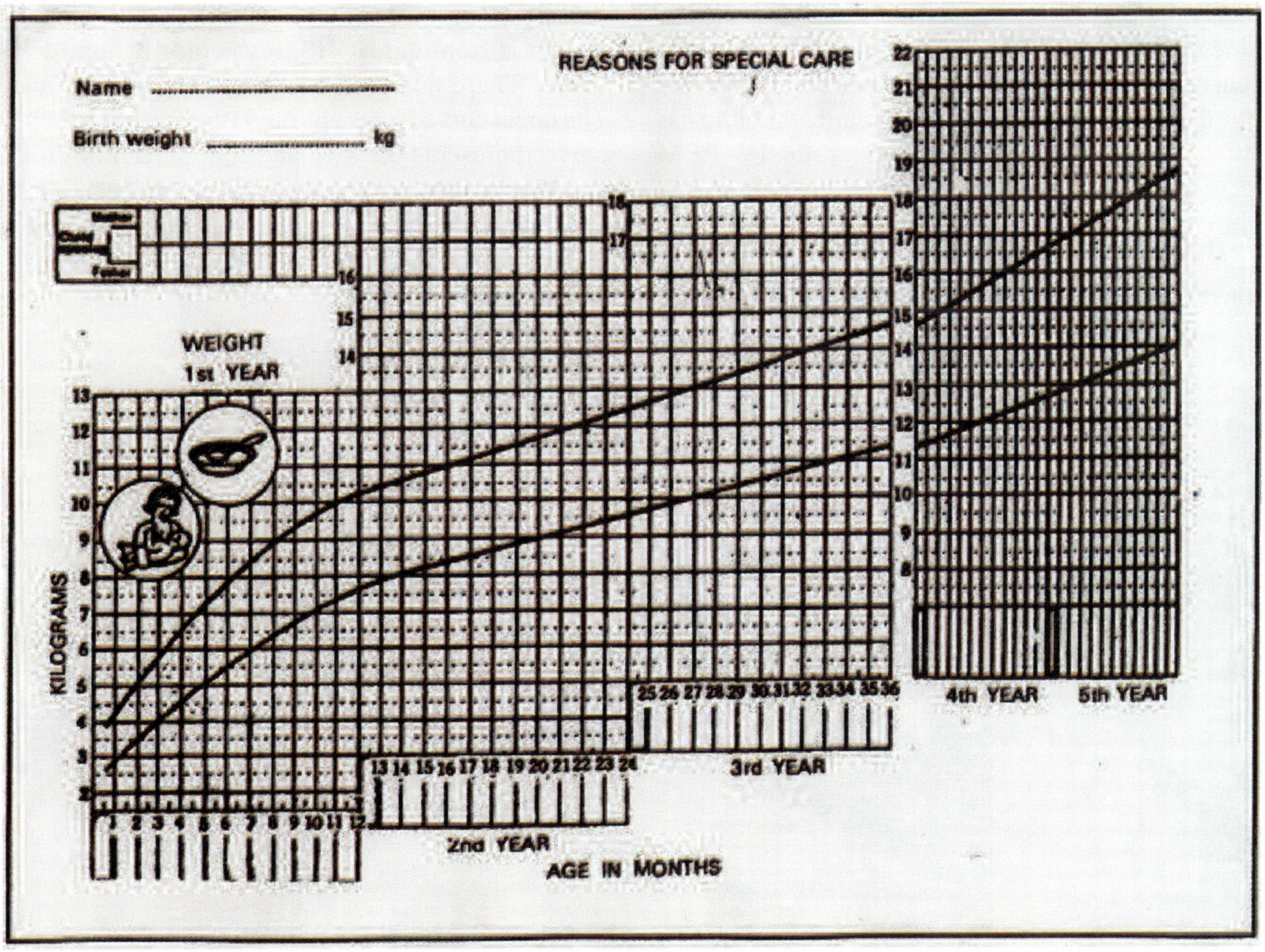

Fig. 5.13: The road to health chart (WHO)

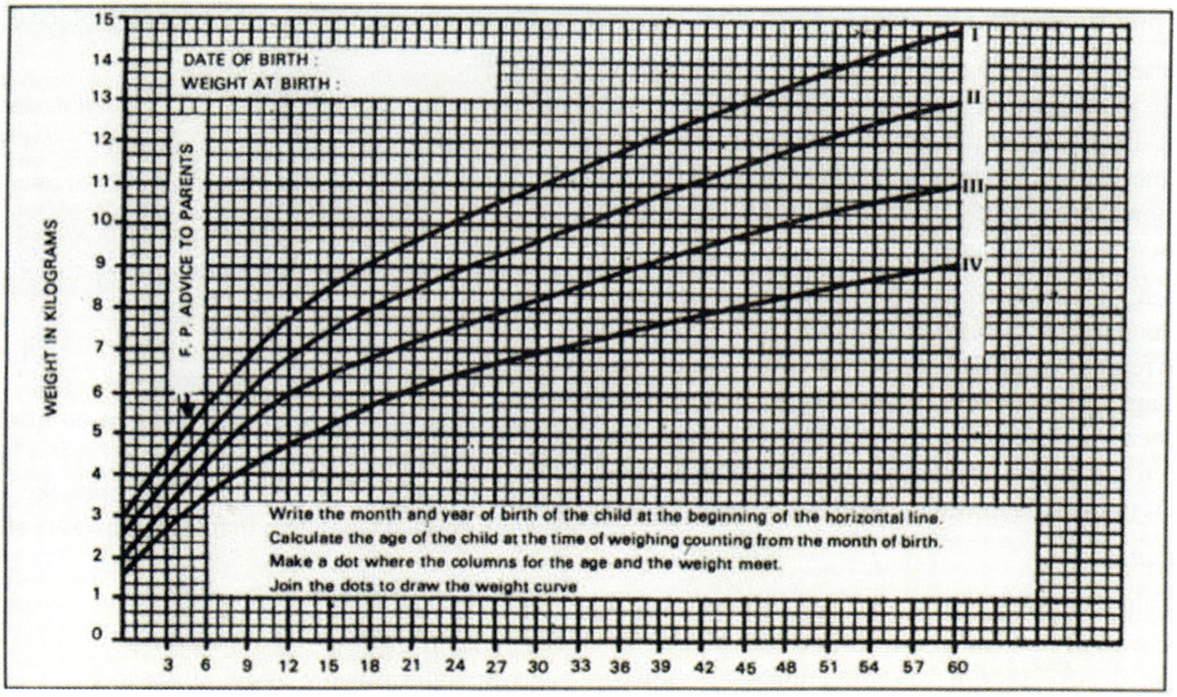

Fig. 5.14: ICDS growth chart

considered to be normal when the weight falls above the first curve. If it falls between the first and second, second and third, third and fourth and below fourth, the child has grade I, grade II, grade III and grade IV PEM respectively.

Growth Chart Adopted by IAP

It is on the lines of the WHO growth chart. The reference weight is from the NCHS. It can also be used for both sexes. There are 3 curves for assessment of weight. The upper curve represents the 95th percentile, the second curve represents the median (50th percentile) for boys and the lower curve represents the 5th percentile for girls. It also has two additional curves which gives idea of the longitudinal growth in head circumference and length.

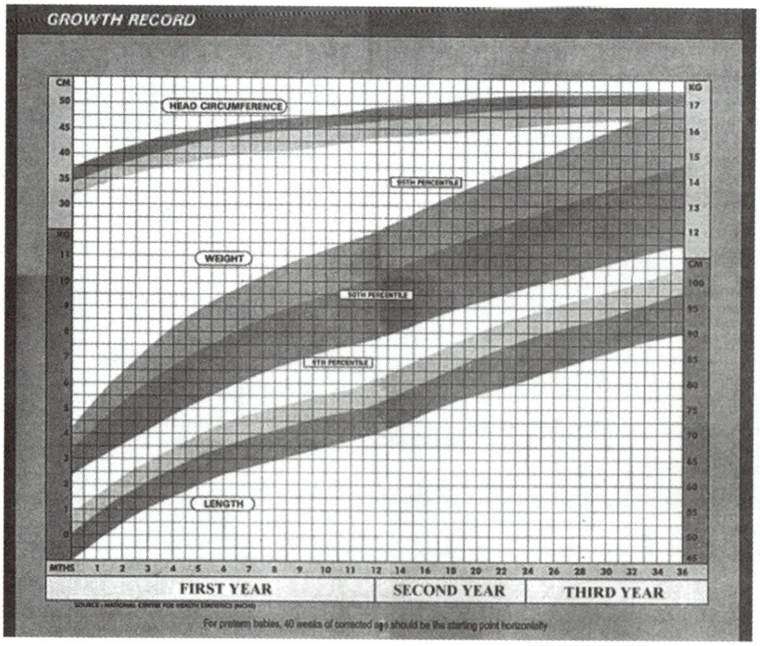

Fig. 5.15: The IAP growth chart

Operation and Interpretation

The child's weight is plotted on the chart corresponding to the age. The child is considered to be normal when his/her weight is between the 50th and 5th percentile curves. Again the direction of the curve is more important than the individual dots. Similarly, the values of the measurement of head circumference and length is plotted and interpreted. For preterm infants 40 weeks of corrected age should be the starting point.

WHO Growth Charts (*See* Appendix)

The World Health Organization (WHO) released a new international growth standard statistical distribution in 2006. It describes the growth of children between ages 0 to 59 months living in environments believed to support what WHO researchers view as optimal growth of children in six countries throughout the world, including the U.S. The distribution shows how infants and young children grow under these conditions, rather than how they grow in environments that may not support optimal growth. These standards were developed using data collected in the WHO Multicentre Growth Reference Study.

At present, IAP suggests using WHO growth charts where India was one of the participating countries in the generation of these charts. The IAP growth charts are available for use now.

Causes of Delayed Gross Motor Development

1. Familial.
2. Mental subnormality.
3. Abnormalities of muscle tone: Hypotonia and hypertonia.
4. Obesity.
5. Neuromuscular diseases.
6. Blindness.
7. Environmental factors viz. children not allowed to practice motor abilities.
8. Lack of confidence of child in motor activities.

Causes of Delay in Speech Development

1. Familial.
2. Presence of hearing defect.
3. Stammering.
4. Mental subnormality.
5. Cerebral palsy.
6. Environmental factors viz. overprotection, child abuse.
7. Defects in articulation.
8. Psychosis, autism, schizophrenia.

Growth and Development in Adolescent Child

The word adolescence comes from the Latin word 'Adolscere' which means "Grow to maturity". It is the period which extends from onset of puberty till the time sexual maturation is completed. The WHO defines adolescence as the period of life from 10–19 years. The adolescent period is divided into three stages:

(a) Early adolescence/Prepubescent stage which includes girls (10–12 years) and boys (12–14 years).
(b) Middle adolescence/Pubescent stage which includes girls (12–14 years) and boys (14–16 years), and
(c) Late adolescence/Post pubescent stage which includes girls (14–18 years) and boys (16–20 years).

Growth and development during adolescence comprises:

1. Physical growth which includes: (i) Adolescent growth spurt; (ii) Changes in body composition; and (iii) Pubertal changes.
2. Cognitive development.
3. Psychosocial development.

Adolescent Growth Spurt

The adolescent growth spurt occurs after around 10 years (8–13 years) age in girls and 12 years (10–15 years) in boys. There is growth of all parts of the skeleton, muscles and most of the internal organs.

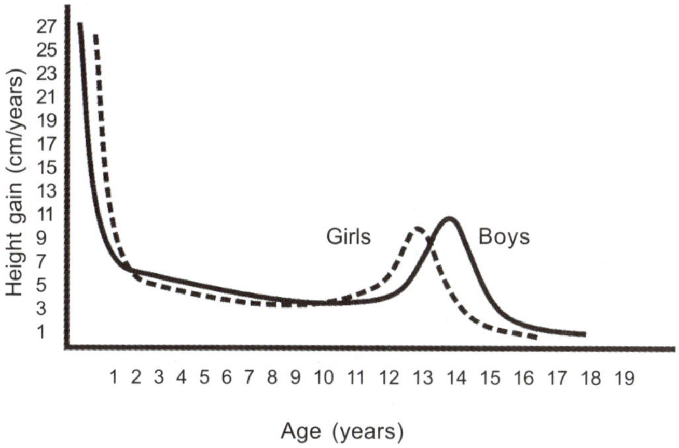

Fig. 5.16: The adolescent growth spurt velocity curve

The adolescent boys and girls gain around 25% of adult height and 50% of adult weight during puberty. However, the age of onset and rate of growth show wide variation. With the pubertal spurt, the boys tend to become more muscular and the girls show fat deposition in characteristic female distribution. The adolescent growth spurt occurs in three phases:

Phase 1: There is moderate increase in height velocity in the pre-pubescent phase.

Phase 2: Both height and weight increase rapidly in the pubescent phase.

Phase 3: In the post-pubescent phase, the velocity of growth decelerates. However, the weight gain continues even after cessation of increase of height due to epiphyseal fusion.

Velocity of Physical Growth

Weight:

10–12 years: 2 kg/year.

13–18 years: 5–6 kg/year.

Height:

10–18 years: 8 cm/year (girls), 10 cm/year (boys).

Arm span:

10–12 years: Height = span.

Above 12 years: Height < span by 2 cm.

Salient Features of Adolescent Growth Spurt

1. The onset of somatic growth is dependent on the degree of sexual maturity rather than the chronological age.
2. The average duration of growth spurt is 2.5–3 years.
3. The boys typically peak 2–3 years later than girls and continue their linear growth for approximately 2–3 years after the girls stop.
4. The boys have a higher peak height velocity of 10.5 cm/year compared to girls with 9 cm/year; hence have a greater ultimate linear growth.
5. The growth spurt is distal to proximal with prominent enlargement of hands and feet followed by arms and legs and lastly trunk and chest. However, most of the height spurt is due to increment in trunk length. The total gain in sitting height in boys and girls is 15.4 cm and 13.5 cm compared to that of leg length of 12.1 cm and 11.5 cm respectively.
6. The major weight gain in boys is due to dominant muscular development; in girls it is due to deposition of fat in the characteristic feminine distribution.

In girls, growth spurt occurs at around 9.5–14.5 years age, starts 2 years earlier than in boys. The peak height velocity occurs 6–12 months before menarche. The spurt lasts for 24–26 months ceasing by 16.5 years may continue maximum upto 19 years.

In boys, the growth spurt occurs later than in girls at around 13.4–15 years with the peak height velocity at around 14.4 years. The spurt coincides or closely follows testicular enlargement and growth of facial hair. Growth ceases by 18 years may continue to maximum 21 years.

Leg length reaches peak followed by trunk length, body breath and lastly shoulder width. The earliest dimensions to reach adult size are head, hands and feet. Growth of legs reaches maximum velocity before that of trunk. The early growth of feet may cause it to look disproportionately large.

Changes in Body Composition

Muscle mass increases with simultaneous loss of fat. Both boys and girls show increase growth of muscles with boys peaking at and girls shortly after the peak height velocity (PHV). As the PHV is reached earlier in girls than boys, initially girls have increase muscle bulk compared to boys of the same age. *Muscle strength* also increases approximately 14 months after PHV and 9 months after peak weight velocity (PWV). Strength per gram is however greater in boys than in girls due to biochemical differences in cells.

There is increase in the width of the dense bony cortex with decrease in the marrow cavity. The limb bone width reaches peak with PHV. The maxilla, mandible, brow, frontal sinuses, middle and posterior cranial fossa enlarge.

Fat distribution is different in boys and girls. There is loss of fat in limbs in boys. Boys have a central distribution whereas the girls have more fat in the lower body. In boys the gain in lean body mass is twice than in girls. Girls finally have 27% fat and boys 18%.

Heart and lung size increase. There is increase in the systolic blood pressure and decrease in heart rate.

The *hemoglobin and RBC mass* increases in boys due to the effect of testosterone. The girls lag behind.

There is little *brain growth* during adolescence as 95% of brain growth is completed by 10 years age. The *pituitary gland* enlarges; more so in girls. The weight of *thymus* reaches a maximum within 11–15 years of age and decreases thereafter. The *lymphatics* in the appendix and the spleen also decrease. There is rapid change in axial dimension of the eyes that may result in myopia.

Endocrinology of Puberty

Puberty is conceived by the onset of gonadal development (gonadarche) and the onset of adrenal dependent secondary sexual characters (adrenarche). Adrenarche precedes gonadarche by few years.

Between early childhood and approximately 8–9 years of age, the hypothalamic-pituitary-gonadal axis is dormant which is reflected by undetectable serum concentrations of luteinizing hormone (LH) and sex hormones (estradiol in girls and testosterone in boys).

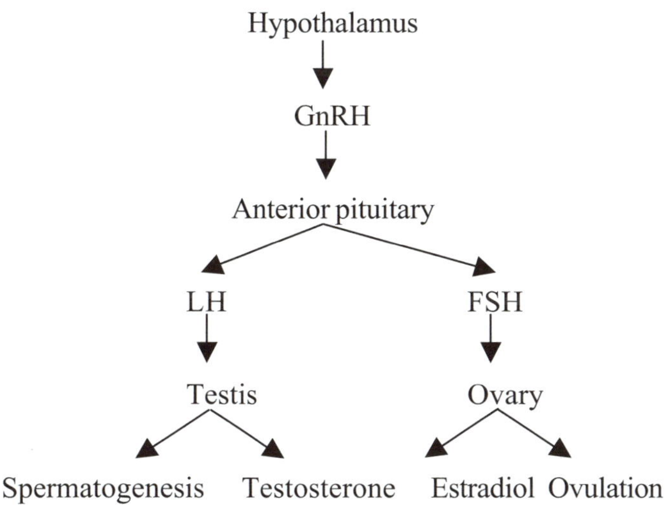

Fig. 5.17: Hypothalamic-pituitary-gonadal axis

The adrenal androgens viz. dehydroepiandrosterone (DHEA) and its sulphate i.e. DHEAS have a role in sexual maturation. The serum levels begin to increase at approximately 6–8 years of age.

One to three years before puberty, LH secretion occurs in pulsatile fashion due to endogenous episodic discharge of hypothalamic gonadotrophic releasing hormone. Nocturnal pulses of LH continue to increase as puberty approaches. This pulsatile secretion is responsible for enlargement and maturation of gonads and for secretion of sex hormones.

During mid or late adolescence, a positive feedback mechanism develops whereby increasing levels of estrogen in mid cycle cause a distinct increase of LH. This results in cyclicity and ovulation in girls.

Changes in the Reproductive System

The sequence of changes in the reproductive system is as follows:

Boys

In boys, the first sign of onset of puberty is an acceleration of the growth of the testes and scrotum. The testes grow from a size of 4 ml at the beginning of puberty to 12 ml, the minimum adult size. The size of the testes can be measured by the Prader orchidometer which consist of a series of wooden or plastic ovoids mounted on a string and numbered according to their volume in milliliter. The size of the testes is compared until one of the nearest size is found. The scrotal development starts with thinning, reddening and wrinkling of the skin. This is followed by the penile growth which starts after about one year, at around 12.5 years of age. The first ejaculation of seminal fluid occurs one year after the onset of accelerated penile growth. Axillary hairs appear around one year after pubic hair growth. The voice breaks late in adolescence. Pubertal gynaecomastia may occur in 40–65% of boys and in around 10% it may be sufficiently enlarged to cause social embarrassment.

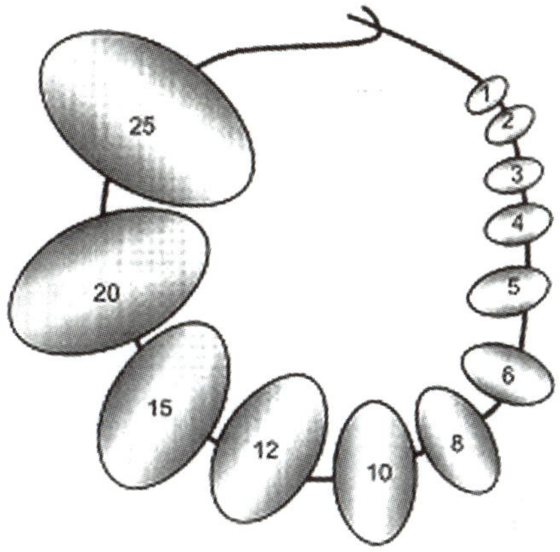

Fig. 5.18: Prader orchidometer

Girls

In girls, the first sign of puberty is an increase in height velocity followed shortly by the appearance of the breast bud. This is followed by gradual enlargement of the breast and areola. As the ovaries develop there is thickening of the vaginal mucosa, labia majora, clitoris and uterus. Menarche is a late event and occurs after the height spurt is passed.

Sexual Maturity

The sexual growth in adolescence has been classified into different stages in boys and girls. The stages of sexual maturation are assessed by the Sexual Maturity Rating (SMR) as follows:

Table 5.3: Sex maturity stages in girls

SMR stage	*Pubic hair*	*Breast*
1.	Preadolescent	Preadolescent
2.	Sparse, lightly pigmented, straight, medial border of labia	Breast and papilla elevated as small mound, areola diameter increased
3.	Darker, beginning to curl, increased amount	Breast and areola enlarged no contour separation
4.	Coarse, curly, abundant but amount less than in adult	Areola and papilla form secondary mound
5.	Adult feminine triangle, spread to medial surface of thighs	Mature, nipple projects, areola part of general breast contour

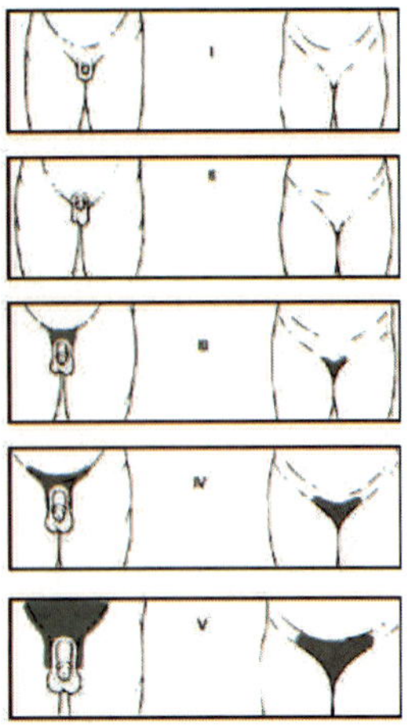

Fig. 5.19a: SMR of pubic hair changes and genitals in adolescent boys and girls

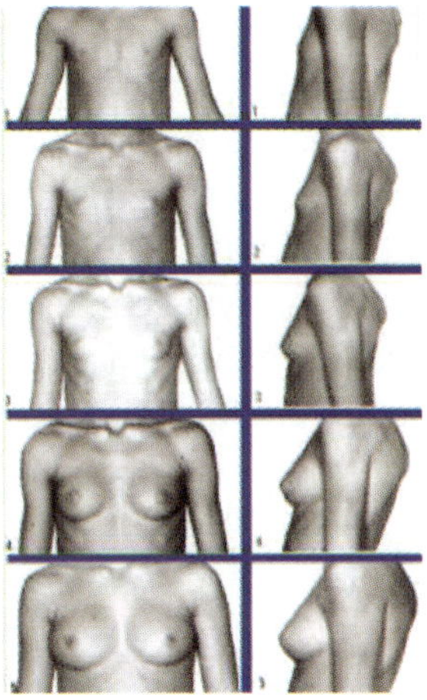

Fig. 5.19b: SMR of breast changes in adolescent girls

Table 5.4: Sex maturity stages in boys

SMR stage	*Pubic hair*	*Penis*	*Testes*
1.	None	Preadolescent	Preadolescent
2.	Scanty, long, slightly pigmented	Slight enlargement	Enlarged scrotum, pink, texture altered
3.	Darker, starts to curl	Longer	Larger
4.	Resembles adult type but less in quantity coarse and curly	Larger; glans and breadth increases in size	Larger, scrotum dark
5.	Adult distribution, spread to medial side of thigh	Adult size	Adult size

Source: Tanner JM: Growth at adolescence, 2nd edition. Oxford, England, Blackwell Scientific Publications, 1962.

Effects of the Physical Changes on the Adolescent

1. They frequently sleep longer. It has been suggested by research work that they require more sleep to allow their bodies to conduct the internal work required for rapid growth. They require on average 9½ hours night sleep.
2. They may be clumsier because of the growth spurts as all body parts do not grow at the same.
3. Teenage girls may become overly sensitive about their increasing body weight during puberty. Adolescent girls may become obsessed with their weight and develop severe eating disorders such as anorexia nervosa.
4. Sometimes teenagers may become concerned because they are not physically developing at the same rate as their peers because some may mature early and others late.

Cognitive and Psychosocial Development

The four main developmental tasks assigned to the adolescent are:

1. Changing from being nurtured and cared for to being able to nurture and care for others.
2. Learning to work and acquire skills to become materially self-supporting.
3. Accepting and becoming proficient in the adult sexual role and coping with heterosexual relationships.
4. Moving out of the family of origin to form a new family or procreation.

Cognitive Development

Early Adolescence

According to the piagetian theory, adolescence marks the transition from the concrete operational thinking characteristic of the school aged children to formal logical operations. This includes ability to manipulate algebraic expression, reasoning, and metacognition which allows individuals to think about how they feel and what they are thinking and develop mnemonic devices for improving learning. However, they may be able to apply formal operations to school work but not to personal dilemmas. Most children in early adolescence perceive right and wrong as absolute and unquestionable. They often question the received morality, embracing the behaviour standards of the peer group. Group membership during this period allows them to avoid guilt feeling for perceived moral refractions by shifting responsibility from themselves to the peer group.

Middle Adolescence

Mid adolescents question and analyze extensively and develop personal codes of ethics. Such codes often appear designed to justify their sexual appetite. In other cases the adolescent may embrace a more strict code than that of their parents. This is perhaps in response to the anxiety engendered by the weakening of the conventional limits.

Late Adolescence

Sexual experimentation decreases as they adopt more stable sexual identities. They seem to be less self-centered, philosophical, with increasing thoughts about concepts like justice, patriotism and history. They are often idealistic but also may be absolutist and intolerant to opposing views.

Effects of Such Changes on the Teenager

1. They demonstrate a heightened level of self consciousness. They tend to believe that every one

is as concerned with their thoughts and behaviour as they are. They believe that they have an imaginary audience of people who are always watching them.

2. They tend to believe that no one else has ever experienced similar feelings and emotions as they have. They become overly dramatic in describing things that are upsetting to them for example put statements like "you will not understand" or "my life is ruined".
3. They tend to exhibit the "it cannot happen to me" syndrome. This belief causes them to take unnecessary risks like drinking and driving (I wont crash the car) or smoking (I can't possibly get cancer).
4. They tend to become very cause oriented and exhibit a justice orientation. They are quick to point out inconsistencies between adults' words and actions. They see little room for error.

Parents should involve the teenagers to discuss their behavioural rules and consequences. They should take an active role in determining how they should behave. One should listen to their ideas. They should be given opportunities to participate in controlled risky behaviour e.g. involving them in supervised extreme sports like parachuting, rock climbing. Teenagers should be provided opportunities to get involved in community services e.g. volunteer at a homeless shelter or take meals to the elderly and then talk with them about the experiences.

Psychosocial Development

The five recognized psychosocial issues during adolescence include: (i) Establishing an identity (self-concept and body image), (ii) Establishing autonomy, (iii) Establishing intimacy, (iv) Becoming comfortable with one's sexuality, and (v) Achievement.

Self-Concept

Early Adolescence

Self-consciousness increases exponentially in response to somatic transformations of puberty. It is normal for early adolescents to scrutinize their appearance and to feel that everyone is staring at them. Girls in particular are at risk for viewing themselves as overweight and may suffer from anorexia nervosa and are at increased risk of depression.

Middle Adolescence

The mid adolescents often experiment with different personae, changing styles of dress, groups of friends and interests from month to month. Intense feelings of inner turmoil and misery are common with philosophical thinkings like "Who am I?" and "Why I am here?" This sometimes may be difficult to differentiate from psychiatric illness. Girls and boys characterize themselves and their peers according to interpersonal relationship e.g. "I am a girl with close friends" whereas a boy as a group may focus on abilities e.g. "I am good at sports".

Late Adolescence

As physical changes slow down during this period, a more stable body image emerges. Relationships increasingly involve love and commitment. An adolescent's self-concept becomes increasingly bound up in the emerging role in society as student, worker and parent. Hence career decisions become pressing.

Relationships With Family, Peers and Society

Early Adolescence

There is a trend towards separation from family with increasing involvement in peer activities. A symbolic expression of this shift is renunciation of family norms of dress and grooming in favour of peer group uniform. Such changes frequently results in conflicts with parents. However, all adolescents do not rebel and all parents do not reject such assertions. Separation from family often involves selecting adults outside of the family as role models. They develop close relationship with particular teachers or parents of other children.

Early adolescents often socialize with same sex peer groups. In one to one friendship, boys and girls may differ. Female friendship may center on sharing confidences, whereas male relationship may focus more on shared activities and competition.

Relationship to society centers on school. There is a shift from elementary to junior high school during this period. This shift entails giving up the protection of the home room in exchange for the additional stimulation and responsibility.

The societal preoccupation with youth and sexuality generates constant exposure to sexually suggestive and explicit images. In addition ready access to pornography on the internet may increase the risk of premature sexual activity or exploitation whereas reliable information about sexuality in general and contraception in particular remains sparse.

Middle Adolescence

Relationship between parents and the adolescents become strained. They become distant from parents redirecting emotional and sexual energies towards peer relationships. Gradually the need to belong to same sex groups declines. Physical attractiveness and popularity remain critical in both peer relationships and self-esteem.

Middle adolescents often begin thinking seriously about what they want to do as adults a question which was formerly hypothetical. The process involves self-assessment and assessment of the opportunities available. The presence or absence of realistic role models opposed to idealistic ones of the earlier period is crucial in this aspect.

Late Adolescence

During late adolescence, the rebellious attitude is replaced by gradual return to the family. They adopt more stable sexual identities. Hence sexual experimentation decreases. Cognition tends to be less self-centered, with increasing thoughts about the concepts like justice, patriotism and history. They are often idealistic but may be absolutist and intolerant of opposing views. Religious or political groups that promise answers to complex questions may hold a great appeal to them.

Effects of Such Changes

1. Teenagers begin to spend more time with their friends than their families. It needs mention that it is within friendship groups than they can develop and practice social skills. They however tend to conform to parental ideals when it comes to decisions about values, education and long-term plans.
2. They may have more questions about sexuality e.g. how one knew that it was time to have sex? Or why one waited to have sex?
3. When they are in their rooms they may lock their bedroom doors. Locking doors is a way to establish privacy. However, as long as they continue to interact with their family, locked doors are usually nothing to worry about.
4. They may become involved in multiple hobbies and clubs. This is an attempt to find out what they are good at by trying different activities.
5. They may become more argumentative and may question adults' values. For example when they don't get their way, they may say "You just don't understand".
6. They may not want to be seen with parents in public. They may want to interact with adults more as equals. They may view their parents as public and ask questions about how a parent was in their teens.

Assessment of Growth and Development in Adolescent Child

1. Physical growth is assessed by weight for age, height for age, BMI, and skin-fold thickness and arm span.
2. SMR, onset of menarche and assessment of size of testis with Prader orchidometer.
3. Skeletal maturation by study of appearance and fusion of epiphysis. An X-ray of left hand and wrist, AP view is adequate for assessment of bone age. Menarche appear to be associated with skeletal maturity (bone age 13–14 years). The *Tanner and Whitehouse* method is the most accurate and reliable method currently available and can differentiate bone age upto 1/10th year. In this method scores are assigned to each of the 20 hand bones including radius, ulna, carpals, metatarsals and phalanges depending on the stage of maturation.
4. Dental growth is assessed by counting the number of erupted teeth. A tooth which has atleast partly emerged through the gum is considered erupted. Boys and girls show similar maturity with respect to primary dentition, but girls are advanced than boys in permanent dentition.
5. Developmental assessment is carried by various tests. A battery of tests is available to assess the cognitive and psychosocial development. It is carried out by experts in the field. A child should be referred when indicated.

Growth Monitoring and Criteria for Referral

The recommended parameters for assessment are anthropometric measurements viz. height, weight, and BMI and SMR. The interval for assessment is once a year during adolescence.

The criteria for referral include the following:

1. Height below 3rd percentile or above 97th percentile on growth chart.
2. Crossing of two major centiles (upwards or downwards) e.g. going from 75th percentile to below 50th percentile on height or weight chart.
3. Below or above mid parental range of height.

4. BMI above 85th percentile at all ages.
5. Arrest at the same stage of puberty for more than 2 years.
6. Micropenis, bilateral or unilateral gynaecomastia in boys.
7. Hirsuitism and menstrual irregularities in girls.
8. Delayed puberty i.e. no breast budding in girls by 14 years or no menarche by 15 years. No signs of puberty by 16 years age in boys.

Problems in Adolescence

The adolescents have a lot of restructuring both physical and psychological and hence this group of population has health problems which are unique. They have both physical as well as psychosocial illness unique for the adolescent age group as well as increased incidence of common illness like acute upper respiratory infection, malnutrition, anemia, poisoning. With rapid growth and maturity, there may be scoliosis, slipped capital femoral epiphysis, goitre. Some diseases regarded as adult diseases may be present during adolescence. They are viz. hypertension, hypercholesterolemia and carcinoma in situ of the cervix.

COMMON HEALTH PROBLEMS

The common health problems include the following:

Gynecological problems: They include dysmenorrhoea, dysfunctional uterine bleeding, vulvovaginitis, pregnancy.

Breast problems: They include fibroadenomas in girls, gynaecomastia in boys, mastalgia.

Dietary problems: They include anorexia nervosa, snacking and obesity.

STDs include gonorrhoea, syphilis, chlamydia, venereal warts, genital herpes, chancroid.

Skin problems include acne.

Dysmenorrhoea

Dysmenorrhoea usually presents as lower abdominal pain or back pain during menstruation. It may be mild, moderate or severe. *Mild dysmenorrhoea* occurs only on the first day of menstrual bleeding and has few associated symptoms. *Moderate type* lasts from second to third day accompanied by malaise, nausea, diarrhoea and headache. *Severe type* is associated with severe crampy pain that lasts from second to seventh day and is associated with gastrointestinal complaints.

Dysmenorrhoea may be primary or secondary. Primary type is common in adolescents but secondary causes should be ruled out before making a diagnosis. It is associated with ovulatory menstrual cycles. There is increased synthesis of prostaglandin which causes excessive uterine contractions as a result of increase in tone of the myometrium and uterine ischemia.

Treatment depends on the degree of dysmenorrhoea and includes the following modalities: (i) Explanation of menstrual process and reassurance, nutritious diet, correction of constipation and physical exercise, (ii) Analgesics like paracetamol, diclophenec and antispasmodics, (iii) Prostaglandin synthetase inhibitors viz. ibuprofen, mefenemic acid, indomethacin, (iv) Contraceptive pills and danazol.

Majority of the cases will respond to non-pharmacological treatment. Some may need analgesics or prostaglandin inhibitors. Severe cases may require hormonal treatment.

Dysfunctional Uterine Bleeding

It is the term used when no demonstrable organic lesion is identified to account for abnormal uterine bleeding. In adolescents, it mostly results from anovulatory cycles. It occurs in the first year of menarche in the age group 9–13 years. The nature of bleeding is one of menorrhagia, polymenorrhoea, metrorrhagia, and continuous bleeding preceded by amenorrhea. A demonstrable organic lesion in the form of ectopic pregnancy, threaten abortion, endometritis and use of hormonal contraceptives may be found in around 9% cases in the 10–20 years age group.

Treatment depends on the severity of the disturbance. In mild cases (Hb level > 11 gm/dL), iron supplementation and maintenance of a menstrual calendar usually suffices. With moderate disturbance (Hb level 9–11 gm/dL), in addition to iron supplementation cycling with oral contraceptives should be considered. Cases with severe bleeding with Hb level <9 gm/dL, does not require hospitalization but can be treated with oral contraceptives. In patients with hemoglobin level <7gm/dL blood transfusion may be required in addition.

Vulvovaginitis

It is a superficial infection of the vaginal mucosa with or without involvement of the vulva, frequently presenting with vaginal discharge. Bacterial colonization without infection can also present with discharge. Sexual activity is also associated with increased frequency of vaginitis. Trichomoniasis, candidiasis and bacterial infection are the causes.

Treatment consists of broad spectrum antifungals or metronidazole.

Breast Cyst and Fibroadenoma

These are the common breast masses in adolescent girls. Carcinoma of the breast is rare in adolescence. The breast masses vary in size over the course of menstrual cycle. A persistent swelling or enlargement over a period of 3 menstrual cycles needs surgical consultation.

Gynaecomastia

Enlargement of the breast can occur in around 30% of males during early to mid puberty. It is a transient phenomenon. The only treatment is explanation of the transient nature and reassurance. However, nonpubertal gynaecomastia with hypogonadism is associated with Klinefelter syndrome.

Mastalgia

Physiologic swelling and tenderness of the breast can occur on a cyclical basis commonly during the premenstrual phase. It is secondary to hormonal stimulation resulting in proliferative changes.

Treatment includes firm breast support, analgesics, hormonal therapy.

Adolescent Pregnancy

Adolescent pregnancy should be prevented and the health practitioners have an important role in the matter. Teenage mothers are more likely to receive inadequate antenatal care, experience more pregnancy related complications as well as complications during labour, and give birth to LBW babies. Further more, early sexual activity can result in higher risks of STDs which can impair future fertility and general health.

Health professionals should discuss decision making with their adolescent patients from a young age regarding issues like sexuality, individual choice, peer pressure, safe sex and methods of contraception in a manner appropriate to the developmental stage. Adolescents of both sexes who are likely to engage in early sexual activity should be counseled in methods of contraception including emergency contraceptive pills.

Anorexia Nervosa

It is a condition mostly seen in adolescent girls who have a feeling that they are overweight and impose dietary restriction on themselves. They become obsessive with weight loss and dieting which results in cachexia and amenorrhea.

Management requires the joint effort of a pediatrician and a psychiatrist.

Snacking

It indicates intake of small meals inbetween regular meals. It is common in urban adolescents. Usually snacks consist of carbohydrates and fats, devoid of fruits and vegetables and hence do not provide a balanced nutrition. As such snacking is not a bad habit when the intake is of nutritious food.

Obesity

Adolescents are prone to obesity due to hormonal changes, growth spurt, erratic dietary habits and psychological conflicts. Obese children face friend's ridicule and parents and peers admonish them. This makes them lonely and outcast and more prone to obesity.

Treatment consists of motivation. Decreasing calorie intake and increasing energy expenditure is the basis of management.

Sexually Transmitted Diseases (STDs)

STDs are significant public health problems, and their significance is further increased by their contribution to HIV transmission. STDs are transmitted by unprotected sex. They include infections like gonorrhoea (caused by N. gonorrhoeae), syphilis (caused by T. pallidum) and chlamydia (caused by chlamydia trachomitis). Girls with gonorrhoea are at increased risk of infection with chlamydia and syphilis.

Gonorrhoea presents with dysuria or increased frequency of micturition, irritant vaginal discharge, rectal discomfort due to proctatitis and low grade fever. Gram stain and culture of secretion clinches the diagnosis. Serological tests for syphilis and rapid diagnostic test for chlamydia should also be done. Both the partners are to be treated simultaneously with any one of the single dose regimen viz. ceftriaxone, 250 mg IM, ciprofloxacin 500 mg PO, ofloxacin 400 mg PO or ampicillin 3 gm with probenecid 1 gm PO.

Syphilis presents with different manifestations according to the stage whether primary, secondary or tertiary. It is discussed in detail in the chapter of infectious diseases.

Chlamydia infection in most cases is non-specific and asymptomatic. It may present with dysuria, dyspareunia, post coital bleeding and intermenstrual bleeding.

Treatment is antibiotic therapy. The drug of choice is erythromycin 500 mg 6 hourly daily for 1–2 weeks. azithromycin 1 gm single dose can also be used.

Venereal Warts

These are small papillary lesions caused by herpes simplex

virus (HSV) seen in moist area of the penis or beneath the prepucial sac and sometimes within the proximal or distal urethra. Urethral lesions present with bloody discharge or hematuria.

Treatment includes local application of podophylline solution in tincture of benzoin. Urethral lesion require 5% solution of 5-HU. Non-responsive or large lesion requires excision and fulguration.

Genital Herpes

It is an infection caused by HSV 1 and HSV 2. It presents as edematous wheal on the penis followed by appearance of tiny vesicles. It produces severe itching.

Treatment includes oral acyclovir (800 mg 4 times a day × 5 days) and local application of cortisone cream several times a day.

Chancroid

A chancroid presents as an erythematous area over the penis which changes into a papule within 24 hours, pustule within 96 hours which finally ulcerates causing pain.

Treatment includes oral sulphonamides and tetracycline and local application of chloramphenicol ointment.

Acne

Development of acne in adolescents is encouraged by increased activity of the sebaceous glands in the skin resulting from rising levels of sex hormones. Acne affects almost all adolescents to some extent. Symptoms of acne are pimples with white heads and black heads. They are deep cystic lesions, painful and hot to touch and can cause scarring. Severe acne can cause emotional problems and lead adolescents to become increasingly shy with inferiority complex.

Treatment consists of cleansing with mild soap and water, proper hygiene and topical application of benzoyl peroxide lotions in mild cases. Severe cases require antibiotics.

COMMON PSYCHOSOCIAL PROBLEMS

The key developmental milestone of an adolescent is gaining autonomy from parents or caretaker. Risk taking behaviour is common among adolescents and is mostly a result of peer pressure to take risk. Experimentation with tobacco, alcohol, drugs and sex are typical. Several mental illnesses also occur in this period. They include major depression, bipolar disorders, panic disorder, and schizophrenia. There is evidence that early stabilization of these illnesses may improve long-term outcome. There is also an increased attempt for suicide. The potential risk factors for attempting suicide include chronic illness, poor self-image, diminished competence, self-identification as homosexual and loss of loved ones.

Social problems include school avoidance, school failure, which is common in lower socio-economic society, and juvenile delinquency. A juvenile delinquent is defined as a young person between10 and 17 years who has been prosecuted and found guilty of an offence that would be classified as 'crime' if committed by an adult. Adolescents are also prone to accidents and injuries because they are impulsive and usually do not conform to standard rules of discipline.

A pediatrician can support the adolescent in gaining autonomy by interviewing adolescents beginning at the time of puberty. The interview should be in absence of the parents so that a sense of privacy is afforded by the adolescent. It also enhances the chances of gaining insight into issues that would not be discussed in front of parents. Confidentiality on the part of the pediatricians is very important. Physical examination also should be carried out in absence of parents unless the adolescent patient requests otherwise.

Each adolescent visit requires a careful social history and an opportunity for discussion about how to make choices regarding tobacco use, alcohol use, drug use and sexual risk taking. A good psychiatric review of symptoms is necessary for cases in which mental illness is suspected.

The adolescent interview requires careful attention to detail. It should be done using a structured format for briefly assessing risk taking behaviour, social stressors, sexual identity and orientation and psychologic adjustment. More adolescent lives will be saved by a good interview and respectful counseling about behaviour.

Disorders of Growth

The disorders of growth include: (i) Tall stature, (ii) Short stature, (iii) Failure to thrive, and (iv) Malnutrition which includes Protein Energy Malnutrition and Obesity (see Chapter 6). Among these short stature, failure to thrive, PEM and obesity are common in children. Tall stature is an uncommon condition.

TALL STATURE AND SHORT STATURE

Normal stature is the result of a complex growth process. Pregnancy, genetic and ethnic influences, nutrition, endocrine function, general health as well as psychosocial well-being are involved in the normal process of growth. The result of this growth process is a height within the range of the 3rd and 97th percentile or a height just deviating from normal resulting in tall or short stature. Hence tall or short stature is primarily a normal variation of height.

Normal height data are required to define tall or short stature. Height data are specific for a certain population and widely vary, especially in ethnic background. They are collected within a defined population from cross-sectional, mixed cross-sectional and longitudinal height measurements or, rarely, from prospective longitudinal studies.

TALL STATURE

Tall stature is defined as a height above 97th percentile or above 2 standard deviation of the mean for the population. This means that 3% of the population has tall stature.

Causes

The most common cause of tall stature is constitutional or familial tall stature. These children and adolescents have parents with tall stature but below the 97th percentile. The mid parental height is at the higher centile for the population. Height measurements in these children should be considered in relation to parental heights; a height above the upper end of the target centile range (> 1.33 SD from the mid parental height) is likely to indicate tall stature for age.

The mid parental height is different for boys and girls. It is calculated as follows:

For boys:

$$\frac{\text{Mother's height} + \text{Father's height} + 13 + 2\ \text{SD}}{2}$$

For girls:

$$\frac{\text{Mother's height} + \text{Father's height} - 13 + 2\ \text{SD}}{2}$$

Table 5.5 : Some causes of tall stature

Tall stature with tall parents
1. Familial/Constitutional
2. Marfan syndrome
3. Homocystinuria
Tall stature with parents with normal stature
1. Sotos syndrome
2. Klinefelter syndrome
3. True precocious puberty
4. Simple virilizing adrenal hyperplasia
5. Pituitary tumors
6. Thyrotoxicosis
7. Nutritional obesity

The diagnosis of familial tall stature can be generally made from previous height measurements which demonstrate growth above but parallel to the 97th percentile and a normal physical examination.

The other causes of tall stature with tall parents are Marfan syndrome and homocystinuria. Both these conditions have tall stature with associated abnormal physical findings. *Marfan syndrome*, with autosomal dominant inheritance, is characterized by tall stature in one or both parents, long, thin extremities, arachnodactyly, scoliosis, pectus excavatum (or carinatum), upward dislocation of lens and myopia with aortic dilatation which may lead to sudden death due to aortic dissection at a later age. *Homocystinuria*, with an autosomal recessive inheritance, is associated with learning disabilities, downward dislocation of lens, cataract, and thromboembolic episodes.

The causes of tall stature with parents with normal stature includes Sotos syndrome, Klinefelter syndrome. *Sotos syndrome* is characterized by macrosomia at birth, dolicocephalic head, prominent forehead, hypertelorism, high arched palate and a pointed chin. *Klinefelter syndrome* is diagnosed by an eunachoid body proportion, behavioural abnormalities, gynaecomastia and appearance of immature genitalia and small testes. Rarely tall stature may be due to excess secretion of growth hormone caused by a pituitary adenoma or by an ectopic GNRH-producing tumour. Transient tall stature is also observed in patients with true precocious puberty. The other causes are thyrotoxicosis, simple virilizing congenital adrenal hyperplasia and nutritional obesity.

Evaluation

A thorough family history and longitudinal assessment of height centiles is the basis of evaluation. It is important to evaluate the pubertal state in all children referred for tall stature.

The investigations required depend on the suspected cause e.g. an echocardiogram when Marfan syndrome is suspected; radiological study of the epiphysis in adrenal hyperplasia, central precocious puberty, thyroid profile for possible thyrotoxicosis, karyotyping in children with suspected chromosomal abnormalities.

Treatment

There is no standardized treatment for progressive tall stature. Prediction of adult height plays an important role in the management of tall stature. Height limitation is considered whenever height gain continues beyond reasonable expectation. One method of treatment says that whenever height predictions exceed 3 SD above the population mean, treatment of tall stature may be considered. The aim of treatment is height limitation which can be achieved with administration of sex steroids, testosterone in boys and estrogen in girls. The sex steroid treatment may be initiated in mid or late puberty in high doses (250 mg testosterone IM, 2–4 weekly in boys and 200 micrograms of ethinyl estradiol orally daily in girls for 4–6 months). This method of treatment with high dose steroids is currently not favoured in view of serious side effects like increase incidence of breast cancer due to exposure to high doses of estrogen. An alternative method is induction of puberty at an age just prior to that of normal puberty with administration of low dose of sex steroids (testosterone 50–100 mg every 4 weeks in boys and 50–100 microgram orally daily in girls for 4–6 months).

SHORT STATURE

Definition

Short stature may be defined as (a) height below third percentile or below 2 standard deviations of mean of national standards, (b) height within normal population percentiles but is excessively short for mid parental or target height, (c) height within normal percentiles for national or parental standards at present, but growth velocity on successive height measurements has been demonstrated to be consistently below 25th percentile over 6–12 months of observation.

Causes

Majority of children with short stature do not have a pathological cause. Almost 50% have a physiological cause which includes familial short stature and constitutional delay in growth. The most common cause of short stature in India is protein energy malnutrition with or without infection. The pathological short stature may be classified on the basis of the body proportion into proportionate (ratio of upper to lower segment normal) and disproportionate (ratio of upper to lower segment is abnormal).

Table 5.6 : Causes of short stature

A. Physiological short stature
   1. Familial
   2. Constitutional delay of growth and puberty
B. Pathological
   1. Proportionate
      a. Intrauterine growth retardation
      b. Chromosomal anomalies e.g. Down's syndrome, Turner's syndrome
      c. Protein energy malnutrition
      d. Gastrointestinal disorders: Celiac disease, chronic diarrhoea
      e. Renal disorders: Chronic renal failure, renal tubular disorders
      f. Pulmonary disease: Asthma, Cystic fibrosis
      g. Cardiac disease: Congenital cyanotic heart disease, chronic congestive heart failure
      h. Endocrine disorders: Hypopituitarism, hypothyroidism, Cushing's syndrome, hypogonadism, Growth hormone deficiency, Diabetes mellitus
      i. Psychosocial
   2. Disproportionate
      a. Skeletal dysplasia: Achondroplasia
      b. Rickets
      c. Congenital hypothyroidism.

Familial Short Stature (FSS)

In this condition the child usually inherit stature equally from both parents. However, the growth pattern may sometimes follow that of the extended family members. It is therefore necessary to elicit the family history of height of the parents as well as the first degree relatives of the parents. In a very small subset of patients abnormalities of growth hormone receptors have been demonstrated.

The child is shorter than the 3rd percentile when evaluated against national standards, but within normal limits when evaluated against the parents' height. Growth velocity is normal and the growth curve follows a line parallel to the 3rd percentile. Body proportions and bone age are normal. The child achieves puberty at an appropriate age.

Adult stature is below normal.

No treatment is necessary.

Constitutional Delay of Growth and Puberty (CDGP)

This is a condition where the child has a delayed onset of puberty and the pubertal growth spurt, but ultimately achieves a normal adult height. The exact cause is not yet clear. Investigations have shown that the normal pubertal rise of growth hormone does not occur in this condition.

Children with CDGP are born with a normal birth weight and growth is normal in the first year of life. Then there is deceleration of growth during the second and third year so as to reach just below the 3rd percentile for height. Thereafter they grow parallel to 3rd percentile with a normal growth velocity throughout childhood. The onset of puberty and adolescent growth spurt occur at an age later than the outer limit of normal. Due to the late onset there is delayed closure of epiphysis and hence linear growth (height) continues beyond the normal time.

There may be a history of delayed puberty in either parent. These children may be slim or have a marginally lower weight for height. The body proportions may range from normal to eunuchoid. The bone age is atleast 2 years below the chronological age but equivalent to height age. No treatment is necessary for this condition.

Psychosocial Short Stature

This is a condition related to the psycho-social environment of the child. There are two types: Type 1 and Type 2. The type 1 occurs in children below the age of two years. It is associated with an unhappy home environment where the child is neglected. This type responds to improved care and nutrition. The type 2 is seen in older children. These children are totally rejected by parents and show abnormal behaviour like taking food from garbage cans or drinks water from toilet bowels or puddles. Biochemically, there is deficiency of growth hormone and ACTH. The hormones become normal when the child returns to a better environment. Growth hormone therapy or improved nutrition does not show any response.

Growth Hormone Deficiency

Growth hormone deficiency may be genetic or acquired. Genetic causes may be growth hormone gene abnormalities and mutations. The acquired causes include pituitary/ hypothalamic tumours, cranial irradiation. There may be growth hormone insensitivity as a result of abnormalities of the growth hormone receptors or by defects in growth factors like GH–IGF 1 axis distal to growth hormone receptors. The clinical phenotype resembles that of growth hormone deficiency.

The child usually presents with short stature, low growth velocity and retarded bone age. There may be facial dysmorphism with frontal and parietal bossing, depressed bridge of the nose, midfacial hypoplasia. Other features include high pitched voice, immature doll like face with prominent cheek fat and abdominal obesity.

Diagnosis: The use of growth factors like GH–IGF 1 and IGFBP–3 may be helpful but not confirmatory for the diagnosis of growth hormone deficiency. The diagnosis of growth hormone insensitivity includes low IGF–1 and IGFBP–3 in presence of normal or high growth hormone level.

Achondroplasia

It is the most common non-lethal chondrodysplasias. It is the result of mutation at the FGFR3 gene codon 380. Achondroplasia behaves as autosomal dominant trait. However, most cases arise from a new mutation. Couples with achondroplasia have a 50% risk of transmitting their condition, heterozygous achondroplasia to each offspring and a 25% risk for homozygous achondroplasia.

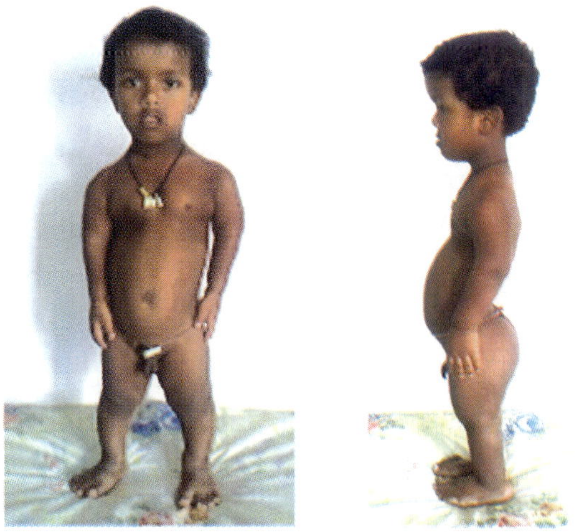

Fig. 5.20: A child with achondroplasia

It typically presents at birth with short limbs, a long, narrow trunk, and a large head with mid facial hypoplasia and a prominent forehead. The limb shortening is greatest in the proximal segments with fingers often displaying a trident configuration. Most joints are hyper extensible except the elbows where extension is restricted. There is a thoracolumbar gibbus. Usually the birth length is slightly less than normal but occasionally may be in the normal range.

As infants they usually exhibit delayed milestones, especially not walking alone until 18–24 months. As the child begins to walk there is an exaggeration of the lumber lordosis.

Infants and children with achondroplasia progressively fall below normal standards for length and height. Bowing of legs is common. Other common problems include dental crowding, articulation difficulties, obesity and hearing loss resulting from frequent episodes of otitis media. The child has a stenotic spinal canal. They may present with neurological complications. These include spinal cord compression at the level of foramen magnum and in the lumbar spine. Virtually all infants and children have a large head, but very few have hydrocephalous. The head circumference should be monitored.

There is no specific treatment. Surgical limb lengthening and human growth hormone treatment have been tried to increase height. Both are controversial. Bowing of legs may need surgical treatment.

Other causes are discussed in specific chapters.

Evaluation of a Child with Short Stature

As in any other condition, the first step in evaluation of a child with short stature is a thorough history and clinical examination including anthropometry followed by appropriate investigation for confirmation of the cause.

History and Clinical Examination

The history taking should target to exclude chronic systemic diseases like congenital heart disease, chronic renal failure, anemia, liver disease, chronic inflammatory bowel disease etc. In addition, antenatal and natal history including birth weight, developmental history, dietary history and psycho-social history are equally important. A family history should include enquiry about presence of consanguinity, height of the family members, and age at onset of menarche in mother.

Records of previous height and weight should be sought for. If charted on a growth chart, it can give an idea of the previous weight status and also the growth velocity.

A general and systemic examination should be carried out to search for signs of chronic diseases. Anthropometry will confirm short stature as well as detect type of short stature: proportionate or disproportionate. The anthropometric measurements required for this purpose are weight, height and body proportion in the child and the mid parental height. The pubertal development must be recorded as per Tanner's sexual maturity rating.

A child can be declared normal when the height corresponds to the national standards and mid parental height and the growth velocity in the preceding year/years is normal. In such cases, the parents should be reassured.

Investigations

In all cases of significant short stature with a low growth velocity or delayed bone age, the following screening tests should be advised:

a. Blood
   1. Hb%, CBC, ESR and peripheral blood smear.
   2. Serum creatinine, blood glucose.
   3. Serum calcium, phosphorous, alkaline phosphatase.
   4. Serum protein, SGPT, venous CO_2.
   5. Thyroid profile in suspected hypothyroidism.

b. Urine for routine, microscopic, pH.

c. Stool for ova and cysts.

d. X-ray wrist and skull in case of rickets and suspected craniopharyngioma respectively, X-ray of limbs for achondroplasia.

If these screening tests are found to be normal, the conditions to be suspected are Turner's syndrome in girls, growth hormone deficiency, malabsorption and renal tubular acidosis. These children should be subjected to specific tests for growth hormone deficiency, malabsorption, renal tubular acidosis and a karyotyping depending on the associated clinical features present.

	Associated clinical features	*Suspected condition*
1.	Failure to thrive, rickets, hypokalemia	Renal tubular acidosis
2.	Anemia, clubbing, vitamin deficiency signs, pain abdomen/loose stools	Malabsorption
3.	A relatively preserved weight for height	Growth hormone deficiency
4.	Female, webbed neck, increased carrying angle	Turner's syndrome

A child with border line short stature and an essentially normal history and clinical examination, normal growth velocity over 1 year observation, but with height below the mid parental height percentile and bone age below chronological age, needs the screening tests. If the screening tests are normal, CDGP should be suspected but growth hormone deficiency should be ruled out because it is sometimes very difficult to distinguish between the two.

Management

Management of short stature is essentially the treatment of the cause. Familial short stature requires counseling. The parents may be advised to highlight the positive points in the child's personality. All cases should be advised regular exercise and balanced diet. A child with CDGP should be reassured regarding attainment of normal height and puberty. In a psychologically disturbed child with CDGP a short course of low dose of testosterone (50 mg testosterone enanthate intramuscularly, every 3 weeks) or estrogen (2.5 microgram of ethinyl estradiol daily) may be given for 6 months only. This will help bring on minimal secondary sexual characteristics and will advance the pubertal growth spurt.

Indications of Growth Hormone Therapy

Trials over the last three or four decades has proved that growth hormone therapy for short stature is ineffective except for the following indications: growth hormone deficiency, in a proportion of cases of Turner's syndrome, and in end stage renal failure. For all other causes of short stature, growth hormone therapy remains experimental.

Limb Lengthening

Limb lengthening may be useful in conditions like achondroplasia. It can give a height increment of 7-14 cm.

FAILURE TO THRIVE (FTT)

Failure to thrive usually refers to growth below the 3rd or 5th percentile or a change in growth that has crossed two major growth percentiles (i.e. from above the 75th percentile to below 25th percentile) in a short time. It is most often observed in infants but also occurs in later childhood.

The causes of insufficient growth include failure of parents to offer adequate calories, and/or failure on the part of the child to take and/or retain sufficient calories. The common reasons why the parent/caregiver may not offer appropriate or sufficient food include lack of knowledge, unusual dietary beliefs and lack of food. Hence a detailed dietary history is particularly important in approach to diagnosis of FTT before looking for an organic cause.

Classification

FTT is classified into organic or non-organic types. Organic FTT is associated with an underlying medical cause which is responsible for the poor growth, while non-organic or psychosocial FTT occurs in a child who is younger than 5 years and has no known medical condition. It is often a result of poverty or poor parent-child relationship. It occasionally occurs with severe stress like child abuse. However, organic and inorganic etiologic factors can occur together.

Causes of Organic FTT

The causes of organic FTT are numerous and may arise from almost any system. Some important causes are enumerated below systemwise:

System	*Cause*
Gastrointestinal	Gastroesophageal reflux, cleft lip/ palate, Hirschsprung's disease, pyloric stenosis, lactose intolerance, milk protein intolerance, malabsorption, hepatitis, cirrhosis, inflammatory bowel disease.
Renal	Urinary tract infection, renal tubular acidosis, chronic renal failure, diabetes insipidus.
Cardiopulmonary	Congestive cardiac failure, asthma, anatomic abnormalities of upper airway, cystic fibrosis, bronchopulmonary dysplasia.
Endocrine	Hypothyroidism, diabetes mellitus, adrenal insufficiency or excess, human growth hormone deficiency, hypopituitarism.
Neurologic	Mental retardation, degenerative disorders.
Infection	Parasitic or bacterial infection of GIT, tuberculosis, HIV.
Metabolic	Inborn errors of metabolism.
Congenital	Chromosomal abnormalities, perinatal infections, fetal alcohol syndrome.
Miscellaneous	Lead poisoning, malignancy, collagen vascular disease, recurrent infection of tonsils and adenoids.

Reference: Nelson Textbook of Pediatrics, 17th edition, 2004.

Clinical Manifestations

The clinical presentation differs in developing and developed countries. In developing countries, the clinical manifestation may vary from failure to achieve standard norms of weight and height for expected age to features of severe protein energy malnutrition (marasmus and kwashiorkor) and recurrent infections. In developed countries, the most common presentation is poor growth in an ambulatory child.

The degree of FTT can be determined by anthropometric measurement viz. weight, height and weight for height ratio as follows:

Degree	*Weight*	*Height*	*Weight for height ratio*
Mild	75–90%	90–95%	81–90%
Moderate	60–74%	85–89%	70–80%
Severe	< 60%	< 85 %	< 70 %

Appropriate growth chart should be used as a reference. Serial measurements are more useful for early detection of FTT. In case of FTT, there is decrease of weight for age followed by decrease of height for age. For premature infants, correction must be made for the extent of prematurity. Corrected age rather than the chronological age should be used in calculations of their growth percentile until the age of 2 years of age.

Laboratory Investigations

A detailed history (including a thorough dietary history) and physical examination usually suggest a diagnosis. Investigations for organic FTT will depend upon the suspected organic cause.

A complete blood count, urinalysis and a bone age determination are useful screening tests. Bone age determination helps in differentiating familial short stature (bone age and chronological age are equal) from endocrine and nutritional abnormalities (bone age is less than chronological age).

Treatment

For organic FTT, the underlying organic medical condition should be treated. In addition, a proper diet has to be planned depending on the degree of FTT and the medical condition diagnosed.

For children with psychosocial FTT, the meal has to be planned with adequate calories for age and growth monitored. A weight gain in response to adequate calorie feedings usually establishes the diagnosis of psychosocial FTT.

The child with severe PEM needs hospitalization for treatment. The other indications for hospitalization include need for diagnostic tests for evaluation, lack of catch up growth. The goals of hospitalization are to obtain sustained catch up growth and educate parents about appropriate foods and feeding styles.

Some Important Disorders of Development

The common and important disorders of development include the following:

1. Autism.
2. Mental retardation.
3. Cerebral palsy.
4. ADHD.
5. Learning disabilities.

AUTISM

Autism is a pervasive developmental disorder characterized by a qualitative impairment in verbal and non-verbal communication, in imaginative activity, and in reciprocal social interactions.

Epidemiology

Western studies show a prevalence rate of 10–20 per 10,000 children. It develops before 36 months of age and is typically diagnosed at 18 months age. It is much more common in males; the male female ratio being 3–4:1.

Etiology

Etiology of autism is multifactorial. Genetic factors have shown to play a significant role. There is a concordance of 60–90% in monozygotic twins and less than 5% concordance in dizygotic twins. The chromosomal anomalies detected are deletions and duplications in chromosome 15. The other theories of causation include pre or perinatal brain injury.

Structural changes in the brain like deficits in reticular activating system, structural changes in cerebellum, forebrain hippocampal lesions, neuroradiologic abnormalities in the prefrontal and temporal lobes and idiopathic macrocephaly have been documented in children with autism. Another significant finding is the anatomical changes in the anterior cingulated gyrus, an area of the brain associated with decision making, and the ascription of feelings and thoughts.

Abnormal neurochemical findings like implication of levels or pathways of dopamine, catecholamine and serotonin have also been associated with autism.

Clinical Manifestations

The symptoms and signs include poor eye contact, little symbolic play, limited joint attention or orienting to one's name and reliance on non-verbal communication with delay in use of words.

The autistic child is often withdrawn and spends hours in solitary play. It is common to have marked need of sameness and a very narrow range of interests. Behaviour is ritualistic which reflects the child's need to maintain a consistent, predictable environment. Disruptions of routine may accompany tantrum like rages. There may be stereotype body movements. Eye contact is minimal or absent even in the older children. There is diminished response to pain and lack of response to sudden, loud noise. There may be echolalia, pronoun reversal, nonsense rhyming when speech is present.

Assessment of intelligence is difficult due to deficits in language and socialization. However, by conventional psychologic testing they fall in the functionally retarded range. Some children perform well in non-verbal tests and those with developed speech may demonstrate adequate intellectual capacity. Occasionally the autistic child may have an isolated remarkable talent.

Treatment

There have been considerable advances in the management of the autistic child. It is now evident that intensive behavioural therapy has been successful in improvement of language capacity and social functioning. Behavioural therapy should be started before the age of 3 years and targeted towards speech and language development. Parent education, training and support are very essential. Pharmacotherapy may be required for certain associated behaviour problems like hyperactivity, tantrums, physical aggression, self injurious behaviour and obsessive compulsive behaviour.

The autistic child requires alternate educational approaches in special schools even when language capacity is near normal. Educational programming should begin by the age of 2–4 years.

Behaviour modification is the major part of the overall treatment in older children. Older children and adolescents, with relatively higher intelligence but poor social skills and psychiatric symptoms viz. depression, anxiety, obsessive compulsive symptoms require psychotherapy, behavioural or cognitive therapy and pharmacotherapy.

Prognosis

Prognosis is better in the group of children with higher intelligence, functional speech, and less bizarre symptoms and behaviour. They may grow upto live self-sufficient, employed but isolated in the community. Others remain dependent on parents for life or they may have to be placed in institutions. Delayed diagnosis is a factor for poor outcome.

MENTAL RETARDATION

Mental retardation implies impairment in intelligence from early in life and inadequate mental development throughout the growth period. It is one of the five most disabling conditions of childhood; the other conditions being cancer, mental illness, heart disease and arthritis.

Definition

A complete and satisfactory definition of mental retardation is still not available. The diagnostic criteria formulated by the American Psychiatric Association are most widely accepted. The criteria are as follows:

1. Significantly subaverage intellectual functioning i.e. an IQ of 70 or below on an individually administered IQ test (in infants only clinical judgement because the available intelligence tests do not yield numerical IQ values).
2. Concurrent deficits or impairments in adaptive functioning (i.e. the person's effectiveness in meeting the standards expected for his/her age by his/ her cultural group) in atleast two of the following areas such as communication, self care, home living, social/ interpersonal skills, use of community resources, self direction, functional academic skills, work, leisure, health and safety.
3. The onset is before the age of 18 years. When impairment occurs after the age of 18 years, it is classified in DSM III as dementia.

Classification

A classification of mental retardation on the basis of the IQ is helpful to evaluate the degree of defect. However, for academic and administrative purposes it is inadequate and not infrequently misleading.

Using suitable tests to assess the intellectual functioning, an IQ is obtained. By assessment of adaptive behaviour, the level of adaptive functioning is determined. Both IQ and adaptive functioning are considered together to make a diagnosis of mental retardation. A child whose IQ is less than 70 and at the same time has a significant deficit or impairment in adaptive functioning is labeled as mentally retarded. If there is impairment in only one area i.e. only IQ or only adaptive functioning, the child is not labeled as mentally retarded.

The result of intelligence testing is expressed as intelligence quotient (IQ). It is calculated as mental age/ chronological age × 100. In infants and young children less than 3 years it is difficult to obtain mental age due to lack of standard tests. Therefore in this age group, assessment of mental maturity is based on developmental tests and the developmental quotient (DQ) is obtained in place of IQ. It is calculated as developmental age/ chronological age × 100.

It should be noted that the IQ of any child may change as much as 20 points, but for most children, the measured intelligence remain relatively stable after 5 years age. Despite limitations, intelligence tests remain the only way of confirming mental retardation.

The severity of mental retardation on the basis of IQ can be done by using the Wechsler's classification as follows:

Mild mental retardation	: IQ 55–69 (Educable)
Moderate mental retardation	: IQ 40–54 (Trainable)
Severe mental retardation	: IQ 25–39 (Dependent)
Profound mental retardation	: IQ less than 25 (life support)

Mild Mental Retardation

This group comprises 85–90% of the total. They are usually capable of reaching the 4th or 5th grade level in a conventional school system. They can make a moderately satisfactory social adjustment. In general they are self-supporting in times of high employment, particularly in jobs not requiring abstract thought. The majority of this group is recognized in the early years of school through their poor academic achievement. As adults, they are able to live an independent life.

Moderate Mental Retardation

This group comprises 5–10% of the total. They are considered trainable and can be capable of their own physical care. They can also make an adequate social adjustment in the home and neighbourhood. Some will achieve some degree of economic usefulness at home or in sheltered type of occupation. They are usually identified during preschool years because of significantly delayed developmental milestones, and may have physical defects. As adults they need to work and live in sheltered environment.

Severe and Profound Mental Retardation

They constitute approximately 5% of the total retarded group. They have minimal response to environment, are generally considered to be nontrainable. The majority is identified during infancy.

The severely retarded are usually dependent on others for most of their care. They are often, but not always physically handicapped.

Profound retardation needs constant care and supervision for survival as they have gross impairment in physical coordination and sensory development. They have multiple disabilities requiring medical diagnosis and special care.

Mental Retardation Severity Unspecified

This is a group where there is a strong presumption of mental retardation but the person's intelligence is untestable by standard tests.

Etiology

Normal mental development depends on genetic endowment, structural and functional integrity of the brain and external stimuli. Abnormalities in any one or more of these areas can be associated with mental retardation. However, in 65–75% cases no cause is identified.

Majority of these cases are thought to result from socio-cultural and environmental deprivation. These children are usually from the lower socio-economic group, generally poorly nourished and subjected to frequent acute and chronic illness. They have lesser opportunity for education and lacks environmental stimulation. They survive but do not thrive. When they reach school they lack the skill, experience and motivation and therefore perform poorly. This leads to negative feeling about learning and finally there is failure.

The proportion of cases due to organic causes is small. Severe malnutrition is usually linked with biologic causes.

Table 5.7 : Etiology of mental retardation

A. Genetic disorders
  a. Chromosomal abnormalities like Down syndrome
  b. Non-chromosomal abnormalities like tuberous sclerosis
B. Prenatal, perinatal and post natal brain insult
  a. Antenatal infections, hypertension, medication, pregnancy

Contd.

Contd.

associated complications like APH, prolonged labour, obstructed labour, aided delivery

- b. Birth trauma and asphyxia, prematurity, LBW, neonatal seizures, neonatal sepsis, hyperbilirubinemia
- c. Postnatal head trauma, encephalitis, meningitis, cerebral vascular disease

C. Organic/systemic diseases
- a. Congenital malformations of CNS like hydrocephalous, microcephaly and porencephaly
- b. Degenerative brain disease
- c. Neuroectodermosis

D. Metabolic disorders
- a. Inborn errors of metabolism like galactosemia, phenyl ketonuria, homocystinuria, mucopolysaccharidoses
- b. Endocrine disorders like hypothyroidism
- c. Lead toxicity

E. Non-pathologic (No well-defined cause or disease entity)
- a. Psychosocial
- b. Idiopathic

Clinical Manifestations

The children who are mentally retarded from or before birth is backward in all fields of development except occasionally in gross motor and rarely sphincter control. They are relatively retarded in speech and show lack of interest in surrounding, lack of concentration, alertness and promptness of response.

If mental retardation starts late, the child initially develops normally and thereafter shows regression of development or development is slowed. Some children are brought to the physician for some other disease and mental retardation is suspected by the doctor. Presence of chromosomal disorder, seizures and hepatosplenomegaly are common findings in these cases.

Mental retardation can be diagnosed early even soon after birth. The features for early diagnosis are as follows:

1. Excessive sleep. Is not active and does not cry much.
2. Feeding difficulties like difficulty in sucking, easy regurgitation and failure to demand feeds.
3. Delayed motor, language and social development.
4. Late in following with the eyes. Blindness may be suspected in such situation.
5. Lateness in responding to sound which may lead to mistaken diagnosis of deafness.
6. Lateness in learning to chew.
7. Persistence of reciprocal kick even after the child starts walking.
8. Persistence of hand regard beyond 24 weeks.
9. Persistence of mouthing beyond 12 months age.
10. Persistence of casting (deliberate throwing of objects on the floor) beyond 15 – 16 months.
11. Tooth grinding when awake almost always indicate mental retardation.
12. Increased latent period between stimulus and cry. Repeated stimulus needed to elicit cry. Voice quality may be different.
13. Lack of interest and concentration. This is the most important point. Fleeting interest in toys, may not do anything with toy if one is offered. If the child drops the toy; does not make any attempt to pick it up.
14. Lack of alert expression and is easily distracted and slower at responding to test situation.
15. Presence of aimless activity as they grow older.

The **physical findings** may include the following:

- a. Presence of major congenital abnormalities.
- b. Signs of cerebral palsy.
- c. Abnormal size/shape of the head.
- d. Facial dysmorphism.

Presence of any significant congenital anomaly carries an increased risk of anomalies in other systems including the nervous system and therefore mental retardation.

Psychometric Evaluation

All cases of suspected or clinically diagnosed mental retardation should be subjected to psychometric evaluation to confirm and determine the severity of mental retardation.

Laboratory Investigations

Investigations should be planned judiciously. Every case does not require all the investigations mentioned below. Investigations are usually indicated in pathological mental retardation i.e. those cases with abnormal physical findings. Priority should be given to tests for preventable causes of inborn errors of metabolism (viz. hypothyroidism, phenylketonuria, galactosemia etc.) for which treatment is available and early diagnosis is necessary to accrue the maximum benefit. The following investigations are useful:

- a. Blood biochemistry for inborn errors of metabolism and hypothyroidism.
- b. Serology for TORCH infection.

c. X-ray skull can detect calcification in neurocutaneous syndromes.
d. CT and MRI scan for cerebral malformation and cases of mental retardation with abnormal physical findings.
e. Chromosomal analysis in those cases where clinical features suggest a chromosomal anomaly.

Differential Diagnosis

Mental retardation may be associated or confused with the following conditions like delayed maturation, cerebral palsy, sensory defects (vision or hearing), effect of emotional deprivation and schizophrenia.

When **delayed maturation** is suspected, the diagnosis of mental retardation should not be made without follow up if no physical anomaly is detected.

Mental retardation is frequently associated with **cerebral palsy** and both may present with delayed milestones. Hence there may be confusion.

Sensory defects like defective vision and defective hearing when undetected may give the impression of mental retardation because they may present with lateness in following with the eyes and lateness in responding to sounds.

Emotional deprivation may lead to retardation in a child. When such a situation is suspected the child should be transferred to a good environment (e.g. from an institution to a good foster home) for about 3 months and the progress is assessed.

Schizophrenia has similar presentations like lack of response, delayed or absent speech and peculiar behaviour. Schizophrenia manifests usually after 4 years age. There is family history and hallucination may be present. Sometimes psychosis is associated with mental retardation and therefore differentiation becomes difficult.

Management

The effective management of a retarded child is a complex problem requiring the physician to become involved as a compassionate, understanding, resourceful person who treats the child, supports the family, and communicates effectively with others in the community.

Where to Treat?

It is generally agreed that most children with mild to moderate retardation should be kept and cared for within their own homes. Serious emotional and behaviour disorders may arise, but the use of behaviour modification techniques is frequently helpful in bringing about more acceptable behaviour. Foster home care or group living in the community may be considered. Supportive care away from home should be considered for the severely affected when home care is completely impossible or unsuccessful. However, the decision for removal of the child from home is a parental responsibility, but the parents should be guided and supported by the physician.

Parent Counseling

Parents should be seen together. Diagnosis should be fully explained emphasizing the abilities of the child rather than the disabilities. Prognosis should be discussed and principles of management should be explained.

Supportive Care

Retarded children require the same general care which is desirable for all children. A good parent-child relationship early in life and a home environment providing adequate learning experience, relative security, love and acceptance as an individual are essential for development of the inherent potential of normal child. These factors are even more essential for the development of the retarded child.

Guidance relevant to the child's functioning e.g. feeding, toileting, schooling, accident prevention and sex education and assessments of relevant issues like examination of teeth in presence of bruxism, thyroid function in children with Down syndrome, vision and hearing tests in all such children are important components of supportive care.

Many children may require physiotherapy, speech therapy, occupational therapy, hearing aids.

The educational programme for these children should be structured and relevant to the child's individual needs. They should be sent to schools with facilities for special education which have curricula developed on an individual basis.

The child's social and recreational needs should also be addressed. They should be encouraged to participate in sports because it offers benefits like weight management, development of physical coordination, maintenance of cardiovascular fitness, and improvement of self image. Social activities should include dances, trips and other usual social events.

Medications

No drug has been found to improve intellectual function.

Medications are however useful to treat associated conditions like epilepsy, behaviour disorders and psychiatric problems.

Prognosis

There may be unexpected improvement in some children with mental retardation but it is chiefly confined to the first years of life. If the IQ is about 50 and there is no associated physical handicap, the child ultimately is likely to be able to earn his living.

Some mentally retarded adults acquire remarkable proficiency in certain skills like arithmetic or music. Some may have a good memory. While discussing the prognosis, therefore both possibilities should be kept in mind that there may be unexpected improvement or rapid deterioration specially if associated with epilepsy.

The final outcome is however determined not only by the level of intelligence but also the behaviour. A quiet, easily manageable child can achieve much more than a hyperkinetic, destructive child. Environment in which the child is brought up is equally important. A child brought up in a supporting atmosphere, achieves much better.

Prevention

Prevention of mental retardation may be primary, secondary and tertiary.

Primary prevention include improved antenatal care, special care of the preterm, prevention of kernicterus, immunization against Rubella, genetic counseling specially in consanguineous marriages, elderly mothers and when first child is retarded, proper management of hypothyroidism and hyperthyroidism in mothers and reduction of teen age pregnancy.

Secondary prevention should deal with newborn screening for phenylketonuria, galactosemia and congenital hypothyroidism, screening for increased levels of alpha feto protein and carrier detection in inherited disorders.

Tertiary prevention includes early detection and intervention and provision of supportive services to the families of the affected children.

CEREBRAL PALSY

Cerebral palsy (CP) is a persistent disorder of posture and/or movement, due to non-progressive damage to the developing brain. The damage may occur in utero, during the birth process or during the first few years of life. The upper age limit of brain insult is not strictly defined but the American Academy of Cerebral Palsy arbitrarily fixed the age at 5 years.

Etiology

The etiology of cerebral palsy is diverse. Genetic factors contribute in about 2% cases. Different studies have shown the following conditions as high risk factors for development of cerebral palsy:

Major Risk Factors

- Prematurity/VLBW.
- Exposure to disrupted brain perfusion/oxygenation in fetal, natal, neonatal period.
- Birth asphyxia.
- Apgar score 3 or less at 20 minutes (250 fold increased risk).
- Postnatal causes, e.g., meningitis, sepsis.

Other Risk Factors

- Mother 40 years or older.
- Mother 20 years or younger.
- Father 20 years or younger.
- First born or 5th or later born.
- Twin.
- Birth weight <1.5 kg.
- Rh or ABO incompatibility.
- IU infection in early pregnancy (German measles).
- 18% of CP is acquired after birth (meningitis, head trauma).

Among the factors, prematurity/low birth weight has been reported to have a significant association whereas birth asphyxia, once considered as an important causal factor has been questioned. Studies have shown that not more than 10% of cerebral palsy was related to asphyxia. The recent thought is that asphyxia may be a consequence rather than a cause of the process that leads to cerebral palsy. Nonetheless a low Apgar score (0–3) at 5, 10, 15 minutes and HIE grade III are associated with an increased incidence of cerebral palsy.

The National Neonatology Forum, India has recommended the following high risk factors for selection of infant for follow-up:

- Birth weight < 2000 grams.
- Asphyxia: i.e. no cry for 15 minutes after birth.
- Hypotonia: Limpness and floppy neonate.
- Feeding difficulties: Not sucking well in first 2 days.
- Respiratory distress in first 2 days.
- Jaundice within first 2 days.
- Convulsion in the neonatal period.

Early Diagnosis

During the past two decades, major advances in maternal-fetal medicine and neonatal care have resulted in unprecedented survival of very preterm (<32 weeks) and extremely preterm (<28 weeks) babies. Despite the advances in prenatal care, neurodevelopmental motor impairment remains a substantial sequelae. To prevent neuromotor impairment and ensure a quality life to these survivors, an early diagnosis is the only answer.

Early Diagnosis of CP is Difficult

Many a time, an adequate diagnosis becomes difficult in the early months of life. The reasons may be more than one as follows:

1. There are different grades of severity of CP. The most severe form can be diagnosed in the neonatal period whereas the mildest forms may be detected as late as 9–10 years with complains of only clumsiness.
2. CP can be of different types with distinct features of its own and different age of onset of signs. For example, the spastic type can be diagnosed in the first few months, the ataxic type by only about 6 months whereas the athetoid type not until the child is about 1–2 years old. A mild degree of spastic type may be detected only by school age with complains of clumsiness.
3. Association of mental retardation complicates diagnosis because mental subnormality itself has affect on developmental pattern.
4. Occasional disappearance of signs of cerebral palsy, as the child grows, may confuse the diagnosis in some cases.

In diagnosis of CP *one should pay more attention to combination of signs rather than single sign*. For example a combination of hypertonia and delayed milestones should be given much more importance than hypertonia or exaggerated reflexes alone.

How is Early Diagnosis Possible?

Early diagnosis is possible if follow-up screening is advised in all babies with established risk factors present at birth. All babies with high risk factors of CP at birth should be followed up till one year of age to declare them normal. Early diagnosis is necessary to start early intervention.

Why Early Intervention?

Advances in the field of neonatology and establishment of special care nurseries, have no doubt, improved the survival chances of many high risk neonates. But atleast some of these survivors are found to be handicapped at a later age–physically, mentally or both in varying degrees. Very often their problems are identified late, may be at school, when nothing much can be done to improve their disability. Early intervention can help to improve the quality of life in these children.

Can Early Intervention Be Really Effective?

Animal studies in neurophysiology have shown that neurones are not regenerable but synapses are regenerable. This indicates that neurotransmission can be improved by selectively stabilizing one impulse at the expense of others. Both these processes can be enhanced by training. This modifiability of the brain at the molecular level forms the basis of early intervention in the high risk infants.

Neurodevelopmental Follow-up for Early Detection of Cerebral Palsy

It is ideal to follow-up all neonates with high risk factors at 2, 4, 8, 12 months and if found abnormal or suspect, additional visits at 18, 24 and 36 months. At one year corrected age it is important to have a definite diagnosis after a detailed assessment in suspected cases.

Over the years several screening methods have been evolved. These are simple and can be practised by doctors, nurses, health workers and mothers as well. They can be followed even in busy clinic practice as well. These consist of the following:

1. Education of the mother about the 4 important milestones.
2. Evaluation of normal developmental milestones.
3. Documentation of early neuromotor behaviour.
4. Use of Trivandrum developmental screening chart.
5. Assessment by Amiel Tison angles.

The babies detected to have any abnormality by any one of these procedures should be subjected to a thorough neurodevelopmental workup by standard tests.

As delayed milestones is one common presentation of cerebral palsy, education to mothers and evaluation of developmental milestones can be adopted as easy methods for early detection so as to facilitate early intervention. Documentation of early neonatal behaviour in the infant is another easy and useful method to predict later development of cerebral palsy.

Education of the Mothers

For ease of follow-up, mothers can be informed, at the time of discharge from hospital after delivery, the four milestones in the first year of life viz. *Social smile (by 2 months), head holding (by 4 months), sitting without support (by 8 months) and standing without support (by 12 months).* It has been shown to be useful in screening at risk newborn. She should be advised to report to the health worker if there is any delay in achieving the milestones. This can help detection of developmental delay as early as 2 months age.

Normal Child Developmental Milestones

A delayed milestone is one of the important presentations of cerebral palsy. Every child should undergo an assessment of milestones during the first year of life whenever they are brought to a doctor or health worker for any reason. For this, knowledge of normal child developmental milestones and its variations is very essential for all health professionals.

The minimum essential developmental milestones to be assessed in a child include the following:

Age	*Milestones*
2 months	Social smile
4 months	Neck holding
8 months	Sitting without support
12 months	Standing without support
13 months	Walking without support, single words
15 months	Feeds self
15–18 months	Domestic mimicry
18 months	10 words with meaning
21–24 months	2 or 3 words together spontaneously
24 months	Speaks short sentences/ understands sentences
3 years	Dresses self, stands momentarily on one foot. Speech 3–4 words sentences

The infant with a deviation of any one of the milestones should be subjected to a thorough neurodevelopmental assessment to exclude cerebral palsy.

Early Neuromotor Behaviour

In all neonates under follow-up emphasis should be made on documentation of early neuromotor behaviours which may predict later development of cerebral palsy. These include certain observations by mothers and some abnormal signs in the infant.

Mother's Observations

- Baby feels stiff, on one side or both.
- Baby keeps one hand clenched, refuses to use one hand.
- Kicks both legs together instead of reciprocal kicking.
- When creeping, one leg trails behind.
- Excessive crying.
- Dissociation of development, i.e., baby may have severe retardation in gross motor development like sitting or walking but is more advanced in other fields viz. the pincer grip may be normal.
- Delayed milestones.

Abnormal Signs

- Reduced head circumference or fall in head growth.
- Constant fisting with adduction of thumb beyond 2 months.
- Delayed social smile.
- Primitive reflexes persisting beyond 6 months.
- Obligatory asymmetric tonic neck reflex (ATNR).
- Delayed appearance of postural reflexes and developmental milestones.
- Persistent tone abnormalities.
- Persistent asymmetry in posture, movement and reflexes.
- Occulovisual problems: Roving eyes, no visual following, nystagmus, persistent squint.
- Lack of auditory response.

Mother's observations may be the chief complain during the visit and the *abnormal signs* may be detected by the attending doctor. Screening for presence of abnormal neuromotor behaviour in the high risk infant can aid early diagnosis of CP to a great extent.

Trivandrum Developmental Screening Chart and Amiel Tison Method of Neurological Assessment (*See* Pages 92-93)

These tests are simple, less time consuming and can be administered with minimal amount of equipment and training. Both have been acclaimed to be useful tools for follow-up of at risk babies.

An infant who is suspected to have developmental delay by TDSC should be subjected to further neuro-developmental assessment by standard developmental tests and an infant who is suspected to have abnormal tone by the assessment of Amiel Tison angles for assessment of passive tone should be subjected to further neurological assessment.

Classification

The clinical classification of cerebral palsy is based on the nature of the observed motor deficit and degree of severity.

(A) Nature of Observed Motor Deficit

1. Spastic cerebral palsy
   a. Quadriplegia
   b. Diplegia
   c. Paraplegia
   d. Hemiplegia
   e. Monoplegia
2. Extrapyramidal/dyskinetic cerebral palsy
   a. Choreoathetosis
   b. Dystonia
3. Atonic cerebral palsy
   a. Atonic diplegia
   b. Congenital cerebellar ataxia
4. Mixed types.

(B) Degree of Severity

This classification is done on the basis of speech problem, activities, requirement of aids, any intervention needed. This classification of cases of cerebral palsy helps in planning management of cases.

Mild Degree

There is no speech defect. The child is independent in activities of daily living and ambulation. No aids and appliances are required. No intervention is needed. Prognosis is good.

Moderate Degree

These children have some speech problems. They are inadequate in ambulation and activities of daily living. May require aids and appliances. Some intervention is required. Prognosis with treatment is fair.

Severe Degree

These children have communication problem. They depend on others for daily activity and ambulation. Aids and appliances may be of help. Intervention is necessary. Prognosis is poor.

Spastic Cerebral Palsy

This is the most common type accounting for 70–75% of all cases. The child usually presents with delayed milestone.

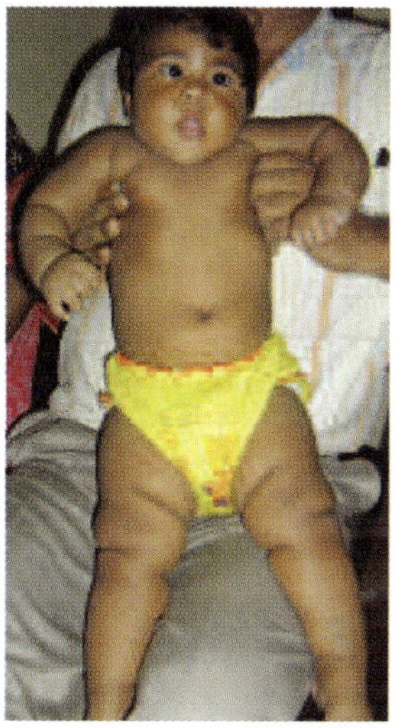

Fig. 5.21: Spastic cerebral palsy

On examination there is hypertonia manifested by tight fisting of the hands due to hyperactivity of the grasp reflex. On vertical suspension of the infant there is arching of the back and rigid extension and adduction and internal rotation of the lower limbs. In case of severe spasticity, there may be scissoring of the legs which may be obvious or may be seen on vertical suspension. In older children, the feet are held in equinovarus position and the child walks on tip toe. The arms are internally rotated, elbows extended or tightly flexed and hands are fisted. All tendon reflexes are brisk, often with a sustained ankle clonus. There is persistence of the primitive reflexes. The plantar reflex is extensor and abdominal reflexes are exaggerated. Spasticity and rigidity become more evident as the child grows and often leads to contractures.

Pseudobulbar palsy is present when spasticity is bilateral leading to difficulty in swallowing and excessive drooling of saliva.

In **spastic quadriplegia,** there is involvement of all the four limbs, the arms being equally or more involved than the legs. One side may be more affected than the other. The term double hemiplegia has been applied to cases where the upper limbs are more affected than the lower limbs and there is pseudobulbar palsy. There are multiple associated abnormalities in these cases. They are seizures, mental retardation, feeding difficulties, and speech problems, visual and hearing defects.

Spastic diplegia refers to the motor deficit that affects all the four limbs but is much more severe in the lower extremities. The involvement of the hands may be minimal, expressing as only clumsiness in grasping, and later with awkwardness of hand movements. There is usually no pseudobulbar palsy or may be limited to a brisk jaw jerk only. Intelligence is often normal or borderline but apraxia is common and may lead to difficulties in learning to draw and to form letters. Spastic diplegia has a strong association with prematurity and periventricular leucomalacia. In the early years there may be hypotonia with brisk jerks which gradually develops into spasticity later.

Spastic paraplegia is a rare form of cerebral palsy where only the lower extremities are involved. In such cases, the possibility of a spinal cord lesion should always be considered and excluded.

Spastic hemiplegia refers to an upper motor neurone involvement of the face, arm and leg on one side of the body. Usually the upper limb is affected more than the lower limb and the right side more than the left. There is often homonymous hemianopia and a hemisensory deficit on the hemiplegic side. Spastic hemiplegia can be suspected below one year of age in children with definite hand preference. Sitting and crawling is achieved in time but walking is delayed. In severely affected older children, the posture of affected side is characteristic. The arm is held adducted, flexed and internally rotated at the shoulders with elbow flexed, forearm pronated, wrist flexed and thumb adducted. The lower limb is adducted at the hip, semiflexed at the knee and planter flexed at the ankle. The gait is characterized by limping, often with circumduction of the affected limb. Mild cases are often missed in the early years and may present around school age with clumsiness or educational problems. Intellectual level will depend on the area of involvement. Convulsions occurring early in life in these children decrease the likelihood of normal intellectual development.

Spastic monoplegia, with weakness confined to one limb and Triplegia i.e. weakness involving three limbs have been reported. They are rare. A careful examination usually reveals an asymmetric diplegia or hemiplegia.

Extrapyramidal Cerebral Palsy

The most important causes of extrapyramidal cerebral palsy are perinatal asphyxia and kernicterus which results in predominant damage of the basal ganglia and extrapyramidal system. This type manifests as hypotonia in early infancy with drooling and feeding difficulties and by choreoathetosis and dystonia later in childhood. The asymmetric tonic neck reflex (ATNR) is prominent and the postural reflexes appear late. The earliest sign is abnormal posturing of hands when the infant, after 6 months of age, attempts to reach an object. Typical choreoathetoid movements (i.e. bizarre writhing movements and facial grimace on attempted movement) develop generally after one year of age, coinciding with hypermyelination of the basal ganglia, a phenomenon called status marmoratus. Involvement of oropharyngeal muscles results in speech problems. Intelligence is often preserved. These children may be mistakenly diagnosed as mentally retarded because of their severe physical and communication disabilities.

Atonic Cerebral Palsy

Atonic cerebral palsy may result from central nervous system damage (Atonic diplegia) or damage to the cerebellum (Congenital cerebellar ataxia). Both types have hypotonia as a common presentation. This type of cerebral palsy needs careful evaluation to exclude neuromuscular disorders.

Atonic diplegia is characterized by hypotonia, easily obtainable or brisk tendon reflexes, in contrast to neuromuscular disease, where jerks are also diminished. Severe mental retardation is usual in this type of cerebral palsy.

Congenital cerebellar ataxia is a rare form. It occurs due to predominant cerebellar damage. There is hypotonia and hyporeflexia during infancy. By second year, the gait is ataxic and there is intention tremor. Nystagmus, however, is rare. There may be associated mental defect, usually of mild degree.

Mixed Types

The common mixed type is a combination of spastic and

1. Abnormal behaviour should begin before the age of 7 years and must be present for atleast 6 months.
2. Behaviours must be statistically abnormal for the child's age and developmental level.
3. Symptoms must be pervasive in nature (present in atleast two or more settings) and impair the child's ability to function normally.
4. Symptoms must not be secondary to another disorder.

DSM–IV Diagnostic Criteria for ADHD

A. Either 1 or 2

1. Six (or more) of the following symptoms of inattention have persisted for atleast 6 months to a degree that is maladaptive and inconsistent with developmental level

Inattention

a. Often fails to give close attention to details or makes careless mistakes in school work, work or other activities
b. Often has difficulty sustaining attention in tasks or play activities
c. Often does not seem to listen when spoken to directly
d. Often does not follow through on instructions and fails to finish school work, chores, or duties in the workplace (not due to oppositional behaviour or failure to understand instruction)
e. Often has difficulty organizing tasks and activities
f. Often avoids, dislikes, or is reluctant to engage in tasks that requires sustained mental effort (such as school work or home work)
g. Often looses things necessary for tasks or activities (toys, school assignments, pencils, books etc.)
h. Is often easily distracted by extraneous stimuli
i. Is often forgetful in daily activities

2. Six (or more) of the following symptoms of hyperactivity-impulsivity have persisted for atleast 6 months to a degree that is maladaptive and inconsistent with developmental level

Hyperactivity

a. Often fidgets with hands or feet or squirms in seat
b. Often leaves seat in classroom or in other situations in which remaining seated is expected
c. Often runs about or climbs excessively in situations in which it is inappropriate (in adolescents or adults may be limited to subjective feelings of restlessness)
d. Often has difficulty playing or engaging in leisure activities quietly
e. Is often "on the go" or often acts as if "driven by a motor"
f. Often talks excessively

Impulsivity

a. Often blurts out answers before questions have been completed
b. Often has difficulty awaiting turn
c. Often interrupts or intrudes on others (butts into conversation or games).

Contd.

Contd.

B. Some hyperactive-impulsive or inattentive symptoms that caused impairment were present before 7 years of age.

C. Some impairment from the symptoms is present in 2 or more settings e.g. school (for work) or home.

D. There must be clear evidence of clinically significant impairment in social, academic or occupational functioning.

E. The symptoms do not occur exclusively during the course of a pervasive developmental disorder, schizophrenia, or other psychotic disorder and are not better accounted for by another mental disorder (e.g. mood disorder, anxiety disorder, dissociative disorder, or personality disorder).

Types of ADHD

1. **ADHD combined type:** If both criteria A1 and A2 are there for the past 6 months.
2. **ADHD predominantly inattentive type:** If criterion A1 is there for past 6 months. Criterion A2 is not met for past 6 months.
3. **ADHD predominantly hyperactive-impulsive type:** If criterion A2 is there for past 6 months. Criterion A1 is not met for past 6 months.

Differential Diagnosis

Impairment of attention and school performance can occur in children as a result of *chronic illness* either because of the disease itself or the medication used for control of the disease. In adolescents *substance abuse* may be the cause.

Sleep disorders frequently result in behavioral and emotional symptoms. Conversely disruption of sleep may be due to such symptoms.

Depression and anxiety disorders may present with many symptoms such as inattention, restlessness, poor organization, inability to focus and concentrate on work and forgetfulness, similar to ADHD.

Obsessive-compulsive disorder may mimic ADHD particularly when persistent and recurrent and interfere with normal daily activities.

Adjustment disorders secondary to major life stresses (e.g. parental divorce, death of a close family member, family violence etc.) or parent child relationship disorders involving conflicts over discipline, overt child abuse and/ or neglect, or overprotection may result in similar symptoms like ADHD.

Treatment

Treatment includes psychosocial interventions, behaviour management training and medications. Stimulant medications are shown to be effective in treating core symptoms of ADHD, whereas psychosocial interventions and behaviour management training are effective in treating many comorbid conditions frequently associate with ADHD.

Medications

The two main classes of stimulants used are methylphenidate and amphetamines and their derivatives. When used sequentially, approximately 80% children respond satisfactorily with relief of major symptoms. Adverse effects are mild and dose related. Common side effects include loss of appetite, initial weight loss, abdominal discomfort, dysphoria, tics and disturbed sleep. Symptoms remit when the dose is lowered. Other agents like tricyclic antidepressants (imipramine and desipramine) and buproprion are considered as second line drugs and are effective when associated with comorbid conditions. Long-term use of these drugs does not result in addiction and drug abuse.

Psychosocial Interventions and Behaviour Management Training

It consists of counseling the parents and the child regarding the effects of the disease on learning, behaviour, self-esteemed, social skills and family function and plan intervention by behaviour therapy. Behaviour therapy should include modification of the physical and social environment as well as the child's behaviour.

Prognosis

With combination of medication and psychosocial and behavioural interventions most children show significant decrease in the symptoms.

LEARNING DISABILITIES

Although for more than hundred years, it has been recognized that seemingly normal children can have impairment of learning to read and write it was only in 1886, Morgan described a 14-year-old boy who was bright and intelligent but had great difficulty in reading. He termed this syndrome as 'congenital word blindness'. The term 'Learning disabilities' was first coined by Kirk in 1962.

Specific learning disabilities (SpLD) are common neurodevelopmental disorders presumed to be due to central nervous system dysfunction. It is an invisible handicap. They are chronic life-long conditions with problems in learning to read, write, spell or do mathematics. Children with SpLD fail to achieve school grade at a level that is commensurate with their intelligence resulting in an impact on self image, peer and family relationship and social interactions.

Definition

Specific learning disabilities (SpLD) is a generic term that refers to a heterogeneous group of neurobehavioral disorders manifested by significant unexpected, specific and persistent difficulties in acquisition and use of efficient reading (dyslexia), writing (dysgraphia) or mathematical abilities (dyscalculia), despite conventional instruction, intact senses, normal intelligence, proper motivation and adequate socio-cultural opportunity.

Characteristics of Dyslexia

Dyslexia is the most common and most comprehensively studied of the learning disabilities. Both sexes are affected equally and affect 5–12% of school children. It is characterized by an unexpected difficulty in reading in children who otherwise possess intelligence, motivation, and opportunities to learn which are considered necessary for accurate and fluent reading. Children with dyslexia read slowly and hesitantly, follow the words with fingers, mispronounce words and confuse letters. Examples of confusion of letters include 'bog' for 'dog', inversion of 'n' for 'u'. They are poor at copying from board and skip or add words when reading loud.

There is no single unified theory to explain the etiology of dyslexia. It is both familial and heritable. Linkage studies implicate loci on chromosomes 1, 2, 6 and 15 for the transmission of phonologic awareness deficits and subsequent reading problems. However, the exact mechanisms by which genetic factors predispose someone to dyslexia are not clear. Neurobiologic investigations viz. postmortem brain specimens, brain morphometry, and diffusion tensor MRI suggest that there are differences in the left temporo-parietal-occipital brain regions between dyslexic and normal readers. In normal children there is a smoothly functioning integrated reading system. In dyslexic children there is disruption of left hemispheric posterior reading systems to function properly during reading with increased activation in frontal region. The dyslexic children attempt to compensate by shifting to other ancillary systems for example anterior sites such as inferior frontal gyrus and right hemisphere sites. This underlies the failure of skilled reading to develop.

It is hoped that future progress in genetics will allow identification of genetic markers for risk of dyslexia, and ongoing neuroimaging studies (MRI, positron emission tomography) in children and adults with dyslexia will help unravel the etiology. Tests to identify children at risk for dyslexia at the time of admission to school are being developed. These would help in early intervention.

Characteristics of Dysgraphia

It is characterized by difficulty in writing. The writing may be very small or large, may be impossible to read. There is use of faulty pressure in writing and written sentences are jumbled with faulty spacing.

Characteristics of Dyscalculia

It is characterized by difficulty in mathematics i.e. calculations, tables and logic. They count numbers on fingers. Mental sums are difficult for these children. They mix up symbols like '+', '=' etc.

Early Diagnosis of SpLD

An early diagnosis is essential to prevent poor school performance and its emotional sequelae. In addition, longer the child is with SpLD at any level of severity more difficult is to treat. Hence all children with learning problems in school should be evaluated for SpLD.

Identification of SpLD is difficult during preschool years. A conclusive diagnosis is not possible until the age of 8 – 9 years. The red flag signs for dyslexia are: (i) History of language delay, (ii) Not attending to sounds of words (e.g. trouble playing rhyming games with words or confusing words that sound alike), (iii) A positive family history.

Evaluation of Suspected SpLD

The child with a learning problem needs a multidisciplinary assessment by a pediatric neurologist, counselor, clinical psychologist, special educator and a child psychiatrist. Every one has their own part to play to arrive at a diagnosis of SpLD.

The *pediatric neurologist* will exclude other causes of poor school performance. The causes include medical (hypothyroidism, chronic lead poisoning), neurological causes (cerebral palsy, Wilson's disease), behavioural causes (depression, conduct disorders, opposition defiant disorders etc). An audiometric and ophthalmic examination should be done to rule out hearing or visual deficit as the cause of the learning problem.

The *counselor* rules out whether any environmental deprivation due to poor home or school environment, or any emotional problem due to stress at home or school, is primarily responsible for the child's poor performance at school.

The *clinical psychologist* will conduct intelligence tests viz. Wechsler intelligence scale for children and rule out mental retardation as a cause of poor school performance.

The *special educator* will assess the child's academic achievements on the basis of standard educational tests and assess child's performance in areas viz. reading, spelling, written language and mathematics. An academic achievement of two years below child's actual school grade placement or chronological age is considered diagnostic of SpLD.

The *child psychiatrist* plays an important role in confirmation of diagnosis of ADHD, a comorbid condition found in around 12–24% of children with SpLD. He also helps in confirmation of diagnosis of depression, behavioural problems as a cause of the learning problem.

Management

Management of child with SpLD includes primarily remedial education and accommodations, counseling and guidance, and treatment of associated problems.

Remedial education is the cornerstone of therapy. It includes understanding of the strengths and weaknesses and providing an individualized educational plan.

Role of *accommodation* is to help the child with SpLD to cope up in regular mainstream school. The treatment of dyslexia in students in high school, college is typically based on accommodation rather than remediation. Accommodations include exemption from spelling mistakes, dropping a language and substituting it with work experience subject, dropping algebra and geometry and substituting them with a lower grade of mathematics.

Other helpful accommodations may be use of laptops, computers with spelling checkers, tape recorders in the classrooms, recorded books, access to lecture notes, tutorial classes and separate quiet room for taking tests.

Outcome

With appropriate remedial education and accommodations, most children achieve academic competence and complete their education in regular mainstream school. Some children need to continue education in special schools as they are unable to cope up in mainstream schools. The outcome however depends on the severity of disability, age or grade when remedial education was started, length and continuity of treatment, presence or absence of associated emotional problems, parental and school support.

Common Behavioural Problems

A child's behaviour problems represent a conflict between his developing personality and that of his parents, teachers and siblings and of other children with whom he/she comes in contact.

PROBLEMS OF HABIT

Thumb Sucking

Babies have always sucked their thumb. Rare instances of babies born sucking their thumbs have been reported. The children normally suck thumb constantly or at the time shortly before going to sleep. This behaviour usually disappears by the age of 5 years. In mentally retarded children, it may persist into school years. It is rare in adolescence. Thumb sucking however is a cause of concern if it persists after the age of 3 years or it starts after a long period without it. It might well be an indicator of some hidden stress factors which need timely intervention so as to forestall future personality derangements.

Thumb sucking has been variously described as a pleasurable and soothing action by the infant and a model of infantile sexual manifestations. About 90% of children with thumb sucking have associated stress factors viz. neglect, overprotection, strictness of parents, parental disharmony, sibling rivalry, loneliness and boredom. It has been related to loss or separation, in which the child symbolically tries to overcome his pain and anxiety by attaining the remembered infantile sensation of being full and satiated. In older children, the thumb may serve the function of an imaginary companion to ward off feelings of loneliness. Turning to thumb sucking in times of stress may represent a withdrawal from a situation which is too frightening to face except through regression to a younger age.

Treatment: Thumb sucking requires no treatment during infancy or when it is practised only in relation to sleep. When thumb sucking is practised during waking hours after the first year of life, it indicates the child is bored, unhappy or fatigued. Therefore treatment should aim at correcting the situation rather than thumb sucking. The child should have adequate rest and ample play activities. The child should be kept busy during the day and the habit will take care of itself.

If the habit persist beyond 5–6 years age, promise of a reward, an appeal to the child's will power, or having the child himself apply a bitter tasting substance or wear gloves as a reminder is usually sufficient to terminate the habit. If the older child is not willing, it indicates a manifestation of general emotional and social immaturity.

It should be noted that the use of devices like mechanical restraints e.g. tying of hands, nagging scolding should be avoided as it may further perpetuate the problem.

Nail Biting

Nail biting has been described as an extension of thumb sucking, in that at about the age of three, thumb sucking tends to disappear and nail biting take its place which increases in incidence upto 6 years age. The incidence again increases at the age of 9 years reaching a second peak from 13 to 15 years age. Approximately 50% give up the habit after 16 years in response to disapproval from peers and is replaced by other habits like gum chewing, cigarette smoking or nose picking. There is no significant difference in gender of nail bitters, although males persist longer in nail biting than do females.

Recent literatures describe nail biting as a tension discharging phenomenon. It is mostly an expression of tension produced by anticipation of a difficult test in school or of a parental punishment or by any kind of excitement. In contrast to thumb suckers who are calm, placid, unemotional children, nail biters are hyperactive, quick, fidgety and energetic. Nail biting may also be observed as the response of a generally compliant child to the myriad of rules, regulations and demand placed on him or her, particularly if the child is not very flexible, does not receive positive support and feedback, or attain success. Disappointment and anger are then expressed as nail biting.

Treatment: Treatment of nail biting basically consists of identification and removal of the causes of tension, responsible for the origin and maintenance of this habit. Treatment is usually not indicated in mild cases, as nail biting is usually replaced by some acceptable activity at a later age. Parents should be advised to seek expert opinion if a child bites the nails continuously or more so without any apparent cause.

Nail biting is said to be lessened when there is opportunity for more vigorous muscular or athletic activity as well as more protection from the avoidable forms of excitements or stress.

The preoccupation with toys and healthy association with other children also help in treatment.

An appeal to the child's pride often gives good result in girls. Threats, punishments, mechanical restraints and application of bitters, chillies etc are harmful and may even make the child more prone to other habit disorders.

Teeth Grinding (Bruxism)

Teeth grinding or bruxism is common during the first five years of life. It seems to be associated with daytime anxiety. The problem may be relieved by helping the child find ways to reduce anxiety. Bed time can be made more enjoyable and relaxed by reading or talking with the child permitting review of fears and angers experienced during day time. Praise and emotional support are also useful. Day time teeth grinding may indicate mental retardation. As commonly believed there is no relation between teeth grinding and worm infestation.

Pica

Pica is an eating disorder characterized by repeated or chronic ingestion of non-nutritive substances. These substances include plaster, charcoal, clay, wool, ashes, paint, hair, earth etc. Some children, especially mentally retarded, show no discrimination and would ingest anything available. Ingestion of fecal matter (coprophagy) indicates either a more severe emotional problem or a seriously retarded and psychotic child. Children normally explore the environment by tasting or mouthing of objects as an infant and toddler. Pica after 2 years of age needs investigation.

Pica may be an accepted cultural practice where the mother indulged in the habit at one stage or other and they often permit or encourage the habit in the child. However, the presence of a strong father figure usually acts as a deterrent in the development or retention of pica.

It may be an expression of an underlying emotional disturbances and consequent to organic etiologic factors. The emotional or stress factors include neglected child, marital disharmony, overprotection of the child, strictness of parents and teachers, sibling rivalry, loss or separation of a parent, birth of another child, and beginning of school. The organic factors associated with pica include mental retardation, autism. Pica appears to be more prevalent in the lower socio-economic classes.

Children with pica are at increased risk of iron deficiency anemia, lead poisoning, and worm infestation. A child with pica therefore needs screening for presence of these conditions. Eating of hair may lead to intestinal obstruction. These children also have constipation, and they are prone to other addictive behaviour like alcoholism, over eating and depression later in their life.

Treatment: Pica disappears promptly in children of normal intelligence with (i) Careful evaluation of the underlying stress factor and appropriate remedy, (ii) Provision of proper diet, (iii) Adequate supervision and training of the child. If the above measures fail then, (iv) Alteration of child's environment, and (v) Behaviour and directive guidance to improve parent-child relationship should be considered.

Triochotillomania

Triochotillomania is a condition characterized by an irresistible urge to pull one's own hair. Some may pull their hair when they are tense. Some may pluck them while others may even eat them. Children usually start this habit first by plucking hair of a furred toy or pet animals, other siblings and later on practise on themselves.

This condition is more common in females and is prevalent from early childhood to adulthood. More than 50% cases present to the physician with some other symptom like itchy alopecia or intestinal obstruction as a result of a hair ball rather than hair pulling.

The causative stress factors broadly include parent-child conflict and mother-daughter relationship. The parent-child conflict is an expression of conflict between the personality of the child with mother and/or father. The mothers of these children, during their childhood could not fulfill their needs and regarded their parents with resentment and disgust. The fathers are usually passive, ineffective, helpless men usually dominated by their wives. The mothers are usually competitive, ambivalent and critical of aggressive behaviour by their children. The mother-daughter relationship is characterized by hostile dependency and mutual fears of separation. The mothers want to use their daughter for their unfulfilled ambitions and this causes an interference with their own autonomy consequently leading to hair pulling.

Treatment: Treatment is directed at the cause, the child's developmental struggles and the disturbed parent-child relationship rather than the symptom itself. Family therapy for removing the identified stress and behaviour modification are found to be very successful in treating this problem.

Fears

All normal children have fears. Fears constitute a normal defense mechanism. The infant is likely to show fear when there is a sudden noise, a sudden falling movement or some sudden unexpected event which he/she cannot understand. At about 6 months age the child may show fear of strangers. Children between the ages 2–3 years develop fear of every day objects e.g. dogs, motor cars, noisy machines and darkness. They may also show fear of being deserted by mother. Girls tend to have more fear than boys and an imaginative child shows more fear. Fear is harmful only when it is exaggerated enough to cause anxiety.

Shyness

The first sign of shyness is observed at about 4 months age when the baby shows shyness when spoken to by strangers. After one year age, the child tends to cover the eyes with the forearm when spoken to, becomes notably quiet, pulls faces and hides behind the mother. The child aged 2–3 years, expresses shyness by crying if mother leaves them with other children, fails to play either alongside or with other children.

Shyness may be inherited from any of the parent. The cause may be in the environment for example the child is likely to be shy if he is never given a chance to mix with adults or other children.

Prevention and treatment: Children should be allowed to mix with others from early infancy. Shyness can be prevented by wise upbringing which gives love, security and self confidence.

It must not be ridiculed and nothing should be said about shyness in front of the child. The child should be encouraged to have friends at home at frequent intervals and also go out to visit friends, at first with his mother. The child should be encouraged to play alongside friends and not be pushed into playing with them.

Stealing

The young child has a natural desire to achieve what he/she wants. With maturity they learn to respect the property of others. Therefore the act is a normal developmental behaviour in a preschool child while in a school child the act will be considered as stealing. The causative factors include dishonesty at home, feeling of insecurity, bad example from friends or other persons, self-indulgence as a result of an anti-social personality, and feeling of inferiority when a child has no pocket money or has less than others. However, the most important aspect is honesty by parents in action as well as in conversation. For example, if a parent picks up a coin when it does not belong to him/her, the child may be expected to do the same.

Treatment: Treatment should be directed towards resolving domestic conflicts particularly between the parent and child. Whenever possible the child should make restitution by restoring whatever he has stolen, however embarrassing and difficult it may be for him.

Lying

A child aged 2–3 years is not expected to be truthful. This is called innocent lying. A child of 5–6 years may indulge in fantasy thinking and narrates stories in all seriousness to the parents. This is called fantasy lying. This fantasy thinking should be distinguished from deliberate or delinquent lying. A child may learn the habit of lying from adults. A child may deliberately lie to win praise, gain prestige, boost ego, and gain friends or to escape punishment or the displeasure of his parents. It is commonly because of lack of love and security at home, excessive religious strictness or domestic friction.

Treatment: Treatment is directed towards the cause. The sense of insecurity should be appropriately dealt with. Punishment for lying should be avoided as it will do more harm.

PROBLEMS OF MOVEMENT

Rocking and Head Banging

Rocking and head banging are rhythmic motor habits, common in infants and toddlers which may occur during sleep or waking state. In *rocking,* the baby gets up on hands and knees and rocks back and forth some time violent enough either to hurt himself or to break the crib. In *head banging,* the child repeatedly strikes his head against a solid subject often the head of the crib or against the mattress.

Both rocking and head banging appear in the later half of the first year of life. It is most commonly seen when the infant is moving from one developmental stage to the other e.g. from sitting to standing or from crawling to walking. Usually these are benign, self limiting conditions and terminate around the second year. In older children, it represents either some stress condition or an organic brain damage. The associated stress factors include separation of mother and child by death, divorce, hospitalization or a working mother, overprotected child, strictness of parents and parental disharmony.

Treatment: In most children, no treatment is necessary as the habit will cease spontaneously. Reassurance to parents that the outcome is favourable is only what is necessary. However, in severe cases the following approaches may be useful:

a. Replacement of the rhythmic movements with a rhythmic auditory stimulus like hand tapping.
b. Replace these activities by more purposeful and acceptable rhythmic motor activities like dancing, swinging etc.
c. Sedatives and tranquillizers in very low doses for violent cases to break the cycle.
d. Helmets for the protection of head and padding of the crib.
e. In chronic cases a complete physical, neurological, psychological evaluation and treatment of primary cause.

Breath Holding Spells

Breath holding spell is a drastic expression of emotional discomfort. It occurs at any time from one to five years of age; rare before 6 months age and after five years. The child throwing a breath holding spell is generally active and energetic who react vigorously to situations. They are of obstinate and resistive nature, attention seeking for winning parent's attention and concern. The parental factors associated include disturbed parent child relationship, overprotective parents, separation from an attached parent and strict parental discipline.

The common precipitating factors of an attack are anger, frustration, fall, pain etc. The sequence of events in this disorder is that the child starts crying after he is hurt, admonished, frustrated and frightened. In the midst of violent crying the child stops breathing and does not resume respiration for about half a minute. During this time the child becomes blue especially around the lips and face. The child may throw the limbs around helplessly and sometimes the eyes turn upwards. There may be twitching and jerks which may be localized or generalized. This attack may last for 5 to 10 seconds and then promptly stop. If the breathing is not reestablished quickly enough, the child may become limp and lifeless in most cases but in some cases may continue crying.

Prevention and treatment: Most of the time the spells are benign and ceases with age. In some cases it may be replaced by other behaviour problems like temper tantrums if the root cause persisted.

During the spell, efforts should be made to prevent injury. The measures like pinching, throwing cold water on the child's face, shaking and slapping are rarely successful. When the spell has originated out of a behavioural problem the parents should be advised to correct their faulty attitude. In persistent cases, the child should undergo a complete physical, neurological and cardiovascular evaluation and the child investigated for detection of iron deficiency anemia. If present should be treated with iron therapy along with changing parental attitude and child's environment.

Temper Tantrums

Temper tantrums are expressions of open resentment and displeasure in small children in the form of dramatic outbursts. It is more common upto five years age and gradually decline thereafter. It is three times more common in boys as compared to girls. The first born child has the problem twice as compared to the later siblings.

The individual outbursts may be precipitated by a variety of situations, basically the same as those which produce feelings of anger in adults. The problem is usually seen in an active, determined, and energetic child. Tantrums represent the confrontation of the child's developing personality with the will of the parents. A child with tantrum may imitate the bad temper of parents or friends. Overprotection or overindulgence is one of the common causes of tantrums as these children are undisciplined and whenever they are denied of anything, they throw a tantrum. Similarly strictness, deprivation, an alcoholic father may produce tantrums. Parental inconsistency may be a cause. For example if one parent forbids a child to do a particular thing and the other permits it, the child may throw tantrum in order to get what the child wants. Sibling jealousy may be another situation which leads to tantrums.

Frequent tantrums are always associated with feeding problems, bed wetting, fear reactions, night terrors, head banging, nail biting, hair plucking etc.

Treatment and prevention: The appropriate steps for managing this problem include:

a. Remedy of underlying insecurity, overprotection, overindulgence, overstrictness and other faulty attitude of the parents.
b. The opportunities for resistance should be cut down to minimum in order to prevent the tantrums. The child should be kept occupied, should have playmates of his own age at his home and go out to visit them in their homes. The child should be encouraged to practise skills and to take pride in what he/she does.
c. The best way to treat tantrums is to ignore it. The child should certainly not be given what he wanted after the tantrum. As soon as the child finds that he/she is achieving nothing by tantrums, he/she will stop having them.
d. Persistent tantrums should be investigated to rule out epilepsy, brain tumours etc.

Tics (Habit Spasm)

Tics are sudden, quick, and involuntary, frequently repeated movements of circumscribed groups of muscles, serving no apparent purpose. It represents discharges of tension related central nervous system electrochemical signals. Tics may be of following types:

a. Motor tics which involves body movements include grimacing, yawning, sighing, protruding tongue, nose picking, scratching, wrinkling the nose, writhing hands, clenching fist, pulling /twisting hair, blinking / winking eyes, manipulating genitals and thigh rubbing.
b. Vocal tics which can be in the form of coughing, hiccoughing, whistling, barking, spitting, repeating words or tunes, uttering obscene words.
c. Other complicated tics include jumping, squatting, and skipping, hitting, kicking touching floor or people etc.

Although quite often only one form is present, the same child may display a combination of tics which are carried out simultaneously, alternate or follow each other.

Tics must be distinguished from petit mal or other non-generalized seizure disorders. Seizure disorders are characterized both by transient inability to interact during periods of eye blinking or lip smacking or amnesia for the event. An EEG may be necessary in some cases for confirmation. Tics can be distinguished from dyskinetic movements and dystonias by their discontinuation during sleep and by the virtue of conscious control that can be achieved for short periods.

Treatment: Most children with simple motor tics do not require any treatment. Some children may have associated problems (viz. stress problems like strict parents, overprotected child, neglected child, parental disharmony and family history of tics), neuropsychological dysfunction, academic underachievement, or low self-esteem. These problems require psychotherapeutic intervention.

PROBLEMS OF TOILET TRAINING

Enuresis (Bed Wetting)

Enuresis is defined as the voluntary or involuntary repeated discharge of urine into clothes or bed after 5 years, the age at which most children achieve bladder control during day and night.

The diagnosis of enuresis is made when the urine is voided twice a week for atleast three consecutive months or clinically significant distress occurs in areas of the child's life as a result of wetting. Enuresis may be classified into nocturnal enuresis i.e. voiding urine at night, and diurnal enuresis voiding while awake.

Nocturnal Enuresis

In majority (75%) of cases enuresis is nocturnal only whereas the rest are wet day and night. Nocturnal enuresis may be primary (75%) where nocturnal urinary control has never been achieved or secondary (25%) when the child was dry at night atleast for few months and then enuresis occurred. Approximately 60% of affected children are males. Family history is usually present in around 50% cases. Nocturnal enuresis affects upto 20% children at the age of 5 years. It ceases spontaneously approximately at the rate of 15% every year. Atleast 2% of children continue bedwetting upto adolescence.

The pathogenesis of primary nocturnal enuresis is multifactorial and includes the following:

- Delayed maturation of the cortical mechanisms that allow voluntary control of the micturition reflex.
- Considered as a sleep disorder. Enuretic children are described as deep sleepers. They are more difficult to arouse than children with normal bladder control.
- Reduced ADH production at night is thought to result in an increased urine output.
- Genetic factors have been described. Genes for enuresis have been localized to chromosomes 12 and 13 q. If one parent was enuretic each child has a

44% risk of enuresis. If both were enuretic, each child has 77% risk.

The organic causes of enuresis include urinary tract infection, hypertrophy of adenoids, thread worm infection, local irritation due to phimosis, adherent prepuce, excoriation of vaginal orifice, diabetes insipidus and diabetes mellitus, congenital anomalies of bladder, distal bladder neck obstruction and deformities of spine.

The child with nocturnal enuresis should be carefully examined to exclude neurologic and spinal abnormalities. Laboratory investigations may be necessary in some cases. Urine analysis for specific gravity or osmolality or both, glycosuria, a microscopic examination and culture to exclude infection. A normal urine examination does not warrant any further investigation. A renal sonogram may be necessary in an older child with enuresis or in children who do not respond appropriately to therapy. An X-ray/CT scan of the spine may be done in suspected cases of myelodysplasia.

Treatment: The first step in the treatment is reassurance to the parents that the condition is self-limiting and advice to avoid punitive measures that may affect the child's psychological development adversely. Nonpharmacologic and pharmacologic treatment has been tried. However, active treatment should be avoided in children younger than 6 years.

Nonpharmacologic Treatment: The nonpharmacologic measures consist of the following:

- Situational manipulations which include restriction of fluid intake in the evening after 6 or 7 o'clock, ascertaining that the child voids at bedtime, waking the child after few hours of sleep to have them void urine. These measures help to have dry nights in some cases. The child should be advised to try holding the urine for longer periods during day time which may help in some cases.
- Conditioning therapy which involves use of an auditory alarm attached to electrodes in the underwear. The alarm sounds when voiding occurs. It is intended to awaken the child to void urine. Conditioning therapy is shown to be effective in older children. Among the nonpharmacologic treatment this is found to be most effective.
- Self-hypnosis is another form of therapy to which some children responds. The primary aim of this therapy is to help the child deal with enuresis psychologically and help motivate arising to void at night.

Pharmacologic Treatment: Pharmacologic treatment of enuresis is intended to treat the symptom. It is not curative. It temporarily stops enuresis and majority will show recurrence after cessation of therapy. Drug treatment should not be started before 6 years age. Drug treatment is best advised to get rid of the symptom when the child is away from home temporarily and stopped as soon as the child is back.

Various drugs have been used. *Imipramine,* in the dose of 25 mg in children aged 6–8 years, 50 mg for 9–12 years and 75 mg for teenagers. It should be given at bedtime. It is a tricyclic antidepressant. The reported success rates are 30–60%. Side effects include dry mouth, anxiety and insomnia. *Desmopressin acetate* is another drug in use. It is a synthetic analogue antidiuretic hormone and reduces urine production over night. It is available as tablets and nasal spray. The tablet is given at a dose of 0.2–0.6 mg and the nasal spray with a dose of 10 microgram (1 spray) to 40 microgram (4 sprays) at bedtime. The lowest effective dose should be used. The effectiveness is around 40%. When effective it should be continued 3–6 months then tailed off. Hyponatremia has been reported with use of nasal spray. The oral preparation should not be used if the child has vomiting and diarrhoea. The nasal spray is ineffective in presence of rhinorrhoea. *Oxybutyrin chloride,* a pure anti-cholinergic agent, has been used in some children with primary nocturnal enuresis, but the response rate is low.

Associated UTI and worm infestations, if present should be treated.

Prevention: The most important aspect of this problem is prevention. The mainstay for prevention is timely bladder training. The bladder training should be best started at 12–16 months of age. For training bladder control, the child should be placed on the toilet at a definite time during the day, preferably in relation to some event in the daily routine e.g. at waking in the morning and after every nap during the day, before and after meals, after coming in from outdoors and at bed time. The toilet seat should be comfortable with adequate back support. No longer than 2–3 minutes on toilet should be permitted. When the infant can sit steadily without support, it is advisable to teach the use of the adult toilet seat. When the infant has learnt to urinate in the toilet at the times mentioned and to remain dry during the intervals, the time between the voiding should be lengthened. As soon as the child is dry during day, pants should be substituted for the diaper. Sometimes, this has a remarkable effect lessening frequency.

Diurnal Enuresis

Diurnal enuresis is more common in girls. It rarely occurs after the age of nine years. The most common cause is micturition deferral i.e. waiting until the last moment to void urine. It is common in a preschool child. Other etiological factors need to be considered include urinary tract infection, chemical urethritis, constipation, diabetes and stress incontinence. Children with voiding difficulties associated with enuresis are likely to have abnormalities of the urinary tract. These children require a thorough investigation to find out the cause and then treated.

Encopresis (Fecal Soiling)

Encopresis refers to repeated, involuntary evacuation of feces into clothing without a gross organic cause after the age of 4 years. Fecal soiling denotes uncontrolled defecation of emotional origin.

Encopresis is classified into primary or continuous which refers to a child who has never achieved bowel control and secondary or regressive which refers to a child who looses previously achieved control in response to stress. In contrast to enuresis, secondary encopresis is more frequent (about 65%). About two thirds of the cases are associated with constipation.

Unpleasant or coercive toilet training is an important etiological factor but it is more common in developed countries. Such children may have the fear of the pot or the toilet. The other factors may be (i) Separation from mother, (ii) Parental neglect, (iii) Dominating nagging mother, (iv) Birth of a sibling, (v) Overambitious parents, (vi) Start of school, (vii) Step mothers or unsatisfactory relationship with family members, and (viii) Hereditary. Personally, the children with encopresis are tense, easily frightened and very prone to anxiety reaction and with poor self-esteem. Physically these children are described as pale, sickly and asthenic.

Primary encopresis is associated with global developmental delay and enuresis. Secondary encopresis is associated with high levels of stress factors and conduct disorders. Encopresis may secondarily affect school performance and attendance as the child becomes the target of ridicule because of the offensive smell.

Treatment: The mainstay of treatment is removal of impacted fecal matter with short term use of laxatives, prevention of constipation with use of laxatives, high fibre diet and toilet training and simple behaviour therapy. This form of treatment is successful in majority of cases.

Prevention: The mainstay of prevention is bowel training at the appropriate age. Most infants can be trained by 12–16 months although many may not be trained until the end of 2 years. When stools are passed at the same time each day, the infant should be placed on the pot at expected time from the beginning. Two to three minutes is long enough to hold the child over the receptacle. If there is no result the child should be removed from the toilet without any comments. If successful, some words of appreciation may be said so that the child learns that he has done what is expected. The child may be merely placed over the receptacle after every feed which will suffice to stimulate defecation. This interval is gradually lengthened e.g. after alternate feeds followed by two times a day. With this the child may get trained by 15–18 months.

PROBLEMS OF SPEECH

Stuttering (Stammering)

Stuttering is a disorder of speech rhythm and fluency caused by intermittent blocking, convulsive repetition or prolongation of sounds, syllables, words or phrases.

Some repetition and hesitation is present in children who develop normal speech. This initial grouping for words has been referred to as physiological stuttering. It is not stuttering but just jumbling of words due to hesitation and repetition when the child starts talking. However, parental disapproval during this stage may produce tension when the child attempts to speak and create a pattern which more and more assumes the qualities of real stuttering.

In most children with stuttering, emotional factors play a vital role. It has been observed that parents of stutterers tend to be perfectionists holding the child to high standards of achievement in all spheres, which they have not enjoyed in their life. Some mothers are very anxious and want to see their child speaking sentences as early as possible. These give the child a lot of tension and anxiety which may be expressed as stuttering. There is no confirmatory evidence that heredity plays a role. However, it is known that parents who are stutterers are prone to be particularly anxious to correct early hesitations and repetitions in their child and thus set of tensions in connection with speech. Stuttering can also be a sequel to mental retardation, deafness etc.

Treatment: Though some children have been observed to acquire normal speech spontaneously after a period of stuttering, every stuttering child past three years age should be treated as it may lead to problems of academic, vocational, social and overall emotional adjustment. It should be noted that only children with repetition and hesitation of speech can recover spontaneously and not the real stutterers.

While treating the preschool child, the main attention should be directed towards the parental attitudes and policies which should be rectified so as to form an environment in which there is minimum anxiety, tension and disapproval. The parents should make the child realize that his speech was approved regardless of how he spoke. A friendly relationship should be created between the parents and the child. The parents should change their policy of criticizing and ridicule.

The school aged child requires a more personal approach. Individual psychotherapy can be instituted so as to allow the child to release tensions and hostility through play or drawing. They need speech therapy when they stutter for several years.

PROBLEMS OF SCHOOLING

School Phobia

School phobia refers to reluctance or fear of a child to go to school. The child has a fear of some aspect of the school. The fear may be the teacher, another child, anticipation of failing an examination etc. This is more evident in nursery school and girls. The oldest and youngest child in the family is more afflicted.

The preschool child has a feeling of insecurity when they are separated from parents, usually mother, while the older child may develop the withdrawal from school mates, defiance, sleeplessness and night terrors, truancy, learning difficulties etc. School phobia may be precipitated after an acute illness or an accident which is experienced by the child as a narrow escape from death. The other factors may be birth of a sibling, physical illness in parents, parental disharmony, parental overprotection or neglect etc.

At the time of departure for school from home, anxiety rapidly rises and may be accompanied by vomiting, headache, abdominal pain, giddiness, leg pains, and even fainting. When the child is allowed to remain at home, the anxiety rapidly abates and the child returns to a seemingly cheerful state.

Treatment: The problem is successfully treated by identifying and removing the precipitating factors. The parents and teachers should be advised to review and revise their faulty attitude.

SLEEP PROBLEMS

Nightmares and Night Terrors

Nightmare is a condition where the child awakens terrified after a horrific dream. The episode lasts for a few minutes. The child is able to describe his fearful dream. He can be reassured and becomes comfortable and may soon go off to sleep. *Night terror* is the condition where the child is obviously living through a horrific experience but he remains asleep and cannot recall the events of his dreams afterwards. The episode lasts for 15 to 20 minutes. There is often profuse sweating during the attack and the eyes are wide open with dilated pupils and a terrified expression on the face. Night terror and nightmare rarely persist into adolescence except in those who have been subjected to severe psychological trauma.

Treatment includes reassurance of the parents about their child's physical and mental well-being. Correction of any obvious psychological stress may be required in some cases.

Suggested Reading

1. Problems of behaviour in children (A practical guide for healthy upbringing) P.K. Singhal and M.S. Bhatia. CBS Publishers and Distributors, 485 Jain Bhawan, Bholanath Nagar, Delhi.
2. Practical Pediatric Problems. James H. Hutchison and Forrester Cockburn, 6th edition, 1986. Published by P.G. Publishing Pvt. Ltd., New Delhi.
3. Nelson Textbook of Pediatrics, 17th edition, 2004. Edited by Behrman, Kliegman and Jenson, Published by Saunders.
4. Matkin N (1984) Early recognition and referral of hearing impaired children. Pediatrics in review 6(5), 153.
5. Specific learning disability: The Invisible Handicap; Editorial Indian Pediatrics 2005; 42: 315–319.
6. The Development of the Infant and Young Child, Normal and Abnormal. Ronald S. Illingworth ELBS 9th Edition. Churchill Livingstone, U.K.

6

Nutritional Requirements in Children and Common Nutritional Disorders

OUTLINES

Nutrition is the basic component of life. It helps to attain normal growth and development as well as maintain good health throughout life. Adequate nutrition is the necessary first step in the improvement of quality of life.

Why Good Nutrition?

Good nutrition helps to prevent acute and chronic illness, to develop physical and mental potential and to provide reserve for stress. Knowledge of nutritional requirements is useful for the diagnosis of deficiency, specifying diet for critical age groups and to set targets for intervention programmes.

Food and Nutrition

It is not strictly correct to use these two terms synonymously. **Food** is a composite mixture of various substances, the quantity of which may vary from a fraction of a gram in certain cases to hundreds of grams in others. The term **foodstuff** is defined as anything which can be used as food. **Nutrition** is a dynamic process in which the food that is consumed is utilized for nourishing the body.

Balanced Diet

A balanced diet is one which supplies all the nutrients in the right quantity and proportion. It is essential for growth, to maintain good health and to prevent deficiencies. Carbohydrate should yield 55-60% of the calories, protein should yield 10-15% of the calories and fat should yield 30-35% of the calories.

A balanced diet in adequate amount and in proper consistency, appropriate for age, is what is necessary for proper growth and development of children.

Constituents of Food

Carbohydrates, fat, protein, vitamins, minerals and water.

Most food contains all the 6 constituents in varying amounts.

Proximate Principles of Food

Proteins, fats and carbohydrates.

Classification of Food

Food is classified on the basis of their predominant function, knowledge of which is necessary to prepare a balanced diet.

1. **Energy yielding food:** Food rich in carbohydrate and fat e.g. cereals, sugar, roots and tubers, oils.
2. **Body building food:** Food rich in protein e.g. milk, pulses, fish, eggs and meat.
3. **Protective food:** Food rich in protein, vitamins and minerals e.g. green leafy vegetables, fruits, protein rich food.

Functions of Food

1. Food provide energy.
2. Food is necessary for body building and repair.
3. It is required for maintenance and regulation of tissue functions.

Normal Requirements

Energy

The energy requirement of an individual is the level of energy intake from food that will balance energy expenditure when an individual has a body size and composition and level of physical activity consistent with good health.

The estimated energy necessary to build body tissue (growth) is the difference between the calories ingested and those expended for other purposes.

a. 1 gram of protein or carbohydrate provides 4 kcal. and 1 gram of fat provides 9 kcal.
b. 1 gram of short chain fatty acid provides 5.3 kcal.
c. 1 gram of medium chain fatty acid provides 8.3 kcal.
d. 1 gram of long chain fatty acid provides 9 kcal.

Critical Period for Energy Intake

There are two particularly critical periods in the early life of a young child as far as the energy requirement is concerned:

a. **At about 4-6 months age:** This is the period, when in most communities, supplements of breast milk are started. It is at this age that weight and height of many children in developing countries starts falling from the desired level.
b. **Between 1-2 years of age:** During this period breastfeeding is often terminated. Even if breastfeeding is continued it is bound to be inadequate as sole source of nutrient. The child, on the other hand, may not be able to partake his full share of the family meal, which may be very starchy and bulky. The child also gets involved into a lot of physical activity. This is the age where highest incidence of Protcin Energy Malnutrition is seen.

Estimated Energy Requirements

The energy requirement of the children depends on the periods of growth. It increases during the periods of rapid growth. A decreasing rate of growth results in decreasing requirements for energy per unit of size (kcal/kg).

Recommended Energy Requirements (Adapted from ICMR Group)

Group	*kcal/kg*	*Boys (kcal/day)*	*Girls (kcal/day)*
0-3 months	116	-	-
3-6 months	99	-	-
6-9 months	95	-	-
9-12 months	101	-	-
1-3 years	100	1287	1193
4-6 years	90	1752	1630
7-9 years	80	2075	1833
10-12 years	-	2194	1965
13-15 years	-	2447	2056
16-18 years	-	2642	2064

Holiday and Segar Formula for Calculation of Calories

- Upto 10 kg: 100 kcal/kg.
- 10–20 kg: 1000 + 50 kcal for each kg above 10 kg.
- Above 20 kg: 1500 + 20 kcal/each kg in excess above 20 kg.
- Expected weight is taken for calorie calculation.

Bedside Calculation of Calories

Age (years)	*Energy (kcal)*
1	1000
2	1100
3	1200
4	1300
5	1400
6	1500
7	1600
8	1700
9	1800
10	1900
11	2000
12	2100
Adolescent girl	2100
Adolescent boy	2400

Additional Energy

1. Allowances for pregnant women for fetal growth.

   1st trimester: 150 kcal/day.

   2nd and 3rd trimester: 300 – 350 kcal/day.

2. Allowances for lactating mothers
   1st 6 months: 550 kcal/day.
   6–12 months: 400 kcal/day.

Water

Human needs for water are related to caloric consumption, to insensible loss and to the specific gravity of urine. Dietary fluid provides the principal source of water. Some water is obtained from the oxidation of food and when needed from body tissues.

In the body, water acts as a solvent for cellular changes, a medium for ions, transport nutrients and waste products, and regulate body temperature.

Depending on the rate of growth 0.5-3% of fluid intake will be retained by the body. On an average, water 5-6 glasses/day in toddlers and 8-10 glasses/day in older children is recommended. Extra water is not recommended in infants.

Carbohydrate

No specific recommendation for intake of carbohydrate has been made as glucose can be synthesized from amino acids and glycerol moiety of fat. 40% of calorie intake in human milk is in the form of lactose. After the first 2 years of life, 55-60% or more of energy requirements should be derived from carbohydrates.

Glucose is the principal fuel for the brain and it is a necessary energy source for certain other tissues, including white and red blood cells. If the dietary carbohydrates do not meet the energy needs of the body to maintain glucose homeostasis, the body uses protein and glycerol from dietary and endogenous sources.

Protein

Protein requirement of an individual is defined as the lowest level of dietary protein intake that will balance the losses of nitrogen from the body in persons maintaining energy balance at modest level of physical activity. In children, the protein requirements include the energy needs associated with the deposition of tissues.

There are 9 amino acids, which the body cannot synthesize and hence are to be supplied in diet. They are called essential amino acids. These are: leucine, isoleucine, lysine, methionine, valine, threonine, tryptophan, phenyl alanine and histidine. Infants require higher proportion of cysteine, tyrosine and perhaps arginine.

Functions of Protein

1. It helps in growth of the child by tissue synthesis.
2. Formation of digestive juices, hormones, plasma proteins, enzymes, vitamins and hemoglobin.
3. It acts as a buffer.
4. It is a source of energy.

Requirements of Protein

Dietary protein must supply the essential amino acids in proper proportion needed by the body; therefore the quality of protein consumed is equally important. The efficiency of utilization of dietary protein depends upon its ability to supply the required amount of essential amino acids. Egg protein is used as a reference protein against which the quality of other protein is compared.

Both essential amino acids and a dietary source of nitrogen are required to maintain the positive balance. All calculations of protein requirement are done in a situation where energy requirements are met and if this condition is not fulfilled estimates of protein requirements will be meaningless since part of it will be utilized to provide energy.

The energy balance of the body is an important factor in determining the nitrogen balance and influences the utilization of dietary protein. A protein energy ratio between 8-12% would meet the protein requirement of any group provided its energy requirements are also met.

ICMR Suggested RDA of Proteins

Age (months)	*Daily req. (gm/kg)*	
0-3	2.3	
3-6	1.85	
6-9	1.65	
9-12	1.50	
Age (years)	*Boys*	*Girls*
1-2	1.81	1.81
2-3	1.67	1.67
3-4	1.61	1.61
4-6	1.52	1.52
7-9	1.48	1.48
10-12	1.46	1.45
13-15	1.40	1.33
16-18	1.31	1.21

Additional Allowances of Protein for Women

1. During pregnancy : 1st trimester: 1.3 gms/day.
   2nd trimester : 6 gm/day.
   3rd trimester : 10 gm/day.
2. During lactation : 1st six months: 15 gms/day.

Fats

Fats are the main dietary source of energy. Dietary source of fat may be invisible fat and visible fat or the added fats and oils. Upto 50% of energy in human milk is from fats.

Fat in the diet is a source of essential fatty acid, which is required for proper membrane function and synthesis of prostaglandin.

It improves the calorie intake by enhancing the energy density of food. This is an important consideration of Indian diet, which is cereal based and bulky. It improves palatability of diet.

It is required for absorption of fat soluble vitamins and for myelination of central nervous system.

Two families of poly unsaturated fatty acids (PUFA) are important viz. omega 6 fatty acid (Linoleic acid and arachidonic acid), omega 3 fatty acids (linolenic acid, eicosapentanoic acid and docosahexanoic acid). Among PUFA, omega-6 to omega-3 ratio of 5:1 is desirable. Cholesterol intake should be limited to 300 mg/day.

Energy to be provided from essential fatty acids:

1. Infants and children : 6% of total.
2. Pregnant women : 4.5%.
3. During lactation : 6%.

ICMR Recommendation of Fat Requirement

The ICMR recommends an intake of 20% of total energy as fat. At least 50% of fat intake should consist of vegetable oil rich in essential fatty acids. About half of total fat consumed comes from invisible fat present in the foods. Intake of fat as energy source beyond 30% is undesirable. Infants should receive minimum of 30% calories from fat (max. 40-50%) and for children > 2 years 30% of total calories from fat.

Group	*Fat intake(gm/day)—visible fat*	*Energy %*
1- 9 years	25	15
10-12 years	22	9
13-15 years	22	9
16-18 years	22	9

Dietary Fibres

Dietary fibres are of two types:

a. Insoluble fibres (cellulose, hemicellulose and lignin) which increases stool bulk and water content thereby the gut transit time.

b. Soluble fibres (pectin, mucillages) which bind bile acids and reduce lipids and cholesterol absorption.

The AAP suggests 0.5 gram dietary fibres/ kg upto 35 gram/day.

Important Minerals (Normal Requirement)

1. Iron : Infants : 1mg/kg, Children: 0.6 mg/kg.
   Adolescents: Boys: 25 mg/day, Girls: 35 mg/day.
   Allowance during pregnancy: 34 mg/day.
2. Calcium: Infants and children: 500–600 mg/day.
   Pregnancy and lactation: 1000 mg/day.

Important Vitamins (Normal Requirements)

1. Vitamin A: Birth to 6 months : 400 micro gram/day.
   Older children: 250–300 micro gram/day.
2. Vitamin D: Infants and children: 400 i.u./day.
3. Folic acid : Infants and children: 50 micro gram/day.
   Allowance during pregnancy: 200–400 micro gram/day.
   Lactation: 50 micro gram/day.

Essential Trace Elements

Elements which are present in the concentration not exceeding 250 microgram per gram of matrix are called trace elements.

Classification

WHO Expert Committee on Trace Elements in Human 'Nutrition and Health' Geneva 1996 has classified trace elements into three groups:

1. Essential elements: Iron, Iodine, Zinc, Selenium, Copper, Molybdenum and Chromium.
2. Probably essential: Manganese, Silicon, Nickel, Boron and Vanadium.
3. Potentially toxic: Fluorine, Lead, Cadmium, Mercury, Arsenic, Aluminum, Lithium and Tin.

Safe and adequate concentration of trace elements is required in the body for optimal function. Every trace element is potentially toxic when this range exceeds, and deficiency occurs when the concentration falls below the requirement. The potentially toxic trace elements are also necessary in small amounts.

Functions

Trace elements catalyze and control biochemical reactions. More than half of the enzymes in the human body have one or more of these trace elements at active sites. For example calcium and magnesium form complexes with enzymes and nucleic acid and act as biological triggers; zinc and copper are essential for enzyme activities and iodine for hormone synthesis.

Etiology

Primary deficiency
• *Inadequate intake:* Zinc, Copper, Iron, Iodine
Secondary deficiency
• *Genetic or inborn errors of metabolism:* Zinc, Copper
• Total parenteral nutrition: Copper, Zinc, Selenium, Iron, Manganese
• *Drugs:* Copper, Zinc, Iron
• *Environmental:* Iodine, Selenium
• *Malabsorption and chronic diarrhoea:* Iron, Zinc, Copper
• *Protein energy malnutrition:* Zinc, Copper
• *Prematurity and LBW (poor stores):* Iron , Copper, Zinc
• *High requirements:* Pregnancy, lactation, rapid growth in preterm infants: Zinc, Iron.
• *Element interaction with other nutrients and elements:* Copper/ Zinc, Iron/Copper, Iron/Manganese.
• *Increased excretion:* Nephrosis, liver cirrhosis, chelating agents, trauma, burns, pica, hemolytic anemia

(Adapted from IAP Textbook of Pediatrics, 1st edition, 1999)

Diagnosis of Deficiency and Excess

Symptoms and signs of deficiency and excess both are non-specific except for severe zinc deficiency. Hence a high degree of suspicion by clinicians is helpful for clinical diagnosis. Current laboratory techniques available for analysis of trace elements are atomic absorption spectrometry (AAS) and neutron activation analysis (NNA). It should be noted that presence of trace elements in laboratory atmosphere, glass ware, water and reagents can contaminate samples if care is not taken.

The trace elements of clinical importance - viz. Iron (*see* Chapter 8), zinc and iodine are described in details.

Zinc

The lean body mass zinc concentration is 30 microgram/ gram. It is chiefly distributed in skeletal muscles (60%) and bones (30%) and plasma (0.1%). However, zinc is present in all organs, tissues, fluids and secretions of the body.

Functions

1. Zinc is essential for stabilization of RNA, DNA and ribosome. It is important for functioning of biomembranes.
2. It participates in synthesis and degradation of carbohydrates, lipids, proteins and nucleic acids.
3. It is a part of many enzyme systems of the body viz. carbonic anhydrase. It is also thought that it has a role in the process of genetic expression.

Sources

Rich sources of zinc include animal sources like lean red meat and pork. Cheese, whole wheat, nuts and legumes also provide zinc. A high bioavailability of zinc is found in a refined diet low in cereal fiber and having a phytate / zinc molar ratio < 5.

Requirements

Children should receive about 10 mg/day. The requirement for adolescent males and females are 15 mg and 12 mg per day respectively. The recommended allowance for pregnant women is 15 mg/day and lactating mothers is 20 mg/day.

Clinical Manifestations of Deficiency Disorders

Mild zinc deficiency is manifested by reduced growth rate and recurrent infection due to impaired body resistance. Severe zinc deficiency is associated with growth retardation, anorexia, alopecia, behavioural changes and increased susceptibility to infection, acrodermatitis enteropathica and hypogonadism. Zinc deficiency in pregnant women has been linked with preterm delivery, IUGR, and neural tube defects in fetus. Relation of zinc with acute diarrhea has been discussed in the chapter of gastrointestinal system.

Zinc levels of plasma, blood cells, hair and urine decrease in severe deficiency state. Zinc supplementation/ fortification of diet have been found to show improvement of symptoms and signs of deficiency.

Iodine

Iodine deficiency in children is classically associated with goitre. Sea foods and vegetables grown on iodine rich soil are good sources of iodine. However, in India the soil in Himalayan region and the Ganges valley has severely low iodine content. Hence iodine deficiency is very much prevalent in these areas.

Requirement

The daily requirement varies with age. It is 50 micrograms (0 - 12 months age), 90 micrograms (1 - 6 years age), 120 micrograms (7 - 12 years age) and 150 micrograms (12 years onwards).

Clinical Manifestations of Iodine Deficiency Disorders

Iodine is an essential component of thyroid hormones. Iodine deficiency in mothers can result in abortions and still birth. It can lead to congenital anomalies, neurological and myxoedematous cretinism, goiter and psychomotor defects in the newborn. In children, it may result in goiter, juvenile hypothyroidism, mental as well as physical and sexual growth retardation. These conditions are discussed in detail in the chapter of endocrine disorders.

Control of Iodine Deficiency Disease

The first step in control of iodine deficiency disorders (IDD) is identification of areas of prevalence. It can be achieved by assessment of (i) goitre rate (ii) urinary iodine concentration or (iii) T4 and TSH levels in the population of the area.

Control of severe IDD requires administration of iodized oil to all women (upto 40 years) and males (upto 20 years) in areas of severe deficiency. The dose is 1 ml (contains 480 mg of iodine). The same dose may be repeated after 3 years if signs of severe iodine deficiency persist.

In mild and moderate IDD, elimination is possible by introduction of community iodine supplementation programme with iodized salt (containing 20 - 40 mg/kg).

Common Nutritional Disorders

The common nutritional disorders include Protein Energy Malnutrition, Vitamin A deficiency, Scurvy, Rickets and Obesity.

The term protein energy malnutrition (PEM) refers to a class of clinical conditions that may result from varying degree of protein lack and energy inadequacy. This nomenclature replaces the relatively older designation, i.e. protein calorie malnutrition (PCM), on the recommendation of the World Health Organization (WHO) and Food and Agriculture Organization (FAO).

The term PEM has been adopted because it is now widely agreed that the major limiting factors in the diet of children, particularly in the third world countries, are energy and protein, usually more of the former. Deficiency of protein is not primary and isolated. Almost always it appears to be due to poor intake of food (energy) as such. There is evidence that if the child's energy is taken care of, it will be difficult for him to suffer from significant protein deficiency. On the other hand, if the energy consumption is poor, whatever protein is taken is likely to be used to provide energy rather than to build tissues.

PROTEIN ENERGY MALNUTRITION

PEM is a clinical syndrome characterized by multiple progressively worsening deficiencies of nutrient. The different clinical forms of PEM constitute a continuous spectrum of the manifestations of malnutrition with common features of growth failure, impaired tissue repair, and energy shortage (WHO, 1973).

Consequences of PEM

1. Delay in motor and mental development e.g. low IQ (Severe PEM), behaviour problems, maladjustment, and learning problems.
2. Increased risk of morbidity and mortality. Severe PEM results in high mortality due to complications while mild to moderate PEM increases morbidity due to recurrent infection.
3. PEM in early years of life results in decreased physical and intellectual capacity as adolescents and adults.
4. An IUGR girl infant results in a stunted woman who again gives birth to an IUGR baby. This cycle continues and difficult to break. She suffers from cephalopelvic disproportion which results in complications during child birth.

Classification

There are several classifications coined by different workers at different times. One of the oldest classifications is Gomez classification. For practical purpose we have included three classifications which are useful for clinical use.

1. Clinical Classification (Jelliffe, 1969)

This classification is based on the clinical presentation of the different types of PEM. It is useful in tropical countries for diagnosis as well as management of cases.

a. Kwashiorkor.
b. Marasmus.
c. Marasmic Kwashiorkor.
d. Under nutrition.

2. Indian Academy of Pediatrics

The Indian Academy of Pediatrics has coined the following classification based on weight for age taking the reference weight as 50th percentile of NCHS. A weight of > 80% of the reference weight is taken as normal. While grading PEM 'K' should be added to every grade when edema is present.

a. Grade I : 70–80% of reference wt.
b. Grade II : 61–70% of reference wt.
c. Grade III : 51–60% of reference wt.
d. Grade IV : < 50% of reference wt.

3. Waterlow's Classification

Waterlow's classification measures the degree of wasting and stunting on the basis of weight for height. It helps to classify PEM as being acute or chronic. In acute malnutrition, weight is primarily affected. A proportionate reduction of weight and height points towards chronic malnutrition. A greater and disproportionate reduction in weight as compared to height indicates acute on chronic protein energy malnutrition. Waterlow's classification is as follows:

Table 6.1 : Waterlow's classification

Parameter	*Value**	*Nutritional status*
Weight for height	>80%	Normal
Height for age	>90%	
Weight for height	>80%	Stunted
Height for age	<90%	
Weight for height	<80%	Wasted
Height for age	>90%	
Weight for height	<80%	Wasted and
Height for age	<90%	stunted

* Reference standard NCHS data

Table 6.2: WHO classification of nutritional status

Signs	*Classify as*
Signs of severe visible wasting or Edema present in both feet or Weight for age < 3rd percentile or MUAC < 11.5 cm (6 months to 5 years)	Severe malnutrition
Reported weight loss or Weight for age < 15th percentile or Confirmed weight loss > 5 % since last visit or Growth curve flattening	Poor weight gain
Child is gaining weight	Growing appropriately

Stunting, underweight and wasting may be defined also as follows:

Stunting

It is defined as a child below 2 standard deviation score (-3 SD for severe stunting) from the median height for age of NCHS reference population.

Under Weight

It is defined as a child below 2 SD (-3 SD for severe under weight) from the median weight for age of NCHS reference population.

Wasting

It is defined as a child below 2 SD (-3 SD for severe wasting) from the median weight for height of NCHS reference population.

Evolution Hypothesis

Two major clinical syndromes, kwashiorkor and nutritional marasmus are widely recognized. These syndromes however, constitute only a tip of the iceberg of the problem of protein energy malnutrition. A vast majority of children suffer from mild to moderate malnutrition while they remain hidden in the community for one or other reason. Again many malnourished children show overlap in the clinical picture demonstrating features of both the severe deficiency states. They are labeled as marasmic kwashiorkor. Several theories have been put forward to explain the etiology of the severe forms of PEM.

Classical Theory of Protein Deficiency

According to this theory kwashiorkor is predominantly a protein deficiency and marasmus an energy deficiency. However, both energy and protein deficiency exist in both the syndromes. Edema in kwashiorkor is caused by hypoalbuminemia secondary to inadequate supply of amino acids.

Gopalan's Theory of Dysadaptation

Gopalan claims that the dietary background of children suffering from kwashiorkor and marasmus has no difference in protein intake. According to this theory marasmus is an extreme degree of adaptation to prolonged inadequacy of proteins and energy in diet. Kwashiorkor, on the other hand is a stage of adaptation failure or dysadaptation. The failure of adaptation may follow two situations: (a) Continued prolongation of the stress of malnutrition; and (b) Sudden precipitation or aggravation by fulminant infection such as measles, pertussis, pneumonia or acute diarrhoea. The theory also concludes that relatively mild effect of adaptation may be responsible for mild to moderate PEM. According to this hypothesis, since kwashiorkor follows dysadaptation in a marasmic child, most cases of severe PEM presents as marasmic kwashiorkor.

Golden's Theory of Free Radicals

The free radical theory, the most recent concept, concludes that kwashiorkor results from an imbalance between the production of free radicals and their safe disposal. The oxidative toxic stress in kwashiorkor leads to excess production of free radicals on one hand and the mechanism of their disposal is compromised on the other. The excess of free radicals cause cell membrane damage that leads to increased permeability resulting in edema. The damage is much more in kwashiorkor than marasmus. The excess free radicals in kwashiorkor are also linked with a fatty liver and the characteristic skin lesions.

Why PEM is Common in the Preschool Years?

The term PEM comprises very closely interrelated clinical syndromes. These syndromes are the result of differences in the severity and duration of deficiencies, the age of the child, and the relative importance of the protein deficiency in regard to that of calories. PEM is most common during the preschool years because of the following reasons:

1. The young child is transitional as regards diet, immunity to infection, and psychological dependence.
2. This is a period of rapid growth with high nutrient needs.
3. At this age, the nonimmune child comes in contact with various infections.
4. Psychological trauma results as a result of separation from mother frequently caused by pregnancy and arrival of another sibling.
5. Infants and preschoolers are dependent for their sustenance on their parents.

An adequate and age appropriate diet and prevention of recurrent infections during these vulnerable years can prevent PEM.

Clinical Conditions of PEM

Mild-Moderate PEM (Undernutrition)

These forms of PEM are mainly manifested by inadequate physical growth. The children look small for their age, and they do not present symptoms and signs of severe malnutrition. The earliest sign is reduced physical activity. At first there is slow gain in weight followed by arrested growth, under weight then stunting. Chest circumference lags behind head circumference after 1 year age. The child has a long body, thin limbs, large head, and winged scapulae, abdomen distended. The bone maturation is retarded and they are also retarded in mental development. Attention span, memory, abstract thinking and inter sensory integration is more affected than language and social development. The child may suffer from kwashiorkor or marasmus subsequently. These children commonly suffer from mild to moderate nutritional anemia, vitamin deficiencies, recurrent infections, worm infestation and chronic infections like tuberculosis.

Severe PEM

Severe PEM includes the conditions of marasmus, kwashiorkor and marasmic kwashiorkor.

Table 6.3 : Essential and non-essential features of the clinical conditions of severe PEM

Marasmus

1. Essential features
   - ❑ Growth retardation: Wasted, wasted and stunted.
   - ❑ Gross muscle as well as subcutaneous wasting.
   - ❑ Absence of edema.
2. Non essential features
   - ❑ G.I. manifestation.
   - ❑ Mineral and vitamin deficiency.
   - ❑ Infection and infestation.
   - ❑ Psychomotor changes viz.irritability, apathy in advanced cases.

Kwashiorkor

1. Essential features:
   - ❑ Growth retardation.
   - ❑ Muscle wasting with some retention of subcutaneous tissue.
   - ❑ Psychomotor changes.
   - ❑ Edema.
2. Non-essential features
   - ❑ Hair changes and skin changes.
   - ❑ G.I. manifestation: Diarrhoea, vomiting, anorexia.
   - ❑ Anemia: Dimorphic type.
   - ❑ Vitamin A, Vitamin D and C deficiency.
   - ❑ Hepatomegaly.
   - ❑ Infection and infestation.

Marasmic Kwashiorkor: Combined features of marasmus and kwashiorkor.

Marasmus

Marasmus of dietary origin, also called primary marasmus, is the commonly observed type. Severe dietary restriction is the primary and most important cause of marasmus in the underdeveloped and developing countries. The diet in these children may be adequate in qualitative terms but very insufficient in total amounts to satisfy the minimum requirements of the rapidly growing child. Under these circumstances, the child survives by utilizing his own tissues to maintain the minimum metabolic functions.

Marasmus is commonly seen in infants fed exclusively on breast milk when it is inadequate, prolonged breast-feeding with inadequate complementary feeds, artificially fed with breast milk substitutes like over diluted cow's milk or infant formula, very thin cereal gruels or other starchy products. Restriction of food, during and after periods of illness viz. diarrhoea, by mothers for fear of aggravation or relapse or severe dietary restriction by doctors/ health workers may be a cause.

Marasmus is more frequent in the first year of life than in older children. This is mainly because of two reasons. Firstly, the infant is rapidly growing and has high energy requirements. When dietary restrictions are severe, they can develop extreme wasting in a relatively short period of time. Secondly, for cultural reasons, the infant is more likely to be subjected to marasmus producing diet. The effects of this diet and early introduction of complementary feeding increase the incidence of diarrhoea in infants. In older children, marasmus occurs usually with associated chronic infection like tuberculosis or malabsorption and often develops to marasmic kwashiorkor.

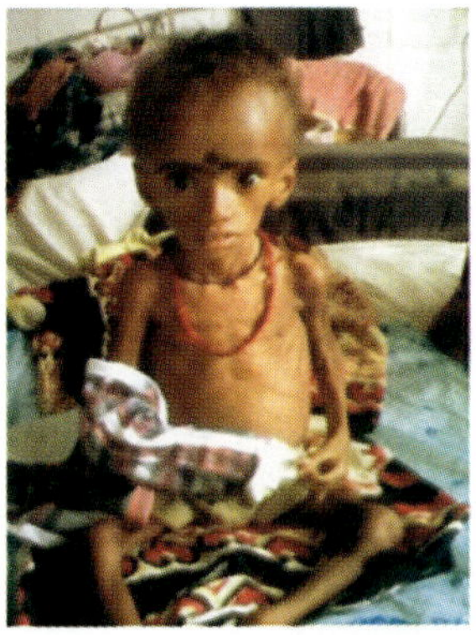

Fig. 6.1: Showing marasmas

Clinical Features

The early feature is arrest of growth followed by wasting of muscles and subcutaneous fat. During this period, the child is hungry, cries continuously and sleeps poorly. The infant is usually constipated or passes frequent small dark green stool of hunger diarrhoea.

If the child is not cared for during this period, the full blown picture of marasmus develops. The child is emaciated, usually weighing less than 60% of the standard weight, with varying degrees of loss of subcutaneous fat depending on the period of illness. Loose folds of skin are prominent over the glutei and the inner side of the thigh due to lack of subcutaneous fat. The buccal pad of fat is preserved till malnutrition is very severe because a higher proportion of saturated fatty acids are stored here and the saturated fat is the last to be depleted. The skin is thin, flaccid, wrinkled, seeming larger than the body it covers, particularly when the wasting has been rapid. The muscles are atrophic. Their shape can be seen under the flaccid skin when contracted. The mucous membrane is usually reddish in contrast to the pale and cold skin particularly of the face and extremities. The bony prominences seem to protrude because of loss of subcutaneous tissue. The abdomen is distended due to wasting and hypotonia of the abdominal wall muscles.

The typical skin lesions and hair changes are not present as seen in kwashiorkor. However, the hair may be thin and dry. The child is usually irritable but alert and gestures with anxiety as if asking for care. All these features make up the typical facies which has been compared to that of an old little wise man or a monkey.

The child may present with diarrhoea and dehydration. The child is usually hungry but cannot tolerate large amounts of food and vomits easily. Mineral and vitamin deficiency are fairly common. There is mild to moderate anemia of varied morphology. Superadded infections and parasitic infestations are common.

Pathological, Hematological and Biochemical Alterations

Pathologically, there is marked atrophy of practically all the organs and tissues of the body. The histological alterations are however minimal.

The hematocrit and hemoglobin levels are slightly reduced except when a superimposed cause is present.

Total serum protein and plasma amino acid levels are slightly depressed but the ratio of essential to non-essential amino acids tends to remain normal, suggesting that muscle amino acids help to maintain a normal composition of the amino acid pools. The serum free fatty acids are elevated indicating lipolysis from adipose tissue. Fasting blood sugar is found low when the period without food is prolonged (6 hours or more) which suggest a low liver glycogen reserve.

Kwashiorkor

The earliest description of kwashiorkor was made in 1933 by Professor Cicely Williams, a British physician. The term kwashiorkor is the local name for the disease in Ghana. It means 'the red boy', because of the characteristic pigmentary changes. Later the term was more aptly interpreted to apply to the disease as it affected the deprived child due to arrival of yet another.

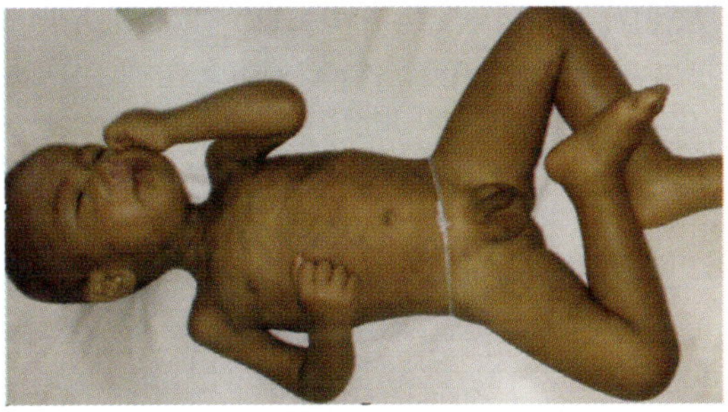

Fig. 6.2: Showing kwashiorkor

The disease is chiefly encountered in the age group of 1–5 years although no age is exempt. It is often a disease of the artificially fed and weaned children. It may however, be seen in breast fed babies who are receiving small amounts of breast milk and additional starch or sugar. In the tropics, the children are usually breast fed during the first year of life; hence kwashiorkor occurs frequently during the second and third year of life. Early introduction of complementary feeds prepones the age of onset of kwashiorkor.

Clinical Features

Apathy and anorexia are the early manifestations. The dietary history reveals that the child is being fed on a very low protein diet, generally based on cereal grains, starch roots and fruits, e.g., sago, barley, ground rice (all cooked in water), banana etc. These children become less lively and refuse to eat. The full blown picture of edematous PEM (Kwashiorkor and marasmic kwashiorkor) ensues after an episode of an infectious disease like diarrhoea, pneumonia, measles from which the child does not recover.

Pitting edema is the main clinical feature of kwashiorkor, on which the diagnosis is based. It is soft, painless, and of varied degree. It may be observed only in the feet and ankles or may be generalized with eye lids swollen and fluid in the peritoneal cavity. The edema usually starts in the lower extremities often spreading to the upper extremities and to the face. The trunk is less frequently affected part of the body.

Psychological changes are constant and very characteristic in kwashiorkor. Most children are apathetic, indifferent to their environment, and have an expression of misery. They resent being disturbed and protest with a monotonous and weak cry to any stimulus even when food is given to them. In some cases, the child is lethargic. The psychological changes are reversible with adequate treatment.

On anthropometric evaluation, there is growth retardation with marked muscle wasting with some retention of subcutaneous fat. Usually both height and weight are affected because kwashiorkor mostly develops in a chronically malnourished child with variable degree of retardation of growth and development.

The four signs viz. growth retardation, edema, psychomotor changes and muscle wasting with some retention of subcutaneous fat are constant features and taken together are sufficient to label a case as kwashiorkor.

Skin lesions are characteristic of kwashiorkor but not always present. Large areas of skin show erythema followed by hyperpigmentation and desquamation to expose raw hypopigmented areas. It gives the appearance of old paint flaking off the surface of wood; hence called 'flaky paint dermatosis'. In some cases the dermatosis can start as small, punctiform areas of hyperpigmentation and hyperkeratosis which grow progressively and become

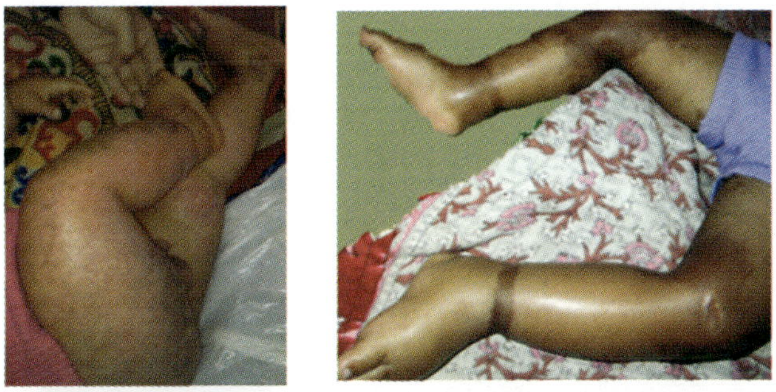

Fig. 6.3a: Skin lesions and edema in edematous PEM

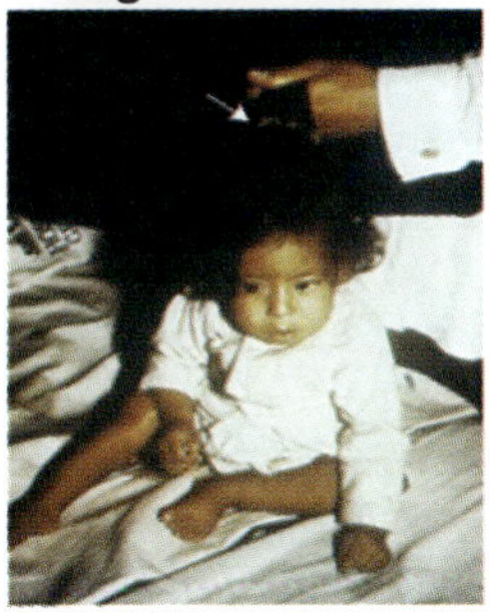

Fig. 6.3b: Figure showing flag sign

confluent. The exposed skin over areas of gross edema or of pressure, are wet and can easily be infected leading to indolent ulcers. There may be petechiae or ecchymosis in severe cases and should be considered as sign of bad prognosis.

Hair changes are characteristic but not a constant sign. The hair becomes dry, thin, lusterless and easily pluckable. When originally curly becomes straight. Black hair may become brown or brownish red. The color change may be uniform through all the length of the hair or may be stripes of different intensity of pigmentation. The depigmented parts indicate periods of malnutrition whereas the more pigmented parts indicate good nutrition. This is described as the 'flag sign'.

Diarrhoea is almost always present on presentation. It may start as an acute episode and then continue as persistent or chronic diarrhoea. Even when diarrhoea is not present, the stool volume is large, a manifestation of intestinal malabsorption. Vomiting may be present especially when the child is forced to eat more than usually accepted.

There is *anemia* of the dimorphic type due to iron and folic acid deficiency. Overt signs of vitamin A deficiency are present in majority of cases. Overt signs of vitamin D deficiency i.e. rickets may manifest during recovery stage once growth starts. Signs of other vitamin deficiencies may be present. The liver is usually enlarged due to fatty infiltration which is reversible after adequate treatment.

Combined Forms

This category of PEM includes marasmic kwashiorkor. In developing countries the common form of PEM is marasmic kwashiorkor where the signs and symptoms of kwashiorkor develop in a child who already has a more or less advanced degree of energy deficiency.

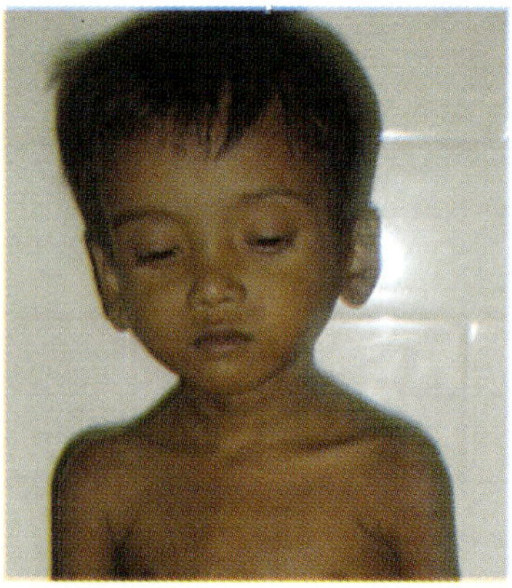

Fig. 6.4: Apathy in edematous PEM

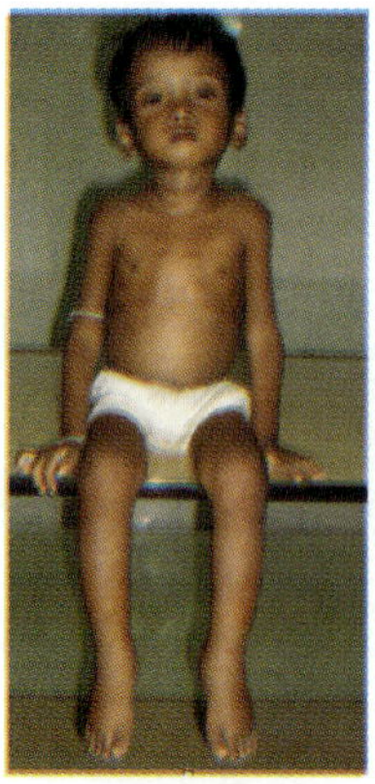

Fig. 6.5: Marasmic kwashiorkor

It is usually seen in a child that has not been growing well for some time and is underweight. This may be because the diet the child is receiving, although sufficiently balanced, is insufficient in total amount. In these children frequent, recurrent, or chronic infections, particularly diarrhoeal disorders act as aggravating factors of the existing state. It is at this time that a more serious attack of diarrhoea, a severe respiratory infection, or measles, or a serious deterioration of diet for socio-economic or cultural reasons, may precipitate the child to acute protein deficiency resulting in development of kwashiorkor in an already marasmic child. When these children are properly treated, the signs and symptoms as well as the pathological and biochemical alterations of kwashiorkor disappear in a few weeks time, leaving behind a grossly emaciated child with or without markedly retarded growth and development.

Clinically, they present with signs and symptoms of a combined form of marasmus and kwashiorkor.

Pathological, Hematological and Biochemical Alterations

Most of the informations about the pathological, hematological and biochemical alterations are obtained from necropsy studies in combined forms of PEM. By comparison of the alterations observed in the combined forms with those observed in pure marasmus, the following are the characteristic alterations in kwashiorkor:

Pathology

In the *liver* there is marked fatty changes with increase in reticulin fibres radiating from the portal tract. These changes are reversible and do not lead to cirrhosis. In the *gastrointestinal tract* there is atrophy of mucosa at the level of the fundus and in the intestine. The brush border of the small intestine is atrophied and disorganized and so the activity of many enzymes which are located in this segment of the cell (i.e. disaccharidases, dipeptidases, lipases) is reduced. In the *pancreas*, atrophy of acini and loss of zymogen granules is the most conspicuous lesion which leads to hypofunction of the gland. In the *kidney* there is fatty degeneration of the cells of the convoluted tubules and hyalinization of the glomerulus. The *thymus* is atrophic with fat replacing the lymphoid tissue. The *heart* is atrophic and cardiac output is low. There are also non-specific ECG changes like T inversion and elevation of ST segment in chest leads. No significant cardiac involvement is observed. The atrophy and hyperkeratosis observed in the *skin lesions* is similar to the dermatosis of pellagra. The skin and hair changes results from deficiency of essential fatty acids, amino acid tyrosine, Vitamin A and zinc.

Hematology

The total red cell mass and total circulating hemoglobin are significantly reduced in relation to body weight even in presence of a normal hemoglobin and hematocrit. The reduction in total hemoglobin is proportional to the marked reduction in active tissue mass. Thus there is no physiological anemia but anemia may rapidly develop during recovery. This is because during recovery there is increase in tissue mass and rapid hemopoetic process takes place to maintain the required hemoglobin concentration. The rate of red cell production during recovery from severe PEM is however, determined by the rate of recovery of active tissue mass as a consequence of protein repletion. The anemia which develops is of the dimorphic type which requires supplementation with iron as well as folic acid. Presence of severe anemia in severe PEM indicates investigation for some other etiology.

Biochemical Alterations

There is *overhydration* in terms of total body water per unit of body weight or body surface which involves all the fluid spaces. There is sodium retention and potassium deficit. *Sodium excess* is primarily extracellular. Intracellular excess are seen in muscles, skin, viscera and brain. *Potassium deficit* is intracellular together with magnesium.

Glucose absorption and handling of intravenous glucose and galactose is abnormal. Absorption of intestinal lactose and occasionally sucrose is reduced because of deficiency of disaccharidases. There is *hypoglycemia* which results from prolonged fasting, decrease glucose-6- phosphatase in the liver and possibly decreased neoglucogenesis.

Fasting circulating insulin levels are low normal and fail to respond adequately to glucose stimulation. In contrast, serum growth hormone is elevated and does not lower on administration of glucose infusion. There is a relatively elevated epinephrine level and free plasma cortisol level which is responsible for the active lipolysis.

Fat absorption in the intestine is reduced. It is further reduced in presence of diarrhoea. Fecal fat is increased even when the diet is free from fat. The reduction of intestinal absorption of fat is due to blunting of the intestinal villi as a result of toxic injury caused by frequent bouts of infective diarrhoea and high concentration of free bile acid through out the small intestine and gallbladder. The fatty liver of kwashiorkor appears to be due to increased fat transport from adipose tissues, to decreased synthesis of lipoproteins hampering the transport of fat from the liver to the tissues and possibly to increased liver lipogenesis. Deficiency of pancreatic lipase is not the limiting factor in fat absorption. The circulating levels of vitamin A are decreased even in presence of adequate amount in the liver because of decreased production of retinol binding protein.

The *total serum protein* level is reduced and it is mainly due to hypoalbuminemia. The total albumin pool is decreased; the intravascular compartment being less affected than the extravascular. The concentration of beta globulins is also decreased while that of alpha 1, alpha 2 and gamma globulins is high. Plasma amino acids are low. The most affected ones are valine, leucine, isoleucine and tyrosine while phenylalanine, lysine, alanine and threonine remain constant. The ratio of essential to non-essential amino acids is altered.

Management

Where to Treat?

Cases of *mild-moderate PEM* do not require hospitalization. Ordinary hospital wards are not suitable for treating these children because all they need is an adequate diet and general attention. They are at risk of infection. Moreover, the general wards are usually meant for children whose hospitalization is imperative for specialized medical care and the nurses and doctors are busy with such children. The result is that recovery may take longer than necessary and even be risky. They can be taken care of either on a complete ambulatory basis with the child living at home or attending a nutritional rehabilitation centre where the child can be fed and taken care of for some hours of the day.

When treatment is planned with the child at home, the mother or the person in charge of the child should be properly instructed as to the child's care and if necessary supplementary food should be provided. The parents should be advised for frequent visits to the hospital. There should also be home visits by qualified personnel. This type of treatment should be preferred because it is cost effective with better results.

Nutritional Rehabilitation Centres

The best place to take care of these children is a nutritional rehabilitation centre where in addition to providing adequate dietary treatment and other medical and general care services, mothers can be educated by direct personal experience, making them participate in the selection, preparation, and administration of food and in the general care of the children under the guidance of qualified personnel. These centres are best suited for children with moderate and uncomplicated severe PEM and for those severe PEM who are discharged from hospital after initial treatment and who are out of danger of death.

The children with *severe PEM* with complications need hospitalization. The criteria for admission to hospital are:

a. Weight < 60%.
b. Age < 1 year.
c. Persistent loss of appetite.
d. Presence of complication.

Treatment

Children suffering from PEM can be divided into two groups, depending upon the type of treatment required. These are mild to moderate cases without complications and severe cases with complications.

Mild and Moderate PEM

All cases of mild-moderate PEM should undergo a thorough physical examination to detect any associated disease. The following investigations should be advised:

1. Hemoglobin, total leucocytic and differential leucocytic count and a peripheral blood smear to study the cell morphology and malaria parasite.
2. Stool examination for ova and cysts.
3. Urinalysis and culture when indicated.
4. Tuberculin test and a chest X-ray when indicated.

Advice on Diet

In case of mild and moderate PEM there is a deficit in normal energy and protein intake. The deficit has to be corrected with supplementation. The parents have to be explained about the inadequacy of the child's intake as well as the quality of diet. They should be instructed how to correct it. The normal requirement of calorie and protein for age has to be calculated and a diet planned for the child. While planning, care should be taken to include locally available, cheap but nutritious food items.

In mild PEM energy and protein intake should be increased according to the requirement for age. In moderate PEM recommended energy intake is 150 kcal/kg body weight out of which 8–10% should come from protein source.

Treatment of Associated Conditions

In addition, the child should receive treatment for existing infection and infestation, and supplementation of iron and folic acid to correct anemia as well as treatment of vitamin deficiencies.

Growth Monitoring

Growth monitoring at frequent intervals till recovery and thereafter at regular interval should be done in all children undergoing nutritional rehabilitation. It is important because appropriate weight gain is by far the best yardstick of adequacy of response to the treatment. Recovery with well organized domiciliary care may take 2–3 months.

Severe PEM (WHO Guidelines for Inpatient Treatment)

The WHO and UNICEF proposed diagnostic criteria for severe acute malnutrition in children aged 6–60 months include any one of the following: (i) Weight for height below–3 standard deviation (SD or Z scores) of the median WHO growth reference (2006); (ii) Visible severe wasting; (iii) Presence of bipedal edema; and (iv) Mid arm circumference below 11.5 cm.

No distinction has been made between the clinical conditions of Kwashiorkor, Marasmus and Marasmic kwashiorkor because the approach to treatment is same.

Children with severe PEM are at risk of several life threatening complications like:

1. Hypoglycemia defined as glucose <3 mmol/l (<54 mg/dl).
2. Hypothermia defined as axillary temp<35° C.
3. Infection including pneumonia, acute gastroenteritis, malaria, tuberculosis.
4. Diarrhoea with dehydration and electrolyte disturbances/shock.
5. Jaundice, bleeding, septic shock.

Prompt and vigorous treatment is necessary in these cases in order to prevent mortality and morbidity. The bad prognostic factors include serum albumin <1 gm/dl, total bilirubin > 6 mg/dl, serum Na <120 mEq/l. Severe PEM carries a mortality of around 20%.

Plan of Management

The plan of management includes the following steps:

1. A quick and thorough history and physical examination to detect complications.
2. Investigations to be done as and when indicated.

(i) In all cases

   a. Blood sugar, electrolytes Na, K, Mg

   b. CBC, Hb% and peripheral blood smear for study of cell morphology and malaria parasite

   c. Tuberculin test

   d. Urine culture

   e. X-ray PA view chest

(ii) When indicated

   a. Liver function test, kidney function test

   b. Blood culture

   c. ECG.

3. Treatment and prevention of complications.
4. Feeding (nutrients and micronutrients).
5. Sensory stimulation.
6. Treatment of associated conditions.
7. Follow-up.
8. Preventive measures.

Treatment of Complications

The most common complications with which the child can present are hypothermia, hypoglycemia, infection and dehydration with electrolyte imbalance.

On admission the child should be separated from infectious children and kept in a warm area (temperature 25–30°C) with no draughts, well covered with cloths. The blood glucose should be checked with dextrosticks, to exclude hypoglycemia (blood glucose < 54 mg/dl). If estimation is not possible child should be treated for hypoglycemia. The temperature should be recorded to detect hypothermia (axillary temperature < 35°C, rectal temperature < 35.5°C). It needs mention that hypoglycemia and hypothermia occur together. They are also signs of infection.

In severe PEM, the usual signs of infection like fever are often not present. Therefore antibiotics to cover both gram positive and negative organisms should be started routinely.

Assessment of dehydration by clinical signs is also difficult in cases with severe PEM. In presence of dehydration, the oral mucosa feels dry to the palpating finger gently rolled on the inner side of the cheek. Presence of thirst, hypothermia, weak pulses and oliguria are signs of severe dehydration. However, in a child with severe PEM, dehydration should be assumed if watery diarrhoea is present.

Treatment of Hypothermia and Hypoglycemia

The child has to be rewarmed till the temperature rises to 35°C. Warming can be done by kangarooing. The child can also be covered with a blanket from head to feet with a room heater nearby. The room should be warmed

General Principles for Routine Care (WHO Recommendation)

Activity	Stabilization Days 1-2	Stabilization days 3 – 7	Rehabilitation weeks 2 – 6	Follow up weeks 7 – 26
Treat or prevent				
1. Hypoglycemia	→			
2. Hypothermia	→			
3. Dehydration	→			
Correct				
4. Electrolyte imbalance	→	→	→	
Treat				
5. Infection	→	→		
6. Micronutrients	Without iron →	Without iron →	with iron →	
Feeding				
7. Initiate feeding	→	→		
8. Increase feeding			→	→
Start				
9. Sensory stimulation	→	→	→	→
Prepare				
10. Follow up	→	→	→	→

with the help of room heaters to maintain the room temperature at 25–30°C.

If the child throws a seizure or become unconscious due to hypoglycemia intravenous infusion of 10% glucose, 5–10 ml/kg should be given. Otherwise a bolus of dose of 50 ml 10% glucose / 10% sucrose solution (1 rounded teaspoonful of sugar in 50 ml water) should be given orally or by N/G tube. The bolus should be followed by 16 ml/feed every 30 minutes to be continued till the child is stable. The bolus dose may be followed by the first feed followed by 2 hourly feeds, day and night, atleast for the first day.

A broad spectrum antibiotic should be started empirically to cover both the gram positive and gram negative bacteria.

Monitoring: The child's temperature should be recorded 2 hourly till the temperature rises to more than 36.5°C or 97.7°F. Temperature should be recorded half hourly if a heater is used.

The blood glucose should be checked after 2 hours. If still low a repeat bolus of 50 ml 10% dextrose or sucrose should be repeated. And feeding continued every 30 minutes.

Prevention: It should be ensured that the child is kept covered at all times. The head should be kept covered with a warm bonnet to reduce heat loss.

- Feeding should be started immediately and continued 2 hourly including night feeds.
- Place the bed of the child in a warm, draught-free part of the ward.
- Wet nappies and clothes and bedding should be changed and bed kept dry.
- Exposure should be avoided during bathing or during physical examination.
- The child should be bedded in with the mother at night to maintain warmth.

Treatment and Prevention of Dehydration

Oral rehydration therapy should be the treatment of choice for dehydration except when the child is in severe dehydration and shock. WHO recommends use of 'ReSoMal' (rehydration solution for malnourished).

Composition of ReSoMal

Component	*Mmol / L*
Glucose	125
Sodium	45
Potassium	40
Chloride	70
Citrate	7
Magnesium	3
Zinc	0.3
Copper	0.045

Mild to Moderate Dehydration

The deficit therapy of 70–100 ml/kg should be given slowly over a period of 12 hours to restore normal hydration. The fluid deficit should be replenished with ReSoMal which should be given orally or by a nasogastric tube @ 5 ml/kg every 30 minutes for 2 hours; thereafter 5–10 ml/kg/hour. Ongoing stool losses should be corrected with 50–100 ml ReSoMal after each watery stool.

Severe Dehydration and Shock

Intravenous route should be used in cases with severe dehydration and shock in the form of Ringers lactate or saline in 5% dextrose in the dose of 30 ml/kg in first 2 hours followed by N/6 saline in 5% dextrose in the dose of 70 ml/kg in next 10 hours. This should be followed by administration of the same solution @ 5 ml/kg/hr in next10 hours. Thereafter, if dehydration is corrected maintenance therapy can be started with N/6 saline in 5 % dextrose in the dose of 75–100 ml/kg/day till feeding is established.

Monitoring: The progress of rehydration should be monitored half hourly for two hours, and then hourly for next 6–12 hours. The following parameters should be checked: respiratory rate, pulse rate, frequency of urine, stool and vomiting. With replenishment of the fluid the child's pulse rate and respiratory rate should decrease and the child should begin to pass urine. Continued fast breathing and rapid pulse rate during rehydration suggest coexisting infection or over dehydration. Return of tears, a moist mouth, less sunken eyes and fontanelle and improved skin turgor are signs that rehydration is proceeding. However, it should be noted that many severely malnourished children will not show such changes even when fully rehydrated.

Prevention: Prevention of dehydration should be in the line of plan A as in case of normal children except that ReSoMal should be used in place of WHO-ORS. It should be noted that in malnourished children it is common to pass small amounts of unformed stool many times a day. This should not be confused with the profuse watery stools and they do not require fluid replacement.

If the child is breast fed, breastfeeding should be continued. Feeding should be initiated and ReSoMal (50–100 ml) should be given after each watery stool to replenish ongoing losses.

Correction of Electrolyte Imbalance

All cases with severe PEM have deficiency of potassium and magnesium which may take two weeks or more for correction. Although the plasma sodium is low there is excess body sodium. Sodium should be restricted to prevent sodium overload and water retension during the initial phase. Food should be prepared without adding salt. No diuretics should be given to treat edema.

All cases should be given extra potassium (3–4 mmol/ kg daily) and magnesium (0.4–0.6 mmol / kg/day) from day 1 for 2 weeks in the form of a mineral/electrolyte mixture. 20 ml of this solution should be added to 1 litre of feed during preparation.

Severe hypokalemia is clinically characterized by weakness of abdominal muscles, skeletal and even respiratory muscles. The muscle weakness is reversible on administration of potassium.

Septic Shock

If a child with severe PEM in shock does not show any improvement with IV fluid therapy after 2 hours, septic shock should be considered. Broad spectrum antibiotics should be started after sending blood for culture. Blood or plasma transfusion should be started @ 10 ml/kg over a period of 3 hours. A central venous pressure line should be inserted and the child should be managed for septic shock in an ICU.

Treatment and Prevention of Infection

Gram negative septicemia should be considered in cases that appear very sick and hypothermic. The common organisms are Klebsiella, salmonella and opportunistic organisms. The other infections include skin and soft tissue infections, pneumonia, meningitis, urinary tract infection, infective diarrhoea etc. Malaria may present with only diarrhoea and no fever. A blood culture, a chest X-ray, peripheral smear/antigen test for malarial parasite and urine culture should be obtained in all very sick cases before starting antimicrobials. If meningitis is suspected, lumbar puncture should be done to confirm diagnosis.

When facilities for such investigations are not available all children with severe PEM should be empirically started on an antibiotic on their arrival in the hospital.

Choice of antibiotics: If the child has no complications, cotrimoxazole: 5ml (2.5 ml if wt< 4 kg) × 5 days. If severely ill (apathetic, lethargic) or has complication viz. hypothermia, hypoglycemia etc, Ampicillin 50 mg/kg/dose IM 6 hrly + Gentamicin 7.5 mg/kg /dose 12 hrly × 7 days. If no response, Chloramphenicol 25 mg / kg IM/ IV 6 hourly × 5 days should be added. Anti-malarial should be given in children with a positive slide. Anti-tuberculous treatment should be given only after diagnosis or when strongly suspected. Tuberculin test may be negative in severe PEM, even in presence of tuberculosis.

All children with severe PEM should be given an anthelmintic after day 7 of admission, in areas of high prevalence even when stool examination is not positive of ova.

Treatment of Micronutrient Deficiency

All cases of severe PEM have vitamin and mineral deficiencies. Although anemia is common, iron should be started usually after the second week when the child has a good appetite and starts gaining weight, because iron can make infections worse.

The following should be given to the child daily from day 1 for atleast 2 weeks:

- A multivitamin supplement, which should not contain iron.
  - Folic acid 5 mg on day 1, then 1 mg per day.
  - Zinc, 2 mg/kg/day.
  - Copper, 0.3 mg/kg/day.
  - Potassium chloride 2 mEq/kg/day per oral.
- Iron, 3 mg/kg/day, from second week for 3–4 months.
- Vitamin A orally on day 1 (< 6 months age: 50,000 IU, 6–12 months: 100,000 IU and older children 200,000 IU).

Feeding

Initial Phase

The child with severe PEM has a fragile physiological state and a reduced hemostatic capacity. So in the initial phase of feeding, a cautious approach is required. Feeding should be started as soon as possible. The essential features to be maintained during the initial feeding include the following:

1. Sufficient energy and protein to maintain physiological needs.
2. Small frequent feeds of low osmolality and low lactose content.
3. Oral or nasogastric feeds may be given. Parenteral preparation should never be used. Oral feeds should

be given from a cup or a bowl or with a spoon, dropper or a syringe.

4. Initial requirement:

   Calorie: 100 kcal/kg, gradually increased upto 200 kcal /kg.

   Protein: 1–1.5 gms/kg /day.

   Fluid: 130 ml/kg/day (100 ml/kg/day if child has severe edema).

5. If the child is breast fed, it should be continued but the scheduled amount of starter formula should be continued.

6. Feeding should be started with a milk based formula such as starter F-75 (75 kcal/100 ml and 0.9 gm protein/100 ml). This is satisfactory for most children. A cereal based Formula, F-75 which partially replaces sugar with cereal flour, has the advantage of lower osmolarity which may benefit some children with persistent diarrhoea but this preparation needs to be cooked.

Schedule of Feeding

A recommended schedule, with gradual increase in feed volume and decrease in feeding frequency is as shown below. Night feeds are essential to avoid long periods without feeds.

Days	*Frequency*	*Vol/kg/feed*	*Vol/kg/day*
1-2	2 hrly	11 ml	130 ml
3-5	3 hrly	16 ml	130 ml
6-7+	4 hrly	22 ml	130 ml

For children with good appetite and no edema, this schedule can be completed in 2–3 days. If the child's intake does not reach 80 kcal/kg/day despite frequent feeds, the remaining part should be given through a nasogastric tube. In the initial phase calorie should not exceed 100 kcal/kg.

Monitoring: During the initial phase, the diarrhoea should gradually diminish and edematous children should lose weight as edema disappears. Monitoring includes the following parameters:

a. Amount of feed offered and left over.
b. Vomiting.
c. Stool frequency and consistency.
d. Daily body weight.

Rehabilitation Phase and Catch-up Growth

The rehabilitation phase starts after about 7 days. The first sign is return of appetite. Aim of dietary therapy is to achieve a weight gain of > 10 gm/day and at the same time be alert to avoid the risk of congestive heart failure, which can occur if the child suddenly consumes huge amounts.

Feeding During Rehabilitation Phase

In the initial period, milk based formula, such as F-100 which contains 100 kcal / 100 ml and 2.9 gm of protein / 100 ml should be given for 2–3 days. Along with porridges, complementary foods with comparable energy and protein contents can be used. Each feed is increased by 10 ml until child consumes about 200 ml/kg/day.

After this transition the child should be given frequent feeds of unlimited amounts with a calorie supply of 150 – 220 kcal /day and protein 4–6 grams /kg/day.

Table 6.4 : Recipes of refeeding formulas F-75 and F-100

	F- 75 starter	*F- 75 starter cereal based*	*F- 100 catch up*
Dried skimmed Milk (gms)	25	25	80
Sugar (gms)	100	70	50
Cereal flour (gms)	-	35	-
Vegetable oil (gms)	27	27	60
Electrolyte/Mineral Solution (ml)	20	20	20
Water upto (ml)	1000	1000	1000
Contents /100 ml			
Energy	75	75	100
Protein (gm)	0.9	1.1	2.9

Table 6.5 : Energy rich food preparations

	Constituents	*Calories/ 100 gm*	*Protein/ 100 gm*
Preparation (1)	Bengal gram flour (1 part) Wheat flour (1 part) Jaggery (1 part) Ghee (1 part)	500	9
Preparation (2)	Milk 750 ml Sugar 100 gm Suji 25 gms Oil 5 gm Water upto 1000 ml	143	2.8
Preparation (3) (Hyderabad mix)	Whole wheat 40 gm Bengal gram 16 gm Groundnut 10 gm Jaggery 20 gm	330/86 gm	11.3/86 gm

Prevention and Treatment of Congestive Heart Failure

Heart failure is unlikely if a gradual transition is followed. However, as a precaution, the early signs of heart failure such as rapid breathing and tachycardia should be monitored. If both the pulse and breathing rates increased (breathing by 5 breaths / minute and pulse by 25 beats / minute) and the increase is sustained for two successive 4 hourly readings then the volume of feed should be reduced to 100 ml/kg/day for 24 hours, then slowly increased as 115 ml/kg/day for next 24 hours, 130 ml/kg/ day for next 48 hours, then each feed increased by 10 ml.

Other treatment include fluid restriction and frusemide 1 mg/kg/dose IV. A single dose of digoxin 5 microgram/kg is indicated if the child does not respond, the jugular venous pressure is elevated and plasma potassium levels are normal. Congestive heart failure may also result from overhydration, severe anemia and high sodium intake.

Assessment of Progress After Transition Period

After transition, the progress is assessed by the rate of weight gain which should be calculated as grams/kg/day every 3 days. The child should be weighed every morning before being fed and the weight plotted on the growth chart. If the weight gain is less than 5 grams/ kg/day, the child needs a full assessment to exclude some other disease. If the weight gain is between 5–10 grams/kg/ day, the intake targets should be checked whether it is met or if there is infection. The rate of weight gain should be 10–20 grams/kg/day.

Response to Dietary Therapy

Features of response in the initial phase of feeding include the following:

1. Initial loss of weight.
2. Return of social smile.
3. Mental changes disappear.
4. Child ask for food.

Failure to response to dietary therapy may be primary or secondary. The features include the following:

1. Primary failure
   a. Failure to gain appetite by day 4.
   b. Failure to start losing edema by day 4.
   c. Failure of disappearance of edema by day 10.
   d. Failure to gain wt. @ 5 gms/kg/day by day 10.
2. Secondary failure
   a. Failure to gain wt @ > 5 gms/kg /day for 3 consecutive days during rehabilitation phase (after 1 week).

The causes of failure may be the following:

a. Infection.
b. Immunological disorders.
c. Inborn errors of metabolism.
d. Malignant disease.

Sensory Stimulation and Emotional Support

In children with severe PEM, there is delayed mental and behavioural development. These children need interaction with other children and adults during rehabilitation. Therefore they should be provided sensory stimulation and emotional support, from day 1 of treatment, in the form of tender loving care, a cheerful stimulating environment, structured play therapy for 15–30 minutes a day, physical activity as soon as the child is well enough. Maternal involvement as much as possible should be encouraged in comforting, feeding, bathing and play. The mother should be taught what to do to stimulate her child effectively and build her self confidence so that she can continue the same at home.

Treatment of Associated Conditions

a. **Vitamin A deficiency:** Children with vitamin A deficiency are likely to be photophobic and have their eyes closed. It is important to examine the eyes very gently to prevent corneal rupture. If any of the eye signs of vitamin A deficiency are present the child should be treated with oral Vitamin A solution on day 1, 2 and 14 (dose < 6 months: 50,000 IU / dose, 6 -12 months: 100,000 IU/ dose, older child: 200,000 IU / dose). If the eyes shows signs of inflammation or ulceration, the following eye care should be given to prevent corneal rupture:
   i. Instillation of antibiotic eye drops 2–3 hourly for 7–10 days.
   ii. Instillation of 1% atropine eye drops, 1 drop 3 times daily for 3–5 days.
   iii. The eyes should be covered with saline soaked eye pads and bandage applied.
b. **Severe anemia** should be treated with whole blood or packed cell transfusion. In severe PEM, transfusion must be slower and of smaller volume than for a well nourished child. A whole blood transfusion is indicated when the hemoglobin is < 4 gm/dl or hemoglobin is between 4–6 gm/dl and the child has respiratory distress. Volume of transfusion is 10 ml/kg slowly over 3 hours with furosemide, 1

mg/kg/dose IV at the start of the transfusion. If the child has signs of heart failure, packed cells, 10 ml/kg should be given. The respiratory and pulse rate should be monitored every 15 minutes. If either increases (respiratory rate by 5 breaths / minute or pulse rate 25 beats /minute) transfusion rate should be further slowed down. After a transfusion, if the hemoglobin is still low, transfusion should not be repeated within 4 days.

c. **Dermatosis of kwashiorkor:** Zinc deficiency is common in kwashiorkor and hence zinc supplementation leads to quick improvement of the skin lesions. In addition, the affected areas should be soaked for 10 minutes a day in 1% potassium permanganate. A barrier cream applied to raw areas and 1% gentian violet or cotrimazole cream applied to the skin sores. The perineum should be kept dry.

d. **Continuing diarrhoea:** Diarrhoea is common but subsides during the first week with cautious refeeding. In the rehabilitation phase, loose, poorly formed stools are not cause of concern, provided the child's weight gain is satisfactory. The causes of diarrhoea may be Giardiasis, lactose intolerance and osmotic diarrhoea. If cysts or trophozoites are present on stool examination it should be treated with metronidazole. *Lactose intolerance* is rare. It should be treated only if it hampers general improvement. *Osmotic diarrhoea* may be suspected if diarrhoea worsens with hyperosmolar F-75 and subsides when sugar content and osmolarity are reduced. In such cases lower osmolar cereal based starter F-75 formulas should be used. The catch up F-100 should be introduced gradually.

e. **Tuberculosis:** Tuberculosis should be suspected in a child with severe PEM if there is a history of contact, poor growth despite good intake, chronic cough or chest infection not responding to antibiotics. A tuberculin test and a chest X-ray should be advised although the tuberculin test is usually false negative. If these are positive or tuberculosis is strongly suspected it should be treated as recommended.

Follow-up After Recovery

A child with severe PEM should be considered as recovered and fit for discharge when the child has achieved 90% of ideal weight for height. This may take 6–8 weeks. However, good feeding practices and sensory stimulation should be continued at home. The mother should be advised to feed the child frequently with energy dense foods and should be also instructed to give structured play therapy. Immunization should be initiated in the unimmunized child. The parent should be asked to bring the child back for regular follow-up at 1, 2 and 4 weeks, then monthly for 6 months.

Discharging the Child Before Recovery

Early discharge may have to be planned in case the parents insist because of some family commitments. Sometimes it may be encouraged to reduce the risk of nosocomial infection in hospital. Home based treatment should be considered only when the following criteria are met:

1. Child is aged 12 months or more.
2. Has completed antibiotic treatment.
3. Has a good appetite.
4. Has good weight gain.
5. Has lost edema.
6. Has taken 2 weeks of potassium, magnesium, and vitamin supplements.
7. The mother or care giver is not employed outside the home.
8. The caregiver has received specific training on appropriate feeding, has been trained to give structured play therapy and has the financial resources to feed the child.
9. The mother /caregiver is motivated to follow the advice given.
10. Local health workers are trained to support home care.

Schedule of Feeding at Home

In children who are being treated at home, the aim is to achieve atleast 150 kcal/kg /day and protein atleast 4 gms/kg/day. This will require foods containing 100 kcal and 2-3 grams protein/100 grams of food. The practical approach is as follows:

1. To give the appropriate meals at least 5 times a day.
2. To give high energy snacks in between meals (e.g. milk, banana, bread).
3. The child should be given food separately and assisted and encouraged to complete each meal.
4. Electrolyte/mineral mixture should be continued, mixed with milk or porridge.
5. Breastfeeding should be continued in the breast fed babies.

Follow-up for Children Discharged Before Recovery

The child should be asked to contact the health facility every week till recovery. The parents may report the OPD in the hospital, a nutrition rehabilitation centre, a primary health centre, or the health worker who regularly visits homes.

A discharge note should be written which should contain the following informations:

1. Any continuing treatment, and the child's weight on discharge.
2. Feeding recommendations.
3. The action the health worker has to take. The child has to be weighed weekly after discharge. If there is failure to gain weight over a two-week period or weight loss between two measurements, the child should be referred back to the hospital.

Prevention of PEM

Principles

1. Optimization of health resources and infrastructure.
2. Perceiving and understanding PEM by all health professionals.

Preventive Approaches

1. Individual and community based integrated approach.
2. Growth monitoring and promotion.
3. Promotion and support of breastfeeding.
4. Immunization.
5. Prompt and adequate treatment of recurrent infection.
6. Hygiene and sanitation.
7. Family and community orientation towards scientific infant feeding practices.

VITAMIN A DEFICIENCY

Vitamin A is a fat soluble vitamin. It is a subgroup of retinoid exhibiting the biological activity of retinol. Naturally occurring retinoid include retinol (Vitamin A alcohol), retinyl ester (Vitamin A ester), retinal (Vitamin A aldehyde) and retinoic acid (Vitamin A acid). Among these, retinoic acid is the most active form of the vitamin.

The source of Vitamin A in the diet is carotene from plant sources and retinol from animal sources. Normally, 90% of ingested retinol and 70% of carotenes are absorbed. Frying of carotenes in oil improves its absorption. Among the carotene pigments, beta-carotene yields the highest amount of retinol. Beta-carotene is also known as provitamin A. It is converted into retinol in the intestinal wall. Retinol and beta-carotenes are fat soluble. Absorbed retinol is stored in the liver as retinyl palmitate. Retinol is transported in blood bound to retinol binding protein.

Dietary Sources of Vitamin A

Colostrum is a rich source of Vitamin A. Breast milk contains adequate amount of Vitamin A. Rich sources of retinol are cod liver oil, shark liver oil and liver. Other sources are butter, ghee and egg yolk. Rich source of carotene is red palm oil. Provitamin A carotenoids are present in green leafy vegetables and yellow red vegetables and fruits like pumpkin, carrots, papaya, and mango. Cooking, canning and freezing of foodstuff results in only small losses of Vitamin A.

Functions of Vitamin A

The major function of Vitamin A is in vision. Retinal is the prosthetic group of the photosensitive pigment in both the photo receptor systems viz. rods and cones.

Retinoids are essential for cell differentiation, membrane stability and activation of retinoic acid responsive genes.

Vitamin A also plays a role in keratinization, cornification, bone metabolism, placental development, spermatogenesis and mucus formation. The characteristic changes of deficiency in the epithelium include proliferation of basal cells, squamous metaplasia, hyperkeratosis, and formation of stratified, cornified squamous epithelium.

Recommended Daily Allowance

Infants: 300 – 400 micro grams/day, Children: 400–600 micro grams/day, and Adolescents: 750 micro gram/day.

Clinical Manifestations

The risk of deficiency is small in healthy children receiving a balanced diet. Dietary deficiency of Vitamin A for a prolonged period can lead to deficiency state. Deficiency state can also result from inadequate intestinal absorption secondary to chronic intestinal disorders or fat malabsorption. A low dietary intake of fat can also result in low Vitamin A absorption. A low dietary protein intake can result in deficient retinol binding protein and hence a low plasma concentration of Vitamin A.

Inadequate Vitamin A status can vary from marginal deficiency without specific clinical signs to early reversible signs, gradually progressing to severe depletion with advanced irreversible signs with a high probability of blindness.

Ophthalmic Manifestations

Ophthalmic manifestations are characteristic and increase in severity with progressive deficiency. These are:

1. **Defective dark adaptation** is the earliest clinical feature followed by night blindness in severe cases. The parents give a history that the child becomes clumsy around dusk.
2. **Conjunctival xerosis:** An early sign, manifests as wrinkled muddy conjunctiva. It is prevalent in 6–36 months old age group, often combined with malnutrition.
3. **Bitot's spot:** Raised, grey, foamy, rough patches on the lateral aspect of the bulbar conjunctiva. These may persist after resolution of deficiency.
4. **Corneal xerosis:** Characterized by ground glass appearance of cornea.
5. **Keratomalacia** or melting of cornea is followed by perforation and anterior staphyloma. Keratomalacia is usually irreversible and results in scar formation or phthisis bulbi.
6. Fundoscopy reveals pale yellow spots near the course of retinal vessels and also in the periphery.

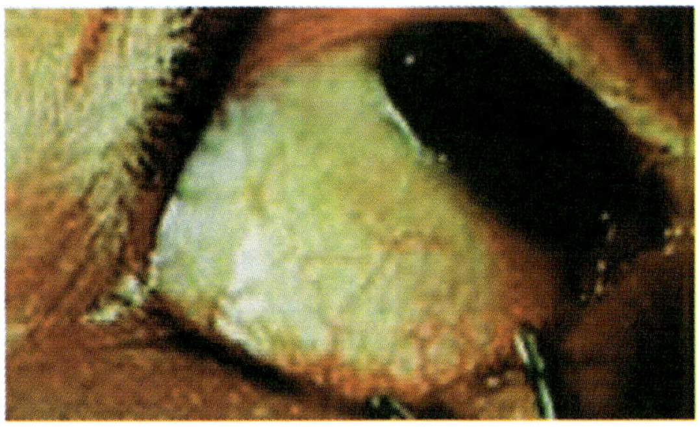
X1A Conjunctival xerosis

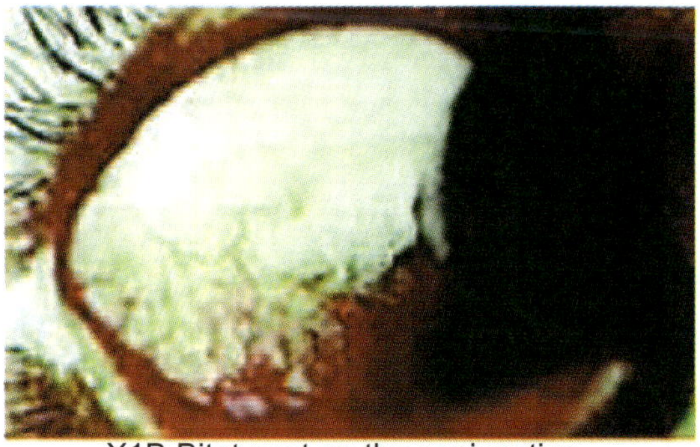
X1B Bitot spot on the conjunctiva

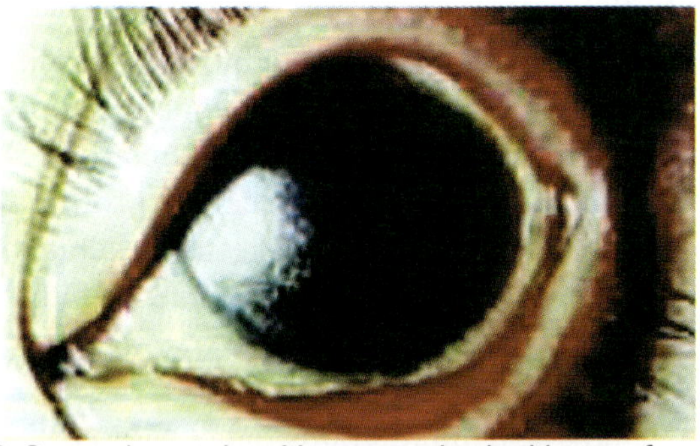
X2 Corneal xerosis with a granular looking surface

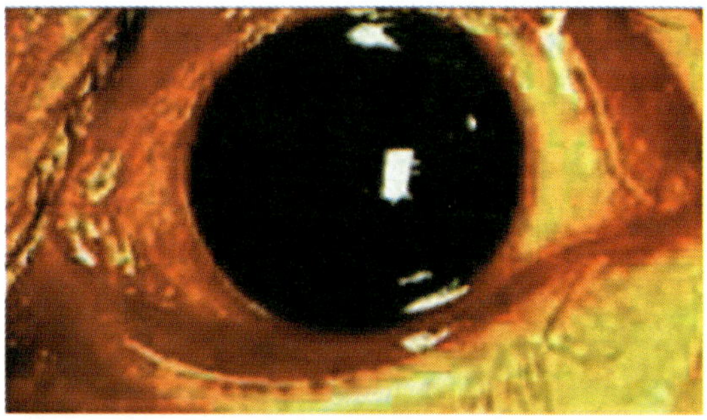
X3A Keratomalacia of less than a third of cornea

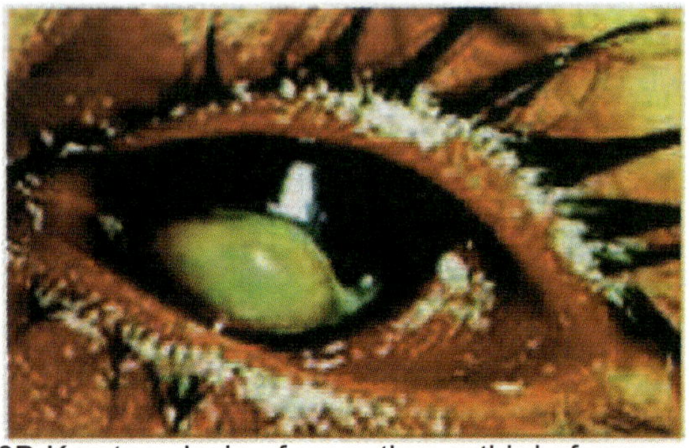
X3B Keratomalacia of more than a third of cornea

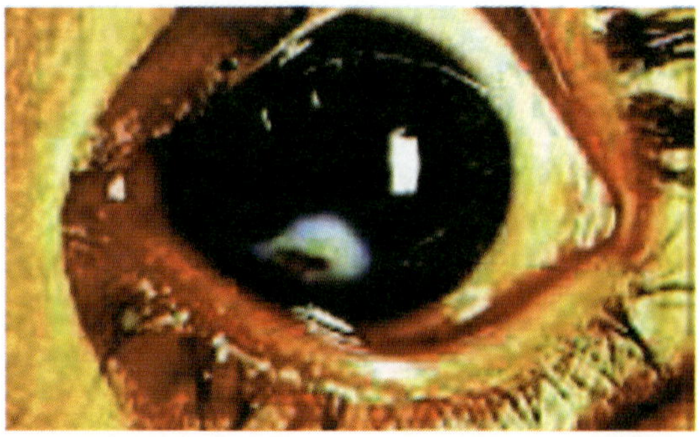
XS Corneal scarring

Fig. 6.6: Ophthalmic signs in Vitamin A deficiency

Other Manifestations

These manifestations are less characteristic but significant signals of Vitamin A deficiency. They are:

1. The child becomes prone to respiratory and gut infections. It is a result of squamous metaplasia of mucosa.
2. Anemia with or without hepatosplenomegaly.
3. Failure to thrive.
4. Skin becomes dry and scaly.
5. Follicular hyperkeratosis which may be found on the shoulders, buttocks and extensor surfaces of the extremities.
6. Pyuria and hematuria as a result of metaplasia of the urinary tract.
7. Increased intracranial pressure with wide separation of sutures may occur. Hydrocephalous with or without cranial nerve palsy is an infrequent manifestation.

Table 6.6 : WHO classification of xeropthalmia

	Primary signs		*Secondary signs*
X1 A	Conjunctival xerosis	XN	Night blindness
X1 B	Bitot's spots	XF	Fundal changes
X2	Corneal xerosis	XS	Corneal scarring
X3 A	Corneal ulceration		
X3 B	Keratomalacia		

Diagnosis

1. Clinical criteria are sufficient to suspect and diagnose Vitamin A deficiency.
2. Conjunctival xerosis can be confirmed by Rose Bengal test. It is done by instillation of 1% Rose Bengal dye in the eye. The areas of xerosis will stain deep pink.
3. Estimation of plasma level of Vitamin A.

Treatment

Vitamin A deficiency is a preventable cause of blindness. It should be treated as an emergency because timely intervention and prompt therapy is the key to final outcome.

1. **Latent Vitamin A deficiency:** A daily supplement of 1500 micro gram (5000 IU).
2. **Clinical Vitamin A deficiency:**

   Oil based preparation of Vitamin A.

   Day 1:

   < 6 months of age: 50,000 IU per oral.

   6–12 months of age: 1,00,000 IU per oral.

   > 12 months of age: 2,00,000 IU per oral.

   Day 2: Same dose.

   After 2 weeks: Same dose.

   Parenteral water soluble Vitamin A may be necessary in cases with impaired absorption, persistent vomiting and severe malabsorption. The doses should be reduced to ½ and ¾ the suggested oral doses in children < 6 months and 6–12 months respectively. Oil based parenteral preparation should not be used for treatment of Xeropthalmia.
3. **A child with severe malnutrition**

   Children with severe PEM are at risk of developing vitamin A deficiency. So they should be treated with the above schedule, even in absence of overt signs of deficiency, from day 1.
4. **Local treatment:**

   Presence of corneal ulcer:
   - Antibiotic ointment or drops 3 times a day.
   - 1% atropine drops or ointment once a day.
   - Padding of the eyes reduces pain and photophobia. It prevents dehydration, further corneal exposure and also enhances epithelial healing.

Prevention

1. All non-breastfed babies should receive supplement of Vitamin A by 2 months of age either 1 dose of 50,000 units or 2 doses of 25,000 units each at 1 month interval in areas of endemic Vitamin A deficiency (i.e. where 2% of the 0–5 year age group of the community shows Bitot's spot in addition to conjunctival xerosis).
2. Every child should be encouraged to eat Vitamin A rich food from the age of initiation of complementary food i.e. 6 months age.
3. Every child should be administered 1 lakh unit of Vitamin A at nine months along with measles vaccine followed by four doses of 2 lakh units each at an interval of 6 months upto 5 years.

4. In endemic areas of Vitamin A deficiency, children suffering from:
   a. Measles should be given two doses of Vitamin A (1 lakh < 1 year and 2 lakh > 1 year) on two consecutive days.
   b. Persistent diarrhea and prolonged febrile conditions should be given 1 dose in each episode keeping at least one month interval between 2 doses.

HYPERVITAMINOSIS A

Hypervitaminosis A can be acute or chronic.

Acute Hypervitaminosis A

Acute hypervitaminosis A may occur in infants after ingesting 100,000 micro gram or more. Clinical features are characterized by:

a. Nausea, vomiting, drowsiness, bulging fontanel (in young infants).
b. Pseudo motor cerebri characterized by diplopia, papilledema, cranial nerve palsies and other symptoms suggestive of brain tumour.

Chronic Hypervitaminosis A

Chronic hypervitaminosis A can result from ingestion of excessive doses for several weeks or months. Clinical features are characterized by:

a. Anorexia, pruritus, lack of weight gain.
b. Irritability, tender swelling of bones with limitation of movements, alopecia, seborrhoeic cutaneous lesions, fissuring of the corners of the mouth, signs of raised intracranial pressure and hepatomegaly may develop.
c. Cranio tabes and desquamation of palms and soles.
d. X-ray long bones: Show hyperostosis in the middle of the shaft.
e. Serum Vitamin A level is elevated.
f. Ingested carotenoids are non-toxic but may result in carotenemia, characterized by yellow discoloration of the skin, sparing the sclera. It is especially likely to occur in children with liver disease, diabetes mellitus, or hypothyroidism and in those who have a congenital absence of enzymes that convert provitamin A carotenoids. Treatment involves simply stopping the use of too much Vitamin A.

SCURVY

Vitamin C is a water soluble vitamin. It is also called ascorbic acid. It is a potent reducing agent. An infant born of a healthy mother with adequate intake of Vitamin C during pregnancy will have adequate store of Vitamin C at birth. Breast milk produced by a mother with sufficient intake of Vitamin C will contain adequate Vitamin C. Low maternal intake of Vitamin C, however, may result in a low breast milk content of the vitamin. Cow's milk contain very low amount of Vitamin C that too destroyed by boiling. Infants fed on cow's milk should receive supplements in order to prevent deficiency state.

Functions of Vitamin C

The most clearly established function of Vitamin C is that it acts as a cofactor in activation of hydroxylation enzymes in oxidation process for hydroxylation of procollagen to collagen. It is important for maintenance of vascular integrity.

It is required for absorption, mobilization, distribution and intoxication of metal ions. It helps in transfer of iron from plasma, transferring into tissue ferritin and thus helps in storage of iron in the bone marrow, liver and spleen.

Vitamin C is a strong antioxidant and protects eyes and lungs against oxidizing agents. It reduces oxidation of low density lipoproteins and prevents deposition of atheromatous plaques.

Dietary Sources

Citrus fruits (viz. orange, lemon) and vegetables including tomatoes, cabbage, green leafy vegetables and germinating pulses are rich sources. Large quantities are also present in liver and kidney but not in meat. Vitamin C is destroyed in cooking.

Recommended Daily Allowance

The recommended daily allowance is 30 mg/day for term infants, 50 mg/day for preterm, 40 mg/day for older children. Requirements are increased during fever, diarrhea, iron deficiency and hypoproteinemia.

Pathogenesis

The deficiency state arising from deficiency of Vitamin C is called scurvy. It is characterized by hemorrhages, bone disease and healing defects in growing children.

Impaired collagen formation results in inadequate support of the walls of capillaries and venules which results in bleeding tendency. Purpura and ecchymosis appear in the skin most prominently along the extensor surfaces of the legs and in the gingival mucosa, particularly at the margins. The loose attachment of the periosteum to bone, together with the vascular wall defects, leads to subperiosteal hematomas and bleeding into joint spaces following minimal trauma. There may be retrobulbar, subarachnoid and intracerebral hemorrhage which may prove fatal.

In the bones, the primary disturbance is in the formation of osteoid matrix. Mineralization or calcification is normal. Both endochondral and membranous bone formation may be severely disrupted. The cartilage cells are formed as usual and are provisionally calcified but there is insufficient production of osteoid matrix. Resorption of cartilaginous matrix fails or slows resulting in cartilaginous overgrowth. The scorbutic bone yields to stress of weight bearing and muscle tension, resulting in bowing of legs, depression of sternum with outward projection of the end of the ribs creating the scorbutic rosary.

Wound healing and localization of focal infections are impaired because of the derangement in collagen synthesis. Anemia is common, most often normocytic normochromic. It results from bleeding into the various tissues and decreased absorption of iron as a result of lack of ascorbic acid in the diet.

Clinical Manifestations

Scurvy can occur at any age. It is unusual in newborn because clinical manifestations require time to develop. The usual age at onset is between 6–24 months.

There is usually a history of exclusive cow's milk feeding during the first 6 months.

In the early stages, symptoms are vague viz. child is listless and fretful, have digestive disturbances with anorexia. As the disease progress, there is evidence of generalized tenderness. It is particularly noticeable in the legs when the infant is picked up or when the diaper is changed. The child cries on being handled.

Pseudo paralysis: The legs are held in frog like position with the hips and knees semi flexed with the feet rotated outwards due to pain. There may be edematous swellings along the shafts of the legs and in some cases subperiosteal hemorrhage can be felt at the ends of femur. The other causes of pseudo paralysis include septic arthritis, acute osteomyelitis, congenital syphilis which may sometimes need to be differentiated.

Gums: Changes in the gums are noticeable after eruption of teeth. The changes include bluish purple, spongy swellings of the mucous membrane especially over the incisors.

Bleeding: Gum bleeds are common during the eruption of teeth. There may be petechiae over the skin. Hematuria, melena, conjunctival or orbital hemorrhage may also occur.

Low grade fever and anemia may be present. Wound healing is slow and apparently healed wounds often break down.

Scorbutic rosary: A rosary at the costochondral junction and depression of the sternum are other typical features. It is a result of laxity of the costochondral junction and depression of sternum.

Diagnosis

The diagnosis of scurvy is based on (a) A history of poor intake of Vitamin C, (b) Characteristic clinical features, (c) Radiological features, in the long bones, (d) Biochemical tests.

The typical *radiological changes* are seen in the distal ends of the long bones. The changes are particularly common in the area of the knee and are as follows:

1. Ground glass appearance of the shaft (trabeculae of the shaft cannot be discerned) with a pencil point cortex.
2. The epiphyseal centres of ossification also have a ground glass appearance surrounded by a white ring described as signet ring appearance (Weinberger sign).
3. The white line of Fraenkal, an irregular, thickened white line at the metaphysis which represents the zone of well calcified cartilage.
4. Zone of destruction/rarefaction is a linear break in the bone proximal and parallel to the white line. A spur or lateral projection of the white line may be present.
5. Sub periosteal hemorrhage is not visible radiographically during active phase. During healing, the elevated periosteum becomes calcified and the affected bones assume a dumb bell shape.

The *biochemical tests* viz. ascorbic acid concentration of WBC / platelet from buffy layer of centrifuged oxalated blood is a good indicator of Vitamin C status. A level of 25–40 mg/100 ml is normal.

Urinary excretion of Vitamin C after a test dose of ascorbic acid is another test. In normal children, 80% of

Radiological Signs of Scurvy

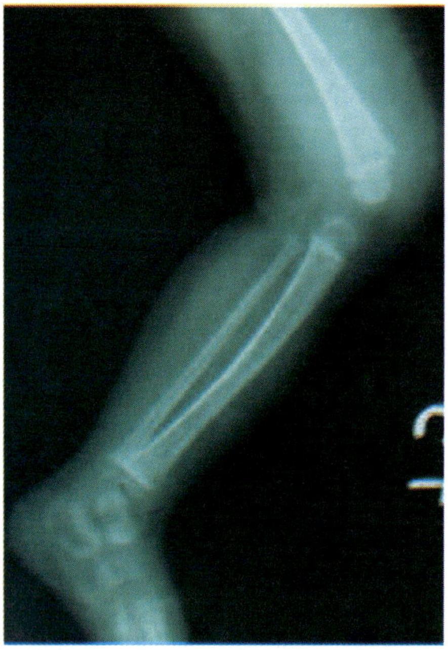

Fig. 6.7: Signs of active scurvy

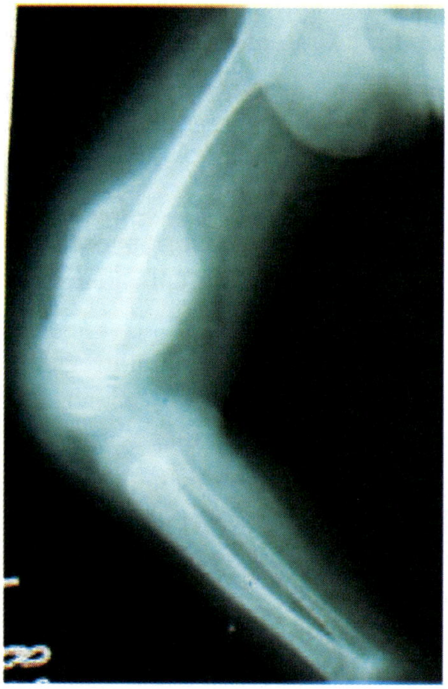

Fig. 6.8: Signs of healing scurvy

the test dose (11 mg/kg) appears in the urine within 3–5 hours after parenteral administration of the test dose.

Treatment

Ascorbic acid 100–200 mg daily orally or parenterally leads to rapid recovery with resumption of rapid growth. A daily intake of 90–120 ml of orange or tomato juice also quickly produces healing but ascorbic acid is preferable. The swelling of the periosteal hemorrhage however, may take months to disappear.

Prevention

Scurvy can be prevented by taking the following measures:

1. Exclusive breastfeeding for first 6 months.
2. Babies fed on cow's milk should be given supplemental Vitamin C.
3. Adequate amount of Vitamin C to lactating mothers.
4. Children of all age groups should be encouraged to eat ample amount of citrus fruits.

RICKETS

Deficiency of Vitamin D results in rickets. It is a metabolic disorder of growing bone resulting in bony deformities. Rickets is characterized by formation of normal collagen and matrix and of osteoid with abnormal mineralization.

The important causes of Vitamin D deficiency, in developing countries are inadequate exposure to direct sunlight, inadequate intake or both. In developed countries, most of the cases result from non-nutritional causes for example malabsorption, defect in metabolism or conditions that disturb calcium and phosphorous homeostasis.

Table 6.7 : Causes of rickets

1.	**Decreased endogenous synthesis of Vitamin D**
a.	Inadequate exposure to sunlight.
b.	Heavy melanin pigment of skin.
2.	**Decreased absorption of Vitamin D in the intestine**
a.	Dietary lack.
b.	Biliary tract, pancreatic, or intestinal dysfunction.
3.	**Enhanced degradation of Vitamin D and 25, (OH) D**
a.	Drugs: Phenytoin, Phenobarbital, Rifampicin.
4.	**Impaired synthesis of 25 (OH) D**
a.	Diffuse liver disease.
5.	**Decreased synthesis of 1, 25 $(OH)_2$ D**
a.	Advanced renal disease.
b.	Vitamin D dependent rickets type I (inherited deficiency of renal alpha 1 hydroxylase).
6.	**Target organ resistance to 1, 25 $(OH)_2$ D**
a.	Vitamin D dependent rickets type II (congenital lack of or defective receptors for active metabolite).
7.	**Phosphate depletion**
a.	Poor absorption–long-term use of antacids, which bind phosphates and render them insoluble.
b	Renal tubular disorder, acquired or genetic, causing increased excretion.

Daily Requirements

The American Academy of Pediatrics recommends daily intake of 400 IU/day for all infants, children, and adolescents beginning in the first few days of life. New evidence supports a potential role for Vitamin D in maintaining innate immunity and preventing diseases such as diabetes and cancer.

Sources of Vitamin D

Eighty percent of body's need of Vitamin D is obtained from endogenous synthesis. Ultraviolet light in sunlight converts the precursor 7–dehydrocholesterol present abundantly in the skin into Vitamin D3. The remainder is obtained from dietary sources such as deep sea fish, plants and grains. In plant sources, Vitamin D is present in its precursor form ergosterol which is converted into Vitamin D2 in the body. Vitamin D3 and D2 undergo identical metabolic transformations and have identical functions. Hence both are referred to as Vitamin D.

Breast milk content of Vitamin D is low. Cow's milk content is even lower. Breast milk content is probably adequate if infant is exposed sufficiently to sunlight.

Full body exposure during summer months for 10–15 minutes in an adult with lighter pigmentation will generate between 10,000 and 20,000 IU of Vitamin D3 within 24 hours. Individuals with darker skin pigmentation require 5–10 minutes more exposure to generate similar amounts.

The amount of ultraviolet exposure available for the synthesis of Vitamin D depends on several other factors like skin pigmentation, body mass, degree of latitude, season and the amount of cloud over, extent of pollution, the amount of skin exposed and amount of clothing.

Metabolism of Vitamin D

The metabolism of Vitamin D can be outlined as follows:

1. Absorption of Vitamin D in the gut or synthesis from precursors in the skin.
2. Transport to liver after binding to plasma alpha 1 globulin.
3. Conversion to 25, hydroxycholecalciferol (25-OH-D) by 25, Hydroxylase in the liver.
4. Conversion of 25-hydroxycholecalciferol to 1, 25-$(OH)_2$ cholecalciferol by alpha hydroxylase in the kidney.

   1-25 $(OH)_2$ cholecalciferol is the biologically active form of Vitamin D. It is regarded as steroid hormone.

Functions of Vitamin D

The essential function of Vitamin D is the maintenance of normal plasma levels of calcium and phosphorous. This involves action on the intestine, bones and kidneys. The active form of Vitamin D.

a. Stimulates intestinal absorption of calcium and phosphorous.
b. Collaborates with parathyroid hormone in the mobilization of calcium from bones.
c. Stimulates parathyroid hormone (PTH) dependent reabsorption of calcium in the distal renal tubule.

VITAMIN D DEFICIENT (NUTRITIONAL) RICKETS

When ossification improves with administration of Vitamin D, the rickets is termed as Vitamin D deficient. If no improvement occurs after administration of conventional dose of Vitamin D, the condition is called Vitamin D resistant or refractory rickets.

Pathophysiology

New bone formation is initiated by osteoblasts and is responsible for matrix deposition and subsequent mineralization. Osteoclasts cause resorption of bone. Osteocytes resorb and redeposit bone. The sequence of normal bone development is as follows:

1. Proliferation of cartilage cells followed by degeneration and formation of osteoid.
2. Capillary penetration and mineralization of osteoid tissue.
3. Resorption and redeposition of bone.

The defect in bone growth in rickets results from retardation of growth of normal epiphyseal cartilage and calcification. These changes result from a deficiency of calcium and phosphorous. The sequence of events in the pathophysiology of rickets is as follows:

1. Cartilage cells fail to complete their normal cycle of proliferation and degeneration. Subsequently there is failure of capillary penetration. The result is a frayed irregular epiphyseal line.
2. Failure of osseous and cartilaginous matrix to mineralize in the zone of preparatory calcification. Deposition of newly formed uncalcified osteoid continues. This results in a wide, irregular, frayed zone of rigid tissue (rachitic metaphysis). This produces flaring of the ends of the bones and rachitic rosary.

3. Preexisting cortical bone resorption continues in the normal manner and it is replaced over the entire shaft by osteoid tissue that fails to mineralize. The shaft becomes soft and rarefied resulting in deformities and fractures.
4. With healing, degeneration of cartilage cells occurs along the metaphyseal-diaphyseal border. Capillary penetration is resumed in these spaces and calcification takes place. It appears as a line of calcification that is clearly visible on radiographs and is called the zone of preparatory calcification. As healing progresses, the osteoid tissue between the line of preparatory calcification and the diaphysis, the osteoid tissues in the cortex and that about the trabeculae in the shaft become mineralized.
5. Biochemical alterations: In presence of Vitamin D deficiency, less calcium is absorbed from the intestine. A low serum calcium level leads to secretion of parathormone which in turn mobilizes calcium and phosphorous from bone thereby calcium concentration is maintained but serum phosphorous is low because parathormone decreases phosphorous reabsorption in the kidneys. The serum alkaline phosphatase is increased due to increased osteoblastic activity.

Clinical Manifestations

Rickets usually appears towards the end of the first year and during the second year. Breast fed infants of Vitamin D deficient mothers may develop within 2 months after birth. The clinical manifestations of Rickets are related to the skeletal system. The osseous changes however cannot be recognized until after several months of deficiency.

The earliest clinical signs are *Cranio tabes, rachitic rosary* (palpable enlargement of the costochondral junctions) and *thickening of the wrist and ankle joints*. Increased sweating, particularly around the head, may be present. *Cranio tabes* is caused by thinning of the outer table of the skull. It can also be detected by a ping pong ball sensation when pressing over the posterior parietal or occipital bones. Cranio tabes also can occur in hydrocephalous and osteogenesis imperfecta.

It is sometimes present in normal infants which tend to disappear by 2–4 months age. Enlargement of costochondral junction can occur in Scurvy (scorbutic rosary) and chodrodystrophy also.

The signs of advanced rickets can be easily recognized.

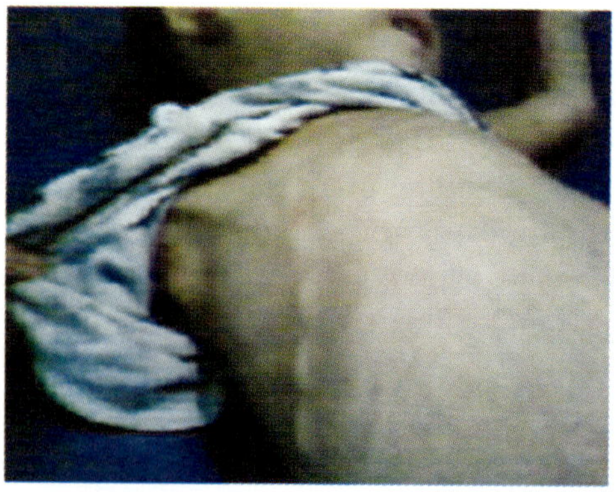

Fig. 6.9: Figure showing rickety rosary

Head: The *anterior fontanel is large and closure may be delayed* beyond 2 years. The softening of the skull bones results in asymmetry of the skull. The thickening of the central parts of the parietal and frontal bones result in a *box shaped skull. Eruption of primary dentition* is delayed and there may be defects of enamel and caries.

The *permanent teeth* which are developing during the period of Vitamin D deficiency are also affected. Usually the incisors, canines and first molars show defects of enamel.

Thorax: Rachitic rosary is not only palpable but becomes visible. The sternum projects forward causing the *pigeon chest deformity*. A groove (*Harrison's sulcus*) develops along the lower order of the chest corresponding to the costal insertions of the diaphragm.

Spinal column: Slight to moderate degree of scoliosis is common. Kyphosis may occur in sitting posture and lumbar lordosis may be seen in erect posture.

Pelvis: The pelvis in rickets is small and continues to be retarded in growth.

Lower limbs show bow leg, knock knee and coxa vera deformities develop in advanced stages after the child starts walking.

Ligaments and muscles: Relaxation of ligaments aids in producing deformities. The muscles are poorly developed and lack in tone. As a result the gross motor milestones viz. standing and walking is delayed. Weakness of the abdominal muscles, weakness of the gastric and intestinal walls aids in production of the pot belly appearance.

Diagnosis

The diagnosis of Vitamin D deficient rickets is based on:

1. History of inadequate intake of Vitamin D or inadequate exposure to sunshine.

2. Clinical features.
3. Biochemical abnormalities viz. normal or low serum calcium, low serum phosphorous (< 4 mg/ dl) and elevation of serum alkaline phosphate.
4. Radiological changes in the bones: An X-ray of the wrist is best for study of characteristic early changes and hence early diagnosis. The changes depend on the stage of rickets.
   a. *Active rickets:* (i) The distal end of radius and ulna becomes widened, concave (cupping) and frayed. (ii) The distance between the distal ends of ulna and radius and the metacarpal bones is increased because of the noncalcified large rachitic metaphysis that does not appear on the X-ray. (iii) The density of the shaft is decreased but the trabeculae are prominent.
   b. *Healing rickets:* Healing is indicated by the appearance of zone of preparatory calcification (ZPC). This ZPC is separated from the distal end of the shaft by a zone of osteoid tissue with decreased calcification. As healing progresses and the osteoid tissue becomes calcified, the shaft grows towards the ZPC until it becomes united with it.

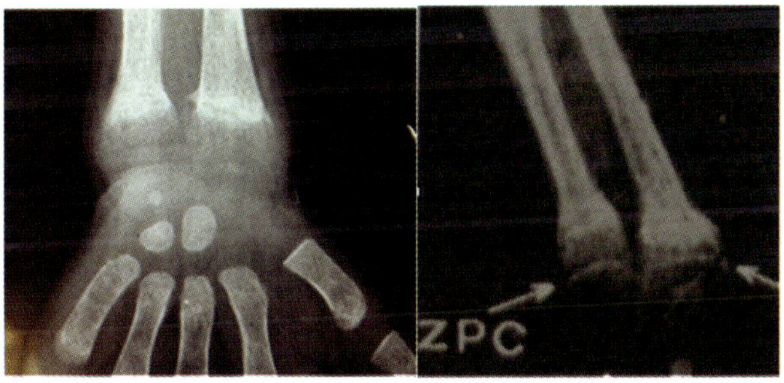

A. Signs of active rickets

B. Signs of healing rickets (Adapted from Nelson Text book of Pediatrics)

Fig. 6.10A and B: Showing signs of rickets

Complications

Vitamin D deficiency may result in:

a. Recurrent respiratory infection, pulmonary atelectasis associated with severe deformities of the chest.
b. Diarrhea or constipation or alternate diarrhea and constipation, and
c. Anemia due to iron deficiency or infections.

Treatment

Spontaneous healing can occur in mild rickets from exposure to sunshine. Severe cases require more energetic treatment with Vitamin D. The regimens for Vitamin D administration are as follows:

1. Single intramuscular/oral dose of 6 lakh IU of Vitamin D. A single massive dose is advantageous because it is followed by rapid healing, early differential diagnosis from resistant rickets and less dependence on parents.
2. Sachets containing 60,000 IU of Vitamin D mixed with water/milk can be given orally, daily for 10 days.
3. A lower dose of 1500–5000 IU can also be used in the same method. It takes a longer time to show signs of healing (upto 4 weeks).

Follow-up

An X-ray of the wrist has to be done after 2 weeks. If no signs of healing are demonstrated, the dose should be repeated and X-ray repeated after two weeks. If still no healing occurs, the rickets is considered to be resistant to Vitamin D.

When rickets is Vitamin D responsive and after healing is complete, a lower dose of Vitamin D 400 IU should be continued.

Course and Prognosis

With adequate doses, healing begins within a few days and progresses until the normal bony structure is restored. The bony deformities viz. epiphyseal enlargement, rosary, bow legs and the deformities of the skull may take months to years after Vitamin D treatment for correction. In advanced cases, deformities viz. bow legs, knock knee, coxa vera, deformities of pelvis and short stature may be permanent.

Rickets itself is not a fatal disease. Intercurrent infections viz. pneumonia, diarrhea, tuberculosis is more likely to cause death in rachitic than in normal children.

Prevention

All babies, term or preterm, breast fed or nonbreastfed require supplementation of 400 IU of Vitamin D beginning at about 5–10 days of age. This can be achieved by exposure to sunlight or by oral administration of Vitamin D. Sunlight as a prophylactic agent can be considered in the tropical countries. In the temperate zones it will be effective only during summer months in haze free areas only. Vitamin D supplement should be advised in pregnant and lactating mothers.

FAMILIAL HYPOPHOSPHATEMIC RICKETS

Familial hypophosphatemic rickets is the most common form of non-nutritional rickets. The common mode of inheritance is X-linked dominant but autosomal dominant and sporadic forms have also been reported. This disorder is typical of pure phosphate deficient rickets.

Pathogenesis

There is defect in the proximal tubular reabsorption of phosphate and in conversion of 25(OH) D_3 to 1,25 $(OH)_2$ D_3. Both these defects have been demonstrated in animal models of this disease. In the X-linked type there is low to normal serum levels of 1, 25$(OH)_2$ D_3 despite hypophosphatemia. Further, phosphate depletion does not stimulate 1,25 $(OH)_2$ D_3 synthesis as it does in normal subjects. The activity of the Na^+ dependent phosphate transporter in the renal proximal tubules is reduced, resulting in excessive urinary phosphate excretion. In addition oral phosphate supplementation alone cannot completely heal bone disease, the correction of rickets requires 1,25 $(OH)_2$ D_3 therapy. Some mothers of affected children exhibit clinical evidence of disease, such as bowing of legs or short stature, whereas others show only fasting hypophosphatemia.

Clinical Manifestations

The clinical features are more prominent in the lower limbs and become evident when the child starts walking. They present with smooth bowing of legs, waddling gait, coxa vara, genu varum, genu valgum and short stature. The typical features of Rickets like rachitic rosary, Harrison's sulcus, myopathy etc are not evident. Dental abnormalities viz. pulp deformities like intraglobular dentine and frequent dental abscesses are common.

Laboratory Diagnosis

The biochemical abnormalities include normal or slightly reduced serum calcium level (9–9.4 mg/dl) a moderately reduced serum phosphate level (1.5–3 mg/dl), elevated alkaline phosphatase activity. Urinary phosphate excretion is increased. The parathyroid hormone level is normal and blood levels of 1, 25 $(OH)_2$ D_3 are low. In potential obligate heterozygotes, serum phosphate level may remain normal for several months of life probably as a result of low GFR. The first laboratory anomaly in such cases is a rise in serum alkaline phosphatase activity.

Radiological changes include metaphyseal widening and fraying and cupping of the proximal and distal tibia and at the distal femur, radius and ulna. The trabecular bone appears coarse.

Treatment

The preferred treatment is oral phosphate supplements together with a Vitamin D analogue. The dose of phosphate is 30–50 mg/kg (total 1–3 gm elemental phosphorous) given 4 hourly. The main side effect of oral phosphate therapy is diarrhoea which usually improves spontaneously.

Vitamin D can be given as 1,25 $(OH)_2$ D_3 in the dose of 50–65 ng/ kg / day (maximum 2 microgram /day) until there is biochemical and radiological evidence of healing of rickets. Periodic monitoring of serum and urine levels of calcium and phosphate is essential for monitoring. A level of serum phosphate greater than 3.0–3.2 is desirable. Increased levels of urinary calcium beyond 4 mg /kg/day necessitate temporary cessation of Vitamin D therapy.

Treatment with phosphates and Vitamin D analogue results in healing of rickets and some increase in the height. Children with severe deformities may require corrective osteotomy after healing of rickets. Growth hormone therapy may benefit children who do not show an adequate increase in height.

VITAMIN D DEPENDENT RICKETS (VDDR)

Vitamin D dependent rickets are autosomal recessive disorders. They are rare and seen in infants between 3–6 months of age who have been receiving doses of Vitamin D (400–600 IU/day) which is appropriate to prevent rickets. Two types have been described. They are VDDR type I or pseudo Vitamin D deficiency rickets and VDDR type II or hereditary Vitamin D resistant rickets.

The VDDR type I is a result of deficiency of enzyme 25-hydroxy Vitamin D 1 alpha hydroxylase as a result of gene mutation leading to non-conversion of 25 (OH) D_3 to 1, 25 $(OH)_2$ D_3. In VDDR type II, there is end organ resistance to 1, 25 $(OH)_2$ D_3.

Clinical Manifestations

The clinical features of VDDR type I are similar to Vitamin D deficiency rickets. The child may also present with convulsion, positive Trousseau and Chvostek sign due to hypocalcemia.

In VDDR type II, there is early onset of rickets. Some patients have alopecia (areata or universalis) and ectodermal defects like oligodontia and epidermal cysts.

Laboratory Diagnosis

Reduced blood levels of calcium, normal to low phosphate and elevated serum alkaline phosphatase activity are characteristic. The blood levels of 25 (OH) D_3 are normal but those of 1, 25 $(OH)_2$ D_3 are markedly reduced despite hypocalcemia.

Hypocalcemia, secondary hyperparathyroidism, elevated blood levels of 1, 25 $(OH)_2$ D_3 are characteristic of VDDR II.

Treatment

The treatment of VDDR type II is administration of calcitriol (1–2 microgram daily) with concomitant therapy with calcium with or without phosphate supplements. In most cases, serum levels of calcium rise and radiological healing occurs within 6–8 weeks.

The response to treatment with calcitriol in VDDR type II is unsatisfactory. A long-term treatment with large doses of oral or IV calcium may show biochemical and radiological improvement in an occasional patient.

Obesity

Obesity is an excess of fat in the body, subcutaneous or internal, that results from a prolonged net positive energy balance i.e. energy consumed has been greater than the energy expended.

Obesity in childhood has reached an epidemic proportion. According to WHO (2000) 20% of children in UK and USA are overweight. In spite of a very high prevalence of undernutrition in our country there has been an increase in the prevalence of overweight and obesity in the affluent urban society in India in the past decade.

Measurements of Obesity

As the body weight is closely related not only to body fat but also to weight, the BMI (weight in kg/height in m^2) is agreed upon as a fairly reliable surrogate of adiposity.

A BMI of more than 95th percentile for the age and sex is considered as obesity and BMI between 85th and 95th percentile is considered as overweight.

Skin-fold thickness (SFT) above 85th percentile for age and sex is also a measure of obesity. The WHO recommends SFT + BMI for accurate estimation of obesity.

Data for age and sex BMI centiles are derived from the National Health and Nutrition Examination Survey III and are available from the Centres for Disease Control and Prevention (CDC). K.N. Agarwal *et al* has described centiles for BMI for Indian children (*See* Appendix).

Predictors of Obesity

The predictors of obesity in childhood are:

(i) Parental obesity, particularly maternal is predictive of childhood obesity; (ii) High birth weight; the most important factor contributing to high birth weight being maternal diabetes and to a lesser degree maternal obesity; (iii) Deficient physical activity; which has been shown to be directly related to hours of television viewing which has significant correlation to weight gain during growing years.

It has been established that blood pressure, blood lipid levels and obesity during childhood track into adulthood. Hence childhood obesity is itself a predictor of adult obesity and of adult morbidity and mortality regardless of presence of overweight in adulthood. There is a rise in obesity related morbidities in youth which is a predictor of more severe problems in the young adults.

Consequences of Obesity

The consequences of obesity may be psychosocial as well as physical. The psychosocial problems include poor self esteem and depression. The physical problems include the following:

1. Cardiovascular: Hypertension, hyperlipidemia (increased total cholesterol, triglycerides, decreased HDL).
2. Insulin resistance syndrome or metabolic syndrome (hypertension, dyslipidemia and impaired glucose tolerance).
3. Cholelithiasis and fatty liver disease.
4. Pickwickian syndrome (Obesity, dyspnea with irresistible urge to fall sleep due to carbon dioxide narcosis) and sleep apnea (presents with disturbed sleep, snoring and lethargy during the day).
5. Orthopedic problems viz. slipped femoral epiphysis, genu valgum, leg and back pain.
6. Gynecological problems viz. polycystic ovary syndrome which presents with menstrual irregularities (usually amenorrhea), hirsuitism and acne.

Causes of Obesity

The causes of obesity may be classified as:

1. Genetic or Constitutional.

2. Secondary:
   a. Dysmorphic syndromes viz. Prader-Willi syndrome, Lawrence Moon Biedl syndrome.
   b. Endocrine causes, viz. Hypothyroidism, Turner syndrome, Cushing's syndrome, Klinefelter's syndrome.
   c. CNS disorders, viz. Trauma, Craniopharyngioma, Hypothalamic tumour.
   d. Medications, viz. antiepileptic drugs, antipsychotic, glucocorticosteroids.
   e. Environmental causes, viz. excess calories, sedentary life-style.
   f. Psychosocial causes, viz. Depression, attention seeking behaviour, psychiatric illness.

Clinical Manifestations

Constitutional Obesity

Constitutional obesity may occur at any age. However, it is more common in the first year, around 5–6 years, and during adolescence. The children are taller and have an advanced bone age. The adiposity is most prominent around the breast, fatty folds at the back and often striae may be present. The external genitalia in boys may appear disproportionately small with the penis embedded in the fat. Puberty may occur early affecting the ultimate height. There is genu valgum and more fat in the upper end of the thigh compared to the rest of the extremities with small tapering fingers.

Secondary Obesity

The characteristics of secondary obesity include short stature, delayed bone age and delayed development of sexual characteristics. These conditions can present with overweight as the initial symptom. All conditions will also have the associated features of the specific cause.

Laboratory Diagnosis

The base line laboratory tests include fasting blood sugar, lipid profile, and thyroid profile and urine analysis. The special investigations which may be required when a specific cause is suspected include urine free cortisol, growth hormone, androgen, serum insulin, karyotyping, imaging of the sela and supra sellar region.

Management

The management of a case of obesity should start with evaluation to exclude a secondary cause. The cornerstones of therapy are diet, exercise and behaviour modification with an aim to achieve weight loss / control and promote a healthy life-style to prevent obesity. The most significant impact on obesity has to be achieved through patient education and prevention.

Evaluation

Evaluation should include a *thorough history* with emphasis on appetite, thirst, school performance, milestones, attainment of puberty, family history of obesity and maternal feeding practices. Enquiry about the life-style of the child regarding diet, amount of physical activity, hours of TV viewing, computer time, hobbies and participation in sports are important. The *physical examination* should include measurement of weight, height, facial features and fat distribution. *Laboratory investigations* should be selected as and when necessary.

Diet

The initial goal should be a 10% reduction in weight for older children. For younger children, severe calorie restriction may result in an unacceptable decrease in height velocity. In many young children simply preventing further weight gain suffices. A balanced hypocaloric diet is the usual advice. This diet is with a calorie deficit of 30–40%, low in fat with high complex carbohydrate, vitamin and mineral supplements. In obesity with significant morbidity, a restricted protein sparing fast diet is needed. This diet should provide 600–700 kcal /day, 1.5–2.5 gm/kg/day of high quality protein, vitamin and mineral supplements and adequate water intake (> 1.5 litres/day).

Exercise

Diet alone without exercise is unlikely to succeed in weight reduction or control. The beneficial exercises are walking, cycling, jogging, tennis. The exercise should be started in a graduated manner and effort should be sustained.

Behaviour Modification

Life-style changes are required in children of all age groups. Behaviour modification is aimed at building self-confidence, self esteem and improving attitude towards food, exercise and body image. In this programme, the entire family should be involved and regular counseling done. The child and the family should be educated regarding the calories and nutritive values of food. There should be a programming for limiting TV viewing and computer time. Over and above these there should be encouragement and rewarding for good performance.

Drugs and Surgery

Drug therapy and surgery are not considered in treatment of childhood obesity except in cases with significant morbidity when other methods are not effective. The drug which is shown to be effective in some children is metformin, a glucose sensitizing agent, which helps obese patients to adhere to a diet has shown promising results.

Surgery may be considered in cases of extreme obesity, only in higher centres. The surgical procedures include gastroplasty (to reduce the volume of stomach) and liposuction (surgery to remove fat). They have been shown to be useful in some patients.

Suggested Reading

1. Diseases of children in the subtropics and subtropics. Edited by D.B. Jelliffe and J.P. Stanfield, Third edition, 1978. The English Language Book Society and Edward Arnold (Publishers) Ltd.
2. Management of the child with a serious infection or severe malnutrition. Guidelines for care at the first referral level in developing countries. Department of child and adolescent health and development. World Health Organization, AITBS Publishers.
3. Price Textbook of Medicine, Edited by Sir Ronald Bodlay Scott, Eleventh edition, 1973, ELBS and Oxford University Press.
4. Nelson's Textbook of Pediatrics, 17th edition, 2004, edited by Berhman, Kliegman and Jenson, Published by Saunders.
5. MME -103 Child Health (Nutrition), Indira Gandhi National Open University School of Health Sciences, Printed and published on behalf of IGNOU by Director, School of Health Sciences, New Delhi.
6. Umesh Kapil and HPS Sachdev. Management of Children with Severe Acute Malnutrition: A national priority. Indian Pediatrics 47: 651– 653, 2010.

7

Neonatology

OUTLINES

Levels of Neonatal Care

Level I or primary care: More than 80% of newborn babies require minimal care at birth. Neonates weighing 2000 grams or more or having a gestational maturity of 37 weeks or more belong to this category. Care can be provided to these babies at home, subcentres, and primary health centres by mothers under supervision of basic health professionals.

Level II or secondary care: Is necessary for babies weighing between 1500 grams to 2000 grams or those between 32–36 weeks of gestation. They form 15–20% of neonates. This care is provided in the district hospitals, nursing homes and medical colleges. These institutions must have adequate facilities including equipment and manned by pediatricians and nurses trained in neonatology.

Level III or tertiary care: Or intensive care is required for babies weighing less than 1500 grams or those born before 32 weeks. These centres should be equipped with modern gadgets of neonatal care and run by skilled nurses and neonatologists specially trained in intensive neonatal care.

Care of Normal Newborn

A normal newborn is one who is born between 37 weeks and 40 weeks of gestation. The average weight of newborn in India is 2.8 kg (male) and 2.75 kg (female). Care of the normal newborn may be domiciliary or institutional. The aim is to provide optimal care based on sound physiological principles. These neonates can be looked after by mothers or family members under the supervision of basic health workers as and when necessary.

The care of the normal newborn can be discussed under the following headings:

1. Care during antenatal period.
2. Care at birth.
3. Care of the skin.
4. Care of the umbilical stump.
5. Care of the eyes.
6. Prevention of hypothermia.
7. Prevention of infection.
8. Feeding.
9. Immunization advice.
10. Normal phenomena and danger signs.
11. Follow-up care.

Care During the Antenatal Period

It is essential that a baby is born mature and healthy and grows optimally. Care of the baby should begin soon after conception. Every pregnancy should be recognized as soon as possible. Pregnancy is a normal event but occasionally complications occur. Early recognition and treatment of complications will ensure safe delivery of a healthy newborn. Thus regular check-up is necessary. A minimum of 5 antenatal check ups is a must for every pregnant woman.

To ensure that a healthy baby with a good birth weight is born, the pregnant women must take adequate food and rest. During the first trimester, the mother should have balanced diet as usual. As far as practicable, she should avoid medication, as a safeguard against development of congenital anomalies. Four months onwards, a pregnant woman needs adequate nutrition with 25% additional calories and 25% additional protein per day. She should take fresh green vegetables, pulses and fruits, milk and milk products in plenty. The requirement of iron is very high during pregnancy. This cannot be met by diet alone. All pregnant women therefore should have supplements of iron for three months. Folic acid deficiency during pregnancy can result in neural tube defects in the fetus. Ideally folic acid should be supplemented from atleast one month prior to conception.

Unimmunized or partially immunized primi gravida women should have two doses of tetanus toxoid. This will prevent tetanus in the mother as well as the newborn in the intranatal and post natal period. An immunized pregnant woman does not require tetanus prophylaxis within 10 years of the vaccination. After 10 years she will require one dose of tetanus toxoid.

During the second trimester, she should be talked about the advantages of exclusive breastfeeding and prepare her mentally, emotionally and physically to offer breast-feeding to the newborn. Any anatomical abnormalities of the nipple or breast should be inspected and mother reassured that such abnormalities have little to affect breastfeeding.

During the third trimester, rest and relaxation is necessary for the pregnant women. The calories conserved by the mother are expended for the growth of the fetus. Every pregnant woman should rest for two hours in the day and eight hours at night.

All women with complicated pregnancies or with bad obstetrical history should be referred, at the earliest to an equipped centre for adequate maternal and neonatal care. It needs emphasis that, for the baby no better transport incubator is available than transfer in utero.

Care at Birth

The care at birth includes a clean delivery, thermal protection, eye, skin and cord care, early initiation of breastfeeding and effective management of complications e.g. birth asphyxia and early onset sepsis.

Delivery should be conducted in a clean, warm, well lighted, draught free, well ventilated room. In domiciliary set up, the room can be kept warm by a fire burning at one corner. The fire should be from burnt wood charcoal or dry wood, so that there is no smoke. In the hospital set up, the labour room temperature should be maintained at around 25°C.

The Five Clean Practices

The *surface*, on which the baby is delivered, should be clean and warm. This can be achieved by using a clean and warm rubber sheet. The *hands* of the birth attendant as well as the perineum of the women should be thoroughly cleaned with soap and water. *Scissors, umbilical tie and gauze pieces* should be sterile. In the community set up, a new blade can be used if the scissors are not available. The umbilical tie and the blade should be boiled for 10 minutes for sterilization. It is advisable to use umbilical cord clips instead of thread ties to prevent delayed bleeding from the umbilical cord due to shrinkage and loosening of the tie. The *cord* should be kept clean and exposed to air till it falls.

Routine Care at Birth

After complete delivery, the baby should be positioned with the neck in slight extension under a radiant warmer.

This position will keep the airway straight and facilitate initiation and maintenance of breathing. If the baby has copious secretions in the nasal and oral cavity, gentle suction may be necessary with the help of a De Lee's mucus trap. Prolonged and vigorous suction should be avoided because it may further depress the baby. The baby should be then dried thoroughly from head to toe with a prewarmed cloth. The wet cloth should be discarded and the baby effectively wrapped by another piece of prewarmed cloth from head to toe keeping the face uncovered. Wrapping the baby by a wet cloth will lead to loss of heat from the baby's body. In community set up, the clothes for the baby can be prewarmed by hanging them over the fire place. After drying and wrapping, the baby should be bedded in with the mother. It helps (a) in provision of warmth (b) in early initiation of breastfeeding and (c) to establish better emotional bonding between mother and baby.

Care of the Eyes

The eyes should be cleaned at birth and once daily thereafter with sterile cotton swabs soaked in sterile water or normal saline. One swab should be used for one eye. Cleaning should be done from the inner canthus to the outer canthus to avoid eye infection with skin bacterial flora.

Care of the Skin

At birth, the baby's skin should be gently cleaned off mucus, blood, meconium and secretions. The vernix gives protection from heat loss. It should be removed over the next few days. The bath should be preferably postponed till the next day when the baby's body temperature has stabilized. It can however be given after 2–6 hours. A bath has to be given immediately after birth in babies born of hepatitis B surface antigen or HIV positive mothers.

In the immediate neonatal period, the baby can be sponged daily with water giving special attention to the axilla, groin and neck. Dip bath should be avoided till the cord has fallen. Lukewarm water at body temperature should be used for the bath. A daily bath is recommended during summer months. In winter, depending on the severity of cold, the baby may be sponged daily and bathed after every 1–2 days.

Steps of Giving Bath

1. The mother should wash her hands with soap and water.
2. The room should be warm and water should be lukewarm. To check the temperature of the water whether it is suitable for the infant, the mother can feel with her elbow or splash some water to the inner side of the wrist. If mother feels hot, it is very hot for the baby.
3. The infant should be quickly bathed and dried with a prewarmed towel.
4. Then the infant should be wrapped with another prewarmed towel and breast fed. Breastfeeding after birth prevents hypothermia firstly by keeping the baby in close contact with the mother. Secondly, breastfeeding increases metabolism and produce heat in the body.

Care of the Umbilical Cord and Stump

The umbilical cord should be cut at 4 cm length from the base and tied with a sterile cotton tie, a rubber band or a clip. The length of around 4 cm is primarily necessary to prevent injury to a persistent uracus or a vitellointestinal duct which may be present in the umbilical cord. A rubber band or a clip is preferred because it prevents delayed bleeding from the cord due to shrinkage or slipped ligature. The cut end of the cord should be checked for bleeding and inspection of the number and position of umbilical arteries and veins. The two umbilical arteries are placed in the 5 and 7 O' clock position whereas the lone umbilical vein at the 12 O' clock position. The arteries have thick walls and are constricted. The vein has thin walls and has a clot. Presence of only one umbilical artery indicates a more serious anomaly to be present in the baby.

The cord should be left open. No bandage or dressing should be applied. The stump will dry and mummify if exposed to air. No antiseptics are needed for cleaning. If soiled, the cord can be washed with clean water and dried with sterile cotton or gauze. The cord usually dries by 24 hours, shrivels by 72 hours and falls by 5–10 days. A delay in falling may be due to infection, umbilical granuloma and polyp, wet cord and immunodeficiency.

Prevention of Hypothermia

The body temperature of a normal newborn is 36.5°C to 37.5°C. The newborn infant is most sensitive to hypothermia during the body temperature stabilization period in the first 6–12 hours but hypothermia can occur at any time during the neonatal period if the environmental temperature is low and thermal protection is inadequate. Hypothermia can occur even at moderate environmental temperature when babies are not well protected.

The measures to prevent hypothermia in the newborn infant include delivery in a warm room, drying the baby quickly and thoroughly soon after birth, wrapping in layers of prewarmed dry cloth, keeping the baby on a warm surface and bedding in with the mother as early as possible. The bath should be delayed till next day although the body temperature stabilizes by 6–12 hours.

Prevention of Infection

The newborn infant is very susceptible to infection as it emerges from a sterile intrauterine environment. Infection can be prevented by adopting the following simple means viz. regularly practising the 5 clean practices while conducting delivery, by early initiation of breastfeeding, not giving prelacteal feeds, by washing hands every time before handling the baby and tetanus immunization during antenatal period. The two most effective and simple ways to prevent infection are exclusive breastfeeding and hand washing. There is no role of preventive antibiotics in prevention of neonatal infection.

Preventive antibiotics increase cross resistance. Unnecessary antibiotics can harm the immature and developing organs of the neonate. The neonate can be infected by an organism which is not sensitive to the antibiotic administered for prevention; hence will be at a greater risk of infection.

Feeding the Neonate

For the newborn baby, the best milk is unquestionably breast milk. Breastfeeding should be initiated as early as possible within 1 hour of birth irrespective of the mode of delivery and in correct position which enables proper latching. The mother should feed on demand till the baby is satisfied and leaves the breast on its own. Prelacteal feeds are harmful and should not be given. During the first 3–4 days there is physiological inadequacy of breast milk production. During this period the baby should be given frequent feeds. Some babies even need round the clock feeding during the first 4–6 weeks. This is normal. The mother should be reassured and explained that the act of sucking is the best stimulus for breast milk production. Adequate milk flow starts from the 4th day.

Adequacy of Breast Milk

During the period of exclusive breastfeeding, the baby should be monitored for adequacy. The criteria for adequate feeding are (a) Passage of urine 2–3 times/day during first 4 days and 6 or more times a day after the 4th day, (b) Baby sleeps or stays awake, contended in between feeds for atleast 2–3 hours, (c) There is adequate weight gain of 20–30 gms/day in the first 4 months 15–20 gms in the second 4 months.

Immunization Advice at Birth

In all babies delivered in hospital BCG, Polio 0 dose and 1st dose of hepatitis B should be advised within 2 weeks of birth.

Identification of Normal Phenomenon

The normal phenomenon should be identified and the mother reassured that they are not harmful to the baby. No treatment is required.They include:

1. The baby passes meconium within 12–24 hours after birth. It may be delayed if the baby has already passed once in utero.
2. The baby normally passes urine within 24–48 hours after birth. It may be delayed if the baby passed urine immediately after birth.
3. Transitional stools. From the 3rd to 10th day, an exclusively breast-fed baby passes greenish yellow watery stool 7–8 times per day. This is called transitional stool and is not diarrhoea. The child is well, feeding normally and has adequate weight gain.
4. Mongolian spots, erythema toxicum, white discharge and bleeding per vagina, mastitis neonatorum, subconjunctival hemorrhage, regurgitation of milk.

Mastitis neonatorum, characterized by swelling of breasts in term babies of both sexes, can occur on the third or fourth day and may last for few days to weeks and spontaneously regress. There is unilateral or bilateral hypertrophy of breast. *Vaginal bleeding* may occur in 25% of female babies after 3–5 days of birth and last for 2–4 days. It is a withdrawal bleeding. Mucoid vaginal secretions are seen in most female babies. Local antiseptic cleaning should be advised. All these conditions are due to transplacental passage of hormones viz. estrogen and progesterone to the baby.

The Danger Signs

The danger signs in the newborn are good indicators of serious illness in the neonatal period. Every mother should be made aware of these signs and advised to report to a health worker in presence of any one of these in the baby. The danger signs include:

- Cold to touch or febrile.
- Poor activity, not arousable, refusal to feed.
- Respiratory rate > 60/minute, chest retractions.
- Apnea/stoppage of breathing or laboured respiration.
- Cyanosis (Blue discoloration of lips/ tongue).
- Jaundice involving palms and soles.
- Convulsion/abnormal movements.
- Bleeding from any site.
- Diarrhea or vomiting or abdominal distension.
- Umbilical discharge or skin boils.

The Target Milestones

All mothers should be made aware of four target milestones viz. social smile by 2 months, head holding by 4 months, sitting without support by 8 months and standing without support by 12 months. A mother's monitoring will help early detection of developmental delay.

Follow-up

All newborn babies should be followed up in the well baby clinic. The follow-up care should include assessment of growth (by anthropometry), advice regarding complementary feeding, immunization, supplementation of iron and remedy for minor problems.

Every baby needs weight record every week in the first two months, monthly for the first year and twice a year from second year onwards.

Advice on Discharge

The mother should be advised in the following line at the time of discharge.

1. Maintenance of warmth throughout the neonatal period.
2. Exclusive breastfeeding upto 6 months age.
3. Follow-up and start vaccination at the earliest contact within 2 weeks and then at 6 weeks age.
4. Monitoring of danger signs. Mother should be made aware of the danger signs during the neonatal period. She should be advised to report if any danger sign appears.
5. The mother should be made aware of the 4 important milestones during the first year of life. She should be advised to report immediately if there is any delay. Babies with delayed milestones need a detail neurodevelopmental examination and early intervention.
6. The mother should be advised about personal hygiene, birth spacing, nutrition (an extra meal over and above the normal food every day), and to continue iron folic acid tablets.
7. Discuss about traditional practices. Promote good traditional practices. Discourage harmful ones and ignore the harmless ones.

Low Birth Weight

A neonate who weighs less than 2500 grams is called a low birth weight baby. In India 30–40% of infants are born low birth weight. Nearly 75% neonatal death and 50% of infant deaths occur among the low birth weight babies. The higher risk of death continues during infancy and even later. Besides the high risk of mortality, these babies often continue to remain more prone to malnutrition, recurrent infection, and neurodevelopmental handicaps. There is increasing evidence that low birth weight infants are at more risk of being prone to diabetes mellitus, hypertension and coronary artery disease in adult life.

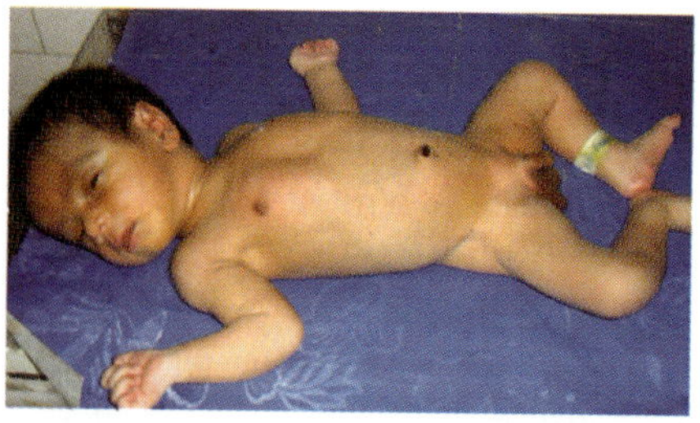

Fig. 7.1: A term infant

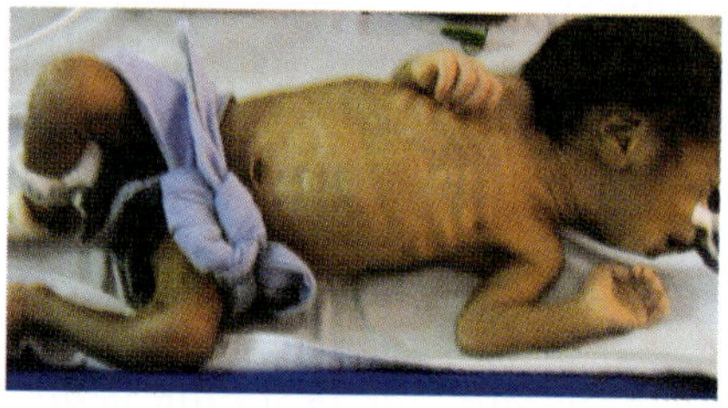

Fig. 7.2: An asymmetric small for date baby

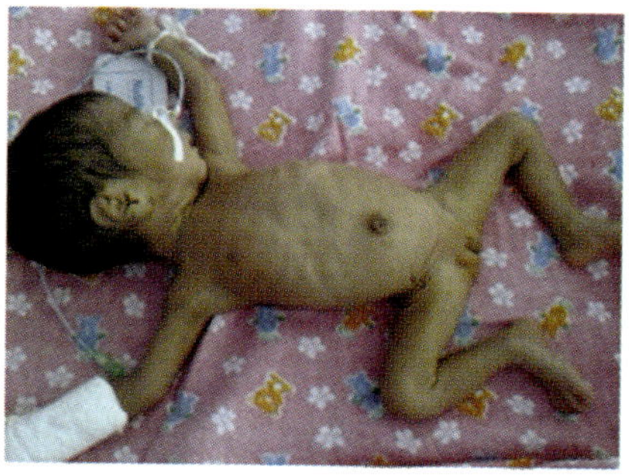

Fig. 7.3: A preterm baby

Types of Low Birth Weight (LBW)

A low birth weight baby may be preterm or small for date and at times both preterm and small for date. 75% of LBW babies born in India are small for date and 25% are preterm a situation which is just the opposite of what is existing in the western countries.

Fetal size and weight are directly related to the period of gestation. If a baby is born early i.e. before completing 37 weeks of gestation, the baby is likely to have a lower weight. On the other hand, the baby may be born at term or preterm but the weight is low as a result of intrauterine growth retardation. This condition is similar to malnutrition but in utero.

A *preterm baby* is one which is born before 37 completed weeks of gestation. A baby is called *small of date* if the weight is less than 10th percentile or less than 2 standard deviation or less than 3rd percentile for the period of gestation. A consensus about the definition of small for date is yet to be reached.

A neonate can be identified as appropriate for date (AFD), small for date (SFD) or large for date (LFD) in relation to gestation by using the intrauterine growth chart.

It will be appropriate to have a locally prepared IUGR chart for precise determination. A baby is said to be AFD if the weight is between 90th percentile and 10th percentile. It is said to be large for date when the weight is above 90th percentile and SFD when the weight is below 10th percentile in relation to the gestation.

Classification of Low Birth Weight

The low birth weight babies may be classified into three categories:

1. *Low birth weight* when birth weight is between 1500 to 2500 grams.
2. *Very low birth weight* when birth weight is below 1500 grams.
3. *Extremely low birth weight* when birth weight is below 1000 grams.

Classification of Small for Date Babies

Small for date babies may be classified into the following three types:

1. **Asymmetric or malnourished:** It results from placental insufficiency during the later part of pregnancy. The baby looks marasmic. Weight is low. The length and head circumference is not affected. The brain weight is unaffected or shows minimal reduction. The other internal organs viz. liver is grossly shrunken. The double skin-fold thickness is reduced. The skin of the buttocks hangs in folds due to lack of subcutaneous fat. The ponderal index is usually less than 2 as compared to more than 2.5 in term appropriate for gestational age. The growth retardation is mainly due to the reduction in size of the cells while the number of cells remaining unaffected. These babies retain the potentiality of normal growth on nutritional rehabilitation. The ponderal index (PI) can be calculated as follows: PI = Weight in grams / $(\text{length in cm})^3 \times 100$.
2. **Hypoplastic or symmetric:** This type is a result of adverse influence of intrauterine infections, certain genetic and chromosomal disorders on the fetus from early embryonic life. There is a reduction in the growth potential. The baby is proportionately small in all parameters including head size. Both cell size and population are reduced which results in permanent mental and physical growth retardation. There is also a high incidence of congenital abnormalities in this type of babies.
3. **Mixed type:** This group of babies is an outcome of adverse effects operating from early or mid pregnancy. They are low birth weight babies for the gestation but they neither look malnourished nor hypoplastic. These babies have varying degrees of reduction in cell size and cell population.

Classification of Preterm

The preterm babies may be classified as follows:

1. *Preterm AFD:* These are babies born preterm but have a birth weight corresponding to gestation.
2. *Preterm SFD:* These babies are born preterm but weight is below 10th percentile for the corresponding gestation.
3. *Preterm LFD:* These babies are born preterm but the weight is above 90th percentile for the corresponding gestation.

The weight corresponding to gestation can be determined from the intrauterine growth chart. Among the low birth weight babies, the preterm SFDs have the worst long term prognosis.

Etiology

The determinants of intrauterine growth retardation as well as prematurity are not fully understood. Some causal factors have been cited for both the conditions.

The factors known to predispose preterm delivery are:

1. Teen age pregnancy, multiple pregnancy.
2. Past history of preterm delivery, cervical incompetence.
3. Fetal abnormalities.
4. Induced preterm delivery.
5. Unknown cause.

The factors known to predispose small for date babies (IUGR) are:

1. Small mother (height < 145 cm, weight < 40 kg).
2. Frequent pregnancies.
3. Pregnancy induced complications viz. Hypertension, pre-eclamptic toxemia, antepartum hemorrhage.
4. Chronic maternal diseases viz. diabetes, severe asthma, chronic renal and cardiovascular diseases, chronic malaria.
5. Multiple pregnancy.
6. Tobacco use.

Clinical Features of the Preterm and Small for Date Babies

Preterm

The appearance and behaviour of the preterm infant is dependent on the degree of immaturity. The baby has a disproportionately large head and abdomen. Lack of subcutaneous tissue results in a thin face, loose skin over the limbs and frequent appearance of visible peristalsis. The infant sleeps more or less continuously and the cry is feeble and infrequent. The respiration is rhythmic but is often jerky or irregular with periodic spells of apnea (periodic breathing). Muscular movements are less frequent and vigorous than in term infant. The ability to suck is absent before 32 weeks of gestation while the coordination between sucking and swallowing develops only after 34 weeks of gestation. Edema may be present at birth and may become more during the next 24–48 hours. Severe edema is a bad prognostic sign. Edema is frequently associated with antepartum hemorrhage, pre-eclampsia and maternal diabetes. In preterm infant, hunger is indicated by crying, restlessness and movements of the limbs. If signs of hunger do not appear within 96 hours, it should arouse suspicion of infection or intracranial hemorrhage. A preterm infant can be diagnosed on the basis of the period of gestation calculated from the last menstrual period. The preterm infant also has some distinct physical features which will help in their recognition in case the last menstrual period is not known accurately.

1. Posture of limbs depends on the degree of hypotonia and the extent of prematurity. The posture may be partially flexed to frog like.
2. Colour of the skin is pink due to lack of subcutaneous fat and relatively thinner skin texture.
3. The hair is fuzzy and scanty. The individual hair can be separated.
4. The external ear is soft and devoid of cartilage. The cartilaginous part does not recoil back promptly on being folded.
5. The breast nodule is less than 5 mm in diameter.
6. In the males, the scrotum is small, light brown to pink in colour, rugaes are absent and testes are not descended into the scrotum. In female babies, the labia majora are widely separated, the labia minora are exposed and clitoris is hypertrophied.

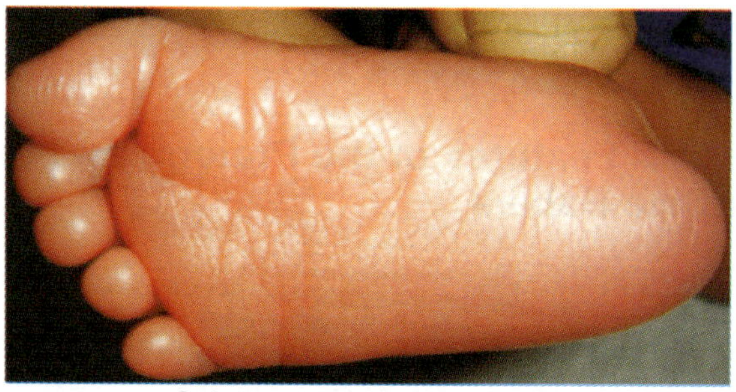

Sole creases (term infant)

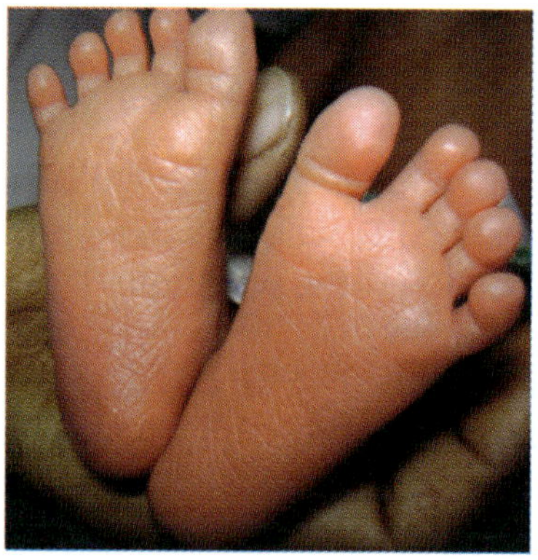

Sole creases (Preterm infant)

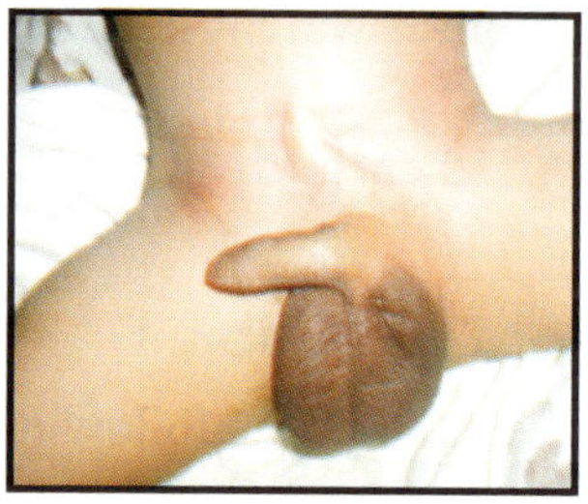

Genitalia male (Term infant)

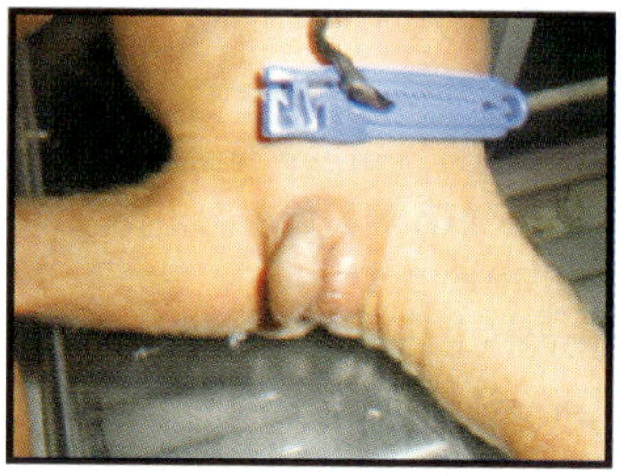

(Preterm infant)

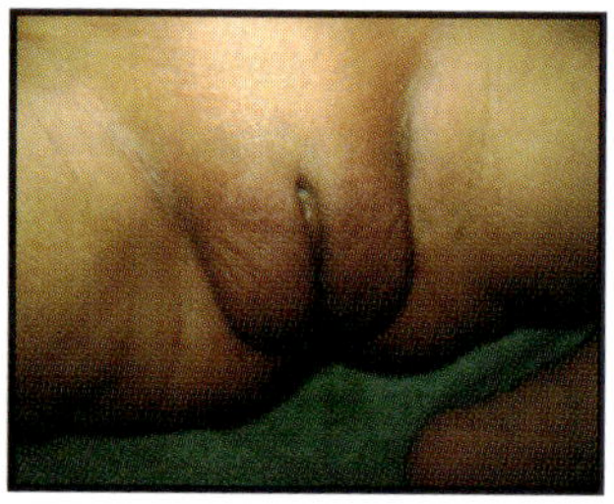

Genitalia female (Term infant)

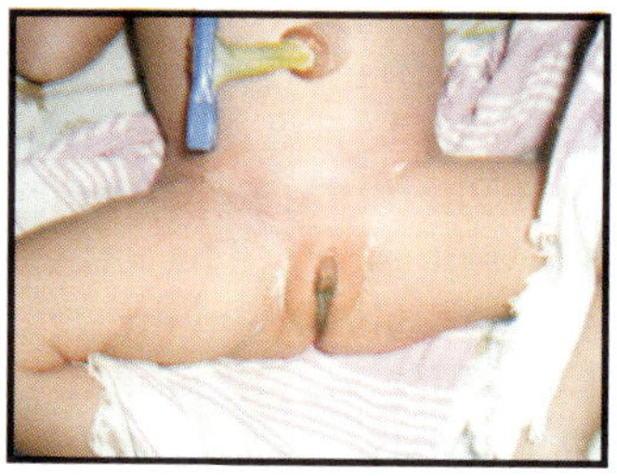

(Preterm infant)

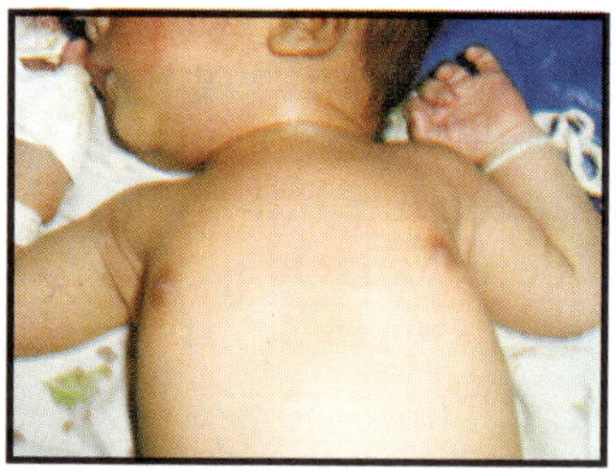

Breast buds (term)

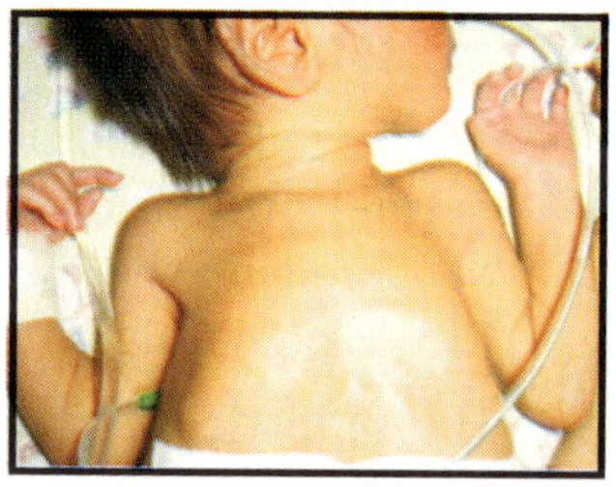

Breast buds (preterm)

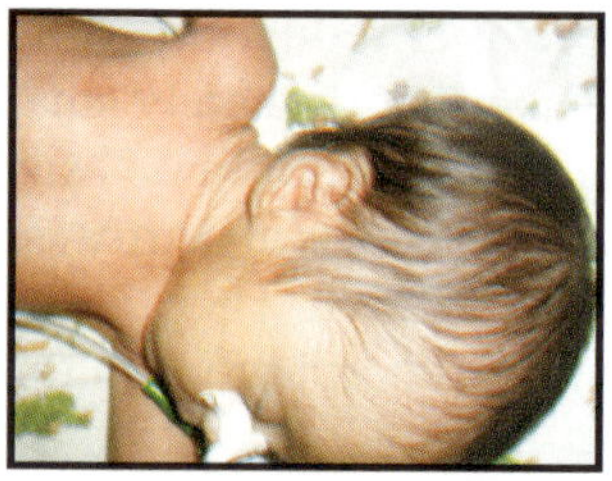

Ear cartilage (term)

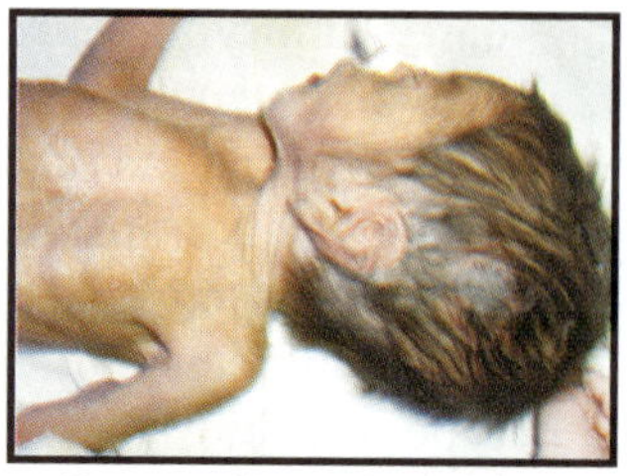

Ear cartilage (preterm)

Fig. 7.4: Some physical features for assessment of gestation

7. The soles are either covered with fine creases all over or show one deep crease in the anterior one third.

Small for Date

The external appearance varies with the degree of placental insufficiency and duration of pregnancy. In postmaturity, the infant looks thin and wasted, often with dry desquamating skin, but length and head circumference are normal. The appearance is that of recent loss of weight. There is frequently meconium staining of nails, skin and umbilical cord. Death due to hypoxia during labour is common in such infants.

In cases with prolonged placental insufficiency, the infant is born term or preterm. All the anthropometric parameters are affected. The length and head circumference are affected more than the weight. The baby looks thin and wasted. The skin is dry and desquamating, often with transverse cracks over the lower chest and abdomen and at the ankles and wrist. There may be meconium staining of the nails and cord. These infants have a characteristic wide-awake expression which is not seen in a preterm infant. These infants have a high risk of pulmonary hemorrhage and a high hematocrit level which is unexplained.

Combined Preterm and Small for Date

These types of babies will have features of both preterm and small for date.

Problems in Low Birth Weight Babies

The low birth weight babies are predisposed to a number of problems. The problems are however different in the preterm and small for date babies.

Problems in the Preterm Baby

Immaturity of the organ systems is the basic underlying feature of the preterm baby. The major problems encountered in management of these babies are:

1 Maintenance of body temperature.
2. Inability to protect against infection.
3. Feeding problems.
4. Vulnerability to complications viz. Asphyxia, RDS, apnea, intracranial hemorrhage, late metabolic acidosis, hyperbilirubinemia, retinopathy of prematurity, necrotizing enterocolitis.
5. Congenital malformations.

Term newborn infants maintain body temperature by active metabolism in brown fat stores. The preterm infant lack brown fat and therefore become hypothermic at usual ambient temperature. They lack an efficient humoral, cellular and mucosal immune mechanism. Thus, being immunocompromised hosts are unable to protect themselves against bacterial infections.

Neonates below 34 weeks of gestation do not have coordinated sucking and swallowing. So direct breast-feeding is not possible. Those less than 30 weeks of gestation may not tolerate enteral feeds initially because of gut immaturity. They are at frequent risk of vomiting, gastric stasis, aspirations, abdominal distension and functional obstruction as a result of immature gastrointestinal digestive and motor function. Late developing digestive enzymes which can compromise nutrition are lactases and lipases often giving rise to lactose and fat intolerance. Enzymes that regulate synthesis of cystine from methionine, taurine from cystine and catabolism of tyrosine are also immature. Therefore, the small preterm is at risk of developing deficiency of some amino acids and potentially toxic accumulation of others.

Preterm babies, especially those less than 34 weeks of gestation have immature lungs which do not expand well at birth and are unable to perform the function of gas exchange efficiently. They develop respiratory distress syndrome. These babies also have a tendency for apneic spells as a result of immature respiratory control mechanism.

Spontaneous bleeding into one or both lateral ventricles is a characteristic complication of a preterm baby. It may be associated with hyaline membrane disease or may develop without lung diseases. This is the result of a immature vascular bed around the brain ventricles. The microvasculature of the germinal layer in the preterm consist of an extensive arrangement of fine capillaries and also of large irregular thin walled vessels which form short connecting channels between arterial and venous trees. These vessels readily rupture when exposed to sudden surges in pressure which can be provoked by both hypoxemia and hypercapnia. The germinal layer involutes from 32 weeks gestation and it is presumed that intraventricular hemorrhage in later gestations arises in the choroid plexus. Intraventricular hemorrhage is common in newborns below 32 weeks gestation but can occur thereafter.

Immature metabolic pathways predispose preterm babies to develop hypoglycemia, metabolic acidosis, and hyperbilirubinemia. Gluconeogenesis is less effective in preterms; therefore glucose administration is rapidly required to prevent significant hypoglycemia. Preterm infants given excess oxygen may develop retinopathy of prematurity resulting in blindness because of damage to the immature retina.

Problems in the Small for Date Babies

The basic problem in these babies is in utero under nutrition and hypoxia. The major problems encountered in management of these babies are birth asphyxia, meconium aspiration, hypothermia, hypoglycemia, infections and polycythemia.

The stress of labour may lead to fetal distress which may lead to passage of meconium in utero and birth asphyxia. As a result of chronic malnutrition in utero, these babies also lack in brown fat and hence are prone to develop hypothermia. Deficient glycogen stores predispose them to develop hypoglycemia. As a result of chronic intrauterine stress on the body immune system, they are prone to infection. Chronic intrauterine hypoxia results in polycythemia. They may also face feeding difficulties although much less than preterm babies.

Identification of Low Birth Weight Babies in Community

Majority of births in our country still take place at homes. These deliveries are attended either by untrained dais or family members. Weighing the baby is the best method to identify low birth weight even in the community. The weight is usually not taken; hence low birth weight babies are often not identified and not referred for proper care. It has been suggested that if the weighing of babies is not possible in the community, the measurements of chest circumference and mid arm circumference can be used to identify low birth weight babies. Studies have shown that both these measurements correlate well with weight. However, there is need for extensive studies before they are accepted as standard methods.

Management

Delivery of the Low Birth Weight Baby

Every effort should be made to avoid the delivery of a low birth weight baby at home because in delivery of such a baby, the full resources of a hospital are desirable. Nonetheless, the low birth weight baby will at times have to be delivered at home. Hence the strategies to increase salvage of these babies shall include:

Identification of mothers at risk and early referral to a centre with adequate facilities for newborn care. Transport in utero should be preferred to transport of the low birth weight newborn, because mother's womb is considered as the best incubator. The mothers at risk of delivering a low birth weight baby are:

1. Young and unmarried mother.
2. Previous history of preterm delivery.
3. Multiple pregnancies.
4. Complications during antenatal period viz—PET, PIH, threatened abortion, APH, cervical incompetence.

If delivery has already taken place, the survival of the baby can be ensured to an extent by early identification and classification of the neonate on the basis of period of gestation and birth weight and suggestion of appropriate level care as shown in the table below:

Wt (gms)	*Gestation (weeks)*	*Care*
Above 2000	Above 34	Level-I
2000-1500	34-32	Level-II
Below 1500	Below 32	Level-III

Place of Delivery

Delivery should always be conducted by trained health professionals, at least one of them should be well trained with the art of neonatal resuscitation. Baby must be provided warmth from the moment of birth. The temperature in the room, where delivery is conducted, should be maintained at 25 degree centigrade, with the help of a heat source like a room heater. The baby should be received in prewarmed cloth (at home) or a pre-warmed resuscitation unit with an overhead radiant warmer. In absence of a warmer, a table lamp with 200 watt bulb can be used which should be kept at a distance of 45 cm over the baby well wrapped from head to foot.

When induction of preterm labour before 34 weeks is planned in a hospital, betamethasone or dexamethasone IM in a dose of 6 mg every 12 hours for four doses or 12 mg every 24 hours for 2 doses should be administered to the mother before delivery. Maternal glucocorticoid therapy lowers the incidence of hyaline membrane disease, bronchopulmonary dysplasia, patent ductus arteriosus and intraventricular hemorrhage. If possible, analysis of the amniotic fluid should be done for determination of phosphatidylglycerol level and lecithin/sphingomyelin ratio.

Irrespective of delivery in a hospital or home, the babies requiring hospitalization and special care include:

i. Gestation less than 34 weeks.
ii. Birth weight less than 1800 grams.
iii. The preterm with complication.
iv. Presence of feeding difficulties, irrespective of period of gestation.

Transportation

Proper care during transport of the baby is very essential since it may determine its ultimate survival. The principles of care during transport include the following:

a. Stabilization before starting the journey.
b. Provision of warmth.
c. Nutrition.
d. Monitoring of vital signs and cardiorespiratory resuscitation during transport.

Details of neonatal transport are discussed in a separate chapter.

Maintenance of Warmth and Prevention of Hypothermia

At home, the newborn infant should be kept dry, effectively dressed in 2-3 layers of non-restrictive and heat retaining prewarmed clothes. The low birth weight baby's scalp constitutes a fairly large part of the total surface area thus heat loss can be minimized by putting a cap or covering with cloth. In summer months, no extra effort is required to maintain the room temperature but in winter months a room heater or a fire place may be required. Room temperature must not fall below 21°C. The baby should lie near the mother to receive maternal warmth. If a baby is maintaining normal body temperature, the trunk feels warm and soles and palm are pink and warm. In early stages of hypothermia (cold stress), the trunk is warm but soles and palms are cold to touch. This is a useful method of monitoring body temperature at home.

At hospital, in the nursery, when under a servo control radiant warmer, the baby should be naked except for the napkin. In order to achieve a thermo neutral environment the nursery temperature should be maintained at 28 ± 2°C and baby's body temperature 36.5°C–37.5°C. Regular monitoring of axillary/rectal temperature (sick babies) should be carried out as soon as the baby is admitted in nursery, then hourly for 4 hours, then 4 hourly.

Feeding

Feeding the low birth weight neonate is a formidable challenge because of greatly increased demands, poor endogenous stores and immature digestive and other organ system. These babies require high protein and energy intake if they are to gain adequate weight.

The first feed in an otherwise hemodynamically stable, non-asphyxiated preterm baby and a small for date baby should be started as soon as possible, within 1 hour after birth. Before the first feed and as soon as after birth as possible, the gastric contents be aspirated. This procedure will exclude esophageal atresia and it seems to lessen the tendency to vomiting.

Early minimal enteral feeding (less than or equal to 10 ml/kg/day) can be given soon after birth to medically stable preterm babies. These feedings, known as trophic feeding are intended to prime the gastrointestinal tract prior to initiation of more substantial enteral nutrition. Trophic feeding has the following advantages:

1. Stimulates and promotes gastrointestinal hormone response.
2. Improves feeding tolerance.
3. Increases weight gain.
4. Decreases hyperbilirubinemia, osteopenia and gastrointestinal residues.

What to Feed?

Breast milk is the ideal food for both preterm and small for date neonates. Those babies who are unable to feed directly from the breast can be given expressed breast milk (EBM) by gavage or from a cup. In case enough EBM is not available from baby's own mother, EBM can be collected from some other lactating women and given to the baby after pasteurization. If this is not possible extra fluid should be replenished by IV fluids for first few days.

It is worth mentioning that breast milk is not only species specific but also baby specific. Milk produced by mothers after preterm delivery contain higher protein and calories and is uniquely suited to provide optimum nutrition to the prematurely born.

If lactation is inadequate in spite of best efforts, the baby should be evaluated for supplementary feeding with top milk. It should be emphasized that a decision to feed a preterm baby with milk other than human milk is a major decision and should not be taken lightly. Moreover, it should be reserved essentially for hospitalized babies and resorted to for the minimum period.

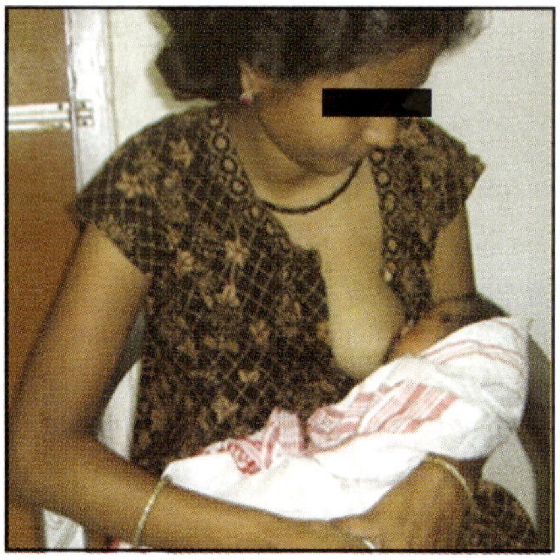

Breastfeeding

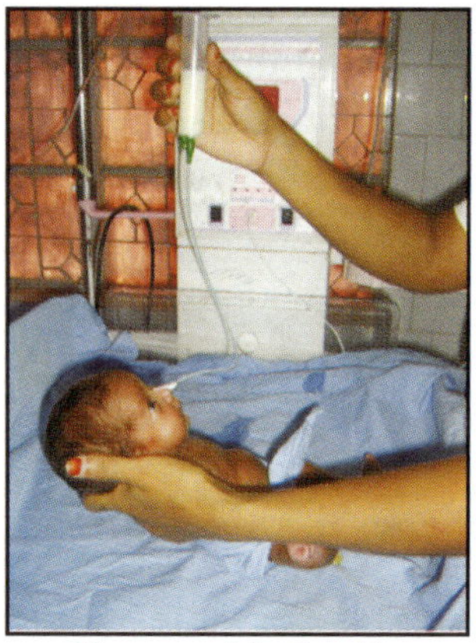

Nasogastric feeding

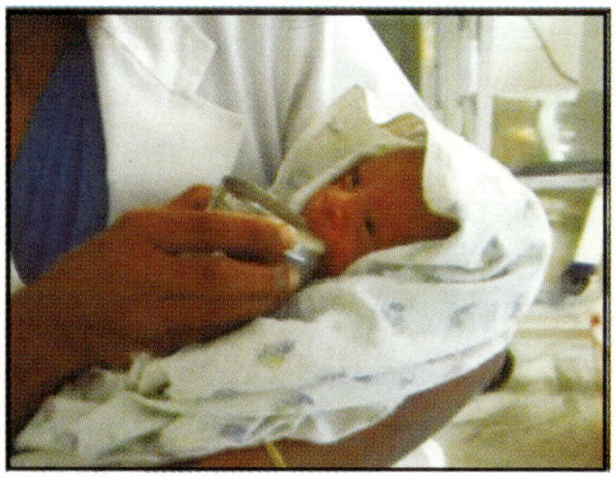

Cup feeding

Fig. 7.5: The modes of feeding

Mode of Feeding

The mode of feeding will depend on the age, birth weight and gestation of the baby as shown in the table below:

Table 7.1 : Guidelines for providing fluids and feeding

Age	*Birth weight and gestation*		
	< 1200 gms	1200 – 1800 gms	> 1800 gms
	< 30 weeks	30 - 34 weels	> 34 weels
Initial	I.V. fluids Try gavage feed If not sick	Gavage feeding	Breastfeeding, if not satisfactory, cup feeding
After 1-3 days	Gavage	Cup feeding	Breastfeeding
Later 2-4 weeks	Cup feeding	Breast feed	Breast feed
4 – 6 weeks	Breast feed	Breast feed	Breast feed

Amount and Frequency of Feed

The total fluid requirements can be estimated from fluid requirements as shown in the table below:

Table 7.2 : Fluid requirements in low birth weight babies

Day of life	*Birth wt. > 1500 grams (ml/kg)*	*Birth weight < 1500 grams (ml/kg)*
1	60	80
2	75	95
3	90	110
4	105	125
5	120	140
6	135	155
7 onwards	150	170

An extra amount of 30 ml/kg/day should be added for babies nursed under radiant warmer and additional 15 ml/kg/day for those receiving phototherapy.

Types of fluid: Intravenous fluid administration when necessary should be given as 10% dextrose in the initial 2 days. Thereafter N/5 saline (prepared by adding 1 part N/S to 4 parts dextrose) with 1 ml kcl/100 ml fluid generally meet the electrolyte demand.

Feeding intervals: Depend on the weight of the baby as shown below:

Weight	Interval
Less than 1000 gms	2 hourly or continuous drip
1000 gms-1500 gms	2 hourly
Above 1500 gms	3 hourly

Volume increment also depend on the weight of the baby

- To begin with 1-2 ml/kg/feed (1ml/kg/hour for continuous feeding).
- For less than 1000 gms increase by 1ml to a maximum of 5 ml/kg/day.
- Between 1000-1500 gms increase by 2 ml to a maximum of 10 ml/kg/day.
- For those above1500 gms increase by 5 ml to a maximum of 25 ml/kg/day.

Feeding Guidelines for Continuous Nasogastric Feeding

Birth weight	Initial rate (ml/kg/day)	Volume increment (ml/kg/day)
Less than 1000 gms	10-20	10-20
1000-1500 gms	20-30	20-30
Above1500 gms	30-40	30-40

Monitoring During Feeding

1. Aspiration of first residual is important. If aspirate is more than 20 ml, than intestinal obstruction should be suspected. If nasogastric tube does not go beyond 8-10 cm, esophageal atresia is suspected.
2. Baseline abdominal girth is noted. Abdominal girth should be measured before each feed. An increase of more than 2 cm than the base line measurement indicates abdominal distension.
3. Prefeed aspiration: 2-3 hourly for intermittent gavage feeding and 4 hourly for continuous gavage feeding should be done.
4. If prefeed aspirate is more than 20% of previous feed, the amount of next feed is reduced by 20%. If prefeed aspirate is more than 50% of previous feed or the abdominal girth is more than 2 cm of baseline, enteral feeding should be stopped and baby monitored on IV fluids till abdominal distension is relieved.
5. The feeding tube should be changed every 2-3 days.
6. The feeding tube size should be 5F(preterm), 6F(term).
7. Stool should be examined for reducing substance daily.
8. Urine should be examined for specific gravity daily.
9. Feeding tolerance is judged by absence of abdominal distension, vomiting, and gastric residue of less than 20% of previous feed, which is nonbilious and non-hemorrhagic.

Monitoring of a Hospitalized Preterm Baby

1. *Temperature:* To be checked 1 hourly for first four hours then 4 hourly.
2. Axillary temperature or human touch methods for otherwise well babies. Rectal temperature to be monitored for the sick babies.
3. Nursery temperature to be maintained at 28±2°C. Baby's body temperature should be maintained at 36.5°C–37.5°C.
4. *Respiration:* To be checked 1 hourly for first 6 hours then 4 hourly. Baby should be closely observed for apnea for 1 week.
5. Blood glucose should be monitored in neonates < 35 weeks, < 1500 grams and SFD at 3, 6, 12, 24 and 72 hours.
6. To look for signs of intraventricular hemorrhage viz. sudden pallor, bulging fontanelle, sudden respiratory arrest.
7. Routine ultrasonography brain to be done in babies < 32 weeks,< 1500 gms on 0-2, 7-10, 21-28 days and close to 40 weeks post conceptional age.

Vitamin and Mineral Supplements

All low birth weight babies should receive:

- Intramuscular Vitamin K (0.5 mg) at birth.
- Vitamin A 1000 IU/day, Vitamin D 400 IU/day, Vitamin C 35 mg/day should be supplemented from 2 weeks of age upto 37 weeks of gestation.
- Iron supplementation (2 mg/kg/day) should be started at 8 weeks of age and continued up to 1 year age.
- A baby below 32 weeks and below 1500 gms also needs to be supplemented with calcium (120 mg/kg/day) and phosphorus (60 mg/kg/day) from birth upto 6 months age.
- Vitamin E 5 IU/day is to be started after 4 weeks and to be continued upto 37 weeks of gestation.
- All babies born below 35 weeks should be given 7.5% sodium bicarbonate (0.5 ml/feed) from birth 37 weeks to prevent late metabolic acidosis, when nursed on artificial milk.

Adequacy of Nutrition

The weight pattern of the baby is the key measure of optimal feeding. A preterm baby looses 1 to 2% of body weight every day amounting to 10 to 14% cumulative weight loss during first week of life. Birth weight is regained by 10 to 14 days. They start gaining weight by the 2nd week of life at the rate of about 10-20 gm per day. The small for date baby's weight remain static for the first 2–3 days. They do not loose weight. They start gaining weight after 2–3 days if adequate feeding is given.

It is desirable to weigh the baby at 2 weeks (to check regaining of birth weight), at 4 weeks (to ascertain a weight gain of at least 200-300 gms, then every month. Hospitalized babies however, should be weighed every day on the same weighing machine.

Milk Fortification

Milk fortification should be continued till the infant is of 3 kg weight. Breast milk continues to be the first choice for feeding. However, when volumes have to be restricted, the nutrients in the breast milk may be insufficient to support adequate growth. In such situations human milk may need fortification. This can be achieved by addition of:

1. Human milk fortifier (recently made in India as dry powder) to increase the protein content and energy content of preterm milk upto 2.8 gm/100 ml and 82 cal/100 ml respectively.
2. *Oil and sugar fortification:* MCT oil and glucose polymer have proven to be the best fortifier as they increase the caloric density without altering solute load or osmolality and easily digested by preterms. Coconut oil (0.25 ml-1 ml/feed) and sugar 2-5 gms/30 ml can be used as fortifiers. Coconut oil contains more than 60% MCT and is cost effective for use in our country.

Immunization

All vaccines are recommended to be administered as per schedule according to the chronological age irrespective of birth weight or period of gestation except Hepatitis B (For details *See* Chapter 3).

Early Detection of Sickness

Anticipation and early detection of complications and sickness is the cornerstone of care of preterm babies. During the neonatal period clinical monitoring of danger signs in newborn is the most important and practical method.

A baby who shows one or more of the danger signs should be immediately referred for hospitalization and prompt management.

During the post-neonatal period prompt recognition and treatment of acute diarrhoeal disorders and ARI is important since the risk of death from these acute diseases is higher in low birth weight babies.

Perinatal Asphyxia

Perinatal asphyxia and birth injuries together contribute to almost 30% of neonatal deaths. It is the most common cause of neonatal mortality in the first 24 hours of life. It is a preventable cause of neonatal mortality.

Definition

The term birth asphyxia has long been used to indicate failure on the part of the newborn to establish spontaneous respiration immediately following complete delivery. The first consequence of failure to breathe is anoxia, rapidly followed by excess accumulation in the blood of carbon dioxide, and by a fall in the blood pH.

The WHO has defined perinatal asphyxia as "a failure to initiate and sustain breathing at birth". The National Neonatology Forum of India has suggested that birth asphyxia should be diagnosed when a baby has gasping and inadequate breathing or no breathing at 1 minute after birth. It corresponds to 1 minute Apgar score of 3 or less. It is a simple definition, which can be used in the community as well as for purposes of estimating the incidence of birth asphyxia.

The National Neonatal Perinatal database also defined moderate asphyxia as slow gasping breathing or an Apgar score of 4–6 at 1 minute and severe asphyxia as no breathing or an Apgar score of 0–3 at 1 minute.

However, the goal is not only to recognize that some degree of asphyxia is present but to identify the degree of asphyxia that pose a serious threat of irreversible neurologic injury. In this context, the American College of Obstetrics and Gynecology and the American Academy of Pediatrics has proposed that the following criteria should be present when perinatal asphyxia with potential for resultant neurologic deficits occurs. They are:

1. Cord umbilical artery pH of < 7.0 with a base deficit of >10 mEq/L.

2. Persistence of Apgar score of 0–3 for longer than 5 minutes.
3. Presence of neonatal neurological sequelae viz. seizures, coma, hypotonia.
4. Evidences of multisystem organ dysfunction (e.g. cardiovascular, renal, gastrointestinal, hematological or pulmonary).

Etiology

Around 90% of asphyxial events occur in the ante partum or intrapartum period as a result of placental insufficiency. The remaining 10% result from post partum events usually due to pulmonary, cardiovascular or neurologic insufficiency in the neonate.

Fetal Anoxia

Fetal anoxia during the ante partum period can occur by the following mechanisms viz. anoxic anoxia, anemic anoxia, stagnant anoxia and histotoxic anoxia.

Anoxic anoxia results from inadequate supply of oxygen to fetus which results from diminution of oxygen tension in the mother's circulation. The conditions responsible include diseases in the mother (e.g. congestive cardiac failure, pneumonia, emphysema), placental insufficiency due to pre eclamptic toxemia, pregnancy induced hypertension, antepartum hemorrhage, and prolonged labour.

Anemic anoxia exists when the fetal blood is so anemic that it cannot carry sufficient oxygen to meet the needs of the tissues. This situation may arise following hemolysis due to Rh incompatibility or fetal hemorrhage associated with twin to twin transfusion.

Stagnant anoxia can arise from compression, prolapse or knotting of the umbilical cord.

Histotoxic anoxia arises when the fetal tissues, specially the nervous system, are so poisoned by drugs or damaged by hemorrhage that the cells can no longer utilize the oxygen delivered to them. The drugs responsible are narcotics. It is particularly important during preterm labour.

Natal and Post Natal Anoxia

Anoxia in the natal and postnatal period may result from failure of the neonate to establish lung inflation and successful transition from fetal to neonatal cardio-pulmonary circulation due to airway obstruction, excessive fluid in the lungs, weak respiratory effort, and drug induced CNS depression, congenital anomalies and birth injury.

Physiology of Asphyxia

The sequence of changes that takes place in asphyxia has been studied in experimental animals. On exposure to anoxia, an initial period of rapid breathing is followed by a period of cessation of respiration called primary apnea.

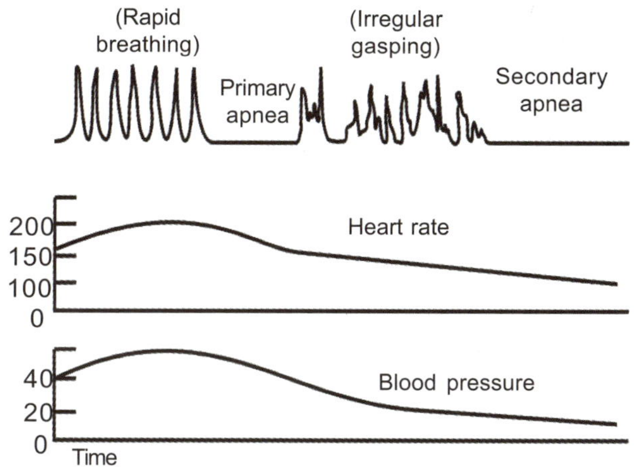

Fig. 7.6: Physiology of asphyxia

During this period, the heart rate begins to fall. Exposure to oxygen and stimulation during this period of primary apnea in most instances induce respiration. If the asphyxia continues, the animal develops deep gasping respiration and the heart rate continues to decrease and blood pressure begins to fall. The respiration become weaker until it takes a last gasp and enters a period of apnea called secondary apnea. In this phase the animal becomes unresponsive to stimulation and positive pressure ventilation is necessary for revival. An important point to note is that in the case of intrauterine asphyxia the fetus may go through the phases of primary and secondary apnea in utero. So all cases of apnea at birth should be considered as secondary apnea and resuscitation must begin immediately. Further, once in secondary apnea, greater the delay in starting ventilation, the longer is the period of secondary apnea. The longer the duration of secondary apnea, the greater is the chance that brain damage will occur.

The changes which occur in an asphyxiated fetus and neonate are probably similar to those observed in experimental animals.

Pathophysiology

When a fetus or neonate is subjected to asphyxia, there is redistribution of blood flow. This is achieved by neurogenic vasoconstriction occurring in the non-vital organs like skin, muscles, gut, liver and kidney in an effort to increase the blood flow to the vital organs – the brain, heart and the adrenals. But under progressive hypoxia myocardial pump failure occur leading to fall in cardiac output and blood pressure ultimately leading to decreased cerebral blood flow. The changes which may occur as a result are as follows:

CNS: Hypoxic ischemic encephalopathy, infarction, intracranial hemorrhage, seizures.

Cardiovascular: Myocardial ischemia, poor contractility, cardiac failure, tricuspid insufficiency, hypotension.

Pulmonary: Persistent fetal circulation, pulmonary hemorrhage, respiratory distress syndrome.

Renal: Acute tubular necrosis or cortical necrosis.

Adrenal: Adrenal hemorrhage.

Metabolic: SIADH, hyponatremia, hypoglycaemia, hypocalcemia, cryoglobinuria.

Skin: Subcutaneous fat necrosis.

Hematological: Disseminated intravascular coagulation.

Hypoxic Ischemic Encephalopathy (HIE)

It is the most important consequence of perinatal asphyxia among all the effects as well as those on the central nervous system.

Pathophysiology

The pathophysiology of HIE has been chiefly studied by creating two experimental states:

1. Prolonged partial asphyxia.
2. Acute total asphyxia.

In *prolonged partial asphyxia* (1 hour or longer) as in placental abruption, at first there is redistribution of fetal blood flow from nonvital to vital organs. As the duration and degree of fetal hypoxemia progresses the fetal blood pressure drops and a second redistribution of blood flow, this time within the brain, occurs. Here the blood flow to the cerebral hemispheres (anterior circulation) is found to decrease relative to blood flow to the thalamus, brain stem and cerebellum (posterior circulation). The cerebral hemispheres then become most vulnerable. In full term neonate, the first areas to be compromised are the parasagittal cortex and the underlying white matter leading to selective neuronal necrosis, parasagittal cerebral injury, status marmoratus and focal and multifocal ischemic brain injury. In preterms, periventricular white matter necrosis occur leading to periventricular leucomalacia.

Often asphyxiated neonates will succumb to dysfunctions of non-brain organs; the CNS showing minimal evidence of hypoxic ischemic brain injury. In such instances the brain was spared in expense of cardiac output to the affected organ (diving reflex). The degree of asphyxia required to cause permanent neurologic impairment is just below that which is lethal for multisystem failure.

In near *total asphyxia* (as in cord prolapse), hypoxia is so abrupt that any compensatory inter organ and intra brain shunting is ineffective and the areas of highest metabolic demand and least reserves–the thalamus and certain brainstem nuclei are the most vulnerable. Cerebral hemispheres are usually spared.

It has been shown that the presence of preceding partial asphyxia followed by total asphyxia results in more rapid physiologic deterioration and neuro-pathological damage predominating in the basal ganglia with variable damage to parasagittal cerebrum, thalamus and brainstem.

Mechanism of Hypoxic Ischemic Brain Damage at Cellular Level

An asphyxia insult precipitates an intricate array of reactions in distinct sequences and they are interrelated on many levels. Under physiologic conditions, levels of cellular ATP, the primary energy source of the cell are maintained stable as energy consumption is balanced by ATP production. When oxygen availability is limited, oxidative phosphorylation ceases and cells shift to anaerobic glycolysis, which is much less efficient than aerobic metabolism. When this also cannot maintain adequate ATP production, existing ATP breaks down. This leads to depletion of high-energy compounds, in turn making it increasingly difficult to maintain intracellular ion concentration and cellular integrity. Failure of the ATP dependent Na^+ - K^+ pump leads to depolarization of cells, allowing the influx of Na^+ and Ca^{++} and there by producing cytotoxic edema. Increased cytosolic calcium, arising from influx across plasma membranes as well as from release of intracellular stores, in turn elicits numerous other intracellular metabolic pathways, including activation of phospholipases, release of prostaglandins, lipases, proteases and endonucleases all of which injure various structural components of the cells, culminating in further cytotoxicity. High intracellular calcium also contributes to the formation of oxygen free radicals.

During reperfusion, a burst of ROS (reactive oxygen species) is generated, mainly by the activity of xanthine oxidase and primarily in endothelial cells. ROS are in high-energy state with the potential to directly damage almost all types of molecules in living cells (phospholipids, sugars, amino acids and nucleic acids). Of the various neurotransmitters, excessive release of endogenous excitatory neurotransmitter glutamate and failure of its reuptake from the synaptic cleft leads to neuronal injury. Glutamate acts through NMDA receptors resulting in influx of sodium and calcium ions into the cells inducing neuronal death from the osmolar load.

In summary, asphyxia triggers a cascade of biologic processes culminating in cell death.

Clinical Spectrum

Hypoxic ischemic encephalopathy has a spectrum of clinical manifestations from mild to severe.

Within 12 hours after the insult, the infants show signs of cerebral dysfunction and are stuporous or comatose, have periodic breathing or irregular respiratory effort, are hypotonic, and have lost all complex reflexes viz. Moro's reflex, sucking reflex etc. They have roving eye movements but the pupillary responses are intact. Subtle, tonic, or multifocal clonic seizures may occur within 6–24 hours in around 50% of cases of moderate or severely asphyxiated infants.

Between 12–24 hours there may be apnea requiring respiratory support.

After 24 to 72 hours following the insult, the severely affected infant may have prolonged apnea, abnormalities of pupillary reactivity, loss of oculometric and caloric responses. Brain death may ensue between 24–72 hours later. In most severe cases, in which the incidence of death or significant neurologic sequelae is greatest, other organ systems inevitably show evidence of asphyxial damage.

Persistent oliguria (<1 ml/kg/hr for the first 36 hours) has been found to be significantly associated with severe HIE and poor outcome. To estimate the severity of asphyxial insult, the Sarnat clinical stages can be used in infants more than 36 weeks of gestation. For practical purpose, the Levine clinical classification of HIE is useful.

Classification of HIE (Levine)

Feature	*Mild*	*Moderate*	*Severe*
Consciousness	Irritable	Lethargy	Comatose
Tone	Hypotonia	Marked hypotonia	Severe hypotonia
Seizure	No	Yes	Prolonged
Sucking/Resp	Poor suck	Unable to suck	Unable to sustain resp

Pathophysiology of Asphyxia in Other Organs

In moderate to severe asphyxia, the non brain organs are doubly compromised. The changes in the different systems are as follows:

Cardiovascular System

Infants with perinatal asphyxia may have transient myocardial ischemia with failure manifested by respiratory distress and cyanosis shortly after birth.

They have signs of congestive cardiac failure viz. tachycardia, tachypnoea, an enlarged liver and a gallop rhythm.

Many infants will have a systolic murmur at the lower left sternal border (tricuspid regurgitation) and some will have a murmur at the apex (mitral regurgitation).

The chest X-ray will show cardiomegaly with or without pulmonary venous congestion.

The ECG may show ST depression in mid precordium and T wave inversion in left precordial leads.

The echocardiogram/Doppler will show normal cardiac structures but decreased left ventricular contractions, especially of the posterior wall and signs of persistent pulmonary hypertension. The ventricular end diastolic pressures are usually elevated. Some infants may show tricuspid regurgitation with right to left shunting at the atrial level. Some may show mitral regurgitation.

Renal Effects

The asphyxiated infant is at risk of acute tubular necrosis and SIADH.

Gastrointestinal System

The asphyxiated infant is at risk of bowel ischemia and necrotizing enterocolitis, early signs of which are intestinal stasis, presence of reducing substances and occult blood in stool.

Hematologic Effects

Disseminated intravascular coagulation (DIC) may occur as a result of damage to blood vessels, failure of the liver to produce clotting factors and bone marrow to produce platelets. Spontaneous bleeding from venepuncture site may be the earliest sign of DIC, followed by bleeding manifestations.

Liver Function

The infant may present with a 'shock liver', i.e., a severely damaged liver unable to provide even the basic functions or signs of liver failure.

Pulmonary Effects

The pulmonary effects of asphyxia include increased pulmonary vascular resistance, pulmonary hemorrhage, pulmonary edema secondary to cardiac failure, and possibly due to failure of surfactant production with secondary hyaline membrane disease (Adult respiratory distress syndrome).

Markers of Perinatal Asphyxia

Clinical Markers

1. *Fetal distress:* Fetal monitoring by intermittent auscultation or continuous electronic fetal monitoring is a useful method for early detection.
2. Meconium staining of amniotic fluid.
3. *Apgar score:* The Apgar scores assigned at 1 and 5 minutes have for long been used to define asphyxia. But persistent low Apgar scores at 10, 15 and 20 minutes have been associated with adverse long-term outcome.

Biochemical Markers

1. Umbilical artery pH < 7.0 is associated with adverse outcome.
2. Elevated serum lactate pyruvate and creatinine kinase brain isoenzyme (CPK- BB > 5 I U), neuron specific enolase.
3. Elevated cord erythropoietin level.
4. Elevated level of hypoxanthine, a breakdown product of ATP, is nowadays being used as the new gold standard for perinatal asphyxia. The recommended cord blood hypoxanthine levels for defining asphyxia is > 16 mmol/L.

Radio Imaging

1. *USG of brain:* Best done during 4-7 days of life. Helps in diagnosis of periventricular and intraventricular hemorrhage and leucomalacia.
2. *CT scan:* It continues to be the gold standard among imaging studies in term neonates with HIE. CT is useful in assessing the degree of edema, when performed early (2 to 4 days after insult) and the extent of cerebral injury (encephalomalacia) when performed late (at least 2-4 weeks after insult).
3. Newer imaging techniques like Magnetic Resonance Imaging (MRI), Nuclear Magnetic Resonance Spectroscopy, Near Infrared Spectroscopy (NIRS), Single Proton Emission Computed Tomography (SPECT) and Positron Emission Tomography (PET) help mainly to prognosticate the disease.

Electrophysiological Study

1. *EEG:* A burst suppression interictal pattern in light sleep and awake stage is ominous.
2. *Evoked responses viz:* Abnormal visual evoked responses (VER) and brainstem auditory evoked responses (BAER) during the first 2 weeks of life have been correlated with poor outcome.

Management

Management of perinatal asphyxia should start in the labour room with resuscitation of all newborns that are unable to initiate spontaneous respiration after complete delivery. The baby who fails to initiate and sustain respiration at birth is at risk of hypoxic ischemic brain injury and needs regular monitoring. All these babies should have a cord blood gas analysis performed. The following babies are to be transferred to the special care newborn unit for observation and treatment:

1. Babies with severe birth asphyxia (Apgar score 0–3 at 1 minute).
2. Babies who required prolonged bag and mask ventilation (> 5 minutes).
3. Babies who suffered from moderate asphyxia (Apgar score 4–6 at 1 minute age) when monitoring is not possible in the postnatal ward.

It should be noted that no specific interventions have yet been shown to improve the outcome following perinatal asphyxia although potential therapies are being evaluated.

Therefore, careful anticipatory supportive management is recommended.

Maintenance of Temperature

The baby should be placed under a radiant warmer and nursed in a thermoneutral environment and temperature monitored.

Check vital signs and record base line data.

An immediate clinical assessment should be made by recording respiration, heart rate, blood pressure/capillary refill time (CRT), temperature, oxygen saturation, urine output.

Fluids

Start intravenous fluids (10% dextrose) in babies with Apgar score < 4 at 1 minute or < 7 at 5 minutes with two third of maintenance fluid.

Check blood sugar, hematocrit and blood gases.

All these parameters should be maintained in the normal range for the first 48–72 hours. Blood gases and acid base status should be maintained in the physiological range (PaO_2 80–100 mmHg, $PaCO_2$ 35–40 mm Hg and pH 7.35–7.45).

Consider Volume Expander

Consider infusion of volume expander (Normal saline/ Ringers lactate10 ml/kg over 5–10 minute, may be repeated if required) if CRT is > 3 seconds, or if there is metabolic acidosis. Blood pressure should be maintained above 35 mm (for term babies).

Poor perfusion may be due to hypovolemia or secondary to myocardial ischemia. If poor perfusion persists after the initial bolus, ionotropes should be started. Dopamine should be started 3–5 microgram/kg/min. The dose should be increased stepwise at the rate of 10 microgram/kg/ min. If perfusion is still poor dobutamine should be added at the rate of 5 micrograms /kg/min. The maximum dose of each drug is 20 microgram /kg/min.

Fluid overload should be avoided. It may exacerbate cardiac dysfunction and cerebral edema or lead to hyponatremia, which increases cerebral irritability and the risk of convulsion.

Fluids should be restricted in the first 24 hours, as oliguria is likely as a result of ADH secretion and renal ischemia.

The markers of normal perfusion are:

a. Normal urine output (>1 ml/kg/hr) and specific gravity.
b. Normal blood pressure. The blood pressure should be maintained at the upper normal range.
c. Capillary refill time normal (< 3 seconds).
d. Absence of metabolic acidosis.

Miscellaneous treatments consist of administration of Vitamin K (1 mg IM) to all infants with perinatal asphyxia. A stomach wash may be performed if there is meconium staining.

Monitoring

Monitoring of the vitals as mentioned above must be continued. An accurate record of urine output is a must. In addition the following should be monitored:

- Blood sugar estimation at 2, 6, 12, 24, 48 and 72 hours of age.
- Hematocrit once a day for first few days.
- Serum sodium, potassium, calcium once a day.
- ABG as often as required.
- Neurological status viz. sensorium, tone, reflexes, seizure, autonomic disturbances every 4–6 hours.
- Special investigations viz. EEG, CT scan, MRI does not help a great deal in the initial management of asphyxia. Their utility is for prognostication.

Maintenance of Oxygenation and Ventilation

Infants with respiratory failure require oxygen and ventilation. Oxygen levels should be kept in the normal range by monitoring of transcutaneous or arterial pO_2 or percent oxygen saturation by pulse oximeter. Blood gases should be monitored with an aim to keep PaO_2 > 60 mm Hg and $PaCO_2$ < 40 mmHg. In babies with adequate spontaneous respiration, oxygenation is maintained by oxygen delivery by an oxygen hood. Assisted ventilation is indicated in presence of apnoea, inadequate spontaneous respiration and continuing hypoxia or hypercarbia. Target PaO_2 is 80–100 torr in term and 60–80 torr in preterm babies. Target $PaCO_2$ is 40–45 torr. Oxygen saturation should be maintained in the range of 90–95 % in term and 90–93% in preterm babies.

Electrolytes

Hyponatremia without excessive urinary sodium loss is likely to be due to excess ADH secretion. It can be managed with fluid restriction.

Hyperkalemia may occur during the acidotic phase. Potassium should not be added to the IV fluids until good urine flow is established.

Hypokalemia may occur as result of secondary hyperaldosteronism. Potassium has to be added to intravenous fluid in time.

Hypocalcemia: Calcium level should be maintained in the normal range. 10% calcium gluconate should be given 4 ml/kg/day for 1–2 days as continuous infusion or as bolus diluted 1:1 under ECG monitoring.

Acidosis: Acidosis should be treated by improving perfusion and maintaining oxygen saturation. There is no evidence that correction of acidosis with buffer improves the condition. However, if problems with perfusion persist despite treatment with fluids and oxygen, then 7.5% sodium bicarbonate should be given in the dose of 2–3 mEq /kg diluted in equal volumes of distilled water.

Blood Glucose

Blood glucose level should be kept at 60–100 mg/dl as hypoglycemia may worsen CNS damage and hyperglycemia may exacerbate acidosis. Blood glucose levels should be monitored and treatment of hypoglycemia should be instituted as and when necessary. Rapid glucose bolus should be avoided. Hence serum glucose levels should be monitored frequently (with Dextrosticks) for adjustments of glucose concentration of the fluid for infusion.

Hematocrit should be maintained at > 40% in ventilated babies. If hematocrit is > 65% it should be brought down to 55% by partial exchange transfusion using normal saline.

Seizures

Seizures are typically focal or multifocal. They occur in about 50% of cases, characteristically on the first or second day, usually in stage II, rarely in stage III, and almost never in stage I HIE. When a seizure is diagnosed it should be treated along the line of neonatal seizure.

When the infant is stable for 3–4 days, all anticonvulscents are weaned except phenobarbitone. All anticonvulscents are stopped by 14 days. Seizures following severe asphyxia are difficult to control and are often resistant to aggressive anticonvulscent therapy in the first 72 hours. It should be noted that once the conventional anti-convulscents are given in the maximum dosage, there is little utility in eliminating every twitch or EEG seizure. For unexplained reasons, even refractory seizures cease after approximately 48 hours.

Cerebral Edema

Cerebral edema and raised intracranial pressure are uncommon concomitants of perinatal asphyxia. They peak at 36 to 72 hours after the insult. They are more properly regarded as an effect rather than a cause of brain damage. They reflect prior cerebral necrosis rather than swelling of intact cells. Their presence indicates a bad prognosis. Present literature has shown that efforts to reduce cerebral edema or ICP do not affect outcome. Hence interventions previously used as anti-edema agents do not have much use. It is believed that the infant's patent sutures and open fontanel are protective of any acute rise of ICP that might occur.

Cardiac Effects

The treatment consists of adequate ventilation with correction of hypoxemia, acidosis and hypoglycemia. Volume overload should be avoided. These babies require continuous monitoring of mean arterial pressure, central venous pressure and mixed venous saturation and urine output. Infants with cardiac collapse will require treatment with dopamine and dobutamine. Some infants in great distress may require afterload reduction with peripheral beta agonist (isoproterenol), a peripheral alpha blocker (e.g. tolazoline), or nitroprusside.

Hepatic, GIT, Hematologic and Pulmonary System Effects

Liver function tests should be monitored. Serum ammonia level should be measured. Serum glucose should be kept at 60–100 mg/dl. Drugs that are detoxified in the liver should be avoided. If used, blood levels monitored. Treatment of liver failure should be done, if present.

It is preferable not to start oral feeds in an asphyxiated infant till 5–7 days. NEC should be treated in the usual lines.

Clotting factors (PTT, PT), fibrinogen, and platelets should be monitored and replaced if need be in case child develops DIC.

Besides oxygenation and ventilation, extracorporeal membrane oxygenation (ECMO) provides a recent therapeutic modality in an asphyxiated infant whose CNS appears otherwise intact.

Newer Treatment Modalities

Opiod antagonist: Post ischemic blood brain barrier disruption and enhanced endogenous opiod have been implicated in the pathogenesis of ischemic neuronal injury.

The potential for use of naloxone is under evaluation.

Free oxygen radical scavengers and inhibitors: It has been shown that super oxide desmutase, Vitamin E, and allopurinol, a xanthine oxidase inhibitor have neuroprotective roles in animal studies.

Calcium channel antagonist: The use of calcium channel blockers like flunarizine and nimodepine could prevent neuronal injury and death by preventing calcium influx into cells.

Excitatory amino acid antagonist: Pre-treatment of animals with agents such as MK801, ketamine and dextromethorphan has produced variable results when used prior to asphyxia.

Selective head cooling has been shown to decrease cerebral energy demands and is an attractive option.

It should be noted that none of these modalities are ready for routine use as yet.

Prognosis

Overall, full term asphyxiated infants have a mortality of 10-20%. The incidence of neurologic sequelae in survivors is 20-45% (approximately 40% of these are minimal; 60% severe). The risk of CP is 5-10% among asphyxiated newborns.

Indicators of poor outcome are low (0-3) extended Apgar score, Saranat Stage III encephalopathy, seizure of early onset and difficult to control, elevated ICP (>10 mm of Hg), persistence of abnormal neurologic signs specially absence of Moro's reflex after 1-2 weeks, persistence of extensive hypodensity on CT, elevated CK-Bb level (>5 IU), persistent oliguria (<1ml/kg/hr) for first 36 hours of life, interictal EEG with extreme burst suppression activity.

Birth Trauma

Birth trauma is physical injury to an infant during birth process. Injuries may occur antenatally, intra partum, or during resuscitation. The following factors contribute to an increased risk of birth injury.

1. Primipara.
2. Short stature in the mother.
3. Maternal pelvis abnormality.
4. Prolonged or unusually rapid delivery.
5. Oligohydramnios.
6. Malpresentation of the fetus.
7. Use of mid forceps or vacuum extraction.
8. Versions and extraction.
9. Very low birth weight/extreme prematurity.
10. Fetal macrosomnia or large fetal head.
11. Fetal anomalies.

Evaluation at Birth

Every neonate at risk should be thoroughly examined at birth to exclude birth trauma. Birth trauma may be minor or major. Minor traumas are asymptomatic and recover spontaneously. Major traumas may require urgent intervention medical or surgical.

Soft Tissue Injuries

Petechiae and ecchymosis: They are common in the skin of head and neck. Treatment is supportive. They resolve within 1 week.

Lacerations and abrasions: These occasionally occur secondary to scalp electrodes, fetal scalp blood sampling or injury during birth. Scalpel injuries can occur during delivery by caesarean section. These injuries are at risk of secondary infection.

Treatment consists of close observation, cleaning of the wound. Deep wound may require sutures.

Subcutaneous fat necrosis: Presents during first 2 weeks after birth. They are sharply demarcated, irregular, firm, non pitting subcutaneous plaques or nodules, present over extremities, face, trunk or buttocks.

No treatment is necessary. They resolve spontaneously in weeks to months.

Head and Neck Injuries

Caput succedaneum: It is a boggy swelling extending over the presenting part of the scalp. It is usually associated with molding. It is a result of subcutaneous, extraperiosteal fluid collection; may be occasionally

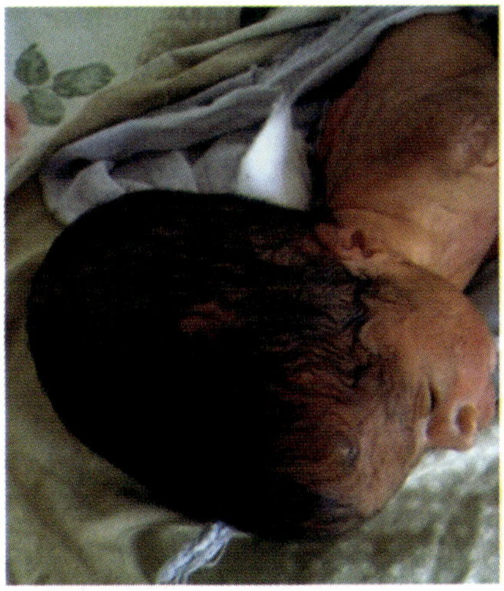

Fig. 7.7: Caput succedaneum

hemorrhagic. It has poorly defined margins and can extend over the midline and across the suture lines. It is present at birth and resolves spontaneously over the first several days.

Cephalhematoma: Is a subperiosteal collection of blood resulting from rupture of superficial veins between the skull and periosteum. The swelling is always confined to the suture lines. It appears 2–3 days after birth. Most cephalhematoma resolve within 8 weeks. Occasionally calcification can persist for several months. An extensive cephalhematoma can lead to hyperbilirubinemia or rarely anemia necessitating blood transfusion. Skull fractures are associated in 5–20% cases. Infection may occur rarely associated with septicemia and meningitis.

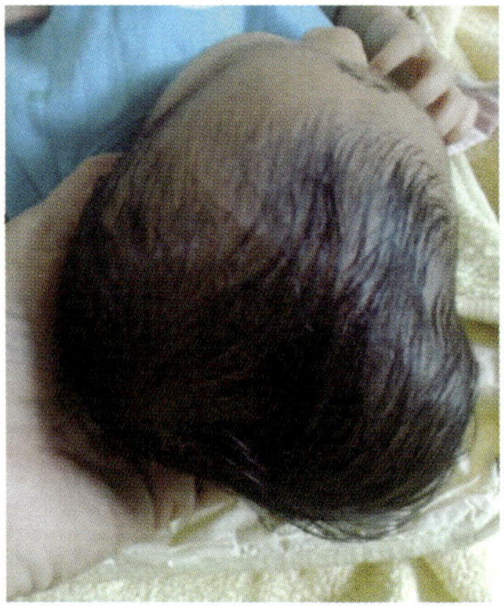

Fig. 7.8: Right parietal cephalhematoma

Management is observation. A CT scan brain should be obtained if there is an associated neurological symptom. Significant anemia and hyperbilirubinemia should be treated in the usual lines. Aspiration of the cephalhematoma is contraindicated because it may introduce infection.

Subgaleal hematoma: Results from hemorrhage under the aponeurosis of the scalp. It may extend across the entire calvarium along the attachment of the aponeurosis from the orbital ridges to the nape of the neck and laterally to the ears.

The clinical presentations include a fluctuant swelling on the scalp, pallor and poor tone. The baby may present with shock in presence of a rapidly increasing hematoma. The blood is reabsorbed slowly. Hypovolemia and hyperbilirubinemia may occur as a result of an extensive lesion.

Management consists of observation. Tests to exclude a bleeding disorder should be considered. Monitoring for hypovolemia, hyperbilirubinemia and infection is important.

Sternocleidomastoid injury: It is also called congenital or muscular torticollis. The exact cause is not known. The most likely cause is thought to be the result of intra-uterine positioning of the fetus. It may also occur as a result of rupture of the sternomastoid muscle fibres due to hyperextension of the muscle during delivery with development of a hematoma and subsequent fibrosis and shortening. Torticollis may be present at birth or more often after 2–3 weeks of age, with a palpable mass 1–2 cm in the sternomastoid region with a head tilt to the side of the lesion. Treatment is initially conservative. Stretching of the muscle should begin promptly and should be done several times a day. Recovery usually occurs within 3–4 months in around 80% cases. Surgery is indicated if torticollis persists beyond 6 months of physical therapy.

Nerve Injury

Brachial Plexus Injury

Three types of injury can occur to the brachial plexus: (a) Duchenne- Erb's palsy, (b) Total brachial plexus palsy, (c) Klumpke's palsy.

a. **Duchenne-Erb's palsy:** It is a result of injury to the upper trunk of brachial plexus (C5, C6 and occasionally C7). As a result of the injury there is weakness or paralysis of the deltoid, infraspinatus, biceps, brachioradialis, and extensors of the wrist and fingers.

   Clinically, the baby present with the affected arm adducted and internally rotated. There is extension and pronation at the elbow and flexion of the wrist and finger with a characteristic posture of policeman tip. The deep tendon reflexes are absent on the affected side. The Moro's reflex is asymmetrical (absent on the affected side) and the Grasp reflex is present. Sensation may be variably affected. There may be diaphragm paralysis in around 5% cases.

b. **Total brachial plexus palsy:** It is a result of injury to the whole brachial plexus. The whole arm is flaccid on the affected side. The deep tendon and primitive reflexes are absent. Sensation is absent. If sympathetic fibres are injured at T1 level, Horner's syndrome may be seen.

c. **Klumpke's palsy:** It is a result of injury to the lower trunk of brachial plexus (C7/C8, T1). Paralysis affects the intrinsic muscles of hand and the long flexors of the wrist and fingers. Deep tendon reflexes are present. The grasp reflex is absent. There is sensory impairment of the ulnar side of the forearm and hand. There is ipsilateral Horner's syndrome due to injury to the sympathetic fibres in T1.

Course and prognosis: Recovery depends on the extent of the nerve injury. If the nerve roots are not avulsed, complete recovery occurs in 90% cases. Notable clinical improvement in the first 2 weeks after birth indicates return of normal or near normal function. Most infants recover by 3 months of age.

Management: A radiograph of the shoulder and upper arm should be ordered if there is suspicion of fracture viz. clavicle, upper humerous or lower cervical spine. These may mimic brachial palsy. The chest should be examined to exclude diaphragmatic paralysis.

Treatment is conservative. No splinting should be advised in Erb's palsy as it may lead to development of contractures of the shoulder girdle muscles. Wrist and finger splints in Klumpke's palsy may be useful. Passive movement of the joints prevents contractures. Physical therapy may be started after 7–10 days when the post injury neuritis has resolved.

In those infants with slow recovery, nerve conduction and EMG will help to distinguish avulsion and stretch injury. These infants may require surgical intervention.

Phrenic Nerve Palsy

Phrenic nerve palsy can occur as a result of stretch injury during breech or forceps delivery. It usually occurs together with brachial plexus injury. Phrenic nerve injury leads to paralysis of the ipsilateral diaphragm.

Clinical features include decreased movement of the affected hemithorax, persistent tachypnoea, cyanosis and decreased breath sounds at the lung base. A chest radiograph may show elevation of the diaphragm of the affected side. The diagnosis is confirmed by demonstration of paradoxical movement of the diaphragm on ultrasonography.

Initially treatment is supportive. CPAP or mechanical ventilation may be needed to avoid atelectasis and pneumonia. Majority of infants recover by 3 months without permanent sequelae. In refractory cases diaphragmatic placation may be considered.

Facial Nerve Palsy

Although it is the most common peripheral nerve injury, most cases are subtle and resolve spontaneously. It results from compression of the nerve by forceps, pressure on the nerve secondary to the fetal face lying against the maternal sacral promontory. Facial nerve injury results in asymmetric crying facies. Both the upper motor and lower motor type of paralysis can occur.

Management is directed towards protection of cornea by using artificial tears, application of eye patch over the open eye. Surgical intervention should not be planned before the first year.

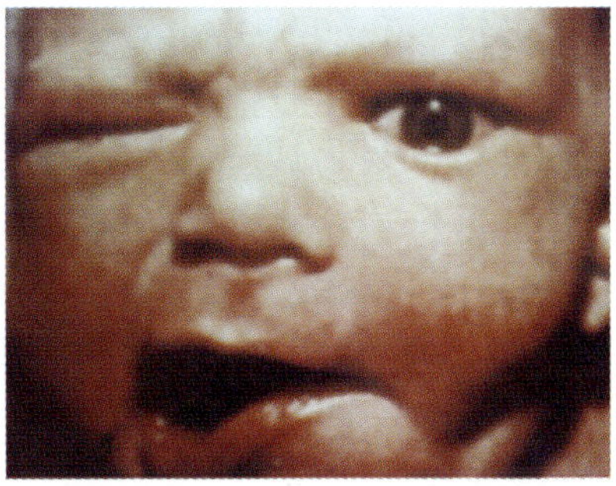

Fig. 7.9: Facial nerve palsy (left side)

The prognosis of acquired facial nerve palsy is excellent with complete recovery by 3 weeks.

Recurrent Laryngeal Nerve Injury

Recurrent laryngeal nerve palsy can occur due to excessive traction on the fetal head during breech delivery or lateral traction during forceps delivery. The left recurrent laryngeal nerve is affected more often because of its long course. Bilateral nerve involvement can occur and is usually due to hypoxia or brainstem hemorrhage.

With unilateral injury, the neonate is asymptomatic at rest. Hoarseness and inspiratory stridor develop during crying. It may be associated with hypoglossal nerve injury which results in difficulty in feeding and secretions. Features of bilateral nerve injury are stridor, severe respiratory distress and cyanosis.

The diagnosis can be confirmed by direct or flexible fiberoptic laryngoscopy.

Unilateral nerve injury usually resolves by 6 weeks of age without any intervention and treatment. Bilateral injury has a variable prognosis.

Spinal Cord Injury

Spinal cord injury can occur during vaginal delivery of an infant with hyperextended head or neck, breech delivery, and severe shoulder dystocia. The manifestations depend on the level of injury.

1. High cervical or brainstem injury present as stillborn or the baby is born with respiratory depression, shock and hypothermia. Death usually occurs within hours of birth.
2. Upper or mid cervical injury present with central respiratory depression, lower motor neuron paralysis of lower extremities, absent sensation of the lower half of the body, urinary retention and constipation.
3. Injury at the 7th cervical vertebra or lower may be reversible.
4. Partial spinal injury or spinal artery occlusion may result in subtle neurologic signs and spasticity.

The aim of management in spinal injury is resuscitation and prevention of further injury. This requires immobilization of head and spine. Neurology and neurosurgical consultations should be advised.

Bone Injuries

Clavicle is the most commonly injured bone during delivery. The humerous fractures occur during difficult deliveries and the femoral are common in infants with congenital hypotonia.

Clavicle Fracture

It usually occurs in large babies, with shoulder dystocia in vertex presentation and in breech deliveries with extended arms.

A green stick fracture may be asymptomatic. The only clinical sign may be a swelling over the clavicle at 7–10 days after formation of a callous. In complete fracture, arm movements are absent because of pain on movement. There is a palpable bony irregularity, crepitus and spasm of the sternomastoid.

A clavicle fracture may be confirmed by an X-ray of the chest.

For treatment, analgesic should be given for pain. The infant's arm on the affected side should be immobilized for 7–10 days until the callous begins to form.

Humerous Fracture

It occurs during difficult deliveries of the arm in breech and shoulders in vertex.

In case of a greenstick fracture, the first sign is loss of spontaneous movement followed by swelling and pain on passive movement. However, it may not be recognized till callous formation occurs. A complete fracture presents with an obvious deformity. Radial nerve injury may be seen. An X-ray confirms the diagnosis.

Treatment is directed towards alleviation of pain with analgesics. Immobilization should be done for 2 weeks. Displaced fractures require closed reduction and casting. Displacement of the epiphysis needs confirmation with an ultrasound examination and immobilization of the limbs for 10–14 days.

Prognosis is excellent with complete healing.

Femur Fracture

It usually occurs following breech deliveries. The injury may not be obvious for a few days until there is a swelling, decreased movement or pain on palpation. Femoral epiphysis separation is confirmed by an ultrasound examination. The diagnosis is confirmed by X-ray.

Therapy includes analgesics for pain and immobilization of the limb for 10–14 days.

Skull Fracture

The skull fractures may be linear or depressed. Linear fractures are seen over the parietal bones. Depressed fractures are seen over the parietal as well as the frontal bones and are associated with forceps delivery. Both types of fractures are asymptomatic unless there is an associated intracranial hemorrhage viz. subdural or subarchnoid. Occipital bone fractures are associated with breech deliveries and may cause cerebellar contusion and significant hemorrhage.

The diagnosis of skull fractures need X-ray evaluation. A head CT should be obtained when intracranial injury is suspected.

An uncomplicated linear skull fracture usually requires no therapy. Depressed fractures require neurosurgical evaluation. If there is CSF rhinorrhoea or otorrhea, antibiotics should be started and urgent neurological consultation should be taken.

Intra-abdominal Injuries

Intra-abdominal injuries during birth are uncommon. The organs affected are the liver, spleen and adrenals. The liver is the most commonly affected organ.

Liver and Spleen

The risk factors, clinical presentation and therapy are similar for injury of both the organs. Risk factors include breech presentation, large babies, hepatic/ splenic enlargement. The etiology is direct pressure over the organs.

Subcapsular hematomas are asymptomatic at birth. The baby develops nonspecific signs of blood loss viz. refusal to feed, pallor, tachypnoea, tachycardia, onset of jaundice during the first 1–3 days after birth. In case of a splenic hematoma, a swelling may be palpable in the left upper quadrant. Rupture of hematoma results in discoloration of the abdominal wall and shock.

Serial hematocrit will suggest blood loss. A coagulation profile may be necessary to exclude coagulation disorder. In case of splenic hematoma, an abdominal radiograph will show displacement of the stomach bubble to the right.

Management includes volume replacement and treatment of coagulation disorder if present. A surgical consultation may be necessary for laparotomy.

Intracranial Hemorrhage

Hemorrhage inside the cranium can occur (i) external to the brain into the epidural, subdural and subarachnoid spaces, (ii) into the brain parenchyma of the cerebrum or cerebellum, (iii) into the ventricles from the subependymal germinal matrix or the choroidal plexus. There is often a combination of two or more types of intracranial hemorrhage e.g. extension of a parenchymal hemorrhage to the subarachnoid space or ventricles.

Clinical manifestation depends on the location of hemorrhage. Diagnosis is usually made on clinical suspicion on the basis of neurological signs viz. seizures, irritability or depressed level of consciousness, focal neurological deficits referable either to cerebrum or cerebellum.

Diagnosis is confirmed by neuroimaging viz. USG or CT scan.

Management varies according to the location and size of intracranial hemorrhage and presenting neurological signs. The modalities include (i) A very large hemorrhage requires surgical intervention for drainage. (ii) A large hemorrhage require volume replacement and or pressor support with dopamine, dobutamine etc. (iii) Symptomatic treatment of seizure and treatment of post hemorrhagic hydrocephalous.

Prevention of Birth Trauma

The following measures can prevent birth trauma:

1. Antenatal diagnosis of at risk pregnancies.
2. Proper monitoring during the antenatal period and prevent conditions like anemia, control of diabetes mellitus, hypertension which may complicate delivery.
3. Early referral of cases.
4. Promotion of institutional deliveries.
5. Delivery should be conducted by skilled personnel. In case of newcomers they should be supervised by doctors more skilled in this field.
6. To avoid instrumental delivery as far as possible (forceps, ventouse).
7. In case of malpresentation and defects in pelvis, cesarean section should be encouraged.
8. A good co-ordination between a gynecologist and a pediatrician in institutional delivery, and wherever possible.

Neonatal Hypothermia

The recognition of importance of thermal control in the present day management of the newborn is essential for improving neonatal survival. A newborn baby is physiologically homoeothermic; but this ability to stay warm may be easily overwhelmed by extremes of environmental temperature. Pierre Budin (1900) first drew attention to the high neonatal mortality among babies allowed to remain cold. The recognition of 'Neonatal cold injury syndrome' in 1957 once again reviewed the earlier observation that cooling is detrimental for neonatal survival. Subsequently optimum thermal conditions for neonates with varying birth weight and gestational age were identified by mid 1960's and means of keeping babies warm were devised.

Neonatal hypothermia and cold injury are now rare in developed countries. In developing countries it still continues to occur and is an important cause of neonatal morbidity and mortality.

Physiology of Temperature Regulation

Heat balance in the body is maintained by the law of conservation of energy according to which

Heat production = Heat loss by convection + radiation + evaporation + conduction.

In the newborn infant, control of body temperature can be achieved only over a narrow range of ambient conditions although they are equipped with a thermostat in the hypothalamus. These thermoregulatory efforts are often insufficient in preterm and low birth weight babies.

Before birth, the baby is warm and well insulated in the aqueous uterine environment. Fetal temperature is slightly higher than maternal temperature with a gradient of the heat flow from the fetus to the mother. After birth, the skin and core temperatures of the body of the neonate fall by 0.3°C and 0.1°C per minute respectively. This fall is faster and greater if the temperature of the delivery room is lower than 25°C.

Heat Production

Non-shivering thermogenesis, which is a result of metabolism of brown fat, is the most important source of heat production in the newborn. The body temperature of the newborn is primarily maintained by this mechanism.

The brown fat is located at the nape of the neck, inter-scapular region, axillae, and groin and around the kidneys and adrenals. It is laid down mostly during the third trimester of pregnancy. It accounts for 4% of the total body fat in a term baby. Brown fat contains more mitochondria; it is more vascular and better innervated.

Mechanism of Heat Production

Prerequisites for effective thermogenesis include integrity of CNS pathways, adequacy of brown fat, and availability of glucose and oxygen.

When the baby is exposed to cold environment, impulses through the afferent nerve fibres reach the heat regulating centers located in the pre optic area of anterior hypothalamus near the walls of the third ventricle. Neurogenic efferents, on reaching the brown fat trigger the release of nor adrenaline which mediates several important thermal responses as follows:

Oxidation of triglycerides to glycerol and fatty acids. The fatty acids are locally consumed for the generation of heat. About 30% of non-esterified fatty acids are oxidized to generate heat and 10% released to the circulation. The areas of brown fat become warm and heat is distributed to various parts of the body through blood stream as brown fat is highly vascular. Approximately 2.5 calories is liberated from 1 gm of brown fat and for this metabolic effort, the body needs extra oxygen and glucose.

The heart rate rises, delivering more oxygen in order to meet the high metabolic needs of non-shivering thermogenesis.

Peripheral vasoconstriction diverts blood from skin towards the organ that drive thermogenesis.

Thus thermogenesis while warming the infant depletes endogenous substrates because of excessive metabolism.

As in older children and adults, muscular activity is not a significant source of heat production in the newborn. The tiny babies cannot shiver to generate heat and are also unable to assume a flexed posture to reduce heat loss. However, during exposure to cold, the baby makes some movements of the limbs but the effort is not sustained. Minimal shivering occurs only when the environmental temperature falls below 25°C.

Heat Loss

After birth, the newborn can loose heat by four mechanisms viz. evaporation, convection, radiation and conduction.

Evaporation

A newborn infant wet with amniotic fluid can loose heat by evaporation as the skin dries. Evaporative heat loss is low in mature infants unless they are sweating in response to heat stress. Preterm infants have high transepidermal water loss due to passive diffusion of water vapour through the thin poorly keratinized immature dermis. Hence loss is high in preterms.

Convection

Heat is lost from the skin surface to the surrounding air by convection. Loss is high if the air is cold, the skin surface is exposed and there is rapid movement of air over the skin. A naked baby in a cold drafty room has a high convective heat loss (Fig. 7.10).

Radiation

Heat is lost from the skin surface to the nearest surface which faces the skin by means of radiation. It varies with the temperature of that surface and its distance from the skin but is independent of the temperature of the intervening air.

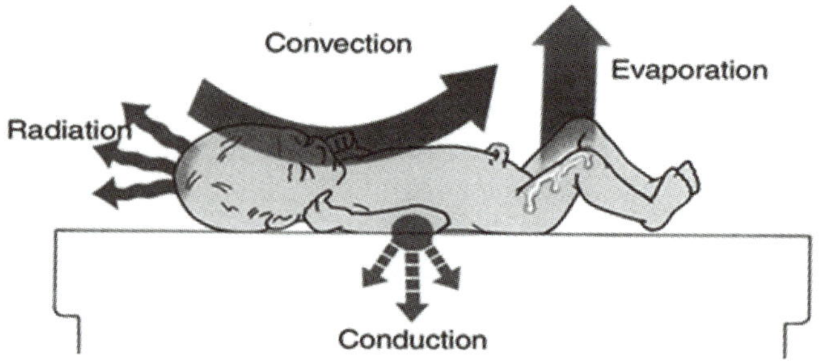

Fig. 7.10: Methods of heat loss

Conduction

By which a newborn looses heat when in contact with cold surfaces like cloth, tray etc.

Thermoneutral Environment

It is the temperature range during which the basal metabolic rate of the baby is at a minimum, oxygen utilization is least and the baby thrives well. For each baby, this range of temperature varies depending on the weight and post natal age.

Why the Preterm Infant is Susceptible to Develop Hypothermia?

The increased susceptibility of the preterm infant to develop hypothermia is due to the presence of certain characteristics like:

- A large body surface area in relation to weight.
- A large head in proportion to the body.
- Decreased subcutaneous fat, with less insulative capacity in low birth weight infants.
- Less developed stores of brown fat in preterm infants.
- Inability to take in enough calories to provide nutrients for thermogenesis and growth in preterm babies.
- Limitation of oxygen consumption in some preterm infants with pulmonary problems.

Effects of Exposure to Cold

Cold Stress

The first clinical situation on exposure to cold is called cold stress. A newborn infant, on exposure to cold environment, responds with peripheral vasoconstriction, causing anaerobic metabolism and metabolic acidosis which in turn can cause pulmonary vasoconstriction leading to further hypoxemia, anaerobic metabolism, and acidosis. Hypoxemia further compromises infant's response to cold. The preterm infant is at greater risk of developing hypothermia. However, their more common problem is calorie loss from unrecognized chronic cold stress, resulting in excess oxygen consumption and inability to gain weight.

Hypothermia

It is usually seen in preterm–low birth weight neonates and term infants with nervous system disorders. It is observed more in home deliveries and when inadequate measures are taken to keep the infant warm and prevent heat loss during delivery, in the post natal ward and during transport. The newborn infant is most vulnerable to develop hypothermia during the first few hours after birth but may develop hypothermia at any time during the neonatal period and beyond if exposed to a cold environment.

Risk Factors of Hypothermia

The risk factors of hypothermia include a cold environment, low birth weight, prematurity and birth asphyxia, use of anesthetic or analgesic drugs during delivery, infection or other illness of the infant, inadequate measures to keep the infant warm before and during transport.

Classification of Hypothermia

The normal axillary body temperature of the newborn is 36.5°C to 37.5°C. By human touch method if the trunk feels warm and the soles are warm and pink, the baby is in thermal comfort.

Hypothermia may be classified as follows:

Cold stress/Mild hypothermia	:	The axillary temperature is between < 36.5°C and 36°C. By human touch method baby's soles are cold, trunk is warm.
Moderate hypothermia	:	The rectal temperature is between < 36°C to 32°C. By human touch method both soles and trunk are cold.
Severe hypothermia	:	The rectal temperature is less than 32°C. By human touch method both soles and trunk are cold.

Effects of Hypothermia

Prolonged hypothermia may lead to impaired growth and increased susceptibility to infection. A vicious cycle occurs in hypothermic newborns because they have poor sucking ability. Impaired feeding will lead to decreased heat production and worsening of hypothermia. Moreover, hypothermia, even if moderate, is associated with an increased risk of death in low birth weight newborns.

Clinical Features

Cold stress is the early stage of hypothermia characterized by pale, cool extremities and warm trunk. The capillary refill time is normal over the sternum but prolonged (> 3 seconds) over the heels which is corrected on warming the infant. The infant fails to gain weight if there is chronic exposure to cold stress.

Continuing exposure to acute cold at this stage makes the infant hypothermic when both the trunk and extremities becomes cold to touch with symptoms and signs of central nervous system depression viz. lethargy, poor feeding, apnoea and bradycardia.

When the core temperature goes below 32°C, the infant has a bright red color. This is a result of failure of oxyhemoglobin to dissociate at low temperature. There may be central pallor or cyanosis. The skin may show edema or sclerema. There is decreased activity, a poor sucking reflex, vomiting, abdominal distension and oliguria. The signs include bradycardia, slow, shallow, irregular respiration, hypotension, and decreased response to stimulus. Hypoglycemia, metabolic acidosis, azotemia and hyperkalemia are present. Sometimes there is tachypnoea, respiratory distress and generalized bleeding, including pulmonary bleeding.

Table 7.3 : Clinical features of hypothermia

a. Peripheral vasoconstriction
• Acrocyanosis
• Cool extremities
• Decreased peripheral perfusion
b. CNS depression
• Lethargy
• Bradycardia
• Apnea
• Poor feeding
c. Increased metabolism
• Hypoglycemia
• Hypoxia
• Metabolic acidosis

Contd.

Contd.

d. Increased pulmonary artery pressure
  - Respiratory distress
  - Tachypnea

e. Sclerema

f. Chronic signs
  - Weight loss

Prevention

Thermal protection of the newborns is very important but not difficult. As cooling of the newborn occurs during the first few minutes after birth, it is important to act quickly to prevent heat loss.

The basic principles are same for home as well as institutional delivery. Satisfactory control demands both prevention of heat loss and promotion of heat gain. The warm chain is a set of interlinked procedures to adopt at birth and during the next few days in order to minimize heat loss in all newborns. Failure to implement any one of these procedures will break the chain and put the newborn at risk of hypothermia.

The ten steps of warm chain are as follows:

(1) Warm delivery room (2) Immediate drying (3) Warm resuscitation (4) Skin to skin contact between baby and mother (5) Breastfeeding (6) Postpone bathing and weighing (7) Appropriate clothing and bedding (8) Mother and baby together (9) Warm transportation (10) Training/ awareness raising of heath care providers.

Warm delivery room: The optimum temperature of the delivery room should be atleast 25°C. It should be clean and free from draught through open windows, doors or fans. If the temperature of the room is less than optimal, a room heater or a fire place should be available to warm the room.

Immediate drying: After delivery, the baby should be immediately dried with a pre-warmed towel from head to feet.

Warm resuscitation: Throughout the resuscitation process warmth has to be maintained. All the resuscitation equipments including the towels for drying should be prewarmed. It is important to keep the baby warm during resuscitation because asphyxiated newborns cannot produce heat efficiently hence are at risk of hypothermia.

The baby should be resuscitated under a radiant warmer or properly wrapped and under a 200 watt bulb kept at 45 cm from the surface of the baby in case of institutional delivery.

Wrapping the baby with a warm blanket with only face and upper part of the chest exposed putting it on a dry warm surface in case of home delivery.

Skin to skin contact: Can be achieved by adopting the Kangaroo method. It is an effective method of preventing heat loss in newborn. The mother's chest or abdomen is the ideal surface to receive the newborn as it is clean and has just the right temperature. Kangarooing helps in the following ways:

- Assists in maintaining temperature of infant.
- Facilitates breastfeeding.
- Helps to increase duration of breastfeeding.
- Improves infant mother bonding.

Breastfeeding: An early and adequate supply of breast milk is essential to provide the newborn with calories to generate heat.

Bathing should be postponed: Postponement of bath helps in conservation of heat. A term baby should be preferably given bath on the second day. In low birth weight babies, bathing should be postponed till the baby weighs 2 kg.

Appropriate bedding and clothing: The bed should be warm and the baby should be wrapped in 4–5 layers of cloth to maintain warmth.

Mother and baby together (bedding in): Babies born at home as well as in institution should be kept with mothers in the same bed under the same blanket 24 hours a day in a warm room. The mother's body warmth will keep the baby warm. Mother is considered as the best incubator.

*Warm transportation:*Temperature maintenance of baby's body as well as environment during transport, is the weakest link in the warm chain. The following are to be maintained during transport:

- The body temperature of the baby should be stabilized as much as possible before transport.
- The mother should be encouraged to accompany and the baby carried by kangaroo method.
- If the mother is unable to accompany, the baby should be carried close to the chest of another adult.
- The baby should be covered properly from head to feet.
- If baby passes urine and stool, then it must be ensured that it does not remain wet.
- Thermacol box, basket padded pouch, polythene covering can be used for ensuring temperature stability during transport.

- The human touch method for assessing the temperature should be taught to the accompanying person and explained to ensure that baby's trunk as well as the soles and palm are warm to touch.
- The baby should be transported to the nearest facility, by the shortest route and by using the fastest possible mode of transport.

Training and awareness raising: All health care providers involved in the process of birth and subsequent care of the newborn need to be adequately trained on the principle and procedures of the warm chain. The family and community need to be made aware of the importance of keeping newborns warm and should be given information on how to do so.

Management

Monitoring of Temperature

a. A low reading thermometer (recording temperature as low as 30°C) should be preferably used in the newborn.
b. Axillary temperature is recorded as the standard procedure, because of safety, hygiene and ease. It is as good as the core temperature recorded by rectal temperature in newborn.
c. Rectal temperature is measured only in sick, hypothermic newborn. It is the best guide for core temperature in these infants.
d. At home the newborn temperature can be assessed by human touch method.

Who Needs Temperature Monitoring?

1. Low birth weight and sick newborn.
2. When there is suspicion that the baby is becoming hypothermic or hyperthermic.
3. When a hypothermic baby is rewarmed or a hyperthermic baby is being cooled down.
4. If a baby needed resuscitation at birth.
5. If it is difficult to maintain the warm chain and provide optimal thermal environment.

Frequency of Monitoring

In healthy newborns, routine temperature monitoring is not necessary. However, to make sure that warm chain is maintained and to identify possible weak links the temperature measurement can be done in early morning hours, when the environmental temperature is its lowest and in the hottest part of the day.

In sick newborns or low birth weight babies the temperature should be initially measured hourly in the first four hours and then 4 hourly or more often if the baby is under the radiant warmer.

During warming of a hypothermic baby, the temperature should be monitored every 15 minutes till the baby is normothermic. If the temperature does not rise within one hour of warming, sepsis has to be suspected, because hypothermia is also a sign of sepsis.

Principles

1. Hypothermia should be confirmed by recording actual body temperature.
2. The baby should be rewarmed as soon as possible.
3. The method of warming will depend on the severity of hypothermia, availability of staff and equipment.
4. The methods of warming in use are as follows:
   - Skin to skin contact (Kangarooing).
   - Overhead lamps and hot water bags.
   - Radiant warmers and incubators.
5. Breastfeeding should be continued.

Kangaroo method care (KMC): It is a simple method of keeping the newborn warm. It is particularly useful in caring for low birth weight infants below 2000 grams.

The benefits of KMC are as follows:

1. *Thermal control:* Prolonged skin to skin contact between the mother and her preterm / low birth

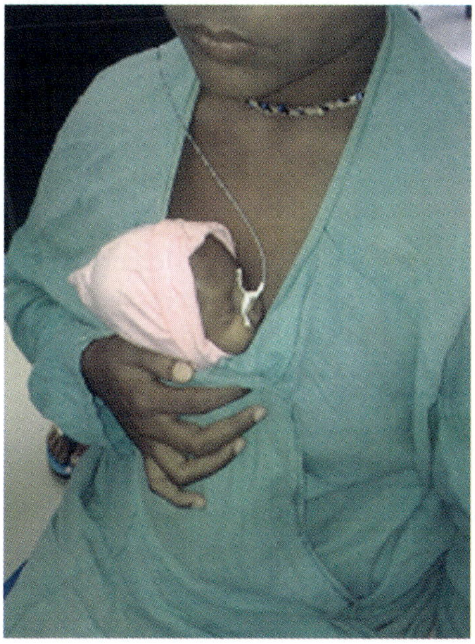

Fig. 7.11: Kangaroo method

weight infant provide effective thermal control and hence associated with reduced risk of hypothermia.

2. *Breastfeeding:* KMC results in increased breastfeeding rates as well as increased duration of breastfeeding.
3. *Effect on growth:* Infants cared for by KMC showed better daily weight gain.
4. *Other effects:* Mothers practising KMC is seen to be less stressed than those mothers whose infant is receiving incubator care. Mothers report increased self confidence, self esteem and feeling of fulfillment with skin to skin contact. Fathers felt more relaxed, comfortable and better bonded while providing kangaroo care.

All newborn infants are eligible for KMC. However, very sick babies needing special care may preferably be cared under the radiant warmer and KMC can be started after the infant is stable. Further, KMC can be initiated in a neonate who is other wise stable but still on intravenous fluids, orogastric feeding or some oxygen administration.

Some guidelines for practising KMC are as follows:

1. In a neonate with birth weight 1800 grams or more, if stable KMC can be started soon after birth.
2. Neonates with birth weight 1200-1799 grams may take a couple of days to become stable before KMC is started. However they may benefit during transport to a special care unit.
3. Neonates with birth weight less than 1200 grams may take days to weeks before the condition allows initiation of KMC. These babies benefit most if they are transported in utero to a special care unit.

The procedure for initiation of KMC is as follows:

- The mother should wear light lose clothing. A convenient time should be discussed with the mother.
- The room should be warm. Mother's wish for privacy should be respected. However, she can ask the other family members to be with her as it helps to lend support and reassurance.
- The baby should be naked except for a cap, socks and nappy.
- The baby should be placed between the mother's breasts in an upright position. The head should be turned to one side and in slightly extended position. This position keeps the airway straight and allows eye to eye contact with the mother and baby. The hips should be flexed and abducted in a frog position. The elbows should also be flexed.
- The mother should be asked to continue breastfeeding and explained that KMC makes breastfeeding easier. Further, holding the baby near the breast stimulates milk production.
- KMC can be started as soon as the newborn is stable. Sessions of less than one hour should be avoided. Where no other means of thermal control is available, the duration should be gradually increased to become as long as possible interrupted only for changing diapers.
- The mother can continue KMC while asleep in a reclined or semi recumbent position about 15 degrees from horizontal. A comfortable chair with adjustable back may be suitable for resting during day time.
- The criteria for discharge of a KMC newborn are as follows:
  1. The baby is well with no disease, feeding well, gaining weight (atleast 15 grams/kg/day for 3 consecutive days) and temperature is stable in KMC position.
  2. Mother is confident of taking care of the infant at home and would be able to come for follow up regularly.
- KMC can be continued at home after discharge when other members of the family can take part. It can be weaned off, once the infant becomes intolerant to the procedure or at 40 weeks of post conceptional age.

Management of Cold Stress/Mild Hypothermia

Cold stress in newborn indicates that the infant needs warming. If not intervened, the infant at any moment may become hypothermic. The steps include measures to prevent heat loss as follows:

1. Cold clothes should be removed, and the infant covered with prewarmed clothes in several layers from head to feet.
2. Heat loss should be reduced from the infant to the environment. This can be achieved by changing the cold bed clothes and replacing with prewarmed clothes. The room should be warmed with the help of a room heater or a smokeless fire place.
3. The baby should be bedded in with the mother in skin to skin contact, under cover of the same blanket.
4. Advise frequent breastfeeding.

Management of Moderate Hypothermia

Moderate hypothermia is an alarming situation. If not taken care of may progress to severe hypothermia. The steps of management include:

1. Measures to prevent heat loss as in case of cold stress.
2. The baby should be provided extra heat till temperature becomes normal. The warming can be done by keeping the baby under a heat source viz. a radiant warmer or a 200 watt bulb. If these are not available, extra heat can be provided with warm packs.
3. Temperature and sucking reflex should be monitored every 15 minutes. If there is no response and hypothermia persist beyond 1 hour after taking adequate measures, sepsis has to be suspected and antibiotics started after sending blood samples for sepsis screen and blood culture.

Management of Severe Hypothermia

Severe hypothermia is a grave situation and should be treated as a medical emergency. The steps of management include:

1. Measures to reduce heat loss as above.
2. The baby should be kept under a radiant warmer. The abdominal skin temperature should be set at 1°C higher than the infant's core temperature (36.5°C–37.5°C) for rapid warming. Rapid warming should be done till the temperature reaches 34°C. After that warming should be slowed down but continued till the temperature is normal. For slow warming, the abdominal skin temperature should be set at 36.5°C.
3. Monitoring:
   - Temperature should be monitored every 15–30 minutes.
   - Sucking reflex.
   - Blood pressure/Capillary refill time and heart rate.
   - Blood glucose.
4. Additional measures:
   - Vitamin K should be given 1 mg intramuscularly for term and 0.5 mg for preterm babies.
   - 10% dextrose 2 ml/kg/dose stat.
   - If CRT is > 3 seconds, a bolus dose of 10 ml/kg/ dose of normal saline should be given.
   - Oxygen administration.
   - Antibiotics should be started to cover both gram positive and gram negative organism if there is slightest suspicion of sepsis after sending blood samples for sepsis screen and culture.

Hyperthermia

Elevation of body temperature beyond 37.5°C (99.5°F) is called hyperthermia in the newborn.

Causes

1. Elevated environmental temperature.
2. Infection.
3. Dehydration.
4. Anoxic brain injury and intracranial hemorrhage.
5. Increased humidity.
6. Excessive clothing.
7. Administration of drugs e.g. belladonna preparation and ephedrine nasal drops.

Effects of Hyperthermia

Hyperthermia increases the metabolic rate and the rate of water loss by evaporation which can cause dehydration. A core temperature of above 42°C can lead to neurological damage.

Differentiation Between An Overheated Neonate and a Febrile Neonate

The following points would help to differentiate a febrile from an overheated neonate:

Features	*Overheated neonate*	*Febrile neonate*
Hands and feet	Warm	Cool
Abdominal skin temp exceeds hand skin temp	by < 2°C	by > 3°C
Color of skin	Pink	Pale
Posture	Extended	Lethargic
Appearance	Healthy	Looks ill

Clinical Features

1. Skin over whole body is hot. Face is flushed. Extremities are red due to vasodilatation.
2. Tachypnoea, tachycardia followed by restlessness and crying.
3. Then gradually become lethargic.

4. In severe hyperthermia, shock, convulsion and coma may occur.

Management

1. When the temperature is 37.5°C to 39°C, the baby should be moved away from the source of heat (shifted to a cool room), undressed partially or fully as necessary.
2. When the body temperature is above 39°C, the baby should be undressed in a cool room and sponging should be done till the temperature come down to <38°C. The water temperature should be approximately 35°C or 2°C lower than the body temperature. Using cooler or cold water is harmful because it may make the baby hypothermic.
3. The infant should be breast fed frequently to treat or prevent dehydration. If baby is unable to breast feed, the baby should be given expressed breast milk by nasogastric tube or even IV fluids as need be.
4. Every hyperthermic baby should be examined for signs of sepsis. With the slightest suspicion of sepsis, a sepsis screen and a blood culture has to be ordered and antibiotics should be started.

Neonatal Hyperbilirubinemia

Jaundice and its underlying hyperbilirubinemia is the most common abnormal finding during the first few weeks of life. Jaundice is clinically appreciable in newborns with serum bilirubin value of 5 mg/dl or more compared to 2 mg/dl in adult. Over 60% of term and 80% of preterm babies develop clinical jaundice and by adult standards almost all newborn babies are jaundiced during the early days of life.

Peculiarities of Neonatal Jaundice

1. The rise of bilirubin in newborns is predominantly of indirect type.
2. In the first weeks of life, the level of total bilirubin is considered as synonymous with indirect bilirubin.
3. The yellow discoloration is first evident over the skin of the face (nasolabial folds and tip of nose).
4. There is always a cephalocaudal progression of the yellow coloration. This is due to relative thickness of skin; being thinnest over the face and thickest over the palms and soles.
5. Jaundice in the neonate is masked by physiological plethora of newborn and can be examined only after blanching the skin.

Assessment of Severity of Jaundice

1. Clinical 2. Icterometer 3. Transcutaneous bilimeter.

Clinical assessment has been acclaimed as the best method of assessment of severity worldwide. It utilizes the principle that clinical jaundice has a cephalocaudal progression as it increases in intensity.

Assessment of jaundice should be done in natural light in a white background. The pulp of the finger or thumb is pressed on the baby's skin, preferably on a bony part, till it blanches. The underlying skin is noted for the yellow color. Extent of jaundice thus detected gives a rough estimate of serum bilirubin on the basis of Kramer's criteria.

Table 7.4 : Kramer's criteria to estimate clinical jaundice

Area of body	*Range of bilirubin*
Face	4–8 mg/dl
Upper trunk	5–12 mg/dl
Lower trunk and thighs	8–16 mg/dl
Arms and lower legs	11–18 mg/dl
Palms and soles	> 15 mg/dl

By experience and with concerted efforts, the observational skills can be sharpened and the accuracy of clinical assessment can be enhanced to within +/- 2 mg/dl. However, serum bilirubin estimation should be done by laboratory test to document bilirubin levels for proper management. Also, it should be emphasized that after phototherapy the skin gets bleached and clinical assessment of severity becomes unreliable and one has to rely on estimation of the serum bilirubin level.

Icterometer assessment is done by matching the skin color with the color codes depicted on the plastic strip. This method can be used by health workers for screening.

Transcutaneous bilimeter work on the principle of computerized spectrophotometry and provide digital display of total bilirubin. The photo probe is pressed against the forehead or sternum to take the reading. Every hospital should have a normogram to compare.

Laboratory Estimation of Serum Bilirubin

Laboratory estimation of bilirubin may be done by the van den Bergh's test or with the help of a microbilimeter. It should be noted that blood samples for bilirubin estimation should be protected from light.

van den Bergh's test is the test carried out in most neonatal unit for estimation of serum bilirubin. Its limitations include large blood sample size, lack of accuracy, reliability etc. The inter laboratory variation in the levels of serum bilirubin range between 10-20% for total bilirubin and upto 25% for conjugated bilirubin.

The microbilimeter requires a micro centrifuged sample of blood in a capillary tube and provides an instant digital read out of the total bilirubin. It should be noted that during the first week of life the total bilirubin is by and large equivalent to the unconjugated fraction for practical purposes. It is a useful equipment for neonatal ICU.

Prediction of Hyperbilirubinemia

In recent years, efforts have gone in to predict hyperbilirubinemia in healthy term babies. Reliable predictors can identify babies at risk of pathological jaundice indicating close monitoring in such babies and reducing hospital stay in babies at low risk.

1. **Universal newborn screening:** A normogram with percentile values of serum bilirubin at different postnatal ages for healthy term babies (Fig. 7.12) is available now. If the value of the serum bilirubin estimated at 24–36 hours after birth is plotted on the normogram, subsequent hyperbilirubinemia can be predicted. For example, if the total serum bilirubin level at this age falls in the high risk zone (> 95th percentile) then chances of subsequent hyperbilirubinemia is around 40%. Whereas, when it falls in the low risk zone (< 40th percentile) there is no measurable risk at all.
2. **First day total bilirubin** level as a predictor for subsequent hyperbilirubinemia has been reported by authors in our country and abroad. Various levels ranging from 3.9 to 6 mg/dl has been shown by different studies to be predictive of subsequent hyperbilirubinemia. If confirmed by more studies these results will suggest babies who will require early follow-up and who will not.
3. **Cord blood bilirubin level:** Raised cord blood bilirubin indicates ongoing in utero hemolysis. A cord blood bilirubin level > 2.5 mg/dl predicts development of pathological jaundice (defined as > 13 mg/dl) with sensitivity of 71% and specificity of 96%.

Anticipation of Hyperbilirubinemia

Hyperbilirubinemia can be anticipated in the following circumstances:

1. Rh negative and O group mothers.
2. Drugs to the mother e.g. large doses of Vitamin K, salicylate, oxytocin etc.
3. Family history of hyperbilirubinemia.
4. Maternal illness suggestive of IU infection viz. febrile illness within 2 weeks of delivery, fever with rash in the early antenatal period.

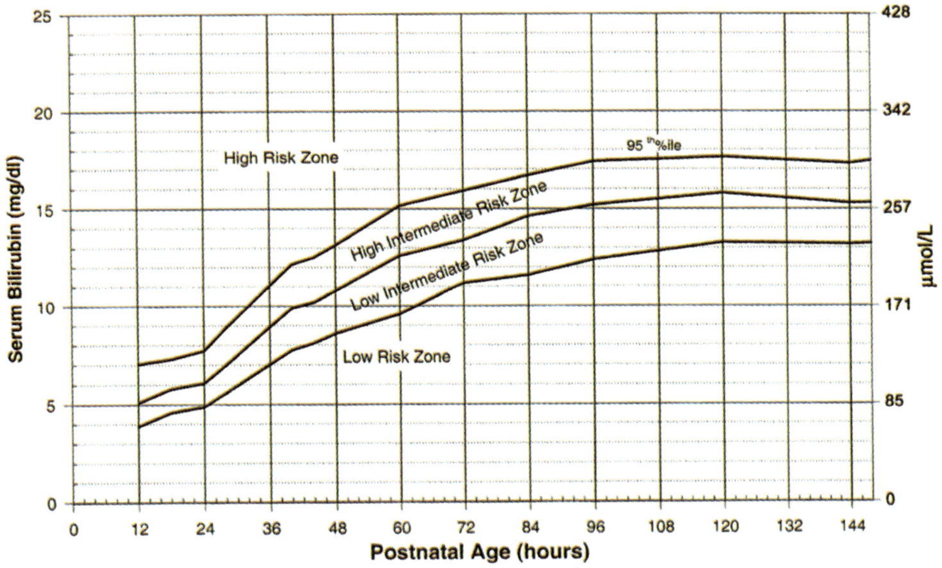

Fig. 7.12: Normogram for risk designation of term and near term well neonates based on their hour spefic serum bilirubin levels (Adapted from AAP subcommittee on hyperbilirubinemia, Pediatrics 2004; 114: 297 - 316)

Anticipation of jaundice in the newborn plays an important role in early diagnosis and proper management. It is an indication of early referral of baby in utero to an institution with facilities for adequate management and prevention of complications of hyperbilirubinemia.

Physiological Hyperbilirubinemia

Physiological hyperbilirubinemia is seen in about 60% of term and 80% of preterm babies. It is now thought that physiological hyperbilirubinemia may provide protection to the newborn against oxygen free radical triggered neonatal disorders because bilirubin is an antioxidant.

Physiologic hyperbilirubinemia is believed to be the result of increased bilirubin production after the breakdown of fetal red blood cells combined with transient limitations in the conjugation of bilirubin in the liver.

Classical Characteristics of Physiological Jaundice

Normally, the level of indirect bilirubin in the umbilical cord serum is 1–3 mg/dl. It rises at the rate of 5 mg/dl/24 hours. Thus in both term and preterm babies physiological jaundice appears on the 2nd to 3rd day of life.

In term babies peak level of 6-8 mg/dl (a rise of upto 12 mg/dl is in the physiological range) is reached by the 4th day of life whereas in preterm babies, the peak may be 10–12 mg/dl on the fifth day of life, possibly rising upto 15 mg/dl without any specific abnormality. In term babies jaundice disappears by 10 days of life and in preterm by10–14 days of life.

Exaggerated Physiological Hyperbilirubinemia

In infants, indirect bilirubin levels rarely rise above 12 mg/dl. In presence of certain variables, hyperbilirubinemia may be exaggerated. The risk factors for an exaggerated physiological indirect hyperbilirubinemia include the following:

- Immaturity.
- Perinatal distress factors (viz. birth asphyxia, hypothermia, acidosis and hypoglycemia).
- Drugs (Vitamin K, salicylates etc.).
- Cephalhematoma, Polycythaemia.
- Congenital hypothyroidism.
- Sepsis, hereditary spherocytosis, red cell enzyme deficiency, minor fetomaternal blood group incompatibility.
- High altitude and Asian race.

Diagnosis and Treatment

Diagnosis of physiological jaundice is usually made by day of appearance, course and exclusion of other pathological causes of jaundice.

Treatment: Physiological hyperbilirubinemia does not require any specific treatment. The presence of risk factors should be sought for and the serum bilirubin monitored clinically as well as by estimation of serum bilirubin when indicated. The mother should be reassured about the benign nature of the condition and advised frequent exclusive breastfeeding.

Pathological Hyperbilirubinemia

Jaundice and its underlying hyperbilirubinemia are considered to be pathological in the following situations:

1. Jaundice appearing in the first 24 hours of life.
2. Serum bilirubin increasing by more than 5 mg/dl/day or 0.5 mg/dl/hr.
3. Total serum bilirubin is more than 12 mg/dl in term and 15 mg/dl in preterm babies.
4. Direct bilirubin more than 2 mg/dl at any time.
5. Jaundice persisting for more than 2 weeks in term and more than 3 weeks in pre-term babies.
6. Stool clay or white colored and urine staining clothes.
7. Treatment is required in the form of phototherapy or exchange transfusion.

Causes of Pathological Hyperbilirubinemia

Pathological hyperbilirubinemia may manifest within 24 hours of birth or after 72 hours. Onset within 24 hours is always suggestive of a serious and rapidly progressive disease.

Onset Within 24 Hours

1. Hemolytic disease of the newborn: Rh, ABO, and minor group incompatibilities between mother and fetus.
2. Intrauterine infections TORCH, Hepatitis B.
3. Congenital hemolytic diseases: (a) Deficiency of red cell enzymes viz. G6PD deficiency, pyruvate kinase deficiency and hexokinase deficiency. (b) Hereditary spherocytosis. (c) Homozygous alpha thalassemia.
4. Administration of large doses of Vitamin K, salicylates etc. to the mother.
5. Crigler-Najjar syndrome and Lucy-Driscoll syndrome.

Onset After 72 Hours and Within 2 Weeks

1. Septicemia.
2. Neonatal hepatitis.
3. Extrahepatic biliary atresia.
4. Intrauterine infection.
5. Breast milk jaundice.
6. Hypertrophic pyloric stenosis and congenital intestinal obstruction.

Kernicterus/Acute Bilirubin Encephalopathy

The most dreaded complication of neonatal hyperbilirubinemia is bilirubin encephalopathy as a result of kernicterus.

Kernicterus is a pathological diagnosis. It literally means yellow nuclei. The term is also used to describe the clinical features of acute bilirubin encephalopathy, the underlying mechanism of which is still uncertain.

Kernicterus refers to yellow staining of the brain by unconjugated bilirubin with evidence of neuronal injury. The cells that are most prone to such injury are those which are metabolically active and receive the largest blood flow. In neonates these are the cells of the basal ganglia and mid brain. Microscopically, there is necrosis, neuronal loss and gliosis.

Pathogenesis

The pathogenesis of bilirubin encephalopathy is still clearly not known. It is multifactorial. It involves an interaction between free bilirubin, albumin binding and free bilirubin passage across the blood brain barrier and neuronal toxicity. The level of bilirubin which will be toxic to an individual infant is unpredictable and the duration of exposure needed to produce toxic effect is also unknown.

Bilirubin entry into the brain occurs as free (unbound) bilirubin or as bilirubin bound to albumin in the presence of a disrupted blood brain barrier. The damage is caused by the free bilirubin in the extracellular fluid. It binds to the neuronal cell membranes with severe and complex biochemical sequelae for the cells. The factors identified to have an increased risk of kernicterus are as follows:

1. Prematurity which is normally associated with a low serum albumin and a more permeable blood brain barrier.
2. Rapidly rising levels of serum bilirubin.
3. Low levels of plasma albumin for bilirubin to bind with.
4. Presence of hypoxia, acidemia, hypoglycemia, sepsis or some other serious illness that might disrupt the blood brain barrier.

The preterms/sick infants are more vulnerable to bilirubin toxicity and low bilirubin kernicterus because the blood brain barrier is more permeable, the binding capacity is less in preterm and sick babies and presence of complications which disrupts the blood brain barrier.

Clinical Manifestations

The clinical manifestation be described as acute or chronic.

Acute bilirubin encephalopathy: The clinical presentation of acute bilirubin encephalopathy can be divided into three phases:

Phase I: Characterized by hypotonia, lethargy, high pitched cry and poor suck.

Phase II: Hypotonia is replaced by hypertonia of the extensor muscles manifested by opisthotonus, rigidity, oculogyric crisis and retrocollis, fever and seizures. Many infants die in this phase. Those who survive this phase develop chronic bilirubin encephalopathy.

Phase III: Hypertonia is replaced by hypotonia after about one week.

Chronic bilirubin encephalopathy: The clinical features of chronic bilirubin encephalopathy include athetosis, partial or complete sensorineural deafness, limitation of upward gaze, dental dysplasia and intellectual deficits.

Early and adequate intervention of neonatal unconjugated hyperbilirubinemia is the cornerstone in prevention of kernicterus and acute bilirubin encephalopathy. Early detection is possible by monitoring of serum bilirubin level and use of BAER (brainstem auditory evoked response).

Measures to Help Prevent Hyperbilirubinemia

The following measures can help prevent hyperbilirubinemia to a large extent. This can be practised at all levels of newborn care:

1. Prevention of Rh isoimmunisation in all unsensitized Rh negative women with prophylactic injection of anti-D immunoglobulin after birth of each Rh + ve baby, after abortion of Rh + ve conceptions, in the situations with increased risk of fetomaternal hemorrhage (e.g. amniocentesis, manual removal of placenta etc).

To further enhance its effectivity it has been recommended to administer anti-D immunoglobulin to all unsensitized women at 28-32 weeks gestation.

2. Prevention of birth trauma and perinatal distress factors, e.g, asphyxia, hypothermia, hypoglycemia and acidosis all of which aggravate jaundice.
3. Avoidance of drugs which may increase or precipitate hyperbilirubinemia, e.g., large dose of Vitamin K, salicylates to mother.
4. Institution of early and adequate feeding. It helps in colonization of gut, reduces enterohepatic circulation, cause effective evacuation of meconium and prevent hypoglycemia and maintain hydration.
5. Early diagnosis of sepsis and treatment or referral.
6. Phenobarbitone administration: Rh sensitized mother should be administered phenobarbitone antenatally at a dose 120 mg daily for 2 weeks prior to delivery.

   The post natal indications for phenobarbitone administration to the neonate include a cord bilirubin > 2.5 mg/dl, difficult or instrumental delivery, oxytocin induced delivery, birth trauma and G6PD deficiency. The dose should be given as 10 mg/kg IM single dose or 5 mg/ kg per oral two times daily for 3 days.

Management

Neonatal hyperbilirubinemia should be treated as a medical emergency. Early referral of a case at high risk of neonatal jaundice, to a centre where facilities for adequate care is available, goes a long way in proper management.

When to Refer a Case?

In utero transfer of the baby should be attempted if jaundice is anticipated. If not possible the baby should be referred at the earliest to a centre with adequate facilities for treatment. The following situations need referral:

- Rh negative mother with previous bad obstetric history.
- History of neonatal jaundice in siblings.
- Appearance of jaundice within 24 hours of birth.
- When a newborn baby's trunk is distinctly yellow stained with yellow tinge of palms and soles.
- Signs of underlying illness (viz. vomiting, lethargy, poor feeding, temperature instability, apnea, weight loss) in any infant with jaundice.
- Persistence of neonatal jaundice beyond 2 weeks in term and 3 weeks in preterm baby.

When to Test for Serum Bilirubin?

1. Onset of jaundice before 24 hours.
2. When upper trunk is yellow and the palms and soles are yellow tinged.
3. When anticipated before delivery to predict significant hyperbilirubinemia.

Other Laboratory Investigations

To be done when there is significant hyperbilirubinemia include the following:

1. Blood groups: Infant and mother.
2. Direct Coombs' test (cord blood or infant's blood).
3. Reticulocyte count, peripheral blood smear and hematocrit.
4. Serum albumin and acid base status, G6PD status.
5. If baby is unwell:
   a. Urine for reducing substances.
   b. Sepsis screen.

Measures to Reduce Serum Bilirubin

1. Phototherapy.
2. Exchange transfusion.
3. Other modalities.

Phototherapy

Phototherapy is widely accepted as a safe and effective method of treatment of neonatal unconjugated hyperbilirubinemia. It is not known whether phototherapy prevents kernicterus or milder forms of brain injury associated with bilirubin toxicity. Hence, when there is an indication for exchange transfusion, phototherapy should not be used as a substitute. Phototherapy is indicated only in unconjugated hyperbilirubinemia. It should not be used in infants with liver disease or obstructive jaundice. If indirect bilirubin is high in presence of conjugated hyperbilirubinemia exchange transfusion is the treatment of choice.

Mechanism of Action of Phototherapy

Phototherapy lowers bilirubin by three mechanism—photooxidation, photoisomerisation and structural isomerisation. The most effective among these is structural isomerism. When bilirubin is exposed to a light source of 450–460 nm emission, bilirubin is converted into stable, water soluble structural isomers like lumibilirubin which are readily excreted in bile, feces and to a lesser extent in urine. The products of photo isomerisation are not stable whereas, photooxidation is a slow process and is shown to be ineffective.

Phototherapy Units

The phototherapy unit consists of a light source. The various light sources used are fluorescent lamps, halogen lamps and fiberoptic lights (pads or blankets).

Fluorescent lamp units are commonly used. Ideal phototherapy unit to be used is a bank of 4 special blue and 4 daylight lamps, which have been found to be most effective. Blue lamps with a peak output at 425-475 nm are most efficient. Fluorescent white light with a peak at 550-560 nm (range 380-700 nm) is used and has been shown to be equally effective. This type of phototherapy unit may be single surface or double surface.

Halogen (halide spot) lamps: It consists of a150 W, 20 V halogen bulb fixed overhead. Light source recommendations are 425-475 nm. It produces intense light that is far brighter than light produced by ordinary fluorescent lamps. It also produces appreciable amount of heat. These lamps are costly and its efficacy is not superior to the renewable fluorescent lamps.

Fiberoptic light source: Light source recommendations are 425-475 nm. Fiberoptic light systems have been developed that deliver light from a high intensity lamp to a fiberoptic pad or blanket (Biliblanket). The pad is cool and can be placed in direct contact with the baby.

LED phototherapy unit: The LED PT delivers blue light with the peak intensity at 455 nm. The light is free of unwanted UV and IR radiation and is produced by LEDs that maintain the intensity level for 20,000 hours.

Procedure

1. Phototherapy should be given continuously until serum bilirubin comes down to safe level or baby is old enough to handle increased levels of serum bilirubin (i.e. 10.7+/-1.2 mg/dl by 7th day in preterm and 13 +/- 0.7 mg/dl by 4th day in term babies). Brief interruption for breastfeeding can be allowed.
2. Infants under phototherapy should be kept naked except for eye patches and diapers. The infants are turned every 2 hours, if under single surface phototherapy. The baby should be kept about 45 cm below the light source. The distance can be reduced to 15–20 cm to provide intensive phototherapy.

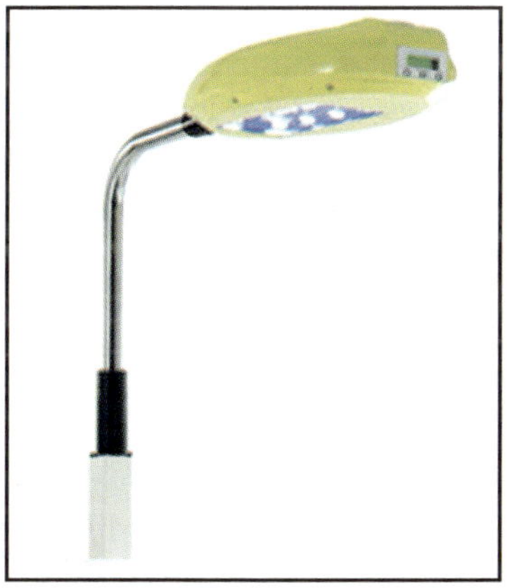

LED phototherapy unit

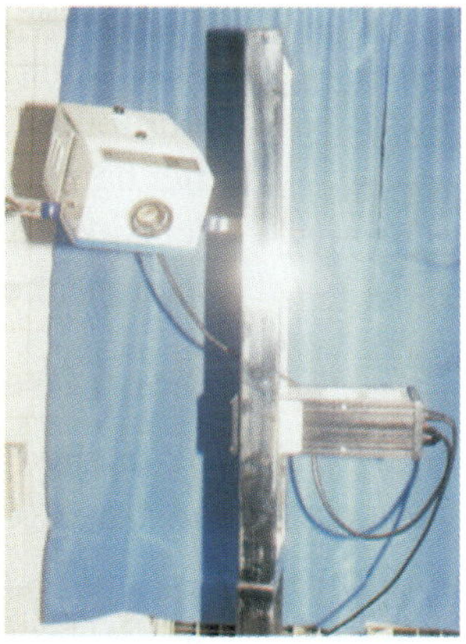

Halogen unit

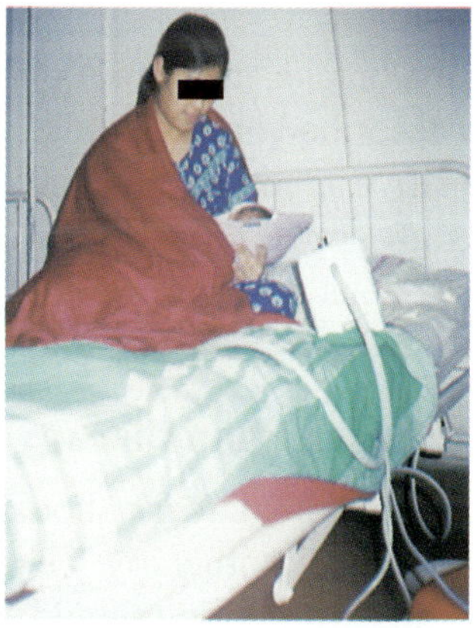

Newborn in biliblanket

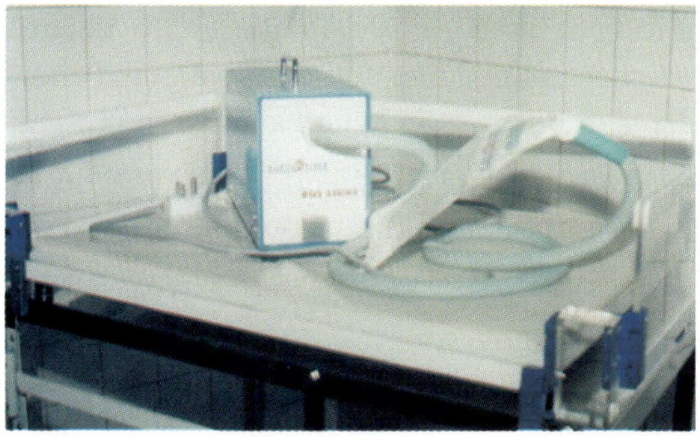

Biliblanket

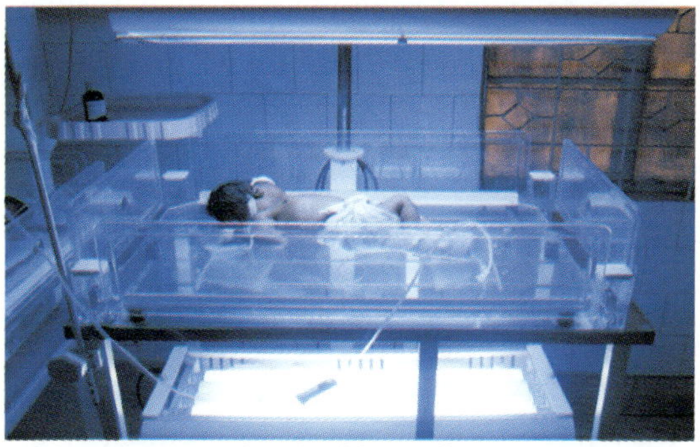

A newborn under double surface phototherapy

Fig. 7.13: Phototherapy units

3. For effective phototherapy, it is desirable that minimum spectral irradiance or flux of 4 - 6 uw/cm2 /nm is available and maintained at the level of infant's skin. The must be checked after every 100 - 200 hours of use to ensure that phototherapy lamps are effective. The flux of phototherapy unit should be checked with a radiometer.
4. Infants should be weighed daily (small infants twice daily). Between 10-20% extra fluid over the usual requirements is required to compensate for the increased insensible water loss. The baby should be kept under a radiant warmer with servo control during phototherapy.

Side Effects

1. Insensible water loss and hyperthermia. It can be avoided by placing baby under a servo control radiant warmer.
2. Watery diarrhoea.
3. Retinal damage as observed in experimental animals. Can be prevented by shielding the eyes.
4. "Bronze baby syndrome" characterized by greyish brown discoloration of skin, urine and serum is seen in babies with cholestatic jaundice undergoing phototherapy.
5. DNA strand breaks, mutations, chromatid exchanges has been described in cell culture. Bilirubin acts as a photosensitive agent for these reactions. Intermittent phototherapy appears to produce more DNA damage than continuous phototherapy. It can be prevented by shielding the gonads with diapers.

Monitoring During Phototherapy

Serum bilirubin and hematocrit should be estimated 6-8 hours after starting phototherapy. Thereafter monitoring every 12-24 hours. Monitoring should continue for at least 24 hours after cessation of phototherapy in babies with hemolytic disease to detect rebound and plan further management. Normally bilirubin should decline by 1-2 mg/dl within 4-6 hours of intensive phototherapy and continue to fall and remain below the threshold level for exchange transfusion.

Exchange Transfusion

It is a widely accepted treatment of hyperbilirubinemia. It is the most effective method for lowering serum bilirubin. It may have to be repeated as frequently as necessary to keep serum levels under the safe level for age and gestation. Repeat exchange transfusion is usually indicated when after early rebound, bilirubin continues to rise over 1 mg/dl/hr or when there is persistent hemolytic anemia in spite of intensive phototherapy.

The normal blood volume of a newborn is 80 ml/kg body weight. A double volume (i.e. 160 ml/kg body weight whole blood) exchange transfusion removes 87% of infant's blood volume and lowers the bilirubin level to about 50% of the pre-exchange levels. However, the bilirubin level increases to 60% of the pre exchange within half an hour due to rapid influx of the bilirubin into the vascular space. This is called rebound. If the rebound is more than 60%, it indicates continuing hemolysis.

Hypoxia, acidosis and hypoalbuminemia if present should be corrected prior to exchange transfusion. However these infants should be put under intensive phototherapy while a decision to exchange is made.

Sick infants who are anemic (hematocrit < 35%) should be given a partial exchange transfusion with packed RBCs to raise hematocrit to 40% before further exchange can be performed for hyperbilirubinemia.

It should be noted that a serum bilirubin approaching a critical level at day 1 or 2 may not be considered so on 4th day in a term baby or on the 7th day in a preterm baby. This is because after this age an imminent fall in bilirubin levels may be anticipated as hepatic conjugating mechanisms become more effective. When taking a decision to perform an exchange one should take into account the age of the baby.

Blood Used in Exchange Transfusion

Blood should be whole blood, collected in citrate phosphate dextrose (CPD).

It should be as fresh as possible (<24 hrs old for hydropic or sick infants and < 72 hrs for all others).

In Rh hemolytic disease of newborn, if blood is collected before delivery, it should be O Rh negative crossed matched against the mother. If collected after delivery, it also can be cross matched against the infant.

In ABO HDN, O Rh specific cells with low titre of anti A and anti B antibodies should be crossed matched with mother or O Rh specific RBCs can be suspended in AB plasma.

For non-immune hyperbilirubinemia blood is typed and cross-matched against the plasma and RBC of the infant.

Other Treatment Modalities

Drugs to increase conjugation: The drug used is phenobarbitone in a dose of 5-8 mg /kg every 24 hours. It has been found to be useful in treating indirect hyperbilirubinemia. It decreases serum bilirubin concentrations to 2-3 mg/dl in 7-10 days. It has to be continued on a long-term basis.

Substances blocking bilirubin reabsorption viz. oral agar in a dose of 500 mg / kg can be used to augment the efficacy of phototherapy.

Substances inhibiting bilirubin production viz. Metalloporphyrins (tin or protoporphyrin). They cause competitive inhibition of hemeoxygenase, the rate-limiting enzyme in heme catabolism and reduce the production of bilirubin. These agents are however not in routine use.

Inhibiting hemolysis with high dose intravenous immunoglobulin (500–1000 mg/kg IV infusion in more than 2 - 4 hours) has been used to reduce bilirubin levels. The mechanism is unknown. It is thought that the immunoglobulin acts by occupying the Fc receptors of reticuloendothelial cells, thereby preventing them from taking up and lysing antibody coated RBCs.

Guidelines of Management

Management of jaundice is directed towards reducing the serum bilirubin level and prevent neurotoxicity.

Guidelines to Treat Hyperbilirubinemia for Babies 35 Weeks or Higher

The current AAP (2004) guidelines are used to treat neonates who are 35 weeks of gestation or higher with phototherapy and/or exchange transfusion. It is provided in the form of normograms which shows hour specific bilirubin level and treatment guidelines for initiating phototherapy and exchange transfusion (Figs. 7.14 and 7.15).

Under these guidelines, neonates with hyperbilirubinemia are divided into 3 groups:

- Infants at lower risk (> 38 weeks and well).

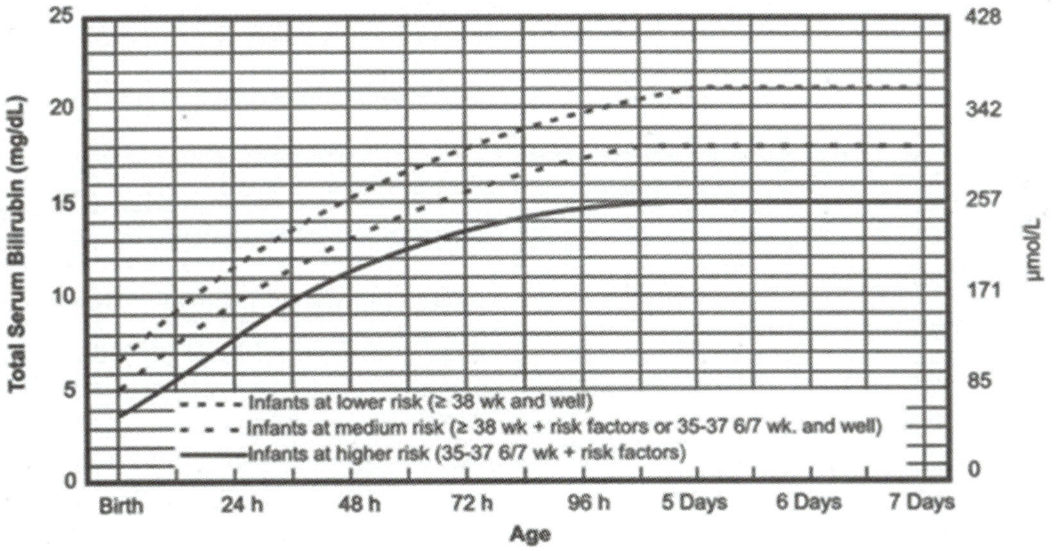

- Use total bilirubin. Do not subtract direct reacting or conjugated bilirubin.
- Risk factors = isoimmune hemolytic disease, C6GPD deficiency, asphyxia, significant lethargy, temperature instability, sepsis, acidosis, or albumin < 3.0 g/dL (if measured).
- For well infants 35-37 6/7 weeks can adjust TSB levels for intervention around the medium risk line. It is an option to intervene at lower TSB level for infants closer to 35 weeks and at higher TSB levels for those closer to 37 6/7 weeks.
- It is an option to provide conventional phototherapy in hospital or at home at TSB levels 2-3 mg/dl (35-50 mmol/L) below those shown but home phototherapy should not be used in any infant with risk factors.

Rebound rise in bilirubin has been reported in about 7% neonates after stopping PT. Neonates with gestation at birth <35 weeks, birth weight <2000 gm and onset of jaundice at <60 h of postnatal age are at higher risk.

Fig. 7.14: Nomogram for initiating phototherapy

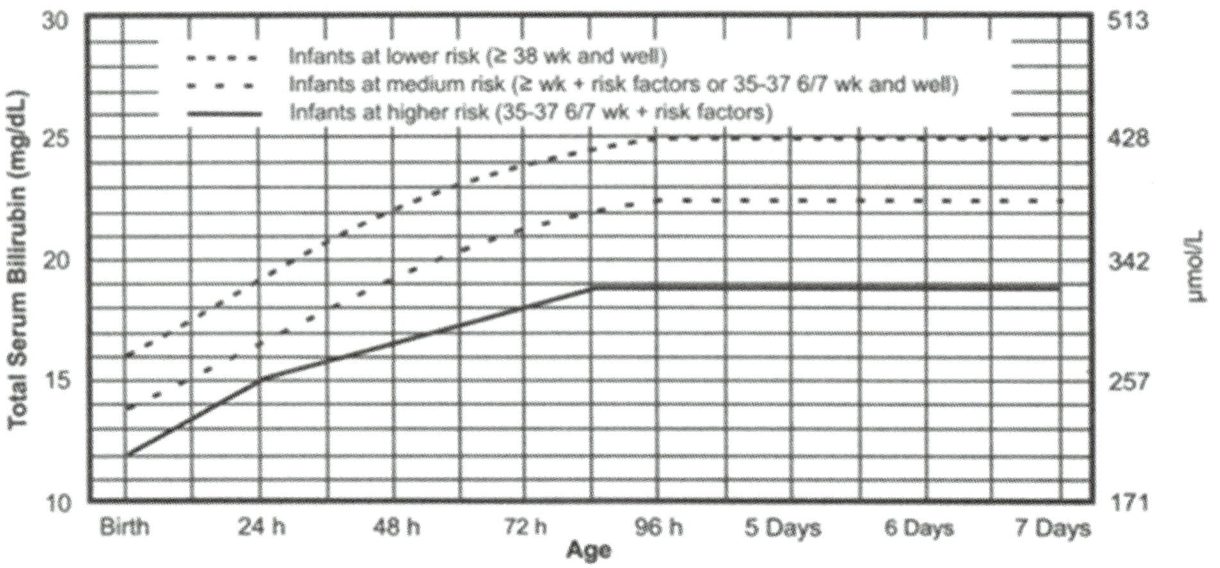

- The dashed lines for the first 24 hours indicate uncertainly due to a wide range of clinical circumstances and a range of responses to phototherapy.
- Immediate exchange transfusion is recommended if infant shows signs of acute bilirubin encephalopathy (hypertonia, arching, retrocollis, opisthotonos, fever, high pitched cry) or if TSB is ≥ 5 mg/dl (85 umol/L) above these lines.
- Risk factors–isoimmune hemolytic disease, G6PD deficiency, asphyxia, significant lethargy, temperature instability, sepsis, acidosis.
- Measure serum albumin and calculate B/A ratio (see legend).
- Use total bilirubin. Do not subtract direct reacting or conjugated bilirubin.
- If infant is well and 35-37 6/7 weeks (median risk) can individualize TSB levels for exchange based on actual gestational age.

Fig. 7.15: Nomogram for instituting exchange transfusion

(Adapted from Training module for Doctors and Nurses, Facility Based Newborn Care)

- Infants at medium risk (> 38 weeks + risk factors* or 35 – 37 weeks and well).
- Infants at higher risk (35 – 37 weeks + risk factors*).

* The risk factors include isoimmune hemolytic disease, G6PD deficiency, asphyxia, significant lethargy, temperature instability, sepsis, acidosis, serum albumin <3.0 gm/dl.

Guidelines to Treat Hyperbilirubinemia in Preterm Neonates (< 35 weeks and < 2500 gms)

Approach to Management

ABO Hemolytic Disease of the Newborn

ABO incompatibility is the most common cause of hemolytic disease of newborn in our country. Infants with ABO incompatibility are considered to have hemolysis if they have anemia (Hct < 45%), an abnormal blood smear (3–4% spherocytes), or if reticulocyte count is 4-5% in first 24 hours, or if reticulocyte count > 1–2% in the first 1-2 weeks.

Birth weight (grams)	*Guidelines for PT* (mg/dl) Healthy infant*	*Guidelines for PT* (mg/dl) Sick infant*	*Consider ET**(mg/dl)*
< 1000 gms	05 – 07	04 – 06	10 – 12
1000 – 1500 gms	07 – 10	06 – 08	12 – 15
1501 – 2000 gms	10 – 12	08 – 10	15 – 18
2001 – 2500 gms	12 – 15	10 – 12	18 – 20

Approach

1. ABO grouping in cord blood should be advised in all babies born to Group O mothers.
2. Serum bilirubin estimation ordered at 12 hours age.
3. If no laboratory facilities are available, clinical assessment of yellow coloration of skin should be done and baby referred.
4. In case of early discharge after delivery mother should be made aware of the possibility of jaundice and advised to report.
5. In term babies with ABO incompatibility with no medical problems *phototherapy* should be started when serum bilirubin is 10 mg/dl at 12 hours, 12 mg/dl at 18 hours, 14 mg/dl at 24 hours or 15 mg/dl at any time.

   Exchange transfusion when serum bilirubin is 20 mg/dl or more. A repeat exchange transfusion may be necessary when after rebound the rise of serum bilirubin is > 1 mg/dl/hour or if hemoglobin level is 11 grams/dl or less after exchange.

Rh Hemolytic Disease of Newborn

Born in Hospital

- Start phototherapy and prepare for exchange. Send blood samples.
- Indications for early exchange include:
  - Cord bilirubin 5 mg/dl or more.
  - Cord Hb 10 gm/dl or less.

Born Outside and Attended Subsequently

When the baby is born outside, the indications for exchange transfusion and intensive phototherapy will depend on the age at which the child attends the health facility.

Exchange transfusion: Indications

- At 24 hours or less with bilirubin level 10 mg/dl or more.
- At 25–48 hours with bilirubin level 15 mg/dl or more.
- >48 hours with bilirubin level 20 mg/dl or more or when the rate of rise of S. bilirubin is 0.5 mg/dl or more/hour.

Intensive phototherapy is indicated when the bilirubin level is 5 mg/dl less than that for exchange transfusion.

Hyperbilirubinemia in Healthy Term Newborn

Guidelines of management on the basis of serum bilirubin levels are shown below in a tabular form:

Age (hours)	*Phototherapy (Serum bilirubin in mg/ml)*	*Exchange transfusion (Serum bilirubin in mg/ml)*
25 – 72	15 or more	20 or more
72 or more	20 or more	25 or more

Points to be Noted

1. Failure of phototherapy is defined as inability to observe a decline in total serum bilirubin by 1–2 mg/dl at 4–6 hours and keep the level below the exchange range.
2. Exchange in a lower bilirubin level is indicated if S. bilirubin increase > 0.5 mg/dl/hour.
3. If at admission bilirubin is in exchange level, start phototherapy and prepare exchange.

   Repeat S. bilirubin after 2 hours. If bilirubin is not declining @ > 0.5 mg/dl/hr, start exchange transfusion. If at admission S. bilirubin is above exchange level start exchange transfusion.

PROLONGED NEONATAL UNCONJUGATED HYPERBILIRUBINEMIA

Definition

Jaundice persisting beyond 14 days in a term baby and 21 days in a preterm is usually considered to be pathologically prolonged.

Causes

1. Breast milk jaundice.
2. Extravasated blood e.g. cephalhematoma.
3. Persistence of hemolysis e.g. Hemolytic disease of newborn.
4. G6PD deficiency.
5. Hypothyroidism.
6. Congenital hypertrophic pyloric stenosis.
7. Functional or organic intestinal stasis.
8. Malaria.

9. Crigler-Najjar type II.
10. Sepsis.

Common Causes

1. Breast milk jaundice.
2. Extravasated blood.
3. Persistence of hemolysis.
4. G6PD deficiency.
5. Hypothyroidism.
6. Infection e.g. urinary tract infection, septicemia.

Workup

As per American Academy of Pediatrics practice parameter, babies with prolonged hyperbilirubinemia should be investigated after 3 weeks provided (1) they are not ill (2) there is no abnormal physical examination and (3) no dark urine or light stools.

1. Careful history and clinical examination.
2. Rule out cholestasis on the basis of birth weight, age at onset, stool color.
3. Investigations: Serum bilirubin and fractions.
   PBS, CBC, Hb%, Rh and ABO grouping.
   Urine RE and culture, reducing substances.
   Thyroid function test (TSH, T_3, T_4).
   X-ray knee joint.
   Sepsis screen.

Breast Milk Jaundice

This condition may manifest as persistence of physiological jaundice or jaundice may appear for the first time at the end of first week. It is seen in term infants. The intensity of jaundice is maximum between 10–14 days. Instead of the usual fall of serum bilirubin by the fourth day, the bilirubin level continues to rise and may reach 20–30 mg/dL by 14 days. If breastfeeding is continued, the bilirubin level will stay elevated and then fall slowly by 2 weeks and return to normal by 4–12 weeks. If breastfeeding is stopped, the bilirubin will fall rapidly in 48 hours. If breastfeeding is started again, the bilirubin level may rise by 2-4 mg/dL but usually will not reach the previous high level. Neonates with breast milk jaundice are well, show adequate weight gain, with normal liver function test results and show no signs of hemolysis. The recurrence rate of breast milk jaundice in future pregnancies is around 70%.

Etiology

The exact cause is still not known. Breast milk jaundice is thought to result from compromised hepatic conjugation of bilirubin due to presence of 3 alpha 20 beta pregnandiol in breast milk in about 1–2% of women. High concentration of unsaturated fatty acids in the human milk due to over activity of lipase may also inhibit hepatic glucoronyl transferase enzyme and Y acceptor protein. The inhibitory substances in breast milk are excreted for about 4 to 10 weeks. Hence breast milk jaundice may last for upto 12 weeks.

In addition, breast fed infants are more likely to have increased entero hepatic circulation because they ingest the beta-glucoronidase present in breast milk. They are also slower to be colonized with intestinal bacteria that convert conjugated bilirubin to urobilinoids, and excrete fewer stools. These may be additional factors.

Diagnostic Features

- Infant in good health, vigorous and feeding well.
- Gaining weight adequately.
- Colourless urine and golden yellow stools.
- Other causes of prolonged jaundice has been excluded.
- Unconjugated hyperbilirubinemia.
- Liver function tests normal.
- No evidence of hemolysis.

Management

- Continue frequent breastfeeding.
- Phototherapy if serum bilirubin is more than 20 mg/dl.
- Reassurance to parents.

Breastfeeding Jaundice

This condition is characterized by an early onset, exaggerated unconjugated hyperbilirubinemia (> 12 mg/dl) in the first week of life in the exclusively breastfeeding babies. It may be due to low production and resulting decreased milk intake leading to dehydration or reduced calorie intake. Supplements of glucose water or plain water to breast-fed babies is also associated with higher bilirubin levels partly due to reduced intake of the higher calorie density breast milk.

Frequent breastfeeding (>10 times/24 hours), rooming in with breastfeeding at night and discouraging glucose water or plain water supplementation can reduce the incidence of this condition.

Management

- Continue frequent breastfeeding.
- Phototherapy if serum bilirubin is more than 20 mg/dl.
- Reassurance to parents.

Cephalhematoma with Hyperbilirubinemia

Aspiration of cephalhematoma may introduce infection; hence contraindicated. Resulting anemia and hyperbilirubinemia should be treated as for hemolytic disease.

Crigler-Najjar Syndrome

It is a condition characterized by unconjugated hyperbilirubinemia due to congenital deficiency of enzyme glucoronyl transferase. There are two types:

Type I: is inherited as an autosomal recessive disorder. Parents of affected children have a partial defect in conjugation but their serum bilirubin concentration is normal.

Diagnostic Features

1. Onset of jaundice is during first 3 days, severe in intensity and rapidly progressing to kernicterus and a fatal outcome.
2. If child survives with treatment, there is persistence of unconjugated hyperbilirubinemia above 20 mg/dl after 1st week without signs of hemolysis.
3. Laboratory test: 1. Bilirubin concentration in bile is < 10 mg/dl (normal 50–100 mg/dl). 2. Absence of bilirubin glucoronide in bile (white bile). 3. Hepatic tissue enzyme assay by closed liver biopsy is confirmatory.

Type II: Is inherited as an autosomal dominant disorder. It is a milder form with onset of jaundice between birth and 10 years.

Diagnostic Features

1. In the neonatal period, onset of jaundice may be in the first 3 days. Serum bilirubin concentration may be in the physiologic range. Kernicterus is unusual.
2. Persistence of unconjugated hyperbilirubinemia beyond 3rd week with bilirubin concentration in the range of 1.5–22 mg/dl.
3. Infants are well.
4. *Lab tests:* (i) Bile bilirubin is normal, (ii) No signs of hemolysis.

Treatment

Oral phenobarbitone, 5 mg/kg/day. Response with a decrease in serum bilirubin concentration to 2–3 mg/dl is shown in 7–10 days. It has to be continued on a long-term basis.

NEONATAL CHOLESTASIS

A newborn is considered to have predominantly conjugated hyperbilirubinemia when the conjugated fraction is greater than 2 mg/dl or 20% of total bilirubin.

Neonatal cholestasis is defined as prolonged elevation of serum levels of conjugated bilirubin beyond the first 14 days of life. Cholestasis in newborn may be due to infectious, genetic, metabolic or undefined abnormalities giving rise either to mechanical obstruction of bile flow or to functional impairment of hepatic excretory function and bile secretion. The clinical features of any form of cholestasis are similar.

Neonatal cholestasis constitutes 30% of hepatobiliary disorders. A multicentric study in India reveals the following causes of neonatal cholestasis:

Hepatocellular Causes

1. Idiopathic neonatal hepatitis.
2. TORCH infection.
3. Sepsis, malaria, UTI.
4. Varied etiology e.g.
   a. Inspissated bile plug syndrome.
   b. Recurrent intrahepatic cholestasis.
   c. Progressive familial cholestasis.
   d. Hypothyroidism.

Metabolic Causes

1. Galactosemia.
2. TPN (Total parenteral nutrition) related.
3. Tyrosinemia.
4. Storage disorders.

Obstructive Causes

1. Biliary atresia.
2. Choledochal cyst.
3. Ductal paucity.

Evaluation

Cholestasis in the neonate may be the initial manifestation of numerous disorders; the clinical manifestations are usually similar and provide very few clues about the etiology. All affected infants have icterus, dark urine, light or acolic stools, and hepatomegaly resulting from decreased bile flow due to either hepatocyte injury or bile duct obstruction. The evaluation of the infant with cholestasis should follow a logical multistep process.

Steps

1. Identification of cholestasis by estimation of serum bilirubin and fractions.
2. Recognition of conditions for which specific therapy is available to prevent further damage and avoid long term complications. These conditions include sepsis, hypothyroidism, panhypopituitarism, metabolic disorders viz. galactosemia, tyrosinemia.
3. Differentiation of neonatal hepatitis and extrahepatic biliary atresia.

The following 4 clinical criteria should be emphasized before planning the laboratory investigations:

- Birth weight.
- Assessment of color of stool for upto 10 consecutive days.
- Age of onset of stool pallor and characteristics of progression.
- Clinical characteristics of hepatomegaly.

A normal birth weight, early persistent stool pallor, and a huge hepatomegaly which is firm to hard in consistency favours extrahepatic obstruction.

A low birth weight baby, gradual onset of change of stool color with waxing and waning of colour and a moderate hepatomegaly which is normal to slightly firm in consistency favours intrahepatic cholestasis.

The other clinical features to look for are splenomegaly, petechiae, chorioretinitis and microcephaly.

Investigations

It should be noted that these four clinical criteria, on their own can differentiate between extrahepatic and intrahepatic cholestasis in 82% cases. Liver biopsy together with the clinical findings enables a differential diagnosis to be made in 85% cases. With addition of HIDA scan, 95% of extrahepatic obstruction can be diagnosed before surgery.

In absence of facilities for liver biopsy and HIDA scan the following laboratory tests may help in differentiating extra and intrahepatic cholestasis.

1. To Confirm Conjugated Hyperbilirubinemia

- *Urine for bilirubin:* Presence of which indicates conjugated hyperbilirubinemia. At the bedside, *foam test* can be done to detect bilirubin in urine. It is a simple, qualitative, valid procedure. When normal urine is taken in a test tube and vigorously shaken, the foam is white. In urine containing bilirubin, the foam will be yellow.
- *Estimation of serum bilirubin and direct bilirubin as well as serial estimation of total serum bilirubin:* Initial high levels, often above 10 mg/dl, is found in hepatitis with a tendency towards an irregular decline with time. In biliary atresia, the levels are initially low with gradually increase with time.

2. To Assess the Degree of Hepatic Dysfunction

a. Gamma glutamyl transpeptidase, enzymes SGPT, LDH, S. alkaline phosphatase, 5, nucleotidase.
b. Serum cholesterol, serum protein and fractions.
c. Prothrombin time.

An increase of SGPT in early stages indicates intrahepatic cholestasis. LDH and 5 nucleotidase are increased in intrahepatic and extrahepatic cholestasis respectively. A 3-fold increase in S. alkaline phosphatase and a serum cholesterol level > 250 mg/dl indicates intrahepatic obstruction. An increased prothrombin time (more than 4 seconds) and INR more than 1.5 indicates hepatic encephalopathy.

3. To Rule Out Definite Causes

- Urine C/S, blood C/S, CSF C/S, Sepsis screen.
- Serological tests for TORCH, hepatitis.
- Urine for reducing substances (Galactosemia, fructose intolerance).
- Coomb's test (HDN).
- TSH, T_3, T_4.

4. To Differentiate between Idiopathic Neonatal Hepatitis and Bile Duct Anomalies, When Other Known Causes have been Ruled Out

a. USG of hepatobiliary system

USG can assess gallbladder size, function, detect dilatation of biliary tract and define choledochal cysts. An USG examination should be done before and after milk feed to assess the function (contraction) of the gallbladder. In infants with biliary atresia, the gallbladder is usually small or absent and CBD is not visualized. A normally contracting gallbladder after a milk feed indicates neonatal hepatitis.

b. Hepatobiliary scans with imido diacetic acid analogs (HIDA).

   In hepatitis, uptake is sluggish, excretion to intestine eventually occurs but in extrahepatic biliary obstruction, uptake is normal but excretion into intestine is absent. Oral administration of phenobarbitone, 5 mg/kg/day for 5 days prior to the study enhances biliary excretion of the isotope in neonatal hepatitis.

c. A less sensitive but simple method for demonstration of biliary patency is aspiration of duodenal contents. Gallbladder contraction is stimulated by administration of fluid and the aspirate is examined for bile. A positive result (i.e. presence of bile in the duodenal contents) rules out biliary atresia. A negative result indicates severe cholestasis consistent with but not pathognomonic of biliary atresia.

d. Liver biopsy provides a precise histological diagnosis. It also helps in enzyme analysis to detect inborn errors of metabolism.

e. An operative cholangiography is indicated in infants in whom the HIDA and liver biopsy indicate extrahepatic obstruction.

Principles of Treatment

1. Prompt recognition of any specific or treatable primary cause of cholestasis e.g. galactosemia, fructosemia etc and institution of appropriate therapy to prevent further hepatocellular injury.
2. Medical management of cholestasis.
3. Treatment of the specific cause.

Medical Management

Nutritional Support

a. In breast-fed babies, continue breastfeeding and supplement medium chain triglyceride (MCT) based diet (use of coconut oil) because they do not require the presence of intraluminal bile acids for absorption. In older infants, diet should be rich in calories (200 kcal/kg/day), rich in MCT with protein (1-2 gms/kg) from vegetable source. At least 2–3% calories should come from essential fatty acids.

b. These infants are prone to develop deficiency of fat soluble Vitamins viz A, D, E, K. They should be monitored and supplemented with water soluble preparations of Vitamin A and D till cholestasis resolves. The Vitamins A, D (water soluble preparations) is recommended in a dose 5 times the normal requirement. Vitamin E supplementation 50–200 mg/day orally. Vitamin K 5 mg/day IM for 3 days and then 5 mg weekly. Water soluble vitamins supplementation in twice the daily recommended doses.

Management of Associated Problems

1. *Pruritus:* Pruritus can be reduced by giving Phenobarbitone (5 mg/kg/day) along with UDCA (10-20 mg/kg/day). Other drugs which can be tried are cholestyramine (4–8 mg/day), terfenedine (1-3 mg/kg/day).
2. *Portal hypertension:* Variceal bleeding should be controlled with endoscopic sclerotherapy.
3. *Ascites:* Bed rest, salt restriction (0.5–1 gm/ day of salt), diuretics (frusemide + spironolactone) and paracentesis in intractable ascites.
4. *Hepatic encephalopathy:* Should be treated in the usual line.
5. *Infection:* Infection should be suspected in the presence of ascites and end stage liver disease. A full work up for infection including ascitic fluid culture and sensitivity should be undertaken. Cefotaxime should be used for peritonitis. If septicemia is suspected amikacin or gentamicin should be added which may be modified later as necessary.

Treatment of Specific Cause

1. Surgical treatment for biliary atresia.
2. *Galactosemia:* Elimination of lactose from diet. Supplementation with soy protein based lactose free formula.
3. *Fructosemia:* Elimination of fructose and sucrose from diet.
4. *Infections:* Treatment of congenital syphilis, toxoplasmosis, sepsis etc.
5. *Choledochal cyst:* Surgery.

6. *EHBA with decompensated liver disease:* Liver transplantation.
7. *Idiopathic neonatal hepatitis:* Supportive treatment.

Prognosis

Prognosis depends on the primary cause of cholestasis. In idiopathic neonatal cholestasis, 60–70% will recover with no evidence of hepatic structural or functional impairment. Approximately 5–10% will have persistent fibrosis or inflammation and a smaller percentage will have more severe disease viz. cirrhosis.

Preventable metabolic causes and infections have a good prognosis with timely intervention. Choledochal cyst has good prognosis with timely intervention.

Patients with biliary atresia usually dies from liver failure before 2 years age when untreated. Even after operative treatment they have persistent inflammation of the intrahepatic biliary tree and in most cases a degree of hepatic dysfunction persist. Around 2/3 of the patients ultimately need liver transplantation.

In the familial variety of cholestasis, 20–30% will recover; 10–15 % will acquire chronic liver disease with cirrhosis.

Neonatal Sepsis

Neonatal sepsis is a major cause of morbidity and mortality in newborns, particularly in the low birth weight. It is the single most important cause of neonatal deaths in the community and may account for around 50% of neonatal mortality. If diagnosed early and treated aggressively, it is possible to save most cases of neonatal sepsis. Neonatal survivors of sepsis can have severe neurologic sequelae due to CNS infection or secondary hypoxemia resulting from septic shock, persistent pulmonary hypertension and severe lung parenchymal disease.

Etiopathogenesis

When pathogenic bacteria gains access into the blood stream, they cause either septicemia (an overwhelming infection without much localization) or a predominantly localized involvement of the lung (Pneumonia), meninges (meningitis) or the urinary tract (Urinary tract infection).

Neonatal sepsis can be classified into early onset sepsis and late onset sepsis. 85% of early onset sepsis present within 24 hours, 5% present at 24–48 hours and a small percentage present between 48 hours and 6 days. Late onset sepsis presents after 72 hours of life.

Early onset sepsis is associated with the organism which colonizes the maternal genital tract. It is acquired during the baby's passage through a colonized birth canal during delivery. The infection may also be transplacental or an ascending infection from the cervix. The organisms implicated are those which colonize the genital tract viz. Group B streptococcus, E. coli, listeria monocytogenes.

Late onset sepsis is acquired from the care giving environment. The organisms implicated include E. coli, klebsiella, coagulase negative staphylococcus, and staphylococcus aureus, pseudomonas, enterobacter, candida, acinetobacter and anaerobes. Preterm and low birth weight babies have increased susceptibility to these organisms. The organisms implicated in meningitis include E.coli, proteus, pseudomonas, klebsiella and staphylococcus. Late onset sepsis with associated pyoderma, cellulitis or umbilical infection and arthritis or osteomyelitis is usually caused by staphylococcus.

Table 7.5 : Difference between early and late onset sepsis

Features	*Early onset*	*Late onset*
1. Time of onset	<72 hours	>72 hours
2. Complications of pregnancy, delivery	Present	May or may not be present
3. Source of organisms	Mother's genital tract	Nosocomial, Community acquired
4. Usual clinical presentation	Fulminant multisystem	Slowly progressive
5. Mortality	30-50%	15-30%
6. Meningitis	Rare	Common
7. Organisms	E.coli, klebsiella, listeria	Staph. aureus, coagulase negative staphylococcus etc.

Risk Factors

The risk factors for *early onset sepsis* are low birth weight, preterm, febrile illness in mother within 2 weeks from delivery, foul smelling liquor, prolonged rupture of membrane (>18 hours), more than 3 unclean vaginal examinations during labour, prolonged and difficult delivery and perinatal asphyxia.

Presence of 3 or more of the above risk factor is an indication of starting an antibiotic.

Presence of 2 or more of the risk factors is an indication for ordering sepsis screen.

The risk factors for *hospital acquired late onset sepsis* include NICU admission, LBW, prematurity, invasive procedures, parenteral fluid therapy, and neonate on ventilator.

The risk factors for *community acquired late onset sepsis* include poor hygiene, poor cord care, bottle feeding, prelacteal feeds and superficial skin infection viz. pyoderma, umbilical sepsis.

These factors enhance the chances of entry of organisms into the body systems of the neonate who are less immunocompetent than older children.

Clinical Manifestations

Early Onset of Sepsis

Early onset sepsis can present as asymptomatic bacteriemia, pneumonia, septicemia and/or meningitis. In majority cases, the clinical signs appear by 24 hours of age. The most common presenting symptom is respiratory distress. The respiratory symptoms may range from mild tachypnea, grunting, with or without supplemental oxygen requirement, to respiratory failure. The features of meningitis include seizure, apnea and depressed sensorium. The baby may present with features of persistent pulmonary hypertension, disseminated intravascular coagulation with purpura and petechiae, and paralytic ileus.

Late Onset Sepsis

Late onset sepsis is caused by the organisms thriving in the external environment of the home or the hospital. The most common way of transmission of the infection is through the hands of the care providers. The onset of symptoms is usually delayed beyond 72 hours after birth. The symptoms and signs at presentation may include those of septicemia, pneumonia or meningitis. 10–15% cases may suffer from overt or covert meningitis. The symptomatology of late onset sepsis is as follows:

A. Features of Septicemia

1. Lethargy, refusal to feed, poor cry, not arousable, comatose.
2. Hypothermia.
3. Diarrhoea, vomiting and abdominal distension.
4. Jaundice.
5. Bleeding.
6. Poor perfusion and shock, renal failure.
7. Sclerema.

B. Features of Pneumonia

1. Tachypnoea.
2. Chest retractions.
3. Grunt.
4. Cyanosis.
5. Apnea or gasping.

C. Features of Meningitis

1. Fever.
2. Seizures.
3. Vacant look.
4. High pitched cry.
5. Excessive crying or irritability.
6. Bulging fontanel and neck retraction.

D. Features of a Low Grade Infection *e.g.* (Urinary Tract Infection).

Failure to gain weight, weight is static or loss of weight in spite of adequate feeding.

The early manifestations of late neonatal sepsis are minimal, vague and non-specific. Therefore a high index of suspicion is necessary for early diagnosis. The most characteristic manifestation is an alteration in the feeding behaviour. The baby who had been active and sucking normally gradually or suddenly becomes lethargic and refuses to suck. Such an observation by the mother or a nurse of the postnatal ward should be never taken lightly. While hypothermia is common, fever is an infrequent presentation. Episodes of apnea or gasping may be the only manifestations of septicemia. In very sick neonates there may be sclerema, poor peripheral perfusion and cyanosis. Sclerema is a diffuse, spreading, waxy hardness of the skin and subcutaneous tissue. It is observed commonly on the thighs, buttocks and trunk. It is a manifestation of shock and insufficiency of peripheral perfusion and is associated with poor prognosis. The critically ill neonate can develop shock, bleeding due to disseminated intravascular coagulation (DIC) and renal failure. In cases presenting with pneumonia, findings on auscultation of chest are non-specific and non-contributory. Meningitis is often missed as it may be masked by the signs of septicemia.

Laboratory Diagnosis

The laboratory investigation and treatment of neonatal sepsis should go simultaneously. It should be noted that early treatment is of critical importance and no confirmatory test is required as a prerequisite to start treatment in presence of strong clinical suspicion.

Cultures and antibiotic sensitivity of blood, CSF, urine and demonstration of micro-organism in a buffy coat smear are necessary to confirm infection. They are useful but take more than 48–72 hours for the result. Moreover in a substantial number of blood cultures (40%) no bacteria are isolated despite strong clinical suspicion of sepsis. An early and objective diagnosis can be made in suspected cases of sepsis with the help of the non-specific septic screening test.

Sepsis screen: It is a simple, side-laboratory test which will indicate infection without identifying the infecting organisms. Such neonates can be treated with the first line antibiotics as per unit's antibiotic policy for sepsis which is essentially based on the profile of organisms isolated in blood cultures in the previous 3-6 months and their sensitivity pattern. The tests included in the sepsis screen are total WBC count, absolute neutrophil count, immature cells (myelocytes, metamyelocytes and band cell) : total neutrophil ratio, micro ESR and C reactive protein level. The cut off abnormal values and the interpretation is given below:

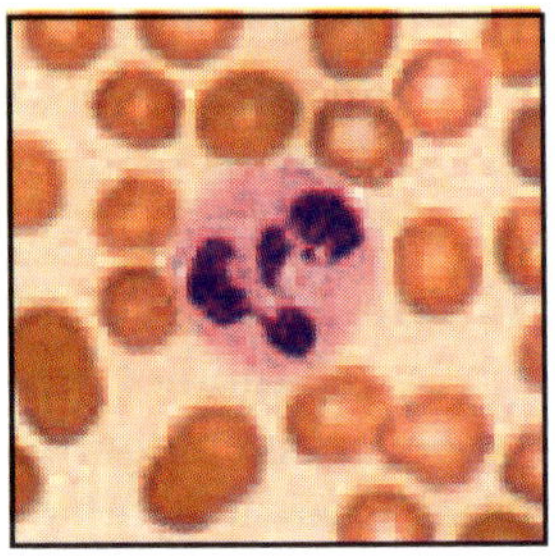

Fig. 7.16a: Neutrophil

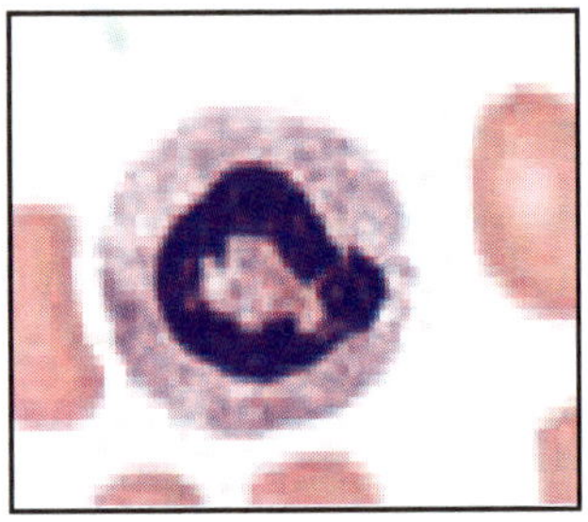

Fig. 7.16b: Band cell

Table 7.6 : A practical sepsis screen

Components	*Abnormal values*
Total leukocyte count	< 5000/cmm
Absolute neutrophil count	< 1800/cmm
Immature/Total neutrophil	> 0.2
Micro-ESR	> 15 mm AEFH
CRP	> 1 mg /dl

If two parameters are abnormal, it should be considered as a positive sepsis screen and infant should be treated with presumptive diagnosis of neonatal sepsis. If none or one test is positive and there is strong clinical suspicion of sepsis, the sepsis screen should be repeated after 12 hours. If the screen is still negative, sepsis can be excluded with reasonable certainty.

Lumbar puncture: A lumber puncture should be done in cases of early onset sepsis with positive blood culture and in all cases of late onset neonatal sepsis as 10–15% cases are associated with meningitis. The detection of meningitis with septicemia has therapeutic implications. A child with associated meningitis needs antibiotics with a high CSF penetration and prolonged therapy.

The normal CSF findings are different in neonates. A knowledge about this is important in interpretation of the CSF analysis findings.

Table 7.7 : Normal CSF picture in neonates

CSF components	*Normal values*
Cells/cumm	8 (0–30 cells)
Polymorph nuclear leukocytes (%)	60%
Protein	90 (20–170) mg/dl
Glucose	52 (34–119) mg/dl
CSF/blood glucose ratio	51 (44– 248)

Radiology

An *X-ray PA view chest* should be done in cases with respiratory distress, apnoea, *and X-ray plain picture abdomen* in presence of abdominal signs (vomiting, feed intolerance, and abdominal distension) or if neonatal necrotizing enterocolitis is suspected.

USG head and CT scan brain is indicated in all cases diagnosed to have meningitis. USG head should be done weekly to monitor for hydrocephalus.

Urine Microscopy and Culture

It is indicated in late onset sepsis especially presenting with unexplained fever, neonates at risk of fungal sepsis, neonates with poor weight gain and unexplained cholestasis.

UTI in neonates is diagnosed in presence of one of the following features: 5 WBCs/high power field, 10^4 organisms/ml in urine obtained by cathterization and any organism found in urine obtained by supra pubic aspiration.

Investigations for Evidence of Multi Organ Failure

A. **Renal function test:** Blood urea, serum creatinine.
B. **Metabolic acidosis:** Blood pH, HCO_3.
C. **Pulmonary function test:** pH, PO_2, PCO_2.
D. **Disseminated intravascular coagulation:** Coagulation profile viz. bleeding time, clotting time, prothrombin time, APTT.

Treatment

The treatment of neonatal sepsis is divided into supportive treatment and specific antibiotic therapy. Both the components are equally important. It should be realized that after the administration of antibiotics, it takes atleast 12–24 hours to show any effect. Supportive care is crucial in the initial period in saving the life of the baby until the action of the specific antimicrobial starts.

Supportive Treatment

The supportive treatment consists of the following:

1. Provision of warmth to maintain thermoneutral environment and avoid hypo or hyperthermia.
2. Intravenous line should be established.
3. Effective management of fluid and electrolyte balance is vital in the treatment of sepsis particularly when the neonate is in shock. The neonate should be first stabilized by infusion of 10% dextrose 2 ml/kg stat. Blood glucose should be maintained between 60–100 mg/dl.
4. Then the CRT is checked. If CRT >3 secs then normal saline/ Ringers lactate should be infused 10 ml/kg over 5–10 minutes. Same dose can be repeated 1–2 times over the next 30–45 minutes, if perfusion continues to be poor. If two boluses of crystalloids fail, inotropic agents should be started. Dopamine (5–20 microgram/kg/min) is the initial drug to be used followed by combined use of dobutamine (5–30 microgram/kg/min) and low doses of dopamine. Epinephrine (0.1–1.0 microgram/kg/min) may be required if there is no response.
5. Vitamin K, 1 mg intramuscularly should be given.
6. If there is cyanosis or grunt, oxygen should be given with hood and oxygen saturation maintained above 92% in term and 88% in preterm.
7. Enteral feed is avoided till baby is hemodynamically stable.
8. Anemia is managed by packed cells,10–15 ml/kg slowly over 2 hours if Hct is below 35–40% and bleeding disorder managed with fresh frozen plasma and /or platelets.
9. Seizures should be treated promptly and effectively.
10. If baby is apneic provide gentle tactile stimulation. If breathing is inadequate, provide positive pressure ventilation and mechanical ventilation as indicated on the basis of the ABG findings.

Antimicrobial Therapy

Indications for starting antibiotics in early onset sepsis are:

1. Presence of 3 risk factors for early onset sepsis.
2. Presence of foul smelling liquor.
3. Presence of 2 antenatal risk factors with a positive sepsis screen.
4. Strong clinical suspicion.

Indications of starting antibiotics in late onset sepsis are:

1. Positive sepsis screen, and
2. A strong clinical suspicion.

There is no role of antibiotics in the following situations:

1. Well preterm neonates with no risk factors for sepsis.
2. LSCS deliveries.
3. Meconium stained amniotic fluid without meconium aspiration syndrome.

Choice of Antibiotics

Each newborn unit should have its own policy regarding the first and second line of antibiotic therapy based on common organism locally prevalent and their sensitivity pattern. Initially two antibiotics should be started to cover both gram positive and negative organisms. Broad spectrum cephalosporins are best avoided because they are particularly prone to encourage the emergence of resistance if used indiscriminately. Antibiotics should be administered intravenously for the entire duration of therapy. Intramuscular route is preferably avoided due to small muscle mass and erratic absorption.

First Line Treatment

a. *Early onset sepsis*

   Ampicillin + Gentamycin

   In case of fulminant infections

   Cefotaxime + aminoglycoside (or as per prevailing unit policy)

   Or, Amoxicillin and clavulanate + aminoglycoside.

b. *Late onset sepsis*

   Pneumonia: Cloxacillin + aminoglycoside

   Or, Amoxicillin and clavulanate + aminoglycoside.

   Meningitis: Third generation cephalosporin + aminoglycoside.

NEC: Third generation cephalosporin + aminoglycoside + metronidazole (for radiologically confirmed cases).

If no clinical improvement in 48 hours, antibiotics have to changed according to the culture sensitivity reports.

Second Line Treatment

Hospital acquired or maternal gram negative infection: Third generation cephalosporin + aminoglycoside.

Pseudomonas infection: Ceftazidime/Piperacillin and tazobactum + aminoglycoside.

*Staph aureus: Cloxacillin/*Amoxicillin and clavulanate + aminoglycoside.

Methicillin resistant staph aureus (MRSA): Vancomycin + aminoglycoside.

Doses of Commonly Used Antibiotics

- Ampicillin: 50–100 mg/kg/dose 8–12 hourly (<7 days).
- Cefotaxime: 50 mg/kg/dose 8–12 hourly (<7 days).
- Gentamycin: 2.5 mg/kg/dose 8–12 hourly (<7 days).
- Amikacin: 7.5–10 mg/kg/ dose 8–12 hourly (<7 days).
- Ceftazidine: 50 mg/kg/dose 8–12 hourly (<7 days).
- Ceftriaxone: 50 mg/kg/dose 12 hourly.
- Vancomycin: 15 mg/kg/day to10 mg/ kg /dose 8 hourly.

Empirically ampicillin with gentamycin can be started. However, resistance to ampicillin is now frequently observed. The third generation cephalosporins viz. cefotaxime, ceftriaxone and ceftazidine are more useful. Vancomycin is suitable in MRSA infection. Aminoglycosides continue to be useful against E. coli, klebsiella and pseudomonas. Antibiotics once started empirically should be modified according to culture and sensitivity reports.

When antibiotics are started only on strong clinical suspicion, it is important to send sepsis screen prior to starting antibiotics. If sepsis screen comes out to be negative, but suspicion is too strong, then after 12 hours a repeat sepsis screen is usually done, if that comes to be negative, antibiotics can be either stopped at this point or can be continued for 5-7 days in case of strong clinical suspicion.

Duration of Antibiotic Therapy

The duration of antibiotic therapy depends on the extent of involvement and is shown in the table below:

Diagnosis	*Duration*
1. Meningitis	21 days
2. Blood culture +ve (no meningitis)	14 days
3. Culture –ve but definite clinical sepsis	10-14 days
4. Culture –ve, clinically probable sepsis, sepsis screen +ve	7-10 days
5. Culture –ve, clinically probable sepsis, sepsis screen –ve	5-7 days

Monitoring

The vital signs should be continuously monitored by using monitors. Clinical monitoring should be done 1–2 hourly in sick neonates and 4–6 hourly in less sick ones. Examination of color, activity, respiratory rate and respiratory distress scoring can be monitored without touching the infant.

Clinical Monitoring

- Temperature should be monitored continuously.
- Weighing, atleast once in 24 hours; 12 hourly in VLBW babies. It helps in assessment of fluid balance.
- Urine output, to keep minimum urine output at 1 ml/ kg/hour.
- Intake output chart should be maintained.
- Phlebotomy losses should be charted.

Biochemical Monitoring

- Blood sugar 4–6 hourly; more frequently if there is hypo or hyperglycemia.
- Serum electrolytes initially once a day; subsequently once in 2–3 days when condition is stable.
- Renal function and liver function tests, bleeding profile as and when indicated.
- Repeat blood / CSF culture if previous tests abnormal till normal reports documented.

Newer Modalities of Treatment

The newer modalities of treatment include exchange transfusion, IV immunoglobulin, G-CSF, and GM-CSF. These are of limited proven or experimental value presently.

Prevention

Prevention is far more cost effective than to treat neonatal sepsis with expensive antibiotics and high cost supportive care. The following measures can promote prevention of infection in the neonate:

Strict Infection Control Measures

1. Avoidance of prelacteal feeds.
2. Hand washing by care givers before and after handling the baby.
3. Exclusive breastfeeding from birth.
4. Asepsis during procedures.
5. Avoiding unnecessary IV fluids, injections, needle pricks, sharing needles, syringes and stock solutions in the newborn unit.
6. Care of umbilical cord and stump.
7. Maintaining proper hygiene of the baby.

Infection Control Policies in the Newborn Units

1. Adherence to written policies for admission into the unit.
2. Following strict antibiotic policies.
3. Regular disinfection policies for wards as well as equipments.
4. Nosocomial infection surveillance.
5. Quick and effective control of outbreak in the newborn unit.
6. Avoid overcrowding and understaffing in the newborn units.

Superficial Infections

Superficial infections are common in newborn. The incidence is related to the standard of hygiene maintained by the caregiver. It needs mention that the newborn is unable to develop sufficient inflammatory response to localize infection, as a result of the immature immune system. Hence superficial infection can readily disseminate to cause systemic infection, especially in low birth weight babies.

The source of infection is contaminated hands of nurses, doctors and family members who may be nasal carriers. The common superficial infections include conjunctivitis, pyoderma, oral thrush and umbilical sepsis.

Conjunctivitis (Ophthalmia Neonatorum)

Conjunctivitis (ophthalmia neonatorum) refers to inflammation of the conjunctiva in the first four weeks of life.

Etiology

The causative agents include topical medications (chemical conjunctivitis), bacteria and herpes simplex virus. Chemical conjunctivitis is most commonly seen with silver nitrate prophylaxis. It requires no specific treatment, and usually resolves within 48 hours. Bacterial causes include Neisseria gonorrhoeae, Chlamydia trachomitis, staphylococcus, streptococci, E. coli and H. influenzae.

Clinical Manifestations and Laboratory Diagnosis

Unilateral conjunctivitis with an onset after 5 days of life is often due to *Chlamydia trachomitis*. *Purulent conjunctivitis* present with unilateral or bilateral eye discharge and is generally diagnosed by culture of eye exudates. *Gonococcal ophthalmia* presents with chemosis, lid edema and purulent exudates beginning 1–4 days after birth. The diagnosis is confirmed by gram stain and culture of conjunctival scrapings which shows intracellular gram negative diplococci.

Treatment

Chlamydia trachomitis should be treated with oral erythromycin ethylsuccinate 40 mg/kg/day divided into 4 doses for 14 days. Topical treatment alone is not adequate, and is unnecessary when systemic therapy is given. Treatment failure may occur necessitating a second course. The infant should be evaluated for chlamydia pneumonia. Treatment is same with additional supportive care.

Purulent conjunctivitis is treated with local antibiotic ointments (erythromycin or gentamycin). Very severe infection caused by H. influenzae may require parenteral therapy and evaluation for sepsis and meningitis. Rarely P. aeruginosa can cause a severe form of conjunctivitis requiring parenteral antibiotics. Purulent conjunctivitis may be associated with dacrocystitis and orbital cellulitis and may need drainage. The infant should be monitored for development of osteomyelitis of the neighbouring bones. Persistence of watery discharge is usually due to a blocked nasolacrimal duct. In such cases, the mother should be instructed to massage the duct area before instillation of the eye drop. If the blockage is not relieved by 3–4 months, probing and dilatation of the duct may be necessary.

If a mother is known to have untreated N. gonorrhoeae infection, the infant should receive ceftriaxone 25–50 mg/kg (not exceeding 125 mg) IV/IM at birth. Uncomplicated gonococcal *ophthalmia* requires a single dose of ceftriaxone (25–50 mg/kg/day IV or IM, not to exceed 125 mg). Additional topical treatment is not necessary.

However, the infant should be hospitalized and screened for invasive disease viz. sepsis, meningitis and arthritis. Complicated cases need treatment with Ceftriaxone (25 mg/kg IV or IM 12 hourly or cefotaxime (25 mg/kg IV or IM 12 hourly for 7–14 days (10–14 days in case of meningitis). The mother and child should also be screened for coincident chlamydia infection. The mother should be treated to eliminate genital gonococci as per standard recommendations.

Prevention

One percent silver nitrate solution, 0.5% erythromycin ophthalmic ointment or 2.5% providone iodine solution, 1 drop to each eye administered within 1 hour of birth are all effective in prevention of ophthalmia neonatorum.

Pyoderma

Pyoderma is more common during summer months. It is characterized by pustules which are commonly seen over the scalp, neck, axilla and groin. The complications which may develop due to spread of the infection include abscess, parotitis, osteomyelitis, septicemia and pemphigus neonatorum. Pemphigus neonatorum results from a life threatening staphylococcal infection and is characterized by marked erythema, bullous lesions and exfoliation giving an appearance of scalded skin syndrome.

Isolated lesions should be treated by puncture and application of triple dye/antibiotic ointment of the punctured lesion. In case the lesions are spreading, erythromycin 50 mg/kg per day in 3 divided doses should be administered for 7 days. The infant should be monitored to detect complications which would require aggressive treatment with parenteral antistaphylococcal antibiotics.

Oral Thrush

Oral thrush is a fungal infection caused by candida albicans. The common source of infection is an infected birth canal. The other sources may be infected feeding bottle nipples and breast nipples, and prolonged antibiotic therapy.

The oral lesions are characterized by discrete white patches or spots over the buccal mucosa and gums. They may be confused with white milk curds. Whereas the curd can be easily removed, white patches due to thrush can be removed with difficulty only leaving a raw red area below it. A white tongue is not due to thrush and does not require cleaning. It is due to a milk layer and clears spontaneously.

With oral thrush, initially the infant is able to suck but swallowing may be difficult due to posterior pharyngeal lesions. Later, the infant may not be able to suck also.

Treatment consists of local application of 0.5% aqueous solution of gentian violet or cotrimazole mouth paint, initially frequently till lesions disappear and then atleast 3 times daily for 5–7 days.

Umbilical Sepsis

The umbilical cord stump is a good portal of entry of organism and it can lead the organism directly into the circulation. Hence umbilical sepsis can be a potent source of septicemia in the newborn. It should be prevented by clean cord care which includes no application to the cord stump and exposure to air for early drying. Umbilical sepsis may follow umbilical catherization and exchange transfusion. An infected umbilical stump should never be catheterized. Spread of infection along the umbilical vein can lead to pyelophlebitis with formation of hepatic micro abscess later followed by portal hypertension, which is however rare.

Umbilical sepsis is characterized by purulent, foul smelling discharge and an inflamed periumbilical area. The presence of a white slimy discharge should not be mistaken for sepsis and a positive bacterial growth from an umbilical swab in absence of pus cells, suggest colonization rather than umbilical sepsis.

Treatment in mild cases consists of frequent cleaning with rectified spirit and application of an antibiotic powder. If paraumbilical inflammation is marked or signs of systemic infection are present parenteral antibiotics should be started in the line of neonatal sepsis.

Neonatal Seizure

A clinical seizure at any age is associated with a paroxysmal burst of electrical activity within the central nervous system.

The newborn is at a particular risk of development of seizures because metabolic, toxic, structural and infectious diseases are more likely to manifest during this period of life. Although it is commonly a manifestion of an acute brain insult or a biochemical abnormality, in about 25% cases no cause may be identified.

The reported incidence of neonatal seizure range from 0.15% in term infants to 20.2% in preterm. The national collaborative project (UK) reported an incidence of 0.5%, preterm and term babies taken together. The precise frequency of neonatal siezures cannot be delineated because many subtle seizures go undetected.

Identification of Seizures in Newborn

It is often difficult to decide whether a neonate has had a seizure or not. It may be impossible to diagnose without witnessing the episode oneself and sometimes even then it may be difficult. This is because unlike older infants, newborn rarely have well organized tonic clonic seizure. Preterms have even less well organized spells than term neonates.

Types of Seizure

In the newborn period at least 5 essential seizure types have been recognized. They are subtle, tonic, multifocal clonic, focal and myoclonic seizures.

Subtle seizures: Constitute 50% of seizures in newborn and often occurs in association with other seizure types. Examples of subtle seizures include:

- Tonic horizontal deviation of eyes or sustained eye opening with ocular fixation or cycled fluttering.
- Repetitive blinking or fluttering of eyelids.
- Oral-facial lingual movements viz. chewing, tongue-thrusting, lip-smacking, drooling, yawning.
- Limb movements, cycling, paddling, boxing jabs.
- Autonomic phenomenon–Tachycardia or bradycardia.
- Apnea may be a rare manifestation of seizure. Apnea due to seizure activity has an accelerated or normal heart rate when evaluated 20 secs after onset.

Subtle seizures are most difficult to identify, are usually not associated with EEG abnormalities and respond poorly to anticonvulscent.

Tonic seizures: May resemble decerebrate or decorticate posturing, often associated with eye deviation and occasionally proceeded by clonic movements or apnea. Most often EEG shows severe abnormalities and prognosis is generally poor.

Multifocal clonic seizures: They are characterized by random clonic movements of limbs similar to those seen in normal babies less than 34 weeks of gestation. The EEG most often is multifocal abnormal.

Focal clonic seizures: In this type movements involve weak localized clonic jerking without loss of consciousness. The EEG is abnormal.

Myoclonic seizures: Manifestations include synchronous single or multiple slow jerks of upper or lower limbs or both.

Neonatal Seizure: Why Poorly Expressed?

The poor expression of seizure in the neonatal period is primarily due to immaturity of cortical organization of neonatal brain. The arborisation of axonal and dendritic synaptic contacts as well as myelination of cortical pathway is incomplete.

Neonatal seizures tend to be brief because immature neurons are unable to sustain repetitive activity for a long period. They are focal or multifocal because the pathway connecting different cortical regions are poorly myelinated and hence seizure discharge cannot readily be propagated throughout the neonatal brain to produce a generalized seizure. Further, the predominance of oral and buccal phenomena as well as ocular motor abnormalities and apnea may relate to the advanced development of limbic structures and their connection to the brainstem and diencephalons in comparison to other forebrain structures.

Movements That Are Not Seizures

Certain movements occur in a newborn, although not seizures may look like and has to be differentiated.

Normal Movements Seen More Commonly in Preterms

- Benign neonatal sleep myoclonus: Occur during REM sleep in preterm.
- Fragmentary myoclonic jerks.
- Eye-movements: Roving or dysconjugate eye-movements with occasional non-sustained nystagmoid jerks.

Neonate in Active REM Sleep With

1. Rhythmic eye jerks with irregular respiration.
2. Sucking movements.
3. Body movements.
4. Twitches of face or limb.

These movements will disappear upon arousing the infant.

Agitation and tremulousness will occur associated with crying when hungry and disappear when the baby is given a feed.

Jitteriness: May be confused with seizures but distinction can be readily made if following points are remembered.

i. Jitteriness is not accompanied by abnormalities of gaze or extra ocular movement.

ii. Jitteriness is provoked by stimulus. Seizures occur spontaneously.

iii. Jitteriness is characterized by rhythmic alternating movements, of equal amplitude at a rate of 5-6/sec. The dominant movement in seizure is clonic jerking i.e. movements have a fast and slow component at a slow rate of 2-3/sec.

iv. Movement of jitteriness can be stopped by flexion of the affected limb. Seizure movement will not stop by this maneuver.

v. Jitteriness is not accompanied by increased blood pressure, tachycardia or bradycardia.

Etiology

The causes of neonatal seizures are diverse. Majority are, however, secondary to relatively few etiologies. It needs emphasis that determination of etiology is highly critical because it helps one to treat specifically and also to make a meaningful prognostic statement.

Table 7.8 : Causes of neonatal seizures

A. Common causes:
1. Perinatal complications
a. Neonatal encephalopathy
b. Hypoxic ischemic encephalopathy
c. Intracranial hemorrhage
d. Contusion
2. Bacterial meningitis
3. Hypoglycemia
4. Early hypocalcemia
5. Idiopathic
B. Less common causes:
1. Developmental defect
2. Subarachnoid hemorrhage
3. Late hypocalcaemia
C. Rare causes:
1. Accidental injection of local anesthetic
2. Hypo and hypernatremia
3. Pyridoxine dependency
4. Other inborn errors of metabolism
5. Hyperbilirubinemia

Diagnostic Work-Up

A search for an etiologic diagnosis should proceed simultaneously with management of the seizure episode. Evaluation of the patient should begin with a careful history, physical examination with emphasis on the following points, because not infrequently the clue for an etiologic diagnosis may become obvious from such pursuits.

Features	*Suspected diagnosis*
1. History of fetal distress, instrumentation, need for resuscitation in labour room with low Apgar score (<3 at 5 min).	1. Perinatal asphyxia
2. Full term baby with history of trauma, difficult delivery, bruise.	2. Contusion, ICH
3. Preterm baby with pallor, Hypotonia, bulging fontanelle, lowering hematocrit.	3. Intraventricular hemorrhage
4. Small for date baby with history of maternal diabetes, PET, LFD or SFD.	4. Hypoglycemia, early hypocalcemia
5. Premature rupture of membrane more than 18 hours.	5. Sepsis
6. History of excess fluid administration during labour.	6. Hyponatremia
7. History of excess and rapid I.V. administration of sod bicarbonate or sod chloride.	7. Hypernatremia
8. Hyperemesis gravidarum with Vitamin B6 therapy.	8. Pyridoxine deficiency
9. Family history of seizure or mental retardation and recurrence of seizure in sibship or unexplained early neonatal death with features of lethargy, vomiting, jaundice etc.	9. Metabolic disorder
10. Dysmorphic facies, microcephaly.	10. Developmental CNS anomaly
11. Hepatosplenomegaly	11. I.U. infection
12. Cutaneous manifestation	12. Neurocutaneous syndrome
13. Top feeding with cows milk	13. Late onset hypocalcemia

The etiology can be suspected also from the day of onset of the seizure as shown below:

Day of onset	*Cause of seizure*
0–3 days	Perinatal complications, metabolic and developmental anomaly.
4–7 days	Sepsis, meningitis, metabolic and developmental defects.

Laboratory Investigations

Initial Investigations: The initial laboratory tests should be directed towards the most dangerous but readily treatable diseases and therefore should include:

1. Estimation of blood sugar, serum calcium, magnesium, sepsis screen, ABG, anion gap.
2. An ECG to rule out hypocalcemia.
3. Lumbar puncture: CSF examination should be done in all cases with the slightest suspicion of meningitis or intracranial hemorrhage, except in severe cardiorespiratory compromise of neonates. It should not be omitted even if another etiology (e.g. hypoglycemia) is present because meningitis may coexist.

Specific Investigations: To be picked up as and when necessary:

1. Serum bilirubin (if jaundice present).
2. Serum sodium, potassium, blood urea nitrogen (BUN), liver function tests to rule out causes and plan fluid therapy.
3. Screen for congenital infections (TORCH) and metabolic screen for inborn errors of metabolism (urine pH, blood pH, blood ammonia, anion gap, urine and serum amino acidogram, serum and CSF lactate/pyruvate ratio).
4. EEG should be done in the interictal period in selected cases. It has both diagnostic and prognostic role in seizure. The value of neonatal EEG has increased with establishment of age related normal and abnormal backgrounds. It has now become unquestionable in the modern management of neonatal seizure. But neither diagnostic procedures nor therapy need to be postponed for an EEG. EEG helps in:
   a. Recognition of subtle seizures.
   b. Recognition of electrical seizures in paralyzed and ventilated newborns.
   c. Prevent over interpretation of abnormal movement and thereby resultant over treatment.
   d. Prognosticate eventual sequelae.
5. Neurodiagnostic studies viz. Ultrasonography and CT scan of brain should be considered depending on the specific clinical features. Ultrasonography would help identify acute lesions like intracranial hemorrhage and also follow-up hydrocephalus. CT scan can also delineate small calcification, developmental defects, infarcts etc.

Treatment

Continuous or recurrent seizures should be treated as an emergency. The treatment can be broadly discussed under the following headings:

1. Treatment of ongoing seizure.
2. Treatment during interictal period.
3. Maintenance and follow-up.
4. Treatment of underlying cause with specific measures in individual cases.

Table 7.9 : Steps of management of ongoing seizure

Step 1:	Stabilize vital functions.
Step 2:	Correct transient metabolic disturbances.
	a. Hypoglycemia (Target blood sugar 70–120 mg/dl): 10% dextrose I.V. bolus 2 ml/kg followed by continuous infusion at 8 mg/kg/minute.
	b. Hypocalcemia: 10% calcium gluconate I.V. at 4 ml/kg (need cardiac monitoring).
	c. Hypomagnesaemia: 50% magnesium sulphate I.M. 0.2 ml/kg.
Step 3:	Phenobarbitone 20 mg/kg I.V. bolus followed by 5 mg/kg (may repeat to total dose of 40 mg/kg), need cardiorespiratory monitoring. Consider continuous EEG monitoring, intubation/ventilation.
Step 4:	Phenytoin 20 mg/kg slow I.V. bolus followed by 5 mg/kg slow IV (may repeat to a total dose of 30 mg/kg).
Step 5:	Lorazepam 0.05 mg/kg I.V. (may repeat to total dose 0.1 mg/kg).
Step 6:	Pyridoxine 50–100 mg /kg I.V. with EEG monitoring.
Step 7:	Other drugs.

After each step, evaluate the infant for ongoing seizure. If seizure persists, advance to the next step.

Steps of Treatment of Ongoing Seizure

1. The first step in successful management of seizure is to nurse the baby in the thermoneutral environment and ensure a patent airway, breathing and circulation.
2. An I.V. access should be secured using a peripheral vein or umbilical vein and oxygen should be started.
3. Dextrostix examination and blood should be collected for sugar and other investigations.
4. A brief relevant history and quick clinical examination should be done.

5. If glucostix shows hypoglycemia or if there is no facility to test blood sugar immediately, 2 ml/kg of 10% dextrose should be given by bolus followed by maintenance infusion of 8 mg/kg/min.
6. If blood sugar is in normal range, an ECG should be done to look for signs of hypocalcaemia (QT interval more than 0.2 seconds in the preterm and more than 0.19 seconds in term babies). A sample for ionized calcium and serum magnesium should be withdrawn and 4 ml/kg of 10% calcium gluconate should be given I.V. under strict cardiac monitoring over 10 minutes. It should be noted that an ECG can be a better alternative to rule out hypocalcaemia. If hypomagnesaemia is associated (usually seen in 50% of cases) 0.2 ml/kg of 50% magnesium sulphate should be given intramuscularly. It should be noted that hypocalcemic seizures are suppressed by anticonvulscent drugs also.
7. If seizure persists, even after correction of hypoglycemia/hypocalcemia, anti-epileptic drugs (AED) should be started. Phenobarbitone is the drug of choice. It is given in a loading dose of 20 mg/kg/dose I.V. very slowly over 20 minutes (not faster than 1mg/kg/min). If seizures persist after completion of this loading dose, repeat dose of phenobarbitone 5 mg/kg/dose may be used every 20–30 minutes till a dose of 40 mg/kg has been given. The maintenance dose is 3–5 mg/kg/day in 1-2 divided doses I.V. or per oral, started 12 hours after the loading dose.
8. Phenytoin is indicated, if the maximal dose of phenobarbitone (40 mg/kg) fails to resolve seizures or earlier, if adverse effects like respiratory depression, hypotension or bradycardia ensues with phenobarbitone. It is given in a loading dose of 20 mg/kg I.V. at a rate of not more than 1 mg/kg/min under cardiac monitoring. A repeat dose of 5 mg/kg may be tried if seizures still persist.
9. Very occasionally in 10-15% of newborns with seizures that do not respond to phenobarbitone and phenytoin, benzodiazepines may be required. Benzodiazepines available are diazepam, lorazepam, midazolum and clonazepam. Diazepam is generally avoided due to its short duration of action, narrow therapeutic index, and presence of sodium benzoate as a preservative which aggravates jaundice. Lorazepam is preferred over diazepam due to its longer duration of action, less cardiovascular adverse effects and wider therapeutic index. Midazolum is faster acting but requires strict monitoring for respiratory depression, apnea and bradycardia. Equipment for resuscitation and assisted ventilation should be available at the bedside of all neonates given multiple doses of antiepileptic drugs.
10. When neonatal seizures prove refractory to the above regimen, pyridoxine dependency should be excluded. The condition can be diagnosed by rapid (within minutes) cessation of EEG seizure after administration of 50–100 mg of pyridoxine I.V. Occasionally apnea and hypotonia may develop. Hence respiratory monitoring is necessary. If the diagnosis is made, maintenance oral dose of pyridoxine should be given at 10–100 mg/day, depending on the response. Infants who fail to respond to adequate doses of anticonvulscents and pyridoxine should be put on a trial of oral folinic acid for 24–48 hours. The starting dose is 2.5 mg twice daily, may have to be increased upto 8 mg/kg/day.

Refractory seizures: Seizures refractory to aforementioned therapy may be due to:

- Cortical dysgenesis, cerebral infarction.
- Severe HIE.
- Intraventricular hemorrhage.
- Inborn error of metabolism, intrauterine infection.
- Narcotic withdrawal.

These cases should undergo investigations in search of a diagnosis and then treated. The anticonvulscent drugs that may be tried in such circumstances are:

- *Lidocaine:* Start with 4 mg/kg/hour I.V. on first day, reduce by 1 mg/kg/hour on each subsequent day. It should not be administered with phenytoin.
- *Paraldehyde:* A dose of 0.1-0.2 ml/kg/dose may be used IM or 0.3 ml/kg/dose mixed with coconut oil in 3:1 ratio may be used by per rectal route.
- *Valproic acid:* Dose is 20–25 mg/kg/day (PO/PR) followed by 5–10 mg/kg every 12 hours.

Other measures: According to the cause.

Doses

- Diazepam—0.25 mg/kg I.V. bolus (0.5 mg/kg rectal); may be repeated 1-2 times.

- Lorazepam—0.05 mg/kg I.V. bolus over 2-5 minutes; may be repeated.
- Midazolum—0.15 mg/kg I.V. bolus followed by infusion of 0.1-0.4 mg/kg/hour.

Treatment During Interictal Period

If a neonate is brought after seizure is over by itself, baby should be subjected to investigations. If dextrostix detects hypoglycemia it should be treated. If normal, other lab tests are carried out to find the cause. The baby is to be kept under observation for recurrence or any abnormality on tests.

Maintenance Treatment

Maintenance treatment after response should be started after 12 hours of bolus. The drugs used are:

- Phenobarbitone: 3-5 mg/kg/day in 1-2 divided doses PO/IV.
- Phenytoin: 3-8 mg/kg/day in 2-4 divided doses I.V.

Recurrence of Seizure During Maintenance

Only life threatening seizures are to be treated with a loading dose of the drug of which the maximum dose has not been used previously, in the same manner as the first seizure. Subtle seizures need no treatment. Maintenance has to be started after 12 hours.

When to Stop Anti-Convulscent?

It is still controversial. The following guidelines may be followed:

1. Single seizure treated with one drug: No maintenance required.
2. Single seizure treated with more than one drug: Stop all drugs if the baby does not have convulsion for 3-4 days or at discharge. If cause of convulsion is HIE continue anticonvulscent for 10 days and then stop. It has been observed that seizures due to HIE tends to subside by itself by 7-10 days.
3. With multiple seizures, treated with more than one drug, baby is reviewed at discharge. If the baby is neurologically normal, all drugs can be stopped, irrespective of the etiology and EEG. If the baby is neurologically abnormal, phenytoin is stopped at discharge and phenobarbitone is continued for 1 month and baby is reassessed after 1 month. If the baby is neurologically normal at 1 month and is seizure free, phenobarbitone is discontinued over 2 weeks. If neurological assessment is not normal, an EEG is done. If EEG is not overtly abnormal, AED is tapered and stopped. If EEG is overtly abnormal, the infant is reassessed in the same manner at 3 months and then 3 monthly till 1 year of age.

Prognosis

The over-all prognosis of neonatal seizure is as follows:

Lower the gestational age higher the mortality. Good recovery occurs in 55%, about 15% die during the first two postnatal weeks and 30% survive with neurological deficits like mental retardation, persistent seizure and cerebral palsy.

Respiratory Problems in Newborn

Respiratory problems are the most common cause of admission of the term and preterm neonates to a special care nursery. It occurs in 4–6% of neonates and contributes significantly to morbidity and mortality during the neonatal period. Mortality can be reduced by timely referral and intervention. Majority causes are preventable. On anticipation, in utero transfer of the baby to secondary or tertiary care, is life saving.

Many neonatal cardiac problems can present with identical clinical signs as respiratory problems. Although the supportive treatment is similar, an early and definitive diagnosis is necessary to plan appropriate treatment. Hence any sign of respiratory distress in a newborn, in the postnatal period is an indication for immediate examination and diagnostic evaluation including a chest X-ray and arterial blood gas determination.

Tachypnoea and Respiratory Distress

The most common presentations of respiratory problems in newborn are tachypnoea and respiratory distress. Tachypnoea alone means an increased respiratory rate of more than 60/minute in a quiet and resting baby. Respiratory distress, on the other hand, includes manifestations viz. tachypnoea, subcostal retractions, grunting, lethargy, poor feeding with or without central cyanosis.

Causes of Respiratory Distress

Respiratory distress may be a result of problems in the respiratory, cardiovascular, central nervous system or gastrointestinal systems. However, pulmonary disease is the most common cause.

Table 7.10 : Causes of respiratory distress

Medical causes:

a. Respiratory causes:
   1. Hyaline membrane disease
   2. Transient tachypnoea of newborn
   3. Aspiration syndromes (meconium, amniotic fluid, blood, milk)
   4. Pneumonia
   5. Pulmonary hemorrhage
   6. Wilson Mikity syndrome.

b. Cardiovascular causes:
   1. Congestive heart failure
   2. Myocardial dysfunction
   3. Persistent fetal circulation.

c. Central nervous system causes:
   1. Asphyxia
   2. Intracranial bleed.

d. Metabolic causes:
   1. Hypoglycemia
   2. Acidosis.

Surgical causes:

1. Diaphragmatic hernia
2. Choanal atresia
3. Esophageal atresia with tracheoesophageal fistula
4. Pneumothorax, pneumomediastinum
5. Pierre Robin syndrome
6. Lobar emphysema
7. Lung cysts, sequestrated lobe
8. Pulmonary atelectasis.

Anticipation of Respiratory Distress

Anticipation of respiratory distress helps in early referral to a center equipped for proper management. Some clinical features which can help in anticipation are as follows:

Clinical features	*Anticipate*
1. Prematurity, history of maternal diabetes	Hyaline membrane disease
2. Prolonged rupture of membrane, history of maternal infection	Pneumonia
3. Asphyxia, history of meconium stained amniotic fluid	Meconium aspiration syndrome
4. History of hydramnios	Tracheoesophageal fistula
5. History of traumatic delivery	Intracranial hemorrhage

Investigation

Investigation in a neonate with respiratory distress would depend on the cause. However, the most important investigation is an *X-ray of the chest*. The other investigations like a *shake test* using gastric aspirate would be indicated in a preterm baby and *examination for polymorphs in gastric aspirate* may help in diagnosis of pneumonia. A *sepsis screen* should be ordered when infection is suspected.

Shake test: It is a simple bedside test to assess fetal lung maturity. It should be done in preterm babies with respiratory distress.

Procedure: Undiluted amniotic fluid is mixed with normal saline of various dilutions and taken in test tubes. The solution in the test tubes is mixed with an equal volume of 95% ethanol and shaken for 15 seconds and allowed to stand for 15 minutes.

Interpretation: The test is said to be positive when a complete ring of bubbles persist at the fluid meniscus. A positive test in dilutions of 1:2 or greater correlates well with mature L/S ratio and absence of HMD.

Another simple test to assess the maturity of fetus is to determine amniotic fluid optical density at 650 nm. An optical density of 0.15 or greater correlates well with mature L/S ratio. However, it has been shown that estimation of phosphatidyl glycerol in amniotic fluid especially in mothers with diabetes mellitus is the most reliable test to assess fetal lung maturity and its presence would assure that the infant would not develop HMD.

Management

The principles of management include supportive and specific therapy. The supportive therapy is very crucial and whatever may be the cause, the same principles apply. Specific therapy is different for different disease.

Care in the Delivery Room

The care of the baby anticipated to have respiratory distress should begin in the labour room. Prompt and effective resuscitation especially in deliveries with a history of meconium stained liquor, and preterm baby will help prevent and reduce the severity of the subsequent respiratory problems. A baby delivered below 30 weeks of gestation may be electively intubated in the delivery room prior to transfer to the neonatal intensive care unit.

Care in the Neonatal Intensive Care Unit

All babies with respiratory distress at birth or those babies anticipated to have respiratory distress should be transferred to a neonatal intensive care unit for close observation and monitoring to facilitate early intervention.

Monitoring: All cases of respiratory distress needs close monitoring from the time of birth for early detection of onset of respiratory distress. A flow chart at the bed side should record observation of vital signs, FiO_2, blood gas results and ventilator settings. A cumulative record of blood taken from the baby for investigation should be recorded.

Clinical monitoring can be done on the basis of the following scoring system:

Clinical Assessment of Severity of Respiratory Distress (Downe's/RDS Score)

Parameters	*Score*		
	0	*1*	*2*
Respiratory rate	< 60/min	60 – 80/min	> 80/min
Cyanosis	None	None with 40% FiO_2	Needs > 40% FiO_2
Retractions	None	Mild	Severe
Grunting	None	Minimal	Obvious
Air entry	Good	Decreased	Very poor

Interpretations

Score > 4 = Clinical respiratory distress. ABG to be monitored.

Score > 6 = Severe respiratory distress.

Score > 8 = Impending respiratory failure.

Investigations

The following investigations should be advised in all cases with respiratory distress:

a. An anterior posterior supine chest X-ray and an abdominal X-ray (if umbilical arterial catheter inserted) should be done.
b. A blood culture should be sent before starting an antibiotic.
c. Blood sugar should be measured every 4–6 hourly.
d. A complete blood count on day 1. To be repeated every 2–3 days.
e. Urea, electrolytes and creatinine should be measured daily.
f. ABG every 4–6 hours during oxygenation.

Steps of Management

1. Baby admitted and put under the radiant warmer in supine position with slight extension of neck and X-ray AP view chest ordered.
2. An umbilical catheter inserted, an I.V. line started and blood samples send for investigations. A nasogastric tube inserted if a surgical cause is suspected.
3. Oxygen saturation is monitored by a pulsoxymeter. If saturation is < 92%, oxygen inhalation started. The FiO_2 and ABG are monitored. If FiO_2 requirements exceed 0.40, CPAP should be started. Mechanical ventilation is indicated when $PaCO_2$ >60 mm Hg and PaO_2 < 50 mm Hg.
4. Treatment of cause.

HYALINE MEMBRANE DISEASE (HMD)

Hyaline membrane disease is a respiratory problem resulting from absence or deficiency of pulmonary surfactant. It is also called respiratory distress syndrome type I.

Etiology

Hyaline membrane disease (HMD) primarily occurs in preterm infants. The incidence is highest in male preterms. Its incidence is inversely proportional to the gestational age. Only 5% of the cases can occur beyond 37 weeks of gestation and it is rare in term infants. The risk of HMD is increased in infants of diabetic mothers, cesarean section delivery, precipitous delivery, asphyxia, cold stress, multiple pregnancy, and history of previously affected infants. The risk is reduced in pregnancies with primary hypertension or pregnancy induced hypertension, prolonged rupture of membrane, maternal opiate addiction.

Pathophysiology

The major constituents of surfactant include dipalmitoyl phosphatidyl choline (lecithin), phosphatidyl glycerol, apoproteins and cholesterol. With advancement of gestational age, phospholipids are synthesized in increasing amounts and stored in the type II alveolar cells. These surface active agents are released into the alveoli, where they reduce surface tension and help maintain alveolar stability by preventing the collapse of the small air spaces at end-expiration. Mature levels of pulmonary surfactant are usually present after 35 weeks of gestation. Absence or deficiency of pulmonary surfactant results in high surface tension and consequent tendency of the affected lungs to become atelectatic. The alveoli collapse during expiration and are difficult to inflate during inspiration. This affects gas exchange and the baby goes to respiratory failure.

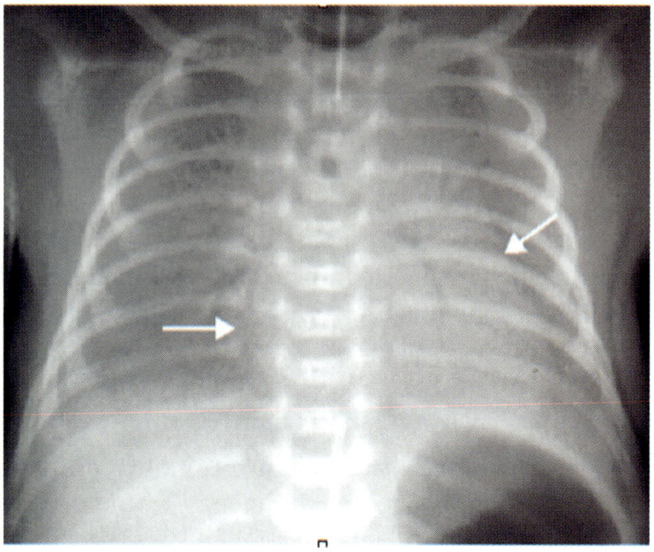

Fig. 7.17: Hyaline membrane disease (reticulogranular pattern with air bronchogram)

Clinical Manifestations

The characteristic clinical features of HMD include tachypnoea, grunting, intercostal and subcostal retraction, nasal flaring and cyanosis. Cyanosis increases and is often relatively unresponsive to oxygen administration. Breath sounds may be normal, diminished or bronchial, with fine rales at the bases on deep inspiration. Onset of symptoms is within 1 hour of birth. The signs may appear within minutes in extremely preterms. An X-ray of the chest has a characteristic but not pathognomonic appearance which includes a reticulogranular pattern in the lung parenchyma with an air bronchogram. The initial X-ray may occasionally appear normal. The typical pattern develops at 6–12 hours.

Prenatal diagnosis can be made by determining the lecithin/sphingomyelin (L/S) ratio in the amniotic fluid. L/S ratio > 2.0 indicates adequate lung maturity. After birth, lung maturity can be tested by *Shake test.*

The natural course of untreated HMD is characterized by progressive worsening of cyanosis and dyspnea. Apnea and irregular respiration are ominous signs. In most cases, the signs and symptoms reach a peak within 3 days, after which improvement starts gradually. Improvement is often heralded by spontaneous diuresis and ability to maintain saturation with low inspired oxygen levels. Death usually occurs between 2 and 7 days. Causes of death include pneumothorax, interstitial emphysema, pulmonary hemorrhage and intracranial hemorrhage.

Differential Diagnosis

The differential diagnosis includes pneumonia, cyanotic heart disease (total anomalous pulmonary venous return), persistent pulmonary hypertension, spontaneous pneumothorax, aspiration syndromes, and diaphragmatic hernia.

All these conditions have typical X-ray features for diagnosis except for pneumonia where X-ray findings may be identical to HMD. Other features of early onset sepsis should be taken into account in such cases.

Investigations

a. An AP supine chest X-ray and an abdominal X-ray (if umbilical arterial catheter inserted) should be arranged.

b. A blood culture should be sent before starting an antibiotic.

c. ABG every 4–6 hours during oxygenation.

Prevention

The measures to prevent hyaline membrane disease include:

1. Prevention of prematurity and preterm delivery.
2. Prophylaxis for lung maturity if preterm delivery is inevitable before 34 weeks of gestation by administration of antenatal steroids. It is the most cost effective perinatal strategies to prevent hyaline membrane disease. It results in 50% reduction of incidence of HMD as well as reduction of incidence of intraventricular hemorrhage and necrotizing enterocolitis. Injection betamethasone/dexamethasone 12 mg I.M./24 hours for 2 doses or 6 mg/I.M. 12 hours for 4 doses, if delivery is planned before 34 weeks of gestation. Optimal effect starts after 24 hours of initiation and therapeutic effect lasts for 7 days.
3. Prophylactic intubation and surfactant therapy is justifiable in very premature infants who have a high incidence of HMD. Early rescue (prior to 2 hours of age) surfactant therapy is preferable to delayed treatment. Early rescue therapy should be administered as soon as diagnosis of HMD is made

and after adequate oxygenation, ventilation, perfusion and monitoring have been established which is usually within 1–2 hours of age. Surfactant therapy should be practised in well equipped centres with skilled staff. Prophylactic or rescue therapy reduces mortality.

Treatment

Supportive Therapy

1. *Maintenance of warmth and prevention of heat loss:* The infant should be nursed in a thermoneutral environment so as to maintain a skin temperature of 36.5°C. The infant should be kept under a radiant warmer or in an incubator.
2. *Minimal handling of the baby:* The baby should be nursed in the prone position. Electronic monitors should be used to record heart rate, respiratory rate, temperature and blood pressure and non-invasive oxygen monitors for PCO_2 or SaO_2. Any disturbance of a sick newborn may precipitate apnea or a fall in blood pressure.
3. *Perfusion and blood pressure:* The peripheral perfusion should be clinically assessed on the basis of skin color, core and peripheral temperature difference and capillary refill time. Hypotension is to be avoided. Blood pressure should be monitored regularly. As a working guide, the mean arterial pressure = gestational age in weeks. If blood pressure is low a plasma expander should be given in the dose of 10–15 ml/kg over 1 hour.
4. *Feeds and fluids:* Oral feeds should be withheld till the baby is stable. A peripheral intravenous infusion should be started according to the fluid requirement and type of fluid recommended for low birth weight babies.
5. *Treatment of acidosis:* Respiratory acidosis may require short-term or prolonged ventilation. Metabolic acidosis can be treated with sodium bicarbonate 1–2 meq/kg diluted with equal volume of distilled water I.V. slowly over 15 to 20 minutes.
6. *Oxygenation:* The aim of giving oxygen is to keep the oxygen saturation (SaO_2) in the range of 85–90% and PaO_2 between 55 and 70 mmHg. Humidified oxygen should be given via a head box and assessment of oxygenation should be done with a pulsoxymeter or a transcutaneous oxygen monitor. During oxygenation, PaO_2, $PaCO_2$, and pH should be measured every 4–6 hours. If the infant needs more than 40% oxygen or respiratory signs persist beyond 4 hours, it is preferable to insert an arterial line into the umbilical artery or a peripheral artery for continuous monitoring of PaO_2. Only measurement of SaO_2 using a pulsoxymeter may lead to unrecognized hyperoxemia or hypoxemia.

   If the PaO_2 cannot be maintained above 50 mmHg at inspired oxygen concentration of 60% or greater it is an indication for application of continuous positive airway pressure (CPAP) at a pressure of 6–10 cm H_2O by nasal prongs. It usually produces a sharp rise of the PaO_2. CPAP prevents collapse of the surfactant deficient alveoli and improves ventilation perfusion matching. Usually, the amount of requirement of CPAP decreases abruptly by 72 hours of age and the infant can be weaned from CPAP.

   If an infant managed by CPAP cannot maintain an arterial oxygen tension above 50 mmHg while breathing 70–100% oxygen, it is an indication for mechanical ventilation.
7. *Surfactant therapy:* Exogenous surfactant is given as rescue therapy as soon as the diagnosis is made and after adequate oxygenation; ventilation and perfusion have been established. Depending on the severity of the disease process, repeat doses may be necessary to be administered. However, there is no clear benefit of giving more than 2 doses of exosurf or 4 doses of survanta. Natural and animal derived surfactants are preferred in view of their higher efficacy.

TRANSIENT TACHYPNEA OF THE NEWBORN

Transient tachypnea of the newborn (TTN) is also called wet lung and occasionally respiratory distress syndrome type II. It is a relatively mild, self limiting disorder, affecting infants born at or near term. It usually follows uneventful vaginally delivery or cesarean section.

The syndrome is believed to be secondary to slow absorption of fetal lung fluid resulting in decreased lung compliance and tidal volume and increased dead space.

The infant with TTN presents with tachypnea (respiratory rate > 80/ minute), sometimes with chest retractions and occasionally cyanosis that is relieved by minimal oxygen (<40%). Auscultation usually reveals good air entry with occasional crackles. An X-ray of the chest shows prominent pulmonary vascular markings, fluid lines in the fissures and hyperaeration with mild to moderate cardiomegaly. The radiographic abnormalities start clearing by 12–18 hours, with complete resolution by 48–72 hours.

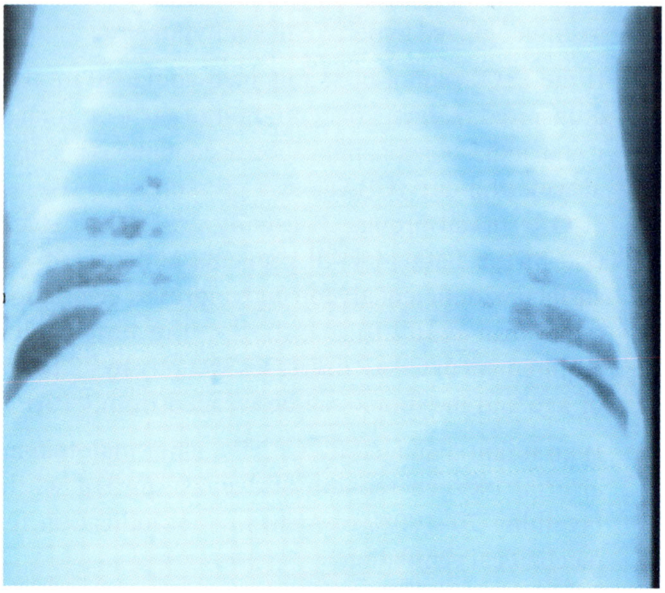

Day 1

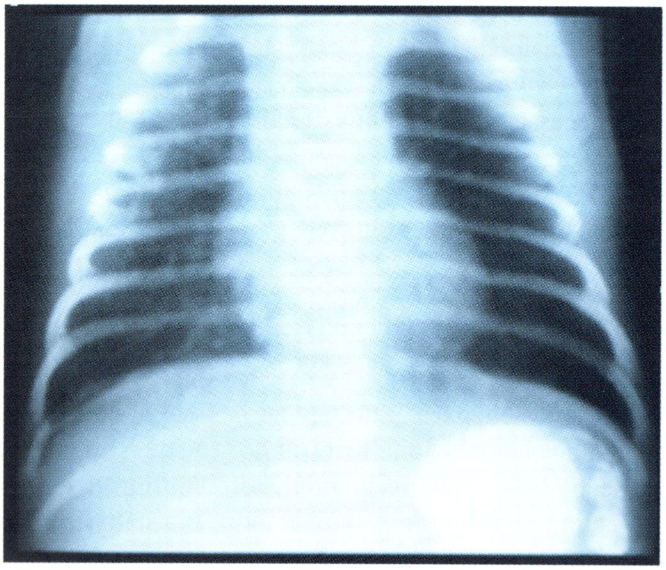

Day 2

Fig. 7.18: Transient tachypnea of newborn. Prominent vascular markings (day 1) followed by complete resolution (day 2)

The symptoms and signs of TTN usually persist for 12–24 hours in mild cases, but can last for upto 3 days. Rarely the course may be protracted.

Treatment is supportive. Supplemental oxygenation should be given to maintain oxygen saturation > 90%. In some infants, CPAP may be required to support lung expansion. In infants with a sustained respiratory rate > 60/minute, oral feeding should be withheld and substituted with nasogastric feeding or intravenous fluid (in case respiratory rate is >80/ min).

The prognosis of TTN is excellent with no residual pulmonary effects.

MECONIUM ASPIRATION SYNDROME

Meconium stained amniotic fluid (MSAF) occurs in 7–15% of live-births. Of such infants, 5% develop meconium aspiration syndrome (MAS). 30% of these require mechanical ventilation and mortality is 5-10%. So, meconium aspiration syndrome is a potentially life-threatening condition.

Definition

The diagnosis of MAS is made on the basis of presence of any two of the following features:

1. Meconium staining of liquor or staining of nails/ umbilical cord/skin.
2. Respiratory distress having onset soon after birth.
3. Radiological evidences of aspiration pneumonia with areas of atelectasis and hyperinflation.

Pathophysiology

Acute or chronic asphyxia can result in the passage of meconium in utero. In such a situation, gasping by the fetus or newly born infant can cause aspiration of amniotic fluid contaminated by meconium. Meconium aspiration leads to 5 major effects:

1. Airway obstruction, 2. Surfactant dysfunction, 3. Chemical pneumonitis, 4. Sepsis, and 5. Persistent pulmonary hypertension.

1. *Airway obstruction:* In infants with significant meconium aspiration, obstruction of large and small airway can occur. Partial obstruction of airway may lead to development of emphysema, pneumothorax, pneumomediastinum or pneumopericardium. Complete obstruction leads to atelectasis and ventilation-perfusion mismatch.
2. *Surfactant dysfunction:* Surfactant dysfunction may occur due to cytotoxic effects of meconium on type II pneumocytes and decreased levels of surfactant. This will result in increased airway resistance and reduced compliance of lungs.

3. *Chemical pneumonitis:* Constituents of meconium (enzymes, bile-salts and fat) also have an irritative and toxic effect on the lining of the airways. There is marked alveolar and parenchymal inflammation and edema with leakage of protein into airways. There is also release of inflammatory mediators like cytokines. All these leads to chemical pneumonitis.
4. *Sepsis:* Meconium adversely affects neutrophil function by inhibiting oxidative burst and phagocytosis with increased risk of infection. Meconium per se is sterile but it can be a good culture medium for microorganisms specially E.coli and Staphylococcus aureus.
5. *Persistent pulmonary hypertension:* Pulmonary vasoconstriction leads to right to left shunt both through foramen ovale and patent ductus arteriosus. This condition is clinically and physiologically similar to fetal circulation and is classified as persistent pulmonary hypertension of newborn (PPHN) secondary to MAS.

Clinical Manifestations

The infant with MAS may be normal term, but are usually post-term or small for date. There may be meconium staining of the umbilical cord, nails and skin. These babies are usually born with severe intra partum or neonatal asphyxia and needs vigorous resuscitation.

After resuscitation, initial apnea is followed by progressive respiratory distress with marked suprasternal, intercostal and subcostal retraction and grunting. Some infants with MAS are well for a few hours after birth before developing progressive respiratory distress. This happens when meconium is aspirated during delivery. The meconium moves progressively downwards with breathing, eventually reaching the periphery of the lung and only then symptoms appear. Tachypnoea reaches 100/min or more and may last from few days to weeks and some time may persist even after complete recovery. On examination of the chest there is a variable percussion note, breath sounds are obscured by coarse bronchial sounds and expiration is prolonged. Frothy yellow green secretions are some time extruded from the mouth.

MAS may exhibit cerebral, cardiac and renal manifestations. Signs of cerebral irritation viz. jitteriness, seizures resulting from cerebral edema, bleeding caused by hypoxia or both may appear soon after birth or later.

Hypotension is found in severely asphyxiated infants. Cardiomegaly, tachypnea, severe cyanosis not responding to adequate ventilation and oxygenation (PPHN) may mimic congenital cyanotic heart disease.

The course of the disease is progressive during the initial 48-72 hours. The condition usually improves within 72 hours. In severe cases, tachypnea may persist for many days or even several weeks. Severe cases requiring assisted ventilation have a high mortality.

Laboratory Investigations

1. *X-ray chest:* An X-ray of chest taken 1-2 hours after birth exhibits mechanical effects of meconium aspiration *i.e.* hyperinflation characterized by a hyper translucent lungs, flat diaphragm (>7 intercostal spaces) horizontal alignment of ribs, and increased cardiothoracic ratio.

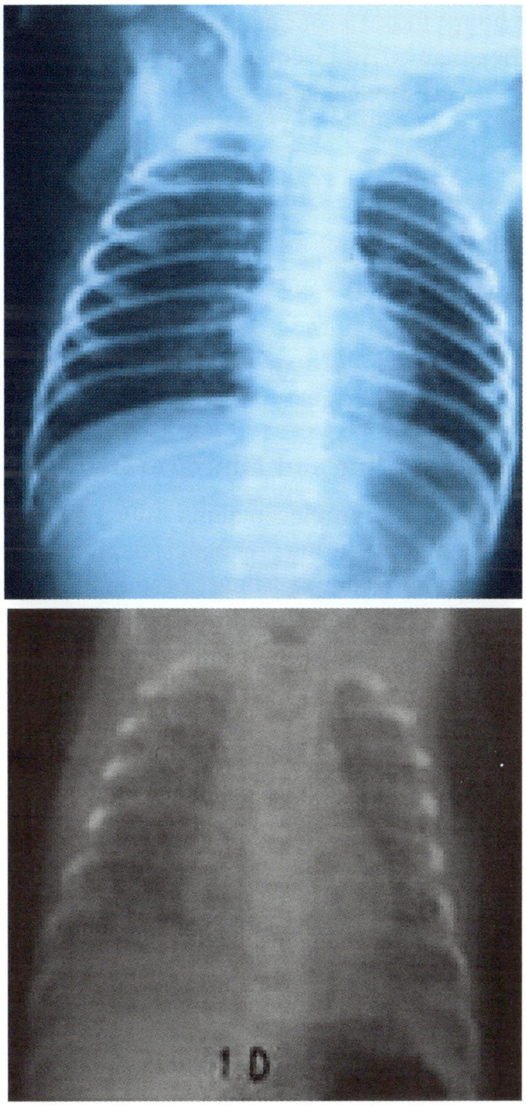

(A)

(B)

Fig. 7.19: Features of MAS at 1–2 hours (A) and after 8–12 hours (B)

An X-ray taken after 8–12 hours age exhibits signs of consolidation and atelectasis characterized by coarse irregular pattern of increased density throughout the lungs, air-leaks, pleural effusion in the transverse fissure.

2. *Sepsis screen:* A sepsis screen should be send to exclude infection.
3. *Arterial blood gases:* Arterial blood gas estimation is necessary for differential diagnosis as well as monitoring. Presence of metabolic acidosis will indicate perinatal stress whereas presence of respiratory acidosis indicates parenchymal disease and PPHN.
4. *Serum electrolytes and hematocrit:* Electrolytes estimation may be required for differential diagnosis. SIADH and acute renal failure with an onset after 24 hours indicate perinatal asphyxia as the cause rather than MAS. Hematocrit must be maintained for O_2 carrying capacity.

Prevention

The risk of meconium aspiration is decreased by:

1. Careful monitoring for fetal distress and timing of delivery.
2. Amino-infusion.
3. Proper care of the baby born through meconium stained amniotic fluid.

Careful Monitoring and Timing of Delivery

Mothers at risk of uteroplacental insufficiency should be carefully monitored during pregnancy and fetal heart rate should be monitored during labour. In addition, fetal scalp blood sampling obtained for pH determination when indicated. In pregnancy continuing beyond 40 weeks, induction as early as 41 weeks may also prevent MAS.

Amnioinfusion

Transcervical amnioinfusion with normal saline may reduce the incidence of meconium aspiration. It is indicated in women whose labour is complicated with meconium stained liquor and repeated fetal heart decelerations.

Proper Care of Infant Born Through Meconium Stained Amniotic Fluid

After complete delivery of the baby if the baby is depressed, the trachea should be intubated under direct laryngoscopy and intratracheal suctioning and toilet should be performed and bag and tube ventilation initiated. If the baby is vigorous, after complete delivery, the baby should be given routine care and kept under observation.

Treatment

Infants who are depressed at birth and have had meconium sucked from the trachea are at risk of meconium aspiration syndrome. These neonates:

1. Should be admitted in NICU and observed for respiratory distress.
2. A chest X-ray taken at this stage may help to determine which infants are more likely to have respiratory distress.
3. A sepsis screen should be ordered to exclude infection.
4. Monitoring of O_2 saturation during this period aids assessment of the severity of infant's condition and allows prevention of hypoxemia.

The treatment plan depends on the severity of MAS.

1. **Mild MAS/Sub-clinical MAS:** Majority of infants suffer from mild MAS. The infant requires less than 40% oxygen for less than 48 hours. These infants improve within 24-48 hours.
2. **Moderate MAS** is a disease requiring more than 40% oxygen for more than 48 hours without air leak. Clinical improvement takes place within 48-72 hours.
3. **Severe MAS** is a disease which requires assisted ventilation for more than 48 hours, often associated with persistent pulmonary hypertension (PPHN).

Supportive Care

1. Maintain an optimal thermal environment and minimal handling of these babies.
2. Prevention and treatment of hypoglycemia and significant metabolic acidosis.
3. Fluid and electrolyte balance to be monitored and corrected.
4. Monitoring of renal function.
5. Management of hypoxemia:
   - Increasing inspired oxygen by monitoring blood gases.
   - CPAP if FiO_2 requirements exceed 0.40.
   - Mechanical ventilation is indicated when $PaCO_2$ >60 mm Hg and PaO_2 < 50 mm Hg.

6. Newer modalities of treatment:
   - High frequency oscillatory or jet ventilation.
   - Exogenous surfactant therapy.
   - Inhaled nitric oxide.
   - Extracorporeal membrane oxygenation.

None of these modalities have been shown to be superior to conventional ventilation in the treatment of MAS. They may be tried in cases refractory to conventional treatment.

Prognosis

Mortality is high. Residual lung problem are rare but include symptomatic cough, wheezing and persistent hyperinflation for 5-10 years. Ultimate prognosis depends on the extent of central nervous system injury from asphyxia, presence of associated problems with persistent fetal circulation.

Neonatal Hypoglycemia

Definition

The normal range of blood glucose is different for each newborn and depends upon a number of factors including birth weight, gestational age, body stores, feeding status as well as presence or absence of disease.

There is no agreed definition of hypoglycemia in the newborn. A recent consensus has been to evolve an 'operational threshold' which defines neonatal hypoglycemia as that concentration of plasma or whole blood glucose at which clinicians should consider intervention. This threshold is currently believed to be a blood glucose value of less than 40 mg/dl (plasma glucose level less that 45 mg/dl) irrespective of the gestational age and age after birth.

Incidence of hypoglycemia is reported to occur in 8.1% of full term large for gestation (LGA) infants, 14.4% of term small for gestation (SGA) infants, 47% of infants of diabetic mothers, 67% and 38% of preterm SGA and preterm LGA infants respectively.

Classification and Causes

It is useful to classify neonatal hypoglycemia as transient and persistent.

Causes of Transient Neonatal Hypoglycemia

1. Small for gestation age (SGA) infants.
2. Prematurity.
3. Birth asphyxia.
4. Hypothermia.
5. Septicemia.
6. Congenital heart disease.
7. Polycythemia.

Hyperinsulinism e.g. Infants of diabetic mothers, erythroblastosis fetalis, maternal drugs, maternal glucose infusion, Beckwith Widemann syndrome.

Causes of Persistent Neonatal Hypoglycemia

1. *Hyperinsulinism:* Insulinoma, nesidioblastosis.
2. *Inborn errors of metabolism:* Glycogen storage disease (type I, III, IV), Galactosemia, maple syrup urine disease, methyl malonic aciduria, hepatic gluconeogenetic deficiencies (fructose 1, 6 diphosphatase, pyruvate carboxylase), mitochondrial fatty acid oxidation defects.
3. *Hormonal deficiencies:* Congenital hypopituitarism, cortisol deficiency states, congenital adrenal hyperplasia, glucagon deficiency.

Screening for Hypoglycemia

Blood glucose should be routinely estimated in the following at risk situations:

1. Very low birth weight babies (< 1500 gms).
2. Small for gestational age (SGA) babies (weight <10th percentile for gestation).
3. Large for gestational age infants (weight > 90th percentile for gestation).
4. Preterm infants (gestation < 35 weeks).
5. Infant of diabetic mother (insulin dependent and gestational diabetes).
6. Rh-hemolytic disease of newborn.
7. History of maternal therapy with terbutaline, propranolol, oral hypoglycemic agents.
8. Neonatal conditions: Perinatal asphyxia, polycythemia, sepsis, shock, hypothermia.

Time Schedule for Screening

Hypoglycemia after the first 2–3 hours is a biochemical symptom and usually means that the baby has failed to make adequate perinatal metabolic adaptation. Hence babies at risk of such metabolic maladaptation should be identified early and managed prospectively. Blood glucose monitoring should be done as follows:

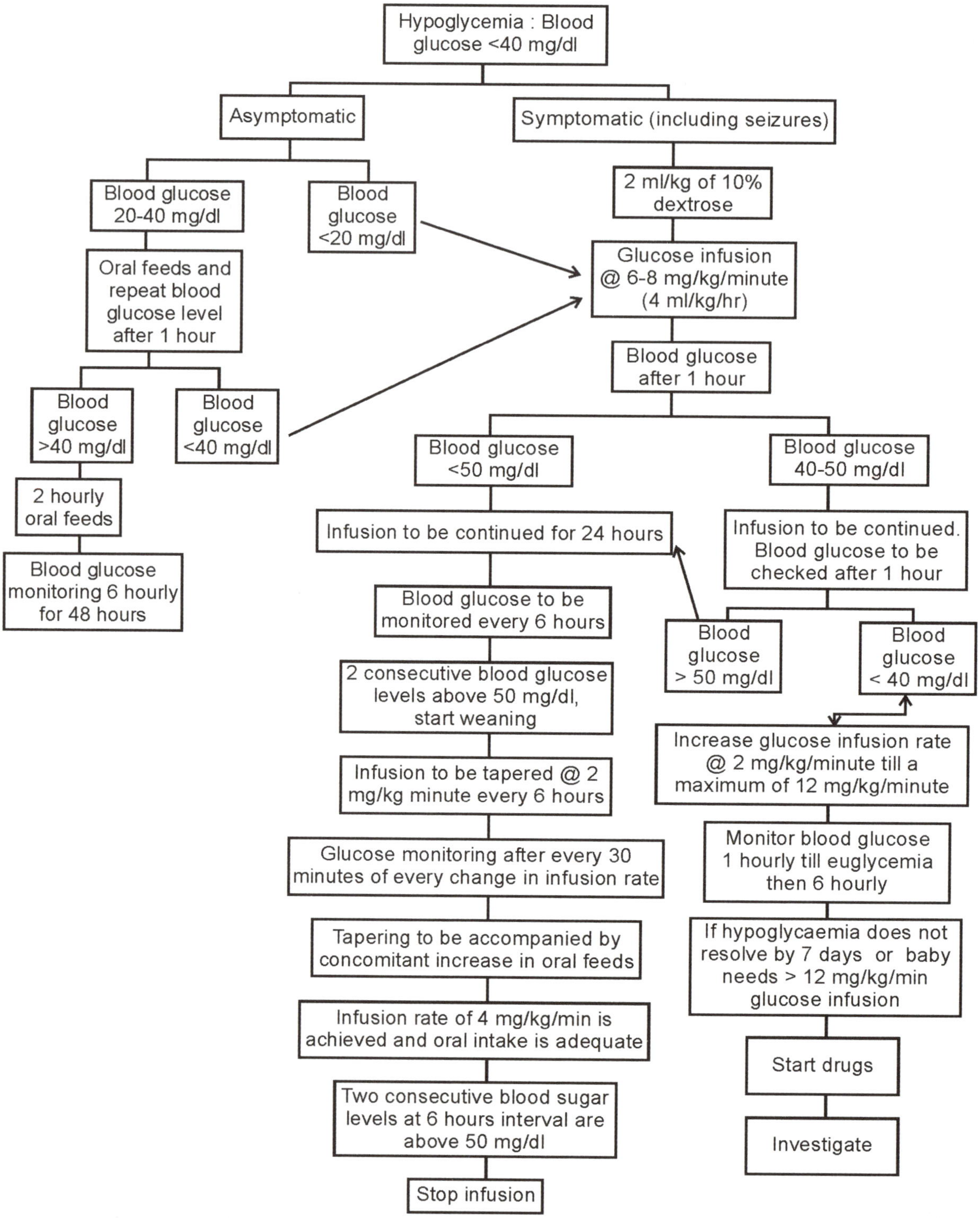

Flowchart for management of hypoglycemia

1. For neonates apparently well but belonging to at risk group at 3, 6, 12, 24, 72 hours.
2. For infants of diabetic mothers and gestational diabetes at 1, 2, 3, 6, 12, 24, 36, 48, 72 hours.
3. After exchange transfusion with CPD blood at 2 hours following exchange.

Point to be Noted

All the readings of blood sugar should be taken prior to feeding as far as practicable.

Screening Should be Stopped When?

1. At the end of 72 hours, an at risk infant has not developed hypoglycemia.
2. An infant on total oral feeds having 2 (two) consecutive blood glucose values >50 mg/dl.

Methods of Glucose Estimation

1. *Reagent strips (Glucose oxidase):* Though popular and widely used, estimation of blood glucose by reagent strips is not accurate especially at blood glucose levels less than 40 mg/dl. Low values should be always confirmed by laboratory estimation before diagnosis of hypoglycemia is made.
2. *Laboratory estimation:* This is the most accurate method. Blood samples should be quickly estimated to avoid erroneously low levels because the glucose level in a blood sample can fall @ 18 mg/dl/hour in a sample that waits analysis.

Diagnosis

Asymptomatic Hypoglycemia

This diagnosis is made when the blood glucose level is below the operational threshold (to be confirmed by laboratory estimation) in the absence of clinical signs.

Symptomatic Hypoglycemia

A diagnosis of symptomatic hypoglycemia is made on the basis of the Whipple's triad viz.

1. Presence of signs attributable to hypoglycemia
   - Lethargy, limpness, stupor, coma.
   - Apnea, cyanosis.
   - Weak or high pitch cry.
   - Poor feeding, vomiting.
   - Seizure, tremor, jitteriness, irritability.
2. Low blood glucose documented by accurate, sensitive and precise method.
3. Resolution of clinical signs within minutes to hours once the blood glucose level is normalized. If the clinical signs are not alleviated by I.V. glucose, then other diagnostic possibilities should be considered.

It is worth mentioning that cerebral fuel deficiency in term babies may be manifested as a reduction in the level of consciousness and/or seizures. Jitteriness is not a useful discriminating symptom in such babies. As the level of consciousness drops, the cry changes, movements decrease, feeding becomes poor, and there are long respiratory pauses or apnea. Infants of diabetic mothers (IDM), are usually quiet and lethargic rather than jittery. Further, the hypoglycemia of most IDM's usually responds to treatment and resolve by 24 hours.

Management

Asymptomatic Hypoglycemia

If blood sugar level < 20 mg/dl, glucose infusion should be started @ 6–8 mg/kg/minute.

If blood glucose level is between 20–40 mg/dl.

Oral feeds have to be started and blood glucose level repeated after 1 hour.

If repeat blood glucose is < 40 mg/dl: Glucose infusion should be started @ 6–8 mg/kg/hour.

If repeat blood glucose > 40 mg/dl, 2 hourly oral feeds should be continued. Blood glucose has to be monitored 6 hourly for 48 hours.

No I.V. glucose bolus is required in asymptomatic infants.

What Oral Feed to be Given?

Breast milk is the best, either direct or expressed (if baby is unable to suck). If breast milk is not available formula feeds in term and SFD babies and IV infusion with 10% dextrose in preterms as per daily fluid requirement can be given.

Symptomatic Hypoglycemia

Treatment consists of a bolus dose followed by continuous infusion.

Bolus Dose

- *For hypoglycemic convulsion:* 5ml/kg of 10% dextrose.

- *For otherwise symptomatic infants:* 2 ml/kg 10% dextrose.

N.B.: Boluses of 25% or 50% glucose should not be used as they are unnecessary and can be dangerous.

Continuous Infusion

- Immediately after the bolus dose, a glucose infusion at an initial rate of 6–8 mg/kg/minute (4 ml/kg/hr) should be started.
- Blood glucose should be checked after 1 hour:
  1. If blood glucose is > 50 mg/dl infusion should be continued for 24 hours. Blood glucose to be monitored every 6 hours. If two consecutive blood glucose levels are above 50 mg/dl, start weaning.
  2. If blood glucose level is between 40 and 50 mg/dl infusion is to be continued. Blood glucose to be checked after 1 hour.

     After 1 hour: If blood glucose is > 50 mg/dl, proceed as (1) If blood glucose is < 40 mg/dl, increase glucose infusion rate @ 2 mg/kg/minute till a maximum of 12 mg/kg/minute.

     Monitor blood glucose 1 hourly till euglycemia then 6 hourly.

When to Start Weaning?

If two consecutive blood glucose values are > 50 mg/kg/minute in or after 24 hours of infusion, the infusion can be tapered @ 2 mg/kg/minute every 6 hours with glucose monitoring after every 30 minutes of every change in infusion rate. Tapering has to be accompanied by concomitant increase in oral feeds.

When to Stop Infusion?

i. When an infusion rate of 4 mg/kg/min is achieved.

ii. Oral intake is adequate.

iii. Two consecutive blood sugar levels at 6 hours interval are above 50 mg/dl.

Recurrent/Resistant Hypoglycemia

This condition has to be considered when there is a failure to maintain a normal blood glucose level despite a glucose infusion rate of 12 mg/kg/minute or when stabilization of blood glucose level is not achieved by 5–7 days of life. In this situation, besides increasing the rate of infusion, investigations have to be considered on the basis of clinical suspicion and drugs may have to be tried in the treatment. One should avoid using dextrose infusion of > 12.5% through a peripheral vein due to the risk of thrombophlebitis.

Investigations

Initial minimum investigations to be ordered:

1. Serum insulin level and serum cortisol level.
2. Urine ketones and reducing substances, ketone bodies in blood.
3. USG upper abdomen, CT scan abdomen (to exclude insulinoma of pancreas).

Other investigations to be done as and when necessary include:

1. Growth hormone level.
2. Blood ammonia.
3. Blood lactate level.
4. Urine and serum amino-acidogram.

Most neonatal hypoglycemia usually resolves in 2–3 days. A requirement of more than 8 mg of glucose/kg/minute suggests increase utilization due to hyperinsulinism. This is usually transient as in infants of diabetic mothers.

If it lasts for more than 7 days, endocrine evaluation may be necessary to rule out excess insulin secretion. Blood samples for insulin estimation should be drawn in presence of hypoglycemia. If the insulin level is high in presence of low blood glucose it will indicate inappropriate secretion of insulin. If the insulin level is normal for the blood glucose level, other causes of persistent hypoglycemia viz. a metabolic disorder (carbohydrate and protein metabolism) and endocrine causes should be considered.

Treatment

Treatment of recurrent or resistant hypoglycemia includes use of drugs and surgery. The drugs include hydrocortisone, diazoxide and glucagon. Rarely epinephrine and growth hormone may be required.

Mother's milk or formula can be started and advanced unless there is suspicion of a metabolic disorder like galactosemia. As the feedings are increased the intravenous infusion is tapered with monitoring of blood glucose levels.

Drugs

1. *Hydrocortisone:* Dose is 10 mg/kg/day in two divided doses IV. Hydrocortisone reduces peripheral glucose utilization, increases neoglucogenesis and increases the effects of glucagons. Before administration of

hydrocortisone, blood samples for estimation of glucose, insulin and cortisol levels should be obtained. Hydrocortisone can be rapidly tapered in a few days after a stable and adequate blood glucose level is achieved. Administration of hydrocortisone usually results in stable and adequate blood level of glucose in the majority of cases.

2. *Diazoxide*: 2–5 mg/kg/dose 8 hourly is given per oral. It inhibits insulin release by acting as a specific adenosine triphosphate (ATP) sensitive potassium channel agonist in normal pancreatic beta cells and decrease insulin release. It may be given in infants who have persistent hyperinsulinemia. A positive response is usually seen in 48–72 hours.
3. *Inj Glucagon:* Dose is 0.025–0.3 mg/kg (max 1.0 mg) I.M. For infants of diabetic mothers, the dose is 0.3 mg/kg (max 1.0 mg). Glucagon is given as an emergency measure until an intravenous access is obtained for glucose administration. It acts by mobilizing glucose and hence should be used in hypoglycemic infants with good glycogen storage. The effect is temporary and glucose level falls by 2–3 hours as the effect of glucagon wanes off.
4. *Epinephrine and growth hormone* are rarely used.

Surgery

A subtotal pancreatectomy may be necessary for insulin secreting tumors.

Prevention of Neonatal Hypoglycemia

1. Antenatal care of diabetic mother:
   a. All pregnant women with a family history of diabetes should have a glucose tolerance test done routinely during pregnancy.
   b. No oral antidiabetic agents should be used to control diabetes during pregnancy or gestational diabetes.
   c. All diabetic pregnant women should maintain a fasting glucose level of less than 105 mg/dl and post prandial level of 120 mg/dl (especially during the 3rd trimester).
   d. Large doses of glucose infusion should not be given to mothers before or at delivery.
2. Drugs such as salbutamol, terbutaline, isoxpurine, and chlorothiazide should be avoided.
3. All small for date babies are particularly at high risk of hypoglycemia and should be carefully monitored.
4. Feeding started early and given frequently (atleast 8 feeds/day). The aim should be for a total of 90 ml/kg/day on day 1. Continuous nasogastric feeds may be considered if the baby is intolerant of volume.
5. During intensive care, clinical detection of hypoglycemia is not possible in sick or preterm babies or babies prone to seizure for some reason other than hypoglycemia. In these conditions routine measurement of blood glucose is the only option. When clinically stable, glucose should be measured once daily but more frequently in the sick or unstable child.

Preparation of Fluid with Required Glucose Concentration

Glucose conc.	*10% dextrose*	*25% dextrose*	*Resultant solution 5% dextrose*
7.5%	435 ml	65 ml	500 ml
9.0%	400 ml	100 ml	500 ml
10%	375 ml	125 ml	500 ml
12.5%	310 ml	190 ml	500 ml
15%	250 ml	250 ml	500 ml
17%	200 ml	300 ml	500 ml
20%	125 ml	375 ml	500 ml

Conversion Table

Glucose (mg/kg/min)	*Fluid ml/kg/min/day*					
	5%	*7.5%*	*10%*	*12.5%*	*15%*	*20%*
4	115	77	58	46	38	29
6	172	115	86	69	58	43
8	230	154	115	92	77	58
10	288	192	124	115	96	72
12	345	230	173	138	115	86

Glucose Rate Calculator

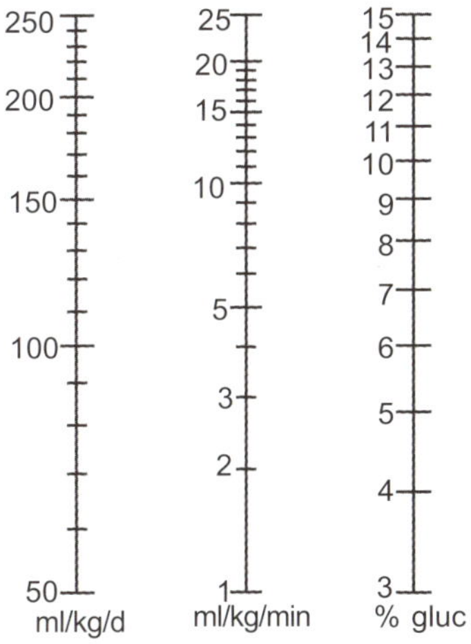

GLUCOSE RATE CALCULATOR

(Use a straight edge to determine the volume required per 24 hours)

Source: Klaus MH, Faranoff AA in care of the high risk neonate, 2nd edition. Philadelphia: Saunders, 1979.

Approach to Anemia in Newborn

Definition

Anemia in newborn is defined as a hemoglobin level less than 12 gm/dl in the first week, or less than 10 gm/dl after the first week.

Embryonic Hematopoesis

Embryonic hematopoesis begins by the 20th day of gestation and is evidenced as blood islands in the yolk sac. In mid gestation, erythropoesis occurs in the liver and spleen. The bone marrow becomes the predominant site in the last trimester. Fetal hemoglobin increases with advancing gestational age. Hemoglobin concentration increases from 8–10 grams/dl at 12 weeks to 16.5 to 18.0 grams/dl at 40 weeks. At term the cord blood hemoglobin is 16.8 gm/dl (14–20 gm/dl). The hemoglobin levels in VLBW infants are 1–2 gms/dl below those at term.

The Normal Hemoglobin Curve

After birth, hemoglobin levels increase transiently at 6–12 hours. Thereafter, in the term infants, there is a decline of the hemoglobin level to 11 gm/dl at 3–6 months. In the preterm babies, those born before 32 weeks, the hemoglobin levels at birth is 1–2 gms/dl lower than in term and the post natal decline of hemoglobin level is more rapid. At 8–12 weeks, the hemoglobin levels reach their nadir. In infants who receive blood transfusion in the neonatal period have lower nadirs than normal because of their higher percentage of adult hemoglobin. The hemoglobin levels in the newborn period differ on the basis of gestation, birth weight and day of life as follows:

Week	*Hemoglobin level (gm/dl)*		
	Term infants	*Preterm infants (1.2–2.5 kg)*	*Preterm (< 1.2 kg)*
0	17.0	16.4	16.0
1	18.8	16.0	14.8
3	15.9	13.5	13.4
6	12.7	10.7	9.7

Source: Avery's diseases of the newborn, 1991, Philadelphia, Saunders.

Hemoglobin Nadir in Infants

The hemoglobin nadir differs according to the gestation and birth weight of the neonate as follows:

Gestation / birth weight	*Hemoglobin level at nadir*	*Time of nadir*
Term	9.5 – 11.0 gm/dl	6 – 12 weeks
Preterm (1.2 – 2.5 kg)	8.0 – 10.0 gm/dl	5 – 10 weeks
Preterm (< 1.2 kg)	6.5 – 9.0 gm/dl	4 – 8 weeks

Source: Avery's diseases of newborn, 1991, Philadelphia, Saunders.

The Type of Hemoglobin

In the fetus, hemoglobin synthesis in the last two trimesters of pregnancy produces fetal hemoglobin (Hemoglobin F). Synthesis of adult hemoglobin (Hemoglobin A) starts immediately prior to term. Hence, the term infant should have some adult hemoglobin. At birth, fetal hemoglobin represents 60–90% of total hemoglobin. The levels of fetal hemoglobin decline to adult levels of less than 5 grams/dl by 3–4 months of age.

Other Hematological Parameters

The blood volume of the term infant is approximately 85 ml/kg. The placenta and umbilical vessels contain approximately 20–30 ml/kg of additional blood. Hence, delayed clamping of the umbilical cord at birth can transiently increase the blood volume and hemoglobin levels for the first three days of life. Delayed clamping increases the risk of polycythemia, increased pulmonary vascular resistence, hypoxia and hyperbilirubinemia but improves glomerular filtration. Early clamping, on the other hand, may result in anemia, poor peripheral perfusion, but lower pulmonary vascular pressures. To avoid both situations, the cord clamping should be done approximately 30 seconds after birth. Immediately after delivery the infant should be placed below the level of the placenta to avoid feto-placental transfusion. If the infant is kept above the level of the placenta, hydrostatic pressure affects blood transfer between the placenta and the infant at birth resulting in an undesired feto maternal transfusion.

Table 7.11 : Other RBC values in term and preterm infants

	Hematocrit (%)	*Reticylocytes (%)*
Term		
Cord blood	45 – 61	< 7
Day 1	58	< 7
Day 3	55	< 3
Day 7	54	<1
Preterm (birth weight < 1500 grams)		
Cord blood	49	< 10
Day 7	45	< 3

Source: Avery's Diseases of Newborn, 2005, Philadelphia, Saunders.

Etiology

Symptomatic anemia in newborn may be a result of:

1. Blood loss.
2. Decreased red cell production.
3. Hemolysis.

Blood loss may be acute following fetomaternal hemorrhage, rupture of umbilical cord, placenta previa and internal hemorrhage. Chronic blood loss may be due to chronic feto maternal hemorrhage, twin to twin transfusion.

Decreased red cell production due to causes like perinatal congenital infections, Diamond Blackfan syndrome, osteopetrosis presents with resistant anemia.

Hemolysis due to causes like ABO and Rh hemolytic disease of newborn, red cell enzyme deficiency e.g. G6PD deficiency, RBC membrane defects e.g. Hereditary spherocytosis etc presents with anemia with associated features.

Table 7.12 : Causes of anemia in newborn

	Blood loss	*Decreased production*	*Hemolysis*
Common	Fetal-maternal bleed	Perinatal congenital infections	Rh HDN
	Placenta previa abruptio placentae Twin to twin transfusion	Anemia of prematurity	ABO HDN Minor gr. HDN
Rare	Vasa previa	Parvo virus infection	RBC enzyme deficiency
	Rupture of cord	Diamond Blackfan syndrome	Hemoglobino-pathy
	Hepatic hematoma	Osteopetrosis	RBC membrane defect
	Splenic hematoma	Congenital leukemia	DIC
	Retro peritoneal hemorrhage	Congenital neuro-blastoma Sideroblastic anemia	SLE in mother

Table 7.13 : Causes according to onset of anemia

Early anemia (within 7 days)

1. Fetomaternal hemorrhage
2. Twin to twin transfusion
3. Placental causes:
   - Placenta praevia
   - Vasa praevia
   - Abruptio placentae
   - Incision of placenta at cesarean section

Contd.

Contd.

4. Fetoplacental transfusion after delivery
5. Hemolysis:
   - Rh and ABO isoimmunistion
   - Alpha thalassemia
   - Intrauterine infection specially rubella, parvo virus
   - Bacterial infection

Late anemia (after 7 days)

1. Hemorrhage:
   - Small perinatal bleeding
   - Excessive blood sampling
   - Hemorrhagic disease of newborn
   - Intraventricular hemorrhage
   - Chronic G.I. bleed
2. Hemolysis:
   - Rh and ABO isoimmunisation
   - Sepsis and DIC
   - Hemoglobinopathies
   - Congenital spherocytosis
   - Vitamin E deficiency
3. Decreased red cell production:
   - Anemia of prematurity
   - Infection (bacterial /viral)
   - Folic acid deficiency
   - Drugs
   - Diamond Blackfan syndrome
   - Congenital leukemia
   - Osteopetrosis

Clinical Manifestation

Anemia at birth can manifest as pallor, congestive cardiac failure or shock depending on the cause and rapidity of blood loss.

Acute blood loss is characterized by pallor, peripheral circulatory collapse and shock. Chronic blood loss presents with marked pallor, heart failure, hepato-splenomegaly with or without hydrops.

Anemia due to decreased red cell production presents at birth with pallor and associated physical signs of the parent disease.

Hemolysis in utero may result in erythroblastosis fetalis or the fetus may be spared and hemolytic disease may appear in the newborn infant. Erythroblastosis fetalis is classically due to Rh blood group incompatibility. ABO blood group incompatibility with sensitization usually does not cause fetal disease except for mild anemia. However, it may produce hemolytic disease of newborn characterized by significant anemia and hyperbilirubinemia. In fact ABO incompatibility is the most common cause of isoimmune hemolysis of the newborn infant.

Table 7.14 : Clinical presentations

1. *Acute blood loss:*
   - Shock
   - No signs of extramedullary hematopoesis, no hepatosplenomegaly
2. *Chronic blood loss:*
   - Marked pallor
   - Signs of heart failure
   - Hepatosplenomegaly
   - Features of hydrops
3. *Decreased red blood cell production:*
   - Pallor at birth
   - Associated physical features of the parent disease
4. *Hemolysis:*
   - Only pallor
   - Pallor with jaundice
   - Pallor with jaundice and hepatosplenomegaly

Severe Anemia with Shock and Severe Asphyxia

Infants born with acute blood loss during or before delivery are often limp, pale, with shock at birth. They need to be differentiated from severely asphyxiated newborns with peripheral circulatory failure.

Table 7.15 : Salient differences between severe asphyxia and anemia with shock

Criteria	*Severe asphyxia*	*Anemia with shock*
Antenatal history	H/o fetal distress	H/o blood loss
Vitals		
• Respiration	Absent or gasping	Tachypnea, gasping/ irregular
• Heart rate	Bradycardia	Tachycardia
• Color	May be blue	Pale
• CVP	Normal	Low/high with CCF
Response to therapy		
• Intubation and O_2	Dramatic response	No response
• PCV/ crystalloids transfusion	No response	Good response

Laboratory Investigations

Screening Tests to be Ordered in Every Case of Anemia

The following tests are to be ordered in every case of neonatal anemia which should be followed by specific tests for individual conditions:

1. Hemoglobin, hematocrit at birth and after 4 hours.
2. Reticulocyte count, MCV, peripheral blood smear.
3. Blood group and Coombs' test.

If blood loss is recent (e.g. at delivery), the hematocrit and reticulocyte count may be normal and the infant may be in shock. The hematocrit will fall later as a result of hemodilution. If the bleeding is chronic, the hematocrit will be low, the reticulocyte increased and the baby is normovolemic.

Other tests: To be picked up as necessary.

1. Apt's test to distinguish between fetal and maternal blood.
2. Kleihauer-Betke test of mother's blood to exclude feto-maternal bleed.
3. Serum bilirubin and fractions.
4. Congenital infection screen.
5. Metabolic disease screen.
6. X-ray long bones to exclude osteopetrosis.
7. Sepsis screen and blood culture.
8. Platelet count and coagulation profile.
9. Stool for occult blood.
10. Urine for microscopic examination.
11. Bone marrow.

Tests for Parents

Complete blood count, peripheral smear, RBC indices, RBC enzymes viz. G6PD, pyruvate kinase.

Table 7.16 : Laboratory findings and diagnosis

Laboratory findings	*Diagnosis*
1. Presence of fetal hemoglobin in vaginal blood	Fetal hemorrhage
2. Positive Kleihauer-Betke test	Feto-maternal hemorrhage
3. Hematological evidences of iron deficiency anemia	Chronic fetal or feto-maternal hemorrhage
4. Hyperbilirubinemia	Hemolytic anemia Perinatal infection
5. Reticulocytosis	Hemolytic anemia Prematurity Small for date Perinatal asphyxia Chronic feto-maternal hemorrhage

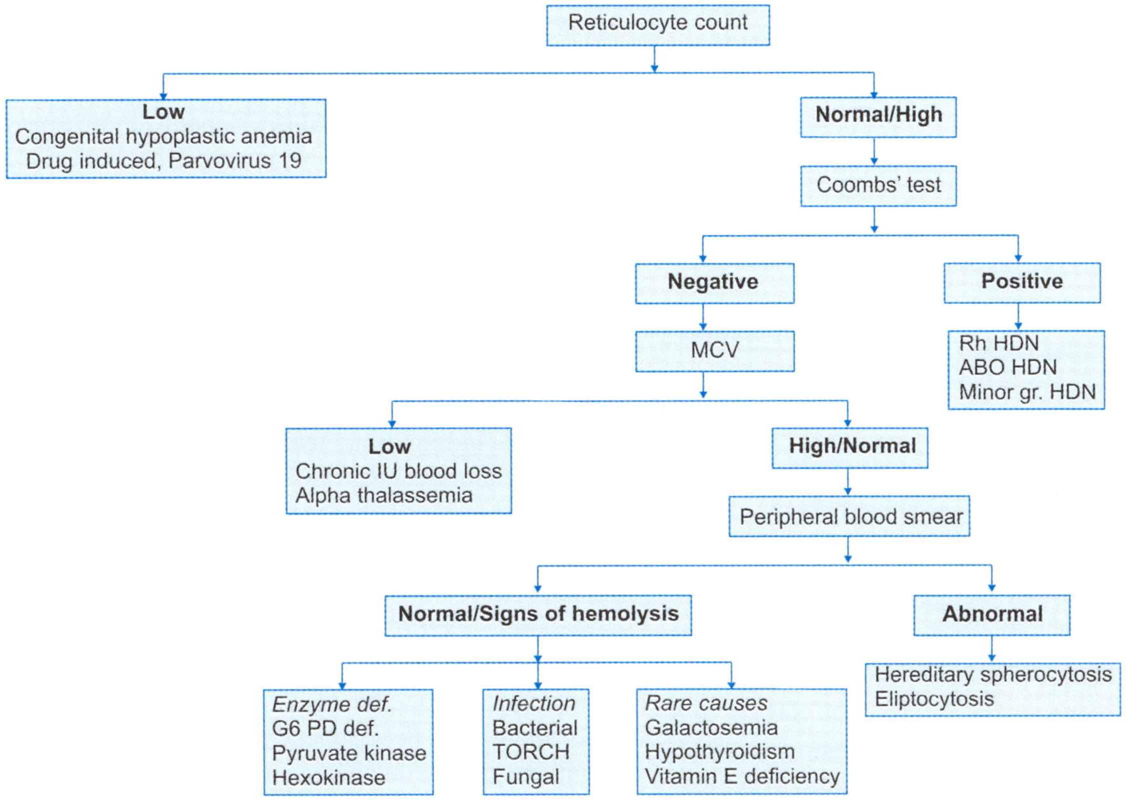

Fig. 7.20: Approach to anemia in newborn

Management

The treatment modality will be different depending on the clinical condition of the child and the cause of anemia. However, a fall of hemoglobin to less than 8 gms/dl (hematocrit < 25%) due to any cause or presence of symptoms viz. poor weight gain, tachypnea, tachycardia, apnea and poor feeding should be treated with transfusion to raise the hemoglobin to 12 gm%. Packed RBCs are usually transfused in the amount 15–20 ml/kg.

Indications of Transfusion

1. *Acute blood loss with signs of peripheral circulatory collapse:* Irrespective of the hemoglobin and hematocrit status these babies will need whole blood transfusion because anemia due to acute blood loss will manifest only after 4–8 hours.

   Type of blood: O Rh negative blood without cross matching.

   Amount: 20–30 ml/kg initially to combat shock.

2. *Infants with severe erythroblastosis:* If the hematocrit is below 30%, a partial exchange transfusion with 50–80 ml/kg packed red cells (hematocrit 70%) should be performed to raise the hematocrit and increase the oxygen carrying capacity before going for the specific treatment e.g. exchange transfusion in Rh incompatibility.

3. *Transfusion in sick babies:* Infants with significant respiratory disease or congenital heart disease (e.g. large left to right shunt) may need their hematocrit maintained above 40%. Transfusion of adult RBCs provides the added benefit of lowered oxygen affinity, which augments oxygen delivery to tissues.

4. *Infants with ABO incompatibility with protracted hemolysis:* These babies may not require exchange transfusion, but may require a transfusion to correct anemia several weeks after birth.

5. *Preterm babies:* Preterm babies may be comfortable with a hemoglobin level of 6.5 to 7 gm/dl. Sick preterms may need transfusion to increase oxygen carrying capacities. In growing preterms, poor weight gain, apnea, tachypnea, poor feeding indicate need for blood transfusion.

6. *A healthy, asymptomatic newborn* will correct mild anemia on its own if iron intake is adequate.

Blood Component Therapy

Transfusion of other blood components should be advised according to need viz.

- Packed RBC 15–20 ml/kg. Larger volumes need to be given in divided doses.
- Platelet transfusion 1 unit every 12 to 24 hours, for thrombocytopenia.
- FFP, 10–15 ml/kg every 12 to 24 hours in suspected coagulation disorder.
- Both FFP and platelet concentrate every 12 to 24 hours in case of DIC.
- Fresh blood in small aliquots (10 ml/kg every 12–24 hours) from a walking donor can be life saving when FFP or platelet concentrate is not available.
- Transfusion of washed platelet packs from mother is the appropriate therapy for replacement of platelet in platelet isoimmunisation.
- Irradiated (5000 rads) or frozen RBCs are recommended in preterm infants weighing less than 1200 grams. Third generation filters helps to deplete leucocyte. Their use reduces the risk of exposure to lymphocytes and cytomegalovirus. For prevention of CMV infection, CMV negative donor blood or blood treated by prestorage leucodestruction can be used.

Drugs

- Vitamin K: Vitamin K_1 and K_2 are preferable because synthetic Vitamin K increases the risk of hyperbilrubinemia. A dose 2 mg daily IM should be given in case of hemorrhagic disease of newborn.
- Diuretics (viz. frusemide) for congestive cardiac failure, cardiotonics (viz. dopamine, dobutamine) in case of shock may be used as and when necessary.

Approach to Cyanosis in Newborn

Cyanosis is a bluish discoloration of the skin and mucous membrane resulting from an increased concentration of reduced hemoglobin. The level of hemoglobin greatly influences the occurrence of cyanosis. Normally, about 2 gms/dl of reduced hemoglobin is present in the venules. Clinical cyanosis is evident when the amount of reduced hemoglobin in the cutaneous veins reaches about 5 grams/dl. Cyanosis usually is recognized when arterial oxygen saturation is 85% or lower. Cyanosis is recognized at a higher level of oxygen saturation in patients with polycythemia and at a lower level of oxygen saturation in patients with anemia. Because the hemoglobin level is often high in newborn and the peripheral circulation often sluggish, cyanosis may occur at oxygen saturation as high as 90% in this age group.

Detection of Cyanosis

Early detection of cyanosis in the newborn is crucial. Mild cyanosis may be too subtle for early detection because of polycythemia and excess of fetal hemoglobin in the early neonatal life. Clubbing of fingers and toes, an associated finding, is not usually manifested until late in the first year of life, even in the presence of severe arterial oxygen desaturation.

Clinically, one can look for cyanosis in the lips, finger and toe nails, oral mucous membrane, and tip of the tongue, conjunctiva and tip of the nose. The tip of the tongue is a good place to look for cyanosis as its colour is not affected by race or ethnic background and the circulation is not sluggish as in peripheral parts of the body. When in doubt, one should obtain the arterial oxygen saturation by a pulse oximeter or arterial pO_2 by blood gas determination to confirm or rule out central cyanosis.

The normal pO_2 in a one day old infant may be as low as 60 mm Hg. In certain congenital cyanotic heart disease with increased pulmonary arterial blood flow, the pO_2 may be more than 60 mmHg and usually does not show a large increase with a hyperoxitest. An arterial oxygen saturation of 90% or above does not completely rule out a cyanotic congenital heart defect. An arterial oxygen saturation of 90% can be seen with a pO_2 of 45 to 50 mm Hg in newborns because of the normally leftward oxygen hemoglobin dissociation curve.

Central and Peripheral Cyanosis

The critical level of reduced hemoglobin in the cutaneous veins may result from either desaturation of arterial blood or increased extraction of oxygen by peripheral tissues. Cyanosis secondary to desaturation of arterial blood is called *central cyanosis*. Cyanosis with normal saturation is called *peripheral cyanosis*. The latter occurs as a result of sluggish flow of blood. Peripheral cyanosis has no clinical significance except when associated with circulatory shock. Central cyanosis, on the other hand, is a significant clinical finding and may be associated with central nervous system depression, lung disease, or cyanotic congenital heart disease. *Circumoral cyanosis* refers to a bluish skin color around the mouth. It reflects a sluggish capillary blood flow and arterial oxygen saturation is normal. It may be seen in healthy infants with vasoconstriction from exposure to cold. Isolated circumoral cyanosis is of no concern unless it occurs with other signs of low cardiac output. *Differential cyanosis* is a condition where the infant present with a pink upper and a cyanotic lower body with accompanying difference in the oxygen saturation and arterial pO_2. It indicates a right to left ductal shunt and suggests persistent pulmonary hypertension of the newborn or obstructive lesions of the left side of the heart e.g. severe aortic stenosis, coarctation of aorta, interrupted aortic arch with a right to left ductal shunt.

Table 7.17 : Causes and clinical features of central cyanosis

1. *Central nervous system depression*
   - Perinatal asphyxia.
   - Heavy maternal sedation.
   - Intrauterine fetal distress.

   Clinical features
   - Shallow irregular respiration.
   - Poor muscle tone.
   - Cyanosis that disappears on stimulation or oxygen inhalation.
   - Increase in pO_2 with oxygen administration.
2. *Pulmonary disease*
   - Parenchymal lung disease viz. hyaline membrane disease, atelectasis.
   - Pneumothorax, pleural effusion.
   - Diaphragmatic hernia.
   - Persistent pulmonary hypertension.

   Clinical features
   - Tachypnea and respiratory distress with retraction and expiratory grunt.
   - Crackles and/or decreased breath sounds on auscultation.
   - Chest X-ray film may reveal cause.

Contd.

Contd.

   - Oxygen administration improves or abolishes cyanosis.
   - Increase in pO_2 with oxygen administration.
3. *Cardiac disease*
   - Congenital heart diseases with right to left shunt.

   Clinical features
   - Tachypnoea with mild or no retraction.
   - Heart murmur may be present on auscultation.
   - Chest X-ray may show an abnormal cardiac silhouette, increased or decreased pulmonary vascular markings.
   - No improvement of cyanosis on oxygen administration.

Clinical Findings of Central Cyanosis

Central cyanosis is a finding with central nervous system depression, pulmonary disease as well as with a cardiac disease. The clinical characteristics are shown in a tabular form.

Hyperoxitest

The determination of arterial blood gas levels clarifies the type of cyanosis–peripheral or central. Hyperoxitest helps to differentiate cyanosis caused by cardiac disease from that caused by pulmonary disease.

Oxygen Dissociation Curve

It is useful to know the oxygen dissociation curve in the newborn before discussing the hyperoxitest. The position of the oxygen dissociation curve is an expression of the affinity of hemoglobin for oxygen. In the newborn, the curve is shifted to the left. This is a result of high percentage of fetal hemoglobin in the newborn which has a high affinity to oxygen but does not allow release of oxygen to tissues. The adult curve is on the right as adult hemoglobin has less affinity for oxygen and allows release of oxygen to tissues. The newborn curve is replaced by the adult curve by 3 months of age.

Clinical findings	*CNS depression*	*Pulmonary disease*	*Cardiac disease*
1. Respiration	Shallow irregular	Tachypnoea, retractions, grunt	Tachypnea without grunt
2. Muscle tone	Poor	Normal	Normal
3. Cyanosis	Disappears on stimulation/O_2 adm.	Improves/abolishes on O_2 adm.	Not much affected
4. Auscultation	Normal	Crackles and/or decreased breath sounds	Murmur may be present
5. CXR	Normal	Reveal cause in lungs	Abnormal heart/pulmonary vasculature
6. Hyperoxi-test	Increases pO_2	Increases pO_2	Little or no increase in pO_2

Steps of Hyperoxitest

1. The arterial pO_2 is measured.
2. Oxygen should be administered through a plastic hood for atleast 10 minutes so that the alveolar oxygen is replaced completely with 100% oxygen administered.
3. The arterial oxygen is measured again and compared.

Interpretation

1. Arterial oxygen concentration rises above 100 mm Hg: indicates pulmonary disease.
2. Rise in arterial oxygen concentration does not exceed 100 mmHg, and the rise is not more than 10–30 mm Hg: indicates significant intracardiac right to left shunt.
3. Arterial pO_2 from the right radial artery is 10–15 mm Hg higher than that from an umbilical artery catheter: indicates right to left ductal shunt.

Points to be Noted

1. The response of pO_2 to 100% oxygen inhalation should be interpreted in the light of clinical picture, especially the degree of pulmonary pathology seen on chest X-ray.
2. Some infants with cyanotic congenital heart defects with a large pulmonary blood flow viz. total anomalous pulmonary venous return, may have a rise in arterial pO_2 to 100 mm Hg or higher.
3. Conversely, infants with a massive intrapulmonary shunt from lung disease (but with a normal heart) may not show rise in arterial pO_2 to 100 mmHg.
4. Arterial blood samples for measurement of pO_2 should be obtained from the upper part of the body viz. radial, brachial or temporal arteries to avoid false low values caused by a right to left ductal shunt. If a low value is obtained from an umbilical artery line or from a lower extremity artery, another sample from the right radial, brachial or temporal should be obtained and should be compared with a simultaneously obtained sample from an artery of the lower part of the body.

Management

The management of a cyanotic newborn includes the following steps:

1. Confirmation of cyanosis.
2. Confirmation whether cyanosis is peripheral or central.
3. Confirm cause: Pulmonary, cardiac or CNS.
4. Laboratory investigations:
   a. An X-ray chest.
   b. ECG.
   c. Arterial blood gas in room air.
   d. Hyperoxitest.

X-ray Findings in Some Common Congenital Cyanotic Heart Disease

	X-ray findings	*Congenital heart disease*
1.	An egg shaped heart with narrow base	D – TGA
2.	Snow man appearance with pulmonary venous congestion	TAPVR
3.	Concave pulmonary segment, boot-shaped heart, oligemic lung fields	TOF
4.	Extreme cardiomegaly	Ebstein anomaly

D-TGA = dextro transposition of great arteries
TAPVR = total anomalous pulmonary venous return
TOF = tetralogy of Fallot.

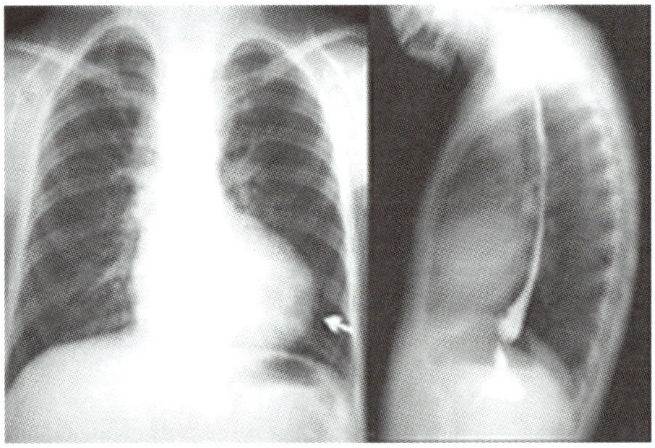

1. Tetralogy of Fallot

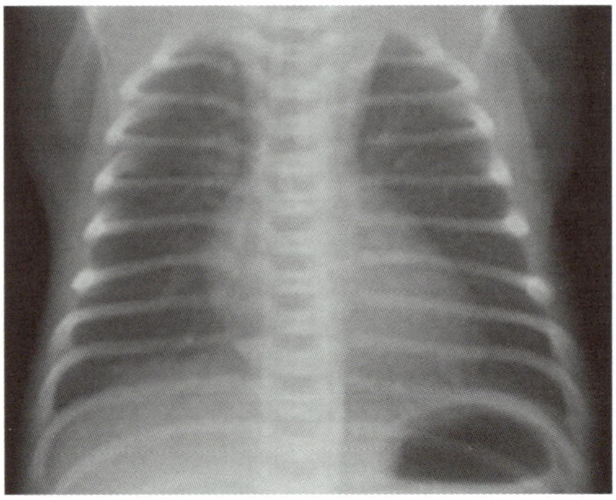

2. D Transposition of great vessels (D-TGA)

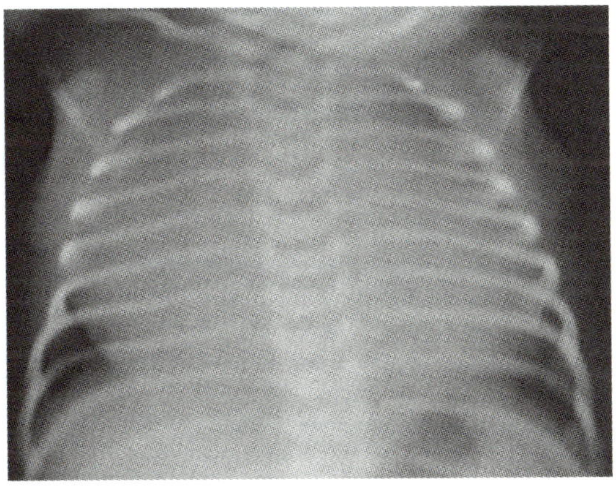

3. Ebstein anomaly

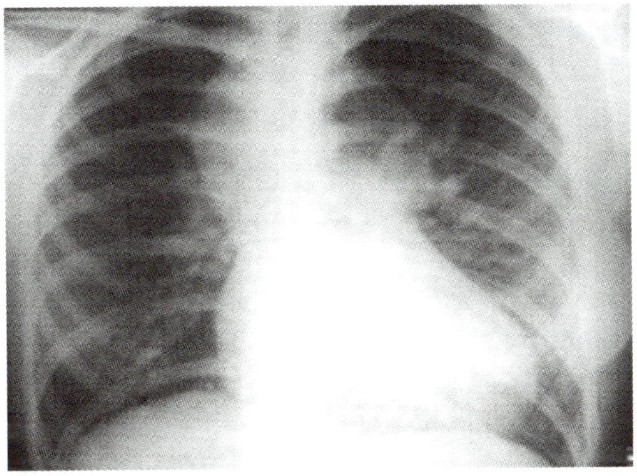

4. Total anomalous pulmonary venous drainage (TAPVR)

Fig. 7.21

Approach to Suspected Congenital Cyanotic Heart Disease

If central cyanosis is present or if the arterial oxygen saturation cannot be raised to a satisfactory level with administration of 100% oxygen, a cardiac consultation, an echo and a Doppler examination will reveal the cardiac lesion responsible for central cyanosis. A physical examination, X-ray PA view chest and ECG do not help as much in diagnosing a cyanotic heart disease as in diagnosing an acyanotic defect. However these tools can be sometimes useful, atleast in reducing the possibilities.

If a congenital cyanotic heart defect is suspected, especially a defect that appears to be ductus dependent (e.g. pulmonary atresia with or without VSD, tricuspid atresia, hypoplastic left heart syndrome, severe coarctation of aorta) prostaglandin E_1 infusion should be started as soon as the diagnosis is suspected or established. The starting dose is 0.05 to 0.1 micro gm/kg/minute which can be increased upto 0.4 micro gm/minute if there is no effect with the initial dose. It should be administered as a continuous intravenous drip. The dose should be reduced step by step to 0.01 micro gm / minute when desired effects viz. increased pO_2, increased systemic blood pressure, improved pH, are achieved.

For respiratory and CNS causes, once the diagnosis is established, treatment of the cause leads to relief of cyanosis.

Hemorrhagic Disease of the Newborn

Hemorrhagic disease of newborn (HDN) is due to the deficiency of Vitamin K dependent clotting factors viz. factors II, VII, IX and X. A moderate decrease of these factors normally occurs in neonates by 48–72 hours after birth with a gradual return to birth levels by 7–10 days of age. This transient deficiency of Vitamin K dependent coagulation factors may be accentuated due to different causes resulting in hemorrhagic disease of newborn.

Types of HDN

There are three forms of hemolytic disease of newborn: Early HDN, Classical HDN and Late HDN.

Early HDN

Early HDN occurs as a result of in utero Vitamin K deficiency precipitated by maternal intake of drugs like phenytoin, phenobarbitone. These drugs given during pregnancy interfere with Vitamin K metabolism and may cause severe deficiency of Vitamin K dependent coagulation factors viz. factors II, VII, IX and X in the fetus. Onset of bleeding may occur in utero or within 24 hours of birth. Bleeding is usually severe and life threatening in the form of concealed hemorrhage in the cranium, thorax and abdomen. Large ecchymoses, subcutaneous hemorrhage, external bleeding may also occur. The prothrombin time is prolonged and may fail to improve with Vitamin K administration.

Classical HDN

This is the most common form of hemorrhagic disease of newborn. It is a result of severe transient deficiency of Vitamin K. Vitamin K stores at birth is very small and rapidly depleted. Breast milk contains small amount of Vitamin K. The amount of milk during the first few days cannot supply adequate amount of Vitamin K. In addition, colonization of gut which is necessary for endogenous synthesis of Vitamin K is delayed. Hence breast fed babies can develop bleeding due to depletion of the factors II, VII, IX and X. Onset of bleeding usually occurs between the 2nd and 4th day of life, may occur from 1-7 days. The bleeding may be in the form of umbilical stump hemorrhage, hematemesis and/or melena, ecchymoses, epistaxis or scalp hemorrhage, bleeding from puncture sites and intracranial. The manifestations are not very severe. The prothrombin time and APTT are very prolonged. The platelet count, thrombin time and fibrinogen level are normal. The factor II, VII, IX and X are significantly decreased. Administration of Vitamin K results in cessation of bleeding, improvement of coagulation defect within a few hours.

Late HDN

The onset of bleeding is after the first week, may be between 2–16 weeks. Bleeding can occur from any site but more commonly from intracranial vessels, mucous membranes, skin and GIT. Intracranial bleed may be a devastating complication which is seen in about one third of cases. Late HDN is often associated with Vitamin K malabsorption as seen in neonatal hepatitis or biliary atresia.

Management

If the baby is in shock, it is evidenced by cold peripheries and a prolonged CRT (> 3 seconds), BP < 35 mmHg and pH < 7.25. The blood pressure usually does not fall until potentially life threatening blood loss has occurred. The hemoglobin may not fall for 2–3 hours. Such a baby requires:

1. A rapid transfusion of 15–20 ml/kg of uncross-matched blood over 5–15 minutes. If the baby is still shocked, another bolus of 15–20 ml/kg should be given over 15–20 minutes.
2. Blood pressure and central venous pressure is to be monitored. Aim is to achieve a blood pressure > 40 mmHg (in term infant) and CVP < 8 cm H_2O.
3. If necessary another transfusion, crossed matched against mother's blood, 10–30 ml/kg over 2–3 hours, accompanied by 1–2 mg/kg frusemide I.V. can be given.

If baby is not in shock

1. Vitamin K should be given as follows:
   i. In classical HDN, 1–2 mg I.V.
   ii. In early HDN, 2 mg I.V.
   iii. In late HDN, 5 mg I.V. every week until the underlying disorder is controlled.
2. If hemoglobin is less than 10 gm%, transfusion of crossed matched packed cells should be given over 2–3 hours with frusemide 2 mg/kg I.V. The amount of packed cells should be calculated on the basis that 10 ml/kg of packed cells will raise hemoglobin by 2–3 gm/dl.

Prevention

Classical HDN can be prevented by administration of Vitamin K, 0.5–1 mg IM to all newborn babies at birth.

An Approach to Neonatal Surgical Emergencies

Surgical emergencies are defined as neonatal conditions which require emergent stabilization and surgical intervention within minutes to hours if severe morbidity and mortality is to be avoided. Most of the conditions are congenital malformations.

The common surgical conditions which may present as emergency include anomalies of the gastrointestinal tract, neural tube defects, diaphragmatic and abdominal wall defects and obstructive uropathy.

The common surgical emergency conditions include:

A. *Gastrointestinal causes*: Intestinal obstruction due to duodenal, jejunal, ileal and anal atresia, congenital diaphragmatic hernia, esophageal atresia, volvulus, bands, Hirschsprung disease, meconium ileus, meconium plug, NEC.

B. *Abdominal wall defects*: Exomphalos, gastrochisis.

C. *Respiratory causes* include bilateral choanal atresia, Pierre Robin syndrome, laryngeal stenosis, congenital lobar emphysema, pulmonary aplasia.

D. *Neural tube defects* e.g. open meningomyelocele, anencephaly.

E. *Urogenital defects* in the form of obstructive uropathy.

Anticipation of Congenital Anomalies

Anticipation of congenital anomalies before birth can help early in utero referral of cases to an equipped centre for proper management. A congenital anomaly can be suspected from the following maternal and fetal indicators:

Maternal Indicators

a. Family history of congenital malformations.

b. Maternal age > 35 years.

c. Antenatal history of ingestion of teratogenic drugs, exposure to radiation, exposure to infection e.g. rubella.

d. History of consanguinity.

e. Mother with history of chronic illness like diabetes.

Fetal Indicators

a. Polyhydramnios is associated with esophageal atresia, duodenal and ileal atresia, congenital diaphragmatic hernia, abdominal wall defects.

b. Oligohydramnios is associated with congenital renal abnormalities.

c. Meconium peritonitis is associated with antenatal perforation of intestinal tract.

d. Dystocia is associated with abdominal wall defects, intestinal obstruction, genitourinary abnormalities and sacrococcygeal teratoma.

Prenatal Diagnosis

Prenatal diagnosis is possible with the help of imaging and biochemical examination in majority of congenital anomalies.

Ultrasonography

The best time for an USG examination is 12–15 weeks of gestation. It can diagnose anterior abdominal wall defects, duodenal atresia, congenital diaphragmatic hernia, esophageal atresia etc.

Maternal Serum Alpha Feto Protein

The best time for estimation of maternal serum alpha fetoprotein is 16–18 weeks of gestation. Elevated levels indicate presence of open neural tube defect, abdominal wall defects. Decreased levels are found in Down syndrome (trisomy 21), Edward syndrome (trisomy 18).

Clinical Manifestation

After birth the following features may lead one to suspect presence of a congenital anomaly:

1. Low birth weight and preterm delivery.
2. Facial dysmorphism.
3. Presence of a single umbilical artery.

Common Congenital Anomalies and Their Clinical Features at Presentation

a. *Baby becomes cyanosed during feeding:* Bilateral choanal atresia.

b. *Increase respiratory distress on bag and mask ventilation, scaphoid abdomen:* Congenital diaphragmatic hernia.

c. *Excessive frothing, choking on feeding:* Esophageal atresia with tracheoesophageal atresia.

d. *Abdominal distension:* Intestinal obstruction.

e. *Bile stained vomiting:* Intestinal atresia, malrotation of gut.

f. *Hematemesis and blood in stool:* Necrotizing enterocolitis.

g. *Gastric aspiration >20 ml:* Upper gastrointestinal obstruction.

h. *Failure to pass meconium within 24 hours:* Imperforate anus, Hirschsprung disease.

i. *Failure to pass urine within 48 hours:* Renal abnormalities.

Management

Principles

1. Early diagnosis of specific and associated abnormalities.
2. Preoperative stabilization and referral to a pediatric surgeon.

The cardinal features of neonatal intestinal obstruction are polyhydramnios in mother, vomiting, abdominal distension and failure to pass meconium. All babies with respiratory distress during neonatal period should have an X-ray of the chest done.

Supportive Treatment and Initial Stabilization is Same For All Cases

i. All babies should be admitted to the intensive care unit, nursed in a thermoneutral environment, an I.V. line set up and blood samples sent for investigation including blood group and cross matching.

ii. The baby should be kept nil orally. Gastric decompression done by 1–2 hourly aspiration. In between the aspiration the tube is allowed to drain freely.

iii. Correction of fluid and electrolyte balance with I.V.

fluid continued according to requirement for age and weight. Urine output should be maintained at > 1 ml/ kg/hour. Hypoglycemia is to be monitored and blood glucose maintained.

iv. Cardiorespiratory support as and when required.

v. *Drugs:* Vitamin K 1 mg I.M., broad spectrum antibiotics covering both gram positive and negative bacteria should be started. Usually a 3rd generation cephalosporin and gentamycin is the choice.

vi. Surgical consultation as early as possible.

Monitoring in the Preoperative Period

Clinical Monitoring

1. Measurement of abdominal girth hourly and observation of gastric aspirate for quantity and nature every 1–2 hourly should be done in babies with intestinal obstruction.
2. Vitals: Heart rate, respiratory rate, temperature and CRT/ blood pressure.
3. Oxygen saturation and ABG monitoring for babies with respiratory distress.

Laboratory

1. Hematocrit, glucose every 6–8 hourly.
2. Serum electrolytes 12 hourly in the first 48–72 hours, then once daily.
3. TLC, DLC, platelet count initially. Repeated once after 48 hours.
4. Acid base status 12 hourly during the initial 48–72 hours.

Nursing

Babies with respiratory distress needs intensive nursing which include:

i. Position of the baby: Babies with retrognathia should be nursed in prone position with the head turned laterally. Babies with tracheoesophageal fistula or congenital diaphragmatic hernia should be nursed in head up position.

ii. Continuous and slow suction in cases diagnosed as esophageal atresia, to prevent aspiration.

iii. If the baby has mild to moderate respiratory distress oxygen inhalation with hood or nasal catheter should be given and ABG monitored.

iv. If there are signs of respiratory failure, the baby will need intubation and assisted ventilation.

Identification, Referral and Transport of High Risk Newborn

A high risk neonate is defined as one who is at an increased risk to die or sustain brain damage. Majority of the neonatal deaths occur in the high risk neonates. Hence early identification of these neonates, timely referral to an appropriate hospital can result in better chances of survival.

Low Risk Neonates

These neonates do not pose any problem and can be looked after by the mother. A low risk neonate should fulfill the following criteria:

1. Born at term by spontaneous vaginal delivery following an uncomplicated pregnancy.
2. Spontaneously breathing at birth without difficulty or need for oxygen administration.
3. Weight above 2500 grams at birth.
4. Have a vigorous sucking reflex and breastfeeding.
5. Free from any major congenital anomalies or illness.

Moderate Risk Neonates

These babies can be managed at home under the supervision of a health worker. However, if they are ill, they will need referral. These include:

1. First born baby.
2. Mother uneducated or in teens.
3. Babies born to high risk mothers.
4. Birth weight 2000 grams to 2500 grams.
5. Babies with superficial infections.

High Risk Neonates

This category of newborn infant need level II/III care in a neonatal unit. Some of these babies weighing between 1800–2000 grams with good sucking can be managed at home under supervision. This group of babies, if sick needs intensive (level III) care. These include the following:

High Risk Neonates Needing Intermediate (Level II) Care

1. Birth weight 1500–2000 grams.
2. Gestation period 33–36 weeks.

3. One minute Apgar score of 6 or less, with 5 minutes Apgar score of 7–10.
4. Babies not sucking well but tolerating tube feeds.

High Risk Babies Needing Intensive (Level III) Care

1. Five minutes Apgar score of 6 or less.
2. Babies with gross congenital malformations.
3. Presence of danger signs.
4. Baby needing I.V. fluid therapy.

Any neonate, irrespective of birth weight and gestation, having the above mentioned characteristics must be considered as high risk babies needing intensive care and immediately transferred to a centre having adequate facilities for intensive newborn care. Most of these babies are at a high risk of brain damage or death and need advanced therapeutic interventions. Besides these, the following categories also need intensive care even if they have no abnormal signs.

1. Birth weight less than 1500 grams.
2. Gestation 32 weeks or less.

Which Newborns to Refer?

In utero transfer of the baby should always be preferred in the event of a high-risk pregnancy. The following neonatal conditions are guidelines to be used when considering the possibility of neonatal transport.

1. Prematurity and/ or birth weight <1500 g.
2. Gestational age <32 weeks.
3. Respiratory distress requiring ventilatory support (CPAP, ventilation).
4. Seizures.
5. Congenital anomalies and/or inborn errors of metabolism.
6. Congenital heart disease or cardiac arrhythmias requiring cardiac services.
7. Severe hypoxemic–ischemic injury.
8. Other conditions requiring neonatology consultation and consideration for transfer viz.
   - Hyperbilirubinemia, possibly requiring exchange transfusion.
   - Infant of diabetic mothers.
   - Severe intrauterine growth retardation.
   - Birth weight between 1500 and 2000 g and gestational age between 32 and 36 weeks.
   - Procedures unavailable at the referring hospital.

Responsibilities of the Referring Hospital

Stabilization

Unless there is a surgical emergency it is preferable to stabilize the child and keep the patient in the referring hospital awaiting the arrival of a trained pediatric transport team.

Thermoregulation: Provide neutral thermal environment. Place under preheated radiant warmer with servo control or under a 200 watt bulb at a distance of 45 cm above a well covered baby or in a preheated incubator.

Respiration: Prevent hypoxia and prevent hyperoxia in premature infants.

- Maintain airway by positioning and suctioning as needed.
- Provide stimulation, bag and mask ventilation and chest compression if resuscitation is required. Intubate if needed for positive pressure ventilation.
- If supplemental oxygen is required, it should be preferably warm, moist and blended.
- The baby is monitored with a pulsoxymeter.

Circulation: Check CRT and maintain blood pressure and perfusion. If CRT > 3 secs.

- Use volume expanders (Normal saline/ Ringer lactate) 10 ml/kg.
- Maintain hydration with intravenous 10% dextrose solution.

Metabolism: Prevent hypoglycemia and acidosis:

- Maintain glucose over 40 mg/dl. Assess blood glucose by reagent strip.
- Treat *hypoglycemia* with 10% dextrose 2 ml/kg bodyweight/dose I.V.
- *Correct acidosis* by treating underlying cause.

  Respiratory acidosis: May require mechanical ventilation.

  Metabolic acidosis: May require sodium bicarbonate 2–3 ml/kg/dose mixed with equal volume of distilled water slow I.V.

First Dose of the Following Drugs

- Inj Vitamin K, 1 mg I.M. stat.
- Inj Ampicillin 50 mg/kg I.M./I.V stat.
- Inj Gentamicin, 2.5 mg/kg stat.

Pretransport Care of the Surgical Neonate

Pretransport stabilization of a surgical neonate includes the following measures:

- Nil per oral and I.V. fluid.
- Bag and tube ventilation in case of suspected diaphragmatic hernia.
- Sterile saline soaked gauge covering for meningocele, Gastrochisis etc.
- Continuous slow naso gastric suction in suspected tracheoesophageal fistula.
- Decompression of stomach in suspected congenital intestinal obstruction.

Communication

- Explain condition of the baby and need for referral.
- Explain care during transport.
- Prepare a note regarding the baby's condition and care.
- Encourage mother to accompany. If possible a health care provider should accompany.

Care During Transport

- Ensure warmth by clothing, kangaroo care, and transport incubator, monitoring temperature by measurement of temperature by human touch method or axillary temperature.
- Keep neck in slight extension. Keep airway clear by suction.
- Check respiration. If apneic, provide tactile stimulation, bag and mask ventilation.
- Give feeds by direct breastfeeding. If not sucking by cup or by NG tube.
- If baby is very sick I.V. infusion with 10% dextrose (in first 48 hours) and 0.45 saline in 5% dextrose (after 48 hours of age).
- The attendant should be taught to count drops and regulate, feed the baby and give stimulations if a health care provider does not accompany.

Organization of Transport

- The baby should be transported to the nearest establishment with adequate facilities.
- The fastest mode of transport and shortest route should be selected.
- The referral hospital should be informed in advance.

Neonatal Resuscitation

The resuscitation techniques described below are laid down by the course based on the guidelines for emergency cardiovascular care of the newborn, by the American Academy of Pediatrics and American Heart Association. The following guidelines apply primarily to newly born infants undergoing transition from intrauterine to extrauterine life. However, they are also applicable to neonates who have completed the initial transition and require resuscitation during the first few weeks to months following birth.

Approximately 10% newborns require some assistance to begin breathing at birth; about 1% needs extensive resuscitative measures to survive. Babies at high risk are those born by cesarean section, asphyxiated, preterm and very low birth weight. Premature babies are at higher risk because they have anatomical and physiological characteristics that are quite different from babies born at term. Some of these characteristics are:

- Their lungs may be deficient in surfactant and, therefore, may be more difficult to ventilate.
- Their thin, permeable skin, large surface area to body mass ratio, and lack of subcutaneous fat make them more likely to loose heat.
- They are more likely to be born with an infection.
- Their brains have fragile capillaries that may bleed during periods of stress.

Physiology of Asphyxia

When a fetus or an infant is deprived of oxygen in utero or following delivery, they manifest either as primary apnea or secondary apnea.

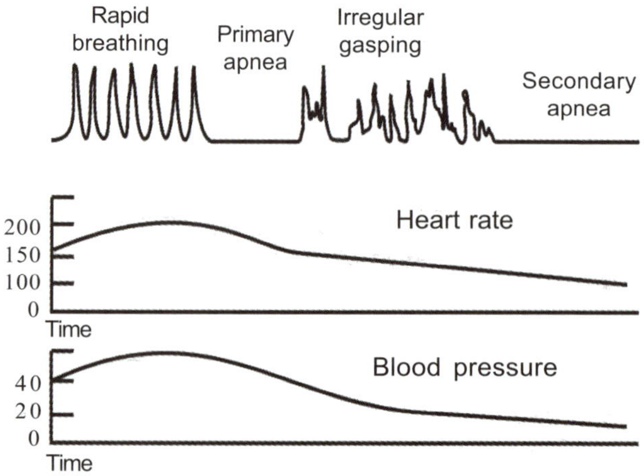

Fig. 7.22: Primary and secondary apnea

Primary Apnea

Exposure to oxygen lack results in an initial period of rapid breathing. If the asphyxia continues, the respiratory movements cease, the heart rate begins to fall, and the infant enters a period of apnea. This is known as primary apnea. Exposure to oxygen and stimulation during the period of primary apnea in most instances will induce respirations.

Secondary Apnea

If asphyxia continues, the infant develops deep gasping respirations, the heart rate continues to decrease, and the blood pressure begins to fall. The respirations become weaker and weaker until the infant takes a last gasp and enters a period of apnea called secondary apnea. The infant is unresponsive to stimulation and positive pressure ventilation with 100% O_2 should be started.

Primary Versus Secondary Apnea

An infant may go through primary apnea into secondary apnea while in utero. Clinically primary and secondary apnea are indistinguishable at birth. In both instances, the infant is not breathing, and the heart rate may be below 100/min. Thus *when an infant is apneic at birth, resuscitation should be started immediately assuming that the infant is in secondary apnea.*

It is important to realize that once the child is in secondary apnea, the longer is the delay in starting positive pressure ventilation, the longer it will take the infant to initiate spontaneous respiration. Further, the longer the infant is in secondary apnea, the greater is the chance that brain damage will occur.

How Does a Baby Receive Oxygen Before Birth?

Oxygen is essential for survival both before and after birth. Before birth, fetal lungs do not function as a source of oxygen or as a route to excrete carbon dioxide. Only a small fraction of fetal blood passes through the lungs. The fetal lungs are expanded in utero but the alveoli are filled with fluid. In addition, the blood vessels that perfuse and drain the fetal lungs are markedly constricted. Most of the blood from the right side of the heart flows through the ductus arteriosus into the aorta. Before birth, the oxygen used by the fetus diffuses across the placenta from the mother's blood. It is only after birth when the baby is separated from the placenta, the lungs take over the function of oxygenation and distribution to the rest part of the body.

What Normally Happens at Birth to Allow a Baby to Get Oxygen from the Lungs?

Following birth, as the infant takes the first few breaths, the lungs expand as they are filled with air. Approximately one third of the fetal lung fluid is removed during vaginal delivery as the chest is squeezed and lung fluid exit through the nose and mouth. The remaining fluid passes through the alveoli into the lymphatics surrounding the lungs. How quickly the fluid leaves the lung depend on the forcefulness of the first few breaths.

At the same time the arterioles in the lungs begin to open, allowing a considerable increase in the amount of blood flowing through the lungs. Blood previously diverted through the ductus arteriosus flow through the lungs where it picks up oxygen to transport to tissues throughout the body. Soon there is no use of the ductus, and it eventually closes.

Problems of Clearing Lung Fluid

Problems in clearing lung fluid occur in infants who do not have forceful first few breaths. They are infants apneic at birth and infants with weak initial respiratory effort viz. premature infants, infants who are depressed as a result of asphyxia, maternal drugs, or anesthesia.

What Happens if There is Asphyxia?

Asphyxia results in hypoxemia with resulting acidosis. In the presence of hypoxemia and acidosis, the arterioles of the newborn's lungs remain constricted, and the ductus remains open. Fetal circulation is maintained with no increase in pulmonary blood flow. Blood that should have been perfusing the lungs continues to flow through the ductus.

It needs mention that merely entry of air into the lungs is not enough to maintain spontaneous respiration. There must be an adequate supply of blood through the capillaries of the lungs so that oxygen can pass into the blood and be carried throughout the body. *Hence, initiation of respiration includes spontaneous breathing and a heart rate > 100/minute.*

Adequate Preparation

The minimum preparation for any delivery, even an expected normal one, should include a radiant warmer, heated and ready for use. All resuscitation equipments should be immediately available and in working order.

In cases of an anticipated asphyxiated infant, all of the equipment should be removed from its packages and kept ready for use. The syringes filled with medications ready for use. Two trained individuals capable of working together to perform all aspects of resuscitation should be available in the labour room/OT.

Universal Precautions

Exposure to blood or other body fluids is inevitable in the delivery room. Universal precautions must be practised by wearing caps, goggles or glasses, gloves and impervious gowns until the cord is cut and the newborn is dried and wrapped.

Resuscitation Equipments

1. Dee Lee's mucus trap.
2. A self inflating infant resuscitation bag with a pressure release valve.
3. Face mask 0 and 1 size.
4. Oxygen source with flow meter.
5. Infant laryngoscope with straight blade 0 (for preterm) and 1 (for term), extra batteries, bulbs.
6. Endotracheal tubes 2.5, 3.0, 3.5, 4.0 mm internal diameter.
7. Oral airway (0, 00, 000 sizes), 8 F feeding tube.
8. Scissors, stylet, adhesive tape.
9. Medications:
   a. Epinephrine (1:10000).
   b. Normal saline, Ringer's lactate.
10. Syringes 1 ml, 2 ml, 5 ml, 10 ml, 20 ml and 50 ml.
11. Radiant warmer.
12. Gloves and 3 pieces of linen measuring 1 square metre.

Preparation of Equipments

1. Ensure that the radiant warmer is on and dry and prewarmed linen/blanket is available.
2. Turn on the oxygen source and adjust flow at 5–8 litres/minute.
3. Test the resuscitation bag for the pop up control and adequate flow. A proper size mask should be available.
4. Make sure that the laryngoscope light is bright and appropriate blade is available.
5. Select the appropriate endotracheal tube for the expected birth weight.
6. If the clinical situation suggest that extensive resuscitation may be necessary the following actions may be required:
   a. Set up an umbilical catheterization tray for venous catheterization.
   b. Draw up 1:10000 epinephrine, sodium bicarbonate and volume expander and keep ready for use.

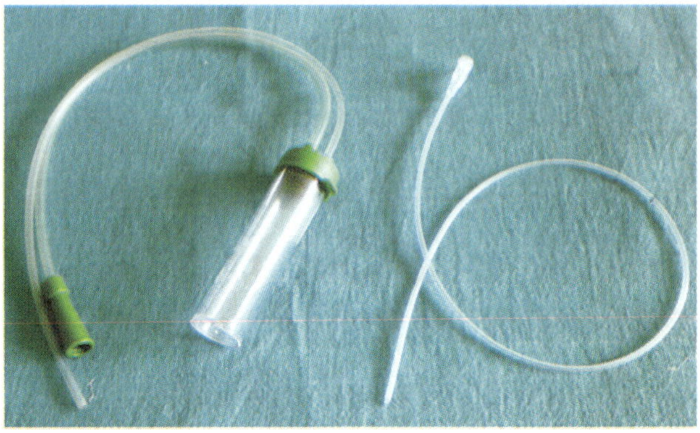

Fig. 7.23: Dee Lee mucus trap and feeding tube

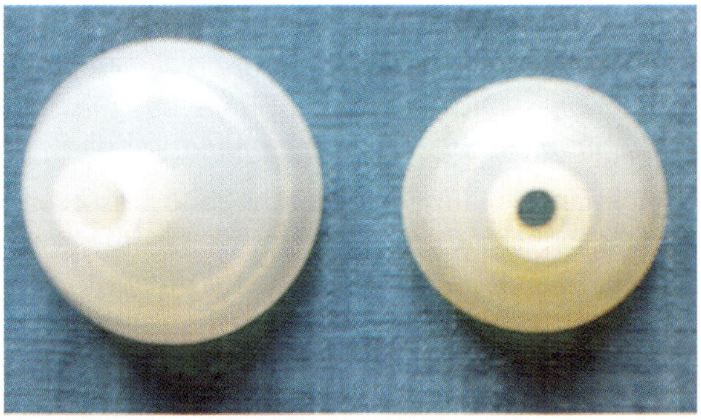

Fig. 7.24: Face mask 0 and 1 size

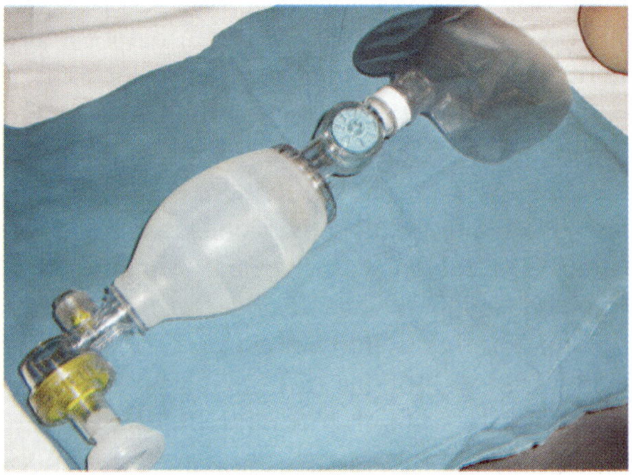

Fig. 7.25: Bag with oxygen reservoir

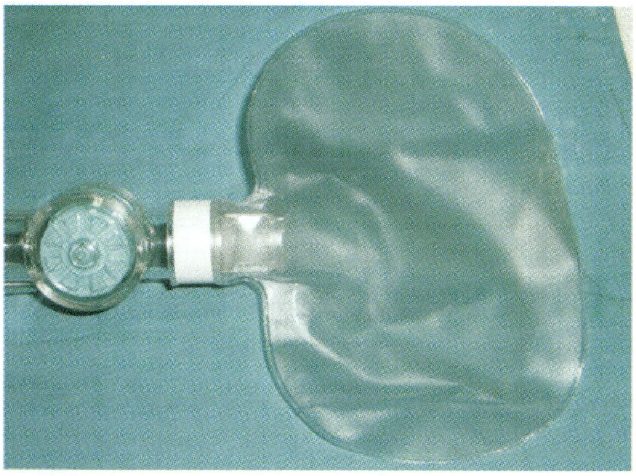

Fig. 7.26: Reservoir (close bag type)

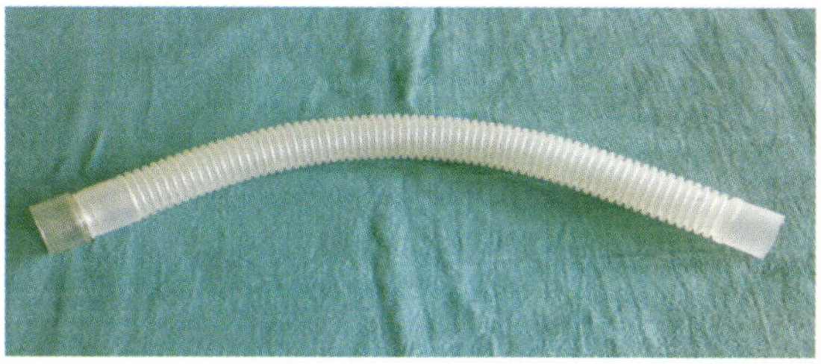

Fig. 7.27: Reservoir (open corrugated rubber tube type)

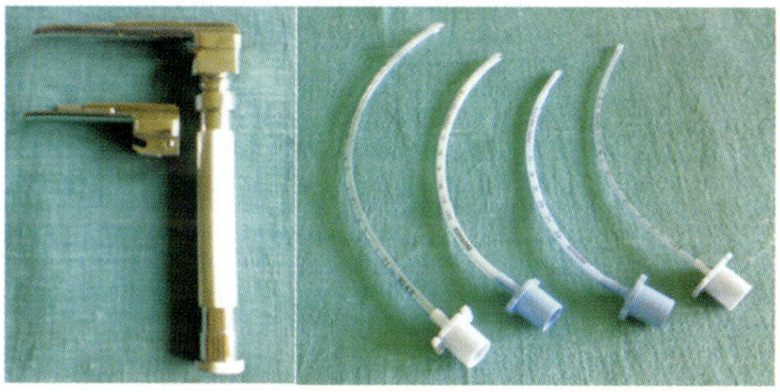

Fig. 7.28: Infant laryngoscope (0 and 1 blades) and endotracheal tubes with connectors

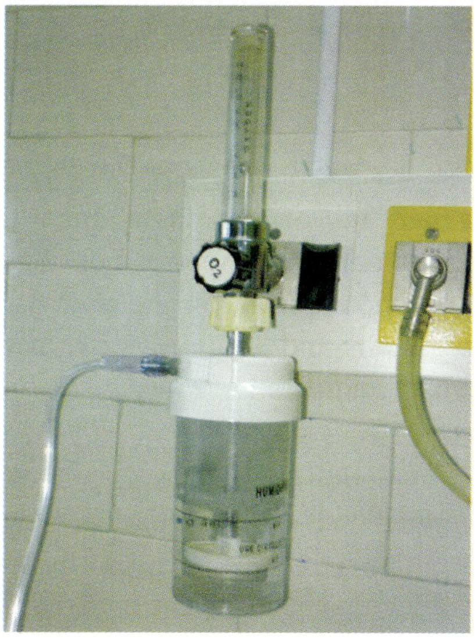

Fig. 7.29: Oxygen source with flowmeter

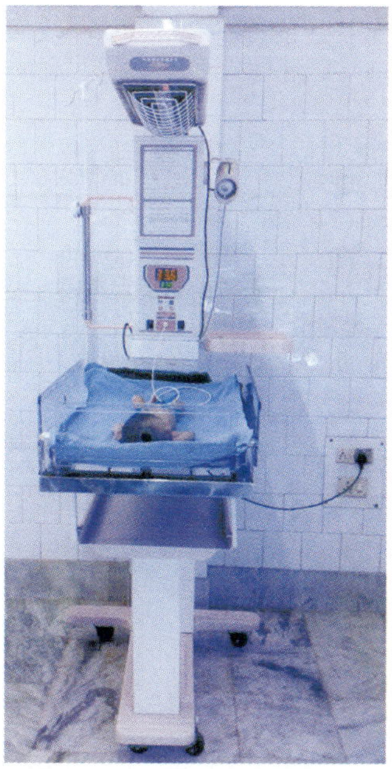

Fig. 7.30: Radiant warmer

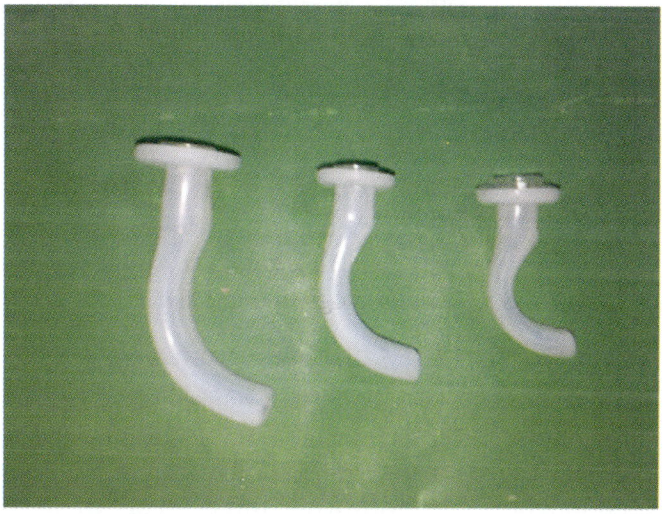

Fig. 7.31: Oral airway sizes 0, 00 and 000

TABC of Resuscitation

T: Temperature, A: Airway, B: Breathing, C: Circulation

T: Maintenance of body *temperature* by keeping the baby under the radiant warmer, using prewarmed linen, warm resuscitation equipments.

A: Establish an open *airway* by positioning, suctioning, intubation.

B: Initiate *breathing* by tactile stimulation, positive pressure ventilation with bag and mask or tube.

C: Maintain *circulation* by chest compression and medications.

Apgar Score in Assessment of Baby at Birth

Apgar Score

	Score		
Sign	*0*	*1*	*2*
Heart rate	Absent	< 100/min	=/> 100/min
Respiration	Absent	Slow, Irregular	Good, crying
Muscle tone	Limp	Some flexion	Active motion
Reflex irritability (catheter in nares, tactile stimulation)	No response	Grimace	Cough, Sneeze, cry
Color	Blue or pale	Pink body, blue Extremities	Completely pink

Points to be Noted

1. Apgar score should be assigned at 1 minute and 5 minutes.
2. When the score is <7 at 5 minutes, additional scores should be scored every 5 minutes upto 20 minutes.

Why is Apgar Score Not Used During Resuscitation?

1. It does not help to take decision regarding resuscitation at birth.
2. There is a poor correlation between Apgar score at birth and future neurological outcome.

What Do You Do After Resuscitation?

Babies who have required resuscitation are at risk for deterioration after their vital signs have returned to normal. The neonatal resuscitation programme has recommended the following three levels of post-resuscitation care:

Routine Care: Nearly 90% of the newborns are vigorous term, infants with no risk factors and clear amniotic fluid. These babies require routine care in the form of provision of warmth, clearing airway if necessary, and drying. They do not need to be separated from their mother after birth. Ongoing observation of breathing, activity and color must be carried out to determine additional intervention.

Supportive Care: Babies who have prenatal or intrapartum risk factors, have meconium staining of the amniotic fluid or skin, have depressed breathing or activity, and/or cyanotic, will need some degree of resuscitation at birth. These babies are still at risk for developing problems associated with perinatal compromise and should be evaluated frequently during the immediate neonatal period.

Ongoing Care: Babies, who require positive pressure ventilation or more extensive resuscitation may require ongoing support, are at high risk for developing subsequent complications of an abnormal transition. These babies should be transported to an intensive care unit for ongoing evaluation and monitoring.

What Questions Should You Ask Before Every Birth?

It is important for the obstetric and newborn health care providers to coordinate care by establishing effective communication. Before every birth, ask the following 4 pre-birth questions:

1. What is the expected gestational age?
2. Is the amniotic fluid clear?
3. How many babies are expected?
4. Are there any additional risk factors?

Based on the responses to these questions, determine if you have assembled the necessary personnel and equipment.

Assessment at Birth

Those newly born infants who do not require resuscitation can generally be identified by a rapid assessment of the following 3 characteristics:

1. Term gestation?
2. Crying or breathing?
3. Good muscle tone?

If the answer to all 3 of these questions is "yes", the baby does not need resuscitation and should not be separated from the mother. The baby should be dried, placed skin-to-skin with the mother, and covered with dry linen to maintain temperature. Observation of breathing, activity, and color should be ongoing.

If the answer to any of these assessment questions is "no", the infant should receive one or more of the following 4 categories of action in sequence: Initial steps, ventilation, chest compressions and administration of epinephrine and/or volume expanders.

Approximately 60 seconds ("the Golden Minute") are allotted for completing the initial steps, reevaluating, and beginning ventilation if required. The decision to progress beyond the initial steps is determined by simultaneous assessment of 2 vital characteristics: respirations (apnea, gasping, or labored or unlabored breathing) and heart rate (whether greater than or less than 100 beats per minute).

Assessment of heart rate should be done by intermittent auscultation of the precordial pulse. When a pulse is detectable, palpation of the umbilical pulse can also provide a rapid estimate of the pulse and is more accurate than palpation at other sites.Once positive pressure ventilation or supplementary oxygen administration is begun, assessment should consist of simultaneous evaluation of 3 vital characteristics: heart rate, respirations, and the state of oxygenation, the latter optimally determined by a pulse oximeter.

Sequence of Resuscitation at Birth

a. Initial steps.
b. Positive pressure ventilation by bag and mask or bag and tube.
c. Chest compression.
d. Medication.

Initial Steps

The initial steps of resuscitation should be performed in the following sequence:

1. Provide warmth.
2. Position the baby.
3. Clear airway.
4. Drying and reposition.
5. Tactile stimulation.
6. Evaluation.

It needs mention that the sequence has to be maintained irrespective of the degree of asphyxia in the baby at birth.

Provide Warmth

The goal is to achieve normothermia and avoid iatrogenic hyperthermia. Warmth can be provided by placing the baby under a radiant warmer.

The term baby should not be covered with blankets or towels to allow full visualization and to permit the radiant heat to reach the baby.

VLBW (< 1500 gms weight) infants are likely to become hypothermic despite use of traditional techniques of decreasing heat loss. Additional warming techniques are recommended for such babies. At present the only properly evaluated method is covering the infant in plastic wrapping and placing under radiant heat. Temperature should be closely monitored for the risk of hyperthermia. Animal studies have indicated that hyperthermia during or after ischemia is associated with progression of cerebral injury. All resuscitation procedures can be performed with this temperature controlling interventions in place.

Position

Position the baby on the back or side with the neck in the position of slight extension. This will bring the posterior pharynx, larynx and trachea in line and facilitate unrestricted air entry. This alignment is also best to assist ventilation with bag and mask and to place an endotracheal tube. Hyperextension or flexion of neck may restrict air entry. To help maintain correct position, a roll of 2.5 cm diameter may be put under the shoulders. This shoulder roll may be particularly useful if the baby has a large occiput resulting from molding, edema, or prematurity.

Clear Airway

Clear airway by gentle suction with a Dee Lee's mucus trap. The following basic rules are important to note during suction:

- Suction mouth first then nose.
- Not more than 2 times in the mouth and 2 times in the nose.
- Give gentle, brief, continuous and negative suction.
- Introduce not more than 2.5 cm of the suction tube into mouth and 1.25 cm into nose.

It is recommended that suctioning immediately following birth should be reserved for babies who have obvious obstruction to spontaneous breathing or who require positive-pressure ventilation (PPV).

Why Suction Should be Gentle, Not Deep and Brief?

Vigorous and deep suction can stimulate the posterior pharynx, which can produce a vagal response causing severe bradycardia or apnea. Brief suctioning is usually adequate to remove secretions in the oral cavity. Prolonged suctioning will cause waste of time.

Drying

Drying should be done starting from head to foot and back with a pre warmed linen. The wet linen should be removed and the baby wrapped with another piece of prewarmed linen. The baby does not require wrapping if under the radiant warmer.

Tactile Stimulation

Tactile stimulation is required if the infant is not able to initiate respiration after drying. The following stimulations should be used:

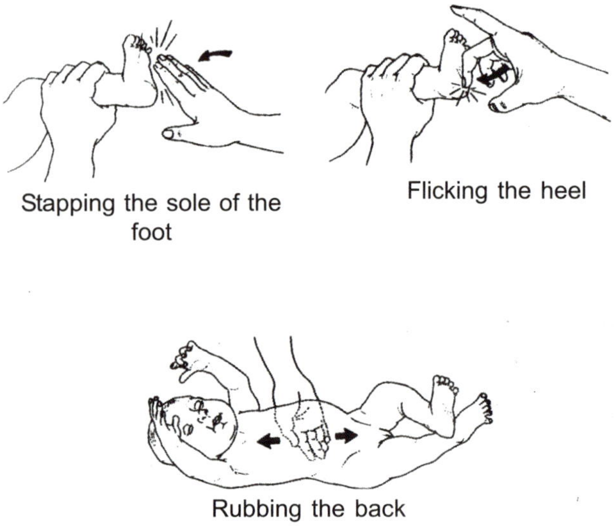

Fig. 7.32: Tactile stimulations

i. Flicking the heal or slapping the sole.
ii. Rubbing the back.

Points to be Noted

- Stimulation should be brief. Not more than 2 times.
- Rubbing of the back should be done if the baby starts breathing but respiration is ineffective.
- If brief stimulation is not effective, continuing stimulation will not help rather harm by prolonging secondary apnea. This baby needs positive pressure ventilation.

Evaluation

Evaluation should be done on the basis of the following criteria maintaining the sequence:

i. Presence or absence of spontaneous respiration.
ii. Heart rate.

Decisions and Actions

1. If the baby has started breathing spontaneously, heart rate is 100/min or more and color is pink / with peripheral cyanosis, the baby is considered to be normal and does not need further resuscitation. Baby should be wrapped in layers of prewarmed linen.
2. *If there is no spontaneous respiration:* Start positive pressure ventilation.
3. If the baby has started breathing but the heart rate is <100/min: Start positive pressure ventilation.
4. If the baby has started spontaneous respiration, heart rate is >100/min but there is central cyanosis: Give free flow oxygen by tube or mask at the rate of 5 litres/min.

SPO_2 Monitoring and Optimal Oxygen Delivery

The state of oxygenation can be suggested by the skin color. Central cyanosis (cyanosis due to low oxygen tension in blood) will appear as blue color of lips, tongue and trunk. Acrocyanosis (blue hue of the limbs and feet) is often due to decreased circulation to the extremities. It is not an indication of low oxygen tension.

The recent recommendation suggests that if central cyanosis is persisting, it would be ideal to attach a pulse oximetry probe to monitor if the oxygenation of the baby is in the abnormal range. If the levels are below the saturation targets for a normal baby during transition, and are not increasing, the baby may need to be provided supplemental oxygen. The accepted ranges of pre ductal oximetry (right hand or wrist) values during first 10 minutes, following birth of uncomplicated babies born at term, are shown in Table 7.18.

Table 7.18: Showing the SpO_2 targets

Pre-ductal SpO_2 Target	
1 min	60 – 65%
2 min	65 – 70%
3 min	70 – 75%
4 min	75 – 80%
5 min	80 – 85%
10 min	85 – 95%

Administration of Supplementary Oxygen

Free flow oxygen can be given to a spontaneously breathing baby by the following delivering methods:

(a) Oxygen mask.
(b) Oxygen tube.
(c) Flow inflating bag and mask.
(d) T piece resuscitator with mask.

N.B. Free flow oxygen cannot be delivered reliably by a mask attached to a self-inflating bag because gas does not reliably flow through the mask unless the bag is being squeezed. However, free flow oxygen may be administered through the open reservoir ("tail") on some self-inflating bags.

When unregulated oxygen is administered to a cyanosed baby or in a baby with oximeter readings lower than the expected range, oxygen levels may increase quickly to levels toxic to the baby at that time. The likelihood of this situation increases in preterm babies. Hence, it is best to use oxygen concentration that can be varied throughout the range of 21% to 100%. This will be possible with availability of a compressed air source and a blender.

Procedure for Delivery of Free Flow Oxygen

A high concentration of free flow oxygen can be achieved reliably with an oxygen mask. The mask should be held close to the face but not so tight that pressure builds. If a mask is not available, try to keep the oxygen concentration around the baby's airway by cupping your hand around the baby's face and oxygen tubing.

How Much Oxygen Should Be Administered?

It is best to give oxygen to maintain the saturation of the newborn in the acceptable ranges with the help of a blender for graded delivery and pulse oximeter for optimal monitoring of oxygen saturation in the early minutes of life. If these facilities are not available in the labour room, it is best to transfer the baby to a SCNU/NICU for further management.

How Long Oxygen Should Be Administered?

Enough oxygen should be provided for the newborn to become pink, i.e., when central cyanosis improves and oxygen saturation is above 85% to 90%. Then supplemental oxygen is gradually decreased till the newborn can remain pink while breathing room air.

If respirations and heart rate are stable, but the newborn continues to require supplemental oxygen, use pulse oximetry to guide the appropriate oxygen concentration. Air and oxygen administered directly from a compressed source is cold and dry. To prevent heat loss, oxygen given to newborns for a prolonged period of time should be heated and humidified.

If the baby has laboured breathing or oxygen saturation cannot be maintained within the target range despite 100% free flow oxygen, one should consider a trial of continuous positive airway pressure (CPAP) or PPV. A trial of CPAP in the delivery room can be given by using a flow-inflating bag or a T-piece resuscitator attached to a mask that is held tightly to the baby's face.

If ventilation is adequate but newborn still remains cyanotic then cyanotic congenital heart disease or persistent pulmonary hypertension of newborn (PPHN) should be considered.

Does the Presence of Meconium-stained Amniotic Fluid Change the Approach to the Initial Steps?

The presence of meconium-stained amniotic fluid may indicate fetal distress and increases the risk that the baby will require resuscitation after birth. The baby is allowed to born completely and then assessed under the radiant warmer.

Meconium-stained Fluid and A Vigorous Newborn

If the baby is vigorous with good respiratory effort and muscle tone, the baby shall receive the usual initial steps of newborn care. Simply use a bulb syringe/Dee Lee's mucus trap to gently clear meconium-stained secretions from the mouth and nose.

Meconium-stained Fluid and A Non-vigorous Newborn

If a baby is born through meconium-stained amniotic fluid and has depressed respirations or poor muscle tone, bring the baby to the radiant warmer and perform the usual initial steps of newborn care. You will use a bulb syringe/ Dee Lee's mucus trap to clear secretions from the mouth and nose. If the baby is not breathing or the heart rate is less than 100 bpm after the initial steps are completed, proceed with PPV. Routine intubation for tracheal suction is not suggested. Previously routine endotracheal intubation and suction immediately was recommended after birth in an effort to reduce the chance of developing meconium aspiration syndrome; however, there is insufficient evidence to continue recommending this practice.

Positive Pressure Ventilation

Ventilation of the lungs is the single most important and most effective step in cardiopulmonary resuscitation of the compromised infant. Positive pressure ventilation can be given either with a resuscitation bag and mask or a bag and endotracheal tube. The principles of ventilation however, are same for both. The ability to perform safe and effective ventilation requires skill and practice.

Equipments

- Self-inflating infant resuscitation bag, oxygen reservoir, mask.
- Oxygen equipment (oxygen source, flow meter, oxygen tubing).
- Orogastric tube No.5 (for term), No. 6 (for preterm).
- Oral airways (size 0, 00 and 000).

Self-Inflating Bag

The self-inflating bag is designed so that it inflates automatically as the grip is released on the bag.

General Characteristics of the Self-Inflating Resuscitation Bag

1. Bags used for newborns should have a volume of 240–750 ml. The tidal volume of a term newborn is 5-8 ml/kg. Bags larger than 750 ml make it difficult to provide such small volumes.
2. The bag should be capable of delivering 90–100% oxygen. This can be achieved by attaching an oxygen source to a self-inflating bag with an oxygen reservoir.
3. The bag should have safety valves to avoid excessive pressure.
4. The mask should be of appropriate size.

Parts: There are 7 basic parts of the self-inflating bag:

- Air inlet.
- Oxygen inlet.
- Patient outlet.
- Valve assembly.
- Oxygen reservoir.
- Pressure release valve/safety valve.
- Pressure manometer attachment site.

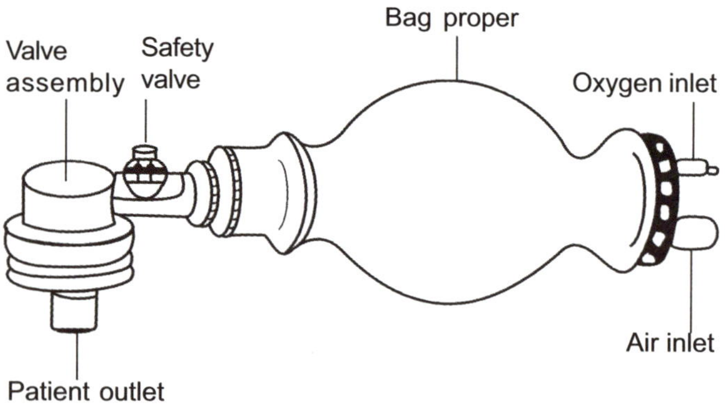

Fig. 7.33: Basic parts of the self-inflating bag

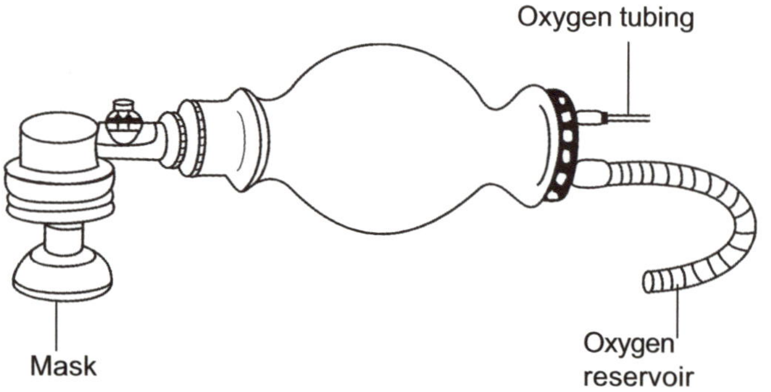

Fig. 7.34: Self-inflating bag with mask, oxygen reservoir and oxygen delivery tube

How to Assemble the Parts of the Bag?

1. The oxygen reservoir should be attached to the air inlet.
2. The oxygen tubing to the oxygen inlet.
3. A mask or endotracheal tube is to be attached to the patient outlet.

The Bag Proper

The bag is usually made of silicon rubber. It is available in three sizes: 240 ml, 500 ml, 750 ml. It has two inlets. The bigger one, called the air inlet, for attaching the oxygen reservoir and a smaller one to attach the oxygen delivery tube. There is an outlet to which the valve assembly is connected.

Valve Assembly

The valve assembly is positioned between the bag and patient outlet. It is a one-way valve. When the bag is squeezed during ventilation, the valve opens, releasing oxygen/air to the patient. When the bag reinflates, the valve is closed. This prevents the baby's exhaled air from entering the bag and being rebreathed.

Pressure Release Valve (Safety Valve)

Self-inflating bags should have a pressure release valve which is generally set to 30–40 cm H_2O. If pressures greater than 30–40 cm H_2O are generated, the valve opens limiting the pressure being transmitted to the newborn. A bag without safety features should never be used for positive pressure ventilation in a newborn.

Pressure Manometer Attachment Site

The attachment site usually consists of a small hole or a projection close to the patient outlet. If a bag has such a site the manometer should be attached or the hole sealed during ventilation. Otherwise, gas will leak through the opening, preventing adequate pressure from being generated.

Oxygen Reservoir

An oxygen reservoir is an appliance, either in the form of a corrugated tube with an open end or a bag with a valve, which can be attached over the air inlet. The function of this attachment is to increase the oxygen concentration in the bag to between 90–100% because both types will allow some air to enter the reservoir.

How Does It Work?

Each time the bag re-inflates during ventilation it will draw air into the bag through the air inlet. The air dilutes the oxygen concentration in the bag even though the 100% oxygen is flowing through the oxygen inlet. As a result, oxygen actually received by the baby is reduced to around 40%. The reservoir allows 100% oxygen to collect at the air inlet, thus preventing the oxygen from being diluted with room air.

No. A self-inflating bag cannot administer free flow oxygen. The amount of oxygen sent to the baby will depend on the relative resistance of the various valves and, therefore may not reach the baby unless the bag is being squeezed. Continuous flow of oxygen to the patient cannot be achieved.

Recommended Oxygen Concentration to Start Positive Pressure Ventilation

It is now established that resuscitation started with 21% oxygen is just as effective as resuscitation started with 100% oxygen. The recent recommendation for the initial resuscitation with PPV is as follows:

- For newborns greater than or equal to 35 weeks gestation, set the blender to 21% oxygen.
- For newborns less than 35 weeks gestation, set the blender to 21 – 30% oxygen.

The oxygen flow meter should be set to 10 litres/minute. Compare the baby's preductal oxygen saturation with the range of target values shown in Table 7.18 and adjust the oxygen concentration as needed.

How to Sterilize the Bag?

The infant resuscitation bag should be disinfected daily and sterilized weekly by cleaning with detergent after dismantling the parts and then immersed in 2% glutaraldehyde for 20 minutes for disinfection and 4 hours for sterilization, then rinsed with clean water and dried with sterile linen. Then the parts are reassembled.

2% glutaraldehyde once prepared is active for 14 days. It should be ensured that glutaraldehyde should be completely rinsed with water from objects before using on infants because these can be damaging to the infant.

How to Test the Self-Inflating Bag?

1. The bag reinflates quickly when you release your grip.
2. Block the mask or patient outlet by making a seal with the palm of your hand. Then squeeze the bag. Look for the following:
   - Do you feel pressure against your hand?
   - Can you force the pressure release valve open?
   - Does the pressure manometer (if present) register 30–40 cm H_2O pressure?

If the answer to any one of these questions is No, it indicates that the bag is not in working condition.

Mask

Masks of two sizes are available 0 (zero) and 1. But the *ideal size of the mask* should be one, which covers the tip of the chin, the mouth and the nose but does not cover the eyes.

How to Sterilize/Disinfect the Mask?

The mask should be disinfected daily and after each use and sterilized every week by cleaning with detergent and immersed in 2% glutaraldehyde for 20 minutes to disinfect and 4 hours to sterilize, then rinsed in clean water. It is then dried with autoclaved linen/sterile linen (washed and sundried).

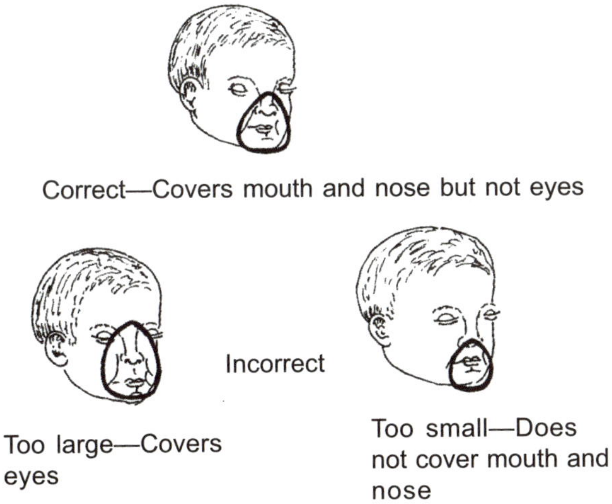

Fig. 7.35: Correct and incorrect size mask

Indications of Positive Pressure Ventilation (PPV)

1. Apnea or Gasping.
2. Heart rate less than 100/min.
3. Baby is breathing, heart rate is greater or equal to 100/minute, but cyanosed/oxygen saturation cannot be maintained within the target range despite free flow oxygen or CPAP.

When indicated, PPV should be started within 1 minute of birth.

How to Suspect Diaphragmatic Hernia?

1. Baby deteriorates with bag and mask ventilation.
2. On examination, abdomen is scaphoid, there is dextrocardia, normal breath sounds absent on the affected side, peristaltic sounds may be heard in the chest.

Rate of Ventilation

40 to 60 per minute.

Pressure

Initially, 30 to 40 cm H_2O pressure followed by 15 to 20 cm H_2O pressure. The preterm baby has a smaller tidal volume but stiffer lungs. So they require higher inflation pressure. Most apneic preterm infants can be ventilated with an initial inflation pressure 20 to 25 cm H_2O. If prompt improvement in heart rate or chest movement is not obtained higher pressures may be needed. If it is necessary to continue positive pressure ventilation, application of PEEP may be beneficial. Continuous positive airway pressure (CPAP) may also be beneficial in spontaneously breathing preterm infants after resuscitation.

Indicators of Proper Ventilation

1. A noticeable rise and fall of the chest is by far the best indication that the lungs are being inflated. The newborn should appear to be taking a normal or easy breath.
2. The presence of bilateral breath sounds and improvement of color are the other indications that the newborn is properly ventilated.

How Long to Ventilate?

30 seconds.

Procedure

1. Select the appropriate size mask.
2. Position the baby's head with slight extension of the neck. Ensure a clear airway. Suction the mouth and nose if necessary.
3. Position yourself at the head end. This position helps to hold the bag and mask comfortably. The sides kept free for two other persons in case needed for chest compression and vascular access via umbilical vein for medication. The bag should be positioned in such a way that it does not obstruct your view of the baby's chest. It is necessary to observe the rise and fall of chest during ventilation.
4. Position the bag and mask on the face. The mask should be placed on the face so that it covers the nose and mouth and the tip of the chin rests within the rim of the mask. The mask should be held on the face with the thumb, index and /or the middle finger encircling much of the rim of the mask while the ring and the little finger bring the chin forward to maintain a patent airway. Once the mask is positioned, an airtight seal can be formed by using light downward pressure on the rim of the mask.
5. Squeeze and release the bag at the rate of 40 to 60/ minute. To help maintain the rate, count loud squeeze —two—three. If you squeeze the bag to make the baby breathe and release while you say two three, probably you are ventilating at a proper rate.

   Continue ventilation for 30 seconds and then evaluate.

How Do You Evaluate Baby's Response to PPV?

The most important indicator of successful PPV is a rising heart rate. Two separate assessments should be made to look for the response.

First Heart Rate Assessment

Check heart rate after 15 seconds of PPV. The baby's heart rate should increase within 15 seconds of PPV.

Heart rate is increasing: Continue PPV and do the second assessment of heart rate after another 15 seconds.

Heart rate is not increasing: Look for chest movement with the assisted breaths.

Chest is moving: Heart rate not improving: Continue PPV and check heart rate after another 15 seconds.

Chest is not moving: Heart rate is not increasing: Perform the ventilation corrective steps until you achieve chest movement with ventilation. Continue PPV with chest movement and check heart rate after 30 seconds.

Second Heart Rate Assessment

Heart rate is greater than or equal to 100/minute: Gradually reduce the rate and pressure of PPV, observe for effective and spontaneous respiration. Discontinue PPV when the baby has a heart rate continuously above 100/minute and sustained spontaneous breathing.

Heart rate is atleast 60/minute but less than 100/minute: Continue PPV as long as the baby is showing steady improvement.

If not improving, reassess ventilation technique. Monitor heart rate, chest movement, respiratory effort, and oxygen saturation. Consider endotracheal intubation/laryngeal mask.

Heart rate less than 60/minute: Despite 30 seconds of PPV with good chest movement. Increase oxygen concentration (FiO_2) to 100% and begin chest compression.

If the baby is breathing spontaneously and has a heart rate atleast 100/minute, but has laboured respiration or low oxygen saturation, CPAP may be helpful. It is administered with a T-piece resuscitator or a flow inflating bag with a mask. The desired CPAP can be achieved by adjusting the PEEP cap in the T-piece resuscitator or the flow control valve on the flow inflating bag. The PEEP cap or the flow control valve has to be adjusted so that the manometer reads 5 cm H_2O pressure. A pressure more than 8 cm H_2O should not be used. If no response PPV may be required.

Causes of Inadequate Expansion of Chest

If the chest does not expand adequately, it may be due to one or more of the following reasons:

1. The seal is inadequate.
2. The airway is blocked.
3. Not enough pressure is being given.

Inadequate Seal: Results in leaking of air around the mask. The most common place for a leak is that between the cheek and the bridge of the nose. Reapply mask and use a little more pressure on the rim of the mask.

Blocked Airway: May be result of improper position of head or secretions in the airway. Reposition baby's head, check the mouth, oropharynx, nose for secretions. Suction the mouth and nose if necessary. If expansion is still inadequate, ventilate with open mouth using an oral airway.

Not Enough Pressure: May result from squeezing the bag with inadequate pressure. So, increase pressure until the pressure release valve actuates. While using a bag with a pressure manometer, check the amount of pressure required to result in adequate chest rise. If adequate chest rise does not occur after increasing pressure, endotracheal intubation and bag and tube ventilation is usually required.

Use of An Orogastric Tube

Newborns requiring prolonged bag and mask ventilation (more than 2 minutes) should have an orogastric tube inserted and left in place.

During bag and mask ventilation, oxygen and air mixture is forced into the oropharynx, where it is free to enter both the trachea and esophagus. Proper positioning of the newborn will transmit most of the air into the trachea and lungs. However, some air and oxygen may enter the esophagus and stomach.

Air–Oxygen forced into the stomach interferes with ventilation in the following ways:

1. A distended stomach puts pressure on the diaphragm, preventing full expansion of the lungs.
2. The air in the stomach may cause regurgitation of gastric contents, which may then be aspirated during bag and mask ventilation.

These problems can be reduced by insertion of an orogastric tube, suctioning of gastric contents, and leaving the tube in place to act as a vent for gas throughout the remainder of the resuscitation.

How to Insert An Orogastric Tube?

Equipments

1. 8 F feeding tube (a larger tube may make it difficult to obtain a seal. Secretions can easily occlude a smaller tube).
2. 20 ml syringe.

Steps

1. Measure the length of the tube. The length should be equal to the distance from the bridge of the nose to the ear lobe and from the ear lobe to the xiphoid process.
2. Insert the tube through the mouth. The nose should be kept open for ventilation.
3. After the tube is inserted for the desired length, the stomach contents should be gently aspirated with a 20 cc syringe.
4. Then remove the syringe and leave the end of the tube open.
5. Tape the tube to the baby's cheek to ensure that the tip remains in the stomach.

Chest Compression

Indications of Chest Compression

Chest compression should be started when the heart rate remains less than 60/minute despite 30 seconds of effective positive pressure ventilation with supplementary oxygen.

Ventilation is the most effective action in neonatal resuscitation. Therefore one should ensure that assisted ventilation is being delivered optimally before starting chest compressions.

Why to Perform Chest Compression?

Babies who have a heart rate below 60/minute, despite stimulation and 30 seconds of positive pressure ventilation, probably have very low blood oxygen levels. As a result, the myocardium is depressed and unable to contract strongly enough to pump blood to the lungs. Therefore, there is need to mechanically pump the heart with simultaneous ventilation of the lungs with 100% oxygen until the myocardium becomes sufficiently oxygenated to recover adequate spontaneous function. This process will also help to restore oxygen delivery to the brain.

It is noteworthy that those who are skilled at endotracheal intubation may choose to intubate at this time to ensure adequate ventilation and facilitate the coordination of ventilation and chest compressions.

What are Chest Compressions?

Chest compressions consist of rhythmic compressions of the sternum leading to:

- Compression of the heart against the spine.
- Increase the intrathoracic pressure.
- Circulate blood to the vital organs of the body.

When pressure on the sternum is released, blood enters the heart from the veins.

How Many People are Needed to Administer Chest Compressions?

Chest compressions are of little value without positive pressure ventilation with 100% oxygen. Therefore, two people are required to administer chest compression. One to compress the chest and one to continue ventilation.

The person performing chest compression should be on one side of the baby while the other performing ventilation should be at the head end.

Methods of Chest Compression

There are two techniques to perform chest compression:

Thumb technique: The two thumbs are used to depress the sternum, while the hands encircle the torso and the fingers support the spine. If the baby is large or your hands are small be sure that the baby is on a firm surface.

Two finger technique: The tips of the middle and either the index or ring finger of one hand are used to compress the sternum. The other hand is used to support the baby's back unless the baby is on a firm surface.

Advantages and Disadvantages

The *thumb technique* is preferred because it is less tiring and control of depth of compression is better. The disadvantages of thumb technique are:

- It is not effective in large babies or if the operator's hand is small.
- Access to the umbilical cord is more difficult when medications are necessary.

The *two-finger technique* is not preferred because:

- It is tiring if chest compression is required for a prolonged period.
- Control of depth of pressure is difficult.

Advantages of the two-finger technique are:

- It can be used regardless of size of baby or size of operator's hands.
- Leaves the umbilicus more accessible in case medications must be administered via umbilical route.

Site of Compression

For chest compression, pressure should be applied to the lower third of sternum. The correct area can be located by running your fingers along the lower edge of the ribs until you locate the xiphoid. Then place your thumbs or fingers immediately above the xiphoid.

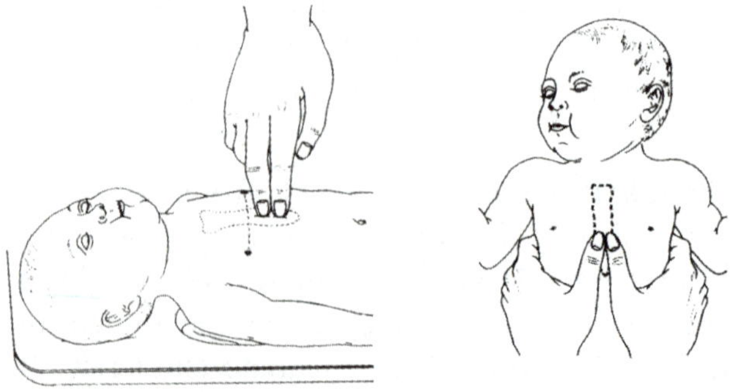

Fig. 7.36: Position for fingers during compression

Thumb Technique

a. The thumbs can be placed side by side or in a small baby one over the other.

b. Only the thumbs will be used to compress the sternum, the other fingers will provide the support needed for the back.

c. The thumb should be flexed at the first interphalangeal joint and pressure applied vertically.

Two Finger Technique

a. The tips of the middle and ring or index finger of one hand are used for compression.

b. The other hand should be used to support the newborn's back.

c. When compressing the chest, only two finger tips should rest on the chest.

d. The pressure should be applied vertically.

How Much Pressure to Use to Compress The Chest?

Controlling the pressure, used to compress the sternum, is an important part of the procedure of chest compression. With the fingers and hands correctly positioned, enough pressure should be used to *depress the sternum to depth of approximately one third of the anterior posterior diameter of the chest.*

Rate of Compression

One cycle of events will consist of 3 compressions and one ventilation. A four-event cycle should take one ventilation interposed after every third compression. It should be remembered that:

- Simultaneous compression and ventilation should be avoided since one will decrease the efficacy of the other.
- A lower ventilatory rate is needed to provide an adequate number of compressions and avoid simultaneous compression and ventilation.

Points to be Noted

1. One compression consists of the downward stroke plus the release.
2. The actual distance compressed will depend on the size of the baby.
3. The duration of down stroke of compression should be shorter than the duration of release for generation of maximum cardiac output.
4. The thumbs or the fingers should remain in contact with the chest at all times during both compression and release. Lifting of the fingers between compressions may lead to:
   - Waste of time in relocating compression area.
   - Loss of control over the depth of compression.
   - Compression of a wrong area—producing trauma to the chest wall and underlying organs.
5. *Chest compression should be accompanied by positive pressure ventilation with 100% oxygen.*
6. The chance of air entry to the stomach is higher while delivering chest compression and PPV. Therefore, endotracheal intubation and bag and tube ventilation is preferable. If not possible, an orogastric tube should be passed to vent the stomach.

Chest Compression: How Long? When to Stop?

After 30 seconds of well-coordinated chest compression and PPV, the heart rate should be counted or pulse felt (umbilical artery, brachial artery) for 6 seconds. The rate obtained multiplied by 10 gives the rate in 1 minute.

- *If heart rate is above 60/ minute:* Stop chest compression but continue PPV till heart rate is above 100/minute.
- *If heart rate is below 60/minute:* Continue chest compression, PPV and start medications.

The Rhythm of Compression and Ventilation and How to Practice it?

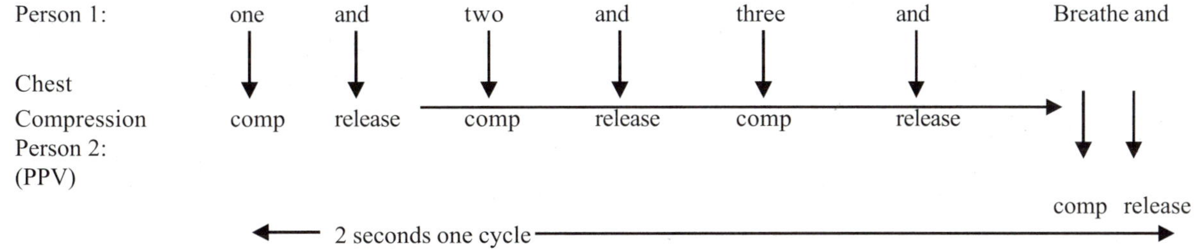

Medications

Drugs are rarely indicated in resuscitation of the newly born infant. Bradycardia in the newborn infant is usually the result of inadequate lung inflation or profound hypoxemia, and establishing adequate ventilation is the most important step to correct it.

Indication

If heart rate remains below 60/minute despite administration of chest compression and PPV with 100% oxygen for 30 seconds, medications are indicated.

Drugs to be Administered

The following drugs should be administered in the sequence as shown below:

1. **Epinephrine:** Despite good ventilation of the lungs with PPV and improved cardiac output from chest compression, a small number of newborn (less than 2/1000 biths) will still have a heart rate of less than 60/minute. The heart muscles of these babies may have been deprived of oxygen for so long that it will not contract effectively despite now being perfused with oxygenated blood. These babies may benefit from receiving epinephrine. Epinephrine increases the rate and strength of cardiac contraction and causes peripheral vasoconstriction. This may play a role in increasing blood flow through the coronary arteries and brain. Epinephrine is the first drug to be used.

   Indication: When heart rate is <60/minute despite 30 seconds of chest compressions and PPV with 100% oxygen.

   Dose and route: The recommended doses of intravenous and intraosseous epinephrine are 0.1 to 0.3 ml/kg (equal to 0.01 to 0.03 mg/kg) and a dose of 0.5 to 1 mL/kg (equal to 0.05 to 1 mg/kg) by endotracheal tube. Epinephrine is given rapidly. The I.V. and intraosseous bolus should be followed with a 0.5 – 1 mL flush of normal saline. The I.V./intraosseous route are the preferred routes. The endotracheal route may be considered while an I.V. access is being obtained. The concentration of epinephrine for all routes should be 1:10,000 (0.1 mg/mL).

   Anticipated effect: Heart rate should increase to more than 60/minute within 30 seconds. If this does not happen, the dose can be repeated every 3–5 minutes. Administration of epinephrine should always be accompanied by effective chest compression and bag and tube ventilation.

2. **Volume expander:** Administration of a volume expander may be indicated if the baby is not responding to resuscitation and there is evidence of blood loss and shock (pale skin, poor perfusion, weak pulse). In shock, the baby may have a persistently high or low heart rate and circulatory status will not improve in response to effective ventilation, chest compression and epinephrine.

   Recommended solutions: The recommended solution for acutely treating hypovolemia is an isotonic crystalloid e.g. Normal saline or Ringer's lactate. In case of very large volume blood loss, O negative blood crossed matched with mother's blood can be used.

   Dose, route and rate of administration: 10 ml/kg by umbilical vein/intraosseous over 5–10 minutes. If the baby shows minimal improvement after the first dose another dose of 10 ml/kg may be given.

   Warning: Preterm babies have a very fragile network of capillaries in the germinal matrix of the brain. Too rapid administration of volume expanders may result in intracranial hemorrhage.

The Newborn is Not Improving After Giving Epinephrine and Volume Expander. What To Do?

1. Positive pressure ventilation and chest compression should be continued.
2. Reassess the quality of ventilation and chest compression.
3. Intravenous epinephrine may be repeated every 3 to 5 minutes.

Procedures

How to Give Epinephrine Through An Endotracheal Tube?

a. The desired dose of epinephrine is diluted with normal saline to a full syringe volume (1 ml) before injection into the endotracheal tube.
b. The full 1ml is injected directly into the endotracheal tube. The medication is then forced into the lungs during PPV.
c. The drug volume can also be injected into a 5 F feeding tube that has been inserted down the endotracheal tube.

How to Give Epinephrine Through the Umbilical Vein?

a. Pre fill a 5 F umbilical catheter with normal saline.
b. Cut the umbilical cord perpendicularly with a sterile scalpel, 1–2 cm from the skin line.
c. Identify the umbilical vein (seen as a large, thin walled structure, usually at the 11 to 12 O'clock position). The two umbilical arteries are thick walled; lie close together in the 4 and 8 O'clock position.
d. Insert catheter into umbilical vein. The tip of the catheter should be located only a short distance into the vein when blood can first be aspirated.
e. The drug volume is then injected.

After resuscitation is complete the catheter is removed and the cord tie is tightened.

Neonatal Resuscitation Medications

Medication	*Concentration to administer*	*Preparation*	*Dosage and route*	*Rate and precautions*
Epinephrine	1:10,000 (0.1 mg/ml)	1 ml	0.01-0.03 ml/kg IV or intraosseous	Give rapidly, may repeat every 3-5 minutes.
Volume expanders	Whole blood, 5% albumin, normal saline, ringer's lactate	Varies	10 ml/kg IV	Give over 5-10 minutes. Repeat as needed.
Sodium bicarbonate	0.5 mEq/ml (4.2% solution)	20 ml or two 10 ml prefilled syringes	2 mEq/kg (4 ml/kg) IV	Give slowly, over at least 2 minutes, may repeat every 10 minutes. Ventilate infant.
Narcan (Naloxone)	0.4 mg/ml	1 ml	0.01 mg/kg (0.25 ml/kg) IV, IM	Give rapidly.

Endotracheal Intubation

Endotracheal intubation may be indicated at several points during neonatal resuscitation.

Indications

1. Prolonged positive pressure ventilation (beyond a few minutes).
2. Bag and mask ventilation is not effective.
3. When chest compressions are performed.
4. Special circumstances viz. suspected congenital diaphragmatic hernia and extreme LBW (< 1000 g).

Equipments

1. Infant laryngoscope with an extra set of batteries and extra bulbs.
2. *Blades:* No.1 (term newborn), No.0 (preterm newborn) No. 00 (optional for extremely preterm newborn. Straight blades are preferred.
3. Sterile, disposable endotracheal tubes with inside diameters of 2.5, 3.0, 3.5 and 4.0 mm.
4. Stylet (optional).
5. Carbon dioxide monitor (optional).
6. Suction setup with 10F or larger suction catheter.
7. Roll tape, ½ or ¾ inch, scissors.
8. Oral airway.
9. Self-inflating infant resuscitation bag and mask with oxygen reservoir.
10. Stethoscope.

Selection of Endotracheal Tube

1. Sterile disposable tubes should be used.
2. Tubes should be of uniform diameter throughout the length of the tube not tapered near the tip. The disadvantages of the tube with tapered end are:
   - During intubation, the view of the tracheal opening is easily obstructed by the wide part of the tube.
   - Tubes with shoulders are more likely to cause trauma to vocal cord.
3. The tube should have a vocal cord guide (a black line near the tip of the tube). While inserting the tube the vocal cord guide should be placed at the level of the vocal cord. This usually positions the tip of the tube above the bifurcation of the trachea (carina). The length of the trachea in a preterm newborn is less than that in a term newborn, 3 cm versus 5 to 6 cm. Therefore, smaller the tube, the closer the vocal cord guide is to the tip of the tube.

Parts of An Endotracheal Tube

- The tube proper.
- A connector. The connectors are made to fit a specific size tubes. They cannot be interchanged.

Preparation of the Endotracheal Tube

1. Select the appropriate size tube.
2. Cut the tube at 13–15 cm length: Remove connector and cut the tube diagonally. Replace the connector.

Table 7.19 : Selection of appropriate tube size on the basis of weight/gestation

Tube size(mm)	*Weight (gm)*	*Gestational age (wks)*
2.5	Below 1,000	Below 28
3.0	1,000 – 2000	28 – 34
3.5	2,000 – 3000	34 – 38
3.5 – 4.0	Above 3000	Above 38

Parts of the Infant Laryngoscope

1. A handle.
2. Blade.

Sterilization/Disinfection

The laryngoscope blade should be wiped with 70% isopropyl alcohol or sterillium after each use. Cidex or glutaraldehyde should never be used.

Preparation of the Laryngoscope

1. Select blade and attach to the laryngoscope handle: No. 0 for preterm and No. 1 for term newborns.
2. Turn on the light to determine that the batteries and bulb are working. Check to see that the bulb is screwed in tightly to ensure that it will not flicker or fall out during the procedure.

Preparation of Suction Equipment

1. Adjust the suction source to 100 mm Hg.
2. Connect suction catheter of size as necessary.

Anatomical Landmarks

The following anatomical landmarks are important to understand the procedure of intubation:

1. *Vallecula:* A pouch formed by the base of the tongue and the epiglottis.

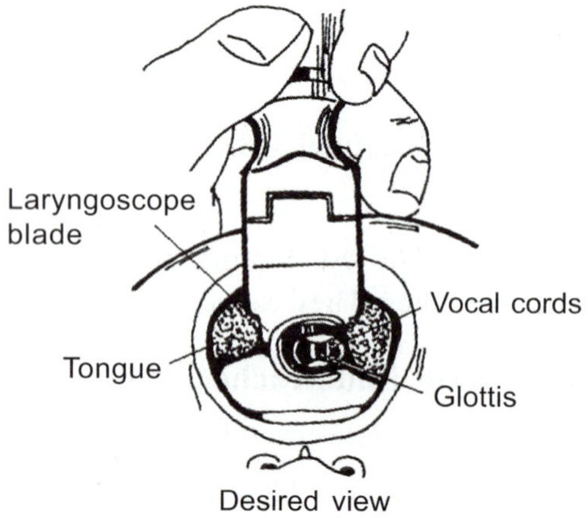

Fig. 7.37: Anatomical landmarks

2. *Epiglottis:* A lid like structure over hanging the entrance to the trachea.
3. *Glottis:* The opening to the trachea; contains the vocal cords.
4. *Vocal cords:* Folds of mucous membrane on both sides of the trachea, just within the glottis.
5. *Esophagus:* The food passage situated just posterior to the tracheal opening.

Steps of Intubation

1. Position the baby with neck in slight extension.
2. Turn on the laryngoscope light and hold the laryngoscope in the left hand between the thumb and first two or three fingers with the blade pointing away from you. The laryngoscope is designed to be held in the left hand by both right and left-handed persons. If held in the right hand, the curved part of the blade will block the view of the glottis, as well as make insertion of the endotracheal tube impossible.
3. Visualization of glottis and insertion of the tube: During actual resuscitation the following steps will need to be completed within approximately 20 seconds. Free flow oxygen should be delivered throughout the procedure.
   a. *Stabilize the baby's head* with your right hand. A second person may be called to hold the head in the proper position.
   b. *Slide the laryngoscope blade from the left angle of the mouth*, over the right side of the tongue, pushing the tongue to the left side of the mouth, and advance the blade until the tip lies in the vallecula, just beyond the base of the tongue. You may need to use your right index finger to open the mouth to make it easier to insert the laryngoscope.
   c. *Lift the blade by raising the entire blade* by pulling up in the direction the handle is pointing, to expose the pharyngeal area.
   d. *Look for the landmarks*: If the tip of the laryngoscope is correctly positioned in the vallecula, you should see the epiglottis at the top, with the glottic opening below. You also should see the vocal cords appearing as vertical stripes on each side of the glottis or as an inverted letter "V". If these structures are not immediately visible, you should quickly adjust the blade until the structures come into view. Applying

downward pressure to the cricoid may help bring the glottis into view. The pressure may be applied with your own little finger or by an assistant. Suctioning of the secretions also may be helpful to improve your view.

e. *Insertion of tube*: Holding the tube in your right hand, introduce it into the right side of the baby's mouth. This will prevent the tube from blocking your view of the glottis. Keep the glottis in view and when the vocal cords are apart, insert the tip of the endotracheal tube until the vocal cord guide is at the level of the cords. This will position the tube in the trachea approximately halfway between the vocal cords and the carina.

f. *If the cords are together,* wait for them to open. Do not touch the closed cords with the tip of the tube. It may cause spasm of the cords. If the cords do not open within 20 seconds, stop and ventilate with bag and mask. After the heart rate and color have improved, you can then try again.

g. *Stabilize the tube* with one hand and remove the laryngoscope with the other. With the right hand held against the face, hold the tube firmly at the lips and/or use a finger to hold the tube against the baby's hard palate. Use your left hand to carefully remove the laryngoscope without displacing the tube. If the stylet was used, remove it from the endotracheal tube.

h. *Check to be sure that the tube is in the trachea:* If the tube is positioned correctly, one should observe:
   - A rise in the chest with each breath.
   - Breath sounds over both lung fields but decreased or absent over the stomach. Use a small stethoscope and place it laterally and high on the chest wall (in the axilla). A large stethoscope or a stethoscope placed too central or too low may transmit sounds from the esophagus or stomach.
   - No gastric distension with ventilation.
   - Vapour condensing on the inside of the tube during exhalation.
   - You can use the tip to lip measurement to estimate if the tube has been inserted the correct distance. Adding 6 to the baby's weight in kilograms will give a rough estimate to the correct distance from the tube tip to the vermilion border of the upper lip. Babies weighing less than 750 gms may require only 6 cm insertion.
   - Detection of presence of CO_2 in the endotracheal tube can serve as confirmatory evidence that the tube is in the trachea by using a CO_2 detector viz. capnograph or a colorometric device connected to the endotracheal tube. However, ELBW babies or babies with very poor cardiac output may exhale insufficient CO_2 to be detected reliably by CO_2 detectors.

To Ventilate the Baby

- Attach an infant resuscitation bag to the tube and resume PPV with 100% oxygen.

What Do You Do If You Suspect That the Tube is Not in the Trachea?

The tube is likely to be not in the trachea if you:

- Do not see the chest rise.
- Do not hear good breath sounds over the lungs.
- Do hear noises over the stomach.
- There is no mist in the tube.
- The abdomen appears to become distended.
- The CO_2 monitor does not indicate the presence of exhaled CO_2.
- The newborn remains cyanotic and bradycardic despite PPV.

If you suspect that the tube is not in the trachea you should:

- Remove the tube, use a bag and mask to stabilize the heart rate and color and then repeat intubation procedure.

How Do You Continue Resuscitation While You Intubate?

It is not possible to continue chest compression and PPV while intubating the baby. Therefore an effort should be made to minimize the amount of hypoxia imposed during intubation. The following will be helpful:

- *Pre-oxygenate before attempting intubation:* Oxygenate the baby appropriately with bag and mask before beginning intubation and between repeated intubation attempts.

- *Deliver free flow oxygen during intubation:* Hold 100% free flow oxygen by the baby's face while the intubator is clearing the airway and trying to visualize the landmarks. If the baby makes any spontaneous respiratory efforts during the procedure, he will be breathing oxygen-enriched air.
- *Limit attempts to 20 seconds:* If you are unable to visualize the glottis and insert the tube within 20 seconds, remove the laryngoscope and attempt to oxygenate the baby with bag and mask ventilation using 100% oxygen. Then try again.

What Can Go Wrong While You are Trying to Intubate?

1. *You may have problems visualizing glottis. The problems may be as follows:*

Problems	*Landmarks*	*Corrective action*
Laryngoscope not inserted far enough	You see the tongue surrounding the blade	Advance the blade
Laryngoscope inserted too far	You see the walls of the esophagus surrounding the blade	Withdraw blade slowly until the epiglottis and glottis are seen
Laryngoscope inserted off to one side	You see part of the glottis off to one side of the blade	Gently move the blade to midline. Then advance or retreat according to landmarks seen

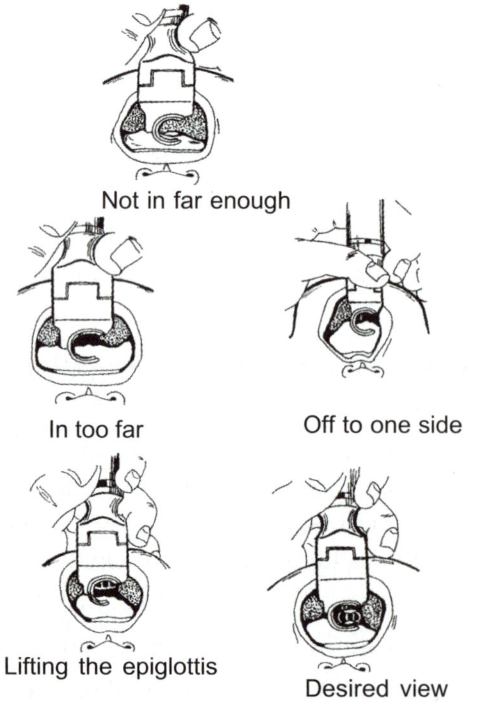

Fig. 7.38

   - Poor visualization of the glottis also may be caused by not elevating the tongue high enough to bring the glottis into view.
   - Pressure applied over the cricoid by the 4th or 5th finger will help to bring the glottis into view.
   - One should practice intubating in the manikin, dead babies enough times to find the correct landmarks quickly, thus allowing one to insert the tube within 20 seconds.

2. *You may insert the tube into the esophagus instead of trachea:* It is worse to have a tube in the esophagus than no tube at all since the tube will tend to obstruct the baby's pharyngeal airway without providing an artificial airway. If there is concern that the tube is in the esophagus, one should visualize the glottis and the tube with a laryngoscope and/or remove the tube, oxygenate the newborn with a bag and mask, and reintroduce the tube.

The signs of endotracheal tube in esophagus are:

- Poor chest movement.
- No breath sounds are heard.
- Hear air entering the stomach.
- Gastric distension may be seen.
- No mist in the tube.
- CO_2 detector fails to show presence of expired CO_2.
- Poor response to intubation (cyanosis, bradycardia etc.).

3. *You may insert the tube too far into the trachea:* If the tube is inserted too far, it usually passes into the right bronchus. It is important to remember to watch the vocal cord guide on the tube and stop inserting as soon as the guide reaches the cord.

If you think that the tube may be in the right main bronchus:

- Check the tip to lip measurement.
- Withdraw the tube slightly while you listen over the left chest to hear if the breath sounds improve.

The signs of the tube being in the right bronchus include:

- Breath sounds heard over the right and not on the left side of the chest.
- Louder breath sounds on the right side than on the left side.

- Lack of improvement in the baby's color or heart rate.

Complications, Possible Causes and Corrective Action of Endotracheal Intubation

Complication	*Possible causes*	*Corrective action*
1. Hypoxia	Taking too long to intubate	Pre-oxygenation, free flow O_2 during procedure, halt intubation after 20 secs.
	Incorrect placement of tube	Reposition tube.
2. Bradycardia/ Apnea	Hypoxia	Pre-oxygenation with bag and mask.
	Vagal response from Laryngoscope/ suction catheter	Free flow O_2 during procedure. Oxygenate after intubation with bag and tube.
3. Pneumothorax	Over ventilation of one lung due to tube in right main bronchus	Place tube correctly. Use appropriate ventilating pressure.
4. Contusions or lacerations of tongue, gums or airway	Rough handling of laryngoscope or tube. Inappropriate rocking rather than lifting of laryngoscope	Obtain additional practice/skill.
	Laryngoscope blade too long or too short	Select appropriate equipment.
5. Perforation of esophagus	Too vigorous insertion of tube. Stylet protrudes beyond end of tube	Handle gently. Place stylet properly.
6. Obstructed endotracheal tube	Kink in the tube or tube obstructed with secretions	Try to suction tube with catheter. If unsuccessful consider replacing tube.
7. Infection	Introduction of organism via hands or equipment	Pay careful attention to clean/ sterile technique.

When to Discontinue Resuscitation?

The persistent absence of heartbeat (Apgar 0) at 10 minutes is a strong, but not an absolute predictor of mortality and serious morbidity in late preterm and term newborns. If there is a confirmed absence of heartbeat after 10 minutes of resuscitation, it is reasonable to stop resuscitative efforts; however, the decision to continue or discontinue should be individualized.

Summary

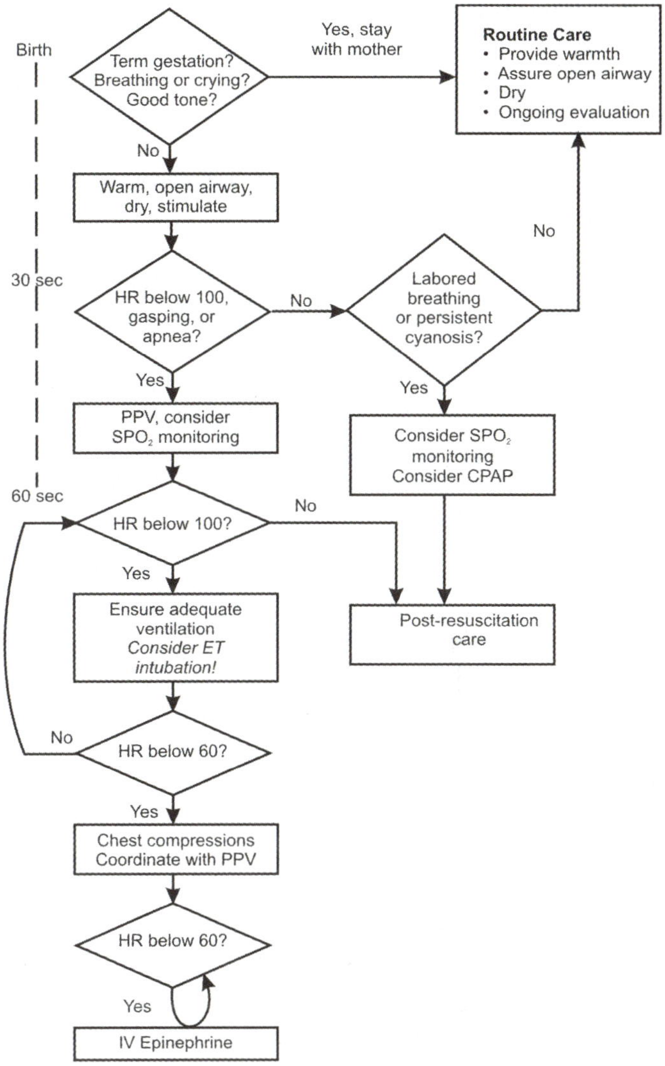

Flowchart: Algorithm of neonatal resuscitation

Suggested Reading

1. Hutchison's Practical Pediatric Problems, 6th edition, 1986. Published by Singapore National Printers.
2. Manual of neonatal care edited by John P. Cloherty, Eric C. Eichenwald and Ann Stark, 5th edition, 2004.
3. Manual of care of critical newborn edited by J.N.Sharma, 1st edition, 2007. Peepee Publishers and Distributors (P) Ltd, New Delhi.
4. Report of National Neonatal Perinatal Database (National Neonatology Forum, India) 2000.
5. American Academy of Pediatrics, American College of Obstetricians and Gynecologists: Guidelines for perinatal care, 3rd edition, Elk Grove Village, Illinois: American Academy of Pediatrics 1992.

6. Neonatal Vade-Mecum edited by Brian Speidel, Peter Fleming, John Henderson *et al.,* 3rd edition, 1998. Published by Oxford University Press Inc., New York.
7. Forfar Arniel's Textbook of Pediatrics edited by Neil McIntosh, Peter Helms, Rosalind Smyth, 6th edition, 2003. Published by Churchill Livingstone.
8. Resource book for training of PHC Medical Officers. Published by WHO Collaborating Centre for Training and Research in Newborn Care, AIIMS, New Delhi.
9. Avery's diseases of the newborn, 8th edition, 2005, edited by Taesch, Ballard and Gleason. Published by Elsevier, New Delhi.
10. Textbook of Neonatology edited by D.Vidyasagar, 1st edition, 1987, published by Imprint, New Delhi.
11. Challenges in Neonatology. Editor Arvind Saili, Jaypee Brothers, Medical Publishers (P) Ltd, New Delhi, 1st edition, 1997.
12. Newborn care training and operationalisation at Primary Health Centres, Resource book. Training of PHC Medical Officers. WHO collaborating centre for training and research in newborn care, AIIMS, New Delhi.
13. Textbook on Neonatal Resuscitation, 4th edition, 2003. Editor John Kattwinkel based on original text by Ronald S. Bloom and Catherine Cropley. American Academy of Pediatrics and American Heart Association.
14. American Heart Association Guidelines for Cardiopulmonary Resuscitation and Emergency Cardiovascular Care: Part 13: Neonatal Resuscitation Guidelines, Circulation 2005: 112: IV 188 – IV 195.
15. Indian J Pediatrics 2001; 68: 963-965.
16. A review of literature. WHO/CHD 1997; 97(1): 1-55.
17. Manual of neonatal intensive care, fourth edition and first Indian edition, 2004,Viva Books Pvt. Ltd., Daryaganj, New Delhi.
18. Text Book of Neonatal Resuscitation, 7th edition. Editor Gary M. Weiner. Published by American Academy of Pediatrics, 2016.
19. Facility based Newborn care: Training module for doctors and nurses (2014).

8

Hematology

OUTLINES

Anemia: Definition and Classification

Definition

Anemia is defined as a reduction of hemoglobin concentration or red cell volume below the lower extreme of normal range for the age and sex of an individual.

For diagnosis of anemia one has to always refer to the normal range of hemoglobin appropriate for age and sex. Otherwise it may lead to a misdiagnosis because an acceptable level in a one year old could represent moderately severe anemia in an adult male.

The red cell count does provide an alternative means of assessment, but it can be in the normal range in children who are anemic on the basis of hemoglobin when the cells are microcytic. Further, the red cell indices can be abnormal when the underlying disorder is not sufficiently severe to cause anemia. Hence the hemoglobin level is employed as the prime arbiter in diagnosis of anemia.

WHO has recommended a hemoglobin cut off point of 11 gm% for children aged 6 months to 6 years and 12 gms % for children aged 6 to 14 years, to define anemia.

Grading of Anemia: WHO Classification

Mild Anemia: > 10 gm/dl to < normal for age.

Moderate Anemia: 7 gm/dl to 10 gm/dl.

Severe Anemia: < 7 gm/dl.

Very Severe Anemia: < 5 gm/dl.

Screening for Anemia

A routine hemoglobin test to detect anemia is recommended in the children of the following age groups:

1. At about 1 year age in term infants and at 6–9 months in preterm infants.
2. Between 2 and 3 years age.
3. At 5 years age and during early adolescence.

These are the periods during which the prevalence of iron deficiency anemia is highest in many populations.

Classification

Anemia may be classified on the basis of the etiology and pathogenesis or on the morphology of the red cells. However, the two classifications are complementary to each other as the clinical investigation of a patient with anemia involves two distinct steps: determination of the morphological type of anemia and determination of the cause of anemia. The morphological type of the anemia frequently gives a lead to the cause of anemia.

Morphological Classification

The morphological classification is based on two features, viz. mean corpuscular volume (MCV) and the mean corpuscular hemoglobin concentration (MCHC). The red cell absolute values (MCV and MCHC) are calculated from the red cell count, the hemoglobin and hematocrit estimations. However, it should be noted that the MCV is subjected to error because of the inherent error of the red cell count from which it is calculated.

In practice, therefore, red cell morphology is usually best determined by the examination of a well made and well stained peripheral blood film. This allows estimation of red cell size as indicated by the diameter of the cells and an assessment of the concentration of the hemoglobin in the individual cells. Further, the examination of the peripheral blood film also gives information about variations in size and shape of the red cells and information about the white blood cells as well as the platelets. The MCHC, however, a reliable estimation, can be determined to confirm the state of hemoglobin concentration as assessed by examination of the blood film. The following morphological types are recognized:

1. The *normocytic anemias,* in which the MCV is within normal range (76–96 cubic micron). Most normocytic anemias are normochromic with a normal MCHC (30–35%), but in some there may be mild hypochromia. The common causes are bone marrow failure, renal failure and chronic infection.
2. The *microcytic hypochromic anemias* in which the MCV is reduced (< 76 cubic micron) and the MCHC is also reduced (< 30%). The common causes include iron deficiency, thalassemia trait, lead poisoning, chronic disease, sideroblastic anemia and HbE hemoglobinopathy.
3. The *macrocytic anemias* in which the MCV is increased (> 96 cubic micron). Most macrocytic anemias are normochromic but in some there may be mild hypochromia. The common causes are Vitamin B_{12} and folic acid deficiency.

Classification on the Basis of Pathogenesis and Etiology

Anemia can result from three fundamental disturbances viz. blood loss, impaired red cell formation by the bone marrow and increased destruction of the red cells. However, more than one factor can contribute to the anemia.

Both acute and chronic *blood loss* can cause anemia. Acute blood loss results in normocytic normochromic or macrocytic normochromic anemia whereas chronic blood loss initially results in normocytic normochromic anemia but later microcytic hypochromic anemia when the body iron stores are exhausted.

Table 8.1 : Classification of anemia on the basis of pathogenesis and etiology

1. *Blood loss:* Acute and chronic
2. Impaired red cell formation
   a. Due to deficiency of substances essential for erythropoiesis viz. Iron, folic acid, Vitamin B_{12}, ascorbic acid, protein.
   b. Due to metabolic disturbance of bone marrow function caused by a systemic disorder viz. Infection, renal failure, liver disease, collagen disease, hypothyroidism, hypopituitarism, aplastic anemia.
   c. Due to infiltration of bone marrow by abnormal cells viz. leukemia, lymphoma, sideroblastic anemia and aplasia.
3. Increased red cell destruction
   a. Hemolytic anemias due to intracorpuscular or intrinsic abnormality.
   b. Hemolytic anemia due to extracorpuscular or extrinsic abnormality.

Impaired red cell formation may result from two types of disturbances (1) Due to deficiency of substances essential for erythropoiesis viz. iron, folic acid, Vitamin $B_{12,}$ uncommonly ascorbic acid and rarely protein. (2) Due to either a metabolic disturbance of bone marrow function caused by a systemic disorder or by disorders associated with bone marrow infiltration with abnormal cells.

Increased red cell destruction which results in hemolytic anemia is common in this part of the country. Hemolysis may result from intrinsic defect of the red blood cells or due to an abnormal hemolytic mechanism.

Physiological Anemia of Infancy

The hemoglobin level at birth is very high, as high as 17 gm/dl from umbilical cord blood, 19 gm/dl from venous blood and 21 gm/dl from skin prick blood. The hemoglobin level falls to 10–11 gm/dl by the age of 8–12 weeks. This decline in hemoglobin level is referred to as physiological anemia of infancy. This condition is seen in both term and preterm infants and the same mechanism is operative in both but exaggerated in the preterm. Hence there is more rapid and more extreme decline of the hemoglobin level in the preterm. In the preterm infant the minimal hemoglobin levels may be 7–9 gm/dl by 3–6 weeks of birth with even lower levels in small premature infants.

Etiopathogenesis

The cause of this anemia is multifactorial. With the onset of respiration, hemoglobin-oxygen saturation increases from 50–95% or more. After birth, the normal developmental switch from fetal to adult hemoglobin synthesis replaces high oxygen affinity fetal hemoglobin with lower oxygen affinity adult hemoglobin, which can deliver a greater fraction of hemoglobin bound oxygen to the tissues. This increase in blood oxygen content and tissue oxygen delivery, immediately after birth, down regulates erythropoietin production resulting in suppression of erythropoiesis. In absence of erythropoiesis, the hemoglobin level decrease because there is no replacement of the aged RBCs as they are normally removed from the circulation. The decrease in hemoglobin concentration continues until tissue oxygen needs are higher than oxygen delivery. This point is reached between 8–12 weeks when the hemoglobin level is 9–11 g/dl. The resultant hypoxia is detected by the hepatic and renal oxygen sensors. Erythropoietin production increases and erythropoiesis resumes.

Treatment

Physiological anemia of infancy does not create any hematological problem and no treatment is required. However, cell transfusion / recombinant human erythropoietin may be necessary in treatment of premature infants. In an otherwise healthy preterm infant, hemoglobin level as low as 6.5 gm/dL is well tolerated. When transfusion is necessary, the recommended value of packed cell volume is 10–15 ml/kg. In very low birth weight preterm infants, use of recombinant human erythropoietin and oral iron (4–6 mg/kg/day) during the first 6 weeks of life has shown to decrease the need of transfusion but the cost of treatment is very high. Parenteral iron may be used in infants who are not able to take oral iron.

Iron Deficiency Anemia

Iron deficiency anemia is the mostcommon nutritional cause of anemia affecting mankind globally. Infants, preschool children, adolescents and women of child bearing age are most vulnerable to develop iron deficiency anemia. In 0–4 years old children, the worldwide prevalence is approximately 40%. In India, prevalence in preschool children is about 60–75% and in the 5–10 years group it is about 50%. In adolescent girls and in pregnant women it is around 75–80%.

The WHO criteria for diagnosis of iron deficiency anemia are hemoglobin less than 11 gm %, red cell distribution width more than 15% and serum ferritin value less than 12 ng/mL.

Sources of Iron

Body Store

At birth, the iron content of the body is directly proportional to the weight. 80% of body iron is present in blood and 20% in the tissues. During the early months after birth, as a result of hemolysis of the RBCs, the hemoglobin level falls from nearly 20 gm% at birth to 10–12 gms% in the third month. This is accompanied by storing of released iron in the body. In full term infant the iron rises in the tissues from an average of 30 mg/kg body weight at birth to 80 mg/kg body weight at 3 months. A low birth weight infant, owing to the decreased period of gestation or being small for date, has less iron stores. It is around 6 mg/kg body weight at birth with a small rise to 25 mg/kg at 3 months. In addition, the rapid growth of a low birth weight infant puts an increased demand on the already poor iron stores.

A term infant has adequate iron stores to meet the post natal growth upto 4–6 months age. A preterm infant has a lower total body iron, although the proportion of iron to body weight is similar. Due to the rapid post natal growth they can develop iron deficiency by 8–12 weeks, unless supplemented with iron.

Dietary Iron

Sources of Iron	
Non Heme sources	*Heme sources*
Green leafy vegetables	Meat, fish, poultry, liver
Jaggery	
Cereals	**Additional sources**
Pulses	Water, cooking in iron pots
Dates, Almond, Nuts	
Ripe banana, Mango, Melon	
Cow's milk and breast milk	

Dietary iron comes from two sources: heme and nonheme. Nonheme iron is the major source and forms 90% of iron in the diet and is found in varying degrees in all foods of plant origin. The absorption is influenced by dietary factors. The remaining 10% of iron in the diet comes from the heme present in meat, fish, poultry and blood products. Heme is better absorbed than nonheme iron and is not influenced by dietary factors. Additional sources of iron in diet include water, cooking food in iron utensils. Breast milk contains low levels of iron (0.8 mg/litre) but has a better absorption and bioavailability, compared to cow's milk iron.

Normal Iron Requirement

Age	*Daily requirement*
Term infants*	1 mg/ kg /day from 4 months of age
LBW babies*	2 mg /kg/day from 2 months of age
Babies < 1000 gms*	4 mg/kg /day from 2 months of age
1000 – 1500 gms*	3 mg/kg/day from 2 months of age
Upto 10 years age	10 mg/day
Males above 11 years	12 mg/day
Females above 11 years	15 mg/day

*In the form of daily iron supplements

Etiology

The highest incidence of iron deficiency anemia is seen among children 6 months and 3 years and between 11 and 17 years of age. It is relatively uncommon in school children. The etiological factors are as follows:

1. Inadequate dietary intake of iron, a major factor which fails to meet the increased demand during the growth periods i.e. infancy and adolescence. Infants on predominantly milk diet and faulty feeding habit in older children are contributory factors.
2. Diminished iron stores at birth as a result of low birth weight, prematurity, perinatal blood loss, severe maternal anemia and multiple pregnancy.
3. Blood loss as a result of hook worm infestation, GI bleed, Meckel's diverticulum, hiatus hernia etc.
4. Some rare causes include idiopathic pulmonary hemosiderosis, congenital transferrin deficiency.

After 6 months of exclusive breastfeeding, the infant depend on the complementary food for supply of iron. The usual problem is that feeding of iron containing food viz. vegetables, eggs, meat etc are commenced too late. The diet mainly consists of milk and carbohydrates i.e. food of low iron content. Such a diet may have adequate calorie content. So the infant is of normal weight or obese but anemic.

Pathogenesis

Stages of iron deficiency
First Stage: Iron deficiency state
• Deficient iron store
• Decrease serum ferritin
• Decreased iron store in liver, spleen and bone marrow
Second Stage: Iron limited erythropoesis
• Low / Normal hemoglobin
• Decrease iron stores
• Low serum iron
• Reduced transferrin saturation
• Increased total iron binding capacity
• No clinical anemia
Third Stage: Iron deficiency anemia
• Presence of pallor
• Low hemoglobin +
• Biochemical alterations

Iron deficiency anemia is the end stage of a relatively long drawn process of deterioration of the body iron status. It has three distinct stages viz:

1. **Depletion of body iron stores:** In this stage, serum ferritin is reduced. Hemoglobin, serum iron, total iron binding capacity (TIBC) and transferrin saturation are normal.
2. **Iron limited erythropoiesis:** In this stage, hemoglobin is normal or slightly reduced, serum iron

and serum ferritin are low, TIBC is increased, and transferrin saturation is reduced.

3. **Iron deficiency anemia**, the third stage is manifested by presence of pallor, low hemoglobin in addition to the biochemical alterations.

In iron deficiency anemia, besides the symptoms of anemia, the more important manifestations are alterations of behavioral development and cognitive performances. The biochemical basis of these alterations are unclear but may be related to functional changes in iron containing enzymes at cellular level e.g. diminished activity of enzyme aldehyde oxidase required for serotonin catabolism resulting in increased levels of serotonin and 6-hydroxyindole compounds and reduced levels of MAO which is also required for catabolism of catecholamine. Recent observations have indicated that iron deficiency anemia at the time of crucial brain growth and development may produce permanent and irreversible abnormalities. Experimental evidence suggests deficiency of D_2 dopamine receptors in iron deficiency in early life which may not be correctable by the subsequent treatment.

Clinical Manifestations

Iron deficiency anemia usually manifests after 6 months of age. Not infrequently, the infants are predominantly on milk feeds. So weight gain is adequate but they are pale. When significant anemia (Hb < 7 gm%) is present below the age of 6 months one should exclude causes like hemolysis, blood loss or bone marrow failure rather than iron deficiency.

The clinical features may be divided into those resulting from low hemoglobin and those resulting from depletion of non-heme iron containing tissue proteins.

Features of Anemia

There may be no symptoms and signs in mild anemia. Mild to moderate anemia is accidentally discovered during routine examination. These children have poor growth, loss of appetite and suffer from recurrent infection and respond to iron therapy.

The features of severe iron deficiency anemia include easy fatigability, breathlessness and signs of congestive heart failure.

Other Features

These features include:

1. Behavioral changes viz. irritability, reduced attention span, decreased scholastic performance, poor academic achievement and conduct disorders.
2. Epithelial changes include angular stomatitis, atrophic glossitis, and malabsorption as a result of mucosal changes in stomach and small bowel.
3. Altered host response affecting both cell mediated as well as humoral immunity with normal phagocytic activity resulting in recurrent infection.
4. Growth retardation manifested by a marked reduction in weight although height seems to be unaffected.
5. Pica and breath holding spells have been linked with iron deficiency anemia. However, a cause and effect relationship has not been established. The present consensus is that iron deficiency anemia is associated in a majority of children who have these manifestations.
6. Mild splenomegaly may be observed in 10–15% cases especially in infants and young children. In these cases it is prudent to order investigations to exclude thalassemia syndrome.

Laboratory Diagnosis

The laboratory investigations include the following:

Complete Hemogram

1. Hemoglobin % to confirm anemia and assess severity.
2. Study of a well prepared and well stained peripheral blood smear.
3. *Red cell indices:* MCV, MCH and MCHC.
4. Red cell distribution width.

Confirmatory Tests for IDA

1. Serum ferritin levels, serum iron and TIBC, transferrin saturation.
2. Free erythrocyte protoporphyrin.
3. Bone marrow examination.

Blood Picture

The degree of anemia is usually mild to moderate, but may be marked, especially in cases due to persistent, severe blood loss. The red cell count is reduced to a lesser degree than hemoglobin and may be normal even when the hemoglobin is reduced to 8–9 gm/dl. The MCV and MCH are reduced. With coexistent Vitamin B_{12} or folate deficiency the MCV and MCH may be normal in spite of iron deficiency. The MCHC is reduced in parallel to MCV.

In the peripheral blood smear, the red cells are hypochromic and there is anisocytosis and poikilocytosis. The majority cells are microcytic. Variation in shape is often marked. Elliptical forms are common. Elongated pencil shaped cells may be seen. Target cells are present in small numbers. Normoblasts occasionally appear in small numbers in severe anemia or after hemorrhage. A small number of macrocytic polychromatic cells are present.

The reticulocyte count may be increased from 2–5% especially if there is hemorrhage. The white cell count and the differential count and the platelet count are usually normal but may be increased, especially in patients who are bleeding.

Red Cell Distribution Width

It is estimated on an electronic counter. Elevation of red cell distribution width (RDW) is probably the earliest sign of iron deficiency and precedes the overt changes in the peripheral blood film.

The classical triad of abnormalities in iron deficiency anemia is:

a. Low red cell count.
b. Reduced MCV < 80.
c. High RDW (normal reference range 11-15%).

Bone Marrow

The characteristic change in the marrow is erythroid hyperplasia; the increase is mainly in the more mature forms. Erythropoiesis is macronormoblastic; the predominant cells being polychromatic normoblasts. Granulopoietic cells and megakaryocytes are present in normal numbers and are of normal appearance. Examination of films stained with potassium ferrocyanide shows that reticuloendothelial iron is absent and sideroblasts are greatly diminished.

It should be noted that marrow examination is seldom necessary for diagnosis, unless there is difficulty in the differentiation of iron deficiency anemia from other causes of microcytic anemia.

Biochemical Findings

Serum ferritin levels is reduced to less than 15 micro gram/L. Serum iron is low (<75 microgram/dl) and TIBC is increased (> 470 microgram/dl). Transferrin saturation is low (cut of for infants and children 12% and 14% respectively). Free erythrocyte protoporphyrin (FEP) is increased. Values of 3–18 microgram of Hb are suggestive of IDA. Estimation of FEP has been used to diagnose iron deficiency before development of overt hypochromic anemia.

Although serum iron, TIBC, serum ferritin estimation are confirmatory tests, they are expensive and should not be ordered routinely. Besides, the results are influenced by factors like (i) improper collection (iron free tubes) (ii) prior therapy e.g. iron/cell transfusion (iii) associated deficiency of folate/Vitamin B_{12}. They may be necessary to diagnose iron deficiency coexisting with congenital hemolytic anemias viz. thalassemia minor, hemoglobin E trait and disease.

Treatment

The treatment consists of:

1. Replenishment of iron stores.
2. General measures.

Replenishment of Iron Stores

Iron therapy is the treatment of choice and oral route is the route of choice in children.

Oral Iron Therapy: Various salts have been used. Ferrous salts are much more effectively absorbed than ferric salts because ferric salts need to be reduced to ferrous form before absorption. Ferrous sulphate is the most frequently used iron salt. It is least expensive, and causes few side effects when given in appropriate doses. Ferric hydroxide polymaltose complex has fewer gastrointestinal side effects, but has not been as effective as other salts.

Table 8.2 : Percentage of elemental iron in some commonly used iron salts

Preparation	*Percentage of elemental iron*
a. Ferrous sulphate	20%
b. Ferrous fumerate	33%
c. Ferrous gluconate	12%
d. Ferrous sulphate (anhydrous)	37%
e. Ferrous sulphate (exsiccated)	30%

Doses: WHO recommends 3 mg/kg body weight per day. Higher doses are unnecessary and may increase side effects, thereby reducing compliance. Single daily dose is effective but 2–3 divided doses are better tolerated in children. Ideally oral iron should be given at least half an hour before meals to ensure maximum absorption. A dose given after 1–2 hours after meals can also be practised because children may not tolerate iron well in empty stomach.

Response to Therapy: A positive response to iron therapy can be described as follows:

- A sense of well being within first 24–48 hours.
- An increase in the reticulocyte count from 48–72 hours which peaks in 5–7 days.

- Hemoglobin level rises at an average rate of 0.15 g/dl per day, usually commencing about 1 week after institution of therapy. Hemoglobin comes to normal level after 2 months of therapy.

Duration of Therapy: The aim of iron therapy is to restore hemoglobin to normal and replenish body iron stores. Iron supplements in therapeutic doses should be continued for at least 3–4 months after initiation of therapy or 2–3 months after hemoglobin is normal or serum ferritin level is 30 microgram/L.

Side Effects: Nausea, vomiting, abdominal discomfort, diarrhea and constipation may occur in some children on iron therapy. These side effects are dose related and can be minimized by adhering to standard doses, gradual increase of dose and administration with or after meals.

Failure to Respond to Iron Therapy (Refractory Anemia)

The causes of failure to respond adequately to iron therapy within 2–3 weeks may be as follows:

1. Inadequate doses and poor compliance.
2. Use of ferric hydroxide polymaltose complex.
3. Hematological disorders e.g. Beta thalassemia minor, lead poisoning, sideroblastic anemia, concurrent folic acid/Vitamin B_{12} deficiency, HbE hemoglobinopathy.
4. Malabsorption e.g. Celiac disease, giardiasis.
5. Chronic blood loss from GIT e.g. Meckel's diverticulum, arteriovenous malformation, trichuriasis.
6. Chronic renal failure.
7. Chronic infection e.g. Tuberculosis, UTI, chronic URTI.

Approach to Diagnosis in Refractory Cases

The patients refractory to iron therapy should undergo proper evaluation which include a thorough history, clinical examination and laboratory investigations keeping in mind the conditions mentioned above. Investigations to be picked up depending on the clinical evaluation may include the following:

a. Stool for occult blood and parasites.
b. Complete blood count.
c. BUN and serum creatinine.
d. Blood lead levels.
e. Hb electrophoresis.
f. Bone marrow examination with iron staining for sideroblastic anemia and dysplasia.

Parenteral Iron Therapy

Parenteral iron therapy is rarely required in treatment of iron deficiency anemia in children. The candidates for parenteral iron therapy include those children with intolerance to oral iron and/or those with impaired iron absorption.

Two preparations are available: Iron dextran and iron sorbitol citrate. Iron dextran contains 50 mg/ml elemental iron and is the preparation commonly used. The dose can be calculated in milligrams by the following formula:

Iron required = Hb deficit × body weight in kg × 3.4 × 1.5

It should be noted that the therapeutic response with parenteral therapy is similar to that attained with oral iron. The side effects include anaphylactic reaction usually seen with intravenous administration. Intramuscular iron administration is very painful and may cause serious allergic reaction and hence not recommended in children.

Red Cell Transfusion

Transfusion is indicated only if there is evidence of impending or overt cardiovascular decompensation. Nutritional deficiency is the most common cause and hemoglobin level decline gradually. Hence these children tolerate even very low hemoglobin levels well.

General Measures

The general measures consist of the following:

1. Deworming at initial diagnosis and then periodically at 6 months interval.
2. Treatment of associated folic acid deficiency which is common with moderate to severe nutritional anemia necessitating supplementation.
3. Improvement of diet with addition of iron containing food.

Prevention

The measures that can be undertaken to prevent iron deficiency anemia are as follows:

1. Exclusive breastfeeding for first 6 months after birth.
2. To start complementary feeding with iron containing food from 6 months age.
3. Every child should be started on iron supplements from 6 months of age and continued upto 5 years age, then in the adolescent period. They should be advised iron supplements (elemental iron 2 mg/kg body weight) for 3 months every year during these years.
4. Control of parasitic infestation.
5. Food fortification with iron.
6. Modification of diet to encourage consumption of iron rich affordable food.

Megaloblastic Anemia

The megaloblastic anemias may be regarded as deficiency diseases, caused by deficiency of either Vitamin B_{12} or folic acid, both of which are essential for the normal development of the red blood cells. In the tropical zones nutritional folic acid deficiency is the most common cause of megaloblastic anemia. In the temperate zones Addisonian pernicious anemia, due to Vitamin B_{12} deficiency is the common cause which is however exceedingly rare during childhood.

Megaloblastic anemia is so named because it is characterized by the appearance of abnormal nucleated red cell precursors, called megaloblasts, in the bone marrow. The mature red cells thus formed from these cells show abnormalities in shape and size, the most prominent being macrocytosis. Hence the term megaloblastic macrocytic anemia more appropriately describes the features of both bone marrow and the peripheral blood.

Nutritional megaloblastic anemia and megaloblastic anemia associated with celiac disease are usually due to folic acid deficiency. Megaloblastic anemia in breast fed babies of vegetarian mothers; juvenile pernicious anemia, congenital intrinsic factor deficiency, familial selective Vitamin B_{12} malabsorption and inherited transcobalamin II deficiency are associated with Vitamin B_{12} deficiency.

Folic Acid Deficiency

Folic acid is a water-soluble B vitamin. It plays an essential role in cellular metabolism and is essential for normal hemopoesis. Chemically it is a molecule of pteroylglutamic acid which contains a pteridine ring, one molecule of glutamic acid and one molecule of para-amino benzoic acid. The term folate is used to refer folic acid compounds naturally occurring in blood and other tissues.

Body Stores

The normal body stores of folic acid can supply only about 2–3 months requirements. Although some folic acid is synthesized in the large gut by bacteria, it is not absorbed because absorption of folic acid occurs in the duodenum and jejunum. The normal body requirements are therefore supplied by naturally occurring folic acid in food.

Normal Requirement and Sources

The normal requirement is around 25–35 micrograms/day in infants and 50 to 100 micrograms per day in older children. The richest sources of folic acid are liver, kidney, green leafy vegetables (spinach and cabbage). Lesser amounts are present in foodstuffs including muscle meat and cereals. Human milk, as well as pasteurized cow's milk and formula milk, if supplemented, contain adequate amount of folic acid. Goat milk is a poor source.

Functions

Folic acid, as such, is apparently not metabolically active in body tissue, and must be converted to its metabolically active form, tetrahydrofolic acid, a coenzyme, which acts as a catalyst in the chemical reaction leading to synthesis of nucleoproteins.

Etiology

The deficiency of folic acid can occur as a result of inadequate intake, intestinal malabsorption, increased demand and presence of folic acid antagonists hampering utilization.

Most cases of folic acid deficiency are due to inadequate intake. Anemia usually become manifest under situation of increase demand viz. growth in infancy, chronic hemolysis and pregnancy. The first abnormality in the sequence of development of deficiency is reduction in serum folate level by 2 weeks, followed by hypersegmentation of neutrophil by 7 weeks, reduction of red cell folate by 18 weeks and finally appearance of megaloblastic anemia by 20 weeks.

Intestinal malabsorption due to chronic diarrhoea or diffuse inflammatory bowel disease can lead to folate deficiency. Certain anticonvulscent drugs like phenobarbitone, phenytoin and primidone can impair folic acid absorption and serum folic acid levels may be very low, but frank megaloblastic anemia is rare and the child responds to folic acid therapy even if the offending drug is continued.

A number of drugs e.g. methotrexate, pyrimethamine, triamterene and trimethoprim have anti-folic acid activity (enzyme dihydrofolate reductase inhibitors) as their primary pharmacologic effect and produce megaloblastic anemia.

Congenital dihydrofolate reductase deficiency has been reported resulting in development of megaloblastic anemia in early infancy.

Clinical Manifestation

The peak incidence is between 5 and 12 months age. However, combined deficiency of iron and folic acid is common in children with malnutrition. Mild megaloblastic anemia has been reported in very low birth weight infants.

Besides clinical features of anemia viz. pallor, irritability, listlessness and anorexia the child may present with respiratory infection, failure to gain adequate weight and chronic diarrhoea and glossitis. In advanced cases there may be bleeding manifestations due to thrombocytopenia. An older child present with symptoms and signs of anemia and the features of an underlying disease which may be responsible for the deficiency.

Laboratory Diagnosis

The anemia is macrocytic (MCV > 100 fL) with variation in RBC size and shape and presence of nucleated RBCs with megaloblastic morphology. The neutrophils are large and more than 5% of these have hypersegmented nuclei (> 5 lobes). The reticulocyte count is low. In long standing cases there is neutropenia and thrombocytopenia. The bone marrow is hypercellular. Giant metamyelocytes with cytoplasmic vacuolization as well as hypersegmentation of the nuclei of the megakaryocytes is seen.

Special tests for diagnosis include serum and red cell folate assays. The red cell folate is a more reliable indicator of the tissue folate stores than the serum folate, which fluctuates widely according to dietary intake. Microbiological or radio isotope assay methods may be used but the latter is preferred. The normal serum folic acid level is 5–20 ng/ ml. With deficiency the level is less than 3 ng/ml. The RBC folate level is a better indicator of chronic deficiency. The normal red cell folate level is 150–600 ng/mL of packed cells. Levels of serum iron and Vitamin B_{12} are normal or increased. Serum LDH is increased. The best diagnostic test is however, the therapeutic test with Folic Acid as in iron deficiency anemia.

Treatment

Folic acid in the dose of 0.5–1 mg /day should be given orally or parenterally and continued for 3–4 weeks until a definite hematologic response has occurred. A response to therapy is usually observed by 72 hours of therapy. The serum folate level returns to normal within days of commencement of therapy. Maintenance therapy with a multivitamin preparation containing 0.2 mg folate is adequate. Cell transfusion is indicated only when anemia is severe or the child is very ill.

Peripheral Blood Smears Picture of Different Types of Anemia

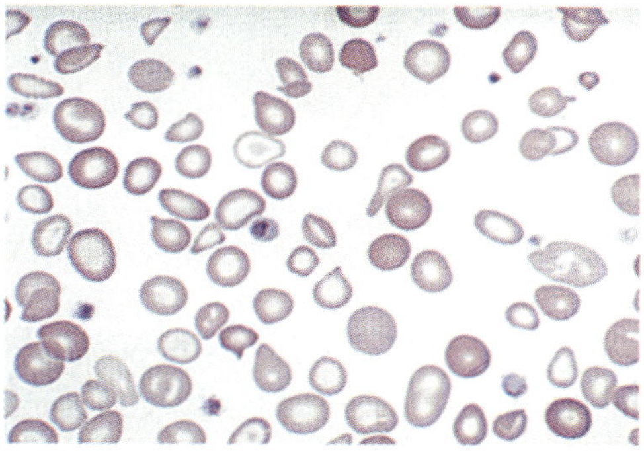

Fig. 8.1: Microcytic hypochromic anemia

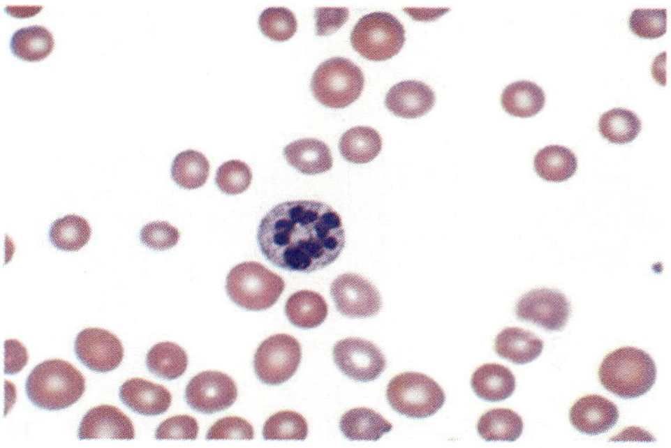

Fig. 8.2: Megaloblastic anemia (hypersegmented polymorph)

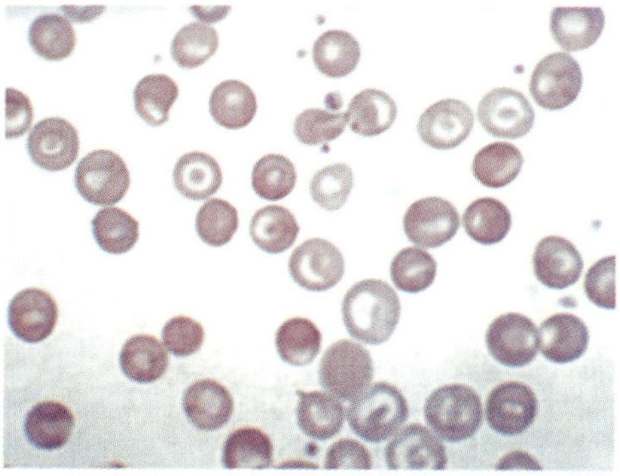

Fig. 8.3: Hemolytic anemia (Target cells)

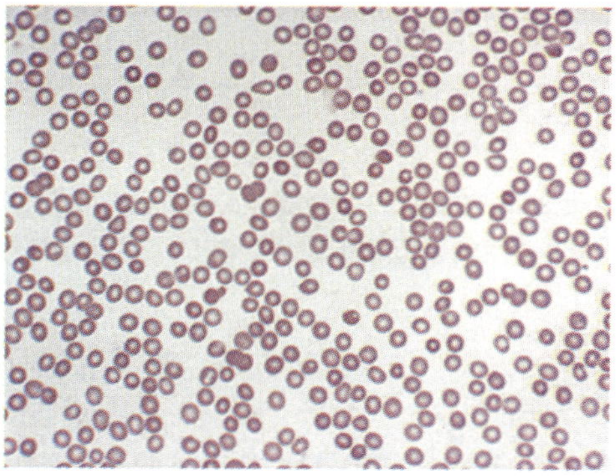

Fig. 8.4: Aplastic anemia

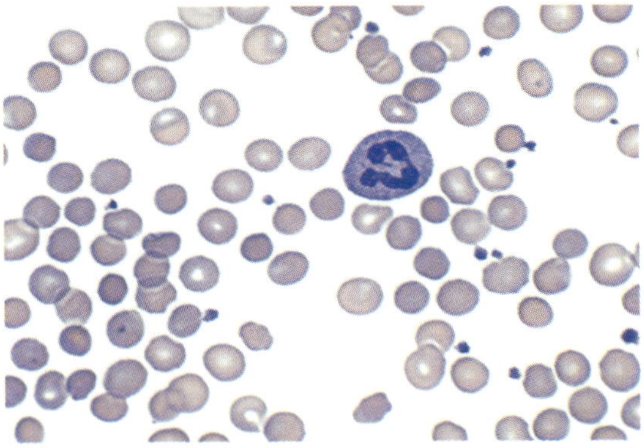

Fig. 8.5: Congenital spherocytosis (Microspherocytes)

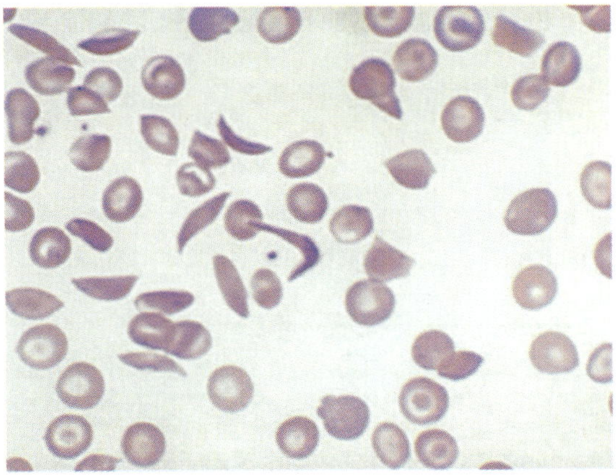

Fig. 8.6: Sickle cell anemia

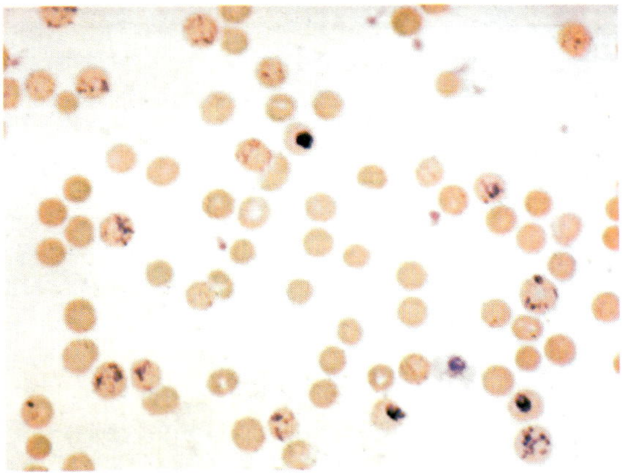

Fig. 8.7: Reticulocytes

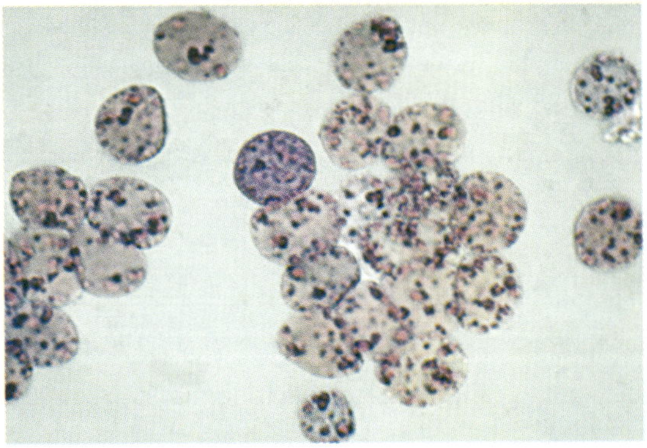

Fig. 8.8: Heinz bodies (Supravital stain)

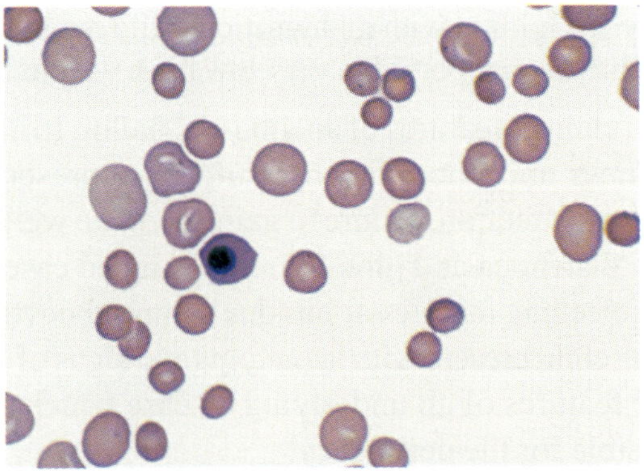

Fig. 8.9: Autoimmune hemolytic anemia

Bone Marrow Smears Normal and Abnormal

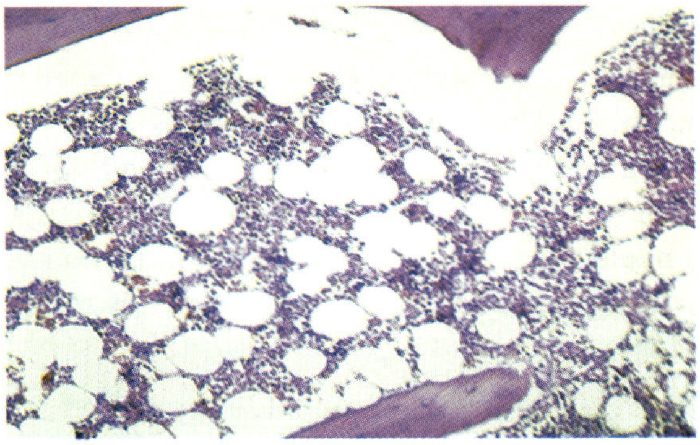

Fig. 8.10: Normal bone marrow

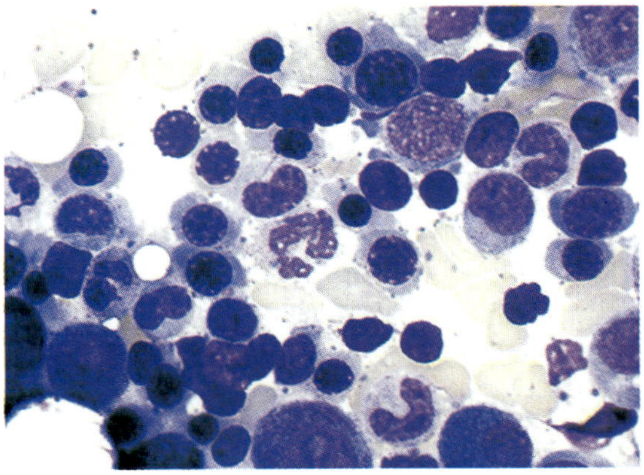

Fig. 8.11: Erythroid hyperplasia

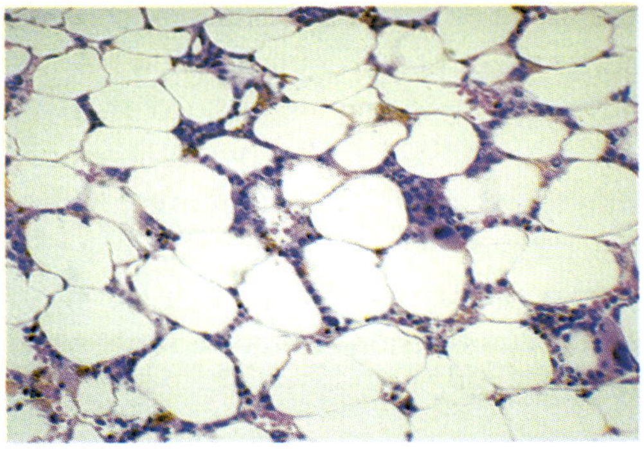

Fig. 8.12: Aplastic anemia

Hemolytic Anemia

The normal RBC survival time is 110–120 days (half life, 55–60 days) and approximately 1% of RBCs are removed each day and replaced by the marrow to maintain the RBC count. Hemolytic anemias result from an increase in the rate of red cell destruction. The normal red cell life span is shortened in hemolytic anemia and in very severe cases it may be only a few days.

The premature destruction of red cells may result from two fundamental defects: an intracorpuscular (intrinsic) abnormality of the red cells where the fault lies in the cells themselves and an extracorpuscular (extrinsic) abnormality due to development of an abnormal hemolytic mechanism.

Hemolytic anemias due to intracorpuscular (intrinsic) abnormality are mainly congenital. The basic defect may be in any of the three main components of the cell–the membrane, the hemoglobin molecule and the enzymes concerned with red cell metabolism. Hemolytic anemias due to extracorpuscular or extrinsic abnormality are usually acquired. The hemolysis may result from either an immune or non-immune mechanism.

Hemolytic disorders always may not present with anemia but show reticulocytosis and erythroid hyperplasia of the bone marrow because compensatory marrow hyperplasia may increase red cell production 6–8 fold and maintain a normal hemoglobin level. Anemia occurs only when marrow hyperplasia is unable to compensate for the increased destruction. Therefore anemia is not invariable in the hemolytic disorders.

CLASSIFICATION

Hemolytic Anemia Due to Intracorpuscular (Intrinsic) Mechanism

Congenital

a. Membrane defect e.g. hereditary spherocytosis, hereditary elliptocytosis, hereditary stomatocytosis.

b. Hemoglobin disorders

   i. Hemoglobinopathies viz. sickle cell anemia, hemoglobin E, hemoglobin C, hemoglobin D.

   ii. Thalassemia syndromes.

   iii. Double heterozygous disorders viz. sickle cell beta thalassemia, hemoglobin E thalassemia.

c. Enzyme defects

   i. Non-spherocytic congenital hemolytic anemia e.g. Glucose 6 phosphate dehydrogenase deficiency, pyruvate kinase deficiency.

   ii. Drug induced hemolytic anemia.

Acquired

Paroxysmal Nocturnal hemoglobinuria.

Hemolytic Anemia Due to Extracorpuscular (Extrinsic) Mechanism

1. Autoimmune hemolytic anemia.
2. Fragmented hemolysis e.g. DIC, HUS, ECMO, prosthetic heart valve, burns.
3. Hypersplenism.
4. Plasma abnormalities e.g. liver disease, infections, Wilson's disease, abetalipoproteinemia.

DIC = Disseminated intravascular coagulation, HUS = Hemolytic uremic syndrome, ECMO = Extracorporeal membrane oxygen.

HEREDITARY SPHEROCYTOSIS

Hereditary spherocytosis is the most common congenital abnormality of the red blood cell membrane. It is not confined to a particular race but it occurs most frequently in the British and northern European stock. It is usually transmitted as an autosomal dominant, less frequently as autosomal recessive and in about 25% cases, patients have no previous family history. However, a careful examination of the blood may show abnormality of the osmotic fragility in one of the parents. Another percentage may be new mutations. Males and females are equally affected.

Etiology

The basic defect in hereditary spherocytosis lies in the red cell membrane skeleton. The red cell membrane is composed of certain specific proteins and lipids viz. band 3 protein, band 4.1 protein, glycophorin and spectrin, phospholipids and cholesterol. The most important constituent, however, is spectrin. The molecules of spectrin are linked together by a specific protein and actin to form a lattice like network which is attached to the internal surface of the cell membrane. This network is a resilient structure which is responsible for the biconcave disc form of the red cells. There exist specific sites on spectrin which serve as points of attachment to molecules of band 4.1 proteins and protein ankyrin which links spectrin to the internal pole of band 3 protein.

A qualitative and quantitative abnormality of spectrin has been demonstrated. The most common finding is reduction in the amount of spectrin; in some patients, the spectrin lacks the ability to attach to band 4.1 protein. This results in the cell being of spherocytic shape. The spherocytes have a decreased surface area to volume ratio and are more rigid and less deformable than normal cells and an associated increase in cation permeability, cation transport, adenosine triphosphate utilization and glycolysis. The decreased deformability of the spherocytic RBCs impairs their passage from the splenic cords to the sinuses, and the spherocytes are destroyed prematurely in the spleen.

Clinical Manifestations

The age at which diagnosis is established is determined largely by the severity of the disorder. Most patients present in the first ten years of life; occasionally in the neonatal period. Mildly affected ones are discovered on routine examination; may remain undetected till adulthood.

The newborn presents as hemolytic disease with anemia and hyperbilirubinemia sufficiently severe to require phototherapy or exchange transfusion.

The presentation in infants and children is variable. Some may be asymptomatic into adulthood; discovered on routine examination with splenomegaly and mild anemia. Others may have severe anemia with symptoms like fatigue, exercise intolerance and jaundice. Jaundice is seldom obvious in the first few years of life, and frequently does not appear until adolescence. Jaundice may be sometimes intermittent. The spleen is enlarged after infancy and pigmentary gall stones may form as early as 4–5 years of age.

The course of the disease is characterized by hemolytic and aplastic crises. They are often precipitated by infection (usually viral) but may sometimes occur without obvious cause. *Hemolytic crisis* is a minor crisis as a result of increase in the rate of hemolysis. The *aplastic crisis* commonly results from a temporary marrow aplasia predominantly affecting erythropoiesis. Human parvovirus B_{19} infection has been recognized as an etiological agent for the aplastic crisis.

Hemolytic crisis results in increase in the depth of jaundice, darkening of the urine and increase in the size of the spleen which may become tender. In the *aplastic crisis,* jaundice may decrease. There may be rapidly increasing profound anemia resulting in hypoxia, high output heart failure, cardiovascular collapse and death.

Laboratory Diagnosis

The *hemoglobin* level is usually 7–14 grams/dl. It may fall below 7 gm/dl during a crisis. The hemoglobin level may be normal when hemolysis is compensated. The RBCs in *peripheral blood smear* vary in size and include polychromatophilic reticulocytes and spherocytes. The spherocytes are smaller in diameter (smaller than the nucleus of the small lymphocytes) and hyperchromic; their central pallor is less than two third of the cell diameter. Depending on the severity of the disease, the spherocytes may be the predominant cells or may be relatively sparse but they usually account for more than 15–20% of the cells in presence of hemolysis. The MCV is normal or slightly reduced. The MCHC is increased to the range 36–38 gm/dl RBCs. The *reticulocyte count* may be increased to 6 – 20 % with a mean of 10 %. *Bone marrow* shows erythroid hyperplasia. The erythroid hyperplasia is also evident on *X-ray of the skull and small bones of the hands* as in thalassemia but to a lesser degree. Other evidence of hemolysis may be presence of gallstones on *ultrasonography*.

Spherocytosis can be confirmed by the *osmotic fragility test.* The RBCs are put in progressive dilution of an iso-osmotic buffered salt solution. Exposure to hypotonic saline causes RBCs to swell and the spherocytes lyse more readily than biconcave cells in hypotonic solutions. This feature can be accentuated by depriving the cells of glucose overnight at 37°C. This is called incubated osmotic fragility.

The mean corpuscular fragility (MCF) is the concentration of saline causing 50% lysis. Normal values range from 4.0 to 4.45 g/litre NaCl. In hereditary spherocytosis the RBCs show an increased tendency to lysis in hypotonic saline solutions.

The specific protein abnormality can be established by RBC protein membrane analysis using gel electrophoresis and densitometric quantitation. It is more evident after splenectomy. Molecular diagnosis is also possible by DNA analysis which shows mutations in the beta spectrin and ankyrin genes in 50% of patients with unaffected parents.

Differential Diagnosis

The differential diagnoses include causes of acquired spherocytosis. An acquired spherocyte is produced by the action of some abnormal extrinsic factor on a previously normal cell. The acquired spherocyte can be distinguished from the congenital spherocyte by presence of the normal central pallor and the irregular cell margin.

The causes include hemolytic disease of the newborn due to ABO incompatibility confirmed by a positive Coombs' test, autoimmune hemolytic anemia with a past history of normal hemoglobin, hematocrit and reticulocyte count. Rare causes of acquired spherocytosis like thermal injury, clostridia septicemia with exotoxinemia, and Wilson's disease have only transient hemolytic anemia.

Treatment

Splenectomy is the mainstay of treatment. Whether all cases should be treated with splenectomy is controversial. Patients with hemoglobin level less than 10 gm %, reticulocytosis more than 10% or those with hypoplastic or aplastic crisis, poor growth, cardiomegaly, splenomegaly should be advised splenectomy after 5–6 years of age to avoid the risk of post splenectomy sepsis.

According to some hematologists, in patients with a hemoglobin level above 10 gm %, reticulocyte count less than 10% splenectomy is not indicated. They should be advised folic acid 1 mg/day to prevent secondary folic acid deficiency.

All patients planned for splenectomy should be administered pneumococcal, meningococcal and hemophilus influenzae B vaccines preoperatively and prophylactic oral penicillin, upto 5 years age, postoperatively.

As the spherocytes in hereditary spherocytosis is almost exclusively destroyed in the spleen, after splenectomy, anemia, reticulocytosis and hyperbilirubinemia resolves while spherocytes remain in the blood with increased osmotic fragility.

GLUCOSE 6 PHOSPHATE DEHYDROGENASE DEFICIENCY

Among the enzyme deficiency hemolytic anemias, hereditary glucose 6 phosphate enzyme deficiency is common. It is associated with two clinical syndromes:

1. An episodic hemolytic anemia induced by certain drugs (Table 8.3), infection (bacterial and viral), rarely fava beans; and
2. A spontaneous chronic non-spherocytic congenital hemolytic anemia.

In the former, the affected are not anemic / symptomatic unless hemolysis is induced while in the latter, which is relatively rare, is associated with lifelong hemolytic anemia.

Table 8.3 : Agents precipitating hemolysis in G6PD deficiency

Medications
a. *Antibacterials*: Sulphonamides, trimethoprim sulphamethoxazole, nalidixic acid, chloramphenicol, nitrofurantoin.
b. *Antimalarials:* Primaquine, pamaquine, chloroquine, quinacrine.
c. *Other drugs:* Phenacetin, Vitamin K analogs, methylene blue, probenecid, acetyl salicylic acid, phenazopyridine.
Chemicals
Phenyl hydrazine, benzene, naphthalene
Illness
Diabetes ketoacidosis, hepatitis, favism

Source: Conn's Current Therapy. Philadelphia, WB Saunders, 1994, p 341.

Episodic Hemolytic Anemia

This disorder is genetically transmitted by a sex linked gene of intermediate dominance which is located on the end of the long arm of the X chromosome. Full expression of the trait occurs in hemizygous males, in whom the single X chromosome carries the mutant gene and in the homozygous females in whom both X chromosomes carry the mutant gene. Intermediate expression is found in heterozygous females, in whom expression is variable. Heterozygous females have been shown to have two populations of cells, one with normal and one with markedly deficient enzyme activity. The relative proportion of the two population results in the G6PD activities that may vary from almost normal to those found in heterozygotes. Most heterozygous females do not have clinical hemolysis after exposure to oxidant drugs. Rarely, the majority of the RBCs are G6PD deficient in the heterozygous females due to random inactivation of the normal X chromosomes.

Clinical Manifestation

The most common precipitating factor is administration of an oxidant substance. Both viral and bacterial infection, diabetes, hepatitis, may cause hemolysis without administration of oxidant drugs and chemicals, or aggravate drug induced hemolysis. In addition, spontaneous hemolysis may occur in preterm babies. Female heterozygotes may have severe jaundice when there is associated Gilbert's syndrome. Hemolytic anemia and jaundice may be apparent at birth when a pregnant woman ingests oxidant drugs which are transmitted through placenta to her G6PD deficient fetus.

The clinical features are those of acute hemolytic anemia. The severity of the hemolytic episode induced by a particular drug is, in general, related to the inciting agent, the dose, and the severity of the enzyme deficiency. Hemolysis starts by 1–2 days after ingestion of the oxidant substance, lasts for about 7 days, and is followed by return of the hemoglobin level to normal by 20–30 days. Some spontaneous recovery of hemolysis may be observed even if the drug administration is continued.

The self limiting nature of hemolysis is because red cell drug sensitivity is a function of cell age. Older cells are destroyed, while the younger cells are resistant. So when the older population of red cells are destroyed, the younger resistant population remain, hemolysis ceases and hemoglobin level returns to normal. However, in some, the hemolysis is not self limiting and needs drug withdrawal. Moreover, resistance of the young cells is also relative. Hence a second hemolysis may be induced if a higher dose of the drug is administered.

Some patients may have only darkening of the urine whereas others more severely affected have constitutional symptoms, hemoglobinuria and jaundice with rapid lowering of the hemoglobin level.

Laboratory Diagnosis

The *red cell morphology* as well as the other blood findings is normal in deficient individuals when not exposed to oxidants substances. In presence of acute hemolysis, there is a fall of the hemoglobin and hematocrit. The *peripheral blood smear* study shows polychromatophilic cells (bluish large RBCs representing reticulocytes), fragmented cells and presence of Heinz bodies. *Heinz bodies* (precipitated hemoglobin) appear 1–2 days after ingestion of the drug and disappear by 3–4 days of illness because the RBCs containing these inclusion bodies are rapidly removed from the circulation. The *reticulocyte count* may be as high as 5–15%.

In severe hemolysis there is reduction of plasma haptoglobins, presence of free hemoglobin in plasma and subsequently in urine.

Screening tests and enzyme assay helps in confirmation of diagnosis. The testing for enzyme level however, should be deferred for 2–4 months for a confirmed diagnosis. This is because immediately after a hemolytic episode reticulocytes and young RBCs predominate in the circulation. These young cells have a significantly higher enzyme activity than do older cells. Hence enzyme activity may show normal levels. However, the enzyme level should be tested in the initial stage. The diagnosis of G6PD deficiency, in the initial stage, can be suspected when the G6PD activity is within normal range in presence of a high reticulocyte count.

Management

When G6PD deficiency is suspected at any age, the following investigation should be sent for:

1. Hemoglobin and hematocrit to assess the degree of anemia.
2. PBS study for RBC morphology.
3. Reticulocyte count.
4. Direct Coombs' test to exclude immune hemolytic disease.
5. Serum bilirubin and fractions to assess degree and type of hyperbilirubinemia.

Treatment of an acute episode of hemolysis is essentially supportive which include the following:

1. Drug withdrawal.
2. Cell transfusion as indicated.
3. Phototherapy and exchange transfusion in newborn along the lines of management of hemolytic disease of newborn.

Prevention of hemolysis constitutes the most important therapeutic measure. Males of the vulnerable group should be tested for G6PD deficiency before oxidant drugs are given. The parents of the neonates with G6PD deficiency should be provided with the list of oxidant drugs and advised to avoid them life long.

Spontaneous Chronic Non-spherocytic Congenital Hemolytic Anemia

Spontaneous chronic non-spherocytic congenital hemolytic anemia is associated with profound deficiency of G6PD caused by enzyme variants, particularly those defective in quantity, activity or stability. This condition is characterized by chronic hemolysis which may be worsened by ingestion of oxidant drugs.

HEMOGLOBIN DISORDERS

The hemoglobin disorders are characterized by impairment of synthesis of normal adult hemoglobin due to genetically determined abnormalities in the formation of the globin moiety of the molecule. These are hereditary disorders and may be classified into two broad groups, the hemoglobinopathies and the thalassemia syndromes. The *hemoglobinopathies* are characterized by production of structurally defective hemoglobin due to abnormalities in the formation of the globin moiety of the molecule. The *thalassemias* are characterized by a reduced rate of production of normal hemoglobin due to absent or decreased synthesis of one or more types of globin polypeptide chains.

The common hemoglobinopathies viz. HbS and HbC are prevalent in tropical Africa. HbE is common in South East Asia and HbD–Punjab in the Indian subcontinent. The thalassemias are widespread with maximum prevalence around the Mediterranean littoral and in South East Asia. However, no ethnic group is totally spared from suffering from the hereditary disorders of hemoglobin.

In India Hb E and HbE-thalassemia is common in the eastern part. HbS alone or in combination with hemoglobinopathy is common among the tea garden labourers. HbD–Punjab is seen in the western part of India.

Normal Hemoglobin Types

Hemoglobin is a conjugated protein in which four haem groups are attached to the protein moiety globin. Human hemoglobin exists in a number of types which differ in the structure of their globin moiety while haem remains identical.

There are three normally occurring hemoglobin types:

1. Normal adult hemoglobin (Hb A) which is composed of 2 alpha and 2 beta chains. 97% of hemoglobin in adult is of this type.
2. Fetal hemoglobin (Hb F) is composed of 2 alpha and 2 gamma chains. This is the predominant type in fetus. At birth red cells contain from 10–30% adult and 70–90% fetal hemoglobin. After birth, the proportion progressively diminishes to 25% by 1 month and 5% at 6 months. The adult level of about 1% may not be reached in some children until puberty.
3. A minor adult hemoglobin (HB A_2) which is composed of 2 alpha and 2 delta chains is present normally in small quantities (about 2–3%) upto adult life.

Hb Gower 1 and Hb Gower 2 are confined to the embryonic stage of development. Hb Portland is detected in trace amount throughout intrauterine life and in the neonates. Hb Bart's is found in small amounts in cord blood.

Abnormal Hemoglobin Types

Among the abnormally occurring hemoglobin types, the common ones are hemoglobin E, hemoglobin S, hemoglobin C and hemoglobin D–Punjab.

HEMOGLOBINOPATHIES

The hemoglobinopathies are characterized by the production of structurally defective hemoglobin due to abnormalities in the formation of globin moiety of the molecule. The hemoglobin is structurally abnormal because of an amino acid substitution. In these disorders, the normal hemoglobin is replaced in varying degree by the structural variants. Hemoglobin E alone or in combination with thalassemia (E-thalassemia) is the most common hereditary hemoglobin disorder in the eastern part of the country followed by hemoglobin S.

HEMOGLOBIN E HEMOGLOBINOPATHY

Hemoglobin E hemoglobinopathy is a hereditary disorder in which the red cells contain hemoglobin E. Hemoglobin E arises from the substitution of lysine for glutamic acid in the 26th position of the beta chain. The conditions include hemoglobin E trait (heterozygous state), hemoglobin E disease (homozygous state) and combination of hemoglobin E and thalassemia or any other structural variants.

Hemoglobin E Trait

Hemoglobin E trait (heterozygous state) is asymptomatic and the hemoglobin level is normal. There is no organomegaly. The RBC count may be elevated. The RBCs are microcytic with mild reduction of MCV and MCH.

Hemoglobin E Disease

Hemoglobin E disease (homozygous state) may also be asymptomatic or may present with mild anemia. No organomegaly. There may be mild jaundice. The red cells are microcytic and hypochromic usually with many target cells. The MCV and MCH are reduced. Affected children may however have low hemoglobin levels during the periods of rapid growth.

Hemoglobin E Beta-Thalassemia

Hemoglobin E Beta-thalassemia is a more severe condition than the former two. The clinical and hematological features resemble those of beta-thalassemia major or intermedia. Occasional patients are less severely affected. Death from infection in childhood is frequent. Some patients may live until adulthood. *Hemoglobin E alpha-thalassemia* is an uncommon condition, but have been described.

Laboratory Diagnosis

Demonstration of hemoglobin E by hemoglobin electrophoresis or HPLC confirms diagnosis of Hemoglobin E trait and disease. In hemoglobin E beta-thalassemia both hemoglobin E and hemoglobin F are present.

Treatment

HbE trait and disease usually do not require any treatment. Because of the microcytic hypochromic blood picture these children may be treated as IDA. Prolonged iron therapy is harmful.

Monitoring of Hb level is important. Presence of concomitant IDA should be treated adequately after confirmation. With low hemoglobin level during periods of rapid growth, a child may require short term red cell transfusion.

Diet is normal for age. Parents should be counselled about the benign nature of the disease and reassured about normal life expectancy. Genetic counselling is important.

HbE thalassemia should be treated in the line of thalassemia major.

HEMOGLOBIN D

Of the 16 variants of hemoglobin D, hemoglobin D-Punjab is seen in 1–3% of western Indians and in some Europeans with a tie to India. Heterozygous D is clinically asymptomatic. Homozygous D produces a mild to moderate anemia with splenomegaly. In association with Hb-S, symptoms are similar to sickle cell disease.

HEMOGLOBIN S HEMOGLOBINOPATHY

The hemoglobin S (HbS) or sickle hemoglobinopathies are hereditary disorders, inherited as Mendelian codominant in which the red cells contain the abnormal hemoglobin S. Hemoglobin S arises from the substitution of valine for glutamic acid in the sixth position of the beta chain. The conditions included in this disorder are sickle cell trait (heterozygous state) and sickle cell disease (homozygous state), and conditions in which hemoglobin S is combined with other structural variants or thalassemia.

Pathogenesis

HbS is much less soluble than adult hemoglobin (HbA). In deoxygenated state, the solubility is 10% of that of HbA. On deoxygenation HbS undergoes changes with the result that cells become markedly deformed, assuming a sickle or crescent shape. This is known as the sickling phenomenon. Sickling has been shown to be due to reorientation of the hemoglobin molecules in the reduced state. The molecules link to form long chains which form tactoids i.e. liquid crystalline masses. Several factors influence the degree of deoxygenation required to produce sickling of red cells containing HbS. They are as follows:

1. Amount of HbS in the red cells. Sickle cell trait which contains less than 50% HbS are less likely to sickle at a particular level of deoxygenation than the cells in sickle cell disease which contain nearly 100% HbS.
2. Presence of associated abnormal hemoglobin like homozygous HbC and HbD potentiate sickling whereas heterozygous states cause moderate sickling. Presence of HbF tends to diminish sickling.
3. Packed red cell volume and proportion of red cells containing HbS are important in determining the increase in blood viscosity resulting from a fall in oxygen tension.

Red cells containing large amount of Hb-S begin to sickle at an oxygen tension of 50–60 mmHg. This tension is experienced by the cells in parts of the microcirculation. If the flow is rapid, sickling does not become fully established and the cells resume normal shape when they are swept back to areas of circulation where the oxygen tension is higher. If the flow rate is slow, and the cells are delayed in areas where the oxygen tension is low the cells sickle and there is further slowing of circulation. Oxygen tension is further reduced; additional sickle cells accumulate and finally blockage of the vessels occurs. Tissue ischemia resulting from such vessel blockage is the basis of the painful crises that are a major clinical presentation of sickle cell disorder.

The sickling of red cells in the circulating blood therefore has two major pathological effects: (i) the distorted and rigid cells block small blood vessels, impairing flow and causing ischemia and infarction and (ii) repeated sickle-unsickle cycles lead to loss of fragments of red cell membrane, and the cells become spherocytic and fragile. They are removed prematurely by the reticuloendothelial system, and to a lesser extent destroyed in the circulation resulting in both extravascular and intravascular hemolysis.

SICKLE CELL TRAIT

Sickle cell trait is the heterozygous state for Hb-S gene where Hb-S comprises 38–45% of total hemoglobin, the rest being Hb-A (55–70%), Hb-A_2 (2–4%) and HbF (<1%). The cells do not contain sufficient Hb-S to undergo sickling at the lowest oxygen tension normally occurring in the body and the red cell span is normal.

Clinical Mainfestation

Sickle cell trait does not cause anemia and in general is asymptomatic although it may occasionally present with hematuria. If anemia is present another cause like iron deficiency should be sought for. Splenic infarction during air travel in non-pressurized aircraft has been described. There is some evidence to suggest that possession of Hb-S gene confers a relative resistance to P. falciparum malaria.

Laboratory Diagnosis

On examination of the peripheral smear the red cells are normal. The MCV and MCH are normal. The red cells are microcytic and MCV and MCH are low if it is associated with alpha thalassemia and a Hb-S concentration of less than 38%. Sickling can be demonstrated by the sickle test. In the sickle test, the red cells containing HbS take on a sickle shape when mixed with a freshly prepared solution of the reducing agent, sodium metabisulphite. This test can detect both heterozygotes and homozygotes of the sickle gene. Demonstration of hemoglobin S by hemoglobin electrophoresis/HPLC is diagnostic.

Treatment and Course

No active treatment is necessary. An associated cause like iron deficiency anemia needs treatment. The life span is normal and complications are rare. The most important aspect is counseling to at risk individuals and families to prevent the condition.

SICKLE CELL ANEMIA

Sickle cell anemia represents the homozygous state for the Hb-S gene. The affected child receives one Hb-S gene from each parent, both of whom show the sickle cell trait. The probability for each child of such a union to have normal hemoglobin only, sickle cell trait or sickle cell anemia is 25%, 50% and 25% respectively. In sickle cell anemia, Hb-S comprises 75–95% of total hemoglobin, the rest being Hb-A (0%), Hb-A_2 (2–5%) and Hb-F (1–20%). In contrast to the sickle cell trait, the red cells contain sufficient Hb-S for sickling to be produced in vivo by the reduction of oxygen tension which occurs in the capillaries. The in vivo sickling is responsible for the clinical manifestation of the disease.

Clinical Manifestations

Manifestations of sickle cell disease usually do not appear till 2–4 months of age when hemolytic anemia gradually develops. It parallels the replacement of fetal hemoglobin by Hb-S. By about 6 months of age, there is functional asplenia in many children making bacterial sepsis the greatest risk of morbidity and mortality and by 5 years of age, 95% has functional asplenia.

Patients with sickle cell anemia experience episodes which are traditionally called crises. These are vaso-occlusive crisis, sequestration crisis, aplastic crisis and hyper hemolytic crisis.

Vaso-Occlusive Crisis

The *vaso-occlusive crisis* presenting as 'hand foot syndrome' due to acute dactylitis is frequently the first overt evidence of sickle cell disease in an infant. Dactylitis is associated with painful, usually symmetric, swelling of the hands and feet. The underlying abnormality is ischemic necrosis of the small bones as a result of occlusion of the small blood vessels with distal ischemia and infarction. Radiologically, there is bony destruction with periosteal reaction. Vaso-occlusive crises become more frequent from 5–10 years age. Some children develop avascular necrosis of the hips. In older patients, the large joints and the surrounding parts become painful and swollen. The child can present as acute abdomen, stroke leaving hemiplegia as a result of infarction in abdominal structures and cerebral vessel occlusion respectively.

Sequestration Crisis

The *sequestration crisis* is only seen in young patients. For unknown reasons large amounts of blood become acutely pooled in the liver and spleen. The spleen becomes massively enlarged and signs of circulatory collapse develop rapidly. This is a frequent cause of death in the infant with sickle cell disease. It may also occur in older patients with sickle cell variants in whom splenomegaly persist into later life.

Aplastic Crises

The *aplastic crises* are transient periods of bone marrow failure characterized by acute life threatening anemia, reticulocytopenia, and markedly decreased numbers of red cell precursors in bone marrow. These episodes are self limiting and last for 10–14 days.

Hyper Hemolytic Crises

The *hyper hemolytic crises* are unusual but may result when a child with homozygous sickle cell disease, who coincidently has G6PD deficiency, ingests an oxidant drug.

In addition to the crises, as a result of severe hemolytic anemia and chronic vaso-occlusive disease, there is progressive impairment of liver function which contributes to the regular presence of jaundice in these patients. Gall stones have been reported in children as young as 3 years of age. There is progressive impairment of renal function due to diffuse glomerular and tubular fibrosis. Nephrotic syndrome can also occur. Initially the spleen is enlarged but there is functional hyposplenism. With repeated episodes of infarction, the spleen becomes small and fibrotic and is rarely palpably enlarged after 5–6 years age. Growth may be initially normal. By later childhood, most patients are underweight and puberty is delayed. The children have a markedly increased susceptibility to pneumococcal meningitis and septicemia and it is a common cause of death in the first two years of life.

Laboratory Diagnosis

There is usually mild to moderate anemia. The peripheral blood smear shows presence of target cells, poikilocytes, hypochromasia, sickled red cells, nucleated RBCs, and Howell-Jolly bodies. The reticulocyte count is increased to around 5–15%. The MCV is normal. The leukocyte count may be normal or high as also the platelet count and the differential leukocyte count may show polymorphonuclear leucocytosis. The diagnosis is confirmed by Hb electrophoresis or HPLC (high pressure liquid chromatography). Bone marrow shows erythroid hyperplasia.

The characteristic radiological findings include mild expansion of the marrow cavities, osteoporosis and sclerosis of long bones and femoral heads. There is alteration of hepatic functions and renal concentrating power is usually decreased.

Treatment

Treatment of sickle cell anemia is directed towards prevention of complications of sickling and maintenance of optimum growth and development.

In addition to the routine vaccines, all children with sickle cell anemia should be immunized with *conjugate pneumococcal vaccine*. *Oral penicillin V prophylaxis* should be started at 2 months of age in the dose of 125 mg two times daily, increased to 250 mg two times a day at the age of 3 years, and continued upto 5 years age. Because of the risk of conditioned folate deficiency, a maintenance dose of folic acid should be given if the dietary intake is inadequate.

Factors that promote sickling and predispose to crises should be avoided. These include hypoxia, dehydration, and acidosis. Excessive fatigue and exposure to cold and stress should be avoided.

Regular blood transfusion may result in increased blood viscosity and are not usually desired. *Cell transfusion* is indicated for stroke, stroke prevention, severe anemia, recurrent crises.

Splenectomy may be indicated in selected patients with recurrent episodes of sequestration crisis or in an occasional patient with hypersplenism. It may result in an improvement of the hemoglobin level.

The principles of *treatment of crises* are to keep the patient warm, to alleviate pain, to rehydrate and to treat infection, hypoxia and acidosis when present. For treatment of pain a nonsteroidal anti-inflammatory drug and an opiate medicine should be given together. The opiate medicine should be weaned after 3–4 days because the patient may have withdrawal symptoms if opiates are abruptly withdrawn.

There is an increased susceptibility to sepsis, meningitis, and pneumonia by streptococcus pneumoniae and hemophilus influenzae, and salmonella osteomyelitis. Any such infection should be monitored, detected early and treated promptly with appropriate antibiotics.

Drug therapy with hydroxyurea has shown encouraging results in children also. Hydroxyurea causes elevation of fetal hemoglobin levels and reduce morbidity. Children with sickle cell complications are usually begun on hydroxyurea at 15 mg/kg/day, and, if tolerated, the dose is increased to a maximum of less than 30 mg/kg/day. The fetal hemoglobin levels, complete blood counts and liver function tests should be monitored monthly for as long as the patient is on medication. An increase in fetal hemoglobin, a decrease in the leucocytic count to low normal and increase in MCV of over 100 fL/dl is an indication of compliance and efficacy. The increase in fetal hemoglobin is usually between 10–25%.

Bone marrow transplantation is the only cure for sickle cell disease but it is an option for children younger than

16 years of age with a HLA-matched sibling. A non-myeloablative method of transplant has been used in few patients with good result. However, long term stability of the graft needs to be proven before this technique is accepted.

THALASSEMIA SYNDROMES

The thalassemias are a group of closely related inherited disorders in which the fundamental abnormality is a defective rate of synthesis of normal hemoglobin. Hence they are also termed as quantitative hemoglobinopathies. Thalassemia is also called Mediterranean anemia because it was originally described in Italians, Greeks and other people of Mediterranean origin. However, it is now realized that it has a widespread geographical distribution. It also occurs in the Middle East, India and South East Asia, some parts of Africa, the West Indies and in American Negroes.

Classification

The alpha and beta chains of hemoglobin are synthesized independently and are under separate genetic control. Therefore there are two groups of thalassemias, one affecting the synthesis of alpha chains and the other affecting the synthesis of beta chains respectively called alpha thalassemia and beta thalassemia.

In beta thalassemia, classically there is an increase in Hb-F and Hb-A_2 and the hemoglobin level is maintained in part by the production of the gamma chain of Hb-F and the delta chain Hb-A_2.

In alpha thalassemia, on the other hand, the level of Hb-A, Hb-F and Hb-A_2 is equally depressed since they all have alpha chains, the structure of which is determined by a single genetic locus. In the absence of sufficient alpha chains, an excess of beta chains and gamma chains are formed which aggregate to form Hb-H ($Beta_4$) or Hb-Bart's ($Gamma_4$). There is no increase of Hb-F or Hb-A_2 in alpha thalassemia.

Pathogenesis

The key feature is that there is a globin chain imbalance. In the bone marrow, the genetic mutations of thalassemia disrupt the maturation of the red cells resulting in ineffective erythropoiesis. In beta-thalassemias, there is decreased rate of beta chain synthesis and consequent reduction of Hb-A in the cell. There is an excess of alpha globin chains relative to beta and gamma globin chains and alpha globin tetramers are formed. These inclusions interact with the red cell membrane and shorten red cell survival, leading to anemia and erythroid hyperplasia. The gamma globin chains and delta globin chains are produced in normal amounts leading to an elevation of Hb-F and HbA_2.

In alpha thalassemia, there are relatively fewer alpha globin chains and an excess of beta and gamma globin chains. These excess chains form Bart's hemoglobin ($Gamma_4$) in fetal life and Hb-H ($Beta_4$) after birth. Presence of these abnormal tetramers leads to extravascular hemolysis.

The inheritance of thalassemia is codominant, and follows Mendelian principles. Both alpha and beta-thalassemia exist in heterozygous and homozygous states.

THE BETA-THALASSEMIAS

Clinically, beta-thalassemia occurs in three forms: Beta-thalassemia major or Cooley's anemia, beta-thalassemia minor and beta-thalassemia intermedia. *Beta-thalassemia major* is a severe illness characterized by major or total suppression of beta chain synthesis and is the homozygous form of the disease. *Beta-thalassemia minor or trait* represents the heterozygous form where suppression of beta chain synthesis is less severe. It is a mild and sometimes asymptomatic condition. Some patients do not fit into these two clearcut clinical categories. Their severity of disease lies between that of major and minor forms and are classified as beta-thalassemia intermedia. *Beta-thalassemia intermedia* encompass a range of interactions between many different thalassemia genes which result in milder defects of beta chain synthesis and globin chain imbalance than which occur in beta-thalassemia major.

BETA-THALASSEMIA MAJOR

Beta-thalassemia major is the homozygous state for either the B^0 or B^+ thalassemia gene or less commonly, the compound heterozygous state for the two genes. It is usually a severe form which, if untreated often results in death during early childhood.

Clinical Manifestations

The newborn infant with beta-thalassemia major is not anemic. The initial manifestation is pallor of insidious onset, which is usually obvious by the first year of life and in severe cases within few weeks of birth. The subsequent course depends on whether the child is entered into a programme of regular transfusion or not.

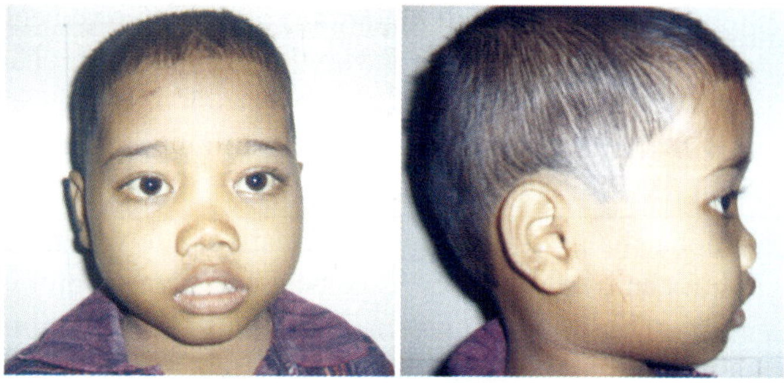

Fig. 8.13: Thalassemic facies

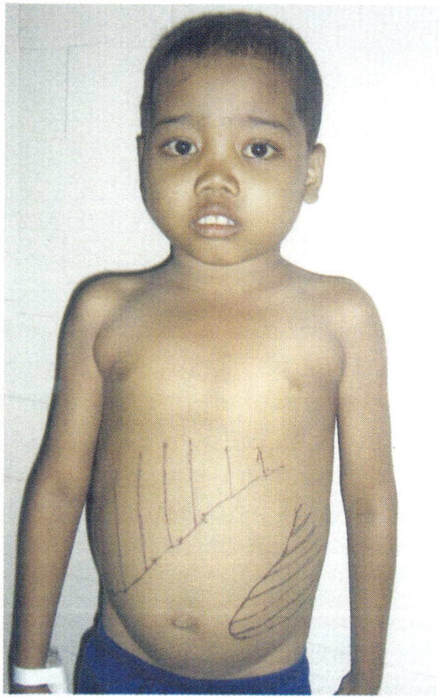

Fig. 8.14: Massive liver and spleen

If the disorder takes its natural course without any therapeutic intervention there is retardation of growth and development in early childhood. Most infants and children have cardiac decompensation when the hemoglobin level is 4 gm/dl or low. Fatigue, poor appetite, lethargy are late findings of severe anemia in an infant and the child.

The classic presentation with thalassemic facies, massive hepatosplenomegaly, pathological fractures, and cachexia is still seen in many children without regular transfusion. These are all features of ineffective erythropoiesis, extramedullary hematopoesis, and high calorie need. Splenomegaly is obvious by the age of three years of age. The spleen may become so enlarged that it causes mechanical discomfort and secondary hypersplenism. Clinical jaundice is uncommon but sometimes may be present in mild degree. Pallor, jaundice and hemosiderosis may combine to produce a greenish brown complexion. The characteristic facies is due to expansion of the marrow in the malar bones.

Children who receive regular transfusions grow and develop normally during the first decade and many of the features mentioned above are less severe or infrequent. However, in both treated and untreated insidious deposition of iron in tissues during late childhood and early adolescence results in organ dysfunction. The increase in body iron is due to the combination of frequent transfusion as well as increased intestinal absorption of iron due to ineffective erythropoiesis and chronic anemia. Iron overload in liver leads to cirrhosis, in the beta cells of pancreas to diabetes, in the pituitary, ovary and testis to growth retardation, hypogonadotropic hypogonadism. Hemosiderosis of cardiac muscles leads to arrhythmias, heart blocks and congestive heart failure and is the main cause of mortality after the first decade. Most of these complications can be avoided by the consistent use of an iron chelator. However, chelation therapy is not without associated complications.

Laboratory Diagnosis

Blood Picture

The *hemoglobin level* is usually 3–9 gm/dl. A *peripheral smear study* shows marked anisocytosis and poikilocytosis. Microcytes predominate but some cells are macrocytic and there are occasional spherocytes. Tear drop cells are often seen. Hypochromia is a striking feature with target cells. Normoblasts are invariably present; some may be in the early stages but often they are small, mature with pyknotic nuclei. They are in large numbers especially post splenectomy. Polychromasia and punctuate basophilia are usually present to a moderate degree.

The *reticulocyte count* usually ranges from 5–20% and is usually higher in splenectomized patients.

The *white cell count* is usually raised, with values upto 15–40 × 10^9 / litre. Neutrophils show a shift to the left and some myelocytes are commonly present. The *platelet count* is normal but may be reduced in presence of massive splenomegaly.

The *osmotic fragility* reveals an increased resistance to hemolysis. The mean corpuscular fragility (MCF) is the concentration of saline causing 50% lysis. Normal values range from 4.0 to 4.45 gm / litre NaCl.

There is mild rise of *unconjugated serum bilirubin.* Eventually there is iron accumulation with an elevated serum ferritin and saturation of transferrin.

Examination of *bone marrow* shows hyperplastic erythropoiesis proportional to anemia. The myeloid erythroid ratio is reduced from the usual figure 3–4: 1 to 1: 1 or even less. The hyperplastic erythroid cells are macronormoblastic. Marrow hemosiderin is normal or increased.

Hemoglobin pattern on electrophoresis is as follows: In thalassemia B^0, Hb-F constitutes 98% of total hemoglobin and Hb-A_2 the rest 2%. In thalassemia B^+, there is 70–90% Hb-F, 2% Hb-A_2 and traces of HbA. The acid elution test demonstrates a heterogenous distribution of HbF in red cells.

Radiological Findings

The radiological findings are a result of bone marrow hyperplasia. They result in the characteristic *mongoloid facies* due to expansion of the marrow in the malar bones and X-ray changes in the skull. In the *skull*, there is broadening of the diploic space, with separation of the tables. The medulla is less dense, giving a ground glass appearance. The tables, especially the outer are thinned. Bony trabeculae may develop at right angles to the tables giving rise to 'hair on end' appearance. These features are seen mainly in the frontal and parietal bones (Fig. 8.15A). In the *tubular bones* of the extremities, marrow hyperplasia results in widening of the marrow cavity, thinning of the cortex, and decreased density of the medulla. The trabecular pattern becomes coarse and exaggerated. With marked changes, the bone diameter is increased. These changes are specially marked in the metacarpals (Fig. 8.15B). After puberty, these changes regress while the changes in the skull persist and progress.

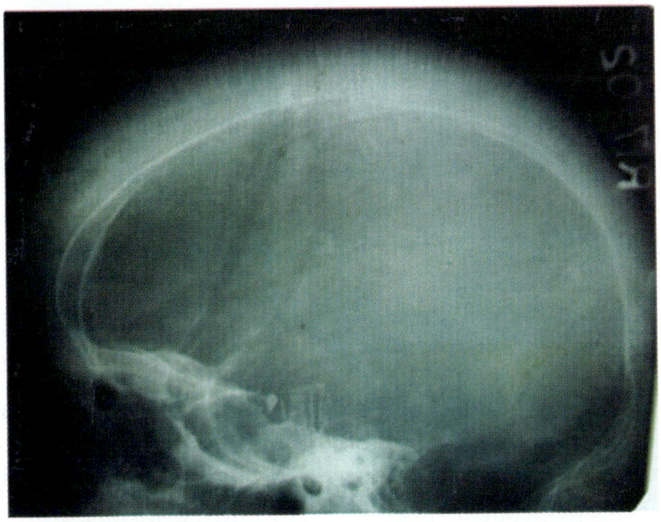

A. X-ray skull showing hair on end appearance

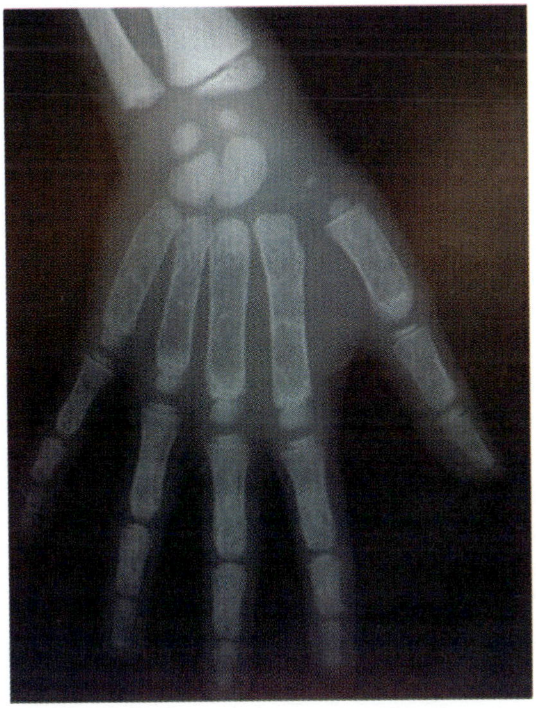

B. X-ray hand showing rectangular shaped small bones with thinning of cortex, increased trabeculation

Fig. 8.15: Radiological changes in thalassemia major

Treatment

The conventional management of thalassemia is based on a program of regular blood transfusion and iron chelation. This treatment modality has progressively transformed thalassemia major from an invariably fatal disease into a chronic disease permitting normal life or atleast prolonged survival. In fact, many patients are now getting married and successful pregnancies have been reported increasingly from all over the world including India. Other alternatives available are bone marrow transplant and gene therapy which have the possibility of cure.

Plan of Transfusion

Regular transfusion is needed for all thalassemic children who cannot maintain the hemoglobin level above 7 gm/dl. The goal of transfusion is to keep the hemoglobin level at a minimal baseline level. Such a regimen is currently universally accepted since maintaining a near normal baseline hemoglobin level suppresses the bone marrow completely preventing its expansion. Maintenance of normal hemoglobin level prevents chronic hypoxemia, hypervolemia, hypersplenism, and promotes normal physical growth and activity. It also checks excess gastrointestinal iron absorption and iron overload.

Transfusion Regimen

The average rate of hemoglobin fall is 1 gm/dl per week. For packed cells, to raise the hemoglobin by 1 gm/dl, the volume required is 3 ml/kg. The current recommendation is to maintain a hemoglobin level of 12 gm/dl. This can be achieved by not letting the hemoglobin to fall below 9.5 to 10 gm/dl for which a 3 weekly transfusion regimen is found to be convenient; hence mostly practised. This regimen can maintain a pretransfusion hemoglobin level of 10.5 gm/dl and a post transfusion level of 13.5 gm/dl to maintain a mean value of 12.0 gm/dl.

Type of Blood

A thalassemic child should receive group and type specific packed red cells ideally infused through a leukocyte filter. This prevents unnecessary infusion of plasma proteins and leukocytes thereby prevent non-hemolytic febrile reaction. The use of filters also minimizes antigenic exposure which is important because of future prospects of bone marrow transfusion.

Prior to transfusion, the blood should be screened to prevent infections like hepatitis B, hepatitis C, malaria, syphilis, cytomegalovirus and HIV. Fortunately, majority of thalassemia patients do not develop red cell antibodies and standard cross matching suffices. Hepatitis B vaccination should be routinely advised to all HbsAg negative thalassemia children.

Amount and Rate of Transfusion

The amount of blood to be transfused varies with different anticoagulants; procoagulant solutions and the hematocrit. In case of CPD-A blood with a hematocrit of 75%, the volume per transfusion is 10–15 ml/kg. The rate of transfusion should be 5 ml/kg/hour of packed cells. When there is heart failure or the hemoglobin level is less than 5 gm/dl it is recommended to give 1–2 weekly transfusion of 5 ml/kg at the rate of 2 ml/kg/hour.

Evaluation and Monitoring

At each transfusion the following evaluation should be done viz.:

1. Pre- and post-transfusion hemoglobin.
2. Weight and hematocrit of the blood transfused.

In addition, growth monitoring, cardiac and endocrine evaluation, serum ferritin and liver function should be done at regular intervals.

Indicators of Appropriate Management

The most important indicators of appropriate management are:

1. Annual mean hemoglobin level i.e. the average of the mean pre and post transfusion hemoglobin.
2. Annual pure red cell consumption (ml/kg/year) which is = Total wt (g) of blood given × mean hematocrit / patient's body wt (in mid year) × 1.08* (* represents density of pure red cells).

Annual red cell consumption should not exceed 180–200 ml/kg/year. An increased value indicates development of hypersplenism or presence of red cell antibodies.

Iron Overload

Iron overload occurs from two sources viz. transfused blood and enhanced gastrointestinal absorption. Each unit of packed cells provides 200–250 mg of iron and by 10 years of age about 20–30 grams of iron gets deposited in various organs of the body. Iron overload leads to liver fibrosis, cardiomyopathy and dysfunction of endocrine organs. The different strategies for reduction of iron overload include:

1. Inhibition of G.I. absorption of iron by:
   - Maintaining pre-transfusion Hb > 9 gm/dl.
   - Avoiding iron rich foods.
   - Consumption of tea with every meal.
   - Food should not be cooked in iron pots.
   - No iron containing medications.
2. Splenectomy for hypersplenism to avoid excessive and more frequent transfusion.
3. Iron chelation therapy.

Evaluation of Iron Overload

The easiest and most widely used method of evaluation of iron overload is estimation of serum ferritin. A sixth monthly estimation is recommended for appropriate monitoring of iron stores. However, the most sensitive method is measurement of iron content in liver tissue obtained by USG guided biopsy. It is specific and gives a quantitative measure of iron burden. MRI can also be used to evaluate iron overload but the results are not very accurate.

Splenectomy

If the currently recommended blood transfusion regimen is followed, splenectomy is usually not needed. If necessity arises splenectomy should be delayed till the child is atleast 5 years of age as there is a risk of overwhelming sepsis below this age. The indications of splenectomy are as follows:

1. Transfusion requirement increases to more than 200–220 ml/kg/year of packed cells (assuming the hematocrit of transfused blood is 75%).
2. Massive splenomegaly causing upper left quadrant pain or risk of splenic rupture.
3. Hypersplenism.

Iron Chelation Therapy

The two chelating agents widely used are desferrioxamine injection and oral deferiprone which are shown to be clinically effective with acceptable toxicity. Other experimental iron chelators include a depot formulation of desferrioxamine, oral chelators like HES-DFO, ICL 670A etc. They are less toxic as well as effective chelators.

The optimal time for starting chelation therapy has not been properly defined yet. The goal is to keep the serum ferritin level below 1000 mcg/L. Chelation therapy may be started when:

1. Serum ferritin approaches 1000 mcg/L.
2. Patient has received 15–20 transfusion.
3. Hepatic iron concentration exceeds 3.2 mg/gm dry weight.

Deferoxamine

The daily dose of deferoxamine is 40–60 mg/kg. It is given subcutaneously as a continuous infusion over a period of 8–10 hours. Vitamin C in a dose of 100 to 200 mg given during infusion helps in increasing iron excretion. The infusion can be given at home with a portable battery operated pump at night for 5–7 days a week.

Trials are on to evaluate the effectiveness of twice daily subcutaneous injection instead of continuous infusion. This will be a cost effective method for developing countries. However, it needs further validation before it is routinely used. Continuous intravenous infusions can be given by using surgical implants. It is usually indicated for patients who are heavily iron loaded with adverse effects like cardiac problems.

The side effects of deferoxamine are mostly local irritation at injection site and febrile reactions which respond well to antihistaminics and antipyretics. Other uncommon side effects include infection with Yersinia and mucormycosis, retinal changes, and cataract and hearing problems.

Oral Iron Chelators

Deferiprone is the only oral iron chelator found to be reasonably effective. Deferiprone is rapidly absorbed when taken orally. When given 2–3 times a day, it causes iron excretion comparable to that caused by a daily dose of desferrioxamine.

The daily dose of deferiprone is 75 mg/kg /day divided into 3 doses given one hour before food. The side effects include agranulocytosis and arthropathy which may necessitate discontinuation of the drug. The transient and reversible side effects include gastrointestinal intolerance, zinc deficiency and alteration of liver enzymes.

Diet and Vitamins

Food rich in iron content viz. meat, liver, kidney, green leafy vegetables and jaggery should be avoided. Food and water storage in iron utensils should not be practised. Iron containing drugs should be avoided. Diet should include food containing high phosphorous or phytates e.g. cereals, bread, milk, moong dal, soyabeans, roasted peas which will inhibit gastrointestinal iron absorption. The child should be advised to take tea with every meal to decrease iron absorption.

In children not on chelation therapy, Vitamin C containing food viz. citrous fruits, guava, amla etc should be avoided. Folic acid should be prescribed to patients receiving no or irregular blood transfusion in the dose of 1 mg / day or 5 mg/week. The patients receiving regular transfusion do not require folic acid supplementation unless actual deficiency occurs.

Alternative Modalities of Treatment

Bone Marrow Transplant

It is at present the only curative treatment for thalassemia major. It is an accepted alternative to life long regimen of transfusion and chelation. In bone marrow transfusion, the patient's marrow is destroyed by help of drugs in a process called conditioning. Marrow is then harvested from a histocompatible donor and infused intravenously to the patient. The stem cells from the donor find their way into the marrow cavity of the recipient and start growing there. As these stem cells are from a normal person, the red cells that are produced will be normal. At present the cure rate of bone marrow transplantation is about 70%.

Stem Cell Transplantation

It is a technique where stem cells are collected either from the peripheral blood of the donor (peripheral blood stem cell transplantation) or from the umbilical cord blood of newborn (cord blood stem cell transplantation).

The advantages of the former technique are easier processing, less expensive, fast marrow recovery and lower risk of graft versus host disease, rejection and infection. The stem cells are collected from the peripheral blood of the donor by stimulating their release from marrow by using certain growth factors.

The advantages of the latter technique are easy availability, less stringent requirement for HLA matching and lesser incidence of graft versus host reaction. In this technique, hemopoetic stem cells present in the cord blood are used for transplantation. However, at present, most of these transplants are carried out in patients suffering from leukemia.

In Utero Transplantation

This technique involves in utero marrow transplantation. The advantages of this technique are requirement of low level engraftment and immunological tolerance of the fetus. However, experience is limited but it may be an important development in future.

Gene Therapy

Thalassemia is a genetic disorder. Hence gene therapy remains the ultimate treatment for providing life long cure. In this mode of therapy, patient's bone marrow is harvested and the beta globin gene is incorporated into stem cell and reinfused in the body system.

Stimulation of Fetal Hemoglobin Synthesis

The aim of this therapeutic modality is to increase gamma globin synthesis and reduce the imbalance of alpha chains and hemolysis. Several drugs have been shown to increase fetal hemoglobin synthesis. Among them hydroxyurea and butyrates have been shown to raise gamma globin level without major side effects. However, large studies are not yet available to prove their utility conclusively. Other drugs shown to increase HbF synthesis are cytosine arabinocide, busulphan, vinblastine and 5-azacytadine. These drugs cause myelosuppression which has limited their use.

BETA-THALASSEMIA INTERMEDIA

As the name implies, this disorder is of a severity intermediate between that of beta-thalassemia major and minor. Hence it is referred to as beta-thalassemia intermedia although the hemoglobin constitution is usually identical to that seen in classical beta-thalassemia major. It is presumed that genetically the condition is due to the interaction of two beta-thalassemia genes, one of which causes complete inhibition of beta chain synthesis while the other causes only partial inhibition. Genetically a family study shows atypical beta-thalassemia trait in one or both parents with raised Hb F, mild microcytosis, borderline Hb A_2 level.

Clinical Features and Laboratory Findings

The intermedia type of the disease is also found in patients suffering from Hb-Lapore thalassemia disease and in certain cases of beta-thalassemia associated with abnormal hemoglobin, e.g., Hb-C, Hb-E and Hb-D.

The spleen is often markedly enlarged. Rarely the child may present with spinal cord compression as a result of extramedullary hemopoetic tissue. Bony changes, nutritional hemosiderosis, and other complications of thalassemia and iron overload can occur in due course of time.

Spinal cord compression with neurological symptoms is a medical emergency which will require immediate local radiation therapy.

Hematologic features include a hemoglobin level of 8 gm /dl or more. The Hb F level is in the range of 10–50%, high Hb A_2 (> 4%) and Hb A in the range of 30%.

Treatment

Treatment of anemia should be in the lines of thalassemia major. Recombinant erythropoietin has been tried in thalassemia intermedia as treatment modality to increase HbF synthesis.

Patient who lead a normal life with a mean Hb level of 8 gm/dl should not be started on regular transfusion.

Persistent clinical problems such as pathological fractures, growth retardation, cardiac failure are absolute indications for regular transfusion (scheme is same as beta-thalassemia major).

Patient may need occasional transfusion if Hb falls below 7 gm/dl.

Hypersplenism may lead to persistent fall in Hb level. Even in such cases appropriate management is splenectomy rather than starting regular transfusion.

Iron reduction strategies should be started as indicated as patient may develop iron overload because of increased GI absorption.

Folic acid 5 mg weekly should be advised as there is continued hemolysis.

BETA-THALASSEMIA TRAIT

This disorder is the heterozygous state for the beta-thalassemia gene, inherited from one parent. It is characterized by a moderate reduction in beta chain synthesis. It should come in the differential diagnosis of a case of anemia with failure to response to iron therapy.

Clinical Mainfestations

The condition is commonly not diagnosed until adolescence or adult life. It may be detected on routine hematological screening or when there is an affected child in the family with thalassemia major or a combination of HbE thalassemia or thalassemia S. It is a very mild disorder with mild or no anemia, no symptoms and a normal life expectancy. The spleen may be palpable.

Laboratory Diagnosis

The *hemoglobin level* is normal or mildly reduced, rarely less than 10 gm%. The *peripheral blood smear* shows mild red cell anisocytosis, microcytosis and hypochromia with variable numbers of target cells. The *RBC count* is normal or increased despite anemia. The *MCV and MCH* is reduced, with values of 63–77 fl and 18–25 pg respectively. *MCHC* is normal or marginally reduced. Red cell distribution width (RDW) is low.

On electrophoresis, the most characteristic finding is an increase in HbA_2 (3.5–7%). In around 50% cases HbF is slightly increased (1–5%). HbA constitutes 90–95%.

Differential Diagnosis with Iron Deficiency Anemia

The main problem in diagnosis is the differentiation of beta-thalassemia minor from iron deficiency anemia.

Clinical features are often not helpful. However, history of a well supplemented diet on one hand and family history of congenital hemolytic anemia on the other may help. Presence of splenomegaly with anemia favours a diagnosis of thalassemia although iron deficiency anemia can also lead to splenomegaly.

Both the disorders have hematological features like microcytosis, hypochromia and reduction in MCV. It is relatively marked considering the normal or absent anemia in thalassemia minor while it is proportionate to the degree of anemia in iron deficiency anemia. Children with beta-thalassemia minor will have a persistently low red cell distribution width.

Estimation of iron, ferritin and transferrin saturation showing normal values, and increase HbA_2 and HbF usually provide a definitive diagnosis of thalassemia minor.

Administration of therapeutic doses of iron shows signs of improvement of hemoglobin and other parameters in iron deficiency anemia. Thalassemia minor can also be associated with iron deficiency anemia in which case the elevated HbA_2 usually falls to normal and returns to a supranormal level when iron stores are replenished.

Treatment

Mild cases do not require any treatment. The parents should be counseled regarding the benign nature and normal life expectancy. Genetic counseling for the future of child should be emphasized. Hemoglobin level should be monitored especially during the growth periods viz. early childhood and adolescence.

Treatment of associated iron deficiency, if present, should be done after confirmation. Confirmation needs estimation of biochemical parameters viz. serum iron, ferritin and transferrin saturation. Therapy is as usual for IDA. Inappropriate iron therapy is harmful. Prophylactic folic acid should be given to all cases.

A normal diet should be advised with advice to take tea after every feed to inhibit absorption of iron.

A low Hb level (< 10 gm %) during early childhood and adolescence may necessitate a short term transfusion regimen.

Prevention of Congenital Hemolytic Anemia

Prospective preventive measures should include population education, mass screening in high risk groups, antenatal diagnosis and genetic counseling.

Screening Tests

Screening programmes have been established in many countries to detect asymptomatic, previously unknown, thalassemic heterozygotes. This helps to provide information and genetic counseling. The commonly used screening tests are described.

The *measurement of red cell MCV*, using a cell counter, has usually been used as the basic test. MCV has a sensitivity of 83% and a negative predictive value of 93%. The disadvantage of using MCV is that it requires a cell counter and is not practical in field studies. *NESTROFT* (Naked Eye Single Tube Red Cell Osmotic Fragility Test) is a rapid, simple and reliable test used for mass screening. The test is based on the principle that the red blood cells in thalassemia trait resist hemolysis more than normal RBCs. It is simple to perform with high sensitivity (83%) and high negative predictive value 89%).

NESTROF Test: Two test tubes are taken. In one 2 ml of distilled water and in the other 2 ml of buffered 0.36% saline is taken. A drop of blood to be tested is added to both tubes and they are left undisturbed for half an hour at room temperature. After half an hour the test tubes are shaken and then held against light.

Interpretation: In normal subjects a line is clearly visible through the contents at the bottom of both the test tubes. It is NESTROFT negative and it indicates that all the RBCs are hemolysed and settled leaving a clear solution. If the line is not clearly visible through the test tube containing 0.36% buffer saline it suggests partial hemolysis of the RBCs and the test is considered positive. Those who test positive on NESTROFT should have an HbA_2 estimation and a diagnosis of thalassemia trait should be made if HbA_2 is >3.5%.

Antenatal Diagnosis

Antenatal diagnosis and selective termination in pregnancy at risk for homozygous beta thalassemia, homozygous sickle cell disease and Hb–Batt's hydrops fetalis are now available in limited number of specialized centres. The two methods use for the purpose is measurement of globin chain synthesis in fetal blood at 18–20th week of gestation and analysis of fetal DNA in amniotic fluid obtained by transabdominal amniocentesis during 15–18th week of gestation. First trimester diagnosis has also been possible by using trophoblastic tissue obtained by transcervical aspiration. This is in experimental stage but it is expected that this method will be increasingly favoured in the future.

Genetic Counseling

Marriage counseling to avoid marriage between two heterozygotes will help in reduction of incidence of homozygous states.

Hemorrhagic Disorders

An Approach to a Bleeding Disorder

The hemorrhagic disorders are a group of disorders with different etiologies, which have in common an abnormal tendency to bleed. This abnormal tendency to bleed is due to a defect in the mechanism of hemostasis.

The diagnosis of many hemorrhagic disorders is largely or wholly clinical and the selection of appropriate laboratory tests required for accurate diagnosis depends on the full clinical assessment. Hence the importance of the history and clinical examination needs emphasis.

The Clinical Approach

When to Suspect a Hemorrhagic Disorder?

A hemorrhagic disorder should be suspected when there is:

1. Spontaneous bleeding into the skin, mucous membrane and internal tissues, joints.
2. Excessive or prolonged bleeding following trauma or surgery.
3. Bleeding from more than one site.
4. Associated family history of abnormal bleeding.

The common forms of bleeding into the skin are petechiae and ecchymosis. The child usually presents with red spots or blue patches on the skin. Red spots appearing and disappearing at different sites all over the body is characteristic of purpura due to platelet abnormality but it must be differentiated from erythematous allergic rashes. The allergic rashes blanch on pressure with a glass slide while purpuric lesion will not disappear on pressure.

Nose bleeds is a common form of mucosal bleeding in childhood and causes may be an abrasion in the little's area, polyp, foreign body as well as a bleeding disorder. The local lesions usually causes unilateral epistaxis whereas a bleeding disorder always results in bilateral epistaxis which is severe, recurrent or both.

A post operative or traumatic bleed may be the first manifestation of a coagulation disorder. It should be noted that although bleeding from more than one site is usual in a hemorrhagic disorder, occasionally an episode of bleeding may be localized to one site. It should also be remembered that abnormal bleeding from a local pathological lesion may be precipitated by an unsuspected hemorrhagic disorder and secondly in a patient with known hemorrhagic disorder bleeding may be precipitated by the development of a local pathological lesion.

Which Component of the Hemostatic Mechanism is Affected?

There are three components of normal hemostatic mechanism: *the vascular, platelet and coagulation components* which act together in a coordinate manner to arrest bleeding. A breakdown in the normal hemostatic mechanism and tendency to bleeding may result from a defect in any one of these three components. Which of the three components of the hemostatic mechanism is affected can be sometimes suspected from the type of bleeding.

In *vascular disorders* the bleeding is usually confined to the skin and may cause petechiae and ecchymoses. The petechiae tend to be pale and often confluent and ecchymoses are usually small. Bleeding is spontaneous and often not severe. When bleeding occurs from wounds it is immediately excessive, persists for less than 48 hours and rarely recurs.

In *platelet disorders* petechial bleeding is common, ecchymoses present are usually not larger than 2 cm in diameter and bleeding from mucous membranes is prominent. Bleeding is spontaneous. When bleeding occurs from wounds it commences immediately, persists for less than 48 hours and rarely recurs.

In *coagulation disorders* petechial hemorrhage is rare. Ecchymoses tend to be larger than in platelet and vascular disorders. Bleeding more frequently occurs in deeper tissues. Bleeding occurs after minor trauma or surgery and is less often spontaneous. Wound bleeding tends to commence after a delay of several hours, to persist for more that 48 hours and to recur after hemostasis has apparently occurred.

It should be noted that although the component involved may be suspected from the type of bleeding it can usually be determined with certainty only after blood tests and consideration of the other clinical features. Further, in some hemorrhagic disorders it is not uncommon for more than one component of the hemostatic mechanism to be involved. It also needs mention that spontaneous bleeding without obvious antecedent trauma reflect severe coagulation disorder (e.g. a level of 0–1% factor VIII) or a platelet disorder with a platelet count < 10,000 / micro litre while hemorrhage occurring only after trauma is suggestive of a milder defect (e.g. a level of 15–25% factor VIII) or a platelet count 10,000–30,000 / micro litre).

What is the Etiology of the Hemorrhagic Disorder?

Having decided that the child is likely to be suffering from a hemorrhagic disorder, the next question is whether the defect is congenital (hereditary) or acquired. The features favoring a congenital disorder are as follows:

1. Family history of a bleeding disorder.
2. Bleeding from umbilical stump, big cephalhematoma after normal easy vaginal delivery, prolonged bleeding after circumcision.
3. History of bleeding from early childhood.
4. Spontaneous hemarthrosis or recurrent hemarthrosis.
5. Frequent and prolonged bleeding after trauma or surgery.

The features of an acquired bleeding disorder are as follows:

1. Family history is absent.
2. Onset later in life.
3. Presence of associated features viz. fever, jaundice, pallor, hepatosplenomegaly, lymphadenopathy, rash.
4. Presence of features of other disorders like autoimmune diseases, lupus erythematosus, septicemia, uremia, liver disorders etc.

It should however be remembered that these points are just guidelines and there are exceptions. For example congenital disorders like mild hemophilia may have the bleeding episode only in adult life.

A detailed family history is an important aspect for diagnosis of a bleeding disorder. A proper pedigree chart must be recorded taking care to enquire about the dead family members also.

Inheritance pattern also help in clinching a diagnosis. For example classical hemophilia and Christmas disease has a sex linked recessive inheritance (where male suffer and female transmit) whereas qualitative platelet disorders, fibrinogen abnormalities, deficiency of factors V, VII, X, XI and XII have an autosomal recessive inheritance where parents do not suffer, both sexes are affected, and there is a history of consanguinity. The examples of autosomal dominant pattern of inheritance are von Willebrand disease and hereditary hemorrhagic telangiectasia.

The Laboratory Approach

The laboratory tests used in the investigation of suspected coagulation disorders belong to 3 groups: essential tests, screening tests and special tests.

1. **Essential investigations** for all cases include Hb%, and red cell morphology, total leucocytic count, differential leucocytic count, and reticulocyte count.
2. **Screening tests** for hemorrhagic disorders include platelet count and examination of blood film for number, morphology and presence of platelet clumping, the skin bleeding time, tourniquet test, prothrombin time (PT), activated partial thromboplastin time (APTT), thrombin time and vWF test.
3. **Special tests** are required to (a) identify the deficient coagulation factor, (b) to determine the degree of deficiency, and (c) to detect and quantitate immune inhibitors. They include prothrombin consumption test, coagulation factor assays and platelet function tests.

A child who has a positive bleeding history or is having active bleeding should have a platelet count, bleeding time, APTT and PT done. If the results are normal, a thrombin time and vWF testing should be considered. If the initial test results are abnormal, special tests should be planned.

Screening Tests

Platelet Count

It is the simple initial test for evaluation of the cellular aspect of hemostasis. It should be preferably done on a cell counter. However, a good peripheral blood smear examination can give a gross idea of the number of platelets by study of clumping of platelets (1 clump is equivalent to 10,000 platelets/mm^3) as well as its morphology. Although there is no absolute relationship between the platelet count and frequency and severity of bleeding, spontaneous bleeding is seen with a platelet count less than 10,000/cumm and serious bleeding after trauma is unusual if the platelet count is more than 50,000/cumm. If bleeding occurs when the platelet count is above 50,000/cumm, a functional platelet disorder should be suspected particularly if clot retraction is also poor.

Bleeding Time

It is the time interval required for hemostasis following standard superficial incision (1 mm deep and 5 mm long) in the skin of the forearm while venous pressure is maintained at about 40 mm of Hg. To maintain the venous pressure a blood pressure cuff is applied to the upper arm and inflated to 40 mm Hg. After the incision, blood is blotted from the margin of the incision at 30 seconds interval until bleeding ceases.

The normal bleeding time is 4 to 7 minutes. The bleeding time assesses the function of the platelets and their interaction with the vascular wall. Prolongation of bleeding time occurs when the platelet count falls below 50,000 / cumm. If the count is below 15,000 / cumm the bleeding time is often more than 15 minutes.

Bleeding time is prolonged in both quantitative and qualitative defect of the platelets and vonWillebrand disease. A prolonged bleeding time disproportionate to the platelet count indicates a qualitative disorder or von Willebrand disease. A prolonged bleeding time may be observed in acquired conditions viz. sepsis, disseminated intravascular coagulation (DIC), and uremia as well as administration of drugs like aspirin and other NSAIDs.

Tourniquet Test

It is performed by placing a sphygmomanometer cuff around the upper arm and raising the pressure to 100 mm Hg for 5–7 minutes. If the systolic pressure is less than 100 mmHg, the pressure is raised to half way between the systolic and diastolic pressure. An area with a 3 cm diameter is marked 1 cm below the cubital fossa. After two to three minutes the cuff is deflated and the number of petechiae is counted in the marked area. In most normal subjects, the number of petechiae is upto 10. More than 20 petechiae are abnormal. In severe thrombocytopenia the number of petechiae is increased upto 100.

Prothrombin Time (PT)

It measures the extrinsic clotting system and the common pathway. The plasma from the patient as well as a normal child should be tested at the same time. The normal prothrombin time is 10–13 seconds. The patient's result is considered abnormal when it exceeds by more than 2 seconds compared to the control result. The preferred method of expression of the result is the INR (International normalized ratio) upper normal limit of which is 1.2.

The PT is prolonged with deficiencies of factors V, VII, X, fibrinogen and presence of certain inhibitors. To distinguish between factor deficiencies and presence of inhibitors, the test is repeated on the patient's plasma after adding a small volume of normal plasma. The PT is corrected completely if the abnormality is due to deficiency of the factors. Prothrombin time is normal with deficiencies of factors VIII, IX, XI and XII.

Activated Partial Thromboplastin Time (APTT)

It detects the abnormality in the intrinsic pathway of coagulation. In this test also the plasma from the patient as well as a normal child has to be tested at the same time. The normal APTT is 35 to 45 seconds. The patient's result is considered abnormal when the patient's APTT is 10 or more seconds longer than the control time. When the prothrombin time is normal an abnormal APTT indicates deficiency of factor VIII or factor IX; but rare deficiencies of factors XII, XI, as well as presence of inhibitors, must be considered.

Thrombin Time

The normal thrombin time is usually between 11–15 seconds. When the patient's thrombin time is more than 18 seconds it is considered as abnormal. Prolongation of thrombin time occurs with hypo or afibrinogenemia, dysfibrinogenemia or by presence of substances that interfere with fibrin polymerization viz. heparin or fibrin split products. *Reptilase time* is prolonged only with hypo or afibrinogenemia. Unlike the thrombin time, it is not sensitive to heparin. Therefore if thrombin time is prolonged but the reptilase time is normal, the prolonged thrombin time is due to heparin.

Table 8.4 : Screening tests profile in bleeding disorders

PC	*BT*	*PT*	*APTT*	*Inference*
N	N	N	N	Vascular disorder, factor XIII deficiency
L	I	N	N	Thrombocytopenia
N	I	N	N	Functional platelet disorder
N	N	N	I	Intrinsic pathway factor deficiency
N	N	I	N	Extrinsic pathway factor deficiency
N	I	N	I	vonWillebrand disease
N	N	I	I	Common pathway deficiency, liver disease, Vitamin K deficiency
D	I	I	I	Disseminated intravascular coagulation.

PC: platelet count, BT: bleeding time, PT: prothrombin time, APTT: activated partial thromboplastin time, N: normal, I: increased, D: decreased

Special Tests

The special tests include thromboplastin generation test, prothrombin consumption test, coagulation factor assay and platelet function tests. These tests are done in few specialized centres.

Replacement Therapy in Coagulation Disorders

The object of replacement therapy is to achieve rapid correction of the deficiency of one or more coagulation factors. Factors may be given in the form of whole blood, fresh frozen plasma (FFP), or factor concentrates. Long term prophylactic replacement therapy in case of severe hemophilia and Christmas disease, may be beneficial but is generally not practised in view of the storage of material and the possible increased risk of development of inhibitors due to antibody formation.

Irrespective of the type of coagulation abnormality, acute blood loss must always be replaced with whole blood or the appropriate fraction (viz. FFP, factor concentrate) when whole blood is not indicated. Only correction of clotting factor deficiency can be usually achieved by transfusion of fresh frozen plasma or an appropriate factor concentrate.

In spontaneous episodes of bleeding following minor trauma, a single transfusion of FFP, 10–15 ml / kg body weight usually arrests bleeding. When there is greater tissue damage or bleeding is from a dangerous site like tongue, it is usual to give twice the amount. In major trauma, including surgery, it is necessary to use clotting factor concentrates to avoid fluid overload. Treatment with factor concentrates should be monitored with factor assays and the amount required adjusted accordingly. The transfusion should be repeated at intervals of 24 hours or less for several days till bleeding stops. It is essential to monitor replacement therapy and adjust the dose and frequency according to the results of laboratory tests. The rate of administration should be rapid in order to obtain high peak blood concentrations of the clotting factor and optimum hemostatic effect.

Complications of replacement therapy with blood components include pyrogenic and allergic reactions, transfusion hepatitis and HIV infection.

Local Treatment at Bleeding Site

Local treatment measures include pressure, topical hemostatics and immobilization. Appropriate local treatment, especially in minor wounds, prevents prolonged bleeding and the need for replacement therapy.

Local pressure can be applied digitally, with pressure dressings and with sutures. In conjunction with topical hemostasis it is more effective.

Topical application of adrenaline solution (0.5–1%) has been found to be both safe and effective. Initially a temporary adrenaline moistened dressing is applied with pressure to the wound for about 5 minutes and repeated at intervals till bleeding has stopped or reduced. Then a permanent dressing is applied. If bleeding tends to recur, an aqueous solution of thrombin (1000 units of thrombin / ml) is applied to the wound after being rendered relatively blood free with vasoconstrictor drugs because natural antithrombins in the spilled blood will rapidly destroy the applied thrombin. Thrombin can also be used dissolved in a solution of adrenaline.

Suturing of wound should be done as and when indicated but bleeding should be controlled with topical hemostatics. Replacement therapy should be given when repeated attempts of local hemostasis fail or in case of a very deep and large wound.

Wounds should remain undisturbed until healing occurs. Immobilization by bandaging, with or without splinting helps to prevent recurrence of bleeding. In case of small wounds of mucus membrane (e.g. tongue) which cannot be immobilized, repeated application of local hemostatics usually prevents recurrence. Initially it should be applied frequently and subsequently several times a day till healing is evident.

In case of hematomas and hemarthrosis, the most useful measures are elevation and immobilization of the part. Aspiration of a hematoma should be done only when loculation is certain. Aspiration of the joint, particularly the knee may help in early ambulation but is not universally recommended. If done, these invasive procedures should be always done after coagulation factor replacement.

General Supportive Measures

The supportive measures viz. relief of pain, anxiety and hypovolemia helps in arrest of bleeding. Correction of iron deficiency anemia resulting from blood loss and physiotherapy when needed help to return to normal activity. Congenital coagulation disorders also require measures to prevent psychological and social complications, education for appropriate emergency care of acute episodes of bleeding and for hereditary counseling.

COMMON HEREDITARY CLOTTING FACTOR DEFICIENCY DISORDERS

Deficiencies

The most common serious hereditary clotting factor deficiencies include hemophilia A (factor VIII deficiency) and hemophilia B (factor IX deficiency) which presents with similar clinical findings. Factor XI deficiency, described as hemophilia C, is a rare defect with no world-wide distribution. von Willebrand disease is another hereditary disorder of hemostasis which clinically resembles hemophilia but with a defect of platelet function and a coagulation defect of factor VIII activity in plasma. This chapter will describe the above mentioned disorders. For the rare coagulation disorders one can consult a recommended book on hematology.

HEMOPHILIA

Hemophilia was the first described hemorrhagic disorder. It is a hereditary bleeding disorder of males transmitted by healthy women.

Two types of hemophilia have been described: Hemophilia A or classical hemophilia and hemophilia B or Christmas disease. The former is due to deficiency of factor VIII and the latter is due to deficiency of factor IX. Hemophilia occurs in approximately 1:5000 males, with 85% having factor VIII deficiency and 10–15% having factor IX deficiency. It is seen in all ethnic groups.

Inheritance

Hemophilia A and hemophilia B are genetically unrelated but both types are inherited as sex linked recessive characters. The genes for the disorders are carried by the sex chromosomes. The females carrying the gene in one of the two chromosomes transmit the gene to 50% of their female offspring and 50% of their male offspring. The female carrying a gene is called a carrier. The male with the gene invariably has the deficiency of the corresponding coagulation factor. Having one X chromosome, the hemophiliac, transmits the gene to all their female offspring, but to none of their male children. The male who inherit a gene for hemophilia invariably have deficiency of the corresponding coagulation factor.

The concentration of the deficient clotting factor in their plasma ranges from complete deficiency to as high as 30% of normal. Related males with hemophilia have a similar and usually identical concentration of the deficient clotting factor in their blood. The concentration does not vary with age.

About 30% of cases of severe hemophilia may be a result of gene mutation. In these cases, the evidence of inheritance is lacking. A small proportion of carriers, especially of hemophilia B, have a very mild tendency to bleed and a subnormal concentration of the relevant clotting factor in their blood.

Genetic analysis using a DNA probe can be used in both carrier detection and in prenatal diagnosis using chorionic biopsy or fetal blood collection. Such probes are available for hemophilia A, hemophilia B and vonWillebrand disease.

Classification

The severity of hemophilia is classified on the basis of patient's baseline level of factor VIII or factor IX because severity of bleeding corresponds to the factor levels. Conventionally, 100 ml of normal plasma has 100 U/ dl (100% activity) of each factor. The hemostatic level for factor VIII is more than 30–40 U/dl and for factor IX, 25–30 U/dl. *Severe hemophilia* is characterized by severe bleeding with the specific clotting factor level less than 1.0 U/dl (<1% activity). *Moderate hemophilia* require mild trauma to induce bleeding with a level between 1–5 U/dl. *Mild hemophilia,* on the other hand, require significant trauma to induce bleeding, have levels greater than 5 U/dl and may go undiagnosed for many years.

Pathophysiology

After injury, the initial hemostatic event is the formation of the platelet plug together with generation of the fibrin clot that prevents further hemorrhage. In the coagulation mechanism, factor VIII and factor IX together with phospholipids and calcium participate to form a factor X activating complex. With the deficiency of factor VIII or factor IX, clot formation is delayed and the clot that is formed may be friable. Hence onset of bleeding is gradual, continues for a long time, and may stop for some time to rebleed with minimal trauma.

Clinical Manifestations

The clinical manifestations vary in severity from patient to patient, but they tend to be same in related hemophiliacs.

The clinical severity is closely but not absolutely, related to the concentration of the deficient factor. Symptoms are usually severe when the concentration is less than 1%, mild when more than 5% except after surgery and severe trauma, and moderate when inbetween 1% and 5%.

There seems to be fluctuation of the bleeding tendency with phases of increased tendency to bleed and phases of reduced tendency to bleed. These phases vary in degree and duration. A phase of increased tendency to bleed commonly lasts for weeks or months and sometimes even years. The cause of the fluctuation is not known.

Both the factors VIII and IX do not cross the placenta. Therefore bleeding symptoms can appear in the fetus or may be present at birth. The bleeding tendency however, usually appears in infancy but may not become apparent until adolescence or adult life in mild cases. 10% of children with severe hemophilia may not be symptomatic till 1 year age.

A neonate with hemophilia may have intracranial hemorrhage. Only about 30% of affected male infants with hemophilia bleed with circumcision. It is only when the child begins to crawl or walk that mobility causes the initiation of easy bruising, intramuscular hematomas and hemarthrosis. Thus if a family history does not alert a physician, the diagnosis in the early infancy, may be missed.

Type and Site of Bleeding

Wound bleeding is the characteristic symptom of all hemophiliacs. It is usually slow and persists for days to weeks in spite of presence of large clots with recurrence of bleeding after hemostasis has apparently occurred.

Tissue bleeding occurs in the form of excessive bleeding from the site of a contusion, ligamentous strain or rupture of muscle fibres. It is most frequently seen in severe hemophiliacs when it may be spontaneous. Bleeding into tissues causes formation of hematomas which may lead to pain, swelling, fever, anorexia, leucocytosis and anemia. Intra-abdominal bleeding may present as acute abdomen. In moderate deficiency, tissue bleeding is infrequent and in mild deficiency it is rare.

Bruise, excessive after a slight injury is seen in all hemophiliacs but spontaneous bleeding into the skin and subcutaneous tissues is common with severe deficiency.

Bleeding from sockets after tooth extraction is common. In mild hemophiliacs it may be the first and sometimes the only presenting feature. Spontaneous epistaxis and bleeding into the muscles of the tongue is not uncommon in severe hemophilia.

Recurrent bleeding into the joint spaces occurs in severe hemophiliacs. It may occur spontaneously but usually result from minor joint strain or injury. In infants the ankle joint is affected. In older children, the knees are most frequently affected. It is less likely in moderate hemophilia and may never occur in mild hemophilia. Chronic arthritis with permanent joint damage usually follows after recurrent joint bleeding. Bleeding into joints was a common presentation before effective replacement therapy was available.

Intracranial hemorrhage can occur commonly after head injury as well as hematuria with ureteric colic can occur spontaneously in severe hemophilia. Hematemesis and melena can occur usually after ingestion of aspirin, as a complication of peptic ulcer or erosion of the mucosa due to an intramural hematoma.

General Features

Pain is the most common and disturbing symptom. It may be local in case of a hematoma, visceral as a result of an intramural intestinal hematoma or referred pain due to pressure effects of a hematoma on peripheral nerves, nerve roots or trunks.

Anemia frequently develops in patients with severe and moderate hemophilia due to blood loss. The *constitutional symptoms* during a bleeding episode include fever, anorexia, and malaise. Fever usually starts within 24 hours of bleeding into tissues and joint spaces and may persist for a week or more.

Laboratory Diagnosis

A moderate leucocytosis may accompany active bleeding, especially into tissues which may lead to a misinterpretation of a septic condition. The results of the screening tests show prolongation of the APTT. In severe hemophilia, the APTT is usually 2–3 times the upper limits of normal. The other screening tests viz. bleeding time, platelet count, PT and thrombin time are normal. The confirmation of diagnosis is done by the specific factor assay.

If there is an unexplained prolongation of the PT, APTT and thrombin time, a mixing study can be performed. Normal plasma is added to the patient's plasma and the PT and APTT are repeated. Correction of PT or APTT by 1:1 mixing with normal plasma suggests the deficiency of the particular factor.

In the newborn of the carrier mother, factor VIII assay can be done from cord blood or heel puncture after a few days. In case of factor IX, the factor assay should be done after 4–6 weeks as factor IX level may be normally low at birth and slow in rising to normal.

Prenatal diagnosis is possible by chorionic villous biopsy or examination of fetal blood.

Treatment

General Care

1. The whole family including the child needs emotional support. Particular care must be taken to avoid measures that could directly lead to loss of the self-confidence.
2. The child with severe hemophilia can go to kindergarten and ordinary schools. Physical activities should not be restricted. However, sports like foot-ball, basket ball, cricket etc should be avoided. On the other hand, sports like swimming, cycling, tennis and walking should be encouraged even in children with severe hemophilia. Good physical condition seems to reduce incidents of bleeding from sudden accidental strains.
3. It is advisable to plan education to enable children with severe hemophilia for sedentary occupation because they are likely to develop some physical disabilities.
4. Parents should be taught emergency medical care and taught to give first aid to control bleeding till treatment is available. A card should be provided to all hemophiliacs with detail informations. The severe hemophiliacs or the parents should be taught self-administration of factor concentrate for minor bleeding episodes. Careful dental hygiene and regular dental check up are important. Vaccination should be given with a fine needle (25 G) and pressure applied to the injection site for atleast 5 minutes. Aspirin and other NSAIDS that effect platelet function should be avoided.

Treatment of Bleeding

1. Infants and small children should be hospitalized and treated although the older children can be managed at home. However, the period of hospitalization should be kept as short as possible.
2. Local hemostatic measures (as described earlier) are enough to control bleeding from accessible and small wounds. Epistaxis can be usually controlled by external digital pressure just below the nasal bones for 5–15 minutes. If bleeding persists, cotton adrenaline pack is carried to the bleeding site and then pressure is applied. Rarely a thrombin–adrenaline pack may be required to arrest intractable bleeding. Vasoconstrictor nasal drops or spray should be used for several days after removal of the pack.

Replacement Therapy

During the mid twentieth century, whole blood or plasma was used for treatment of hemophilia. It was followed by discovery of cryoprecipitate in 1964 that contained factor VIII and subsequently both factors VIII and IX. In 1984, when the genes for both the factors were cloned, recombinant factors VIII and IX were developed to treat hemophilia A and B. This helped to avoid the infectious risk of plasma derived transfusion transmitted diseases.

When bleeding occurs, levels of factors VIII or IX must be raised to hemostatic levels (35– 40 U/ dl). For major or life threatening bleeding the level should be raised to 100 U/dl. The different type of blood products which can be used includes fresh frozen plasma (FFP) which supplies all coagulation factors, cryoprecipitate of factor VIII, and factor concentrates of recombinant factors VIII and IX. Whole blood can be used when the diagnosis is uncertain in congenital coagulation disorders.

Early administration of factor concentrate after the onset of bleeding is the best step in management. Advice for home therapy is the best method of ensuring early therapy.

The indications of concentrates include (a) home therapy, (b) severe bleeding episodes especially CNS bleeding, (c) failure of response to FFP or severe allergic reaction, and (d) prophylaxis for surgery. The dose of recombinant factor VIII and factor IX can be calculated as follows:

Factor VIII (U/dl)

Dose = (% U/dl desired rise in plasma factor VIII) × wt. in kg × 0.5.

Factor IX (U/dl)

Dose = (% U/dl desired rise in plasma factor IX) × wt. in Kg × 1.4.

If cryoprecipitate or factor concentrate is not available, FFP is safe and effective in most instances of spontaneous and mild bleeding. In acute hemarthrosis and hematomas, a dose of 10–15 ml/kg given over a period of 30–60 minutes often effectively arrests bleeding. This dose normally needs to be repeated at intervals of 12–24 hours until the episode of bleeding is fully controlled. The disadvantages of FFP are the large volume required, and frequent allergic reactions. It is advisable to give an anti-histaminic intravenously at the beginning of infusion and corticosteroids should be available if required. The APTT should be done soon after a dose of FFP.

Life long prophylactic therapy with factor concentrate can be advised to prevent spontaneous joint bleeding. Usually it should be started with the first joint bleeding. It helps in reducing the problems of chronic arthropathy.

Other Therapeutic Measures

With mild factor VIII deficiency, administration of desmopressin acetate can release the endogenously stored factor VIII. With moderate to severe factor VIII deficiency, the stored levels are inadequate; hence desmopressin therapy is ineffective. Desmopressin is not effective in the treatment of factor IX deficiency.

A nasal spray preparation of desmopressin may be used in the doses 150 microgram for children weighing < 50 kg and 300 microgram for children and young adults weighing > 50 kg.

Androgen therapy, danazol has been shown to raise the levels of factor VIII and factor IX in some cases of hemophilia A and B.

Surgery in Hemophilia

Major surgery should be avoided whenever possible. When necessary it should be performed in a centre where facilities for monitoring the response to replacement therapy are available. Factor concentrates should be given at 12 hourly intervals in hemophilia A and 24 hours intervals in hemophilia B. The dose must be adequate to increase the levels to normal range (0.5–1.0 U/ml) during surgery and to maintain levels of 0.4 U/ml until wound healing is complete.

Minor procedures including tooth extraction should be carried out in hospitals with provision for special care for hemophiliacs. Replacement therapy is usually not required except occasionally it may be indicated for lumbar puncture because of the risk of CNS bleeding. Tooth extraction is a common minor procedure in children which can be managed by pre extraction replacement therapy with FFP (10–15 ml/kg), local anesthesia, gentle extraction, insertion of catgut suture and local pressure. Moderate bleeding may occur which should be accepted by the doctor and parents reassured that it is without danger.

Physiotherapy, Orthopedic Care

The use of physiotherapy and orthopedic care has been greatly reduced with early replacement therapy. However they are necessary in presence of muscle and joint deformities.

VON WILLEBRAND DISEASE

von Willebrand disease is a disorder of hemostasis with clinical resemblance to hemophilia but inherited as an autosomal dominant character (occasionally recessive) affecting both sexes. It is characterized by a defect in platelet function giving rise to a prolonged bleeding time and a coagulation defect due to deficiency of factor VIII activity in plasma.

Pathophysiology

The von Willebrand factor (vWF) is a large multimeric glycoprotein that is synthesized in the platelets and endothelial cells. During normal hemostasis, vWF adheres to the subendothelial matrix after vascular damage. When vWF binds to the subendothelial matrix, it causes platelets to adhere to vWF through their glycoprotein IB receptor. These platelets are then activated which in turn causes the recruitment of additional platelets to cause platelet aggregation. vWF also serves as the carrier protein for plasma factor VIII. In contrast to hemophilia where there is factor VIII deficiency with normal or increased vWF, in von Willebrand disease both factor VIII and vWF vary together. A severe deficiency of vWF may cause a secondary deficiency in factor VIII, even though the gene of factor VIII is normal.

Depending on the mutations in different loci that code for different functional domains of the vWF protein, different variants are described. Hence it is classified as type I where vWF antigen is quantitatively reduced but not absent, type II, where vWF antigen is qualitatively abnormal and type III, where vWF antigen is very low or absent.

Table 8.5 : Variants of von Willebrand disease

Type I (classical)	Factor VIII activity low, vWF antigen low, vWF: Rc low
Type II A	Factor VIII activity normal or low, vWF antigen low or normal, vWF: Rc* very low
Type II B	As above, vWF: Rc normal or low, platelet low
Type II N	Factor VIII activity low, vWF antigen normal or low, vWF: Rc normal or low
Type II M	Factor VIII activity normal, vWF antigen normal or low, vWF: Rc very low
PT-vWD	Factor VII activity normal, vWF antigen low, vWF: Rc low, platelet low
Type III (Severe)	As in type I but all activities very low or absent

vWF: Rc = Ristocetin cofactor

Clinical Manifestations

The symptoms of mucocutaneous bleeding like excessive bruising, epistaxis, menorrhagia and post operative hemorrhage particularly after mucosal surgery e.g. tonsillectomy or tooth extraction are the common presenting features.

In case of excessive menstrual bleeding in an adolescent girl, one should take a detailed history of easy bruising, and other bleeding. It is helpful to recommend vWD testing on all teenage females with menorrhagia before initiating hormonal therapy or oral contraceptives. Stress increases the level of vWF because it is an acute phase reactant. Therefore they do not bleed in operative procedures which incur major stress e.g. appendectomy, cesarean section.

In type 3 von Willebrand disease, bleeding symptoms are much more profound. They may present with severe epistaxis or menorrhagia that results in major blood loss and sometimes shock. They are diagnosed early in life. Rarely, there may be joint hemorrhage or spontaneous central nervous system hemorrhage.

Laboratory Diagnosis

The laboratory features include a prolonged bleeding time, and an increased APTT. The platelet count is usually normal but in type II B variant there may be life-long thrombocytopenia. The bleeding time and APTT are normal in type 1. Confirmation can be done by quantitative assay of vWF antigen, vWF activity, plasma factor VIII activity and determination of vWF structure. There is defective or absent platelet aggregation and normal or decreased vWF and normal or decreased factor VIII.

Treatment

Treatment of von Willebrand disease is directed towards increasing the levels of von Willebrand factor and factor VIII. Elevation of plasma level of vWF will result also in increase in factor VIII because the gene for factor VIII is normal in patients with von Willebrand disease.

The modalities available are desmopressin and vWF (von Willebrand factor) infusion. The type I vWD responds to desmopressin while the other types do not. They require vWF infusion.

The dose of desmopressin is 150 microgram for children weighing less than 50 kg and 300 microgram for those weighing more than 50 kg by intranasal route. If bleeding is severe, desmopressin should be used intravenously in the dose of 0.3 microgram/ kg. It will increase vWF and factor VIII by 3–4 folds.

Current replacement therapy uses plasma derived vWF that also contain factor VIII. Purified vWF concentrates or recombinant vWF (containing no factor VIII) are not available at present. When available it will be useful in presurgical or prophylactic management. However, when used for acute bleeding vWF concentrates may need to be supplemented by an infusion of recombinant factor VIII for the first infusion, because if only vVF is replaced, the endogenous correction of factor VIII level takes 12–24 hours. Dental extraction and epistaxis can be managed with desmopressin and an antifibrinolytic agent.

DISSEMINATED INTRAVASCULAR COAGULATION

Disseminated intravascular coagulation (DIC) is a disorder that results in consumption of clotting factors, platelets, and anticoagulant proteins resulting in widespread intravascular deposition of fibrin leading to tissue ischemia and necrosis, generalized hemorrhagic state and microangiopathic hemolytic anemia.

Etiology

DIC most frequently accompanies a severe systemic disease. It may be triggered by a number of life threatening processes including hypoxia, acidosis, tissue necrosis, shock and endothelial damage.

A large number of conditions have been reported to be associated with DIC. They include septic shock (especially as a result of gram negative septicemia and meningococcemia), incompatible blood transfusion, snake bite, purpura fulminans, giant hemangioma, rickettsial infection, and malignancies especially acute promyelocytic leukemia.

The initiating event is an excessive activation of the clotting that consumes both the physiologic anticoagulants (viz. protein C, protein S and antithrombins) and procoagulants resulting in a deficiency of factor VIII, factor V, prothrombin, fibrinogen and platelets. The result is clinical symptoms of hemorrhage. The hemostatic dysregulation results in widespread intravascular thrombosis, ischemia and organ damage especially in the skin, kidneys and brain.

Clinical Manifestations

Bleeding is the most common clinical presentation of DIC. It frequently first occurs from sites of venepuncture or surgical incision. The skin may show petechiae and ecchymoses.

The effects of ischemia due to thrombosis may manifest as infarction of large areas of skin, and subcutaneous tissue. Renal failure may be a serious complication. It is considered to be due to a combination of hypotension and deposition of fibrin in the small renal vessels. Hemolysis as a result of microangiopathic hemolytic anemia may result in rapidly developing anemia.

Laboratory Diagnosis

There is prolongation of prothrombin time, partial thromboplastin time and thrombin time. The hemoglobin is decreased, platelet count may be profoundly decreased and fibrin degradation products appear in blood. The peripheral blood smear contain fragmented RBCs, burr cells, helmet shaped RBCs.

Once the precipitating cause disappears, the clotting factor activities return to normal levels within 24 hours. Thrombocytopenia may persist for several days. The fibrin degradation products remain detectable in blood for 12–24 hours.

Treatment

The principles of treatment include:

1. Treatment of the trigger factor that caused DIC.
2. Restoration of normal hemostasis by correction of shock, acidosis and hypoxia.
3. Replacement of the coagulation factors and platelets.
4. Inhibition of the clotting process.

If the triggering condition can be controlled, bleeding quickly ceases. There is improvement of the abnormal laboratory findings. Blood component therapy is required in patients with hemorrhage e.g. platelet infusion for thrombocytopenia, cryoprecipitate for hypofibrinogenemia, and/or FFP for replacement of coagulation factors.

Heparin infusion has been found to be effective in children with DIC associated with purpura fulminans and acute myeloblastic leukemia (M_3). It may be indicated in DIC associated with other causes when thrombosis is present. Heparin is usually started together with replacement of clotting factors and platelet, as a continuous infusion starting with a low dose of 5–10 U/kg/hour. Otherwise it will result in profound hemorrhage. The duration of therapy and its effectiveness is judged by serial measurement of platelet count, fibrinogen level and fibrin degradation products.

Thrombocytopenia

Thrombocytopenia is defined as a reduction in the peripheral blood platelet count below the lower normal limit of $150 \times 10^9/l$.

Thrombocytopenia may result from impaired platelet production, accelerated platelet destruction, or dilution and/or splenic sequestration. Thrombocytopenia is associated with a number of disorders which may be acquired or congenital. The common causes are shown in the table below:

Table 8. 6 : Common causes of thrombocytopenia

Acquired
Common causes
ITP
Drugs and chemicals
Leukemia
Aplastic anemia

Contd.

Contd.

Hypersplenism
SLE

Less common causes

DIC
Massive blood transfusion
Liver disease
Megaloblastic anemia
Infections including HIV

Rare causes

Thrombotic thrombocytopenia
Post transfusion thrombocytopenia
Hemangioma
Food allergy
Idiopathic cryoglobulinemia

Congenital and neonatal

Immune

Autoimmune: Mother with chronic ITP
Isoimmune: Platelet group incompatibility

Infections

TORCH

Drugs to mother

Thiazide for prolonged periods (upto 3 months) during pregnancy, Associated with immune drug induced thrombocytopenia in the mother

Hereditary

Aldrich's syndrome

Congenital leukemia

Giant hemangioma

Congenital megakaryocytic hypoplasia

IDIOPATHIC THROMBOCYTOPENIC PURPURA

Idiopathic thrombocytopenic purpura (ITP) also known as immune thrombocytopenic purpura is one of the most common bleeding disorders encountered in children. It is a disorder characterized by skin and/or mucosal bleeds in a healthy child with isolated thrombocytopenia (platelet count < 150×10^9/L). It is not a hereditary or familial disorder, although in occasional cases there is a family history of easy bruising or even of frank bleeding viz. epistaxis.

Classification

There are two clinical types namely acute and chronic. *Acute ITP* is common in children aged 2–5 years and accounts for majority of cases in children. In most cases, bleeding ceases spontaneously after a period varying from few days to 12 weeks. In the remainder it usually ceases by 6 months. In around 10% cases it persists beyond 6 months and runs the course of chronic ITP. *Chronic ITP* is commonly a disease of young and middle aged women. The onset is usually less abrupt; symptoms are often intermittent with remissions lasting for weeks, months, or even years.

Pathophysiology

The mechanism of acute idiopathic thrombocytopenia is not well understood. In about 75% of cases, there is a history of preceding viral infection or live viral vaccination and antibody formation resulting from some reaction between the virus and platelets. Platelets with bound antibody are removed by the reticuloendothelial system particularly in the spleen but with the tendency that increasing platelet antibody load increases hepatic sequestration. There is also a small percentage of intravascular platelet lysis. It may be that the thrombocytopenia represents a hypersensitivity reaction to the infection. The antibodies are identified to be IgG antibodies in the majority of cases and bound complement in some.

Clinical Manifestations

The usual presentation is acute onset of mucocutaneous bleeds in a healthy child i.e. in absence of fever or any systemic abnormality. It occurs in children between 2 and 10 years of age and the peak age is 2–5 years. The sex incidence is approximately equal in children upto the age of 12 years. Thereafter females are affected 3–4 times more than males.

There may be a history of a viral illness 1–4 weeks preceding the onset or a history of live viral vaccination (especially MMR) in the recent past.

The bleeding commonly occurs spontaneously but may occur following trauma, surgery or dental procedures. Bleeding from wounds tends to occur at once, ceases within 48 hours and does not recur.

The most common site of bleeding is the skin and it may be the only site in mild cases. The hemorrhage may take the form of multiple petechiae and ecchymoses. The *petechial spots* vary from the size of a pin point to a pin head or even larger. They are not raised and do not blanch on pressure. When fresh they are pink in colour but with time they pass through colour changes of absorbing blood. They appear in crops and especially seen in abundance in the arms and legs, the neck and upper part of the chest. *Ecchymoses* may appear with petechiae or alone. They vary in size, initially purple in colour.

Bleeding from mucous membrane is common and occasionally may occur in absence of skin bleeding. Epistaxis and bleeding gums are the most common forms but hematuria, menorrhagia and melena are not infrequent. Hemoptysis and hematemesis occur less commonly. Bleeding into internal organs especially intracranial hemorrhage may occur but is very rare. Few precipitating factors of intracranial hemorrhage include aspirin ingestion, trauma, and hypertension and platelet count $< 20 \times 10^9$/L.

Table 8.7 : Clinical grading of acute ITP (UK survey, 1997)

Asymptomatic	Incidentally detected low platelet count.
Mild disease	Bruising, petechiae, minor epistaxis, very little or no interference with daily living.
Moderate disease	Skin bleeds more severe, some mucosal bleeds, more troublesome epistaxis and menorrhagia.
Severe disease	Bleeding episodes (epistaxis, melena, hematuria, and/or menorrhagia) requiring hospitalization and/or transfusion, symptoms seriously interfering with quality of life.

On examination, the outstanding feature is absence of physical findings except those due to bleeding viz. petechiae, ecchymoses. Subconjunctival hemorrhage and retinal hemorrhage are relatively common. Anemia is proportionate to the blood loss. There may be a just palpable spleen in 10% cases.

Laboratory Diagnosis

The outstanding feature in examination of the blood picture is thrombocytopenia which may vary from values ranging from just below normal to less than 10×10^9/L. The platelet size is normal or increased. The bleeding time is prolonged upto 30 minutes and the tourniquet test is positive. There is anemia which is proportional to the degree of blood loss. Initially it is normocytic normochromic type. With prolonged bleeding (e.g. menorrhagia) it may be microcytic hypochromic as a result of iron deficiency. The total leukocyte count, differential leukocyte count is normal. The total leukocyte count may be increased in presence of bleeding. The ESR is normal.

The bone marrow examination shows a normal granulocytic and erythrocytic series. The megakaryocytes are normal or increased in number and some of them appear to be immature which reflects an increased turnover. A routine bone marrow examination is not necessary for diagnosis. It may be done before starting steroid therapy.

An antinuclear antibody (ANA) test is positive, more in adolescents with ITP and may indicate a higher likelihood of eventual chronic ITP.

Treatment of Acute ITP

Most children with ITP do not have serious bleeding and can be watched with sensible advice to the parents without giving pharmacological therapy to raise the platelet count. Most children remit spontaneously within 6–8 weeks and have only cutaneous or mild bleeding symptoms even with very low platelet count ($<10 \times 10^9$/ L). This is because the few platelets available function more efficiently and secondly platelet counts obtained by automated machines are inaccurate at these low levels.

Children with acute ITP and mild clinical disease should be managed with supportive advice.

Supportive Advice

- The parents and child should be explained the nature of the disease, the rarity of severe bleeding and good outcome.
- The child should not be excluded from school. Restriction of activity should be minimal and confined to avoidance of contact sports (football, kabbadi etc), use of helmets to prevent injury. Swimming, cycling and other noncontact sports should continue.
- Certain antiplatelet drugs like aspirin, phenacetin, antihistaminics, phenothiazines and NSAIDS are to be avoided.
- Deep intramuscular injections should be avoided and if it has to be given, then pressure over the injection site should be maintained for 10 minutes continuously.
- Immunization with live viral vaccine preferably avoided during the period of severe thrombocytopenia.
- Parents should be advised when they should report to the hospital.
- The full blood count should be repeated within 7 days of diagnosis to exclude a serious marrow disorder.

Indications of Hospitalization

The American Society of Hematology recommends that hospitalization is appropriate in the following situations:

1. A child with severe life threatening bleeding regardless of the platelet count.
2. With a platelet count $< 20 \times 10^9$ / l and mucus membrane bleeding that may require intervention.

3. With platelet count > 20×10^9 / l in a child who may be inaccessible or noncompliant or whose parents request hospitalization.

Emergency Intervention

The appropriate intervention in case of severe life threatening bleeding include platelet transfusion, high dose parenteral corticosteroids (30 mg/kg body weight methyl prednisolone for 3 days) and IVIg. Severe bleeding is characterized by the following bleeding manifestations:

1. Suspected internal hemorrhage/documented intracranial hemorrhage.
2. Repeated, continuous and/or profuse epistaxis requiring more than 15 minutes pressure.
3. Continuous active bleeding from gums, lips, buccal mucosa or posterior pharynx.
4. Extensive petechiae and >5 bruises of >3 cm in diameter.

Indications for Therapy

Cases presenting with only skin bleeds and having a platelet count > 20×10^9/L may be given no therapy but should be monitored closely. Once mucosal bleeds occur or there is suspicion of intracranial bleed they will require intervention. Therapy is recommended in the following situations:

1. Platelet count <20×10^9/L.
2. Patient with significant mucosal bleeds viz. epistaxis, gastrointestinal or genitourinary.
3. Patients requiring surgical procedure.

Modalities of Treatment

The modalities of treatment include (a) drugs, and (b) blood component therapy. The drugs used are (i) oral prednisolone, (ii) methyl prednisolone, (iii) IVIG. All these drugs are effective in increasing the platelet count and in shortening the duration of thrombocytopenia.

Oral steroid is recommended as the first line therapy in acute ITP. The mechanism of action of steroids in treating thrombocytopenia involves multiple factors. They are:

1. Reduction of antibody production in spleen and bone marrow.
2. Decreased consumption of antibody coated platelets by spleen or bone marrow.
3. Increase production of platelets by bone marrow.
4. Reversal of endothelial thinning towards normal. Experimental studies have shown that there is thinning of endothelium with development of fenestration in ITP.

The aim of drug therapy is to achieve a safe level of platelet i.e. > 20×10^9/L. The different drug regimens recommended for treatment of acute ITP include the following:

Conventional dose oral prednisolone, 1–2 mg/ kg body weight for 2–3 weeks followed by tapering the dose in the next week. Some patients may develop a drop in their platelet count during the tapering without clinical deterioration. This is usually transitory and is not an indication to step up the dose. Therapy with conventional doses of prednisolone increases the platelet count faster than in those without treatment but takes about 8–10 days before significant changes are noticed.

High dose oral prednisolone is usually indicated in severe cases as well as in cases with extensive cutaneous and mucosal bleeding. Prednisolone is given in a dose 4 mg/kg body weight for 4 days followed by reduction in the dose to conventional levels and tapering and cessation of therapy by 3 weeks. The same dose have shown to produce good results when used as a short course for only 4 days; the platelet count rising to > 20×10^9/L at 72 hours.

High dose methyl prednisolone produces a more rapid rise in platelet count than conventional oral steroids. This is nearly as rapid as that seen with IVIG. It is therefore, useful in cases with life threatening bleeds. 30 mg/kg/day for initial 3 days followed by 20 mg/kg/day for 4 days is the recommended dosage schedule.

Intravenous IgG is usually effective in raising the platelet count to safe levels within 24–48 hours. However the peak effect is 9 and 12 days in IVIG and steroids respectively, which is not significant. The recent recommendation of a single dose of 0.8 gm/kg body weight is often adequate. If this dose does not produce a desired effect it may be repeated. Another regimen is 1 gm/kg body weight for 2 days but with no added advantage. IVIG should be reserved for emergency treatment of patients who have active bleeding and do not respond to corticosteroids. It is an appropriate treatment to enable essential surgery and dental extractions when a platelet count of 50×10^9/L is desired. However, IVIG is a pooled blood product and has significant side effects. Besides severe headache, fever, chills, vomiting it can transmit hepatitis B and C, cytomegalovirus infection, HIV and possible risk of infection with unknown viruses like variant Creuzfeld-Jacob virus.

Table 8.8 : Commonly used drugs and doses in acute ITP

Drugs	*Dosage schedule*
1. Conventional prednisolone	1–2 mg /kg body weight/day for 2–3 weeks, tapering off in another week.
2. High dose prednisolone	4 mg/kg/day for 4 days, reduction to 1–2 mg/kg for 2–3 weeks and tapering off in another week.
3. Methyl prednisolone	30 mg/kg/day I.V. for 3 days, followed by 20 mg/kg/day for 4 days.

Intravenous anti D globulin use in the initial therapy of acute ITP is under investigation. It has been shown that given at a dose of 60–75 microgram/kg (to Rh + ve individuals only) have demonstrated a rise in platelet count to levels above 20×10^9/L within 2 days. It can be given as an infusion. Enough data in children is not available for recommendation of its routine use.

Management of Epistaxis and Menorrhagia

Epistaxis should be managed with local measures and fibrinolytic agents. Menorrhagia can be managed with oral fibrinolytic agents (like tranexamic acid) taken for first few days of the period or with hormonal control.

Table 8.9 : Types of presentations and treatment of acute ITP

Presentations	*Platelet count*	*Treatment*
Life threatening bleeds	Any platelet count	Plate transfusion + IVIG + High dose methyl-prednisolone
Extensive cutaneous mucosal bleed	Any platelet count	High dose prednisolone/conventional prednisolone
Only skin bleeds	$> 20 \times 10^9$ / L	Supportive advice
Essential surgery and dental extraction	Desired level > 50×10^9 L	IVIG

Blood Component Therapy

Platelet transfusion has little role in acute ITP because the platelets are being destroyed by an immunological process. Platelet transfusion may be helpful in intracranial hemorrhage or in life threatening bleeding to tide over the crisis. It should follow IVIG infusion. Platelet transfusion should be given in much higher doses than for marrow failure. Packed cell transfusion is indicated only if the bleeds have been significant enough to result in moderate anemia.

Monitoring of Platelet Count

In a stable child with acute ITP without any mucosal bleeding, a repeat count should be done after 7 days to know the response or evolution of any occult disease in the bone marrow. An immediate platelet count should be done if there is any fresh mucosal bleeding. In a child with severe bleeding, platelet count may be repeated within 24–48 hours. Once there is adequate rise in platelets, monitoring and repeat counts should be guided by clinical manifestations.

Splenectomy

Splenectomy is considered as a therapeutic option in acute ITP refractory to all medical modalities of therapy and having repeated significant mucosal bleed or life threatening bleeds.

Prognosis

Around 80–85% of children with acute ITP recover spontaneously or after therapy. The remainder pursues a chronic or recurrent course. Children with chronic ITP have infrequent bleeds in spite of very low platelet count ($< 10 \times 10^9$ /L).

Treatment of Newborn of Mother with ITP

The platelet count should be done 3–4 days after birth. A USG of brain should be done if the platelet count is $<50 \times 10^9$/L.

Newborn with USG evidence of intracranial bleed and a platelet count $<20 \times 10^9$/litre should be treated with combined IVIG and corticosteroids. If the platelet count is $<20 \times 10^9$/litre without any evidence of intracranial hemorrhage, the newborn should be treated with only IVIG. Platelet counts between 20–50 $\times 10^9$/litre do not necessarily require IVIG treatment. The newborn with platelet count $> 50 \times 10^9$/litre need no treatment. There is no contradiction to breastfeeding the infant.

Treatment of Chronic ITP

Chronic ITP which is characterized by a platelet count of less than 150×10^9 / L persisting for more than 6 months from the onset of illness is common in older children, especially in adolescent girls. An underlying disease may be present and should be sought for.

Therefore investigations to be done should include a bone marrow examination to exclude causes of bone marrow suppression, and antinuclear antibody titre to screen autoimmune disorders. One should also keep in mind the association of HIV infection and hepatitis C and investigate when necessary.

Optimal management of Chronic ITP continues to be controversial and heavily debated. Most patients have minimal or no symptoms even with low platelet counts. Only a small subset (around 5%) is symptomatic with severe thrombocytopenia (platelet count $< 20 \times 10^9$/L) at one year or longer. Hence the aim of treatment should be *"treat the patient and not the platelet count"*. Those children who have only skin bleeds must be only observed irrespective of the platelet count. Such patients may show recovery even after as long as 10 years since the onset.

The parents are to be explained about the nature of the disease, reassured and explained the plan of treatment. It should be clarified that the primary target of any therapeutic modality for this condition is to keep the patient with a safe level platelet count and not to achieve complete remission or a normal platelet count.

Splenectomy is undoubtedly the most effective treatment modality for chronic ITP. Splenectomy should be considered after atleast 2 years have elapsed since diagnosis giving a fair chance for spontaneous remission or partial recovery. Splenectomy should be preferably planned in children above 5 years of age. The overall sustained remission can be expected in 75–80% patients. Appropriate pre and post operative prophylaxis should be advised.

Alternatives to splenectomy should be considered only for splenectomy failures. Various therapeutic options are available but merits of the individual therapies are difficult to assess because of paucity of randomized controlled trials. The options available are:

1. Long-term corticosteroids.
2. IV immunoglobulin G.
3. Pulse dexamethasone.
4. IV anti-D globulin.
5. Immunosuppressive drugs: Cyclosporin, azathioprine, vinca alkaloids, cyclophosphamide.
6. Rituximab.

Long-term steroids, IVIG, anti D globulin, dexamethasone pulse therapy none of these can produce sustained remission.

Those who initially responded to *steroids* may be continued on long-term low dose steroids (5–10 mg on alternate day).

IVIG in a dose of 250 mg/kg/day for 2 days every 4 weeks shows a good response in 75% cases with a platelet count $> 50 \times 10^9$/l or twice above the base line with control of clinical bleeding but the response is sustained in only 30–40% cases.

Pulse dexamethasone therapy is no longer recommended because high doses have to be continued for a long time with side effects but no sustained effect.

Anti Rh D globulin can be given to only Rh + ve children. It is ineffective in post splenectomy cases, requires repeated doses every 4 weeks and its effect is not sustained. It can cause intravascular hemolysis which may be fatal.

Immunosuppressive drugs viz. cyclosporin, azathioprine, vinca alkaloids and cyclophosphamide are potentially toxic drugs, tried mostly in adults. The overall effectiveness has been variable and remission achieved is short lived. About 2% of children do not respond either to splenectomy, IVIG or steroids and continue to bleed with a platelet count of less than $10–30 \times 10^9$/L. In these children immunosuppressive drugs may be an alternative.

Rituximab is a relatively newer modality which has been reported to be successful with prolonged remission. The recommended dose is 375 mg/m^2 given weekly for upto 6 weeks. Early cases where not much treatment has been given and non-splenectomized patients have a better and early response. Rituximab is well tolerated, apart from fever and skin rash in some patients. This drug seems to be beneficial in children with severe chronic ITP.

Course and Prognosis

Long-term followup of children with chronic ITP has shown that remissions continue to occur over a prolonged period even 10 years after diagnosis. The predicted spontaneous remission rate is 61% after 15 years. Hence essentially treatment of childhood chronic ITP consists of supporting the patient and the parents until there is spontaneous cure. Such families need help and sensible advice concerning living with the disorder rather than a series of potentially toxic treatments, which may be more harmful than good for the child.

Pancytopenia

Pancytopenia is characterized by simultaneous presence of anemia, leucopenia and thrombocytopenia. The presenting symptoms are usually attributable to anemia or thrombocytopenia. Leucopenia is an uncommon cause of initial presentation but when present is life threatening.

A wide variety of conditions can cause pancytopenia. The causes are shown in the table below:

Table 8.10 : Causes of pancytopenia

Aplastic anemia
Subleukemic leukemia, preleukemia
Hypersplenism
Administration of cytotoxic drugs and antimetabolites
Radiotherapy
Megaloblastic anemia
Systemic lupus erythematosus
Severe sepsis
Bone marrow infiltration or replacement as in Hodgkin's and non-Hodgkin's lymphoma
Paroxysmal nocturnal hemoglobinuria

It should be noted that the frequency with which each of the above mentioned condition is associated with pancytopenia differs considerably. Pancytopenia is invariably present at some stage in the course of aplastic anemia, very common in subleukemic leukemia, and relatively uncommon in lymphoma.

APLASTIC ANEMIA

Aplastic anemia is a term used to describe a disorder characterized by anemia, leucopenia, and thrombocytopenia resulting from aplasia of the bone marrow. The fundamental pathological feature is a reduction in the amount of hemopoetic tissue, causing an inability to produce normal numbers of mature cells for discharge into the blood stream. However, the marrow is not uniformly hypocellular and patchy areas of normal cellularity and hypercellularity are sometimes interspersed between the areas of hypocellularity. It is a rare disorder.

Classification

Aplastic anemia is classified into constitutional and acquired. The acquired type may be primary/idiopathic or secondary. The *constitutional type* is associated with inherited defects in DNA repair e.g. Fanconi's anemia. The group of cases where the etiology is unknown is termed as *idiopathic*. The most common cause of *secondary aplastic anemia* is exposure to drugs and chemicals.

Table 8.11 : Classification and causes of aplastic anemia

Constitutional
Fanconi's anemia
Acquired
Primary / Idiopathic
Secondary
– Exposure to radiation
– Exposure to drugs and chemicals e.g. Benzene, chloramphenicol and gold salts
– Virus infection
• Cytomegalovirus
• Ebstein-Barr
• Hepatitis B, hepatitis C
• Human immunodeficiency virus (HIV)
• Parvo virus B_{19}
• Herpes
– Immune diseases
• Thymoma
• Hypoimmunoglobulinemia
– Paroxysmal nocturnal hemoglobinuria
– Marrow replacement
• Preleukemia, subleukemic leukemia
• Myelodysplasia
• Myelofibrosis

Etiology

Apart from the uncommon constitutional type i.e. Fanconi's anemia, aplastic anemia most commonly develops as a response to extrinsic factors like drugs and chemicals, which are normally tolerated by majority of the population.

Fanconi's anemia is associated with a diminished capacity for DNA repair and increased breakage of chromosome during mitosis. The resulting aberration may serve as an initiating event in the development of aplastic anemia or of leukemia. There may be associated abnormalities such as patchy brown cutaneous pigmentation and neurological, renal, or skeletal malformations.

The most notable agents causing aplasia are benzene, chloramphenicol and gold. The severity and duration of the pancytopenia is dependent on the extent of exposure to these agents. A genetic predisposition may exist and may increase the likelihood of pancytopenia after exposure.

Chloramphenicol produces two distinct patterns of toxicity: dose dependent reversible hemopoetic depression and idiosyncratic aplastic anemia.

The *reversible toxic effect* takes the form of an arrested erythropoiesis and consequent depression of the reticulocyte count when the serum chloramphenicol levels

Table 8.12 : Common drugs causing aplastic anemia

Anticonvulsants	*Antibacterials*	*Antirheumatic*	*Tranquilizers*	*Miscellaneous*
Methusuximide	Chloramphenicol	Diclofenec	Chlorpromazine	Chlorothiazide
Methylhydantoin	Sulphonamides	Phenylbutazone	Chlordiazepoxide	Acetazolamide
Carbamazepine	Isoniazid	Indomethacin	Promazine	Hydralazine
	Arsenicals	Gold salts		

are sustained at 15– 20 microgram/ml for atleast several days. There may be depressed production of platelets also. Bone marrow reveals decreased proportions of erythroid precursors. These changes are normal pharmacological responses to relatively high blood levels of chloramphenicol. Recovery of erythropoiesis and thrombocytopenia normally takes place in a matter of days when the drug is withdrawn. Such an effect is not observed with conventional therapeutic doses (50 mg/ kg/ day).

The *idiosyncratic type* is dose independent. There may be a previous history of exposure to Chloramphenicol. The majority of instances follow administration of chloramphenicol for several days at conventional doses. Symptoms may not become evident for weeks or months. The incidence of aplastic anemia following administration of chloramphenicol appears somewhat fewer than 1 in 10,000. However, even such a risk is not acceptable when alternative antibiotics with less severe side effects are available.

As regards other drugs there is currently no evidence of a mechanism to account for the idiosyncratic response. It is difficult to ascertain whether these represents chance relationship or otherwise.

Benzene is a cyclic hydrocarbon employed as a solvent in glues. It can also be found in paint removers and adhesive and cleaning solutions. Aplasia has also been reported following exposure to insecticides gama benzene hexachloride, chlordane, chlorophenothane (DDT) and trinitrotoluene.

Aplastic anemia can occur as a sequel of viral hepatitis A in young children. It develops as an apparent idiosyncratic phenomenon after recovery has taken place.

Pathology and Pathogenesis

The hallmark of acquired aplastic anemia is peripheral pancytopenia coupled with hypoplastic or aplastic bone marrow. The severity of clinical disease is related to the degree of myelosuppression. On the basis of the degree, it may be classified as severe aplastic anemia (SAA) and non-severe aplastic anemia.

Severe aplastic anemia is defined as a condition in which two or more cell components have become seriously compromised viz. an absolute neutrophil count < 500 / mm^3, platelet count $< 20 \times 10^9$ /L, a reticulocyte count $< 1\%$ after correction for the hematocrit, in a patient whose bone marrow is moderately or severely hypocellular.

Non-severe aplastic anemia is characterized by a hypoplastic bone marrow with pancytopenia but fulfilling only one of the above mentioned criteria.

Bone marrow failure can result from several mechanisms. It may be a consequence of a direct cytotoxic effect on the hemopoetic stem cells from a drug or chemical or may result from either cell mediated or antibody dependent cytotoxicity. Many cases of aplastic anemia are also caused by an immune mediated process with increased circulating activated T lymphocytes producing cytokines (e.g. interferon gamma) that suppress hematopoesis.

Clinical Manifestations

Both idiopathic and secondary types of acquired aplastic anemia present with similar symptoms and signs. In majority of cases, the onset is insidious with symptoms of progressively worsening anemia and associated bleeding manifestations. Some may have an apparently acute onset with bleeding and infection.

The prominent symptoms of *anemia* include easy fatiguability, lassitude and dyspnea on exertion. The *bleeding manifestations* include petechiae, ecchymosis, and epistaxis, bleeding from gums and alimentary tract and menorrhagia. Cerebral hemorrhage is not uncommon and is a fatal complication. Features of infection include malaise, sore throat, fever with chills, ulceration in the mouth and pharynx, and recurrent chest infection with pneumonia and septicemia as a common complication and cause of death.

The outstanding feature in clinical examination is the absence of significant objective findings. There is pallor.

The spleen is rarely palpable. The liver may be palpable as a complication of severe anemia with heart failure. Regional lymph glands draining infected lesions may be enlarged.

Laboratory Diagnosis

There is a normocytic normochromic anemia with anisocytosis. Poikilocytosis can occur. The MCV can be elevated. Hemoglobin level is often as low as 7 gm /dl. The reticulocyte count may be normal, low or slightly increased. The absolute reticulocyte concentration is usually low. A relatively high reticulocyte count is a good prognostic factor. The ESR is usually elevated, sometimes to high values.

There is leucopenia, particularly neutropenia, and thrombocytopenia. Red and white cell precursors are absent.

Presence of red and white cell precursors suggests an alternative cause of pancytopenia viz. leukemia or bone marrow infiltration. The Ham's acid serum test is occasionally positive in the absence of overt features of paroxysmal nocturnal hemoglobinuria. Flow cytometric analysis of erythrocytes for CD48 and CD59 is the most sensitive test for diagnosis of PNH.

Presence of fetal hemoglobin suggests a constitutional aplastic anemia but is not diagnostic. A chromosomal breakage analysis should be performed to evaluate for Fanconi's anemia. A bone marrow examination shows that the cellularity of the hemopoetic elements can vary substantially in different sites. A dry tap in which there is blood but no bone marrow particles is not uncommon. In such circumstances a bone marrow trephine biopsy has to be performed in order to assess bone marrow cellularity.

In the aplastic and hypoplastic particles, the proportion of fat cells increases with corresponding decrease in hemopoetic cells varying from moderate to complete absence. In the cellular particles, there is reduction of fat cells and an increase proportion of hemopoetic cells. It contains all cell series, but sometimes one cell type may predominate. Erythropoiesis is normoblastic but often dyserythropoetic features are present, particularly in more mature erythroblasts. Megakaryocytes are commonly in reduced numbers even in cellular regions. The iron content is usually normal or increased.

Management

Management of acquired aplastic anemia is discussed under the following headings:

1. Identification and elimination of exposure to a causative agent if present.
2. Supportive treatment
   a. Prevention and treatment of infection.
   b. Prevention and treatment of hemorrhage.
   c. Treatment of anemia.
3. Measures to accelerate recovery of pancytopenia
   a. Bone marrow transfusion.
   b. Antithymocytic globulin.
   c. Administration of anabolic agents and corticosteroids.

Identification and Termination of Exposure

If there is history of exposure to any drug or toxins, prompt measures should be taken to identify the agent and terminate exposure. This will help to lessen the ultimate severity of aplasia.

Prevention and Treatment of Infection

When the patient is at risk of infection because of neutropenia or because of steroid administration, infection may be prevented by taking the following measures:

- Avoidance of areas of microbial contamination such as hospitals, where resistant organisms are common.
- Use of topical antiseptics to reduce load of nasal and oral bacteria in patients with severe neutropenia.
- Isolation of patients with severe neutropenia in specialized low microbial environment is impractical because in aplastic anemia little change in the condition may occur for prolonged periods.
- Prophylactic antibiotics are not recommended as it tends to alter the microbial flora to resistant organisms.
- Concurrent administration of non absorbable antifungal drugs with high dose of steroids should be considered. It helps to suppress such organism in the mouth and GIT and thereby prevent candida infection.
- Infection appears to be a serious threat to severely neutropenic patients with aplastic anemia.
- Infection can also result in worsening in the degree of thrombocytopenia and if already thrombocytopenic can precipitate fatal bleeding.
- Infection, once detected, should be treated promptly and vigorously according to guidelines for treatment of neutropenia.

- Oral antibiotics may be appropriate for minor episodes of infection in less severely neutropenic patients.
- In severe neutropenia broad spectrum intravenous antibiotic is indicated to prevent overwhelming sepsis.

Prevention and Treatment of Hemorrhage

A simple but important measure to prevent bleeding is avoidance of the use of non-steroidal anti-inflammatory drugs. They affect in two ways: diminution of the functional capacity of platelets, and production of erosions in the upper GIT. Menorrhagia can be a serious problem. The most practical way to contain it is uninterrupted administration of hormonal agents that prevent menstruation.

Random donor platelet transfusion as a measure to prevent fatal bleeding has not been found to be suitable in aplastic anemia. The major reason being the development of isoantibodies to allogenic platelets which occurs in response to repeated platelet transfusion over weeks and months. This ultimately renders random donor platelet transfusion ineffective. Therefore platelet transfusion should be reserved to treat clinically significant bleeding only. Around 6–8 units of random donor platelets can improve the hemostatic defect due to thrombo cytopenia for upto several days.

Red Cell Transfusion for Anemia

The object of transfusion is to raise the hemoglobin to a level at which symptoms of anemia are alleviated and a comfortable life can be lead for a reasonable period before the next transfusion. Individual transfusion requirements vary from patient to patient. Transfusion should be planned when the hemoglobin level has fallen to around 7–9 gm/dl. Most patients remain comfortable for 6–8 weeks after the hemoglobin level is raised to about 12–14 gm/dl, provided that no bleeding occur inbetween. In patients with marked bleeding, transfusion requirements may be sometimes massive. Transfusions tend to become progressively less effective and are therefore required at increasingly shorter intervals. This is thought to be due to development of isoantibodies and increased destruction of transfused cells in the spleen. Transfusion reactions are common in patients receiving repeated transfusions sometimes as a result of development of red cell isoantibodies. This can be detected by careful cross matching. Such reactions can be prevented by using leukocyte filters.

Bone Marrow Transfusion

Bone marrow transfusion has achieved a considerable success in the treatment of young patients with aplastic anemia. Most recipients survive the initial pancytopenia but in atleast 50% of survivors there is development of host versus graft reaction. Immunosuppression also leads to infections such as pneumonia due to cytomegalovirus, yeasts, fungi, pneumocystis carinii which are often fatal. Hence, at present, bone marrow transfusion is restricted to subjects with severe aplastic anemia.

Antithymocyte Globulin (ATG)

Antithymocyte globulin provides a potentially beneficial treatment for patients with aplastic anemia in whom bone marrow transfusion cannot be performed because of lack of a suitable donor. ATG is given at 15 mg/kg/day. Administration of antithymocyte globulin for 1 week is associated with improvement in hematological indices in 50% of the treated subjects. Cyclosporin in the doses upto 12–15 mg/kg/day for 6–12 months when used in combination with ATG has shown to produce remission rates of about 70%.

Anabolic Agents and Corticosteroids

Anabolic agents do not appear to decrease mortality in severe aplastic anemia but are undoubtedly beneficial in less severely affected cases. They can produce a delayed increase in the cellular elements of blood. The most dramatic effect is on the hemoglobin level and may terminate dependence on transfusion. *Oxymetholone* is the commonly administered anabolic agent. The dosage is 100 mg per day or more. In some responders it can be withdrawn after 6 to 12 months. In others where the hematological indices deteriorate after withdrawal, further courses or maintenance therapy at lower levels may be required. The major side effects include hepatic damage and virilization in females. *Nandrolone decanoate* in the dose of 5 mg/kg/week IM for 3 months can be used with the advantage that this preparation is free of hepatotoxicity. Administration of large doses of corticosteroids is shown to be effective in patients treated within few weeks of diagnosis. *Methyl prednisolone* has been used with response rates varying from 38–50%. The regimen used is 20 mg/kg/day × 3 days, 10 mg/kg/day × 4 days, 5 mg/kg/day × 4 days, 2 mg/kg/day × 9 days, 1 mg/kg/day × 10 days. If steroids fail then ATG can be used subsequently with benefit.

Course and Prognosis

Left untreated, severe aplastic anemia has an overall mortality of approximately 50–80% within 12 months of diagnosis. The major causes of morbidity and mortality are infection and hemorrhage. Majority of children with acquired aplastic anemia, however, respond to allogenic bone marrow transplant or administration of antithymocyte globulin leaving them with normal or near normal blood counts. Those children who do not respond to the first line treatment, prognosis is poor. Spontaneous recovery rarely occurs.

CONSTITUTIONAL PANCYTOPENIAS

The common constitutional pancytopenias, which are inherited bone marrow failure syndromes, include Fanconi anemia (autosomal recessive), dyskeratosis congenita (X-linked/autosomal recessive), Shwachman-Diamond syndrome (autosomal recessive) and amegakaryocytic thrombocytopenia (X-linked/autosomal recessive). Fanconi anemia is the most common disorder. These genetic syndromes may be associated with a number of congenital anomalies especially of the bones, kidneys and heart. Fanconi anemia present with hyperpigmentation and café-au-lait spots, skeletal abnormalities (especially absent or hypoplastic thumbs, absent radius), short stature etc.

The hematologic manifestations of these inherited disorders may not manifest until the first years to even decades. The hematologic manifestation may be pancytopenia with aplastic bone marrow (Fanconi anemia and dyskeratosis congenita), neutropenia with hypocellularity or myeloid arrest in bone marrow (Shwachman-Diamond syndrome) and thrombocytopenia with absent or small megakaryocytes in bone marrow (amegakaryocytic thrombocytopenia).

The major complications related to the congenital pancytopenias include the consequences of bone marrow failure, a high risk of leukemia and other cancers and organ complications that are specific to the primary defect e.g. liver problems in Fanconi anemia and malabsorption in Shwachman-Diamond syndrome.

The treatment of congenital pancytopenias includes steroids and androgens (oxymethalone or nandrolone) alone or in combination. These therapies have been shown to prolong life by approximately 2 years. Encouraging results have been reported with administration of GM-CSF, multiple cytokines (erythropoietin, IL 3, IL6) in patients with Fanconi anemia and pancytopenia. The curative therapy till date is stem cell transplantation. With further understanding of the molecular defects, gene therapy may become a feasible treatment.

The prognosis is poor in all the types. Although presently available treatment offers some hope it does not overcome the risks of subsequent cancer or other organ complications. Antenatal diagnosis is possible hence genetic counseling is important.

Blood Component Therapy

The main constituents of blood are red blood cells (erythrocytes), white blood cells (leukocytes) and platelets (thrombocytes) suspended in a medium, the plasma. Each of these constituents has a role to play, i.e., the red cells in carrying oxygen to tissues, white cells in the body defence mechanism and platelets in hemostasis. Deficiency of each constituent leads to different disorders. For example reduction of red blood cells lead to anemia, a low platelet count leads to spontaneous bleeding and lowering of white cell count makes the child vulnerable to infection.

Transfusion practice for the neonatal and pediatric population requires an understanding of the physiologic changes that accompany the transition from fetus to neonate, neonate to infant, and throughout childhood. Hematologic values, blood volume, and physiologic response to stress such as hypovolemia and hypoxia exhibit wide variations. The most dynamic changes occur during the perinatal period and early infancy. Consequently, pediatric transfusion concerns are usually divided into two time periods: from birth through 4 months and older infants (> 4 months to 1 year) and children.

Selection of the appropriate patient is important so that no child is unnecessarily exposed to the hazards of transfusion. Ill neonates are more likely to receive red cell transfusion than hospitalized children of any other age group. Components should be tailored to satisfy the specific needs of very low birth weight and extremely low birth weight babies whose small blood volumes and impaired organ functions provide little margin of safety. Children with gradual onset anemia may remain asymptomatic despite a very low hemoglobin level. Treatment of underlying disease or nutritional supplementation is likely to correct anemia in such cases. On the other hand, abrupt onset anemia with signs of impending heart failure requires volume replacement with component therapy to correct anemia and anoxia.

General Principles of Transfusion

1. One should obtain an informed consent before

transfusion. The informations about the procedure of transfusion, the component to be transfused, length of transfusion and the expected outcome should be described to the parents.

2. Minimal requirements should be available for management of anaphylaxis.
3. Blood group should be reconfirmed on the day of transfusion. Donor's blood should be screened for hepatitis B and C viruses, cytomegalovirus and HIV, and malaria parasite.
4. Pre-transfusion day, time and vitals should be recorded. Transfusion should be avoided, if possible, in febrile patient (Temperature > 38°C).
5. After preparation of the infusion site, the IV line should be secured and the patency checked. A 22 or 23 G IV cannula and standard straight or Y type infusion set with an inline micro filter should be used for transfusion.
6. Warm blood in a thermostatically controlled water bath should be used. If not immediately used the blood component should be returned to the blood bank. If left at room temperature or in an ordinary refrigerator for more than 30 minutes it becomes unsuitable for use.
7. For the first 20 to 25 ml, infusion should be started at the rate of 5 ml/min under strict observation. Subsequently if all goes well, the drip rate should be adjusted for the unit to run over 2–4 hours.

Specific Component Therapy

Whole Blood

Whole blood contains all cellular elements, plasma which contains albumin, globulin, stable clotting factors and coagulant. One unit of whole blood consists of approximately 450 ml blood with 65 grams of hemoglobin. Each unit of red cells elevates hemoglobin by about 1 gram and the hematocrit by 3 points. The self life of whole blood with anticoagulant ACD is 21 days, with CPD is 28 days and with CPD-A is 35 days. Whole blood should be stored at 1–6°C.

The average dose of transfusion is 20 ml/kg.

Indications

1. Shock following acute massive blood loss (> 10 % of normal blood volume).
2. Exchange transfusion in neonates.
3. Partial exchange transfusion in hyperleukocytosis as in acute leukemia or hyperviscosity states like congenital cyanotic heart disease.
4. Replacement of iatrogenic blood loss in neonates.

Packed Red Blood Cells

Packed red blood cells are separated from whole blood by centrifugation at 5000 rmp for 5 minutes at 4–6°C. Two types of packed cells are available: (a) RBCs with CPD-A with hematocrit more than 80% and volume 250–300 ml/unit, and (b) RBCs with 100 ml additive solution with hematocrit 55–60% and volume 300–350 ml/unit. Self life with CPD-A is 35 days, with additive solution 42 days.

Indications

1. Deficiency anemia with a hemoglobin < 5 gm % or with signs of incipient or overt congestive heart failure.
2. Bone marrow failure syndrome and malignancy when hemoglobin < 7 gm %. Transfusion may be given even in absence of symptoms, during or following intensive cycle of chemotherapy or during radiotherapy.

Red blood cell transfusion should not be used for the following situations:

1. To enhance general well-being.
2. To hasten wound healing.
3. Preoperatively, independent of hemoglobin level.
4. In place of hematinic.
5. For volume expansion.

Amount of Transfusion

The transfusion volume of packed RBCs in a hemodynamically stable patient is 10–15 ml /kg infused at the rate of 5–10 ml/ kg/hour. The standard protocol is 10 ml/kg at the rate of 2–5 ml/kg/hour. In patients with impending heart failure, the rate of infusion should not exceed 2 ml/kg/hour. In severe anemia, a partial exchange transfusion is advisable or the child should receive 2–3 aliquots of 3–5 ml/kg over 2–3 hours.

Leukocyte Poor or Washed Red Blood Cells

This is a unit of packed RBCs in which the leukocyte number has been reduced to $< 5 \times 10^8$ in the final product and where atleast > 80% of RBCs remain. Self life is 24 hours. Dosage schedule is same as for packed RBCs.

Indications include: (a) Symptomatic anemia with history of repeated non-hemolytic febrile transfusion reaction in multitransfused patients e.g. thalassemia, (b) To prevent HLA alloimmunization in patient who require long-term platelet support or may require transplant, (c) To minimize virus transmission e.g. cytomegalovirus.

Platelet Concentrate

Platelet concentrate is prepared from whole blood within 6 hours of collection. A platelet unit prepared from a unit of whole blood may be of two types:

1. **Random donor platelet (RDP):** It is from a random donor. One unit of RDP contains a minimum of 5.5×10^{10} platelets, 50 ml of plasma, trace to 0.5 ml of RBCs and, depending upon the preparation technique, varying number of leukocytes (predominantly monocytes and lymphocytes) upto level of 10^8/unit.
2. **Single donor platelet (SDP):** It is prepared from a designate single donor using apheresis procedure. A unit of SDP contains a minimum of 3×10^{11} platelets, approximately 25–30 ml of plasma, trace to 0.5 ml of RBCs and, depending on the apheresis technique or instrument, 10^6–10^9 leukocytes/unit.

Apheresis is the selective removal of blood components during the donation process where the remaining elements are recombined and returned to the donor. It is used for the selective collection of platelets, RBCs, plasma or granulocytes from the donor. A single apheresis platelet product is equivalent to approximately 6 units from random donors. It decreases exposure to multiple donors and minimizes alloimmunization.

Both RDP and SDP can be stored for upto 5 days at 20–24°C on a constant agitator which prevents agglutination of platelets which will otherwise make the platelets inactive. Post transfusional platelets survive upto 6–7 days. It should be transported quickly and infused over 20–30 minutes rapidly. No glass ware should be used.

Random donor platelet, given in the dose of 1 unit/10 kg body weight will raise the platelet count by $10–30 \times 10^9$/L. One unit of SDP is equivalent to 6–7 units of RDP.

Calculation of Doses

The number of units required (n) is calculated by the following formula:

n = desired PLT count – initial PLT count × body surface area/10.

Indications

1. Decreased platelet production with or without increased destruction e.g. leukemia, aplastic anemia, chemotherapy and irradiation.
   a. Platelet count $<50 \times 10^9$/L with bleeding.
   b. Platelet count $<50 \times 10^9$/L with invasive procedures e.g. trephine biopsy, intrathecal injection).
   c. Platelet count $<20 \times 10^9$/L with marrow failure.
2. Prophylactically when platelet count is < 50,000 / cumm in sepsis, DIC, NEC.
3. Abnormal platelet function.
4. Treatment of bleeding after exchange transfusion, cardiopulmonary bypass, massive transfusion.

Granulocyte Transfusion

Granulocyte concentrates can be obtained by centrifugation of refrigerated whole blood but they are of poor function and generally yield inadequate doses. The maximum yield can be obtained by centrifugation leukopheresis from a preconditioned donor. The preconditioning can be done by pretreatment of the donor with granulocyte-colony stimulating factor (G-CSF) and dexamethasone to increase the yield.

Granulocytes should be stored in the same donor's citrate-anticoagulated plasma at room temperature without agitation. They should be administered within 12 hours of preparation. A transfusion of 1 unit of granulocyte concentrate 2–3 times per day is considered as an effective dose. It should be Rh and ABO compatible and irradiated, CMV negative. The optimal duration of therapy is unclear.

Indications for granulocyte transfusion:

1. Severe sepsis with absolute neutrophil count $< 0.5 \times 10^9$/L not responding to antibiotics.
2. Neonates with severe sepsis with absolute neutrophil count $< 3 \times 10^9$/L (in first week of life) or $< 1 \times 10^9$/L thereafter.

However, these situations can be treated with administration of G-CSF and currently it is not clear which of these approaches is more effective. There is no evidence to support the use of prophylactic granulocyte transfusion.

Fresh Frozen Plasma

Plasma frozen within 8 hours of donation contains atleast

0.70 unit/ml of factor VIII and is referred to as fresh frozen plasma (FFP). One unit of FFP has a volume of 160–250 ml if obtained by plasmapheresis. FFP can be stored for 12 months at less than –18°C. FFP should be used immediately. If there is a delay in transfusion or if the indication to use is not hemophilia, FFP can be stored at 4°C upto 24 hours. It is still best used within 4 hours. The dose is 10–15 ml/kg body weight over a period of 30–60 minutes and repeated every 12–24 hours. The APTT should be measured after an infusion.

The indications of FFP transfusion are as follows:

1. DIC with bleeding.
2. Sick children with coagulopathy.
3. Liver disease with abnormal coagulation profile as prophylaxis or to control bleeding.
4. Hemorrhage in hemolytic disease of newborn.
5. Dilutional coagulopathy following surgical bleeding and massive transfusion.
6. Thrombotic thrombocytopenic purpura for exchange transfusion.
7. Factor deficiency when factor concentrates not available.

Cryoprecipitate

Cryoprecipitate contains 80–100 units of factor VIII, 100–250 mg fibrinogen, 40–60 mg of fibronectin, and 40–70% of von Willebrand factor and 30% of factor XIII present in the original unit of plasma.

It is the precipitate formed when FFP is thawed at 4°C and then refrozen within 1 hour in 10–15 ml of the donor plasma. It can be stored at –18°C or less for a period upto 1 year.

The indications for transfusion of cryoprecipitate are as follows:

1. Factor deficiencies viz. fibrinogen, factor VIII, factor XIII.
2. von Willebrand disease.
3. DIC.
4. Massive bleeding or massive transfusion.

The thawed precipitate should be stored at room temperature and transfused immediately or within 4 hours if used as a source of factor VIII. ABO compatible units are preferable for transfusion.

The number of units of cryoprecipitate required is based on the amount necessary to obtain a hemostatic level of fibrinogen level > 0.8–1.0 gram/L. If the units are carefully pooled this can usually be accomplished by the transfusion of 2 units/10 kg body weight of recipient.

Transfusion Reactions

In the majority of carefully prepared and properly supervised transfusions, there are no untoward effects. However in around 5–6% cases complications may occur even when all precautions are taken.

Classification

The reactions following transfusion of blood components may be classified as follows:

Acute

a. Mild reactions include fever, allergic rash.
b. Moderately severe reactions include urticarial rash, non-hemolytic febrile transfusion reaction (NFHTR) due to white cells/platelets/proteins, bacterial contamination/pyrogen.
c. Life threatening reactions include acute intravascular hemolysis, sepsis, fluid overload, anaphylactic reaction, transfusion related acute lung injury (TRALI).

Delayed

a. Delayed hemolytic transfusion reaction (HTR).
b. Transfusion transmitted infections.
c. Iron overload.
d. Transfusion associated graft versus host disease (TA-GVHD).

Acute Hemolytic Transfusion Reaction

Causes

1. Transfusion of ABO incompatible RBCs.
2. Accidental heating or freezing of bag.
3. Injection of water into circulation.
4. Contact of red cells with 5% dextrose in vivo.

Clinical Features

Symptoms include chills, chest/back pain, restlessness, flushing, sweating, pain in the transfusion site, abdominal discomfort, nausea/vomiting.

Signs include fever, rigors, tachycardia, dyspnea/tachypnea, hypotension, pallor/cyanosis, hemoglobinuria, oliguria/anuria, shock/DIC.

Workup

1. Check compatibility report, labels, blood bag.
2. Repeat blood grouping and cross matching; perform direct Combs' test and antibody screening.
3. Other investigations:
   a. Serum bilirubin, plasma hemoglobin, urine hemoglobin/blood.
   b. Complete blood count, peripheral blood smears for spherocytes, crenated cells.
   c Fibrin degradation products.
   d. Coagulation screen (PT, PTT) every 12 hourly.
   e. Electrolytes every 12 hourly.

Management

1. At the first suspicion transfusion should be stopped immediately and fluid continued to maintain blood volume and to ensure diuresis.
2. Provision of cardiorespiartory support, if necessary ionotropes.
3. Monitoring of blood pressure, heart rate and maintenance of adequate airway.
4. Reporting about reaction to blood bank. Samples send for further testing.

Febrile Non-Hemolytic Transfusion Reaction

Febrile reactions are common in patients who have received multiple transfusions. It is a result of development of antibodies to leukocytes or platelets.

It is characterized by fever with chills, nausea / vomiting, hypotension, shock.

It is managed by slowing the transfusion, giving a warm drink, antipyretics for fever. If reactions are recurrent, leukocyte reduced red cells may be used.

Allergic Reactions

The allergic reactions are rare. They range in severity from small urticarial wheals to life threatening circulatory collapse. In most cases, allergic reactions are characterized by sudden onset of wheals surrounded by erythematous areas; usually occurring shortly after the commencement of transfusion. In some there may be headache, nausea, vomiting, dyspnea, edema of face, and swelling of mucous membrane also. Laryngeal edema is uncommon. Rarely, an anaphylactic type of reaction occurs with shock and peripheral circulatory collapse.

When the allergic reaction is limited to only a few wheals, the transfusion is slowed and an antihistaminic administered. With more severe reactions, the transfusion is stopped and adrenaline is given subcutaneously or if necessary intravenously. The reactions may be prevented in patients with past history of allergic reactions by using washed red cells, administering antihistaminics and corticosteroids before transfusion.

Prevention of Circulatory Overload

Circulatory overload resulting in pulmonary congestion and acute heart failure is the most important complication of transfusion. It is probably the most common cause of death following transfusion. The risk of circulatory overload is particularly high in children with chronic anemia, cardiac and pulmonary disease and in the very young ones.

The common clinical presentation is that of acute pulmonary edema. Less commonly, there is an insidious onset of cardiac failure with progressive dyspnea, cyanosis and development of crepitations at the lung bases over 12–24 hours.

Circulatory overload can be prevented by using packed red cells, pedipacks, and use of small aliquots at a time, slow rate of transfusion, keeping the patient warm and use of diuretics.

The transfusion should be immediately discontinued and the patient is propped up in bed and oxygen administered. A rapid acting diuretic viz. frusemide and morphine should be given. If there is no response, rotating tourniquets or venesection should be used. In desperate cases intubation and positive pressure ventilation may be necessary.

Suggested Reading

1. De Gruchy's Clinical Hematology in Medical practice. Editors Frank Firkin, Colin Chesterman, David Pennington and Bryan Rush, 5th edition, 1989, Reprinted 2006, Blackwell Science Ltd.
2. Practical Pediatric Hematology. Reference Manual National Training Project, Editor Anupam Sachdeva, 1st edition, Published by Indian Academy of Pediatrics.
3. PHO Review Volume 1–10, 1988–1997. Compiled and edited by Bharat Agarwal, 1996.
4. Nelson Text Book of Pediatrics edited by Behrman, Kliegman and Jenson, 17th edition, 2004. Saunders, Philadelphia, Pennsylvania.

9

Respiratory System

OUTLINES

Upper Respiratory Tract Infections

Upper respiratory tract infections are those infectious processes primarily affecting the structures of the respiratory tract above the larynx. It should be noted that most respiratory infections affect the upper and lower respiratory tracts simultaneously or sequentially.

Most of the upper respiratory infections are caused by viruses and some by mycoplasma. With the advent of modern methods of virology, it has been clearly established now that Group A beta hemolytic streptococci and C. diphtheria are the only bacterial agents capable of causing primary nasal and pharyngeal disease.

The common upper respiratory infections include the following:

1. Acute nasopharyngitis (Common cold).
2. Acute sore throat (Acute pharyngitis, acute pharyngotonsillitis).
3. Acute otitis media.
4. Acute purulent sinusitis.

ACUTE NASOPHARYNGITIS (COMMON COLD)

Acute nasopharyngitis is a self limiting viral illness. Young children have an average of 6–7 episodes of common cold per year. Around 10–15% of children have atleast 12 episodes per year. The incidence decreases with age to 2–3 episodes per year in adulthood.

Etiology

More than 200 viruses can cause most common cold. However, the common causative viruses are rhino and corona viruses, respiratory syncytial virus (RSV), parainfluenza and influenza viruses. The viruses are transmitted by direct contact. In children below 6 months age and in children with protein energy malnutrition, purulent complication due to secondary bacterial infection is common. The common secondary bacterial infections are acute otitis media, acute mastoiditis, acute lymphadenitis and pneumonia.

Clinical Manifestations

Acute nasopharyngitis is the most common upper respiratory tract infection, most common during the second and third year of life and is virtually endemic in nursery schools. The child has the highest number of episodes during the first year at school.

The clinical presentations differ according to the age of the child. *Infants below 3 months age* present with running nose and block nose and are afebrile. In children *above 3 months to 3 years*, the initial manifestation is sudden onset of fever, often in the range of 39°C to 40°C (102°F to 104°F) which may last for few hours to around 3 days. The other manifestations include irritability, restlessness, sneezing, mucoid nasal discharge, nasal block which may interfere feeding and cause respiratory difficulty. A few infants may have diarrhea and vomiting. Recurrence of fever after initial remission indicates a purulent infection. In *older children*, the initial symptoms are dryness and irritation of nose and/or throat, followed within a few hours by sneezing, chilly sensation, muscular aches, thin nasal discharge and sometimes mild cough. Headache, malaise, anorexia, low grade fever and nasal obstruction may be present. The acute phase may last for 4–14 days or more.

ACUTE SORE THROAT

Etiology

More than 80% of sore throat is caused by viruses viz. RSV, parainfluenza, influenza and adeno virus. The rest is caused by group A beta hemolytic streptococci and mycoplasma. Other bacteria viz. S. pneumoniae, H. influenzae, and S. aureus, which are commensals of the throat, may proliferate during an acute viral respiratory illness and hence may be cultured from the pharynx of a child suffering from a viral sore throat. There is however no epidemiological data to suggest that they are capable of producing acute sore throat.

Clinical Manifestations

Acute sore throat is uncommon in children below 1 year of age. The peak incidence is between 4 years and 7 years age, but the disease continue to occur throughout childhood. Among the two, viral sore throat is a self limiting disease and does not require any specific treatment. Streptococcal sore throat, on the other hand, can lead to complications which may be suppurative viz. retro-pharyngeal abscess, peritonsillar abscess and cervical lymphadenitis or non-suppurative viz. acute rheumatic fever and acute post streptococcal glomerulonephritis. Hence early diagnosis and treatment with anti-microbials is necessary to prevent these complications.

The clinical features somewhat differ depending on whether streptococcus or virus is the offending organism.

Though the clinical features are overlapping, it is possible to distinguish between the two.

Features Common to Both

a. Pharyngeal inflammation may be mild to severe with small ulcers on the soft palate and posterior pharyngeal wall.
b. Exudates may be present over the tonsils, palate and post pharyngeal wall.
c. Presence of enlarged, tender cervical lymph nodes.

Features Peculiar to Viral Sore Throat

a. Onset of illness is gradual with mild to moderate fever, malaise and anorexia.
b. Presence of two or more of the following features viz. rhinitis, conjunctivitis, hoarseness and cough.
c. Period of illness is usually not more than five days.
d. Can occur at any age but common in age group less than 3 years.
e. Does not respond to antimicrobials.

Features Peculiar to Streptococcal Sore Throat

a. Onset of illness is acute with high fever (as high as 40°C/104°F). The child is toxic. The fever may continue for 1–4 days or upto 2 weeks in severe cases.
b. Absence of signs viz. rhinitis, conjunctivitis, hoarseness and cough.
c. Period of illness may be upto 2 weeks.
d. Most commonly seen in the age group of 5 to 15 years.
e. Patient may become afebrile within 24 hours after an appropriate antimicrobial in adequate doses, unless there is a complication.

Atypical Presentation of Acute Streptococcal Sore Throat

Acute streptococcal sore throat can sometimes present with atypical features when diagnosis may be missed if the throat examination is not done. The atypical clinical presentations may be:

a. High fever with headache, vomiting and abdominal pain.
b. With earache as a predominant symptom which can be either due to referred pain or co-existent acute otitis media.

ACUTE SUPPURATIVE OTITIS MEDIA

Acute otitis media and acute purulent sinusitis are generally complications following viral upper respiratory infection as a result of secondary infection by bacteria viz. S. pneumoniae, H. influenzae, and Moraxella catarrhalis. Recent studies have also shown an increase in the incidence of infection by betalactamase producing H. influenzae and multidrug resistant S. pneumoniae. It occurs several days after the onset of a viral upper respiratory infection.

More than 60% of children less than 3 years of age have atleast one episode of acute otitis media. There is a bimodal age distribution of occurrence of ASOM; one between 12–24 months and the other between 5–6 years age.

Pathogenesis

Viral upper respiratory infection enables pathogenic bacteria in the nasopharynx to ascend the eustachian tube into the middle ear by impairing local host defenses or by eustachian tube dysfunction. Atleast 50% of uncomplicated ASOM have spontaneous resolution within 24–48 hours. So antibiotics should be started when symptoms continue for more than 48 hours.

Clinical Manifestations

Several types of acute otitis media may be encountered in children.

Acute suppurative otitis media (ASOM): The best way to diagnose ASOM is by pneumatic otoscopy which shows decreased mobility and bulging of the ear drum which is hyperemic and red with loss of landmarks. It should be noted that mild redness of the drum is not a sufficient evidence of ASOM.

When an **otoscope** is not available ASOM may be suspected when a child with history of upper respiratory infection for several days develop sudden persistent pain in the ear. In an infant, it may be indicated by inconsolable crying, head shaking or rubbing the affected ear. The child may also present with discharge of pus from the ear for less than two weeks.

Recurrent acute otitis media: Acute otitis media is labeled as recurrent when a child suffers from 3 episodes of ASOM in 6 months or 4 episodes in one year.

Otitis media with effusion: Represents eustachian tube obstruction following viral upper respiratory tract infection or it may be a resolved ASOM. It spontaneously resolves in one to two months.

Chronic otitis media: It is diagnosed when there is discharge of pus per ear for more than two weeks.

Complications

The complications of ASOM may be intratemporal or intracranial. The intratemporal complications include mastoiditis, petrositis, facial paralysis and labyrinthitis. The intracranial complications include meningitis, lateral sinus thrombosis, extradural, subdural and brain abscesses.

ACUTE PURULENT SINUSITIS

Acute purulent sinusitis is uncommon in children below 5 years of age. In younger age however, sinus involvement is present with acute nasopharyngitis which resolves with recovery of the primary disease. It is a common illness in children and adolescents with significant morbidity and potential for serious complications.

Around 2% of viral upper respiratory infection is complicated by acute bacterial sinusitis. The other predisposing factors include conditions that impair mucociliary transport viz. exposure to smoke, cold and dry inspired air, allergic rhinitis, gastro esophageal reflux and conditions that cause nasal obstruction viz. foreign body, polyps, enlarged adenoids, deviated nasal septum, tumors.

Pathogenesis

Acute purulent sinusitis typically follows a viral upper respiratory infection. Viral rhinosinusitis causes inflammation and edema which block sinus drainage and impair mucociliary clearance. Bacteria enter from the nasopharynx and grow profusely as growth conditions are favorable in the sinus cavities.

Clinical Manifestations

The clinical manifestations of acute purulent sinusitis include persistent fever, purulent nasal discharge for more than 14 days, tenderness over the sinuses and facial bones or periorbital edema.

The complications of acute purulent sinusitis include periorbital and orbital cellulitis, meningitis, cavernous sinus thrombosis, subdural empyema, epidural abscess and brain abscess. There may be osteomyelitis of the frontal bone.

Investigations

X-ray of paranasal sinuses may show complete opacification of the sinuses, mucosal thickening of 4 mm or more, or air fluid level.

CT scan of sinuses may be indicated in case there is complication of acute bacterial sinusitis, in cases with persistent or recurrent symptoms and there is no response to therapy.

Sinus aspirate culture is the most accurate method for diagnosis but not practical for routine use. It is indicated in life threatening conditions, cases unresponsive to therapy, and in immunocompromised host.

TONSILS AND ADENOIDS

The tonsils and adenoid together with the other lymphoid tissues in the Waldeyer's ring serves as a defence against infection but it may become a site of acute or chronic infection. The principal disturbances of the tonsils and adenoid are infection and hypertrophy.

Etiology

Group A beta hemolytic streptococci is the most common organism causing infection of tonsils and adenoids. Other bacteria isolated are S. aureus coagulase positive, Klebsiella pneumonie. The common anaerobes detected are peptostreptococcus and veillonella. Except Ebstein Barr virus, exclusive viral etiology is considered uncommon.

An enlarged adenoid is the most common cause of nasopharyngeal obstruction in children. The increase in size is due to either infection or hyperplasia. Nasopharyngeal obstruction due to adenoids is rare below one year age. It is most common between 3 and 6 years age because the adenoids outstrip the growth of nasopharynx from 3 years to 5 years after which there is spontaneous regression.

Clinical Features

The diseases affecting the adenoids are:

Acute Adenoiditis

Acute adenoiditis occurs as a part of common cold. The clinical features are same as of acute rhino-sinusitis. Hence normally remain undiagnosed.

Recurrent and Chronic Adenoiditis

The criteria for diagnosis of this condition are:

a. More than four episodes of acute adenoiditis in one season.
b. Persistent or recurrent otitis media, chronic cough.
c. Nocturnal cough and malodorous breath.

Obstructive Adenoid Hyperplasia (OAH)

The diagnostic triad for OAH includes:

a. Snoring and mouth breathing.
b. Hyponasality of voice.
c. Chronic rhinorrhoea accompanied with snoring.

Clinical evaluation of the child is the mainstay of diagnosis. An X-ray lateral view of the soft tissue of the neck may be advised to assess possible OAH in presence of nasal mucosal disease or when history and examination of the child are not consistent.

The disease affecting the tonsils may be:

Acute Tonsillitis

It is characterized by sore throat, fever, dysphagia and tender jugulodiagastric gland with erythema/exudates over the surface of the tonsils.

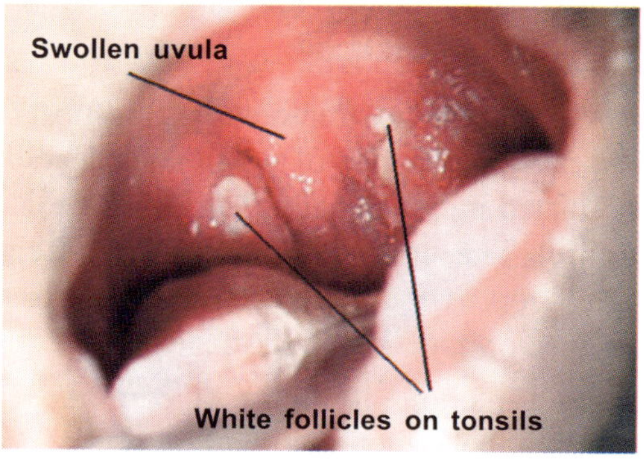

Fig. 9.1: Acute tonsillitis with white follicles on the tonsils and swollen uvula

Recurrent Acute Tonsillitis

This condition is diagnosed in presence of four to seven attacks of acute tonsillitis per season, five attacks per year for last two years or three attacks per year for last three years.

Chronic Tonsillitis

This condition is characterized by presence of chronic sore throat, foul breath, persistent tender jugulodiagastric glands, persistent hyperemia of the anterior pillars and tonsillolith.

Obstructive Tonsillar Hyperplasia (OTH)

This condition is characterized by loud snoring, apnea or irregular breathing, enuresis, nocturnal cough and choking and restless sleep.

MANAGEMENT OF UPPER RESPIRATORY TRACT INFECTIONS

The management of upper respiratory infection may be described under the following heads:

1. Antibiotics.
2. Surgical treatment.
3. Symptomatic treatment and home care.
4. Preventive measures.

Antibiotics

The majority of cases of upper respiratory infection in children are a result of a viral infection. Hence there is no role of treatment with antibiotics. In most cases symptomatic treatment and home care is sufficient. Antibiotics are recommended only in the following conditions:

a. Acute supportive otitis media and acute purulent sinusitis.
b. Acute streptococcal sore throat and its complications.
c. Acute tonsillitis.

Prophylactic antibiotics should not be given in the following conditions of upper respiratory infection:

a. Acute nasopharyngitis and acute viral sore throat.
b. Only high fever or only purulent nasal discharge.
c. Chronic supportive otitis media.
d. Tonsil and adenoid hyperplasia.

Antibiotics are not recommended in the above conditions because of the following reasons. The above mentioned conditions are not bacterial infection; hence antibiotics are not effective. Unnecessary administration of antibiotics causes side effects while providing no clinical benefits. It also increases antibiotic resistant strains.

The antibiotics used in different types of upper respiratory infection differs according to the condition:

1. *Acute streptococcal sore throat:* Penicillin is still the drug of choice. Oral penicillin or intramuscular benzathene penicillin is the drug of choice. Amoxicillin can be given if penicillin is not available. In case of penicillin sensitivity, erythromycin is the drug of choice.
2. *Acute suppurative otitis media:* The drug of choice is amoxicillin. If there is no response within 72 hours, a second line drug viz. amoxicillin clavulinic acid or ceftriaxone should be started. In resistant cases a double dose of amoxicillin is also shown to be effective.
3. *Acute and acute recurrent tonsillitis:* Is treated in the same line as acute streptococcal sore throat.
4. *Acute and recurrent adenoiditis:* It is mainly treated with antibiotics against betalactamase producing organism.

Drugs and Dosage Schedule

1. *Penicillin V:* Oral 125 mg (less than 5 years) and 250 mg (5 years and above) 8 hourly for 10 days.
2. *Amoxicillin:* Oral 30–40 mg/kg/day 8 hourly for 10 days.

3. Benzathene penicillin deep IM single dose 6 lacs IU for children < 27 kg weight and 12 lacs IU for children > 27 kg after negative skin test with benzyl penicillin.
4. Erythromycin 30–40 mg/kg body weight 6 hourly for 10 days.
5. Amoxicillin + clavulinic acid orally 30–40 mg amoxicillin/kg/day 8 hourly for 10 days.
6. Ceftriaxone injection IV 50 mg/kg single dose for 10 days.

Surgical Treatment

1. Tympanocentasis is indicated in ASOM:

a In a critically ill child.
b. With poor response to antibiotics.
c. When suppurative complications are suspected.
d. For confirmation of diagnosis.

2. Adenoidectomy: The indications of adenoidectomy are:

a. Presence of signs of nasopharyngeal obstruction viz.
   i. Presence of obligate mouth breathing, nasal speech and adenoid facies.
   ii. Repeated attacks of otitis media with effusion with conductive deafness.

3. Tonsillectomy: The indications of tonsillectomy are:

a. Peritonsillar abscess.
b. Obstructive tonsillar hyperplasia with obstructive sleep apnea, dysphagia.
c. Recurrent acute tonsillitis i.e. 6 genuine attacks of acute tonsillitis per year for two consecutive years. In such attacks it is important to note that the attacks are those of acute bacterial tonsillitis and not upper respiratory viral infections.

Symptomatic Treatment and Home Care

Treatment of Fever

Paracetamol should be given if the axillary temperature is 39°C (102°C) or more. Dose is 10–15 mg/kg body weight per dose every 6 hours or four hourly if there is a history of febrile convulsion. A sponge bath with tap water (Lukewarm water if below 1 year of age) may be necessary if the temperature goes above 104°F, 45 minutes after giving paracetamol. The child should be kept in a cool room with minimal clothing.

Nasal Obstruction

Nasal obstruction causes most of the distress in a child with upper respiratory viral infection. The small infant is unable to suck breast and sleep. Relief permits the child to sleep and eat well. The infant should be placed in a prone position in a humidified environment. This provides substantial relief. If the nose is blocked with dry or thick mucus, normal saline nasal drops can be useful. It relieves nasal congestion by liquefying the thick and dry mucus. Injudicious use of medicated nasal drops should be discouraged to prevent rebound congestion and rhinitis medicamentosa. When used should be done methodically for proper effect. The effectiveness of oral antihistamines and decongestants is doubtful and should be discouraged. The method of using nasal drops is as follows: The child should be put in supine position with the neck slightly extended. The nasal drop should be dropped into each nostril and the child kept in the position for some time and then allowed to change position.

Washing the Ear and Wicking in Chronic Suppurative Otitis Media

A chronically draining ear will heal only when it is dry. Antibiotic therapy has no role. The ear can be washed with the help of a G8 feeding tube and a syringe. The *steps of washing* are as follows: The feeding tube is cut to a length of 2.5 cm and attached to a 2 ml syringe. 0.5 ml clean water at room temperature is drawn into the syringe. The cut end of the feeding tube is put gently into the child's ear and the water is injected. The water and pus is sucked and thrown away. The procedure is repeated until no pus comes out. This maneuver can be done daily once for 5 days. The mother should be advised how to keep the ear dry by wicking at home. The *steps of wicking* are as follows. A piece of clean, absorbent cloth or sterile cotton is rolled into a wick. The wick is inserted in the child's ear and left in the ear for 1 minute. Then it is removed and replaced with a clean wick. Wicking should be done at least 4 times a day, until the wick stays dry. No ear plug should be applied in-between. The child should not go swimming until the ear is dry.

Treatment of Cough

In mild cough, soothing agents viz. lime water, honey, ginger, tulsi and warm water can be used. These should be administered in small amounts frequently. Commercially available cough syrups or cold remedies do not alter the duration of cough and cold. These are usually combinations of antihistaminics, antitussives and even expectorants. They may sedate the child and interfere with feeding and the child's ability to clear secretions from throat. In case of harassing dry cough, dextrometorphan can be used in a dose of 1–2 mg/kg/day 2 times a day till cough subsides. Some children may have bronchial hyperactivity or bronchospasm after a viral infection. They may have severe cough with or without bronchospasm and require bronchodilators to control. They do not respond to safe cough home remedies. These children respond to salbutamol 1 mg (for less than 10 kg weight) and 2 mg (for 10–20 kg weight) or 0.1 mg/kg/dose, 8 hourly for 5–7 days.

Diet and Fluids

Feeding should be continued during acute respiratory infections to prevent malnutrition or aggravation of existing malnutrition. Loss of appetite is common. The child refuses solid food. Hence child should be encouraged to eat small frequent meals. If the child has fever, lowering of temperature may help some children to eat. Food should be nutritious and calorie dense but low in bulk. The recommended food is cereals + beans or cereals + fish/meat cooked in oil. During recovery, an extra meal per day should be advised for 10–15 days. This will help the child to regain lost weight. In exclusively breast fed babies breastfeeding should be given more frequently. Children with respiratory infection loose more fluids than usual, especially when there is fever. The child should be advised to take more fluids. Encouraging taking extra fluid will prevent dehydration. Extra fluids may include clean water, juices, soups etc.

Maintenance of Warmth

A thermoneutral environment is necessary. The mother should be advised not to over heat the room and overdress the child. The young infants should be protected from chilling. The child can be bathed daily.

Home Care Advice

The mother should be asked to watch for the following signs and bring the child back to the health facility if:

a. Breathing becomes fast.
b. Breathing becomes difficult.
c. Child is not able to drink or has stopped feeding well.
d. Child has become sicker.

The child with any one of these signs may be suffering from pneumonia.

Preventive Measures

1. The child should be immunized according to the national immunization schedule.
2. Measures to be adopted to reduce the incidence of low birth weight babies because the risk of acute respiratory infection is three times higher in this group of babies.
3. Every newborn baby should be exclusively breast fed upto 6 months of age.
4. Prevention of protein energy malnutrition by introduction of complementary feeding in the proper age. The morbidity and mortality from respiratory illness is higher in cases suffering from protein energy malnutrition.
5. Young infants should be protected from chills in cold weather.

Cough, Stridor and Croup

Cough, wheeze and stridor are symptoms of the respiratory tract in children which may occur frequently and/or may persist for prolonged periods. Determining the cause is often difficult particularly for two reasons. Firstly, because these symptoms may be caused by a rapid succession of unrelated acute respiratory infections or by a single pathophysiological process. Secondly, there is paucity of easily performed, specific diagnostic tests for many acute and chronic respiratory conditions.

A systematic approach to the diagnosis and treatment should be a top priority and should consist of the following steps:

1. To determine whether symptoms are a manifestation of a minor problem or a life threatening one.
2. To determine the most likely underlying pathogenic mechanism.
3. To select the most effective therapy, which many a times may be only symptomatic therapy.
4. To evaluate the response to therapy.

Failure of this approach will signal the need of more extensive, perhaps invasive procedures like bronchoscopy for the diagnosis of the condition.

COUGH

Cough is a reflex response of the lower respiratory tract to stimulation of irritant or cough receptors in the mucosa of the airways. It is a protective reflex response for keeping the airways clear; self limiting but sometimes very harassing.

Cough may be acute or chronic. Cough continuing beyond one month is called chronic cough. Cough may be recurrent or persistent. *Recurrent cough* are episodes of cough lasting for a few days to a few weeks with completely asymptomatic periods in-between. *Persistent cough* is a cough of many months or even years. There may be a temporary clearance of the cough with medication, but it rapidly recurs with cessation of treatment.

It needs mention that besides the lower respiratory tract mucosa, cough receptors are also present in the pharynx, paranasal sinuses, stomach and external auditory meatus. Hence the source of a persistent cough needs to be sought for beyond the lungs.

Causes

a. Recurrent Cough

1. Asthma.
2. Recurrent viral respiratory tract infection.
3. Post nasal drip from upper airways.
4. Aspiration syndromes.
5. Idiopathic pulmonary hemosiderosis.

b. Persistent Cough

1. Asthma.
2. Foreign body aspiration.
3. Viral respiratory infection.
4. Mycoplasma pneumoniae infection.
5. Recurrent aspiration due to tracheo-esophageal fistula, tracheo-laryngo-esophageal cleft, pharyngeal incompetence.
6. Gastroesophageal reflux with or without aspiration.
7. Pertussis syndrome.
8. Extrinsic compression of tracheobronchial tree by enlarged lymph node, vascular ring, neoplasm, lung cyst.
9. Endobronchial tuberculosis, endobronchial or endotracheal tumours.
10. Inhaled irritants including tobacco smoke.
11. Irritation of external auditory canal.
12. Chronic sinusitis.
13. Bronchitis, tracheitis due to infection and smoking (in adolescents).
14. Bronchiectasis including cystic fibrosis, primary ciliary dyskinesia, immunodeficiency.
15. Tracheomalacia and broncomalacia.
16. Psychogenic cough.

The most common causes of recurrent cough are however, viral respiratory infection and asthma. The common causes of persistent cough include post viral infection, whooping cough, foreign body inhalation, segmental or lobar collapse after an acute respiratory infection, tuberculosis, smoker's cough in adolescents and history of exposure to smoke. Bacterial infection of respiratory tract do not present with cough.

Evaluation

A detail and careful history taking, giving stress on pertinent points and a careful physical examination can give enough information pertaining to the cause of cough. The type of cough itself can aid in distinguishing the site of origin and even the possible etiology (Tables 9.1 and 9.2).

Table 9.1 : Type of cough and site of origin

	Type of cough	*Site of origin*
1.	Dry, persistent, irritating, increase on lying down	Pharynx
2.	Dry, painful, persistent associated with hoarseness, stridor	Larynx
3.	Dry, associated with retrosternal pain and stridor	Trachea
4.	Paroxysmal spasmodic cough, more at night/ early morning, associated with vomiting	Bronchioles

Table 9.2 : Some characteristics of cough and possible etiology

	Characteristics	*Possible etiology*
1.	Associated with stridor	Laryngeal obstruction
2.	Associated with wheeze	Asthma
3.	Associated with vigorous exercise	Exercise induced asthma, cystic fibrosis
4.	Most severe on awakening in the morning	Cystic fibrosis, bronchiectasis
5.	Cough several times per minute with regularity, disappears with sleep	Psychogenic cough
6.	Paroxysmal with history of choking	Foreign body
7.	Posterior pharyngeal drainage with night cough	Sinusitis

Physical Examination

It is important to detect a spontaneous cough during the examination. A child by 4–5 years age can cough on request. If there is no spontaneous cough, a child can be asked to take a deep breath and forcefully exhale repeatedly which usually induces a cough. A child can be asked to run for 5–6 minutes which usually induces cough with wheeze in a child with bronchial hyperactivity.

Examination of the sputum can give important clue to the cause of cough. Every effort should be made to obtain a specimen of sputum. The older child can comply. A specimen of sputum can be picked up with a throat swab inserted into the lower pharynx while the child coughs with protruded tongue.

Clear mucoid sputum is often associated with an allergic reaction or asthma. *Cloudy sputum* suggests increased cellularity as a result increased polymorphs (respiratory infection) or eosinophil (asthma). *Purulent sputum* is characteristic of bronchiectasis. In cystic fibrosis, the sputum is purulent but rarely foul smelling. Foul *smelling sputum* indicates anaerobic infection of the lungs.

Laboratory Investigations

The following investigations can help in evaluation of chronic cough.

Initial Tests

1. Microscopic examination of sputum and nasal smear.
2. Complete blood count.
3. A trial of bronchodilators.

More Specific Diagnostic Procedures

1. Imaging of paranasal sinuses and chest.
2. Tuberculin test.
3. Serum IgE level.
4. Bronchoscopy.
5. Tests for gastroesophageal reflux.
6. Special microbiologic studies viz. rapid viral tests, evaluation of ciliary morphologic features.

Eosinophilia in sputum or nasal smear suggests an atopic disease while presence of polymorphonuclear reaction in sputum suggests a bacterial infection. Sputum macrophages can be stained for hemosiderin content which is diagnostic of pulmonary hemosiderosis. Sputum culture is not very useful because it can be by the throat flora. If asthma is suggested by history, a trial of bronchodilator may be diagnostic. The significant finding in blood examination may be anemia. The X-ray of the chest is useful in diagnosis of tuberculosis, bronchiectasis, foreign body etc.

The child should be subjected to the initial tests and therapy instituted. If there is no response of cough to the initial therapy, the more specific tests should be advised based on the clinical diagnosis.

Management

The single most important aspect of management is to make a diagnosis and explain the nature of cough to the parents. Specific therapy should be instituted as soon as the diagnosis is clinched.

For symptomatic relief, mild cough can be treated with simple home remedies like tulsi and honey, steam inhalation, hydration and elevation of head end.

Dry cough is a result of viral infection or irritation of pharyngeal, laryngeal, and tracheal mucosa. It is self limiting. It should be treated to comfort the child, parents as well as the doctor. The drug of choice is a cough suppressant. Expectorants are harmful. Antibiotics have no role.

A spasmodic cough results from mild bronchospasm and edema of respiratory mucosa. There is history of presence of triggers viz. viral infection, temperature variation, exposure to dust, pollens. Drug of choice is a bronchodilator and response is dramatic. Antibiotics have no role. Treatment of mild bronchospasm is important because it is self limiting but damages bronchial mucosa and causes remodeling of bronchial mucosa with resultant recurrent attacks and permanent changes in the bronchial mucosa.

A simple cough suppressant such as *dextromethhorphan* (2–3 mg/kg/day 12 hourly × 7 days) may be used in children with dry exhausting cough associated with severe vomiting. *Bronchodilators* (e.g. Salbutamol, upto 10 kg wt 1 mg, 10–20 kg, 2 mg and above 20 kg, 0.1 mg / kg / dose 8 hourly × 7days) are the drugs of choice if there is indication of presence of bronchial hyperactivity or a history of atopy in the child or family.

There is no place for expectorants and mucolytics in the treatment of cough. A child below 5 years age is unable to expectorate. The *cough expectorants* will cause accumulation of secretions, increase irritation of the mucosa and thereby increase the cough. *Mucolytics* will dislodge the mucus plugs in the bronchioles, block the bronchioles and increase the respiratory distress.

STRIDOR

Definition

Stridor is a harsh, high pitched respiratory sound, usually inspiratory but may be biphasic, produced by turbulent air flow due to upper airway obstruction.

Why Stridor is Common in Young Children?

The resistance to airflow in the airways is inversely proportional to the radius of the airway to the fourth power (r^4) when the flow is laminar and to the fifth power (r^5) when flow is turbulent. The upper airway in infants and children is short and narrow. Hence a small amount of narrowing of an already small airway can greatly compromise flow. Secondly, the bronchial sub mucosa is loose and conducive to accumulation of edema fluid, but the confines of the airway are rigid and cartilaginous. Therefore any accumulation encroaches on the lumen of the airway. The final factor contributing to the vulnerability of the infant to upper airway obstruction is the short distance between the pharynx and the trachea. A compromise of the airway, which in an adult, can be localized to a relatively short portion of the upper airway, may appear more generalized in the very young infant.

Evaluation of Stridor

Laryngeal stridor is a high pitched, crowing, inspiratory sound which is aggravated by coughing. It may be produced by a foreign body lodged between the vocal cords, laryngeal spasm, exudate or edema related to acute viral or bacterial infection.

Tracheal stridor is a low pitched sound; best heard during inspiration, is accentuated by coughing and is accompanied by respiratory distress. Stridor may also be produced by partial obstruction of one or both main bronchi.

If stridor is suspected, the child should be asked to cough and then breathe deeply in and out with mouth wide open. If one listens carefully close to the child's mouth during the first few breaths after coughing, one can confirm the presence of stridor at an early stage.

Causes of Stridor

Stridor is a sign and not a disease. The most common cause of stridor is croup. Foreign bodies and trauma can also cause acute stridor. A small number of children however, suffer from recurrent or persistent stridor with an onset from the early days or weeks of life. Most congenital anomalies of the large airways that produce stridor become symptomatic soon after birth. The common congenital anomaly presenting with stridor is laryngomalacia.

Causes of Recurrent Stridor

1. Allergic or spasmodic croup.
2. Respiratory infection: Viral or bacterial.
3. Laryngomalacia.

Causes of Persistent Stridor

Laryngeal obstruction

1. Laryngomalacia, laryngeal webs.
2. Laryngeal papilloma, cysts and tumour.
3. Foreign body.
4. Bilateral abductor paralysis of the vocal cords.

Tracheobronchial disease

1. Tracheomalacia.
2. Subglottic tracheal webs.
3. Endotracheal and endobronchial tumours.
4. Subglottic tracheal stenosis.

Extrinsic masses

1. Mediastinal mass.
2. Vascular ring.
3. Lobar emphysema.
4. Bronchogenic cysts.
5. Enlargement of thyroid.
6. Esophageal foreign body and tracheoesophageal fistula.

Miscellaneous

1. Gastroesophageal reflux.
2. Macroglossia, Pierre Robin syndrome.
3. Hysterical stridor.
4. Hypocalcaemia.
5. Cri-du-chat syndrome.

Laryngomalacia

Laryngomalacia is the most frequent cause of stridor in infants and children. Stridor results from the collapse of supraglottic structures inwards during inspiration. Symptoms usually appear within the first 2 weeks of life and increase in severity for upto 6 months, although gradual improvement may occur at any time. Typically, the child presents with stridor which is inspiratory, low pitched and exaggerated by exertion viz. crying, agitation and feeding. The diagnosis is confirmed by flexible laryngoscopy.

Most infants need observation only because symptoms resolve spontaneously. In patients with severe obstruction and complications like failure to thrive, cyanosis, corpulmonale require surgical intervention.

CROUP

The term croup refers to a heterogeneous group of mainly acute and infectious processes that are characterized by a bark like or brassy cough and may be associated with hoarseness, inspiratory stridor and respiratory distress.

It is the most common form of acute inflammatory upper respiratory tract obstruction in children. Inflammatory conditions involving the vocal cords and the structures below the cords include:

1. Laryngitis.
2. Laryngotracheatis.
3. Laryngotracheobronchitis.

Inflammation of the structures above the glottis is called supraglottitis; the most common condition being acute epiglotitis. Diphtheria, another cause of bacterial croup has become uncommon after proper implementation of the universal immunization programme.

Laryngotracheobronchitis

Laryngotracheobronchitis is the most common form of upper respiratory obstruction in children presenting with stridor. The term refers to the infection of the glottic and subglottic regions.

Epidemiology

Most patients with laryngotracheobronchitis are between the ages of 3 months and 5 years with peak incidence in the second year of life. The incidence is higher in males. It occurs most commonly during the winter season but may occur throughout the year. It can occur recurrently but the recurrences decrease, with growth of the airway, by 6 years of age.

Etiology and Pathology

Laryngotracheobronchitis is primarily a viral disease. Parainfluenza virus type 1, 2, 3 accounts for approximately 75% of cases. The other viruses implicated are influenza A and B, adenovirus, respiratory syncytial virus, and measles virus. Influenza A has been associated with severe form of laryngotracheobronchitis. Measles virus as the cause is more common in developing countries.

There is inflammatory swelling of the vocal cords and the subglottic portion of the larynx.

Clinical Manifestations

Onset is gradual with symptoms of upper respiratory tract viral infection viz. rinorrhoea, mild cough, sore throat and low grade fever for 1–3 days. The child then develops the characteristic barking cough, hoarseness and inspiratory stridor. The low grade fever may continue or temperature may reach 39°C–40°C (102.2–104°F). Some children may remain afebrile. The child prefers to sit up in bed or be held upright. In majority of cases, physical examination reveals a hoarse voice, normal to moderately inflamed pharynx and a mild increase in the respiratory rate. Symptoms and signs are aggravated by crying and agitation and characteristically worsen at night.

The upper airway obstruction may progress and give rise to increasing respiratory rate, nasal flaring, suprasternal, infrasternal and intercostal retractions and continuous stridor. With complete obstruction of the upper airway, the child may become cyanosed or pale or obtunded. These children require immediate airway management. However, most patients progress as far as mild dyspnea before they start to recover and usually signs and symptoms resolve completely within a week.

Direct laryngoscopy reveals erythematous edema and destruction of epithelium of the respiratory tract, larynx and below.

X-ray study of the neck: Acute laryngotracheobronchitis is a clinical diagnosis. An X-ray PA view of the neck show a subglottic narrowing of the trachea, called the 'steeple sign'. It needs mention that steeple sign is not diagnostic. It may be present as a normal variant and may be absent in laryngotracheobronchitis. An X-ray is useful to differentiate severe laryngotracheobronchitis and epiglottis where clinical differentiation is difficult. An X-ray, if necessary, should be advised only after airway stabilization.

Differential Diagnosis

Acute laryngotracheobronchitis has to be differentiated from spasmodic croup, acute infectious laryngitis, diphtheria and acute epiglottitis.

Spasmodic Croup

It is a condition with a similar presentation as acute laryngotracheobronchitis. The age group affected is 1–3 years. Frequently, there is no history of viral prodrome either in the child or in the family. The cause may be viral in some cases but allergic and psychological factors may be responsible in others. The exact pathogenesis is not known. It may represent an allergic reaction to viral antigen.

Onset of symptoms is sudden. The symptoms occur more frequently in the evening or night time. The child suddenly has a barking, metallic cough, noisy inspiration and respiratory distress and appears anxious and frightened. The patient is usually afebrile. The severity of symptoms diminishes within several hours and the following day, the child becomes normal except for mild hoarseness and cough. Similar episodes, often less severe, may recur for another night or two. Direct laryngoscopy shows pale watery edema with preservation of the epithelium of the respiratory mucosa.

Acute Infectious Laryngitis

It is a common illness caused by viruses in majority of cases. Diphtheria may be the bacterial cause, which is now uncommon. The onset is characterized by an upper respiratory catarrh with hoarseness and loss of voice disproportionate to the systemic signs and symptoms. The illness is usually mild. Respiratory distress can occur in infants.

Direct laryngoscopy demonstrates inflammatory edema of the vocal cords and subglottic tissue.

The viral illness is self limiting. Treatment is symptomatic consisting of voice rest, saline nasal drops, paracetamol and rest. The infants with respiratory distress may require hospitalization for oxygenation. Diphtheria should be treated with ADS and benzyl penicillin.

Treatment

The treatment of laryngotracheobronchitis is essentially airway management. It should be given priority over investigation. Most children can be treated at home safely. The child should be hospitalized in presence of any of the following situations:

1. Progressive stridor.
2. Severe stridor at rest.
3. Respiratory distress, cyanosis, depressed mental status.
4. Need for reliable observation.

The different modalities in treatment include:

1. **Cool Mist:** Cool mist can be provided through a tube held in front of the patient by the parent. Children with associated wheeze, however, should not be treated with this modality because it may result in aggravation of wheeze on exposure to cool mist.
2. **Corticosteroids:** Corticosteroids act by decreasing edema in the laryngeal mucosa by its anti-inflammatory action. Steroids can be used orally, parenterally or by inhalation. Oral or intramuscular dexamethasone and nebulized budesonide have similar clinical effect. The dose of dexamethasone as low as 0.15 mg/kg, single dose, is shown to have similar effect when compared to high doses (0.6 mg/kg, single dose).
3. **Nebulized Epinephrine:** Both racemic epinephrine (1:1 mixture of *d* and *l* isomers of epinephrine) and *l* epinephrine are equally effective. The latter does not carry the risk of additional side effects as thought earlier. Epinephrine acts by constricting the precapillary arterioles through the alpha adrenergic receptors which causes fluid resorption from the interstitial space and a decrease in the laryngeal mucosal edema. Racemic epinephrine can be given in a dose of 0.25 to 0.75 ml of 2.25% solution in 3 ml of normal saline and can be given every 20 minutes by nebulization. *l* epinephrine (1:1000 dilutions) can be given in the dosage of 0.01 ml/kg to a maximum of 0.5 ml/dose administered subcutaneously. The indications are moderate to severe stridor at rest, need for intubation, respiratory distress, and hypoxia and when stridor does not respond to cool mist. The duration of action of nebulized epinephrine is around 2 hours. A symptom free child can be discharged after 2–3 hours. Nebulized epinephrine should be used cautiously in patients with tachycardia, congenital heart diseases viz. tetralogy of Fallot and ventricular outlet obstruction.

Acute Epiglottitis

It is a bacterial infection of the epiglottis which usually results in a medical emergency warranting immediate treatment with an artificial airway. The causative organism is H. influenzae type B.

Clinical Features

An otherwise normal child suddenly develops sore throat and fever. Within a matter of hours, the child becomes toxic, swallowing becomes difficult, and breathing laboured. The neck becomes hyper extended in an attempt to maintain the airway and there is drooling. The child assumes a typical position of sitting up and leaning forward with chin up and mouth open while bracing the arms. A brief period of air hunger with restlessness may be followed by cyanosis and coma. Stridor is a late manifestation and suggests near complete airway obstruction.

Sometimes, an initial lack of respiratory distress may deceive the attending physician. The child may not appear in grave danger because the airway obstruction is masked by the measures the child adopts to protect the airway by observing the typical posture as described earlier. The airway may however, suddenly occlude if the protective mechanisms are interfered with; for example when the child is provoked to cry or if any attempt is made to change the posture.

The diagnosis is confirmed by laryngoscopy which reveals a large, cherry red, swollen epiglottis. Occasionally, the other supraglottic structures may be more involved than the epiglottis itself. If epiglottitis is suspected, a throat examination or a laryngoscopy should be done in the operation theatre or an intensive care unit. If epiglottitis is thought to be possible in a patient with upper airway obstruction, the patient can undergo lateral X-ray of the upper airway. The classic X-ray will show the 'thumb sign'. If necessary, the child can then undergo laryngoscopy for further confirmation.

Management

Upon making a clinical diagnosis of acute epiglottitis, the patient should be directly taken to the operation theatre or intensive care unit for examination under anesthesia. This should be done irrespective of the degree of respiratory distress in the child.

If epiglottitis is confirmed, an airway has to be established by nasotracheal intubation or tracheotomy in all cases regardless of the degree of apparent distress. In general, the child has to be intubated for 2–3 days till response to antibiotics is obvious. Samples for blood culture, epiglottic surface culture and blood count has to be sent and intravenous antibiotics started. The antibiotic of choice is ceftriaxone (100 mg/kg /day), cefotaxime (100–150 mg/kg/day) or ampicillin sulbactum (100 mg/kg/day) IV, which may need change after the culture report is obtained. Antibiotic should be continued for 7–10 days. Rifampicin prophylaxis (20 mg/kg orally once a day for 4 days; maximum dose 600 mg) should be given to all household members, if there is a child younger than 4 years of age who is incompletely immunized or if there is an immunocompromised child in the household.

Foreign Body in the Airway

Foreign body aspiration is common in older infants and toddlers. It is most commonly seen in children below 3 years of age. It is so because in this period of life, children use their mouth to explore their surroundings. Hence they take everything to their mouth.

The clinical features of foreign body aspiration depend on the shape and size of the foreign body as well as the site of obstruction. Globular food objects viz. grapes, nuts and candies can cause complete obstruction of the airway. This is the most serious complication of foreign body aspiration. It can be recognized in a conscious child as sudden respiratory distress followed by inability to speak or cough. In the other types of foreign body aspiration, three stages of symptoms can be recognized. Immediately after aspiration, there are violent paroxysms of cough, choking and gagging. It is followed by an asymptomatic period. The foreign body becomes lodged, reflexes fatigued and the initial irritating symptoms subside. This accounts for a large number of delayed diagnoses. This is followed by a stage of complication which includes fever, cough, hemoptysis, pneumonia, atelectasis and localized wheeze.

Treatment

The treatment of choice for airway foreign body is prompt endoscopic removal usually on the same day the diagnosis is first considered.

Wheeze

Wheeze is the second most common clinical presentation in a child with respiratory disease next to cough. Unlike cough, if a child presents with wheeze, it invariably requires treatment.

Definition

Wheeze is a musical sound produced by airflow obstruction in the lungs and be generalized or localized. It is a non-specific physical sign associated with restriction of airflow through narrowed airways and is generated by turbulent airflow and subsequent oscillation of the bronchial wall.

Types of Airway Obstruction

Children with wheeze may have two types of airway obstruction in relation to airway tone: episodic and fixed. The differentiating points between the two types are shown in the tabular form:

Table 9.3 : Differentiating points between episodic and fixed wheeze

Features	*Episodic*	*Fixed*
1. Onset	Gradual	Abrupt
2. Severity	Mild	Severe
3. Duration of attacks	Short	Long
4. Rhonchi between attacks	Absent	Present
5. Response to bronchodilator	Quick	Slow
6. Course	Outgrow with 1–2 attacks	Continue as wheezer

It is important to understand this aspect in wheezing children because it is essential to prognosticate the affected child regarding future attacks and also to advice the parents on prevention of future attacks.

Mechanism of Production of Wheeze

Narrowing of the small airways is produced as a result of infection or an allergic response by two mechanism viz. bronchospasm and inflammation and edema of bronchial mucosa.

Why Wheezing is More Frequent in Children Below 3 Years?

There are certain distinct features which lead to the increase incidence and severity of wheezing in young children. They are as follows:

a. The airways are narrow in the younger child, hence easily blocked.

b. The surface area of the bronchial tree is minimal because airways are short and narrow.

c. Mucosal glands are numerous in the respiratory tract. In the event of irritation of the tracheobronchial tree due to factors viz. infection, allergens, there is mucosal edema and copious mucus secretion which causes clogging of the airways in a short period.

d. There is minimal bronchospasm, because smooth muscles are scanty resulting in ineffective mucosal clearance.

Etiology

Wheeze in children may result from either a structural cause (5%) or functional (95%) abnormality of the respiratory tract. The children with structural abnormality have prolonged wheeze relieved only by surgical correction. Functional wheeze results from a transient functional derangement of the respiratory tract manifesting as attacks of reversible obstructive airway disease under the influence of various precipitating factors.

The common structural abnormalities which causes wheeze include:

1. Foreign body.
2. Tracheoesophageal fistula (H-type).
3. Tracheal stenosis or web.
4. Bronchial stenosis.
5. Tumour.
6. Vascular ring.

The precipitating factors of wheeze may be:

1. Infections:
   a. *Viral:* RSV, Rhino, parainfluenza, adeno virus, influenza virus.
   b. *Bacterial:* Staphylococcus, S. pneumoniae, H. influenzae.
2. Infestations: Ascariasis, giardiasis.
3. Psychological factors: Emotional imbalance.
4. Environmental factors like exposure to cold air, noxious fumes e.g. tobacco smoke, wet paint and allergens like mites, pollen, animal dander, food feathers.
5. Exercise.
6. Drugs: NSAIDS, aspirin, propranolol.

Clinical Conditions Producing Wheeze in Relation to Age

An age related clinical classification of wheeze is possible in children and may be a useful guide in clinical practice.

Causes During Infancy

1. Bronchiolitis.
2. Pneumonia.
3. Congenital malformation of upper gastrointestinal and respiratory tract.
4. Aspiration syndromes.
5. Cystic fibrosis.

Causes in Older Children

1. Asthma.
2. Wheeze associated lower respiratory infection (WALRI).
3. Foreign body (localized wheeze).
4. Tropical eosinophilia.
5. Visceral larva migrans.
6. Tuberculous lymph nodes pressing a bronchus (localized wheeze).

Clinical Symptoms and Signs of Bronchospasm in Early Childhood

Although wheeze is the cardinal sign of bronchospasm, a child with acute bronchospasm in early childhood may present with varied symptoms and signs, viz.

1. Recurrent spasmodic cough, worse during sleep/night or after exercise, often associated with vomiting, which responds to bronchodilators.
2. Only tachypnoea/rapid breathing.
3. Exercise induced cough, chest pain/tightness.
4. Nocturnal cough.
5. An effort in breathing out.
6. Cyanosis, difficulty in breathing with over inflated silent chest or poor air entry with appearance of rhonchi after bronchodilator therapy.
7. Chest indrawing.
8. A prolonged expiratory phase.
9. Generalized polyphonic rhonchi.
10. Only abnormal pulmonary function tests.

Principles of Treatment

The treatment of wheeze depends on the grade. The grading may be done on the basis of presence of wheeze on auscultation and associated features.

Table 9.4 : Grading of wheeze and treatment

Grade	*Associated clinical features*	*Treatment*
1.	Normal respiratory rate	Oral bronchodilators
2.	Increased respiratory rate	Inhalation bronchodilators
3.	Presence of dyspnea	Inhalation bronchodilator, corticosteroids
4.	Presence of dyspnea with audible wheeze	Oxygen inhalation, inhalation bronchodilators, corticosteroids
5.	Presence of dyspnea with audible wheeze with increased work of breathing	Oxygen inhalation, inhalation bronchodilators, corticosteroids, ipratropium bromide, assisted ventilation.

Course and Outcome

Several factors influence the recurrence of wheeze in a child. They are as follows:

Age of Onset

With onset below 3 years of age, 90% children may outgrow the tendency to wheeze in near future. 10% may continue. Out of which 40–50% may turn out to be asthmatics during the 3rd or 4th decade. In children with onset of wheeze after 3 years of age 80% outgrow the tendency. 20% continue to wheeze and majority becomes asthmatics during the 3rd and 4th decade.

Duration of Wheezing Attacks

The children who have one of the following characteristics may continue to wheeze for the rest of the life:

a. An attack for more than 7 days.
b. Experience nocturnal cough or disturbed sleep for a longer period than an attack.
c. Have wheeze on auscultation inbetween attacks.

Frequency of Episodes

If a child has less than 4 episodes of wheezing per year there is a better chance of outgrowing the tendency to wheeze.

Severity of Wheezing Episodes

Frequent severe attacks indicate that the child may continue to wheeze. However, one severe attack in the child does not indicate that the child may continue to wheeze.

Common Wheezing Conditions

The most commonly encountered wheezing conditions are:

1. Acute bronchiolitis.
2. Asthma.
3. WALRI.
4. Gastroesophageal reflux.
5. Foreign body inhalation.
6. Pneumonia.

Acute Bronchiolitis

Acute bronchiolitis is a common disease of the lower respiratory tract occurring mostly in infants but can be seen in children upto 2 years of age with the severe form more common in the age group 1–3 months. It is a seasonal disease, with a peak incidence during winter and early spring. It is more common in males, in those who have not been exclusively breast fed and in those who live in overcrowded conditions. The older family members who suffer from a mild respiratory catarrh are a common source of infection.

Etiology

Acute bronchiolitis is predominantly a viral disease. The most common virus implicated is respiratory syncytial virus. Other agents include parainfluenza and adeno virus, and mycoplasma. A bacterial cause has not yet been found but sometimes bacterial pneumonia may be clinically confused with acute bronchiolitis. Acute bronchiolitis may be followed by secondary bacterial infection.

Pathophysiology

Acute bronchiolitis is an obstructive airway disease characterized by bronchial obstruction due to mucosal edema, mucus and cellular debris. Air flow is affected by increase resistance in small air passages both during inspiration and expiration. Because the radius of an airway is smaller during expiration, a ball valve respiratory obstruction results. This leads to early air trapping and over inflation. In case obstruction is complete, there is resorption of trapped air and there is atelectasis of the lungs.

At the cellular level, there occurs a complex cellular dysregulation which includes a complex immune response to the RSV infection, release of inflammatory mediators viz. interleukin 8, macrophage inflammatory protein etc, and altered regulation of surfactant proteins A and B.

The pathologic and cellular processes impair normal pulmonary gas exchange leading to hypoxemia as a consequence of ventilation-perfusion mismatch early in the course of the disease. With severe disease there is hypercapnia.

Clinical Manifestations

There is usually a history of exposure of the child to an older member of the family with minor respiratory catarrh within 7 days of onset. Onset is gradual with features of mild upper respiratory tract infection with sneezing and clear rhinorrhoea; may be accompanied by fever of 38.5°C–39°C (101–102°F) and loss of appetite. The temperature however, may range from subnormal to severe degree. This is followed by gradual onset of respiratory difficulty with paroxysmal spasmodic cough, dyspnea and irritability which interferes with feeding. In very young infants, apnea may be a more prominent symptom than wheezing, early in the course of the disease.

There is tachypnea and wheeze. Tachypnea does not always correlate with the degree of hypoxemia or hypercarbia. So it is essential to use pulse oximetry and non invasive carbon dioxide determination for monitoring. With increasing respiratory distress, there is increase in the work of breathing with nasal flaring and retractions. Auscultation of the chest may reveal fine crackles and wheeze. In severe disease with nearly complete bronchiolar obstruction, with poor air entry into the lungs, the breath sounds may be barely audible. The liver and spleen may be palpable due to over inflation of the lungs.

Laboratory Diagnosis

The white cell count and the differential counts are normal without lymphopenia as seen with other viral illness.

Sepsis evaluation should be done in a febrile infant to confirm viral bronchiolitis.

Viral tests viz. rapid immunofluorescence, polymerase chain reaction and viral culture have a debatable utility.

An X-ray of the chest reveals hyperinflated lungs, sometimes with patchy atelectasis. The X-ray chest is particularly indicated in the very young and the sick child to exclude pneumonia.

Differential Diagnosis

The diagnosis of acute bronchiolitis is essentially clinical; characterized by a previously healthy infant presenting with a first time wheezing episode during a community outbreak.

The commonly confused conditions with acute bronchiolitis are early onset asthma and pneumonia both of which can present with wheeze.

Early Onset Asthma

The first attacks are difficult to differentiate. A family history of atopy and good response to salbutamol may be helpful in suspecting asthma. Subsequently history of repeated episodes of wheezing without a preceding viral prodrome and a family history of atopy or asthma clinches the diagnosis of early onset asthma.

Pneumonia

Concurrent pneumonia with acute bronchiolitis is highly unlikely. Secondary bacterial infection can occur after initial recovery from acute bronchiolitis after an interval of few days. If the child is very ill, toxic with high fever, a blood count shows polymorphonuclearleucocytosis; pneumonia is the cause not bronchiolitis.

Course and Prognosis

The highest risk of respiratory compromise is during the first 48 hours after the onset of cough and dyspnea. The causes of death are apnea, uncompensated respiratory acidosis, and or severe dehydration. After the critical period, symptoms may persist upto 10–12 days. Acute bronchiolitis in infants with conditions like congenital heart disease, bronchopulmonary dysplasia and immunodeficiency are often more severe with high morbidity and mortality.

Epidemiologic studies have shown that there is higher incidence of wheezing and asthma in children with a past history of acute bronchiolitis, unexplained by family history or atopy.

Management

The mainstay of treatment of acute bronchiolitis is supportive. An assessment of degree of severity is essential to institute supportive treatment. The infant may present with mild, moderate or severe form which can be determined on the basis of the following parameters:

Table 9.5 : Grading of bronchiolitis

Parameter	*Mild*	*Moderate*	*Severe*
Respiratory distress	Absent	Some present	Marked
Fluid intake	Normal	Decreased	Markedly decreased
Oxygen saturation	No demand for supplemental O_2 > 92%	< 92%	Requires FiO_2 5 or more to keep O_2 saturation > 92%

Need for Hospitalization

Cases with mild bronchiolitis can be treated at home. Fluid intake should be monitored. Young infants even with mild symptoms should be preferably admitted.

Infants with respiratory distress should be hospitalized. The cases of moderate bronchiolitis can be treated in the ward whereas those of severe degree should be admitted to the intensive care unit.

Ward Management

1. Maintenance of a thermoneutral environment.
2. Minimal handling of the infant.
3. Comfortable position e.g. sitting with head and chest elevated at a 30° angle with neck extended.
4. Monitor colour, pulse, respiration and oxygen saturation, oral fluid intake.
5. Administration of supplemental oxygen by oxygen hood or tent to maintain saturation > 92%.
6. If unable to feed orally and to avoid aspiration of oral feeds due to tachypnea and difficult breathing nasogastric feeds can be given.
7. If the child deteriorates transfer to ICU.

Intensive Care Unit Management

1. Start supplemental oxygen to keep oxygen saturation > 92%.
2. Start intravenous fluid with 75% of maintenance and child to be kept nil orally.
3. Monitor colour, respiration, heart rate.
4. Consider ABG (arterial blood gas) estimation.
5. Consider nasal or endotracheal continuous positive airway pressure or artificial ventilation as indicated.
6. Sepsis evaluation should be done and empirical antibiotics which should cover both gram positive and gram negative organism (e.g. Cefotaxime 100 mg/kg/day IV 6 hourly + Amikacin 15 mg/kg/day IV 12 hourly) started, awaiting a blood culture, if the child is severely ill.

Proposed Adjunctive Therapy

A number of drugs have been proposed as adjunctive therapy in acute bronchiolitis with conflicting results. *Bronchodilators* viz. salbutamol by inhalation or epinephrine by nebulization has been tried. Epinephrine is found to be more effective. A trial dose of bronchodilator may be given with further therapy decided on the response in the individual patient. *Corticosteroids* have been used by all routes without any definite results. Corticosteroids are however not indicated in previously healthy infants with RSV infection. *Ribavirin*, an antiviral drug administered by aerosol showed no convincing evidence of positive result. Antibiotics have no role unless there is bacterial pneumonia. There is also no effect of RSV immunoglobulin administration during an acute episode of RSV bronchiolitis.

When to Discharge a Patient?

The infant is fit for discharge when it has not received supplemental oxygen for 10 hours, has minimal or no chest retraction, and is feeding adequately, without the need for intravenous fluids.

Prevention

Administration of pooled hyper immune RSV intravenous immunoglobulin is effective in preventing severe RSV disease when given before and during RSV season. It can be used in high risk infants below 2 years age viz. preterm babies, presence of chronic lung disease (bronchopulmonary dysplasia) and cyanotic congenital heart disease. The best approach for prevention in this group of the population is still under investigation. Meticulous hand washing is one established measure to prevent nosocomial infection in these children.

Asthma

Definition

Recurrent wheezing, breathlessness, chest tightness and cough, particularly at night and/or early morning reversible either spontaneously or with treatment is described as asthma. One should also consider the diagnosis of asthma if a child presents with recurrent lower respiratory infection or recurrent pneumonic infiltrates.

Recurrent refers to more than 3 episodes beyond the first year of life. Recurrent isolated cough of unclear etiology may be the sole manifestation of asthma. Nocturnal cough may also be the sole manifestation of asthma. In children under treatment for asthma, persistence of nocturnal symptoms suggests the need for better control. Recurrent pneumonic infiltrates in a chest X-ray is defined as more than two episodes in a year or more than 3 episodes over any period of time. Asthma should be considered in the differential diagnosis if the infiltrates recur in different lobes.

Etiopathogenesis

Asthma, whatever the severity, is now recognized as a chronic inflammatory disorder of the airways. Airways inflammation is strongly linked to hypersensitivity of airways smooth muscles (airways hyperresponsiveness) to irritant exposures viz. cold air, dry air, strong odours and smoke. Over time, the basement membrane of airways may become scarred and thickened. There is subepithelial collagen deposition, hypertrophy and hyperplasia of smooth muscle and mucus gland. This process of chronic remodeling resembles an aberrant tissue repair process in response to persistent tissue injury and lead to less reversible airways changes.

Inhaled allergen challenge tests have revealed two distinct phases of airflow obstruction in asthma: An early phase and a late phase. The *early phase* occurs within 15–30 minutes and consists of bronchoconstriction. The *late phase* occurs 4–12 hours after allergen exposure. It consists of tissue inflammation, immune cellular infiltration into the airways, airways edema and excess mucus production. The late phase is also associated with airways hyperresponsiveness that can persist for several weeks.

Inflammation and intermittent constriction of the airways give rise to symptoms of cough, wheeze, chest tightness and shortness of breath. The early phase can be prevented by pretreatment with β_2 agonist. In contrast, the late phase can be prevented with anti-inflammatory agents (e.g. steroids) and not by bronchodilators.

Wheezing is considered as the cardinal sign of asthma in children but all children with asthma do not wheeze. Wheeze is a non-specific physical sign associated with restriction of airflow through narrowed airways and is generated by turbulent airflow and subsequent oscillation of the bronchial wall. Since flow rates in the small airways are too slow to generate oscillations in the audible range, wheezing reflects airflow obstruction in larger airways. Wheezing also can be produced by obstruction of small intrapulmonary airways as the associated hyperinflation produces dynamic compression of the large airways and subsequent wheezing.

A generalized intra luminal or extra luminal airway involvement which is associated with polyphonic wheezing is typical of asthma. The signs suggestive of generalized airflow obstruction are: (a) generalized rhonchi, (b) prolonged expiration, (c) chest hyperinflation.

Early Adverse Exposure of Lungs and Subsequent Development of Wheeze

A proportion of wheezing illness in infancy and early childhood appears to be associated with impaired airway function, in contrast to later childhood where atopy is a major determinant of wheezing illness.

The most clearly identifiable adverse intrauterine exposure is maternal smoking. Several studies have shown reductions in lung function indices that reflect airway function in asymptomatic infants exposed to the products of cigarette smoke in utero. Studies on effect of maternal diet during pregnancy are going on.

The possibility that the RSV or other viruses encountered in early life interact with the immature immune and respiratory system and initiate complex mechanism leading to asthma has been a subject of considerable study and debate. It is thought that RSV triggers the asthmatic process in subjects who are predisposed either by their genetic background or by events occurring before their first encounter with the virus.

Although early environmental exposures were shown to influence the development of allergen sensitization, a causal link between allergen exposure and the subsequent development of asthma is not established. Allergen avoidance in early life can delay rather than prevent subsequent sensitization.

Protective Factors

A high dietary n-3: N-6 fatty acid ratio may reduce the development of airway inflammation.

There is also trial and circumstantial data suggesting that high anti oxidant intakes (including Vitamin C and selenium) mainly provided as fresh fruits and vegetables may be associated with decreased bronchial hyper responsiveness and reported asthma.

Risk Factors for Asthma Persisting into Adulthood

The risk factors for asthma persisting into adult life include male sex, presence of eczema, onset after 3 years of age, severe disease, parental history of atopy / asthma, maternal smoking.

Clinical Manifestations

The diagnosis of asthma can be made easily in children over 5 years of age who present with cough, wheeze and dyspnea. The diagnosis is difficult in younger children. But in order to establish early intervention strategies to avoid chronic pulmonary disease in later life and thereby improve quality of life, physical and psychological development in asthmatic children, it is important to make the diagnosis of asthma as early in childhood as possible.

More than three episodes of airflow obstruction with presence of one or more of the qualifying features listed below are typical of asthma.

1. Onset after about 3 years of age.
2. Afebrile episodes.
3. History of personal atopy.
4. History of atopy/asthma in parent/sibling.
5. Exercise/activity induced symptoms.
6. Trigger induced symptoms.
7. Seasonal exacerbations.
8. Relief with bronchodilators with or without a short course of oral steroids.

Points to be Noted

Presence of *fever* indicates an infectious cause. However, prolonged cough and/or wheeze after a viral respiratory infection may suggest asthma. If a child has other *manifestations of atopic disease*, the risk of asthma increases. Flexural dermatitis, eczema and allergic rhino-conjunctivitis are other atopic manifestation to be looked for in the child. *Atopy/Asthma in parents / sibling* doubles the risk of asthma in the child. If both parents have asthma the risk is more than 3 times. In a young child, exercise/activity viz. crying, playing, running or laughing may provoke symptoms. *Triggers* are usually inhaled irritants or aeroallergens. They are to be looked for because prevention of exposure is an important part of management. *Relief with bronchodilator* with or without a short course of oral steroid is a clinical indicator of reversible air flow obstruction.

Cough as a Sign of Asthma

In infants and young children, with acute mild bronchospasm, the most common symptom is cough, which usually follows a viral upper respiratory infection. The implied infective origin of the episode results in inappropriate administration of repeated courses of antibiotics and failure to administer a bronchodilator. It is worth mentioning that mild attacks of bronchospasm are usually relieved by 5–7 days even without a bronchodilator.

So in such a situation, the child apparently gets relief after a course of antibiotics. But recurrence is common in such children and permanent changes in the bronchial mucosa are not prevented.

Early Onset Asthma (Below 3 Years Age)

Early onset asthma is characterized by afebrile episodes of recurrent wheezing, may be triggered by viral infection, with more nocturnal symptoms. There is a history of personal atopy, a family history of asthma/ atopy and a predictable good response to bronchodilators.

Special Situations That Merit Follow-up

A child with less than 3 episodes of symptoms of airflow obstruction with a personal history of atopy or a family history of asthma/atopy needs follow-up. They should be advised to maintain a diary of symptoms, identify and avoid trigger factors. The acute episodes should be treated and other qualifying features looked for to assign the diagnosis of asthma. An overtime assessment of severity will help to plan the long-term management strategy in these children.

A child between 6 months and 3 years with frequent airflow obstruction, who wheezes frequently, is often a management dilemma. WALRI and early onset asthma are the common causes of wheezing in this age group. While children with asthma do benefit from a preventer drug regime, preventive therapy in WALRI continues to be a subject of debate. The child who has features of early onset asthma or has overlapping features of WALRI and early onset asthma should be graded and put on a trial of suitable preventive therapy. If the child is better, preventive therapy should be continued. If there is no response reasons for poor control should be looked for. If none are found an alternative diagnosis should be reconsidered.

Need for Investigation

Diagnosis and grading of severity of asthma is essentially clinical but in a newly diagnosed case the following tests should be carried out:

1. Blood count with absolute eosinophil count to exclude tropical eosinophilia (absolute count > 3000/cu mm).
2. X-ray chest, X-ray paranasal sinuses, X-ray nasopharynx (lateral view) in the event of suspected sinusitis and enlarged adenoids.
3. Pulmonary function tests viz. Spirometry, PEFR when clinical diagnosis of asthma is in doubt.

Long Term Treatment Plan

Goals of Therapy

The aim of long-term treatment in asthma is two-fold:

1. Freedom from (a) symptoms, including nocturnal cough, (b) acute exacerbation and emergency doctor/ hospital visits, (c) frequent school absenteeism, and (d) adverse drug effects.
2. Normal (a) daily activities and sports participation, (b) growth, (c) peak expiratory flow/spirometry.

Steps to Achieve These Goals

1. Assessment and categorization of patient.
2. Starting preventive therapy wherever indicated.
3. Monitoring the child for response to therapy.
4. Step up and step down depending on response.
5. Decision to stop therapy.
6. Supportive therapy.

Assessment of the Child

The clinical pattern of the child's asthma is the key to determine the need for preventive therapy. A thorough and accurate clinical assessment of the child's asthma is essential especially at times when the child is between attacks and thought to be well. The following specific questions are to be asked to the patient. These have been found to be helpful in assessing the need for preventive therapy.

1. The number of days on which symptoms of airflow obstruction occurred between attacks.
2. The number of night sleep disturbed due to asthma.
3. The number of days β_2 agonist were required.
4. Limitation of activity during acute exacerbation.

Grading of Asthma

On the basis of the answers to the above questions asthma may be graded as Grade 1: Intermittent, Grade 2: Mild persistent, Grade 3: Moderate persistent, Grade 4: Severe persistent. Grading severity of asthma helps to decide the optimal preventer regime for long-term control.

Table 9.6 : Grading of asthma

Grade	*Symptoms of air-flow obstruction**	*Night symptoms*	*PEFR*
1.	< once a week Asymptomatic and normal between attacks	< twice a month	> 80% of personal best. < 20% diurnal variation
2.	> once a week but < once a day	> twice a month	> 80% of personal best. 20 – 30% diurnal variation
3.	> once a day Symptoms affect activity	> once a week	> 60% - < 80% of personal best. > 30% diurnal variation
4.	Continuous symptoms. Limited physical activity	Frequent	< 60% of personal best. > 30% diurnal variation

Grade 1 = Intermittent asthma, Grade 2 = Mild persistent
Grade 3 = Moderate persistent, Grade 4 = Severe persistent

Points to be Noted

1. The nature of symptoms of airflow obstruction and night symptoms may be wheeze, difficulty in breathing or cough which responds to bronchodilator therapy.
2. In the event of overlapping criteria, it is appropriate to label the patient as belonging to the higher grade.
3. Since asthma is a dynamic condition, the grade of severity may change overtime.

When to Commence Preventive Therapy?

In general preventive therapy should be started when a child has features of persistent asthma (mild, moderate or severe). The Australian National Asthma Council recommends that preventive therapy should be commenced also in the following situations:

1. Asthma attacks occur more than every 6–8 weeks.
2. Attacks are infrequent but severe or life threatening
3. Spirometry (in those old enough) shows reversible airflow obstruction between attacks.

Long-Term Treatment Plan

Asthma is a chronic/recurrent disease. The child usually needs treatment for prolonged periods which vary with the individual child. The principles of long-term treatment of asthma includes the following:

1. The treatment regime consists of managing acute exacerbations and instituting a long-term preventive action plan. This is implemented with a suitable regimen of reliever drugs for acute episodes and preventive therapy for long-term control.
2. The inhaled route is the preferred route of drug delivery. Oral drugs have a limited role in modern management of asthma. However, it can still be used in cases with intermittent asthma with infrequent attacks.
3. Parental education regarding benefits of inhaled therapy and methodical use of the different inhalation devices. Inhalation therapy works best only when administered by the proper procedure.

The Stepwise Approach in Long-Term Preventive Therapy

Step I: Intermittent Asthma (Grade 1)

1. Treatment of acute exacerbation according to severity.
2. No long-term preventive therapy is necessary.
3. Child to be kept under observation and instituted preventive therapy when indicated.

Step II: Mild Persistent Asthma (Grade 2)

Preferred treatment is low dose inhalation steroids. Alternatively sodium chromoglycate inhalation or leucotrine receptor antagonist (Montelukust) may be used.

Step III: Moderate Persistent (Grade 3)

1. Preferred treatment is low dose inhaled steroid + salmeterol/formoterol or medium dose inhaled steroid. Alternatively low dose inhalation steroid + Montelukust/slow release theophylline.
2. If there is recurring acute severe exacerbation then preferred treatment is medium dose inhalation steroids + salmeterol/formoterol. Alternatively Montelukust may be used instead of salmeterol/formoterol.

Step IV: Severe Persistent (Grade 4)

1. Preferred treatment is high dose inhaled steroid + salmeterol/formoterol.
2. If still symptomatic, daily oral steroid (2 mg/kg /day) with an attempt to reduce dose of oral steroids and maintain child on inhalation high dose steroids.

INHALED THERAPY AND DRUG DELIVERY SYSTEM

The inhaler route of drug delivery can be considered as one of the most important recent advances in asthma management. This has made asthma therapy in children simple, effective and safe to administer. The inhaled medicines or aerosols are available through a variety of devices viz. metered dose inhaler (MDI), dry powder inhaler (DPI) and nebulizer.

The Drug Aerosol

A drug aerosol is basically a suspension of a drug (either solid particle or liquid droplets) in a gaseous medium. For aerosol therapy to be effective, the drug must reach the lower airway. This requires a particle size of diameter less than 5 micron. If particles are larger they will be mainly deposited in the larger airways or swallowed.

It should be mentioned that even with a particle size of < 5 micron only 10–15% of the inhaler drug reaches the lower airway, but this small amount is sufficient for a clinical response.

Advantages of Inhaler Route

The major advantages of the inhaler route compared to the oral route of medication are:

1. The desired pharmacological effect is achieved with much smaller dose of the drug. For example while a syrup formulation of salbutamol contain 2 mg (2000 mcg)/ 5 ml, the inhaler salbutamol provides only 100 mcg.
2. Drug delivery occur directly to the desired site i.e. lungs. The onset of action is rapid. When given orally it takes hours in comparison to minutes in case of inhalation.
3. Systemic side effects of inhalation drugs viz β_2 agonist and steroids are significantly minimized because systemic absorption is minimum.

Preventer Medications

The long-term controller medications include inhaled corticosteroids (ICS), long acting beta 2 agonists (LABA), leucotrine modifiers, and sustained release theophylline (theophylline SR). An anti IgE preparation, omalizumab has been approved by FDA for children 12 years age and above as an add on therapy for patients with moderate to severe allergic asthma.

Inhaled corticosteroids (ICS): It is viewed as the first line therapy for persistent asthma because it can achieve all of the goals of asthma management. The available ICS include beclomethasone, budesonide, and fluticasone all available in MDIs and DPIs. Fluticasone and to a lesser extent budesonide are considered second generation ICSs because they have increased anti-inflammatory potency and reduced systemic bioavailability for potential adverse effects, owing to extensive first-pass hepatic metabolism. Only higher doses (> 1000 microgram /day) and frequent administration (4 times/day) are more likely to cause local and systemic side effects. The most commonly encountered side effects are oral thrush and dysphonia.

Long acting inhaled beta agonist (LABA): The available LABA medications include salmeterol and formoterol. The onset of action of salmeterol is around 1 hour whereas that of formoterol is within 5–10 minutes. Both medications have a prolonged duration of atleast 12 hours. Their major use is as an "add on" agent in patients who are not adequately controlled on ICS therapy alone. A combination of ICS and LABA has been shown to be superior to doubling the dose of ICS in these patients. They are also useful in preventing exercise induced asthma. For want of clinical data, at present, salmeterol should be used in children beyond 4 years of age and formeterol above 6 years.

Leucotrine receptor antagonist (LTRA) agents: Two LTRAs are FDA approved for use in children– Montelukust and zafirlukast. The former is FDA approved for use in children 1 year age or more while the latter for use in children 5 years or more. LTRAs have bronchodilator and targeted anti-inflammatory properties and reduce exercise, aspirin and allergen induced bronchoconstriction. LTRAs appear to be less effective than ICS in moderate persistent asthma.

Nonsteroidal anti-inflammatory agents: Cromolyn and nedocromil are the two agents in this group. The NAEPP guidelines recommend both drugs as alternative anti-inflammatory drugs for children with mild persistent asthma. However, they are nearly not as effective as ICS or LRTA for preventive therapy. They can be used in exercise induced asthma in place of short acting beta agonist especially in children with adverse effects like tremor and tachycardia.

Theophylline: It is a mild bronchodilator as well as an anti-inflammatory agent. In young children absorption and metabolism is erratic. So it is not recommended to be used as a first line drug to control mild persistent asthma. Theophylline has a narrow therapeutic window. Therefore when used serum theophylline levels should be monitored especially if the patient has a viral illness associated with fever or is placed on a medication which delays theophylline clearance like macrolides, ciprofloxacin etc. Theophylline overdoses and elevated theophylline levels have been associated with headache, vomiting, cardiac arrhythmias, seizure and death.

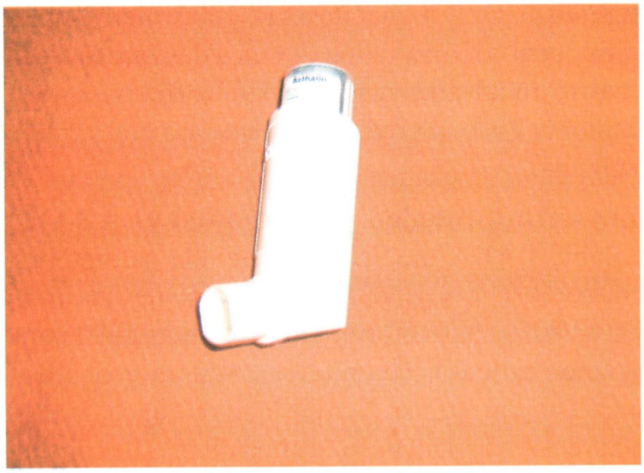

Fig. 9.2: Meter dose inhaler

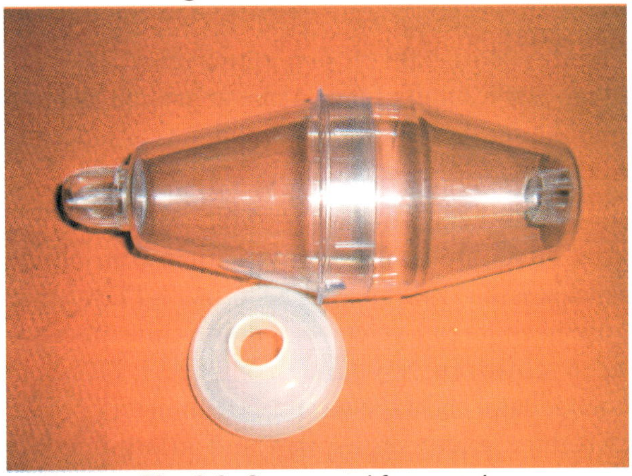

Fig. 9.3: Spacer and face mask

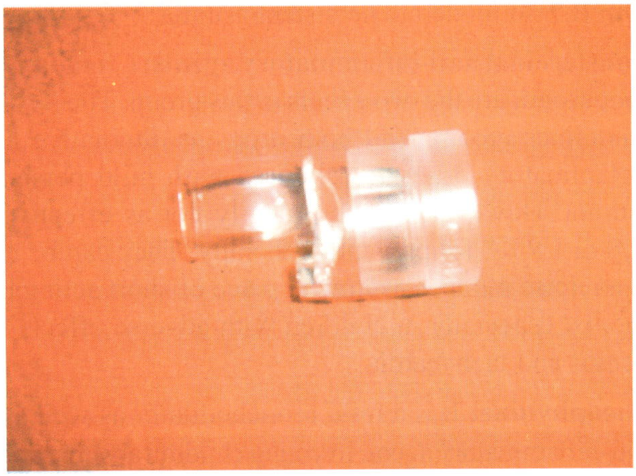

Fig. 9.4: Dry powder inhaler

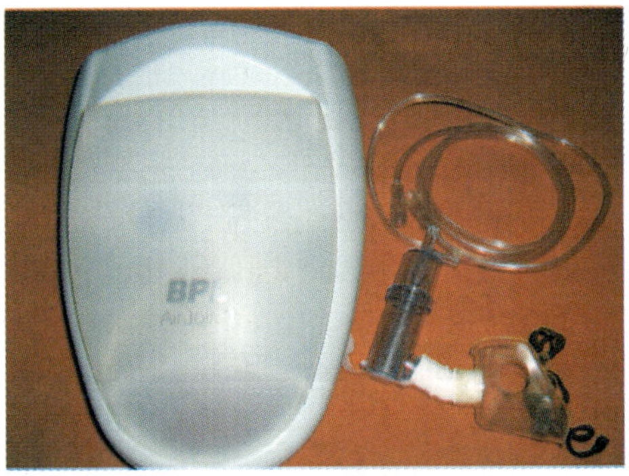

Fig. 9.5: Nebulizer

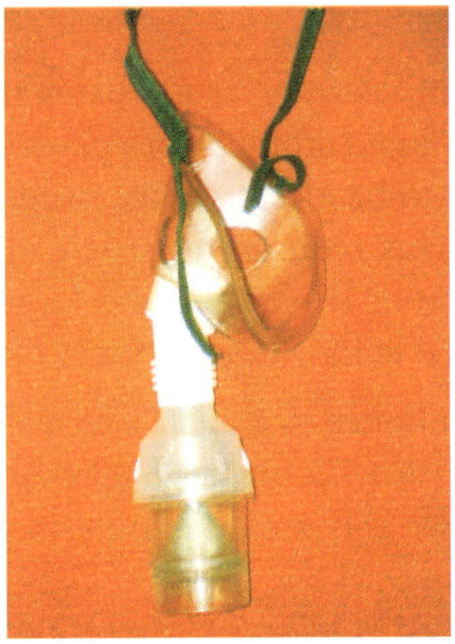

Fig. 9.6: Nebulizer chamber and mask

Inhaled Drug Delivery Systems

The different devices available for inhaled therapy are:

Metered Dose Inhalers (MDI)

The MDI is compact, easy to carry and is the most widely used inhalation device for asthma today. Difficulty with coordination of actuation and inhalation precludes the usage of this device without a spacer in the pediatric age group. Further, direct usage causes deposition of more than 80% of actuated dose in the oropharynx in any age group.

Spacers

Spacer devices are inhaler aids used as accessories to MDIs. In smaller children who are unable to understand or cooperate, a face mask can be attached to the mouth piece of the spacer.

Dry Powder Inhaler (DPI)

For optimal drug delivery, using a DPI, the child must be capable to generate an appropriate inspiratory flow of 30–90 L / min and breathholding for 5–10 seconds. A lower or higher rate leads to either oral or pharyngeal deposition. A child can be trained to do so by the age of

7 – 8 years. Hence a DPI can be advised for drug delivery only after this age. The different types of DPI available are rotahaler, acuhaler, turbuhaler. Its use is limited to preventive therapy only. During an acute exacerbation, the child may not be able to generate the required flow and lead to suboptimal drug delivery. This prevents its use in acute exacerbations.

Cleaning of Spacers and Dry Powder Inhaler

Polycarbonate spacers, DPI should be wiped with soft cotton cloth after every use and washed once a week with a mild soap water solution, and allowed to drip dry.

Nebulizer

A nebulizer is a device which is used to administer solution of drugs in the form of a fine mist. This mist can be inhaled easily either through a mouth piece or by using a mask while the child breathes tidally.

The drug aerosol is delivered to the patient's lungs using compressed air or oxygen. It can be used to deliver higher doses of drugs than MDIs and DPIs. During severe attacks, bronchodilators and anticholinergics can be mixed and given. The nebulizer is therefore mainly reserved for use in treatment of acute severe asthma in hospital. It has been shown that use of nebulizer for preventive therapy is not cost effective. For preventive therapy and even treatment of acute exacerbation at home, MDI with spacer has been shown to give results comparable to nebulizer. A drowsy child, irrespective of age would require drug delivery through a nebulizer. A child on a ventilator needs to have the nebulizer chamber interposed in the tubing.

It is advisable to use free flow oxygen at the rate of 6–7 litres/minute to run a nebulizer, instead of compressed air initially in treatment of an acute severe exacerbation. Use of compressed air may precipitate anoxia and further deteriorate the condition of the asthmatic child.

Steps of Using Different Delivery Devices

How to Use the Meter Dose Inhaler?

1. Remove cap of MDI and shake inhaler in vertical direction. Ask child to keep neck in slight extension. This makes the airway straight and patent.
2. Ask the child to breathe out gently. Put mouth piece inside the mouth and at start of inspiration press the canister down and ask to breathe in slow and deep. Then hold breath for 10 seconds or as long as possible and then breathe out slowly.
3. Wait for few seconds before taking the second dose.

How to Use Meter Dose Inhaler With Spacer With or Without Mask?

1. Remove cap of MDI and shake inhaler in vertical direction and inset into the spacer. Ask child to keep neck in slight extension.
2. Place the mouth piece of the spacer inside the child's mouth. Ask child to breathe in and out gently for some time until breathing pattern is established. Then press the canister at the start of inspiration and ask the child to breathe 3 – 4 times (tidal breathing).
3. Remove the spacer; wait for 30 seconds before giving the second dose.
4. In case of a child below 2 – 3 years of age, the face mask has to be fitted to the mouth piece of the spacer. The other steps are same.

How to Use Rotahaler?

1. Insert the rotacap into square hole, making sure that the top of the capsule is at level with the top of the hole. Ask the child to keep neck in slight extension.
2. Split the capsule into two by twisting the barrel of the rotahaler in clockwise and anticlockwise direction.
3. Ask the child to breathe out gently and put the mouth end of the rotahaler inside the mouth and take a deep inspiration and hold the breath for 10 seconds or as long as possible. Then remove the rotahaler from the mouth. Wait for few seconds before taking the second rotacap.

How to Use the Nebulizer?

1. Connect nebulizer to the mains. Put measured amount of drug in the nebulizer chamber and add normal saline to make the volume upto 2.5 – 3 ml.
2. Connect the nebulizer chamber to the compressor. Switch on the compressor and observe the aerosol coming out. In case of a severe attack of asthma the nebulizer chamber should be connected to an oxygen source with flow meter to form the mist.
3. Fit the face mask to cover the nose and mouth of the child. Ask the child to take tidal breathing with open mouth.

Selecting a Device

For treatment of acute exacerbation:

- For acute mild and moderate episode: MDI + spacer with or without mask.
- For acute severe episode: Nebuliser / MDI + spacer with or without mask.

For preventive therapy:

- DPI / MDI + spacer with or without mask.

Age Appropriate Delivery Device

Age	*Device option*
Less than 2–3 years	MDI + spacer + mask
Above 3 years	MDI + spacer
Above 7–8 years	MDI + spacer/DPI
Above 10–12 years	MDI + spacer/MDI alone may be tried

Drug for Preventive Therapy

(a) Inhalation Steroid

Drugs	*Budesonide (mcg)*	*Beclomethasone (mcg)*	*Fluticasone (mcg)*
Mild Persistent	100 – 400	100 – 400	50 – 100
Moderate Persistent	400 – 800	400 – 800	100 – 200
Severe Persistent	800 – 1000	800 – 1000	200 – 400

(b) Long Acting B2 Agonist

Salmeterol (above 4 years) 50 mcg 12 hourly

Formeterol (above 6 years) 12 mcg 12 hourly

(c) Montelukast

Dose: 2 – 5 years age: 4 mg, 6 – 14 years: 5 mg, > 14 years age 10 mg once daily at bed time.

Steps of Asthma Control with Prophylactic Inhalation Steroids

In gaining initial control of asthma there are two appropriate alternative approaches viz. step down approach and step up approach.

Step down approach: Here therapy is started at a level higher than the patient's grade of severity to gain rapid control. Once this is achieved, therapy should be stepped down to the lowest level in which child is asymptomatic.

Step up approach: Here therapy is started appropriate to the patient's grade of severity at the time of evaluation and doses stepped up if control is not achieved.

Choice of approach: There are no studies comparing the two initial approaches. The step down approach has the advantage of gaining quick control. This gains the patients / parents confidence and is likely to improve compliance.

Steps of control: The lung condition should be stabilized first starting inhaled steroids by step down (preferable) or step up approach. The child should be assessed 2–8 weekly for good control.

According to the GINA 2014 recommendation preventive therapy once started should be continued life time.

Criteria for Good Control

a. For grade 1and 2
  - No symptoms.
  - No nocturnal symptoms.
  - Minimal infrequent exacerbation.
  - No limitation of activities during exercise.
  - PEFR > 80% of predicted best.
  - Minimal or no adverse effects of drug.

b. For grade 3 and 4
  - Least possible symptoms.
  - Least possible exacerbation.
  - Least possible limitation of activities.
  - Least possible variation of PEFR.
  - Least adverse side effects of drugs.

If at 3–6 months, good control continues drug doses should be tapered by approximately 25% every 2–3 months to the lowest dose in which the child's symptoms are under control. If good control continues, on low dose steroid, for 3–6 months stopping of preventer regime can be considered. However, after stopping preventive therapy, the child should be advised to continue trigger avoidance. A home management plan should be advised for use in case of an acute episode. The child should be followed up 3–6 monthly for a period of 1–2 years. The parents should be counseled regarding possible future resumption of preventer regime in case of recurrences.

Poor Controlled Asthma

In case of poor response to preventer treatment, as a first step one should try to rule out an alternative diagnosis, try identification of correctable issues viz. ascertain compliance, check technique of usage of inhaler device, check trigger elimination.

The second step includes identification and treatment of medical conditions viz. allergic rhinitis/ sinusitis, GE reflux that may be responsible for poor control.

Thirdly, when the previous steps do not show any defect, a short course of steroid (1–2 mg/kg/day, maximum 60 mg/day for 3 to 10 days) is often effective to regain control. If it does not control symptoms, or is effective for a short period (less than 1–2 weeks) or needs to be repeated frequently then preventer dose should be stepped up but after objective assessment of daily trends in peak flow. Suitable regimens may be:

1. Addition of long acting β_2 agonist viz. salmeterol (preferred regime), or
2. Double the dose of steroid.

If poor control still persists one should consider:

1. Complications viz. bronchopulmonary aspergillosis or bronchiectasis.
2. The above steps may be repeated and other treatment options viz. methotrexate, immunotherapy may be considered. The child may be referred to a pediatric pulmonologist for such treatment.

Treatment of Concurrent Medical Conditions

Concurrent medical conditions like allergic rhinitis/sinusitis may be responsible for poor control of asthma. Asthma and allergic rhinitis usually co-exist. Similarly asthma and gastroesophageal reflux each may worsen the other.

Allergic Rhinitis/Sinusitis

Allergic rhinitis is suspected in a child with afebrile episodes of rhinorrhoea, sneezing, stuffiness of nose, signs of upper airway obstruction and nocturnal cough, nasal mucosal edema, hyperemia, clear nasal discharge, post nasal drip, cobble stone pharyngeal wall and Dennis-Morgan lines.

Allergic rhinitis is treated with intranasal steroid sprays viz. Budesonide 100 mcg two times a day or Fluticasone 50 mcg once a day or Mometasone once a day.

The dosage of nasal steroids should be added to that of inhaled steroid in order to compute the total dose of steroid therapy. Leucotrine receptor antagonist viz. Montelukust in daily once doses has been also found to be effective.

Gastroesophageal Reflux (GER)

GER worsens asthma by a vagally mediated reflex bronchospasm and micro aspiration. GER may be aggravated by asthma by increased trans-diaphragmatic pressure gradient due to coughing and laxity of the lower esophageal sphincter caused by bronchodilators.

Treatment consist of anti reflux treatment and avoidance of oral bronchodilator/theophylline.

Management of Special Situations

Seasonal Asthma

Daily preventer regime should be initiated prior to the anticipated onset of symptoms and continued throughout the season. The child should be encouraged indoor activities during such seasons.

Exercise Induced Asthma

In about 30% children with asthma, exercise produces symptoms of an acute attack viz. cough, wheeze or dyspnea. Typically, symptoms appear within 5–10 minutes of exercise and subside within 30–60 minutes.

Children with exercise induced asthma remain undiagnosed because they do not have any auscultatory findings in between attacks. A particularly useful way to help in diagnosis is to have the child exercise by running hard for 5–6 minutes. Provided the child has not received any bronchodilator medication in the previous 6–8 hours, this will induce a brief attack of asthma in a large majority of asthmatic children.

Management: The children should be taught to practice nose breathing and slow deep breathing during exercise. They should avoid outdoor exercise on winter mornings, advised short periods of warming up within one hour of main activity. The school teacher should be notified and informed about the need of inhaled medication prior to activity.

The child should be advised a suitable preventer regime after grading of severity. If EIA symptoms persist, an additional drug should be added as necessary. The drugs used are:

a. Inhaled salbutamol given 15–30 minutes before exercise. It is helpful for 2–3 hours.
b. Inhaled salmeterol given 2–3 hours before exercise. It is helpful for 10–12 hours.
c. Inhaled formoterol given 1 hour before exercise. It is helpful for 10–12 hours.

Perioperative Steroids in Risk Situations

Children with asthma are at risk of complications during and after surgery. Acute bronchoconstriction may be triggered by intubation, impaired cough reflex, atelectasis or respiratory infection. The likelihood of these complications depends upon the severity of bronchial hyper responsiveness, mucous hyper secretion and airflow obstruction.

Management: Symptoms and medications used in the child should be reviewed. In those children who have received systemic steroids for longer than 2 weeks duration during the past 6 months, the child should be started on intravenous hydrocortisone 8 hourly on the day of surgery, reducing the dose within 24 hours following surgery. For others, lung function has to be optimized with oral steroid prior to surgery.

Supportive Treatment in Asthma

Supportive treatment of asthma is as important as therapy with anti-inflammatory drugs. Even if the patient has a mild disease not requiring prophylactic therapy, the need for supportive treatment is still very much there.

Parental Counseling

The success of asthma management hinges on patient education. Besides parents, the child and other care givers should also be involved in the discussion. At the first consultation, *'give the patient your time more than your prescription'*.

The parents should be clearly told about the diagnosis. It should be discussed that asthma is a chronic disease with exacerbations and that certain grades of asthma requires preventive therapy should be explained.

It should be emphasized that the drugs used will control but do not cure. The parents should be reassured that a majority of children outgrow their symptoms.

Myths and misconceptions regarding inhaled therapy should be cleared and merits of inhaled route should be emphasized.

Concern regarding use of steroid should be addressed. The steroid regimen selected for the child should be discussed with the parents.

The usage and maintenance of the inhaler devices should be discussed.

The parents should be informed about the approximate time taken to note improvement after starting preventive therapy. The need for proper compliance should be emphasized.

The parents should be advised to maintain a diary of events and carry it at every visit. They may record days with events like day time cough, nocturnal cough, wheeze, reliever medicines used, doctor/hospital visits.

Every child should be provided with a crisis plan for management of acute exacerbation at home prior to doctor contact.

Advised regarding dealing with triggers/precipitants. It should also be emphasized that diet has a small role in causation of symptoms.

First visit for follow-up should be 4 weeks after starting preventive therapy or earlier if there is an acute exacerbation. Subsequent visits may be planned 2–8 weekly depending on the severity or earlier in case of a recurrence.

Group education reassures parents that they are not alone and helps them interact.

Environmental Control

Environmental control is directed to advise avoidance of allergens, irritants, precipitants, drugs and diet. Inhaled allergens, irritants and viral infections are the most important triggers. All patients with asthma should be advised avoidance of triggers and what action has to be taken for that.

Triggers	*Special action to be taken*
Allergen	
• Dust mite antigen	Remove carpets, sun the room, use cotton sheets, no woollen blankets to be used. Mattresses should be periodically dusted and exposed to sunlight. Mattresses and pillows may be encased in plastic covers. Soft toys should be kept away from the sleeping area and washed weekly with hot water.
• Molds and spores	Damp walls and leakages should be attended to. Air conditioners cleaned every month.
• Cockroach antigen	Hygienic measures to limit cockroach population. Insecticide spraying to be done when the child is away.
• Animal dander (pets)	Pets to be avoided. Pets should not be allowed in the sleeping area. Pets should be bathed weekly.
• Pollen (flowers)	Flowering plants should be avoided in indoors. Staying indoors during harvesting/flowering season.
Irritants	
• Smoke (cigarettes, agarbattis, incense sticks, fumes from stoves, crackers, fire places)	Make house free from smoke. Use may be restricted to area where child is not exposed.
• Mosquito repellant mats	Should be avoided. Use of mosquito nets should be encouraged instead.
• Chalk, fine dust, spray	Exposure should be avoided.
• Weather and climats changes, iced drinks, cold bath	Should be avoided.
• Cottage industry at home e.g. carpet weaving, bidi making, flour mill, cow shed/hay stack very near home.	Should be avoided.

Contd.

Contd.

Precipitants	
• Viral infections	a. Short acting β_2 agonist, oral or inhaled should be started at the onset of respiratory symptoms. b. If a child is on a preventer regime of inhaler steroids, dose should be doubled for 5–7 days. c. If the exacerbation is severe or if there is a previous history of severe exacerbation consider rescue steroids.
Drugs	
• Aspirin/NSAIDs,	Total avoidance is necessary only in those children having the triad syndrome –aspirin sensitivity, nasal polyposis/sinusitis and asthma. The triad syndrome is very rare below 8 years of age. Paracetamol is a safe option.
• Propranolol	Has limited indication in children.
Diet	
• Food additives (Sulphites, benzoates, monosodium glutamate, Tartrazine)	Food allergy should be confirmed by avoidance and challenge.
• Eggs, nuts, chocolates, sea foods	Make child aware, list possible foods. Warn about situations with high risk e.g. party and restaurant eating. Educate regarding management of acute episodes.

Other Treatment Modalities

Role of Skin Prick Test and Immunotherapy

The role of skin prick test lies only in detecting the allergic nature of asthma and sometimes in identifying a specific allergen. These tests are not required for diagnosis of asthma.

Immunotherapy is not a method of treatment because of high efficacy of presently available pharmacotherapy. The course of allergen immunotherapy is typically of 3–5 years duration. There is also a danger of life threatening hypersensitivity reaction. However, in severe and poorly controlled cases where only one or two allergen have been identified immunotherapy can be tried as an adjunct to preventer therapy in children above 5 years. However, it is important to have asthma relatively stable when starting immunotherapy because reactions to immunotherapy like bronchoconstriction are more frequent among patients with poorly controlled asthma. It should be tried in a hospital set up with all full resuscitative measures available, by an experienced person.

Immunomodulator Drugs

Methotrexate and gold salts have the best evidence for positive effects. Immunomodulators can reduce the oral systemic steroid dependence. It should be used as an adjunct to preventer therapy and practised in hospital setting by experienced personnel. Indications for use of these drugs are:

1. Poorly controlled asthmatics on optimal preventer therapy with good compliance and elimination of triggers.
2. Poorly controlled asthmatics in whom side effects of oral steroids are not tolerable.

Complementary Medicines

Includes yoga, acupuncture, homeopathy, herbal medicines. No confident data exists till date to support use of these complementary medicines in treatment of asthma.

ACUTE EXACERBATION OF ASTHMA

Acute exacerbations of asthma are episodes characterized by a progressive increase in symptoms of shortness of breath, cough, wheezing or chest tightness and progressive decrease in lung function.

Exacerbations may occur in patients with pre-existing diagnosis of asthma or occasionally as the first presentation of asthma. Exacerbations usually occur in response to exposure to an external agent and/or poor adherence with controller medicine. A subset of patients can present more acutely and without exposure to risk factors. Severe exacerbations can occur even in patients with mild and well controlled asthma.

Asthma exacerbation is often worse between 12 midnight and 8 am when inflammation and hyperresponsiveness in the airways are at the peak.

Risk Factors for Acute Exacerbation

Acute exacerbations usually occur in response to exposure to a trigger. Hence when an asthmatic child reports of a worsening of symptoms the following trigger factors should be considered:

1. An acute viral respiratory infection.
2. Exposure to pollen and pollution.
3. Incorrect inhaler technique and/or poor adherence.
4. Exposure to smoke, change of environment, presence of obesity and eosinophilia.
5. Uncontrolled asthma symptoms having 1 or more severe exacerbations in past 1 year.
6. Low FEV1.

7. High SABA use. Increased mortality is seen if more than one 200 dose canister use per month.
8. Previous history of intubation for asthma.
9. Emotional stress, more often seen in severe or brittle cases.

Identifying Patients at Risk of Asthma Related Death

Some features are specifically associated with an increase in asthma related death. Presence of any one or more of these risk factors should be quickly identified so that they can be encouraged to seek urgent medical care early in the course of an exacerbation. The factors that increase the risk of asthma related death are:

1. A past history of near fatal asthma requiring intubation and mechanical ventilation.
2. Hospitalization or emergency care visit for asthma in the past one year.
3. Currently using or having recently stopped using oral corticosteroid.
4. Not currently using inhaled corticosteroid.
5. Overuse of SABAs, especially use of more than 1 canister (200 doses) of Salbutamol monthly.
6. A history of psychiatric disease or psychosocial problems.
7. Irregular control due to poor adherence with asthma medications and/or poor adherence with (or lack of) a written asthma plan.
8. Food allergy in a patient with asthma.

Assessment of Symptom Control

Assessment of symptom control in the preceding 4 weeks of an acute exacerbation is important because irregular control in a child with preventive therapy can be a trigger (Table 9.7).

Need for Investigations

An acute exacerbation, of any degree, is primarily a clinical diagnosis. Investigations are necessary if (a) the child is unusually ill or if one suspects infection, viz., pneumonia, then a *WBC count, DLC and band cell count* should be ordered to look for polymorphonuclear leucocytosis and band cells. (b) *Estimation of serum electrolytes, viz., potassium* is necessary if there is a history of taking Salbutamol for a long period or in high doses. (c) *A chest X-ray* is indicated when diagnosis is in doubt or if there is suspicion of a foreign body, pneumonia or complications, viz., pneumothorax, atelectasis, pneumo mediastinum.

Management of Acute Exacerbation in Children 5 Years and Younger

Assessment

The updated GINA guidelines (2015) has suggested a simple classification to assess severity of acute exacerbation in children up to 5 years of age as well as management of exacerbations (Table 9.8).

Table 9.7: Assessment of symptom control in preceding 4 weeks (GINA 2014)

Symptom control in the past 4 weeks	*Well controlled*	*Partially controlled*	*Uncontrolled*
1. Daytime asthma symptoms > twice a week 2. Any night waking due to asthma 3. Reliever needed for symptoms > twice a week 4. Any activity limitations due to asthma	None of these present	1–2 of these present	3–4 of these present

Table 9.8 Assessment of acute exacerbation in children 5 years and below

Symptoms	*Mild/Moderate*	*Severe*
Altered consciousness	No	Agitated, confused, drowsy
SaO_2 at presentation	>95%	<92%
Speech	Sentences	Words
Pulse rate	<100 beats/min	>200 beats/min (0 – 3 years) >180/min/min (4 – 5 years)
Central cyanosis	Absent	Likely to be present
Wheeze intensity	Variable	Chest may be quiet

Where to Treat?

A *severe exacerbation* should be started treatment with controlled oxygen, SABA, and systemic steroids and continued while arranging for urgent transfer of the patient to an acute care facility where monitoring and expertise are readily available.

Mild/moderate exacerbations can be treated in a primary care setting depending on resources and expertise.

Management

A. Mild Exacerbation

1. Controlled or titrated oxygen therapy to maintain SaO_2 of 94–98%.
2. Short acting B2 agonist (SABA): Salbutamol inhalation 100 mcg 2 puff with MDI + spacer (above 2 years) spacer + mask (below 2 years age) or 2.5 mg salbutamol by nebulizer every 20 minutes for 1st hour.
3. If good response after 3-4 hours continue SABA intermittently on demand.

If symptoms appear within 3–4 hours:

1. SABA 100 mcg 2–3 puffs every hour till response then intermittently on demand.
2. Prednisolone 2 mg/kg max 20 mg (0–2 years) and max 30 mg (2–5 years).

B. Severe Exacerbation

1. Controlled or titrated oxygen therapy to maintain SaO_2 of 94% to 98%.
2. Salbutamol 100 mcg 6 puffs by MDI + spacer (with or without mask) or 2.5 mg Salbutamol by nebulizer every 20 minutes for 1st hour.
3. Prednisolone 2 mg/kg, max 20 mg (0–2 years) and max 30 mg (2–5 years).

Additional options in the 1st hour in severe exacerbation:

1. Ipratropium bromide 2 puffs (80 mcg) or 250 mcg by nebulizer every 20 minutes for one hour only.
2. $MgSO_4$: Consider isotonic $MgSO_4$ infusion. 25–75 mg/kg, max dose 2.5 gms IV over 20– 60 minutes.

Management of Acute Exacerbation in Children Above 5 Years and Adolescents

Assessment

A brief focussed history and relevant physical examination should be done concurrently with initiation of treatment.

Table 9.9: Assessment of acute exacerbation in children above 5 years and adolescents

Mild/Moderate	*Severe*	*Life threatening*
Talks in phrases	Talks in words	Drowsy, confused or silent chest
Prefers sitting to lying down	Sits hunched forward	
Not agitated	Agitated	
Respiratory rate increased	Respiratory rate >30/min	
Accessory muscles not used	Accessory muscles in use	
Pulse rate 100–120/min	Pulse rate >120/min	
Oxygen saturation (on air) 90–95%	Oxygen saturation (on air) <90%	
PEF >50% predicted or best	PEF =/<50% predicted or best	

Where to Treat?

In *severe or life threatening exacerbation*, treatment with controlled oxygen, SABA, and systemic steroids, as described in primary care, should be started and continued while arranging for urgent transfer of the patient to an acute care facility where monitoring and expertise are readily available.

Mild/moderate exacerbations can be treated in a primary care setting depending on resources and expertise.

Management

A. At Primary Care Level

- Start treatment with Salbutamol 4–10 puffs with MDI + spacer or 2.5 mg Salbutamol by nebulizer. Repeat every 20 minutes for 1 hour + controlled oxygen inhalation with mask with target SaO_2 94–98% + Prednisolone 1–2 mg/kg (maximum dose 40 mg).
- If condition worsens: Transfer to acute care facility. Continue Salbutamol during transport.
- If condition improves: Continue Salbutamol. Assess response after 1 hour and assess for discharge.

B. At Emergency Department

1. Initial assessment: Look for presence of life threatening features.
2. If absent: Start treatment for severe exacerbation as follows:

- Controlled low flow oxygen should be administered by nasal cannula or mask to maintain SaO_2 94–98%.
- Salbutamol inhalation continuously by nebulization till response then intermittently or on demand.

  Systemic corticosteroids (Prednisolone 1–2 mg/kg, max 40 mg): Oral route is as effective as intravenous route. Oral route is preferred because it is quick, less invasive and less expensive. Oral corticosteroids require about 4 hours in producing a clinical improvement. For children a liquid formulation is preferred to tablets.

  Corticosteroids by IV route is indicated when patient is too dyspnoeic to swallow, if patient is vomiting or when patient requires non-invasive ventilation and intubation.

Additional options in the first 1 hour include:

- IM Epinephrine is indicated in addition to standard therapy (Salbutamol + Steroids) for acute exacerbations associated with anaphylaxis and angioedema.
- Ipratropium bromide: 100 microgram every 30 minutes for 3 doses then 6 hourly for 48 hours and stop.
- $MgSO_4$: Consider isotonic $MgSO_4$ infusion. 25–75 mg/kg, max dose 2.5 gms IV over 20–60 minutes.
- Inhaled corticosteroids given in large doses within 1st hour of admission in the emergency room have shown that it reduces the need for admission. However, the agent, dose and duration of treatment still remain unclear.

Table 9.10: Showing drugs used in acute severe exacerbation and doses

- **Salbutamol:** 200 microgram per inhalation as required by MDI + Spacer (for primary care) or 2.5 mg in 3 ml sterile normal saline by oxygen driven nebulization (preferred in hospital setup).
- **Prednisolone:** 1–2 mg/kg (maximum dose 40 mg/day) in 1–2 divided doses.
- **Inj. Hydrocortisone:** 10 mg/kg stat, 5 mg/kg IV 8 hourly.
- **Inj. Epinephrine (1:1000):** 0.01 ml/kg per dose (max 0.5 ml per dose) IM. Repeat the dose after 15 – 20 minutes.
- **Ipratropium:** 100 micrograms every 30 minutes for 3 doses, then 6 hourly for 48 hours and stop.
- **Magnesium sulphate:** 25–75 mg/kg, max dose 2.5 gms IV infusion over 20–60 minutes.

About the Additional Drugs

1. *Ipratropium Bromide:* The results of addition of Ipratropium bromide to Salbutamol are conflicting. Hence not used routinely now. May be used in cases not responding to standard treatment.
2. *IV Magnesium Sulphate* is indicated in children who fail to respond to initial treatment and have persistent hypoxemia and in children in whom FEV_1 fails to reach 60% predicted after 1 hour with inhaled corticosteroids. It is not recommended for routine use.
3. *Helium Oxygen Therapy*: Systemic review studies suggest that there is no role in routine care, but it may be considered for patients who do not respond to standard therapy.
4. *IV Aminophylline and Theophylline*: In view of their poor efficacy and safety profile both these drugs are not used.

Reviewing for Response

- Clinical status and oxygen saturation should be assessed frequently and further treatment should be titrated according to the patient's response.
- Lung function should be measured after 1 hour, i.e., after 3 doses of Salbutamol inhalation.
- Patients who deteriorate after 3 inhalations of Salbutamol and systemic corticosteroids should be evaluated for transfer to ICU.

Measurement of Lung Function

This is strongly recommended without unduly delaying treatment. FEV_1 and PEF should be recorded before treatment is initiated. Spirometry, however, may not be possible in children with acute asthma. PEF can be measured in children above 5 years.

Lung function should be monitored at 1 hour after starting treatment and at intervals until a clear response to treatment has occurred.

Assessment of lung function 1 hour after initial treatment and actions:

(a) FEV_1 / PEF 60–80%: Symptoms improved: Discharge plan.

(b) FEV_1 / PEF < 60% and lack of clinical response: Continue same treatment and reassess frequently.

(c) Signs of life threatening attack: Transfer to ICU.

Monitoring of Oxygen Saturation

Severe airflow obstruction should be treated with administration of supplemental oxygen as the first line therapy. B_2 agonist therapy without oxygen can result in increased pulmonary blood flow through obstructed, unoxygenated areas of the lungs, causing ventilation perfusion mismatch and hypoxemia.

Oxygen saturation should be closely monitored preferably by pulse oximetry. This is especially useful in children if they are unable to perform PEF. In children, oxygen saturation is normally > 95%. A saturation < 92% is a predictor for need for hospitalization. Saturation < 90% signal the need for aggressive therapy. Saturation should be assessed before starting oxygen therapy or 5 minutes after oxygen is removed or when saturation stabilizes.

Arterial blood gas (ABG) measurement should be considered for patients with PEF or FEV1 < 50% of predicted or those who do not respond to initial treatment or are deteriorating. Supplementary oxygen should be continued while blood gases are obtained.

A PaO_2 of < 60 mm Hg and normal or increased $PaCO_2$ (> 45 mm Hg) indicate respiratory failure and transfer to ICU. Fatigue and somnolence suggest that $PaCO_2$ may be increasing and airway intervention may be needed. ABG measurement is routinely not required.

C. Treatment in the ICU

The child admitted into ICU with signs of life threatening features should continue treatment in the line of acute severe asthma with close monitoring and put on mechanical ventilation when indicated.

Indication of ABG Analysis

When oxygen saturation is not maintained at 91% with 100% oxygen in absence of fever, agitation or other condition that increase the demand of oxygen in presence of normal hemoglobin and good cardiac output.

Indications of Mechanical Ventilation

1. Deteriorating respiratory status despite oxygen and nebulization therapy.
2. Anxious, sweaty, lethargic child with deteriorating mental status.
3. Respiratory arrest, recurrent apnea, irregular breathing or excessive work of breathing.
4. PaO_2 =/< 60 mm Hg and/or $PaCO_2$ 50 mm Hg or more despite 100% oxygen. It needs mention that clinical indications are more important for deciding the indication of respiratory support. One should not wait for ABG analysis in presence of clinical indication to start mechanical ventilation.

Mechanical Ventilation in Asthma

Mechanical ventilation in asthma is designed to support oxygenation and assist ventilation until airway obstruction has improved. It needs mention that mechanical ventilation in obstructive airway disease may produce hyper-ventilation, auto-peep and secondary hypotension. Hence careful attention is necessary to balance cycle, inspiratory and expiratory times (I : E ratio). The initial tidal volume (VT) should be 8 to 10 ml/kg and the minute ventilation adjusted to normal pH. The flow rate should be set to an optimal expiratory time (I : E ratio) so as to allow complete exhalation.

In diseases with airway obstruction (e.g., Asthma), longer expiratory time is required. A typical I : E ratio in such cases is 1: 4. PEEP should be avoided.

While the patient is supported with mechanical ventilation, airway obstruction should be aggressively treated. As the airflow obstruction improves, the VT can be increased and time prolonged as the child will tolerate higher VT levels and longer inspiratory times.

Monitoring Course and Response to Therapy

Clinical monitoring: The following parameters should be looked for: mental status, respiratory rate, chest retraction, quality of breath sounds, distal air entry, wheeze, grunting and cardiovascular status.

ABG analysis: It may indicate improving, static or deteriorating gas exchange. Lab parameters which indicate adequate gas exchange are PaO_2 60–80 mm Hg, $PaCO_2$ 50–60 mm Hg, SpO_2 85–90% (in absence of fever, agitation or other condition that increase the demand of oxygen in presence of normal hemoglobin and good cardiac output).

Supportive Treatment

Oxygenation and reversal of airflow obstruction are the

main goals of therapy in acute exacerbation of asthma. Achieving these goals primarily requires bronchodilator drugs and steroids. However, supportive measures are not to be forgotten while the main drugs are instituted.

Position of the child: The child should be in a comfortable position if necessary on the mother's lap.

Oxygen supplementation, sedative and antipyretic: Hypoxia occurs due to ventilation-perfusion mismatch. *Oxygen supplementation* should be the primary therapy in acute severe asthma. Oxygen saturation should be maintained > 91% during salbutamol nebulization.

A *mild sedative* viz. chloral hydrate may be given to quieten the child, if the child cannot be comforted despite comfortable position and oxygen. Sedatives as such should be avoided because they may depress the respiratory drive, suppress the cough reflex and mask the vital signs of deterioration of sensorium.

Antipyretics (Paracetamol 40–50 mg/kg/day 4–6 hourly) should be given when oral temperature is 101° F (axillary) or more.

Intravenous fluid: A child with acute exacerbation may be dehydrated because he/she may not be taking enough fluid orally due to respiratory distress or because of increased insensible loss. Moreover, dehydration leads to viscid secretion and mucus plugs. An attempt should be made to keep the child well hydrated which will make the mucus less viscous. IV fluid should be administered according to the degree of dehydration. The amount of fluid required reduces when the patient is ventilated. SIADH must be anticipated especially if the patient is on positive pressure ventilation. Maintenance fluid should be adjusted to two third of normal requirement.

Antibiotics: Antibiotics are routinely not required as acute exacerbations are triggered mostly by viral infections. However, mycoplasma and bacterial infection may rarely precipitate an acute attack. Antibiotics should be considered if:

- There is strong clinical suspicion of a bacterial infection (pneumonia), i.e., child is toxic, not responding to the bronchodilators.
- There is laboratory evidence of infection, viz., polymorphonuclear leucocytosis, and increased band cells.
- There is radiological evidence of consolidation.

An oral antibiotic like Amoxicillin/Cephalexin in appropriate doses is usually sufficient. IV antibiotics may be used only in those children who are on IV fluids and very sick.

Cough expectorants and mucolytics: Hydration is the best mucolytic agent. Children with acute exacerbation should be encouraged to take plenty of fluids. It makes respiratory secretions less viscid and easy to expectorate.

Expectorants are not necessary because with bronchodilation children above 5 years can expectorate. Children below 5 years age cannot expectorate. Hence expectorants are not useful. *Mucolytics* may dislodge thick secretions and increase airflow obstruction.

Discharge Plan

Assess

- Symptoms improved. Not needing SABA.
- PEF improving and >60–80% of personal best or predicted.
- Oxygen saturation >94% at room air.
- Resources at home adequate.

Arrange

- Reliever (Salbutamol) as and when needed.
- Prednisolone to continue 5–7 days.
- Review compliance, trigger elimination, preventer drug use.
- Initiate or step up controller therapy as needed.
- Check inhaler technique and adherence.
- Provide personalized action plan*.
- Follow up within 2–7 days.

Personalized Action Plan*

1. To start Salbutamol inhalation with MDI + Spacer with or without mask, 2 inhalations every 20 minutes for 3 such.
2. If no response to start first dose of rescue steroid (Prednisolone 1 – 2 mg/kg orally, max dose 40 mg in above 2 years and max dose 30 mg below 2 years age); and
3. Transport child to emergency room. Salbutamol should be continued as and when necessary during transport.

Wheeze Associated Lower Respiratory Infection (WALRI)

WALRI is a common cause of wheezing in the age group between 6 months and 3 years. It is characterized by recurrent episodes of wheeze induced by viral infection. It is associated with fever. There is no history of personal atopy, no family history of asthma / atopy. Response to bronchodilators is variable.

There exists a group of infants who are born with anatomically small airways. This predisposes them to wheeze with viral infection. Each viral infection results in an inflamed hyperactive airway and further narrowing of airway caliber. As these infants grow older, the airways grow in size and the symptoms progressively abate by 3–5 years.

Most of these children respond to bronchodilators (oral or inhalation) and steroid. Parents of children with WALRI can be reassured that the episodes of wheezing will disappear and that they will not be future asthmatics.

Gastroesophageal Reflux Disease (GERD)

Gastroesophageal reflux means the retrograde movement of gastric contents across the lower esophageal sphincter into the esophagus. It is the most common esophageal disorder in children of all ages. Gastroesophageal reflux may be physiological in infants, characterized by regurgitation. It is pathological when the episodes are more frequent or persistent, produce symptoms of esophagitis or respiratory sequelae.

Pathophysiology

Normally the lower esophageal sphincter is supported by the crura of the diaphragm at the gastroesophageal junction and the esophagogastric junction anatomically has a valve like function. They together form the anti-reflux barrier.

A transient lower esophageal sphincter relaxation (TLESR) is the major primary mechanism allowing reflux to occur. Gastric distension is the main stimulus for TLESRs. Whether GERD is caused by a higher frequency of TLESRs or by a greater incidence of reflux during TLESRs is debated. Both are likely in different individuals. Straining during a TLESR makes reflux more likely, as do positions that place the gastroesophageal junction below the air fluid interface in the stomach. Other factors influencing gastric pressure-volume or hyper-osmolar meals and increased respiratory effort (e.g. coughing, wheezing) may have the same effect.

Clinical Manifestations

Reflux in infants commonly manifests as post prandial regurgitation and signs of esophagitis viz. irritability, arching, choking, gagging and feeding aversion. Symptoms resolve spontaneously in the majority by 12–24 months. In the preschool age complain is regurgitation. During later childhood and adolescence complaints of abdominal and chest pain supervene.

The respiratory manifestations are also age dependent. GERD in infants can present as obstructive apnea or with stridor. When complicated with laryngomalacia or bronchopulmonary dysplasia it may present as lower airway disease. In the older children respiratory manifestations are more frequently related to asthma or to sinusitis or laryngitis.

Differential Diagnosis

The important causes to consider in the differential diagnosis of an infant or child presenting with chronic vomiting are milk and other food allergy, pyloric stenosis, intestinal obstruction (malrotation of gut and intermittent volvulus), inborn errors of metabolism, increased intracranial pressure, hydronephrosis and bulimia.

Laboratory Diagnosis

A thorough history and physical examination usually suffice to reach a diagnosis in most cases of GERD.

Investigations like a *barium contrast study* of esophagus and upper gastrointestinal tract is performed in children with vomiting and dysphagia to exclude achalasia, esophageal strictures and stenosis, hiatus hernia and gastric outlet obstruction. *Extended esophageal pH monitoring* of distal esophagus provides a quantitative and sensitive documentation of acidic reflux episodes. However, the most important indications for esophageal pH are to assess efficacy of acid suppression during treatment, and to evaluate atypical GERD presentation like chronic cough, stridor and asthma. *Endoscopy* allows diagnosis of erosive esophagitis and complications like strictures. *Esophageal biopsy* may diagnose histologic reflux esophagitis in the absence of erosions. *Radionucleotide scintigraphy* may demonstrate aspiration and delayed gastric emptying. *Empirical antireflux therapy*, using a time limited trial of high dose proton pump inhibitor, which has been demonstrated as a cost effective strategy for diagnosis in adults, has been applied in older children with good results. However, a formal diagnostic evaluation is indicated in case the child needs a prolonged therapy or fails to respond.

Management

The management of GER includes general measures, pharmacotherapy and surgery as and when indicated.

General Measures

In breast fed/formula fed infants, the thickening of milk feeds with a cereal may result in fewer regurgitation episodes. A short trial of hypoallergenic diet may be tried by exclusion of milk from diet. Older children should be advised to avoid acidic foods like tomatoes, chocolates and beverages. Weight reduction for obese children and elimination of smoke exposure are other measures at all ages.

Positioning measures are particularly important for infants who cannot control their position on their own. During awake periods, prone position and upright carried position have been shown to minimize reflux. In older children, some evidence suggests a benefit to the left side position and head elevation during sleep. The elevation should be done by elevation of the head end of the bed rather than with pillows which will cause abdominal flexion and compression which may worsen reflux.

Pharmacotherapy

Pharmacotherapy is directed at reducing the gastric acidity for which antacids, histamine–2 receptor antagonists, proton pump inhibitors and prokinetic agents have been tried. Antacids are the most commonly used anti-reflux therapy but they provide rapid and transient relief of symptoms. Proton pump inhibitors like omeprazole, lansoprazole, pantoprazole, rabeprazole etc are the most potent antireflux therapy. Dose of omeprazole in children is 0.7–3.3 mg/kg/day. H-2 blockers like ranitidine (1-5 mg/kg/day 6-8 hrly PO/IM), cimetidine, famotidine etc are also beneficial in mild to moderate reflux. Prokinetic agents like metoclopramide have not demonstrated much efficacy for GERD.

Surgery

Surgery viz. fundoplication with or without gastrostomy is an effective therapy for intractable GERD. It is indicated particularly in presence of refractory esophagitis, strictures, and those at risk of significant morbidity from chronic lung disease. Preoperative accuracy of diagnosis of GERD and the skill of the surgeon are two of the most important predictors of successful outcome.

Pneumonia

Pneumonia refers to inflammation of pulmonary parenchyma and is associated with consolidation of the alveolar spaces.

It is a significant cause of mortality in childhood throughout the world, particularly in the developing countries.

Classification

Pneumonia may be classified as simple and complicated pneumonia.

Simple pneumonia can be bronchopneumonia with patchy involvement of the lung which can be unilateral or bilateral and lobar pneumonia which involves almost whole of a single lobe.

Complicated pneumonia refers to a condition where the pulmonary parenchymal infection is complicated by parapneumonic effusion, empyema, necrotising pneumonia, abscess or cavities, pneumothorax or bronchopleural fistula.

Another reasonable epidemiological classification is community acquired pneumonia and hospital acquired/ nosocomial pneumonia.

Community acquired pneumonia (CAP) is an acute infection of the pulmonary parenchyma in a previously healthy child acquired outside of a hospital setting. The patient should not have been hospitalized within 14 days prior to onset of symptoms or has been hospitalized less than 4 days prior to onset of symptoms.

Nosocomial pneumonia may be hospital acquired pneumonia (HAP) or ventilator acquired pneumonia (VAP).

Hospital acquired pneumonia is the pneumonia which is acquired within the hospital environment, that occurs 48 hours or more after admission, which was not incubating at the time of admission.

Ventilator acquired pneumonia refers to pneumonia that occurs more than 48 – 72 hours after endotracheal intubation.

HAP and VAP may be early onset or late onset. Time of onset of pneumonia is an important epidemiologic variable and risk factor for specific pathogen and outcomes.

Early onset HAP and VAP occurring within first 4 days of hospitalisation usually carry a better prognosis and are more likely to be caused by antibiotic sensitive bacteria.

The *late onset* types which occur 5 or more days after hospitalisation are more likely to be caused by multidrug resistant (MDR) pathogens and are associated with high mortality and morbidity.

However, it should be noted that patients with early onset HAP who have received prior antibiotics or who have had prior hospitalisation within the past 90 days have greater risk for colonization and infection with MDR pathogens and should be treated similarly as patients with late onset HAP or VAP.

Etiology

Pneumonia may be caused by a variety of infectious agents (virus, bacteria, parasite, fungus and rickettsia), inflammatory process (SLE, Sarcoidosis and Histiocytosis), and toxic substances that are inhaled and/or aspirated (hydrocarbons, smoke, moulds, dust, chemicals, gases, gastric contents).

The most common cause of pneumonia in children of developed countries is a viral infection; bacterial infection accounting for 10–30% of childhood pneumonias. In contrast, bacteria cause a large proportion of pneumonia in developing countries. A mixed infection due to virus and bacteria is not uncommon.

The common etiological agents causing pneumonia in different age groups are as follows:

Age	*Organisms*
0 – 3 months	Gram negatives Group B Streptococcus Streptococcus pyogenes Chlamydia Viruses (CMV, RSV, Influenza, Parainfluenza)
3 months – 5 years	Streptococcus pneumoniae H. influenzae Viruses (RSV, Adeno, Influenza) Staphylococcus Streptococcus pyogenes Mycoplasma pneumoniae
>5 years	Streptococcus pneumoniae Mycoplasma pneumoniae Chlamydia pneumonia Viruses (Influenza, Varicella) Staphylococcus Streptococcus pyogenes H. influenzae

Causative Organisms in Special Situation

Children with immune system dysfunction, malnutrition or defects in normal defence mechanisms of the lungs are susceptible to pulmonary infections. The causative agents are unusual opportunistic organisms, viz., Pneumocystis carinii, gram negative enteric bacteria, fungi (aspergillosis, histoplasmosis), mycobacterium, anaerobes and viruses (Varicella, measles, CMV).

Nosocomial Infection: The pathogens include gram negatives, viz., Ps. aeruginosa, K. pneumoniae, Acinetobacter and gram positives, viz., coagulase negative S. aureus usually MRSA, Enterobacter and enterococci.

WHO Criteria for Diagnosis of Pneumonia in Children Under 5 Years of Age

A child with cough or difficulty in breathing could be suffering from pneumonia. However, cough or difficulty in breathing may also be caused by common cold, blocked nose, croup, wheeze etc. Therefore, a careful assessment is necessary to exclude pneumonia.

Assessment

Before beginning the assessment, the mother should be asked not to wake up the child, if the child is asleep, and not to undress or disturb the child. It is important to keep the child as calm as possible because a child who is crying and upset may exhibit signs that may confuse with signs of illness.

Ask the mother or caretaker the following questions:

1. How old is the child?
2. Is the child coughing? For how long?
3. Is the child (for child aged 6 months to 5 years) able to drink?
4. Has the young infant (age less than 6 months) stopped feeding well?
5. Has the child had fever? For how long?
6. Has the child had seizures?

Look, Listen

It is important to look and listen to the child to find out whether the child has any one of the danger signs (viz., abnormally sleepy (drowsy) or difficult to awake, not able to drink/stop feeding well, has fever/hypothermia), has difficulty in breathing such as chest indrawing, fast breathing, stridor or wheeze as well as check for signs of severe PEM. It is important to look and listen to the child's breathing only when the child is quiet and calm.

Abnormally Sleepy (Drowsy) or Difficult to Wake

An abnormally sleepy child is drowsy most of the time when the child has to be awake and alert. A child who is difficult to wake may continue to sleep even with the mother's voice or a loud clap. Even a very young infant, who sleeps a lot, should awaken naturally with these disturbances, or when the mother begins to undress the child. In all age groups it is a danger sign and indicates hypoxia, sepsis or meningitis or other infections like malaria.

Not Able to Drink/Stop Feeding Well

A child usually stops taking solid food when ill but continues to take fluids. If a child above 6 months age is not able to drink can have severe pneumonia, sepsis, meningitis, a throat abscess etc. It is a danger sign. Similar conditions can affect a child who is less than 6 months age and stops feeding well, i.e., feeds less than half of the usual amount of breast milk.

Fever/Hypothermia

Fever (38°C or more) is uncommon in the first two months of life and more often indicates a serious bacterial infection than in older children. In addition, fever may be the only sign of a serious bacterial infection. Young infants can also respond to infection with hypothermia.

Counting the Respiratory Rate

Counting the respiratory rate may be done by observation of any part of the child's chest or abdomen. The mother should be asked to lift the child's shirt/frock to view the part. As children grow, the respiratory rate slows down. Therefore, the cut off for fast breathing will depend on the age as follows:

If the child's age is	*Consider fast breathing when the respiratory rate is*
Less than 2 months	60 breaths/min or more
2 months upto 12 months	50 breaths/min or more
12 months upto 5 years	40 breaths/min or more

Methods of Counting the Respiratory Rate

The following three methods are found to be useful:

1. Use a sounding timer that sounds after one minute. Count the child's respiratory rate in one minute.
2. Use a watch with a second hand or a digital watch. Ask another person to tell you when one minute has passed so that you can watch the child's chest. You can also put the watch where you can glance at the second hand while looking at the child's chest to count the breaths.
3. Use a watch with a second hand, or a digital watch. Count to the respiratory cut off for the age of the child. Then look back at the watch to see if this took more than one minute.

In case of a young infant (<2 months age) if the respiratory rate is 60/minute it has to be repeated. If the repeat count is < 60/minute, the young infant does not have fast breathing. If the second count is also 60/minute, the young infant has fast breathing.

A child who is exactly 12 months old would have a fast breathing if the respiratory rate is 40 breaths/minute or more.

The respiratory rate should be counted for 1 minute because in young children the rate is irregular.

Chest Indrawing

In normal breathing, when the child breathes IN, the whole chest wall and the abdomen move OUT. With chest indrawing, when the child breathes IN, the lower chest wall moves IN, while the upper chest wall and abdomen move OUT. So the child is said to have chest indrawing if the lower chest goes in during inspiration.

Chest indrawing is same as subcostal indrawing or retraction. The best place to look for chest indrawing is the upper part of the abdomen and lower part of the chest. A clear groove appears every time the child breathes in. Chest indrawing is only significant if it is present all the time and definitely visible.

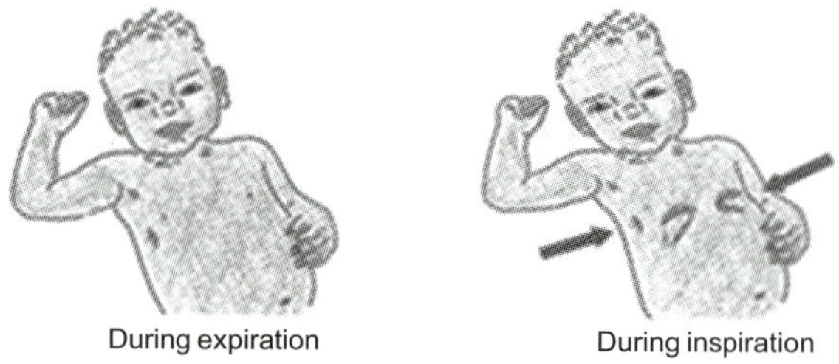

Fig. 9.7. Showing chest indrawing

Stridor

A child who is not very ill will have a stridor only when the child is crying or upset. So one should examine for stridor in a calm child. Sometimes a wet sound may be heard when the nose is blocked. This sound is present in both inspiration and expiration and disappears when the nose is cleared.

Wheeze

If the child has a wheeze, the mother should be asked if there is a past history of such attacks.

Check for PEM

This can be done by clinical examination and anthropometry. Undernutrition is a danger sign in an older child but may not be so in a young infant because 30–40% of our babies are low birth weight.

Classification and Treatment of Childhood Pneumonia at Health Facilities (Revised WHO Guidelines, 2012)

In early 1980's, in view of the high incidence of pneumonia as well as high mortality, pneumonia classification and management guidelines had been developed. In the intervening time, new evidence has emerged which prompted the development of revised guidelines.

The revisions include changing the recommendation for the first-line antibiotic and re-defining the classification of pneumonia severity. The data show that oral amoxicillin is preferable to oral cotrimoxazole for the treatment of "fast breathing pneumonia" and is equivalent to injectable penicillin/ampicillin in cases of "chest indrawing pneumonia". Hence, in a programmatic context, the distinction between previously defined "pneumonia" (fast breathing) and "severe pneumonia" (chest indrawing) loses its significance. The new classification is therefore simplified to include only two categories of pneumonia; "pneumonia" with fast breathing and/or chest indrawing, which requires home therapy with oral amoxicillin, and "severe pneumonia", pneumonia with any general danger sign, which requires referral and injectable therapy.

Revised WHO Classification and Treatment of Childhood Pneumonia (2 Months to 59 Months)

Signs	*Classification*	*Treatment*
Danger signs	Very severe pneumonia/Very severe disease	Urgent referral Hospitalization Antibiotics Supportive treatment
Chest indrawing/ Increased Respiratory rate	Severe pneumonia	Oral antibiotics Supportive treatment
No chest indrawing/ No increased respiratory rate	No pneumonia: Cough and cold	Home care and supportive care

WHO Classification and Treatment of Childhood Pneumonia for the Young Infant (Age Less Than Two Months)

Special Characteristics in the Young Infant

1. The young infant can become sick and die very quickly from serious bacterial infection.
2. Young infants are less likely to cough with pneumonia.
3. Mild chest indrawing is normal in young infant because their chest wall bones are soft. However, in young infants, severe chest indrawing (very deep and easy to see) is abnormal.
4. The *danger signs* in young infants include stopped feeding well, abnormally sleepy/difficult to wake, convulsion, stridor in calm infant, wheeze in calm infant and fever or hypothermia.
5. The fast breathing cut off rate is different and only presence severe chest indrawing is classified as severe pneumonia.
6. Any pneumonia in young infant (0 – 2 months) is considered to be severe. They need hospitalization or referral treatment with parenteral antibiotics. They cannot be treated at home.

On the basis of the assessment the child can be put into one of the three classifications:

Signs	*Classification*	*Treatment*
Danger signs	Very severe pneumonia/severe disease	Urgent referral/ hospitalization Investigations Antibiotics Supportive treatment

Contd.

Contd.

Severe chest indrawing	Severe pneumonia	Hospitalization/urgent referral Oral antibiotics Supportive treatment Follow up
No severe chest indrawing	No pneumonia, cough and cold	Home care Symptomatic treatment

Reassessment After 2 Days

All cases of pneumonia should be assessed 2 days after starting treatment. Depending on the condition of the patient decision can be taken regarding further management.

Condition	*Intervention*
1. Worse: With appearance of danger signs	Hospitalisation/Urgent referral
2. Remaining same	Review antibiotics
3. Improving	Complete antibiotics for 5 days

Treatment

Children (2 – 59 months) with fast breathing pneumonia with no chest indrawing or general danger sign should be treated with oral amoxicillin: at least 40 mg/kg/dose twice daily (80 mg/kg/day) for five days. In areas with low HIV prevalence, amoxicillin can be given for three days. Children with fast-breathing pneumonia who fail on first-line treatment with amoxicillin should have the option of referral to a facility where there is appropriate second-line treatment. The earlier use of cotrimoxazole has been revised by WHO.

Infants (0–2 months) with chest indrawing pneumonia should be treated with oral amoxicillin: at least 40 mg/kg/dose twice daily (80 mg/kg/day) for five days.

Children aged 2–59 months with severe pneumonia should be treated with parenteral ampicillin (or penicillin) and gentamicin as a first-line treatment. — Ampicillin: 50 mg/kg, or benzyl penicillin: 50,000 units per kg IM/IV every 6 hours for at least five days — Gentamicin: 7.5 mg/kg IM/IV once a day for at least five days. Ceftriaxone should be used as a second-line treatment in children with severe pneumonia having failed on the first-line treatment.

VIRAL PNEUMONIA

Viral pneumonia is most commonly caused by respiratory syncytial virus, parainfluenza virus, adenovirus or enterovirus. Less commonly, rhinovirus, influenza and herpes simplex virus have also been recovered from children with pneumonia. The peak attack rate of viral pneumonia is between the ages of 2 and 3 years and decrease slowly thereafter.

Pathogenesis

Viral pneumonia usually results from spread of infection along the airways, accompanied by direct injury of the respiratory epithelium which results in airway obstruction from swelling, abnormal secretions and cellular debris. The small caliber of the airways in young infants makes them particularly susceptible to severe infection. Airway obstruction is often accompanied by atelectasis, interstitial edema and ventilation perfusion mismatch causing hypoxemia. Viral infection of the respiratory tract also can predispose to secondary bacterial infection by disturbing the normal host defense mechanism.

Clinical Features

Most viral pneumonias are preceded by several days of respiratory symptoms, including rhinitis and cough. Often, other family members are also ill. Although cough and fever are prominent features, temperature is generally lower than in bacterial pneumonia. Dyspnea and subcostal retraction may be seen commonly in young children and infants. Physical examination may be surprisingly unrevealing although rales and wheeze are present late in illness. It is sometimes difficult to differentiate viral pneumonia from bacterial pneumonia on clinical grounds.

Laboratory Diagnosis

The *white blood cell count* is usually under 20,000/cumm and lymphocyte is the predominant cell type. The *chest X-ray* shows diffuse, streaky infiltrates of bronchopneumonia especially in perihilar regions. In some cases, transient lobar infiltrates may also be present. Hyperinflation is common. Effusion may occur.

Certain viruses viz. RSV, influenza, parainfluenza, adenovirus may be identified by culture, polymerase chain reaction, or immunofluorescent staining of infected cells washed from the nasopharynx. Cytomegalovirus and enterovirus can be cultured from nasopharynx, urine or bronchoalveolar lavage fluid.

Treatment

There is no specific treatment for viral pneumonia. Many patients are given antibiotics initially if bacterial infection is suspected. Failure to respond to the antibiotic is another evidence for viral etiology. Usually only minimal supportive measures are required, although some patients may require hospitalization for I.V. fluids, oxygen, or even assisted ventilation.

Course and Prognosis

Majority of children with viral pneumonia recover uneventfully and have no sequelae. The course may be prolonged in infants. In addition, infants may develop some complication like bronchiolitis obliterans and unilateral hyperlucent lung. Adenovirus seems to be the most dangerous agent in this regard. It also has been reported to cause a fatal acute fulminant pneumonia. Presence of X-ray changes for 6–12 months is not unusual.

BACTERIAL PNEUMONIA

Etiology

The common nonviral pathogens causing pneumonia in children in developing countries include S. aureus, S. pneumoniae and H. influenzae type B. Other organisms include Gr. A streptococcus, mycoplasma pneumoniae and clamydia pneumoniae.

Children who are immunosuppressed or who have an underlying disease are at risk of specific pathogens e.g. Pseudomonas and Klebsiella pneumoniae. The most common combination of pathogens is streptococcus pneumoniae with either respiratory syncytial virus or mycoplasma.

Pathogens in Pneumonia

Common Pathogens

S. aureus, S. pneumoniae, H. influenzae

Others

Group A streptococci, Mycoplasma pneumoniae, Chlamydia pneumoniae

In immunocompromised/with underlying disease

Pseudomonas, Klebsiella

Combination

S. pneumoniae with RSV or Mycoplasma

Pathogenesis

The lower respiratory tract is normally kept sterile by the physiologic defense mechanism including the mucociliary escalator, the properties of normal secretions viz. secretory IgA and clearing of the airway by coughing. The immunologic mechanisms of the lung that limit invasion by pathogenic organisms include macrophages in the alveoli and bronchioles, and immunoglobins viz. secretory IgA.

The most common event disturbing the defense mechanisms of the lung is a viral infection which alters the properties of normal secretions, inhibits phagocytosis, modifies the bacterial flora, and may temporarily disrupt the epithelial layer of the respiratory passages. A viral respiratory disease usually precedes development of bacterial pneumonia by a few days.

An underlying disorder should be considered if a child experiences recurrent bacterial pneumonia. The defects to consider include cleft palate, congenital bronchiectasis, and tracheoesophageal fistula, congenital heart disease with increased pulmonary blood flow, deficient gag reflex, agammaglobulinemia, or ciliary dyskinesia.

Certain lesions are commonly produced by specific causative agents. For example, S. pneumoniae produces an inflammatory lesion of the mucosa and an alveolar exudate, usually without destruction of mucosal cells or extensive involvement of interstitial tissues. The gross lesion is consolidation of all or part of a lobe in the lobar variety or of scattered lobules in the bronchopneumonic variety. In contrast, viruses and H. influenzae invade or destroy the mucous membrane and may produce principally bronchiolitis, peribronchitis, and interstitial lesion. Both staphylococcus and klebsiella tend to destroy tissue and to produce small abscesses.

STREPTOCOCCUS PNEUMONIAE PNEUMONIA

Streptococcus pneumoniae is the most common bacteria accounting for the majority of cases of pneumonia in children. It is a sporadic disease and occurs in late winter and early spring. The highest attack rates occur during the first 4 years of life. It is uncommon below one year of age. Epidemics may occur in closed communities (e.g. orphanages, schools) following widespread viral respiratory disease.

Pathogenesis

The organisms are probably aspirated into the periphery of the lung from the upper airway or nasopharynx. Initially, there is reactive edema which helps in proliferation of the organisms and spread into adjacent portions of the lung resulting in lobar involvement. The involved lobe undergoes early consolidation, stage of red hepatization characterized by polymorphonuclear leucocytes, fibrin, red blood cells, edema fluid and organisms filling the alveoli. This is followed by the stage of grey hepatization characterized by deposition of fibrin over the pleural surfaces, and the presence of fibrin and polymorphonuclear leucocytes in the alveolar spaces. In the stage of resolution, there is appearance of increasing number of macrophages in the alveolar spaces. The polymorphonuclear leucocytes degenerate, the fibrin threads and remaining bacteria are digested and disappear.

In the untreated cases a clinical crisis occurs about the 7th day of illness, and resolution and reexpansion require 1–3 weeks. If antibiotics are given in the first few days of illness, the course is interrupted and the characteristic stages are not seen.

Usually one or more lobes or part of lobes are involved. Infants may have a more patchy and diffuse disease that follows a bronchial distribution. Permanent injury is rare.

Clinical Manifestations

The clinical manifestations differ in infants and older children.

Infants

A mild upper respiratory illness for several days precedes the onset of pneumonia which is characterized by abrupt onset of fever of 39°C or higher, restlessness, apprehension and respiratory distress. Cough is unusual initially but may be noted later. The child appears ill with moderate to severe air hunger and often cyanosis. Respiratory distress is manifested by tachypnoea, subcostal, intercostal and supraclavicular retraction, flaring of alae nasi, grunting and tachycardia.

There may be dullness on the affected side. Stony dullness on percussion indicates presence of pleural effusion or empyema. Auscultation of the chest may reveal diminished breath sound and fine crackling rales on the affected side. Breath sounds may be exaggerated and bronchial.

In addition, there may be abdominal distension reflecting gastric distension due to swallowed air or to paralytic ileus. It may suggest an acute surgical emergency. The liver may be palpable due to downward displacement of the right diaphragm or superimposed congestive heart failure. Nuchal rigidity without meningeal infection (meningismus) may be present especially with involvement of right upper lobe.

Children and Adolescents

In children and adolescents, the symptoms and signs are similar to those in adults. After a brief, mild upper respiratory infection there is often onset of shaking chill followed by fever as high as 40.5°C. This is accompanied by drowsiness with intermittent periods of restlessness, rapid respiration, a dry, hacking, unproductive cough and occasionally delirium. There may be circum oral cyanosis. Many children lie on the affected side with knees drawn up to the chest, to splint the affected side to minimize pleuritic pain and improve ventilation.

The findings on physical examination include signs of respiratory distress. The abnormal findings on examination of the chest depend on the stage of pneumonia. In the early stages, diminished breath sounds, scattered crackles and rhonchi are commonly heard on the affected side. By 2nd–3rd day of illness, the classical signs of consolidation appear and are characterized by restriction of movement on the affected side, trachea in normal position, increased vocal fremitus, dullness on percussion, bronchial breath sounds and increase vocal resonance and disappearance of rales and rhonchi. As resolution starts, moist rales are heard and signs of consolidation disappear. The initial dry, hacking cough loosens and becomes productive of large amounts of blood tinged mucous material.

If there is associated pleural effusion or empyema, there are restricted movements on the affected side and exaggerated excursion on the normal side. Examination reveals dullness, diminished vocal fremitus and breath sounds. Bronchial breath sound is often heard above the fluid level and on the unaffected side.

Laboratory Diagnosis

The *white cell count* is usually elevated to 15,000 to 40,000 / mm^3, with preponderance of polymorphonuclear cells. White blood cell counts below 5000/mm^3 are often associated with a grave prognosis. The hemoglobin level is usually normal or only slightly low. Arterial blood samples usually show hypoxemia without hypercapnia.

The definitive diagnosis of pneumonia requires identification of the causative organism which can be obtained by the following methods:

Culture of lung aspirates provides the most reliable method of a bacterial diagnosis in children. Sputum is not easily obtained in children. Blood culture is useful but the yield is much less than those with lung aspirate culture. Bacterial agents can be identified by antigen detection from blood or pleural fluid by countercurrent immunoelectrophoresis.

Invasive procedures such as bronchoscopy and bronchoalveolar lavage, lung aspiration or lung biopsy may be necessary to obtain culture specimens. These invasive procedures are to be employed in special instances like pneumonia in immunocompromised host or when the clinical picture is unusual.

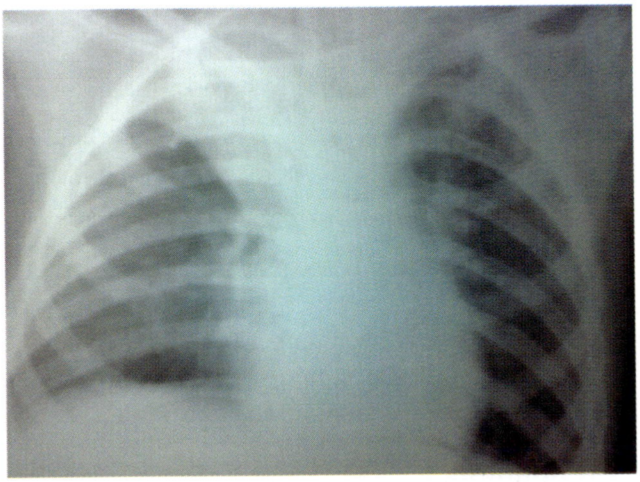

Fig. 9.8: X-ray showing consolidation collapse right upper lobe

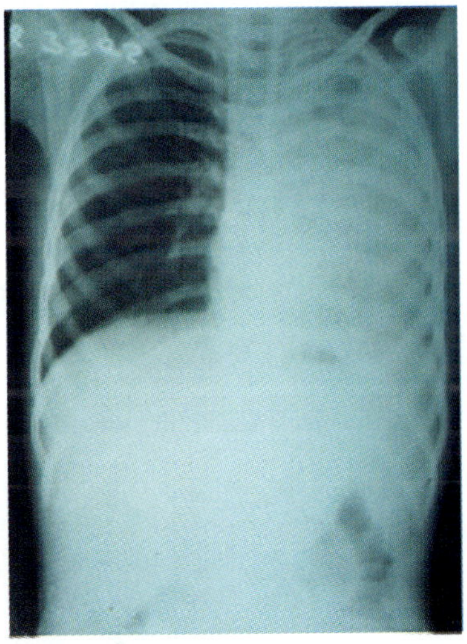

Fig. 9.9: X-ray showing consolidation left lung

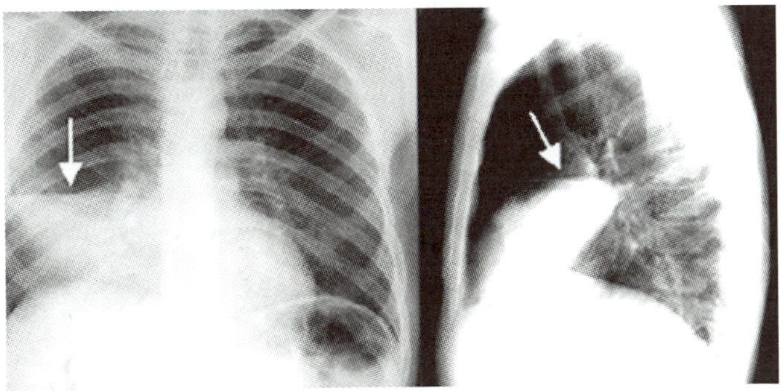

Fig. 9.10: X-ray showing consolidation of middle lobe right lung

The *X-ray changes* of consolidation (non-homogenous opacity with trachea in normal position) may be demonstrated before it is detectable by physical examination and resolution of the infiltrate may not be complete until several weeks after the child is clinically well. Lobar consolidation is a common finding in older children. In infants it is more of patchy and diffuse distribution. Pleural reaction with presence of fluid may be seen early in the disease but does not necessarily indicate empyema. Persistence of infiltrate beyond 3–4 weeks after disappearance of all symptoms suggests an underlying process like foreign body or immunologic deficiency.

Complications

Empyema and lung abscess can occur but is uncommon. It occurs most commonly in the young infant who has received medical attention late in the course of illness or who has been inadequately treated. Persistent pneumatoceles may occur which usually do not require treatment.

Treatment

Treatment consists of antibiotic therapy, drainage of collected pus and symptomatic treatment.

The drug of choice is penicillin as S. pneumoniae is still sensitive to penicillin. In infants and young children, initial therapy should be parenteral penicillin G in a dose of 50,000 units/kg/day. In older children, a single intramuscular injection of procaine penicillin, 600,000 units, followed by oral penicillin V, 50,000 units/kg/day is usually adequate outpatient treatment. The treatment should be given for 7–10 days in uncomplicated cases. In case of penicillin resistant S. pneumoniae, high doses of amoxicillin (80–90 mg/kg/day) should be prescribed. Other alternatives are amoxyclav (40–80 mg/kg/day or cefotaxime (200 mg/kg/day). The duration of treatment is 7–14 days.

STAPHYLOCOCCAL PNEUMONIA

Pneumonia caused by staphylococcus aureus is a rapidly progressive infection which, unless recognized early and treated appropriately, is associated with a high mortality and prolonged morbidity.

Staphylococcus aureus is commonly found on the normal skin and mucous membrane, but serious disease is comparatively rare. Nearly 90% of normal infants become nasal carriers in the neonatal period. This declines to around 20% during the first two years of life and then rises to adult rate of 30–50% by 4–6 years of age. Like other bacterial pneumonias, it occurs in late winter and early spring. It is frequently preceded by a viral upper respiratory infection, which may play a significant role in promoting dissemination of the staphylococcus among infants and in converting colonization to disease. It may occur at any age, 70% cases are however seen below one year age.

Pathogenesis

Staphylococcal infection of the lung parenchyma cause confluent bronchopneumonia which is often unilateral or prominent on one side than the other. It is characterized by presence of extensive areas of hemorrhagic necrosis and irregular areas of cavitation. The pleural surface is covered by a thick layer of fibrinopurulent exudates. Multiple abscesses occur. Rupture of a small sub pleural abscess may result in pyopneumothorax, which in turn may erode into a bronchus producing a bronchopleural fistula.

Clinical Manifestations

The child is usually below one year of age. There is often a history of staphylococcal skin infection in the child or in a family member. There is also a history of an upper or lower respiratory tract infection for several days to one week after which abruptly the child has high fever, cough and respiratory distress in the form of tachypnoea, subcostal indrawing, grunt, nasal flaring, cyanosis. The infant gradually becomes lethargic but becomes irritable upon arousal and appears toxic. Some infants have associated gastrointestinal disturbances like vomiting, anorexia, diarrhoea and abdominal distension secondary to paralytic ileus. A rapid progression of symptoms is characteristic of staphylococcal pneumonia.

The physical findings depend on the stage of pneumonia. In the early stages breath sounds are diminished with scattered rales and rhonchi over the affected lung. With the development of effusion, empyema and pyopneumothorax, there is diminished movement and dullness on percussion on the affected side as well as diminished breath sounds and vocal resonance. Physical findings may, however be misleading, particularly in the young infant with findings disproportionate to the degree of tachypnoea.

Laboratory Diagnosis

Blood Examination

In the young infant, the *white blood cell count* may remain within normal range. In the older infant and the child there is leucocytosis of 20,000/mm^3 or more with polymorphonuclear leucocytosis. A count less than 5000/mm^3 is a poor prognostic sign. Mild to moderate anemia is common. *Blood culture* may be positive. However, finding of staphylococcus in the nasopharynx is of no diagnostic value.

Pleural Fluid Examination

Pleural fluid examination reveals an exudate with a protein level above 2.5 gm/dl, a sugar level low relative to the blood level. The polymorphonuclear cell counts ranges from 300–100,000/mm^3. Gram stain frequently reveals gram positive cocci in clumps and culture is often positive.

X-ray Studies

Early in the illness, there is evidence of non-specific bronchopneumonia. The infiltrate soon become patchy or become dense and homogenous and involve an entire lobe or the hemithorax. The right lung alone is involved in around 60% cases. Bilateral involvement is seen in less than 20% of patients. In most patients, a pleural effusion and a pyopneumothorax will be noted during the course

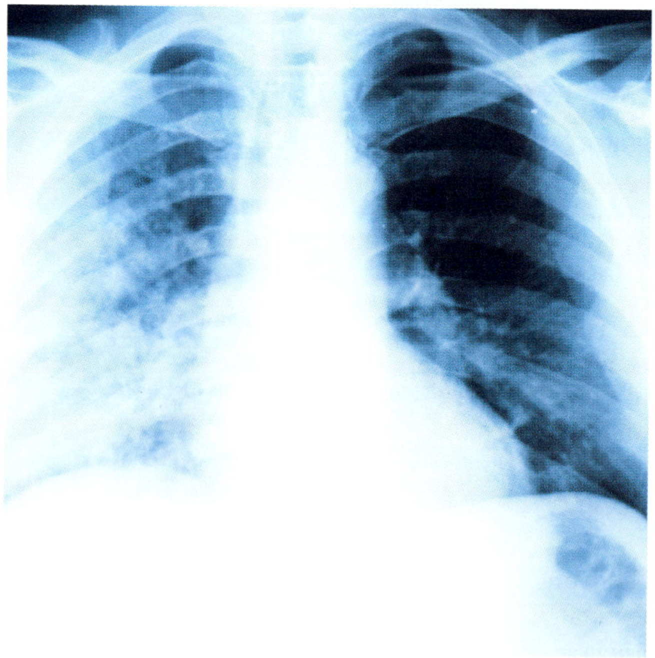

Fig. 8.11: X-ray showing early changes of staph pneumonia

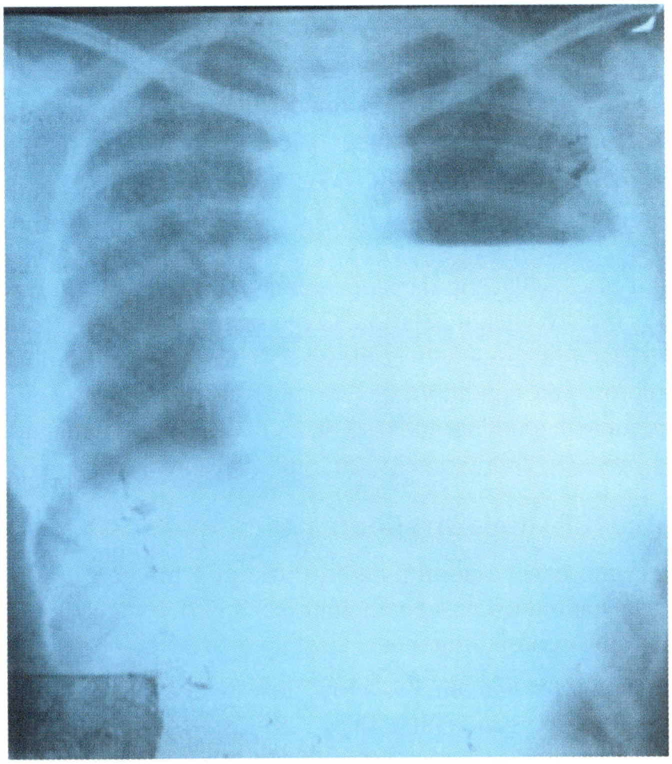

Fig. 8.12: X-ray showing pyopneumothorax

of illness. Pneumatoceles of varying sizes are a common finding.

The X-ray findings are not diagnostic. However, progression over a few hours from bronchopneumonia to effusion with or without pneumatoceles is highly suggestive of staphylococcal pneumonia. Hence chest X-rays should be obtained in frequent intervals if early staphylococcal pneumonia is suspected. Clinical improvement usually precedes radiological clearing by days or weeks. Pneumatoceles may persist in an asymptomatic patient for months.

Complications

Septic lesions outside the respiratory tract viz. pericarditis, meningitis, osteomyelitis and multiple metastatic abscesses in soft tissue can occur in young infant. Metastatic infection after the initiation of appropriate antibiotic therapy is rare.

Course and Prognosis

The course of disease is usually prolonged with hospitalization of 6–10 weeks. The resolution of the process is slow and little improvement may occur for as long as 2 weeks. The antibiotic course should be for 3–4 weeks. With adequate therapy, prognosis is excellent for complete recovery with normal pulmonary function.

It is advisable that all infants with staphylococcal pneumonia should be screened for immunodeficiency state and tested for cystic fibrosis if indicated.

Treatment

Therapy consists of administration of appropriate antibiotics and drainage of collection of pus along with symptomatic treatment.

The effective antibiotics include a combination of cloxacillin (200 mg/kg/day IV/IM 6 hourly for 3–4 weeks) and gentamycin (5 mg/kg/day IV/IM 8 hourly for 10 days), amoxyclav (40–80 mg/kg/day IV/IM 8 hourly initially then per oral for a total of 3–4 weeks) and vancomycin (60 mg/kg/day 6 hourly IV infusion for 10 days). The child can be started on cloxacillin + gentamycin or amoxyclav as the initial therapy. The antibiotic can be changed if necessary after obtaining the culture report. If the response is inadequate or the pus is putrid smelling, anaerobic coverage should be added. Vancomycin is indicated in cases of pneumonia caused by methicillin resistant staph aureus infection or in cases where there is no response to the usual antibiotics.

Although patients with staphylococcal pneumonia may occasionally recover completely without chest tube drainage, it is recommended even if only a small amount of pleural effusion or empyema is present in order to reduce the chance of bronchopleural fistula and the necessity for repeated pleural taps. The tube should be removed once the child begins to improve and drainage is less than 30–50 ml fluid/day.

HEMOPHILUS INFLUENZAE PNEUMONIA

Hemophilus influenzae type B infection is still an important cause of pneumonia in developing countries. In developed countries, routine use of effective vaccine has led to a significant decline of H. influenzae infections. Like other pneumonias, H. influenzae pneumonia is common during late winter and early spring. Males are affected slightly more than females. It is common in preschool children but can occur in older children also.

Pathogenesis

H. influenzae pneumonia is usually lobar in distribution with occasionally 2 or more lobes affected. However, disseminated disease has also been described. The involved areas show a polymorphonuclear or lymphocytic inflammatory reaction with extensive destruction of the epithelium of the smaller airways, interstitial inflammation, and marked edema which is often hemorrhagic.

Clinical Manifestations

It may be difficult to distinguish clinically from pneumonia due to S. pneumoniae. It is more often insidious in onset. Onset is preceded by a nasopharyngeal infection. The child is febrile, has a dry cough and signs of respiratory distress. The child may be already suffering from acute suppurative otitis media and receiving treatment. On physical examination there may be localized dullness to percussion and rales and bronchial breath sounds. Empyema is common especially in the young infant.

Laboratory Diagnosis

There is usually moderate *leucocytosis* with a relative lymphopenia. *Blood culture* is particularly helpful for diagnosis in the small infants.

Examination of pleural fluid as in case of S. pneumoniae pneumonia is helpful in diagnosis. Gram stain and culture will show the organisms. Lung aspirate or bronchoscopic washings can also be examined. Early diagnosis can be possible by counterimmunoelectrophoresis on tracheal secretions, blood, urine or pleural fluid.

X-ray findings are similar to S. pneumoniae pneumonia.

Complications

Complications are frequent, particularly in young infants and include bacteremia, pericarditis, cellulitis, empyema, meningitis and pyoarthrosis.

Treatment

Treatment consists of administration of antibiotics, drainage of collection of pus and symptomatic treatment. The effective antibiotics include chloramphenicol (100 mg/kg/day, 6 hourly IV/IM initially then per oral), ampicillin 200 mg/kg/day 6 hourly IV/IM initially followed by per oral), amoxyclav (40–80 mg/kg/day 8 hourly IV/IM initially then per oral), ceftriaxone 100 mg/kg 12 hourly IV. The duration of treatment is 10–14 days.

SYMPTOMATIC AND SUPPORTIVE TREATMENT IN PNEUMONIA

The specific therapy for pneumonia has been described with the individual pneumonias because the antibiotics necessary differ for different organisms. The symptomatic and supportive treatment however is same. It is equally important as the specific therapy.

Oxygen Therapy

It is an important supportive treatment in pneumonia. All cases however do not require oxygen therapy. Young infants with pneumonia have a higher risk of apnea and respiratory failure if they are not given oxygen when it is required.

Indications

All cases with central cyanosis and inability to drink must be given oxygen inhalation. Oxygen inhalation may also be given in cases with restlessness (if oxygen inhalation improves the condition), severe subcostal retraction, young infant with grunting, and respiratory rate 70 breaths / minute or more (in children between 2 months and 5 years).

Mode of Administration

Oxygen can be administered through a oxygen mask, nasal cannula, a nasal catheter (size 8 FG), oxygen hood and non-rebreathing mask.

A *simple oxygen mask* is a low flow device that delivers 35–60% oxygen with a flow rate of 6–10 L/min. The maximum oxygen concentration is approximately 60% because inspiratory entrainment of room air occurs between the mask and the face and through exhalation ports in the side of the mask. A minimum oxygen flow rate of 6 L / minute must be used to maintain an increased inspired oxygen concentration and prevent rebreathing of exhaled carbon dioxide.

A *partial rebreathing mask* consists of a simple mask with a reservoir bag. It reliably provides an inspired oxygen concentration of 50–60%. Rebreathing of exhaled carbon dioxide from the mask is prevented if the oxygen flow rate into the bag is consistently maintained above the patient's minute ventilation. An oxygen flow of 10–12 litres is generally required.

A *non-breathing mask* consists of a face mask and a reservoir with the following additions: (a) a valve incorporated into one or both exhalation ports to prevent entrainment of room air during inspiration; and (b) a valve placed between the reservoir bag and the mask to prevent flow of exhaled gas into the reservoir. An inspired oxygen concentration of 95% can be achieved with an oxygen flow rate of 10–15 litres / minute and the use of a well sealed mask. The oxygen flow into the mask is adjusted to prevent collapse of the bag.

A *venturi-type mask* is a high flow system designed to reliably and predictably provide controlled, low to moderate (25% to 60%) inspired oxygen concentrations.

A *nasal cannula* is a low-flow oxygen delivery device suitable for infants and children who require only low levels of supplemental oxygen. While administering oxygen through the nasal cannula, the nasal prongs should be cut off and the holes positioned directly under the nose and cannula taped to the cheek bones. The child's nose should be kept clean and free of mucus. This can be done by

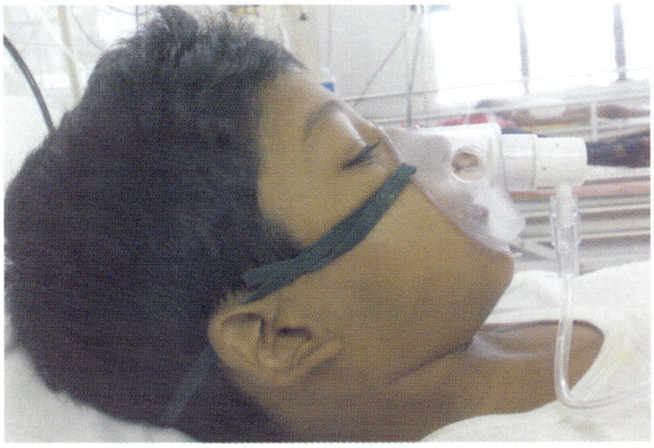

Fig. 9.13: By simple oxygen mask

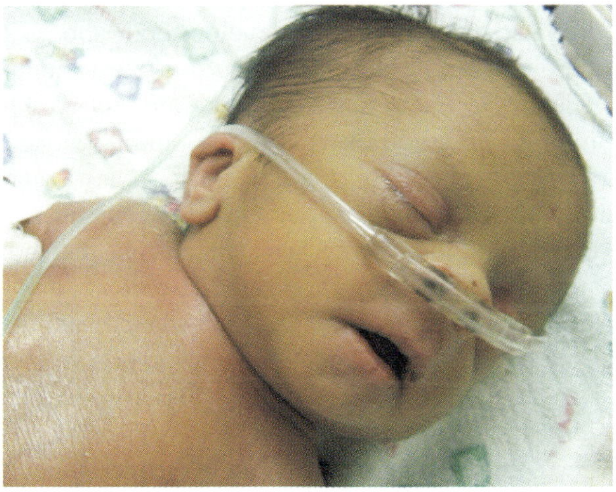

Fig. 9.14: By nasal cannula

Methods of administration of oxygen

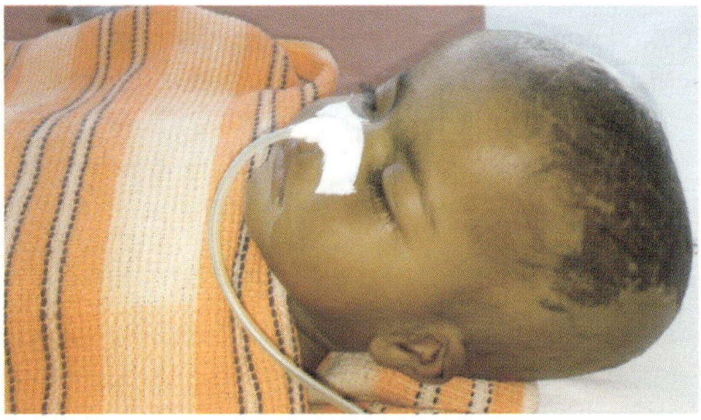

Fig. 9.15: By nasal catheter

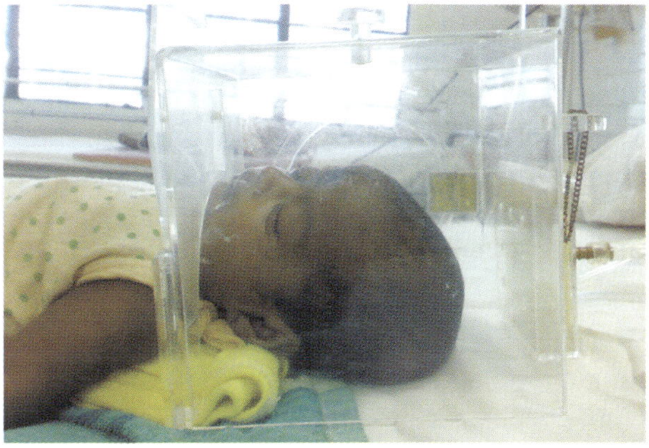

Fig. 9.16: Oxygen hood

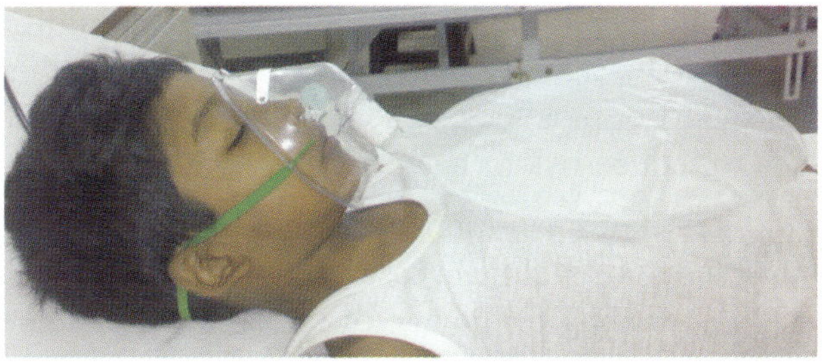

Fig. 9.17: By non-rebreathing mask

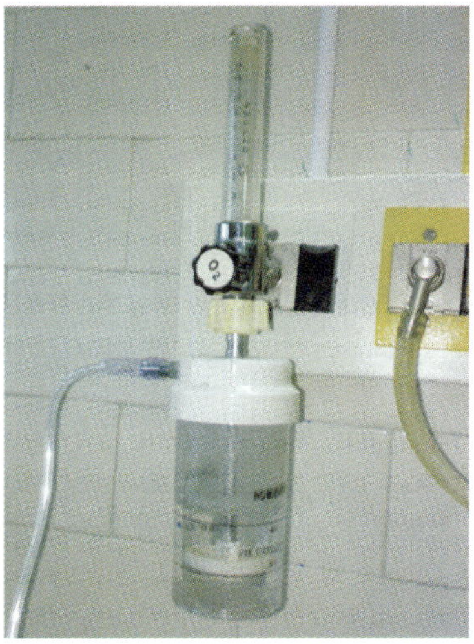

Fig. 9.18: Oxygen flow meter

placing 2–3 drops normal saline in each nostril and clearing the nose with a wick of soft cloth. If necessary, the nose can be suctioned before feeding and sleeping.

If oxygen is administered by a *nasal catheter*, the 8 FG catheter is inserted in one nostril to the depth equal to the distance from the side of the nose (alae nasi) to the front of the ear (tragus). If a nasogastric tube is required for feeding, it should be inserted through the same nostril. The other nostril should be kept clear of mucus. The catheter should be daily removed and cleaned.

An oxygen hood is a clear plastic hood that encompasses the patient's head. It requires a high flow of oxygen (10–15L/minute or more). It can deliver a higher concentration of inspired oxygen than the nasal catheter or cannula. An inspired oxygen concentration of 80 to 90% can be achieved. However, a hood is too small to use in children older than 1 year age.

A *flow meter* should be used to adjust the oxygen flow. If a flow meter is not available the oxygen flow through the cannula should be adjusted so that it can just be felt on your cheek. Nasal catheters should not be used without flow meters. Humidification of the oxygen is not necessary when oxygen is administered through the nasal cannula but desirable with the catheter. The humidifier water should be changed daily. The container, the tubing and the catheter must be cleaned and dried atleast twice a week to reduce risk of bacterial contamination.

For oxygen administration by nasal catheter or nasal cannula, the oxygen flow in case of pneumonia should be adjusted according to the age of the child as indicated below:

Age	*Litres per minute*
Under 2 months	0.5 litre/minute
2 months and older	1.0 litre/minute 2.0 litres/minute may be needed when using cannula

Treatment of Fever

A moderate elevation of body temperature may improve body defenses against infection. A high fever, however, increases oxygen consumption, interferes with feeding and may cause febrile convulsion. The most effective way for reduction of temperature is administration of paracetamol. Paracetamol should be given when the axillary temperature is 39°C (102°F) in a dose of 10–15 mg/kg/dose. The antipyretic should be given every 6 hours and every 4 hours when the child has a past history of febrile convulsion. Sponging with tepid or cold water should be discouraged because it increases oxygen consumption and carbon dioxide production, which may precipitate respiratory failure in a child with pneumonia.

Treatment of Wheeze

Wheeze may be an associated feature in pneumonia. It should be treated with bronchodilator as in cases of asthma according to the degree of airflow obstruction. The bronchodilator of choice is salbutamol. It may be administered orally, by MDI with spacer or by nebulization according to necessity.

Food and Fluids

Food

Children with acute respiratory infection are anorexic especially when fever is present. Children with severe pneumonia may have difficulty in eating because of fast breathing or difficulty in breathing. The child should be encouraged to take small frequent energy dense food. Breastfeeding should be continued. If the child is ill to suck the breast, breast milk should be expressed and given by cup or nasogastric tube. Feeding should be avoided if the child is very ill because it may cause aspiration. These children should be administered intravenous fluid.

Fluids

There is increased fluid loss during acute respiratory infections especially when there is fast breathing and fever. The fluid loss in such situations consists mainly of water. Therefore to replace fluid in absence of diarrhoea, feeding of breast milk, clean water, and home available fluids is sufficient.

Children with pneumonia can develop septic shock. It is also important to note that children with severe pneumonia may secrete an inappropriately large amount of ADH and are at risk of fluid overload and pulmonary edema. Therefore, when the child is not in shock, intravenous fluid should be avoided. In children with pneumonia who are dehydrated, but do not have concurrent diarrhoea, the rate of fluid administration should be slower and the sodium content of the fluid lower than when dehydration is caused by diarrhoea. Once dehydration is corrected a fluid regimen of 70% of the normal maintenance requirement should be advised. In children with concurrent diarrhoea, fluid management should be as recommended for acute diarrhoea.

Secretions

Many infants do not normally breathe through the mouth. A blocked nose may cause respiratory distress and some difficulty in breastfeeding. Nose can be cleared with normal saline drops if it is blocked with dry mucus. Secretions in the nose can be cleared by gentle suction with a plastic syringe or a bulb syringe.

Maintenance of Thermal Environment

Heat and cold stress both can increase a child's oxygen consumption two to three-fold, increase carbon dioxide production and precipitate respiratory failure. A neutral thermal environment minimizes oxygen consumption.

It is important not to over heat or chill a child who has pneumonia. The child should be nursed lightly clothed, in a warm room with a temperature around 25°C. The thermo-neutral environment is especially important for the neonate.

AN APPROACH TO SLOW RESOLVING PNEUMONIA

Typically, patients with uncomplicated community acquired pneumonia respond to therapy with clinical improvement (i.e. improvement of fever, cough, dyspnea and chest pain) within 48–96 hours of initiation of antibiotics. Therefore changes in empirical antibiotic therapy should be delayed for 2–4 days unless the condition of the patient worsens. Radiological evidence of improvement generally occurs within 4–6 weeks but the time to complete resolution varies depending on the etiologic organism. For example pneumococcal pneumonia often requires 1–3 months, staphylococcal pneumonia and enteric gram negative may require 3–6 months for complete radiological resolution. Viral pneumonia may have positive radiographic findings for many months. On the other hand, mycoplasma pneumonia tends to clear more rapidly with radiological improvement occurring within 2 weeks to 2 months.

Slowly resolving pneumonia refers to persistence of symptoms or radiographic abnormalities beyond the expected time course.

The factors to be considered in a case of slowing resolving pneumonia include the following:

1. *Inadequate therapy:* due to inappropriate antibiotic choice, inappropriate dose or poor compliance are common causes of slow or lack of improvement.
2. Development of *resistant strains* of organisms.
3. *Impaired host resistance*: Immunodeficiency, ciliary dyskinesia, or other coexisting diseases.
4. *Foreign bodies, pulmonary sequestration, post infectious bronchiectasis and cystic adenomatoid malformation.*
5. *Nonbacterial causes:* Virus, fungus, parasites and mycobacterium).
6. *Noninfectious causes:* Bronchiolitis obliterans, eosinophilic pneumonia, and aspiration and Wegener granulomatosis.
7. *Obstructing endobronchial lesions:* Congenital and acquired.

Evaluation

1. A thorough history should be obtained to confirm adequacy of treatment.
2. Identify the offending organism with the help of the following investigations: Blood, sputum, pleural fluid, bronchoalveolar lavage, or lung biopsy for gram stain, culture and sensitivity as and when necessary. If these do not provide an explanation then.
3. Chest CT scans (thin cut and /or high resolution) flexible fiberoptic bronchoscopy, lung biopsy and serologic testing like anti-neutrophil cytoplasmic antibodies (ANCA) for Wegener granulomatosis may be helpful.

Pleurisy

Pleurisy is an inflammatory condition of the pleura. It is usually divided into three types: dry or plastic pleurisy, serofibrinous pleurisy and purulent pleurisy or empyema.

DRY PLEURISY

Etiology

It is a condition characterized by inflammation of the pleura. Dry pleurisy may be commonly associated with acute bacterial pneumonia, pulmonary tuberculosis and rheumatic fever.

Pathology

There is deposition of small amounts of yellow serous fluid over the visceral pleura and adhesions may occur between the pleural surfaces. Occasionally, fibrin deposition and adhesion may be severe enough to produce a fibrothorax and markedly inhibit the excursions of the lung.

Clinical Manifestations

The principal symptom is pain in the chest which is aggravated by deep breathing, coughing and straining. Pain with breathing is responsible for grunting and guarding of respiration. The child often lies on the affected side to decrease the respiratory movements. Occasionally, the pain is described as a dull ache over the chest and referred to the shoulder or the back.

On examination a leathery, rough, to and fro friction rub may be audible. The rub usually disappears rapidly. Occasionally, there may be dullness on percussion and diminished breath sounds if the layer of exudate is thick.

Pleurisy may be asymptomatic and detected only on X-ray which shows a diffuse haziness at the pleural surface or a dense, sharply demarcated shadow.

Differential Diagnosis

Dry pleurisy must be distinguished from pleurodynia, fracture rib, herpes zoster, gallbladder disease, dorsal root ganglia lesions.

Treatment

Therapy includes treatment of cause and some symptomatic measures like cough suppressants and drugs to relieve pain. Immobilization of chest may be sometimes necessary for relief of pain.

PLEURAL EFFUSION

Pleural effusion may result from serofibrinous pleurisy and empyema.

Serofibrinous Pleurisy

Serofibrinous pleurisy is characterized by accumulation of fluid in the pleural space. It is usually preceded by dry pleurisy.

Etiology

It is usually associated with inflammatory lesions of the lung, abdomen and mediastinum. It is also found with connective tissue disorders like lupus erythematosus, polyarteritis nodosa and rheumatic fever. Occasionally it is seen in primary or metastatic neoplasm of pleura or mediastinum where it is associated with hemorrhagic pleural fluid.

Clinical Manifestations

The early symptoms and signs are those of dry pleurisy. As fluid accumulates, pleuritic pain disappears. If the fluid accumulation is very small, the child may become asymptomatic or may have the symptoms of the underlying disease. On the other hand, if the accumulation is large, there may be cough, dyspnea, retractions, tachypnoea, orthopnoea and cyanosis. The physical findings are those of pleural effusion and depend on the amount of effusion.

Investigations

Investigations are required to determine the cause such as physical, chemical and microscopic examination of the pleural fluid. Special investigations include pleural fluid for LDH (acute bacterial), ADA (tuberculosis), and malignant cells (malignant disease of pleura or mediastinum) and ANA when connective tissue disorders are suspected.

Treatment

Treatment consists of mainly treatment of cause. Massive effusion may require therapeutic thoracocentesis.

PURULENT PLEURISY (EMPYEMA)

Purulent pleurisy or empyema is characterized by presence of pus or microorganisms in the pleural fluid. The microorganisms may be seen on smear examination or on culture. In absence of microorganism the diagnosis of empyema is made with the following findings on examination of pleural fluid: pH <7.0, LDH $>$ 1000 IU/L, Glucose $<$ 40 mg/dl or lactate $>$ 45 mg/ml.

Empyema is called *simple* when pleural fluid is frank pus, free flowing with a single locule and *complex* when it is frank pus and multiloculated.

Etiology

It is most commonly associated with staphylococcal pneumonia and less frequently with S. pneumoniae, H. influenzae pneumonia and streptococcus pyogenes. It may also be produced by rupture of a lung abscess into the pleural space, introduction of infection from trauma and thoracic surgery or sometimes by mediastinitis or extension of intra-abdominal abscess.

Frank tuberculous empyema may occur rarely in about 2% cases of tubercular pleurisy. It represents a chronic active infection of the pleural space that contains large number of tubercle bacilli. Rare organisms causing empyema include E. coli, pseudomonas and klebsiella. Anaerobes and enterobacter are common in mixed infection. Anaerobes are common after 6 years of age.

Pathology

Purulent pleurisy is a process which results in formation of series of loculated areas involving a large portion of one or both pleural spaces. There is thickening of the parietal pleura. If the pus is not drained, it may dissect through the pleura into the lung parenchyma producing bronchopleural fistula and pyopneumothorax or into the abdominal cavity. The pus may dissect through the chest wall. This condition is called empyema necessitans. Pockets of loculated pus may eventually develop into thick walled abscess cavities or as the exudate organizes, the lung may collapse and become surrounded by a thick, elastic envelope which is called 'peel'.

Three stages have been described in the formation of empyema thoracis: exudative, fibrinopurulent and organizing.

The *exudative stage* is an immediate response with outpouring of thin fluid with low cellular content. The pleura and lung are mobile. The pleural fluid pH, glucose and LDH are normal. Gram stain and culture are negative for microorganism. This stage usually lasts for 1–3 days.

The *fibrinopurulent stage* is characterized by accumulation of large amount of pus in the pleural cavity posteriorly and laterally. The fluid thickens and there is formation of loculations and the lungs become progressively less expandable. The pleural fluid pH is <7.0, glucose <40 mg/dl and LDH > 1000 IU/ L. Gram stain and culture is positive for micro organism. This stage usually lasts for 4–14 days.

The *organizing stage* which occurs after 14 days is characterized by growth of fibroblast into the exudate on both the visceral as well as the parietal pleura producing the membranous peel. With increasing fibrosis, the lung is entrapped and unable to expand leading to the stage of chronic empyema. Early intervention can prevent such chronic disease.

Clinical Manifestations

Empyema is most frequently encountered in infants and preschool children. The initial symptoms and signs are primarily those of bacterial pneumonia followed by respiratory distress. The older child is more ill with greater respiratory distress than the infant. Patients who are treated for pneumonia inadequately or with inappropriate antibiotics may have an interval of few days between the clinical pneumonic phase and development of empyema.

Empyema should be suspected in a child with pneumonia when there is no response to appropriate dose of antibiotics after 48 hours and in a child with coexisting staphylococcal infection of the skin (boils, infected scabies), arthritis etc.

The physical examination findings include fullness of the intercostal spaces with restriction of chest movement on the affected side. The trachea/mediastinum are shifted away from the affected side, chest expansion is restricted and vocal fremitus is diminished. The percussion note is dull to stony dull. On auscultation, the breath sounds and vocal resonance are diminished in intensity. These signs may shift with the position of the patient. However, with loculated effusion, there is no shifting of the signs. The above mentioned physical signs depend on the amount of effusion.

In infants, the findings are non-specific and may present with features of sepsis such as lethargy, poor feeding, irritability and rapid breathing.

Laboratory Diagnosis

X-ray PA View Chest

It is the primary investigation of patients with pleural disease. In a PA view chest, small effusions may cause obliteration only of the costophrenic or cardiophrenic angles or a widening of the interlobar septa. A large effusion shows a homogenous density obliterating the normal markings of the underlying lung. The trachea and mediastinum are shifted to the opposite side. The costophrenic and cardiophrenic angles are obliterated.

The PA view chest film should be taken with the patient in the supine and upright positions to demonstrate a shift of the effusion with a change in position. Finding no shift of fluid with change of position indicates a loculated empyema. A PA view chest can also show an encysted pleural effusion. A lateral decubitus X-ray film can give an idea of the amount of fluid in the pleural cavity. A

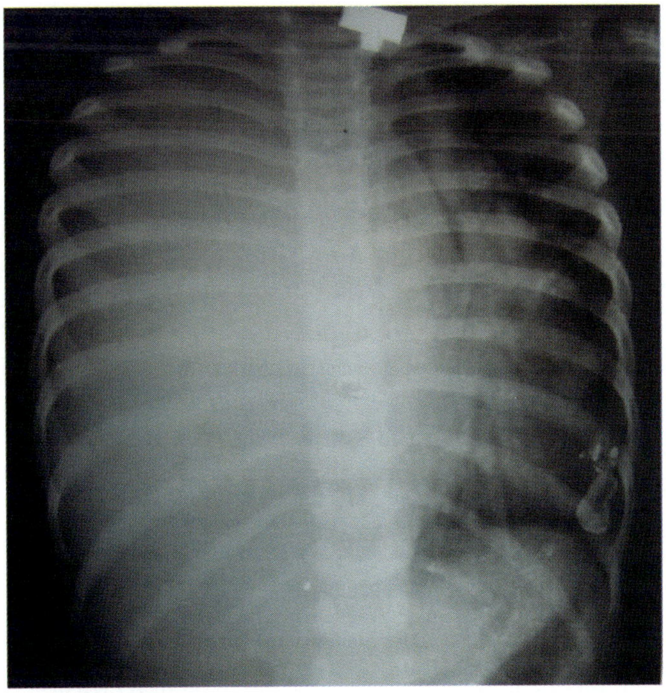

Fig. 9.19: X-ray showing massive pleural effusion

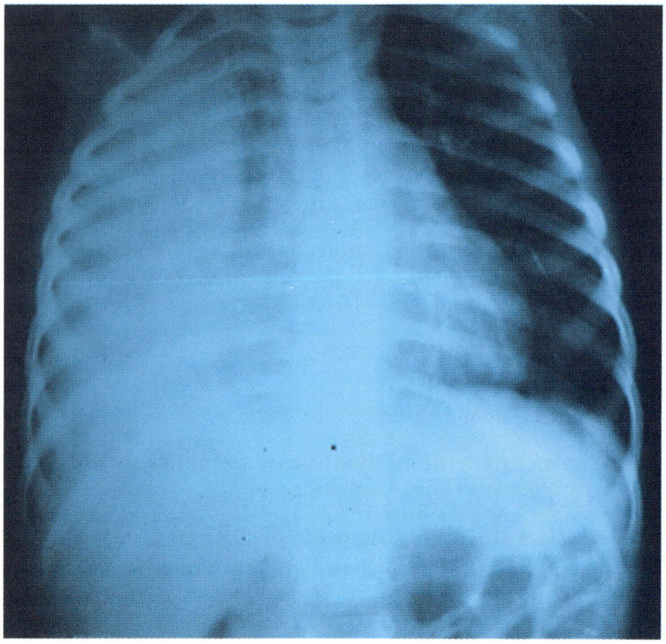

Fig. 9.20: X-ray showing encysted pleural effusion

fluid thickness of more than 10 mm on a lateral decubitus film indicates need for chest tube drainage.

Ultrasonography of Chest

Ultrasonography can differentiate between pneumonia and empyema in an opacified chest better than a plain X- ray. It gives information regarding the size of effusion, presence of adhesions and loculations and echogenecity of the pleural fluid. Transudates are usually anechoic, whereas exudates are usually echoic (rarely anechoic). It also helps in ultrasound guided thoracocentesis and chest tube insertion.

CT Scan

A CT scan shows the "split pleura sign" of empyema which is characterized by interposed empyema fluid between the visceral and parietal pleura. It helps in differe-ntiating empyema from lung abscess and consolidation. A calcified ring surrounding loculated pleural fluid is characteristic of tuberculous empyema. However, CT scan should not be advised routinely as most information regarding diagnosis and treatment decisions can be obtained by X-ray and ultrasonography. It should be avoided in view of exposure of the child to high dose of radiation.

Thoracocentesis and Examination of Pleural Fluid

Thoracocentesis should be done when pleural effusion is present or suspected except when effusion is very small and the patient has classic findings of lobar pneumonia. Thoracocentesis can differentiate serofibrinous pleurisy and empyema, hydrothorax, hemothorax and chylothorax. Examination of pleural fluid will differentiate whether the fluid is an exudate or transudate.

The serofibrinous fluid is clear or cloudy and that of empyema is purulent. The exudative pleural fluid is indicated by a pH less than 7.2, protein levels greater than 3 gm/dl, lactic dehydrogenase (LDH) values higher than 200 IU/L. Complicated parapneumonic effusion is characterized by pH less than 7.1, glucose less than 40 mg/dl, proteins more than 3 gm/dl and LDH more than 1000 IU/L.

Cytological examination may reveal large numbers of leucocytes and some red blood cells. A gram stain and culture of the fluid should be done for the presence of microorganism. The rate of isolating an organism varies from 8% to 76%. Overall rate of culture positivity is decreasing because of widespread use of antibiotics.

Blood Examination

Leucocytosis with increase in polymorph count is characteristic of acute bacterial infection. A raised ESR may indicate acute bacterial infection. A blood culture has a high yield.

Treatment

All children with empyema need admission to hospital. Therapy is basically of the underlying condition and drainage of fluid when indicated. Small parapneumonic effusions may respond to antibiotic therapy alone. Symptomatic effusions need drainage. Assessment of the fluid level in a lateral decubitus film of the chest can determine the type of treatment.

With an empyema of thickness < 10 mm on lateral decubitus film, administration of antibiotics is sufficient.

With a thickness > 10 mm, antibiotics should be started and thoracocentesis and fluid analysis should be done. If the fluid is frank pus, biochemical parameters indicate pleural fluid pH < 7.1, glucose < 40 mg/dl, LDH > 1000 IU/L, gram stain and culture positive, an ultrasonography of the chest should be ordered to look for loculations.

If there are no loculations, treatment will consist of antibiotics and tube thoracostomy. If multiple loculations are found (2 or more loculations without communication), in addition to antibiotics and tube thoracostomy, fibrinolytics may be used.

If there is no response or if there is a thick peel the child shall need decortication in addition to antibiotics.

Closed drainage is usually continued for about a week and removed when the amount of fluid draining is less than 30 to 50 ml/day.

Antibiotic Therapy

The empirical antibiotic therapy should take into account the likely prevalent organism. The first line empirical antibiotics suggested are combination of Cloxacillin and Gentamycin or Ceftriaxone/Cefotaxime and Co-Amoxyclav alone. It can be changed later on the basis of culture and sensitivity report. Anaerobic coverage with metronidazole or clindamycin is indicated when pus is putrid smelling, if multiple loculations are revealed or when response is inadequate.

It should be noted that children continue to be febrile for 7 days after starting therapy in cases of S. pneumoniae and H. influenzae infection and for 10–14 days in staphylococcal infection. The response to therapy is indicated by general well-being, decrease in fever, decrease in drain volume, normal WBC count, normal CRP, clearing in chest X-ray.

In case of non-response after 96 hours of antibiotic therapy which is indicated by high spiking fever and persistent drainage, second line treatment should be instituted. The second line empirical antibiotics suggested are a combination of vancomycin and ceftazidine (150 mg/kg/day).

Parenteral therapy should be continued till the child is afebrile or atleast till the chest tube is removed. Subsequently oral antibiotic therapy should be continued until the patient is afebrile, WBC count is normal, tube thoracostomy yield is less than 30–50 ml/day and radiography shows considerable clearing. It may take 3–4 weeks depending on the organism.

Fibrinolytics

Streptokinase (2.5 lakh units) or urokinase (50,000 to 1 lakh units) in 100 ml normal saline is to be instilled through the chest tube and clamped for 3 hours. It is recommended in multiloculated empyema with thick fluid. It increases the drainage and shortens hospital stay. The treatment however is expensive and has side effects which can be serious.

Supportive Therapy

1. Oxygen inhalation should be started when the SaO_2 is less than 92%.
2. IV fluids when the child has severe dehydration or is unable to drink.
3. Adequate analgesia should be given especially when the child has a chest tube. It aids mobilization and prevents scoliosis.
4. Antipyretics such as paracetamol (10–15 mg/kg/dose) should be judiciously used in presence of fever.
5. Physiotherapy should be started once toxemia has subsided. It consists of breathing exercises in the form of balloon blowing, flute playing to increase breathing efficiency.
6. Food rich in protein and calories should be given as frequent feeds in small amounts.

Table 9.11: Guide to antimicrobial therapy against the common organisms

Infecting organism	*Drug, dosage*	*Duration*
Staphylococci	Cloxacillin 200 mg /kg/day 6 hourly IV/IM	3 – 4 weeks
	+ Gentamycin 5 mg/kg/day IV/IM	10 days
	Amoxyclav 40 – 80 mg/kg/day IV/IM initially then orally	3 – 4 weeks
	Vancomycin 60 mg/kg/day 6 hourly IV infusion	10 days
H. influenzae	Amoxyclav 40 – 80 mg/kg/day IV initially then orally	7 – 14 days
	Ceftriaxone 100 mg/kg/day IV 8 – 12 hourly	7 – 14 days
	Cefotaxime 200 mg/kg/day 8 hourly IV/IM	7 – 14 days
S. pneumoniae	Penicillin G 1 lakh – 4 lakh units/kg/day 6 hourly	7 – 14 days
Anaerobes	Metronidazole 15–35 mg/kg/day 8 hourly	6 – 12 weeks
	Clindamycin 40 mg/kg/day 6 – 8 hourly	6 – 12 weeks

Indications of Surgical Treatment

Surgical management is indicated in cases with persistent sepsis, not responding to medical therapy, and large collection beyond 10 days. The other indications are chronic empyema with symptomatic child who will need decortication (multiloculation and peel formation) and those with a bronchopleural fistula.

Pneumothorax

Pneumothorax, an uncommon condition during childhood, is accumulation of air in the pleural cavity.

Etiology

Pneumothorax often results from leakage of air from within the lung. Air leaks can be primary which is not associated with trauma or an underlying lung disease or secondary which arises as a complication of an underlying lung disorder but without trauma.

Pneumothorax can be spontaneous, traumatic, and iatrogenic. It can be closed, open or tension pneumothorax. A pneumothorax is said to be closed when it is airtight or open when there is free communication with the bronchial tree (bronchopleural fistula). A tension pneumothorax may develop when a valve mechanism allows air to enter the pleural space during inspiration especially during the inspiratory phase of coughing, and prevents escape of air during expiration. This causes progressive and often rapid shift of the mediastinum to the normal side, which impedes ventilation not only on the affected side but of the contralateral lung and may obstruct the venous return to heart and thus eventually compromising cardiac output.

Primary spontaneous pneumothorax with or without exertion (valsalva) occasionally is seen in teenager males who are tall and thin. Children with Ehlers-Danlos disease and Marfan syndrome are prone to develop pneumothorax. Secondary spontaneous pneumothorax can occur in pneumonia with empyema, pulmonary abscess, infarct, and gangrene, rupture of a lung cyst or emphysematous bleb. It can occur with foreign body, lymphoma or other malignancies. It is a serious complication of cystic fibrosis.

Leakage of air into the pleural space can result from external chest or blunt trauma and penetrating injury which can tear a bronchus or abdominal viscus.

Iatrogenic pneumothorax can occur as a complication of tracheotomy, subclavian line placement, thoracocentesis, and transbronchial biopsy.

Pneumothorax may be associated with serous effusion (hydropneumothorax) or purulent effusion (pyopneumothorax).

Clinical Manifestations

The clinical presentation depends on the extent of collapse of the lung and the pre existing lung disease.

Symptoms: In spontaneous pneumothorax due to rupture of an apical bleb, there is sudden pleuritic chest pain and breathlessness. The pain is short lived for a few hours only.

Serious and distressing breathlessness may often develop if spontaneous pneumothorax is superimposed upon acute severe asthma.

Severe breathlessness is also a feature of tension pneumothorax. It is accompanied by cyanosis, tachycardia, hypotension and cold extremities. The jugular veins are distended and there is a marked shift of the trachea and mediastinum away from the affected side. If this condition is not immediately relieved, cardiorespiratory failure may rapidly cause death. Mild to moderate pneumothorax may cause little or no displacement of the intrathoracic organs and few or no symptoms.

Physical Signs: On inspection, the affected side is fixed and hyperinflated. On palpation, there is restriction of chest movement on the side of the lesion and deviation of trachea away from the affected side. Percussion reveals tympanitic note. On auscultation, breath sounds are diminished in intensity or absent. The coin test is positive.

When fluid is present, there is usually a sharply limited area of tympanitic note above a level of dullness. An open bronchopleural fistula is suggested by presence of amphoric breathing, gurgling sounds synchronous with respiration and presence of fluid. The presence of air and fluid is indicated by presence of a splash in addition to signs of pleural effusion.

It is important to make a rapid diagnosis of tension pneumothorax because of its life threatening effects. A shift of mediastinal structure may not occur in case of bilateral pneumothorax and when both lungs are stiff. In such situations, a diagnosis of tension pneumothorax is made only on the basis of evidence of circulatory compromise or the evidence of an audible "hiss" of rapid exit of air under pressure with the insertion of the thoracostomy tube.

X-Ray Studies: The chest radiograph shows a clear zone without lung markings separating the lung margin from the chest wall. This is more clearly seen on expiration. A small pneumothorax may only be seen on an expiratory film. With large collection of air, the underlying lung collapses down to a small opacity adjacent to the hilum and the mediastinum tends to shift to the normal side especially when there is tension pneumothorax (Fig. 9.21). Presence of bullae is indicated by line shadows within the lung. Presence of fluid is indicated by an airfluid level (Fig. 9.22).

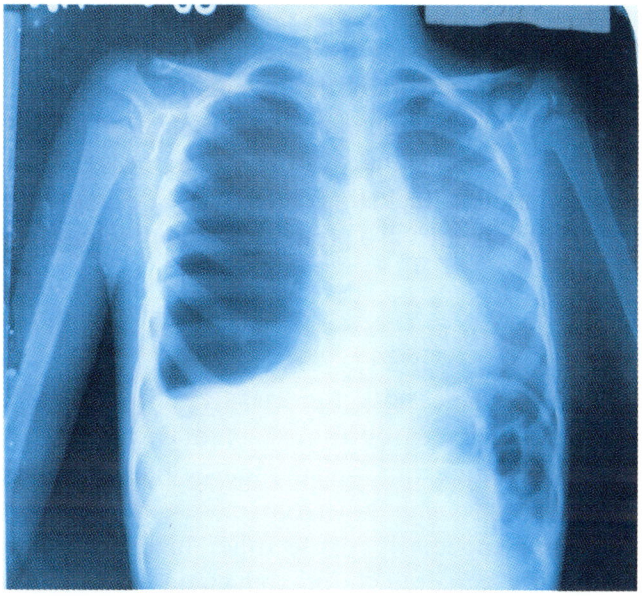

Fig: 9.21: X-ray showing tension pneumothorax (right)

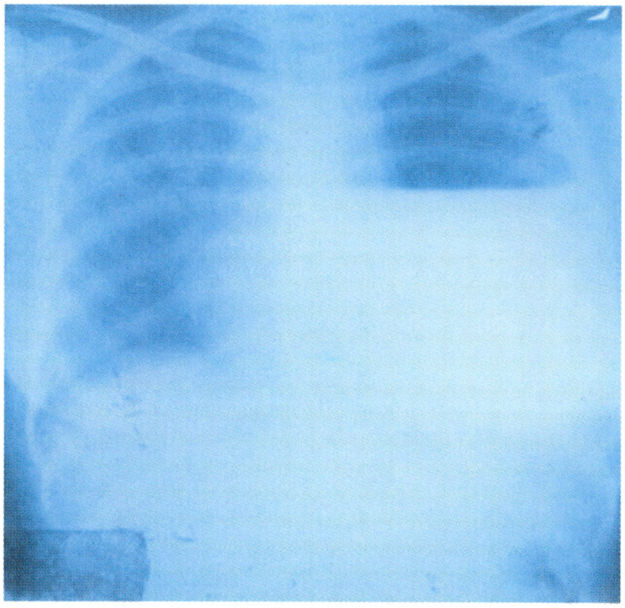

Fig. 9.22: X-ray showing open pneumothorax (left)

Treatment

Small pneumothorax in which the lung remains more than 70% inflated does not require active treatment. These patients should be kept under observation and examined regularly. The lung usually reexpands over 2–4 weeks. With considerable deflation of lung and persistent symptoms, an intercostal tube should be inserted in the axilla and attached to an under water seal. The lung usually expands rapidly within 12–24 hours. The tube should be then clamped and if a radiograph shows that the lung remained re-expanded, the tube should be removed. Thoracotomy is indicated if the lungs fail to re-inflate. A tension pneumothorax demands immediate insertion of any needle or tube, if possible connected to under water drainage. This should be replaced as soon as possible by an intercostal catheter.

Treatment of the underlying pulmonary disease should continue simultaneously. Some cases may develop recurrent or chronic pneumothorax. The treatment of choice in such cases is pleurectomy. Chemical methods like instillation of silver nitrate; tetracycline or talc into the pleural space is often unsuccessful in preventing recurrent pneumothorax.

Course and Prognosis

In 70–80% of spontaneous pneumothorax, there is rapid absorption and no recurrence. The prognosis in chronic pneumothorax is guarded, especially when it complicates chronic respiratory disease. Tension and bilateral pneumothoraces, on occasions may prove rapidly fatal, but if the condition is recognized and dealt with immediately the prognosis is good.

Atelectasis

Atelectasis or collapse is a condition in which the volume of the lung is diminished due to failure of, or reduction in, aeration. Atelectasis may be of two types: congenital and acquired.

Congenital Atelectasis

Congenital atelectasis is said to exist when the fetal lung fails to inflate at birth and remains totally or partially airless. Example is hyaline membrane disease.

Acquired Atelectasis

Acquired atelectasis results from complete obstruction of intake of air into the alveolar sacs. The obstruction should persist sufficiently long to permit absorption of alveolar air into the blood.

Acquired atelectasis is of two types: relaxation/compression collapse and absorption collapse. In the former external pressure directly acts on the lung parenchyma resulting in expulsion of air from the lung by elastic retraction. In the latter, there is external compression or intraluminal bronchial or bronchiolar obstruction resulting in absorption of air from the lung parenchyma distal to the obstruction.

Causes of external compression causing relaxation collapse are pleural effusion, pneumothorax, intrathoracic tumours and diaphragmatic hernia.

External compression of a bronchus completely obstructing entry of air can be caused by enlarged lymph glands, tumours and cardiac enlargement. The right middle lobe is especially likely to become atelectatic because of extrinsic pressure from the lymph nodes that encircle its bronchus. Segmental and subsegmental collapse is prevented by collateral ventilation through alveolar pores and communications between terminal bronchioles and adjacent alveoli. Such communications are limited by connective tissue septa which are more frequent in the middle lobe and the lingula segment of left upper lobe. These segments are therefore more liable to collapse. Intermittent middle lobe collapse occurs in association with acute exacerbation of asthma. Tuberculous glands are another cause of middle lobe collapse.

Complete internal obstruction of a bronchus may be produced by a foreign body, granulomatous tissue, neoplasm or by secretions. Obstruction of one or more bronchioles may be produced by the above mentioned causes. Widespread bronchiolar obstruction is produced by bronchiolitis, asthma and interstitial pneumonia. In these conditions, as the disease progress, bronchioles may become completely obstructed resulting in interspersed areas of atelectasis and emphysema. In pneumonia, varying degrees of shrinkage of lung parenchyma accompanies consolidation without necessarily any bronchial occlusion.

Clinical Manifestations

Symptoms: The symptoms depend on the mode of onset and the extent of atelectasis. A gradual onset atelectasis may be asymptomatic. If, however, underlying function is impaired or parts of lung larger than segments suddenly collapse then breathlessness may be a feature. There may be transient cyanosis. Recurrent hemoptysis from the damaged branches of the middle lobe bronchus may be a presenting feature of middle lobe collapse.

Massive collapse of lung is usually sudden in onset. There is pain in the lower thorax behind the sternum, severe dyspnea, cyanosis and restlessness.

Signs: Signs of atelectasis of segments and lobules may be difficult to elicit. If a lobe is involved and is adjacent to the surface, there may be shift of the mediastinum towards the abnormal side with bronchial breath sounds.

Signs of massive collapse include tachypnoea, tachycardia. The affected side is immobile, the trachea and mediastinum is displaced towards the affected side and there is dullness to percussion. Breath sounds are either diminished in intensity or there is bronchial breathing, bronchophony and whispering pectoriloquy.

A radiograph of the chest establishes the diagnosis. A posterior anterior view (PAV) of the chest shows a homogenous shadow of the atelectatic lungs. The other signs like displacement of the fissures, elevation of the diaphragm and deviation of the trachea and heart towards the side of the collapse are also helpful. If the atelectasis persist after the bronchial occlusion has been removed, an air bronchogram will be seen within the abnormal lung shadow.

Complications

Atelectasis, especially the massive type, may be complicated by infection. Atelectatic areas are susceptible to infection because mucociliary clearance is impaired and cough is ineffective. Respiratory failure may occur especially if the other lung is already functionally impaired. In an atelectatic lung there is bronchial dilatation beyond the obstruction due to

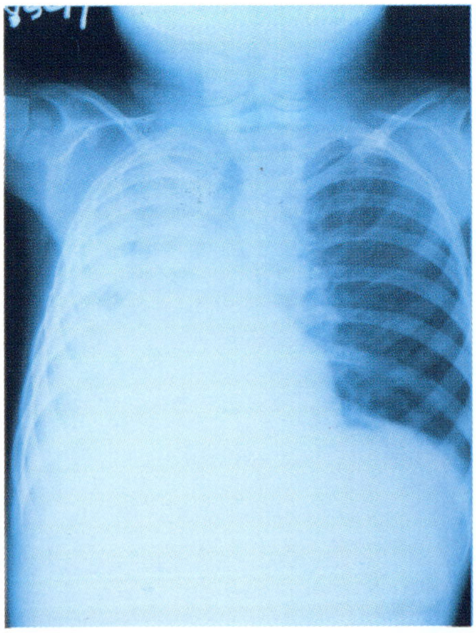

Fig. 9.23: X-ray showing absorption collapse (right) (Trachea deviated to the right, heart shifted to the right, a nonhomogenous opacity on the right side)

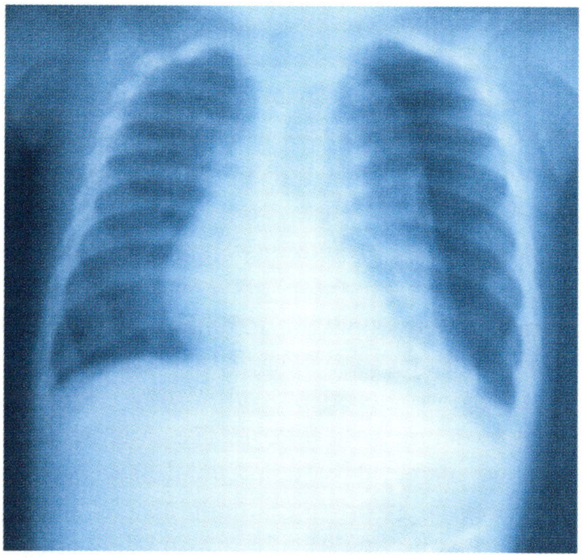

Fig. 9.24: X-ray showing compression collapse (left) (Trachea and heart shifted to right side. Collapse lung margin is seen on the left side with clear zone without lung markings)

distension with mucus. If the obstruction is relieved bronchial caliber may be restored to normal. If unrelieved or if infection develops then permanent bronchiectasis can occur even if the obstruction is relieved later. Pulmonary abscess is occasionally a complication.

Treatment

Therapy will depend on the cause of atelectasis. Hence priority should be given for diagnosis. A bronchoscopic examination is indicated immediately when foreign body or any other bronchial obstruction is suspected to be the cause. It is also indicated when an isolated area of atelectasis persists for several weeks. If no anatomic abnormality is detected and no material obtained by suctioning, a saline wash is taken for culture and cytological examination.

Postural drainage and deep breathing is beneficial. Antibiotics are indicated when there is infection. In cases with asthma bronchodilators and steroids may accelerate atelectasis clearance. Respiratory failure, if present, should be treated in the usual lines.

A lobectomy is indicated if chronic infection poses a threat to the remainder part of the lung, bronchiectasis is demonstrated radiologically, or by systemic symptoms like persistent anorexia or fatigue. Occasionally, the atelectatic part becomes fibrosed. In such cases no further treatment is required.

Acute Respiratory Failure

Respiratory distress is a primary diagnosis in nearly 50% of admissions in pediatric intensive care unit and a common cause of cardiopulmonary arrest in children.

Definition

In general terms, acute respiratory (ARF) failure is defined as inability of the respiratory system to fulfil the exchange needs of the body resulting in hypoxemia and/ or hypercapnia. Using lab parameters, ARF is diagnosed when PaO_2 <60 mm Hg with FiO_2>0.6 and/or $PaCO_2$>50 mm Hg.

From management point of view, one must rely on the pathophysiological definition rather than laboratory parameters, because (i) Lab studies are time consuming and can delay initiation of treatment; (ii) Underlying conditions like congenital cyanotic heart diseases and chronic lung diseases can alter blood gases without intrinsic respiratory impairment; (iii) If the child is breathing increased inspired O_2 concentrations, lab parameters may be normal even in presence of substantial derangement of gas exchange.

Classification

Acute respiratory failure may be classified as follows:

Type I or oxygen failure or hypoxemic respiratory failure with low PaO_2 with normal or low $PaCO_2$.

Type II or ventilation failure or acute hypercarbic failure with low PaO_2 with elevated $PaCO_2$.

Pathophysiology

Four basic derangements viz. hypoventilation, diffusion defect, intrapulmonary shunting and ventilation perfusion mismatch can result in respiratory failure.

Hypoventilation may occur due to mechanical, neuromuscular or central control dysfunction. Increasing FiO_2 helps in such cases. *Diffusion Defect,* a relatively unimportant cause in children, is associated with thickening of alveolocapillary membrane such as in interstitial fibrosis, pulmonary alveolar proteinosis *Intrapulmonary shunting* where alveoli are perfused but not ventilated. Mixed venous blood goes to systemic arterial circulation without coming in contact with oxygen. Increasing cardiac output helps in such cases. *Ventilation perfusion mismatch* where there is increase in dead space ventilation i.e. areas are ventilated but not perfused. It can be corrected by increasing minute ventilation.

Etiology

Upper airway causes	*Lower airway causes*
Epiglottitis	Asthma
Croup	Bronchiolitis
Laryngotracheomalacia	Foreign body aspiration
Subglottic stenosis	
Foreign body aspiration	
	Alveolar and pleural causes
Vocal cord paralysis	Pneumonia (Empyema, pleural effusion)
Vascular ring	CCF (pulmonary edema)
Angioedema	Pneumothorax
	Tracheoesophageal fistula
Neurological causes	**Causes of ARDS***
Central hypoventilation:	*Respiratory causes*:
Spinal cord trauma	Pneumonia
Tetanus	Toxic gas inhalation
Guillain-Barré syndrome	Aspiration
Poliomyelitis	*Non-respiratory causes*:
Myasthenia gravis	Trauma
Botulism	Sepsis
	Shock
	Near drowning
	DIC
	Massive transfusion

* Acute respiratory distress syndrome.

Mechanics of Respiratory Failure

The disease process directly interferes with the exchange of oxygen or carbon dioxide or both. Mismatch of ventilation and perfusion causes shunting of pulmonary blood through the lung leading to hypoxia and to a lesser extent hypercarbia e.g. asthma, bronchiolitis or aspiration pneumonia. The disease process decreases lung compliance or increases airway resistance or both, resulting in increased work of breathing and increase oxygen consumption that exceeds delivery e.g. pneumonia, ARDS or asthma.

Clinical Manifestations

The basic clinical manifestations depend on the level of involvement. In *upper airway obstruction* major clinical signs are during the inspiratory phase viz. stridor, hoarseness, inspiratory retractions, use of accessory muscles and nasal flaring. The respiratory rate is often only mildly elevated.

In *lower airway obstruction,* major clinical signs are during expiration viz. wheeze, prolonged expiration. Respiratory rate is usually elevated, particularly in infants. Retractions become prominent; it means the lower airway obstruction impairs both inspiration and expiration, requiring increasing effort.

In parenchymal lung disease, the child's lungs are stiff requiring increased respiratory effort in both inspiration and expiration. Retractions are common and hypoxemia is often marked due to alveolar collapse or increased oxygen diffusion caused by pulmonary edema and inflammatory debris in the alveoli. The child frequently attempts to counteract alveolar and small airway collapse through increased effort to maintain an elevated end expiratory pressure, this usually manifests as grunting respiration. Children with *impending respiratory failure* present with tachypnea, exaggerated use of accessory muscles, supraclavicular, intercostal and subcostal retraction.

Brain, brainstem injury or drug overdose is indicated by an abnormal pattern of breathing. There are periods of increased effort alternating with decreased effort and later continuously inadequate causing hypoventilation.

When a child is progressing in respiratory distress, it is important to recognize the early signs of respiratory failure viz. tachypnea, agitation, nasal flaring, grunting, retractions and act rather than waiting for lethargy, cyanosis and bradycardia, the signs close to cardiorespiratory arrest.

Management

Management of acute respiratory failure includes treatment of respiratory failure and treatment of the cause. Investigations to find out the status of the patient as well as the cause and therapeutic intervention should go simultaneously. The child can be treated in the ward initially but transferred to the PICU in the following situations:

1. Lethargic child.
2. Deteriorating mental status.
3. Severe respiratory distress, tachypnea and chest retractions.
4. Oxygen requirement more than 50% to maintain saturation above 90%.
5. ABG showing hypoxemia, hypercarbia or metabolic acidosis.

A pulse oximeter probe should be placed to check saturation. Oxygen therapy by mask, nasal cannula or head box should be initiated.

A comfortable position of the child such as a sitting position or in the mother's lap should be maintained. Nothing should be done forcefully like making the child lie down for examination or taking an X-ray of the neck or chest. This will increase respiratory obstruction, cyanosis, bradycardia and chances of cardiac arrest.

If airway and breathing is maintained, salbutamol can be started if there is wheeze or adrenaline nebulisation if there is stridor.

If respiratory distress is severe or airway is not maintained, the airway should be opened with jaw thrust or head tilt and chin lift maneuver followed by bag and mask ventilation with 100% oxygen. Endotracheal intubation should be performed after transfer to PICU or in the operation theatre especially if upper airway obstruction is suspected due to acute epiglottitis, severe croup or bacterial tracheatis. A tracheostomy kit and an ENT surgeon should be available during the procedure of intubation because an emergency tracheostomy may be required.

Once the airway has been secured, an intravenous line should be established. Blood samples collected for CBC, blood culture, serum sodium, potassium, urea and creatinine and ABG. The I.V. line should be kept in situ for drug therapy as indicated according to the cause.

If the patient is relatively stable, a portable upright chest and airway, anterior posterior and lateral view X-ray may be obtained.

If history is suggestive of foreign body inhalation followed by respiratory distress, bronchoscopic removal may be required under anesthesia.

Indications of Mechanical Ventilation

The indications of mechanical ventilation are essentially clinical. ABG though important is not an absolute necessity. Intubation and ventilation is indicated in the following situations:

1. Deteriorating respiratory status despite oxygen and nebulisation therapy.
2. Anxious, sweaty, lethargic child with deteriorating mental status.
3. Respiratory arrest or recurrent apnea.
4. Severe shock even if arterial blood gases are within acceptable range.
5. In acute neurologic compromise for inadequate or absent ventilation, for loss of protective reflexes (cough and gag) or for therapeutic hyperventilation.
6. $PaO_2 < 55$ mm of Hg or/and $PaCO_2 > 60$ despite 100% oxygen.

Monitoring Course and Response to Therapy

Clinical monitoring include mental status, respiratory rate, chest retractions, quality of breath sounds, distal air entry, wheezing, grunting, perfusion and cardiovascular status.

ABG analysis may indicate improving, static or deteriorating gas exchange. Lab parameters indicative of adequate gas exchange are PaO_2 60-80 mmHg, $PaCO_2$ 50-60 mmHg, SpO_2 85-90% (in absence of fever, agitation and other conditions which place increase demand of O_2 in presence of normal hemoglobin and good cardiac output).

Treatment of Cause

After stabilization and initiation of treatment of respiratory failure, the cause of respiratory failure should be managed.

Suggested Reading

1. Asthma by consensus. Consensus statement on the diagnosis and management of Asthma in children. IAP Respiratory chapter. December 2001.
2. Global Initiative for Asthma. Global strategy for asthma management and prevention 2014. Available from www. ginaasthma.org.
3. Asthma by consensus. Consensus statement on the diagnosis and management of Asthma in children. Updated 2015. Available from www. ginaasthma.org.
4. National Asthma Education and Prevention Programme (NAEPP) guidelines for the diagnosis and management of Asthma–Update on selected topics, 2002. Washington, DC (NIH Publication No. 02-055075).
5. Basic Pediatric Intensive Care, 3rd edition. Sunit Singhi. Peepee Publishers and Distributors (P) Ltd, New Delhi.
6. Drugs and dosages in Children, 8th edition by Meherban Singh and Ashok K Deorari. Sagar Publications, New Delhi.
7. Acute respiratory infection in children. Case management in small hospital (Doctor's manual). Government of India, Ministry of Health and FW, New Delhi.
8. Management of the child with a serious infection or severe malnutrition. ATTBS Publishers, Department of child and adolescent health and development, WHO.

9. Hutchison's clinical methods edited by Michael Swash, 21st edition 2002.
10. Macleod's Clinical Examination, 10th edition. Churchill Livingstone 2001.
11. Price's Textbook of the Practice of Medicine edited by Sir Ronald Bodley Scott, 11th edition, 1973, printed in Great Britain by Morrison and Gibb Ltd, London.
12. Nelson Textbook of Pediatrics, 10th edition, 1975. Editors Victor C. Vaughan, R. James McKay and Waldo E. Nelson. WB Saunders Company, Philadelphia, London, Toronto.
13. Nelson Textbook of Pediatrics, 12th edition, 1983 edited by Richard E. Behrman, Victor C. Vaughan and Waldo E. Nelson. WB Saunders Company, Philadelphia, London, Toronto.
14. Nelson Textbook of Pediatrics, 17th edition, 2004 edited by Richard E. Behrman, Robert M. Kliegman, Hal B. Jenson. WB Saunders Company.
15. National Asthma Education and Prevention Program (NAEPP) guidelines for the diagnosis and management of asthma – Update on selected topics, 2002. Washington, DC (NIH Publication No. 02-05-5075).
16. PALS provider manual. American Heart Association
17. Principles of Pediatric and Neonatal Emergencies. Second edition, 2004. A publication of Indian Pediatrics. Published by Jaypee Brothers, Medical Publishers, N. Delhi.
18. Childhood Asthma: A modern approach to diagnosis and treatment. Guest author Dr. R.P. Khubchandani. Published by Medical Division Cipla Ltd.
19. Asthma by consensus: A consensus statement on diagnosis and management of asthma in children, December 2001. IAP Respiratory Chapter.
20. RTI Facts. IAP Action Plan 2006. IAP consensus guidelines on rational management of respiratory tract infections in children.
21. The Hospital for Sick Children. Hand book of Pediatric Emergency Medicine. Edited by Amina Lalani and Suzan Schneeweiss. First edition 2007. Jones and Bartlett Publishers. Sudbury, Massachusetts.

10

Gastrointestinal System, Liver and Pancreas

OUTLINES

Diarrhoeal Disorders

Diarrhoeal diseases are a leading cause of morbidity and mortality in the developing countries. 10–15% of all episodes of acute diarrhoea among children under five years of age are due to dysentery.

Definitions

Diarrhoea is defined as the passage of 3 or more loose or watery stools in a 24 hours period. However, it is the recent change in consistency and character of the stools rather than the number of times that is more important. A *loose stool* is one that takes the shape of the container. One bout of watery stool in a large amount can cause severe dehydration amounting to death.

Diarrhoea may be classified into acute and persistent.

In *acute diarrhoea,* onset is acute and most episodes terminate within 7 days. A small percentage may persist upto 14 days.

Acute diarrhoea may be classified as acute watery diarrhoea and dysentery.

Acute watery diarrhoea is characterized by passage of frequent watery stools associated with vomiting and fever. It is referred to as acute gastroenteritis.

Dysentery is defined as a syndrome characterized by presence of blood and pus in stool, abdominal cramps, fever and rapid weight loss.

Persistent diarrhoea is defined as passage of 3 or more stools of presumed infectious etiology, starting as an episode of acute watery diarrhoea or dysentery and persisting for more than 14 days.

What is Not Diarrhoea But Sometimes Misdiagnosed As Diarrhoea?

1. Passage of frequent formed stool.
2. Passage of frequent golden yellow colored, semi-loose, curd like stool mixed with water by breast fed babies.
3. Passage of frequent, loose greenish yellow stools from the 3rd and 4th day of life. It is commonly known as transitional diarrhoea. It may continue upto 10–15 days. There is no dehydration; baby is well and feeding normally.
4. Passage of stool during or immediately after feeding. It is due to the initiation of the gastro colic reflex.
5. It should be noted that microscopic examination of stool, in exclusively breast-fed babies, normally show presence of WBCs and macrophages. They are normal constituents of breast milk. Therefore, they do not indicate infection.
6. A toddler may pass stool of normal consistency, several times a day. The child is not sick and feeding normally.

Acute Diarrhoea

Etiopathogenesis

Acute diarrhoea is usually caused by ingestion of contaminated water or food.

Risk Factors

The factors that increase the risk of diarrhoea include:

1. Failure to breast feed exclusively for the first 6 months.
2. Unhygienic infant feeding practices.
3. Storing cooked food at room temperature for prolonged periods of time.
4. Drinking water which is contaminated with fecal bacteria.
5. Failing to wash hands after defecation, before taking food.

The Organisms

The organisms most frequently associated with acute diarrhoea are rotavirus, enterotoxigenic E. coli (ETEC), vibrio cholera, shigella, campylobacter jejuni, and non-typhoidal salmonella. Watery diarrhoea is mostly caused by rotavirus and enterotoxigenic E. coli while dysentery is caused by shigella. Amoebic dysentery is rare in a young child.

In diarrhoea due to *rotavirus infection*, the virus replicates within the villous epithelium of the small bowel, causing patchy epithelial cell destruction and villous shortening. The absorptive villous cells get replaced by secretary crypt cells, leading to secretion of water and electrolytes and secretory diarrhoea. It accounts for 20–40% of hospitalized cases of acute diarrhoea.

Diarrhoea due to *enterotoxigenic E.coli* accounts for 10–20% of acute diarrhoea. ETEC produce toxins which alter the epithelial cell function. These toxins decrease the absorption of sodium by the villi and increase the secretion of chloride by the crypts, resulting in net secretion of water and electrolytes.

Vibrio cholera produces non-invasive diarrhoea mediated by cholera toxin resulting in profuse secretion of water and electrolytes in the small bowel. Vibrio cholera serotype 01 has 2 serotypes—classical and Eltor. The latter subtype has been responsible for most of the outbreaks of cholera. It also causes a high proportion of asymptomatic infections. Most cholera infections are mild and patients may have no symptoms or mild diarrhoea. In a minority, there is acute onset of severe watery diarrhoea and vomiting leading to rapidly developing severe dehydration.

Shigella, campylobacter jejuni, enteroinvasive E.coli and rarely nontyphoidal salmonella cause acute diarrhoea with blood and mucus by destroying and invading mucosal epithelial cells mostly in the colon and distal part of ileum. Invasion may be followed by formation of micro abscesses and superficial ulcers resulting in the presence of red and white blood cells or frank blood in stool. In addition, toxins produced by these organisms cause tissue damage and possibly also mucosal secretion of water and electrolytes.

Pseudomonas infection is a very rare cause of diarrhoea. It results in green coloured stool and a very sick child. The other common causes of green coloured stool include transitional stool in the neonatal period, severe acute gastroenteritis (bile flow down due to intestinal hurry), and marasmus/starvation.

Consequences of Acute Diarrhoea

The main cause of death due to acute diarrhoea is dehydration. A substantial portion of such deaths however, occurs as a result of malnutrition consequent to recurrent diarrhoeal episodes. Malnutrition is associated with nearly two thirds of diarrhoeal deaths. Malnutrition increases the risk of diarrhoea, particularly its severity. In malnourished child, diarrhoea lasts longer, loss of weight is more severe and the risk of death is almost 15–20 times greater than in the well nourished.

Diarrhoea cause malnutrition and worsen existing milder forms of malnutrition by the following mechanisms:

1. Impaired intestinal absorption resulting in loss of macro and micro nutrients.
2. Increased catabolism due to infection.
3. Loss of appetite.
4. Restriction of food intake during and after diarrhoea.
5. Lack of emphasis by health professionals on the need of continuing feeding during diarrhoea and correction of faulty feeding practices.

Laboratory Diagnosis

Acute diarrhoea is a clinical diagnosis in most instances. Laboratory investigations do not have much role. The following investigations however need discussion.

1. Stool routine examination.
2. Stool culture.
3. Serum electrolytes.

Stool Microscopic Examination: Fecal leukocyte counts of more than 10/ high power field suggest invasive diarrhoea requiring antibiotic therapy. Such a finding may be present in acute watery diarrhoea due to viral infection also. Stool examination therefore is not helpful in diagnosis of acute diarrhoea.

Stool examination may be helpful in a suspected case of watery diarrhoea caused by giardiasis or diarrhoea with blood and mucus caused by entamoeba histolytica. These conditions should be suspected when there is no clinical response to therapy for presumed viral diarrhoea or shigellosis. Here stool samples may show presence of cysts or trophozoites of entamoeba histolytica and giardia lamblia.

Stool culture is of little value in routine management of acute diarrhoea. The clinical presentation of shigellosis and cholera are more useful than culture. E. coli is often reported on stool culture but most laboratories lack the ability to identify whether they are pathogenic or non-pathogenic.

Serum electrolytes estimation is not required for routine management of acute diarrhoea and some dehydration. Electrolytes estimation is useful in cases of severe dehydration, altered sensorium, seizures, and abdominal distension.

Assessment of a Child with Acute Diarrhoea

For planning an appropriate treatment, a child with acute diarrhoea should be assessed for the following:

1. Degree of dehydration.
2. Signs of extraintestinal infections.
3. Presence of malnutrition.

Assessment of Degree of Dehydration

Dehydration occurs during diarrhoea as a result of increased loss of water and electrolytes (sodium, potassium, chloride and bicarbonate) from the body through stools and vomitus.

Clinical Evaluation of Dehydration

Mild dehydration (3–5% body weight loss)

Increased thirst, decreased urine output, normal/ increased pulse, normal physical examination.

Moderate dehydration (7–10% body weight loss)

Decreased tears, irritable/lethargic, oliguria/anuria, sunken eyes and fontanel, dry mucous membrane, mild tenting of skin, delayed capillary refill, cool and pale skin.

Severe dehydration (10–15% body weight loss)

Drowsiness/lethargy, anuria, no tears, very sunken eyes and fontanel, rapid and weak pulse, decreased blood pressure, parched mucous membrane, tenting of skin very delayed, prolonged capillary refill, cold and mottled skin.

The WHO guidelines have classified dehydration into no dehydration, some dehydration and severe dehydration on the basis of the symptoms and signs present. The classification clubs mild and moderate dehydration as some dehydration, since the distinction between the two was always arbitrary.

The diagnostic clinical features of the different types of dehydration as described by WHO for use by community health workers are shown in a tabular form:

Clinical features	*No dehydration*	*Some dehydration*	*Severe dehydration*
General condition	Well, alert	Restless, irritable	Lethargic/ uncon-scious
Eyes	Normal	Sunken	Very sunken, dry
Tears	Present	Absent	Absent
Mouth and tongue	Moist	Dry	Very dry
Thirst	Not thirsty Drinks normally	*Thirsty Drinks eagerly	**Not able to drink
Skin pinch	Goes back quickly	*Goes back slowly (2 secs)	**Goes back very slowly (> 2 secs)

Interpretation

1. *Some dehydration:* When the patient has 2 or more signs including at least one *sign.
2. *Severe dehydration:* When the patient has two or more signs including at least one ** sign.

Fallacies

The signs of dehydration cited above have fallacies in the interpretation. Hence a combination of signs should be taken into consideration rather than one sign.

1. In some infants and children, the eyes normally appear sunken. It is therefore helpful to ask the mother whether the child's eyes are normal or more sunken than usual.
2. The mouth can be dry in a child who is a habitual mouth breather. The mouth may be wet in a dehydrated child who has recently vomited.
3. The skin pinch test is less useful in children with Marasmus. It will be false positive because of lack of subcutaneous fat. It will be false negative in edematous malnutrition because of presence of fluid or in infants and obese children because of abundance of subcutaneous fat.
4. Whether a baby is lethargic or sleepy should be properly looked for. A lethargic child's mental state is dull and the child cannot be fully awakened. There is no eye contact either with the mother or the examiner.
5. The amount and frequency of urination is an important feature of assessment of dehydration. In a child with no dehydration, urination is normal. With some dehydration, the frequency and amount is less than normal. In severe dehydration, there may be oliguria or anuria. It is not included as diagnostic criteria.

Signs of Extra Intestinal Infections

Many extraintestinal infections in children can present with acute diarrhoea. This type of acute diarrhoea is also called *parenteral diarrhoea*. The common conditions are acute suppurative otitis media, upper respiratory viral infection, pneumonia, septicemia, meningitis and urinary tract infection. These children should be carefully examined for the presence of these conditions and specific treatment advised, if present. The diarrhoea subsides with treatment of the conditions.

Assessment of Malnutrition

Assessment of malnutrition should be done in all cases of diarrhoea with the help of anthropometric measurements viz. weight for age, height for age or mid arm circumference (in 1–5 years age) and degree of malnutrition determined on the basis of IAP classification of malnutrition or the Waterloo classification.

Management

The management of acute diarrhoea should be planned under the following headings:

1. Prevention and treatment of dehydration.
2. Drug therapy.
3. Nutritional management.
4. Management of special situations.

Prevention and Treatment of Dehydration

All cases of acute watery diarrhoea should be started on oral fluid from the first episode of diarrhoea. The WHO recommended treatment plan A should be followed for the child with acute diarrhoea with no dehydration.

Treatment Plan A–Prevention of Dehydration

Patients with acute diarrhoea who show no physical signs of dehydration require fluids to prevent dehydration. This can be achieved by:

a. Provision of normal daily fluid requirement i.e. breast milk for those who are breast-fed, full strength artificial milk for the top fed. Other fluids and plain water normally taken by the child should be continued.
b. Replacement of ongoing losses due to diarrhoea and vomiting can be possible by:
    i. *Home available fluids:* Examples of such fluids are plain water, lemon water, coconut water, curd water, rice kanji, dal without salt etc.

       Most of these fluids lack a glucose precursor or salt or both. Therefore these are likely to be effective only in presence of continuing feeding which provide starch and protein to promote luminal sodium absorption. Home available fluids together with food should be started from the first loose stool.

       Soft drinks, sweetened fruit juices and tea do not contain salts, therefore are unsuitable and potentially dangerous. Plain glucose water without salt may cause osmotic diarrhoea.

ii. *Food based solutions:* Examples are rice water (50 grams of rice in litre of water) and dal mixed with salt, lassi with salt, and soups with salt. The salt amount should be a 2 finger pinch (0.8 gm) per 200 ml. These solutions contain acceptable amounts of starch and sodium and are suitable.

iii. *Sugar salt solution:* It is a home-made mixture of 1 two finger pinch (0.8 grams) of salt, one heaped teaspoon (8 gm) of sugar to be mixed in one glass (200 ml) of water. Properly prepared and consumed in adequate quantities, it makes a scientifically sound replacement when ORS is not available. However, it has been shown that solutions prepared have high sodium concentration despite proper instruction sometimes causing hypernatremia.

iv. *Oral rehydration salts (ORS):* ORS is appropriate for both prevention and treatment of dehydration. Preparation is easier than the home formulae mentioned above.

Composition of ORS

The composition of standard ORS and the low osmolarity ORS recommended by WHO is as shown below:

Ingredients	*Standard ORS*		*Low osmolarity ORS*	
	Gm/L	*mmol/L*	*Gm/L*	*mmol/L*
Sodium chloride				
Sodium	3.5	90	2.6	75
Chloride		80		65
Trisodium citrate				
dehydrate	2.9	10	2.9	10
Potassium chloride	1.5	20	1.5	20
Glucose, anhydrous	20	111	13.5	75
Total osmolarity		311		245

The recent recommendation by WHO is ORS with a reduced osmolarity (224 mOsmol /litre). This reduction of osmolarity is achieved by reducing the osmolarity of both sodium and glucose respectively to 60 mmol/litre and 84 mmol/litre. Another low osmolarity ORS (245 mOsmol/litre) has been tried with equal results in noncholera diarrhoea. The second composition is made to preserve the strategy of a single formulation for cholera and noncholera diarrhoea. Cholera cases treated with this formula however, had a higher incidence of asymptomatic hyponatremia.

Preparation of ORS

ORS is available in powder form in packets of two sizes– a small and a large. The mother should be asked to wash her hands with soap and water before preparation of the solution. A small packet should be mixed thoroughly in 200 ml of water and a large packet in 1 litre of water. The powder should be stirred properly so that there is no residual powder at the bottom of the container. It should be kept covered. Once prepared it should be used within 24 hours or discarded.

Procedure for Feeding ORS

ORS should be fed slowly. One teaspoonful should be given every 1–2 minutes for a child under 2 years. For an older child frequent sips from a cup.

If the child vomits, wait for 10 minutes. Then start more slowly e.g. one spoon every 2–3 minutes.

Amount of ORS to be Given, After Every Loose Motion, for Prevention of Dehydration

Age	*Amount after every loose stool*
Less than 2 years	50 to 100 ml
2 years to 10 years	100 to 200 ml
10 years or more	As much as desired

Advice to the Mother as Regards When to Call on the Doctor

The mother should be advised to call on the doctor or a health worker if the child does not get better in 5 days or immediately, if the child develops any of the following danger signs:

1. Many watery stools.
2. Repeated vomiting.
3. Marked thirst.
4. Eating or drinking poorly.
5. Fever.
6. Blood in stool.

Treatment Plan B: Rehydration Therapy for Patients with Physical Signs of Some Dehydration

All cases with signs of dehydration should be admitted to a hospital and treated. The child should be given ORS. It should be started as early as possible.

Components of Oral Fluid Therapy

1. Deficit therapy which consist of correction of existing fluid and electrolyte deficit.

2. Replacement of ongoing loss due to continuing diarrhoea or vomiting.
3. Provision of normal daily fluid requirement.

Amount of Fluid to be Given

The amount of fluid to be given includes the fluid which the child has already lost (deficit therapy) + replacement of ongoing losses for continuing diarrhoea and vomiting + the normal daily maintenance fluid.

1. Deficit therapy: 75 ml of ORS/kg in the first 4 hours. However, if the child wants more ORS than the calculated amount, it should be given.
2. Replacement of ongoing losses:
   a. ORS, 10–20 ml/ kg body weight after every liquid stool.
   b. Plain water inbetween ORS.
   c. Breastfeeding should be continued in breast-fed babies.
3. Normal daily requirement should be calculated according to the age of the child (*See* Chapter 2, Table 2.1).

Monitoring and Assessment

The child should be closely monitored every 1 hour and assessed. After 4 hours if the child still continues to have some dehydration, another 4 hours treatment with ORS should be repeated. If dehydration increases to severe degree, the child should be treated with Plan C.

Causes of Refusal to Take ORS

The child may refuse to accept ORS for the following reasons:

1. If there is no fluid or salt loss and dehydration is corrected.
2. If salt loss is corrected but fluid loss continues, the child will accept only plain water.
3. If preparation is not correct.
4. If the child is drowsy and unable to drink.

Treatment Plan C: Rehydration Therapy for Children with Physical Signs of Severe Dehydration

All cases with signs of severe dehydration should be treated with rapid I.V. rehydration for correction of existing water and electrolytes deficits. However, while the I.V. drip is setup, the child should be started on ORS.

The steps of I.V. rehydration are as follows:

1. Amount of fluid: 100 ml/kg body weight to be infused in 4 hours.
2. Nature of fluid: Ringer's lactate with 5% dextrose is the best. 0.9% sodium chloride (normal saline) can be used if Ringer's lactate is not available. Ringer's lactate is preferred because it contains potassium and lactate which helps to correct hypokalemia and acidosis in addition to sodium and chloride. Severe dehydration usually has hypokalemia and acidosis.
3. Amount and rate of therapy:
   a. Age less than 12 months: 30 ml/kg body weight in 1 hour (can be repeated if the radial pulse is weak or not palpable), then 70 ml/kg body weight in 5 hours.
   b. Older children: 30 ml/kg body weight in 30 minutes (can be repeated if the radial pulse is weak or not palpable), then 70 ml/kg body weight in 2½ hours.

Evaluation and Action

1. The child should be assessed every 15–30 minutes until a normal radial pulse is present. If there is no improvement, the rate of I.V. fluid infusion should be given more rapidly.
2. All children should be started on ORS solution 5 ml/ kg body weight/hour when they are able to drink properly during the time they are getting I.V. fluids.
3. If I.V. infusion is not possible, rehydration therapy can be started with ORS using a nasogastric tube at the rate of 30 ml/kg/hour (total of 120 ml/kg body weight) in 4 hours. If there is repeated vomiting, the rate should be slowed down. If there is no improvement after 3 hours, I.V. fluid should be started. This method may be used in children with severe dehydration during transport to a higher facility for management.
4. If the signs of severe dehydration are still present after 4 hours of deficit therapy, the treatment Plan C is repeated.
5. If the child shows signs of some dehydration after 4 hours, I.V. fluid administration should be discontinued and ORS solution should be given for 4 hours as in Plan B.
6. If there are no signs of dehydration after 4 hours, ORS should be given as in Plan A. The child should be observed in the hospital for 6 hours and if the hydration is maintained, child can be discharged.

Drug Therapy in Acute Diarrhoea

Antimicrobial drugs are not required for treatment of acute watery diarrhoea, because majority is caused by virus or enterotoxigenic E. coli which produces diarrhoea by producing enterotoxin. The specific indications for antibiotic therapy are cholera, dysentery and associated extraintestinal causes.

Cholera: In India, cholera still accounts for 5–10% cases of acute diarrhoea. It is endemic in some parts and may occur in outbreaks. The onset is sudden with large volume watery stool (rice water stool). The child very rapidly progresses to severe dehydration within hours. Mortality is very high. Oral rehydration therapy should be started promptly and cases should be timely referred for intravenous fluid therapy.

Cotrimoxazole is the drug of choice in children. Tetracycline is equally effective but should be used in children above 7 years. Erythromycin or chloramphenicol may be used if the above recommended drugs are not available or where V. cholerae is resistant to them.

Antibiotics	*Dose*	*Duration of treatment*
1. Trimethoprim +	5 mg/kg	12 hourly × 3 days
Sulphamethoxazole	25 mg/kg	
2. Tetracycline	12.5 mg/kg	6 hourly × 3 days
3. Erythromycin	12.5 mg/kg	6 hourly × 3 days
4. Chloramphenicol	20 mg/kg	6 hourly × 3 days

Dysentery: The clinical features of dysentery include continuous, high fever of sudden onset followed by frequent passage of stool with mucous initially, then blood and mucous. If left untreated the child may pass only blood. There is pain abdomen, tenesmus and the child is toxic and ill. The number of stools may be upto 15–20 times. The response to antibiotic therapy is seen by 48 hours with remission of fever, decreased blood in stool, decreased frequency, improvement of appetite and general well being. However, the child may continue to pass stool with mucus upto 7 days.

Most episodes of severe diarrhoea with blood and mucus are caused by shigella. As shigella invades the intestinal mucosa and multiplies within the mucosa, systematically effective antimicrobials should be used.

Antibiotic Therapy in Dysentery

Currently Shigella strains are resistant to cotrimoxazole. Hence it should be started empirically only if the strain is known to be susceptible (e.g., in an outbreak from a defined strain).

In view of the frequent occurrence of resistant organisms, optimal empirical therapy should include azithromycin, nalidixic acid, a third generation cephalosporin or ciprofloxacin. First and second generation cephalosporins are inadequate for treatment of Shigella. Ciprofloxacin is now the drug of choice recommended by the WHO for all patients with bloody diarrhoea irrespective of age. However, some experts recommend that these agents be reserved for seriously ill children with bacillary dysentery caused by organism that is suspected or known to be resistant to other agents. It should be noted that although risk of joint damage in children appears to be minimal, overuse of quinolones promotes development of resistance to these drugs.

Drugs	*Dose*	*Duration of treatment*
First line		
Nalidixic Acid	55 mg/kg /day	6 hourly × 5 days
Ciprofloxacin	20 – 30 mg/kg/day	12 hourly × 5 days
Azithromycin	12 mg/kg / day on 1st day Followed by 6 mg/kg/day	Daily × 5 days
Trimethoprim + Sulphamethoxazole	5 mg/kg 25 mg/kg	12 hourly × 5 days
Second line		
Ceftriaxone	50 mg/kg/day IV or IM	Single daily dose × 5 days
Cefixime	8 mg/kg/day	Daily or 12 hourly × 5 days

Steps of Therapy

1. Start with Nalidixic acid/Azithromycin/Ciprofloxacin.
2. Look for signs of response* after 2 days. If better, complete the course of 5 days.
3. If no response, exclude Amebiasis by examination of stool for trophozoites. If present, treat for amoebic dysentery.
4. If there is no evidence of Amebiasis, the second line drugs should be started.
5. If the child has risk factors**, the second line drug should be started in place of the first line. Rest will be same.

Amebic dysentery: Amebic dysentery is a very infrequent cause of diarrhoea with blood and mucus in children. In a child with acute bloody diarrhoea, one should consider amoebic dysentery as a cause when use of two antibiotics usually sensitive to Shigella does not show signs of clinical response. A microscopic examination should be done to demonstrate trophozoites of entamoeba histolytica. Metronidazole is the drug of choice.

Disease	*Drug of choice*
Amebic dysentery	Metronidazole 10 mg/kg/dose, 3 times daily × 5 days (10 days for severe disease)

Supportive Treatment of Dysentery

Supportive treatment is as essential as antibiotic therapy and should go simultaneously. It consists of the following measures:

a. Treatment of dehydration.
b. Continue feeding with calorie dense food.
c. Treatment of associated features viz. fever, hypokalemia, rectal prolapse etc.

Acute Gastroenteritis

It is the most common cause of acute diarrhoea in children. The most common organism is rotavirus. The peak incidence of rota viral diarrhoea is reported to be in cooler months in temperate regions. In our country it has been shown to occur throughout the year. It is characterized by watery diarrhoea of acute onset. The child presents with vomiting and fever. The fever may be associated with respiratory catarrh. The vomiting stops and fever subsides after 2–3 days and the child starts passing loose watery stools. The number of stools may be as high as 15–20 times.

The child should be treated with adequate amount of ORS solution and referred for I.V. fluid therapy when indicated. There is no role of antibiotic therapy in acute gastroenteritis as it is caused by a viral infection. Treatment with antibiotics may prolong the course. The normal course of the disease may be 7–14 days.

Acute watery diarrhoea can be caused by enterotoxigenic and enteropathogenic E. coli with similar presentation and should be treated in the same line as rota viral diarrhoea. Antibiotic therapy have shown not to alter the course of these bacterial diarrhoea; hence not recommended.

Zinc Supplementation in Acute Diarrhoea

It has been shown that zinc deficiency during diarrhoea results in decreased brush border activity, enhanced secretory response, altered intestinal permeability. Zinc supplementation causes reversal of these effects. Hence recent recommendations advocate zinc supplement during acute diarrhoea. Zinc given in the dose of 20 mg/day (10 mg/day below 6 months age) for 10 to 14 days reduces duration and severity of the episode. Zinc supplementation also lowers the incidence of diarrhoea in the following 2–3 months.

Associated Extra Intestinal Infections Presenting With Acute Diarrhoea

Examples of extra intestinal infection presenting with acute diarrhoea are pneumonia, septicemia, meningitis, and urinary tract infection. The presence of these conditions should be carefully looked for particularly in infants below 3 months and those severely malnourished. They should be treated with specific therapy according to the disease present.

Drugs Which Are Not Effective in Acute Diarrhoea

The following drugs, though commonly used in the treatment of acute diarrhoea, are found to be ineffective and cause side effects. These include:

1. *Adsorbents* e.g. Kaolin, pectin have been found to be of no value. They are not available at present.
2. *Motility suppressants* e.g. loperamide. These drugs decrease intestinal peristalsis and delay the elimination of the causative agents. In infants they can cause paralytic ileus, abdominal distension, and bacterial over growth and sepsis.
3. *Stimulants* (adrenaline, nikethamide) and corticosteroids. There is no role of these drugs in management of shock following acute diarrhoea and severe dehydration. Shock should be treated with appropriate I.V. fluid therapy.
4. *Combination drugs* e.g. combinations of antibacterials or combinations of antibacterial and antidiarrhaeal and antimotility agents offer no extra benefit than a properly selected single anti-bacterial. Combination therapy increases complications e.g. overgrowth of harmful resistant bacteria and the antimotility agents may delay excretion of the invasive pathogen.
5. *Lactobacilli and saccharomyces boulardii:* Studies with formulations containing lactobacillus in acute diarrhoea have shown no reduction either in diarrhoeal duration or severity. Limited controlled

studies with saccharomyces have shown some benefit in antibiotic induced diarrhoea. No effect has been shown in treatment of acute diarrhoea.

Nutritional Management of Acute Diarrhoea

Facts About Nutritional Intake and Absorption During Diarrhoea

Feeding during diarrhoea facilitates mucosal recovery and correct malabsorption. It does not worsen diarrhoea. Some malabsorption of macro nutrients does occur. 80–95% of carbohydrates, 70% of fat and 75% of protein are actually absorbed from mixed diet based on common foods when taken during diarrhoea. Children receiving recommended calorie requirement from the first day of diarrhoea absorb more nutrients, retain more nitrogen, gain more weight compared to children receiving half the recommended calories. Resting the bowel during or after diarrhoea further reduces the digestibility of food in the intestine. It is more dangerous in children with PEM. Affected children consume a higher than the recommended intake during convalescence. This should be allowed as it facilitates catch up growth.

Recommended Dietary Intake

Feeding during diarrhoea is physiologically sound and prevents or minimizes the deterioration of nutritional status that usually accompanies. Type of feeding differs according to the age of the child.

1. *Exclusively breast-fed baby:* Breastfeeding should be continued uninterrupted even during rehydration with ORS. Breastfeeding in infants during diarrhoea causes better weight gain and prevents malnourishing persistent diarrhoea.
2. For *babies on top milk*, cow or buffalo milk can be given undiluted after correction of dehydration.
3. For *a baby on mixed diet*, staple food enriched with oil or sugar e.g. Khichri with oil, rice and dal with oil, rice with curd and sugar, mashed banana with curd, mashed potatoes with lentil and oil can be given. Foods with high fibre content e.g. coarse fruits and vegetables should be avoided.
4. *Lactose free milk* e.g. soya milk formula is not required routinely during acute diarrhoea. It may be required in very few infants in whom diarrhoea persists beyond 8–10 days with progressive weight loss and presence of 1% or more of reducing substances in stool.
5. During convalescence, an intake of atleast 125% of normal calories should be attempted with nutrient dense foods. It should be continued till the child reaches the pre illness weight and ideally until the child achieves normal nutritional status. It may sometimes take 6–8 weeks time.

Management of Special Situations in Diarrhoea

Acute Diarrhoea in Infants Under 2 Months

Complications like septicemia, severe electrolyte disturbance are common in this age group. In young infants born low birth weight with diarrhoea must be presumed to have sepsis. They should be admitted to hospital and treated with appropriate systemic antibiotics.

In babies of normal weight with diarrhoea, after correction of dehydration, systemic antibiotics should be considered if any one of the following danger signs is present: Not feeding well, fever or hypothermia, lethargy, fast breathing, chest indrawing, nasal flaring or grunting, convulsion, bulging fontanelle, signs of bacterial infection at local sites.

These babies should be discharged only after the following criteria are fulfilled:

i. They have received 5 days of systemic antibiotics.
ii. They are accepting feeds.
iii. Mothers are conversant with the method of preparation of ORS.
iv. Mothers are aware of the danger signs.
v. The malnourished have a consistent weight gain over several days.

Management of Electrolyte Disturbances

It should be noted that extreme lethargy, floppiness, and inability to drink ORS can be signs of electrolyte disturbance as well as severe dehydration. Thus in a child with relatively milder dehydration, presence of changes in mental status should alert one to think of a possible severe electrolyte disturbance. The following electrolyte disturbances may occur in acute diarrhoea:

Hypernatremia: Can occur especially in infants when they are given oral fluids that are hypertonic e.g. improperly prepared ORS, fruit juices etc.

Children with hypernatremic dehydration are extremely thirsty which is out of proportion to the other signs of dehydration. Other signs which may be present are doughy feeling of skin, woody tongue, brisk tendon reflexes and convulsion.

The diagnosis can be confirmed by estimation of serum sodium which is > 150 mEq/litre. Hypernatremic dehydration is treated with WHO low osmolarity ORS solution. This usually causes the serum sodium to come down to normal by 24 hours. Hypernatremic dehydration can be prevented by teaching the mothers to prepare the ORS solution properly and prevent the child with dehydration to drink fruit juices and soft drinks.

Hyponatremia: Can occur if a child with diarrhoea consumes large amount of water or drinks which contain very little salt. Clinically, the hydrated child is lethargic or have convulsion. The serum sodium is below 130 mEq/litre. Hyponatremia is treated with ORS solution. IV fluid may be required in children with altered sensorium or convulsion.

Hypokalemia: Can occur as a result of insufficient replacement potassium losses during diarrhoea. The clinical features include muscle weakness, paralytic ileus, renal impairment and cardiac arrhythmia. Hypokalemia can be corrected by using ORS solution for rehydration and feeding potassium rich food viz. bananas and green coconut water. Intravenous potassium therapy may be required when serum potassium levels are very low i.e. equal to or less than 2 mEq/litre which is clinically characterized by marked muscle weakness, abdominal distension and weak respiration.

Causes of Seizure in Acute Diarrhoea

1. Febrile seizure.
2. Hypoglycemia.
3. Hypo or hypernatremia.
4. Cavernous sinus thrombosis.
5. Meningitis.
6. Shigella infection.

Acute Diarrhoea in a Child with PEM

Children with mild to moderate malnutrition should be managed as children without malnutrition with greater emphasis on feeding.

Children with severe malnutrition (Weight for age < 60% of the median of NCHS reference values or presence of symmetrical edema of atleast the feet) should be admitted to a hospital for treatment.

Dehydration in Severe PEM: The reliable signs of some dehydration include eagerness to drink (manifested as irritability in infants). The signs of severe dehydration are weak or absent radial pulse and decreased or absent urine flow. The signs of dehydration, seen in normal children are fallacious in children with severe PEM.

Fluid Therapy: Whenever possible oral rehydration should be the practice in a dehydrated child with severe PEM without shock. Intravenous fluid therapy may cause overhydration and heart failure particularly in those with edematous malnutrition.

In Some Dehydration

Deficit therapy: ORS, 70 ml/kg over a period of 8–10 hours instead of 4–6 hours as in well nourished children. The child should be assessed every 1 hour.

For ongoing losses: After initial dehydration is corrected, WHO-ORS should be given 5–10 ml/kg after every loose stool. The child should be allowed plain water ad libitum.

In Severe Dehydration

Correction of severe dehydration requires intravenous fluid therapy followed by oral rehydration.

For I.V. infusion, the fluid of choice is Ringer's lactate in 5% dextrose. If not available, half normal saline in 5% dextrose can be used.

Steps

1. Ringer's lactate should be given @ 15 ml/kg/hour for the first hour.
2. Monitor pulse, respiratory rate, and CRT every 5–10 minutes. Assess after 1 hour.
3. If there is no improvement, pulse rate increases by 25 beats/minute or the respiratory by 5 breaths/minute consider septic shock or fluid overload.
4. If there is improvement i.e. pulse rate slows/CRT is faster, repeat 15 ml/kg in 1 hour.
5. Assess after 1 hour again.
6. If the child has signs of some dehydration and accepts orally, treat as some dehydration.
7. If the child is clinically improving but still not accepting orally, continue I.V. fluid 10 ml/kg/hour till patient accepts orally. If further I.V. fluid is required, maintenance fluid should be given at 4–5 ml/kg/hour until oral fluids are accepted.

Treatment of Septic Shock

Patients with septic shock should be treated as follows:

1. Whole blood/plasma expanders, 10 ml/kg slowly over 3–4 hours should be given. The I.V. fluid infusion should be continued till blood/plasma expanders are available.
2. If the patient has signs of myocardial dysfunction, the infusion rate should be reduced to 4 ml/kg/hour and ionotropic drugs, dopamine (5–20 microgram/kg/minute) and dobutamine (5–20 microgram/kg/min) should be administered. The signs of myocardial dysfunction include increasing heart rate, respiratory rate, and liver size, crepitations and rhonchi, following rapid intravenous infusion.

Identification and Treatment of Overhydration

The signs of overhydration are increasing respiratory and heart rate, or increasing edema and puffy eyelids. If these signs occur, oral or I.V. fluids should be stopped and the child assessed after 1 hour.

In a severely malnourished child, even when fully rehydrated there is no return of tears, no improvement of sunken eyes or skin turgor and mouth remains dry. So it is important to assess at regular intervals for signs of overhydration.

Persistent Diarrhoea

Definition

WHO has defined persistent diarrhoea as a diarrheal illness with passage of 3 or more stools of presumed infectious etiology, starting as an episode of acute watery diarrhoea or dysentery and persisting for more than 14 days. This condition is usually seen in infants with more than 60% episodes occurring in infants below 6 months and 90% before one year of age. 3–20% of acute diarrheal episodes (average 10%) tend to become persistent. These episodes are generally associated with growth failure, inadequate weight gain or loss of weight.

When persistent diarrhoea is associated with some or severe dehydration it is classified as severe persistent diarrhoea. It is usually associated with signs of malnutrition and often with serious non-intestinal infections like pneumonia. Children with severe persistent diarrhoea require hospitalization and treatment.

The term persistent diarrhoea is now the standard nomenclature for what was previously referred to as protracted or intractable diarrhoea. Persistent diarrhoea should not be confused with chronic diarrhoea, which is recurrent or long lasting diarrhoea (> 14 days) due to non-infectious causes, such as gluten sensitivity or inherited metabolic disorders.

Etiopathogenesis

The exact cause as to why an episode of diarrhoea may get prolonged is not known. A variety of risk factors have been identified which seem to predispose the child to the possibility of developing persistent diarrhoea. They include the following:

Risk Factors in Persistent Diarrhoea

Table 10.1

Host factors	*Age < 1 year*
	Malnutrition
	Impaired cell mediated immunity
	Previous persistent diarrhoea
	Recurrent acute diarrhoea
Pre-illness feeding practices	Recent introduction of animal milk
Stool pathogens	Enteroadherent or enteroaggregative E. coli
	Enteropathogenic E. coli, Shigella
Drugs used in acute phase	Antibiotics

Hypothesis of Interplay of Risk Factors

The young child has increased intestinal mucosal permeability. Early introduction of top feeds leads to absorption of foreign proteins and hypersensitivity resulting in mucosal damage and disaccharidase deficiency.

Early introduction of top feeds in the form of diluted milk leads to malnutrition. Malnutrition predisposes the child to gut and systemic infection resulting in mucosal damage and malabsorption which aggravates malnutrition. Diarrhoea causes anorexia resulting in decrease food intake and contributes to development of malnutrition.

The prevailing practices of diarrheal management viz. indiscriminate use of antibiotics, withholding of food or feeding diluted milk, can lead to further compromise of nutritional status and thus initiating the vicious diarrhoea-malnutrition-diarrhoea cycle, leading to ultimate development of persistent diarrhoea.

Enteropathogens and Persistent Diarrhoea

No definite enteropathogen has been implicated in the causation of persistent diarrhoea. Recent findings of higher incidence of enteroadhesive and enteroaggregative E. coli in cases of acute diarrhoea, which later prolonged, suggest that atleast certain strains of E.coli may be responsible for the prolongation of diarrheal episodes in some children. Shigellosis has also been blamed for persistent diarrhoea. In shigellosis, after blood disappears from stool after 2–3 days of starting antibiotic, it may take upto 3–4 weeks for stool frequency to return to normal. However, during this period, the child is usually active, non-anorexic and able to maintain hydration and nutrition if fed properly.

30–50% of children hospitalized for persistent diarrhoea may have some systemic infections at the time of admission. The usual infections are urinary tract infection, pneumonia and septicemia. As most of the hospitalized children are severely malnourished (body weight < 60%), the systemic infection is usually asymptomatic, and require careful screening for diagnosis. However, presence of systemic infection at the onset of acute diarrhoea is not responsible for prolongation of diarrheal episodes.

Common Underlying Etiologic Factors

The common underlying factors include: PEM, Vitamin A deficiency and zinc deficiency, lactose intolerance, colitis and antibiotic colitis, cow's milk protein intolerance.

Malnutrition – Diarrhoea – Malnutrition Cycle

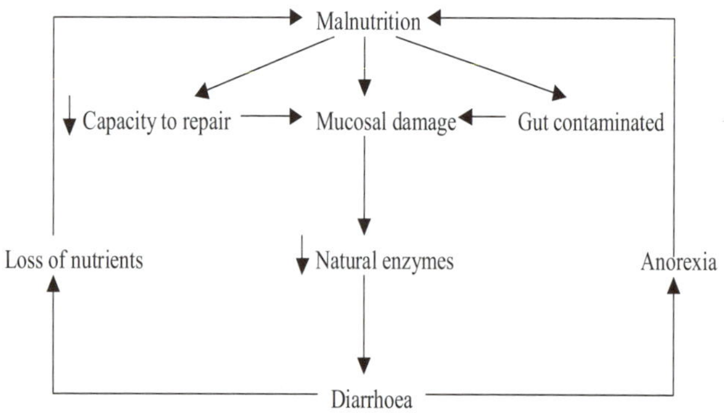

Acute diarrhoea causes mucosal damage. The child with malnutrition has a decreased capacity of mucosal repair. There is increased gut contamination due to proliferation of nonspecific bacteria and decreased mucosal enzymes resulting in prolongation of diarrhoea. Malnutrition prolongs the duration of diarrhoea and diarrhoea worsens malnutrition. These children also have multiple vitamin and mineral deficiencies. Zinc deficiency is believed to be a major causative factor in prolonging diarrheal episode.

Lactose Intolerance

Lactose intolerance is the most common sugar intolerance seen in children with persistent diarrhoea. This is because lactase enzyme is present in the most superficial layers of jejunal mucosa and hence most vulnerable to damage. There may be mild and transitory lactose intolerance in the first 2–3 days of a watery diarrheal episode which does not warrant any milk withdrawal. Lactose intolerance appearing after 5–7 days usually warrants active management.

Colitis and Antibiotic Associated Colitis

Colitis is infective in origin in most cases. Severely malnourished children or infants aged below 3 months usually require systemic antibiotics for treatment.

The common offending antibiotics for antibiotic associated colitis are ampicillin, chloramphenicol and cephalosporins although almost any antibiotic may be responsible. The cause of this type of colitis has been traced to the overgrowth of an anaerobic bacteria, clostridium difficile and liberation of an enterotoxin by this organism.

Antibiotic associated colitis can be suspected when a child's diarrhoea, after initial improvement, increases or becomes invasive (i.e. puscells/red cells in stool) after 4–5 days use of antibiotics. If appropriate action is not taken, the child becomes moribund, refuses to feed and develops abdominal distension and pass blood and pus in stools.

The diagnosis can be established by either demonstrating the toxin in the serum or stool or growing clostridium difficile in the stool. As both of these facilities are rarely available, the entity has to be considered and diagnosed on clinical grounds.

Cow's Milk Protein Intolerance (CMPI)

Cow's milk protein intolerance can be suspected when the diarrheal episode in a top fed child exceeded more than 2–3 weeks, causing failure to thrive. The diarrhoea does not respond to low lactose diet (curd, khichri). A trial of milk withdrawal and substitution of diet with non-milk protein sources (rice–dal–oil diet or soya milk) results in remission of diarrhoea but reintroduction of milk in diet causes recurrence of diarrhoea.

Laboratory Investigation and Treatment

Most children with no dehydration or malnutrition can be

treated at home with proper feeding advice and monitoring. The child needs hospitalization if there are signs of:

1. Severe dehydration.
2. Blood in stool in spite of proper treatment.
3. Refusal to feed.
4. Severe pneumonia.
5. Other extraintestinal infection like sepsis, urinary tract infection, oral thrush, otitis media and meningitis.

After admission it is necessary to take a detailed history. The physical examination of the child should include assessment of nutritional and hydration status and careful screening for associated infections viz. otitis media, pneumonia, UTI and pneumonia.

The preliminary investigations should include stool examination for pus cells, ova, cysts, red cells, pH and reducing substances, urine examination and an X-ray chest. Stool osmolarity and electrolytes should also be done. A stool osmotic gap [total osmolality–(2 × sodium content)] of less than 50 is suggestive of secretary diarrhoea, which may require treatment of sepsis and prolonged parenteral nutrition.

Most children with persistant diarrhoea presents in a moribund state with fluid, electrolyte and nutritional imbalance and their management should be started immediately while investigation reports are awaited.

A Stepwise Approach

Step I: If the clinical examination and preliminary investigations fail to reveal any evidence of infection, oral feeds and all antibiotics should be stopped for 24–48 hours and hydration should be maintained with intravenous fluids. In most cases diarrhoea subsides with these measures and oral feeds can be started gradually with ORS followed by gradual increase in milk feeds. If the diarrhoea does not settle down, it suggests secretory diarrhoea and a trial of systemic antibiotics may be warranted.

Step II: If diarrhoea recurs on reintroduction of milk feeds, it indicates lactose intolerance besides possibility of a systemic infection. The child should be investigated for a systemic infection and treated appropriately. The child should be given a low lactose diet (diet A Table 10.2) and the same continued for 3–5 days. If the child tolerates the diet and starts gaining weight, the amount can be increased slowly.

Step III: If the child fails to respond to lactose free diet then the clinical setting suggests possibility of CMPI besides possibility of a systemic infection. These children should be treated with a complete milk free diet (diet B Table 10.3) besides treating systemic infection. Around 97% of these cases responds, leaving 1–2% which fail to respond.

Once the child responds to completely milk free diet, then it is advisable to maintain the milk free diet for atleast 4–6 weeks. Occasionally these infants may require milk free diet for as long as 8–12 months. If no response after 7 days, diet C should be started.

Step IV: If the child is unable to tolerate step III diet and continues to have diarrhoea, then the child would require parenteral nutrition.

Modalities of Treatment

The modalities of treatment of persistent diarrhoea include recognition and treatment of dehydration, feeding and medications.

Recognition and Treatment of Dehydration

The child should be assessed on the basis of signs of dehydration and rehydration should be advised according to Plan B or C, as appropriate. In children with glucose malabsorption, administration of ORS will increase stool volume, develop signs of dehydration and stool contains large amount unabsorbed glucose. These children will require I.V. fluid until ORS is tolerated.

Feeding

Appropriate feeding is an essential component of treatment of persistent diarrhoea. Besides giving energy and nutrition to the child, feeding helps in gut recovery.

Diet for Infants Aged Less Than 4 Months

In infants aged <4 months, exclusive breastfeeding should be continued. If the child is not breastfeeding, a breast milk substitute that is low in lactose such as yoghurt or lactose free milk can be given. However, the breast milk substitute should be given with a cup. A feeding bottle should not be used. Simultaneously, the mother should be helped to reestablish lactation. The total intake should be atleast 110 calories/kg/day. The infant may not feed adequately in presence of a systemic infection. So in the initial period, the infant may require nasogastric feeding for the first 24–48 hours until the serious infection has been treated.

Diet for Infants and Children Above 4 Months

The two types of diet recommended for infants above 4 months age and children are diet A i.e. a starch based reduced milk concentration (low lactose) diet (Table 10.2) and diet B which is a no milk with reduced cereal diet (Table 10.3).

The diet A is given first for 7 days. Around 60–70% children will improve with this treatment. If there are signs of dietary failure (increase in stool frequency usually > 10 watery stools/day, often with signs of dehydration shortly after the new diet is begun or a failure to establish daily weight gain within 7 days), or if the child is not improving after 7 days of treatment, the diet A should be stopped and the diet B should be given for 7 days. If no response, diet C (Table 10.4) should be given similarly for 7 days. Poor outcome with diet C may be due to transient glucose malabsorption which should be treated with parenteral nutrition.

Table 10.2 : Diet A: Starch based, reduced milk concentration (low lactose) diet

Constituents	*Amount*
Full fat dried milk	11 grams
Or whole liquid milk	85 ml
Puffed rice powder*	15 grams
Vegetable oil	3.5 grams
Cane sugar	3.0 grams
Water to make	200 ml

* Can be substituted with cooked rice or suji.

This diet provides 83 k calories/100 gms, 3.7 gm lactose/kg body weight/day and 11% calories from protein.

Table 10.3 : Diet B: No milk (lactose free) diet with reduced starch

Constituents	*Amount*
Egg white*	64 grams
Puffed rice powder**	3 grams
Vegetable oil	4 grams
Glucose	3 grams
Water to make	200 ml

* Can be substituted with finely ground cooked chicken (12 grams) to provide 70 kcal/100 grams.

** Can be substituted with cooked rice.

This diet provides 70 kcal/100 grams, and 10% calories as protein.

Table 10.4 : Diet C: A monosaccharide diet

Constituents	*Amount*
Egg white or chicken	12 grams
Glucose	25 grams
Vegetable oil	4 grams
Water to make	100 ml

This diet provides 60 kcal/100 grams and 3 grams protein/100 grams.

Supplementary Micronutrients

All children with persistent diarrhoea should receive daily supplementary micronutrients for two weeks. The micronutrients include folate, zinc, Vitamin A, iron, copper and magnesium.

Antimicrobial Therapy and Other Drugs

Antimicrobial therapy is indicated in the following situations:

1. In presence of gross blood in stools and Shigella infection is suspected.
2. Presence of associated infections like pneumonia, UTI, otitis media, or meningitis.
3. Isolation of group B salmonella in stool.
4. Identification of trophozoites or clinical suspicion of amebiasis or giardiasis.

Other drugs viz. antimotility and antisecretory agents, lactobacilli and saccharomyces boulardii have not shown significant clinical benefit.

Criteria for Discharge

The criteria for successful treatment include the following:

1. Adequate food intake.
2. Weight gain.
3. Diminished number of diarrheal stools (2 or less stools/day for 2 consecutive days).
4. Absence of fever.

The most important criterion is weight gain. Many children will loose weight for 1–2 days, and then steadily gain weight as the infections get under control and the diarrhoea subsides. There should be atleast 3 successive days of increasing weight before one can conclude that weight gain is occurring.

After 7 days of treatment with the effective diet they should resume an age appropriate diet, including milk, which will provide atleast 110 kcal/kg/day. Children may be discharged but followed up regularly to ensure continued weight gain and compliance with feeding advice.

Follow-up

The child should be called for reassessment after 5 days or earlier if diarrhoea worsens or other problems develop. The child should be assessed for presence of dehydration or signs of infection and readmitted if necessary. Those who have gained weight and who have less than 3 stools per day may resume normal diet for age.

Constipation

What is Constipation?

If a child has fewer than three bowel movements per week and they are hard and difficult to pass, it should be treated as constipation.

What is not Constipation?

A normal child may have a soft stool only every second or third day without difficulty; this is not constipation. An infant on exclusive breastfeeding passes normal stool infrequently. The duration may be as long as 10 or more days.

Etiology

Constipation may result from non-organic/functional and organic causes. Functional constipation is caused by the passage of painful bowel movements with voluntary withholding of feces to avoid the painful stimulus.

Following are the causes of constipation:

Non-organic/Functional

Organic

Anatomical causes viz. anal stenosis, imperforate anus, intestinal stricture, anteriorly placed anus.

Abnormal musculature: Gastrochisis, Prune Belly syndrome, Down syndrome.

Intestinal muscle or nerve abnormalities: Hirschsprung disease, visceral myopathy/neuropathy, intestinal neuronal dysplasia.

Spinal cord defect: Spinal cord trauma, spina bifida.

Drugs: Anticholinergics, narcotics, antidepressants, vincristine, lead, Vitamin D intoxication.

Metabolic disorders: Hypokalemia, hypercalcemia, hypothyroidism, diabetes mellitus.

Intestinal disorders: Celiac disease, cow's milk protein intolerance, cystic fibrosis, inflammatory bowel disease (stricture), tumour.

Connective tissue disorders: SLE, scleroderma.

Other disorders: Anorexia nervosa, depression, ADHD, cerebral palsy, mental retardation.

The most common cause in a child older than 18 months is their willful avoidance of the toilet (for various reasons). For example, toddlers are often so involved in their play that they lack time or patience for toilet breaks. At school they may be concerned with lack of privacy or the cleanliness of the bathroom. They may have had a prior painful or frightening experience that makes them want to avoid defecation. Over time, their brain learns to ignore repeated urges by the colon to visit the bathroom. As stool remains in the colon, the colon will absorb water out of the stool, making it hard and dry. This hard stool is even more difficult or painful to pass, which causes the child to continue "holding it".

The nature of diet as well as changes in diet affect bowel habits. In adults, high-fiber diets have been shown to improve bowel function. In children, however, high-fiber diets have not been proven to improve constipation. Infants and children who eat well-balanced meals typically are not constipated. Teenagers and toddlers who eat a lot of sugar and desserts are prone to difficult passing of their stools.

Any intense change in a child such as illnesses causing fever, a long time in bed, eating less, or dehydration may decrease frequency of stools or may harden stools.

The majority of children with constipation does not have a medical disease or disorder causing the constipation. Rarely, a secondary disorder causes infants and children to have significant problems moving their bowels.

Pathogenesis

Infants and children with constipation should be treated differently than adults because patterns of bowel movements change from the time they are born until they reach the age of 3 or 4 years.

Constipation may arise from defects either in filling or emptying of the rectum. *Defective filling* occurs when colonic peristalsis is ineffective (e.g. hypothyroidism, intestinal obstruction, Hirschsprung disease). This results in stasis in the colon which leads to excessive drying of the stool and a failure to initiate the reflexes from rectum that normally trigger evacuation. *Emptying the rectum* by spontaneous evacuation depends on a defecation reflex initiated by pressure receptors in the rectal muscle. So stool retension can result from lesions affecting the rectal muscles, the sacral spinal cord afferent and efferent fibers, or the muscles of the abdomen and pelvic floor as well as disorders of anal sphincter relaxation.

Hard stools in the rectum become difficult and even painful to evacuate leading to more retension and a vicious cycle ensues. Distension of the rectum and colon lessens the sensitivity of the defecation reflex and the effectiveness of peristalsis. Eventually, watery content of the stool from the proximal colon may percolate around the hard retained stool and pass per rectum. This condition is called encopresis and it should not be mistaken for diarrhoea.

Constipation may lead to urinary stasis in severe long standing cases. It may generate anxiety and have a marked emotional impact on the patient as well as the family.

Clinical Manifestations

Children commonly show the following symptoms when they suffer from constipation:

- Difficulty in passing stools or infrequent bowel motions.
- Pain and discomfort when passing stools.
- A heated sensation in the stomach, generally after eating a meal.
- An uncomfortable feeling of fullness in the stomach after having meals.
- Lethargy and wanting to lie down on the bed for a long time, even after just having woken up in the morning.

Children with constipation often exhibit characteristic behaviors while trying to keep away from having a bowel movement. Infants having painful bowel movements may extend their legs and squeeze their anal opening and buttock muscles to prevent passage of stool. Toddlers often rise up on their toes, rock back and forth, and hold their legs and buttocks stiffly.

Physical examination often demonstrates a large amount of stool palpated in the suprapubic area. Rectal examination demonstrates a dilated rectal vault filled with stool.

Different medical disorders mentioned as causes of constipation, will have the associated features of the primary disease besides constipation. One such example of true constipation in infants and children that may be present since birth is Hirschsprung disease. Most infants with this condition display symptoms within the first few weeks of life. They may be underweight or small for date. They may vomit and pass small stools, which are described as ribbon-like. A spinal pathology may be suggested from presence of a tuft of hair over the spine, spinal dimple or failure to elicit a cremasteric or anal reflex.

Investigations

Children with no abnormalities on physical examination rarely require any investigations. In refractory cases the following special tests may be considered:

1. Tests to rule out hypothyroidism, hypocalcemia, lead toxicity and celiac disease.
2. A barium enema to study structural abnormalities.
3. MRI of spine to identify an intraspinal process.
4. Motility studies to identify underlying myopathy or neuropathic bowel abnormalities.

Management

The management of functional constipation includes patient education, relief of impaction, and softening of stool.

The parents should be made to understand that fecal soiling with overflow incontinence is not a willful act. It is a result of loss of normal sensation. A regular bowel training programme as well as keeping track of the frequency of the bowel movements should be emphasized. This helps in developing a proper bowel habit. The body has a natural reflex called the gastrocolic reflex. After a meal, the colon undergoes peristalsis and attempts to clear the bowels. Taking the advantage of the gastrocolic reflex, the child should sit on the toilet for 5–10 minutes after meals. It is often easier for the child if the feet are on the floor or on a footstool.

If an impaction of stool is present in the initial examination, the impaction should be cleared by an enema. Bowel softeners should be advised as maintenance medicine. These include lactulose, mineral oil, milk of magnesia, polyethylene glycol preparations. All these softeners are locally acting drugs. Milk of magnesia (2–3 ml/kg/day) and lactulose (infants 2.5–10 ml/day in 3–4 doses, children

40–90 ml/day in 3–4 doses) are the commonly used drugs. They are safe. The dosage should be adjusted according to the need to enable the child to pass a soft stool every day. Maintenance therapy is generally continued until a regular bowel pattern has been established for several months. Children with behaviour problems that are interfering with successful treatment should be referred to a psychiatrist.

A change in the behaviour and diet is also important. Positive reinforcement is the first step in giving children the desire to begin regulation of their bowels. It is important to remove any negative thoughts about being constipated, especially if fecal soiling is present. A well-balanced meal consisting of cereals, fruits and vegetables and plenty of fluids with less candy and dessert also helps.

The management of constipation as a result of an organic cause requires a detailed investigation and management according to the cause.

Vomiting

Vomiting is a coordinated reflex process that is usually preceded by increased salivation and involuntary retching. During the act, there is violent descent of the diaphragm and constriction of the abdominal muscles with relaxation of the gastric cardia which actively force the gastric contents back up the esophagus.

Vomiting is a symptom not related to GI disease only, but may be associated with diseases of the central nervous system, respiratory system, urinary system as well as with any infection or emotional stress. Vomiting with an organic GI disease is characterized by a bile stained vomitus and associated with nausea and weight loss. Early morning, projectile vomiting without nausea indicates increased intracranial pressure. In respiratory disease, the child has an episode of severe cough followed by vomiting. Metabolic derangements may lead to severe persistent vomiting.

Conditions that Resembles Vomiting

Regurgitation or effortless movement of stomach contents into the esophagus and mouth should be differentiated from vomiting. With regurgitation, the child is well and is often hungry immediately after the episode. It is a result of gastroesophageal reflux or in infants an immature lower esophageal sphincter. It is a developmental process and resolves spontaneously with maturity.

Rumination resembles vomiting. It consists of repetitive, effortless regurgitation of recently ingested food into the mouth followed by rechewing and reswallowing or expulsion. The pathophysiology of rumination is not clear. It is commonly seen in children with mental retardation, neglected children, untreated GER, in association with bulimia and anorexia nervosa. Behaviour modification is the most effective treatment.

Table 10.5 : Showing causes of vomiting

Infant	*Child*	*Adolescent*
Common	**Common**	**Common**
Gastroesophageal reflux	Gastritis	Gastroenteritis
Over feeding	Gastroenteritis	Gastritis
Intestinal obstruction	Pertussis	Systemic infection
Gastroenteritis	Systemic infection	Migraine
Systemic infection	Sinusitis	Sinusitis
Pertussis syndrome	Otitis media	Gastroesophageal reflux (GER)
	Gastroesophageal reflux	Appendicitis
Rare	**Rare**	**Rare**
Adrenogenital syndrome	Reye's syndrome	Reye's syndrome
Inborn errors of metabolism	Increased intracranial pressure	Hepatitis
Renal tubular acidosis	Pancreatitis	Peptic ulcer
Increased intracranial pressure	Migraine	Pancreatitis
	Peptic ulcer	Increased intracranial pressure
	Inborn errors of metabolism	Biliary colic
		Renal colic
		Migraine
		Middle ear disease

(Adapted from Nelson Textbook of Pediatrics, 17th edition, 2004)

An Approach to Diagnosis

While taking the history of vomiting one should give stress on the following points: onset, number, character, timing, contents and colour of the vomitus and associated symptoms.

Physical examination should include

- Examination of hydration status
- Systemic examination of the abdomen, respiratory system and central nervous system.

Table 10.6 : Showing associated signs and symptoms

Associated symptoms and signs	*Etiology*
Jaundice	Hepatitis, cholecystitis, cholangitis
Loose stools	Acute gastroenteritis
Headache, seizure and fever	Meningitis
Seizures and vomiting without nausea, diplopia, ataxia	Intracranial space occupying lesion
Dysuria and increased frequency	Urinary tract infection
Right iliac fossa pain, fever	Acute appendicitis
Vertigo, tinnitus and deafness	Vestibular pathology
Pain abdomen, distension	Intestinal obstruction

Complications of Vomiting

1. Mallory-Weiss tear.
2. Failure to thrive.
3. Dehydration.
4. Electrolyte imbalance viz. hyponatremia, hypokalemia.
5. Alkalosis.
6. Peptic esophagitis.

Danger Signs

- Child has fever.
- Child's vomiting is getting worse.
- Child will not drink the rehydration fluid (ORS) or keeps vomiting up the ORS.
- Child has projectile vomiting (forceful bursts of vomit) after a feed.
- Child's age is less than four months and has vomiting that is different than regular spitting up.

Indications for Hospitalization

- Vomiting up all liquids that are given.
- Dehydration.
- Hematemesis.
- Very sick.
- History of consumption of poisonous food, plant, or substance.
- Altered sensorium, a stiff neck, or very bad headache.
- Severe abdominal pain that does not feel better after vomiting.
- Dysuria.
- Difficulty in breathing.

Investigation

All cases should have the screening tests done. The specific tests should be done as and when necessary.

Screening Tests

1. Complete blood count.
2. Urine routine analysis and culture.
3. Stool examination for parasites, occult blood.
4. Urine for bile salts and pigments/ALT to exclude an icteric hepatitis.
5. Blood urea nitrogen (when chronic renal failure is suspected).

Specific Tests

Selection of the specific tests will depend on the findings of history and physical examination.

1. A plain X-ray abdomen (erect posture) in suspected intestinal obstruction.
2. Barium studies in suspected gastroesophageal reflux, malrotation of the gut and hypertrophic pyloric stenosis.
3. USG in hypertrophic pyloric stenosis.
4. Upper GI endoscopy in GER, biopsy for H. pylori, examination of duodenal aspirate for giardia.
5. CT scan/MRI for intracranial space occupying lesions.
6. ABG and metabolic screen for inborn errors of metabolism in neonates.

Management

Symptomatic Treatment

Vomiting is symptomatically treated with antiemetics. The commonly used antiemetics are metoclopramide, domperidone and odansetron.

Metoclopramide act centrally in the emetic centre through antagonism of the dopamine D2 receptor. It also acts as an antroduodenal prokinetic agent. Metoclopramide may cause extrapyramidal side effects if the dose is not calculated properly. It is useful in post-operative nausea and vomiting, chemotherapy and radiotherapy induced vomiting and GERD. The dose is 0.5 to 2 mg/kg/day 6 - 8 hourly per oral/IM.

Domperidone is a weaker antiemetic compared to metoclopramide. It acts primarily as a peripheral dopamine D2 receptor antagonist. It also decreases proximal gastric relaxation and facilitates gastric emptying. Its main use is in the management of GERD. The dose is 0.3 mg/kg/dose per oral/IM may be repeated after 8 hours.

Odansetron is a highly selective 5HT3 antagonist. It is usually well tolerated but may cause headache, constipation and dizziness. It is a useful drug for preventing nausea and vomiting in children receiving chemotherapy and radiotherapy. The dose is 0.15mg/kg orally or IV given 30 minutes before chemotherapy.

It needs mention that antiemetics should be prescribed in children after knowing the cause. They are contraindicated in vomiting secondary to diarrhoea, structural abnormalities of GIT, acute appendicitis and increased intracranial tension.

Antiemetic use is recommended in the following: Chemotherapy/radiotherapy induced vomiting, post operative vomiting, cyclic vomiting and vomiting due to motility disorders.

Supportive Treatment

Fluid: The treatment of dehydration resulting from persistent vomiting should be in the recommended line of treatment. The best fluid to be used for correction of severe dehydration is normal saline. Ringer lactate should not be used. A child with persistent vomiting develops hyperchloremic hypokalemic alkalosis. Ringer lactate can cause aggravation of alkalosis because lactate is converted to bicarbonate.

Food: Normal food for age given in small frequent feeds. This tends to minimize the tendency to vomit.

Specific Treatment

The specific treatment should be directed to the cause of vomiting.

Pain Abdomen: Approach to Diagnosis

Abdominal pain is a very common symptom for which a child is brought for consultation. Abdominal pain can result from the following reasons:

1. Inflammatory lesions of intra abdominal structures.
2. Distension of hollow viscus where discomfort is often felt as pain.
3. Increased peristaltic activity of hollow organs.
4. Referred from extra abdominal structures like pleura, spine etc whose dermatomes are represented in the abdominal region. Examples of conditions with referred pain in the abdomen are basal pneumonia and caries of thoracic vertebra.

Abdominal pain is usually felt in the same dermatome which shares the neurological supply with the underlying organ. For example, pain arising from stomach is felt in the epigastric region; while that arising from bladder is felt over the supra pubic region. Intestinal pain is usually felt at the umbilical region.

Classification

Pain abdomen may be acute and recurrent. Acute abdominal pain may be due to medical and surgical causes.

In case of acute abdominal pain, a careful evaluation should be made to rule out an underlying surgical cause and in recurrent abdominal pain, an organic cause has to be excluded before making a diagnosis of psychogenic pain. A strong consideration of an underlying surgical cause should be made if pain is the first symptom in the triad pain, vomiting and fever. On the other hand, in similar circumstances when fever and vomiting precede the onset of pain, the underlying cause is more likely to be medical in nature.

Recurrent abdominal pain is defined as occurrence of more than two episodes of pain abdomen over a period of 3 months. Recurrent abdominal pain may be organic or non-organic or psychogenic. The features suggesting an organic cause of recurrent abdominal pain are as follows:

1. Age below 3 years.
2. Consistent, well localized pain, away from the umbilicus.
3. Presence of tenderness/rigidity on local examination.
4. Associated features viz. fever, rash, joint pain, jaundice, hypertension.

Table 10.7 : Causes of acute abdominal pain

Child below 2 years age	*Child above 2 years age*
Medical Causes	**Medical Causes**
Acute gastroenteritis	Acute gastroenteritis
Basal Pneumonia	Intestinal worms
Hepatitis	Inflammatory bowel disease
Spontaneous bacterial peritonitis	Acute hepatitis and pancreatitis
Urinary tract infection	Mesenteric adenitis
	Urinary tract infection and renal calculi
Surgical Causes	Henoch-Schönlein purpura
Acute appendicitis	Lead poisoning, Diabetes ketoacidosis
Incarcerated inguinal hernia	Peptic ulcer disease
Volvulus, intussusception and malrotation	Liver abscess
Necrotizing enterocolitis	Congestive heart failure
Choledochal cyst	Rheumatic pericarditis
	Crisis in sickle cell and hereditary spherocytosis
	Acute hepatic porphyria
	Surgical Causes
	Acute appendicitis
	Meckel's diverticulum
	Intestinal obstruction
	Cholecystitis
	Peritonitis
	Incarcerated inguinal hernia
	Trauma

Approach to Diagnosis of Acute Abdominal Pain

A child presenting with acute pain abdomen should be thoroughly evaluated to exclude a surgical cause and then decide whether the child needs admission or can be treated as an outpatient.

Features of a surgical cause	*Indications of hospitalization*
Acute onset pain	Child appears ill, lethargic
Bilious vomiting	Rolling about with pain
Blood in stools	Alert but lying still
Diarrhoea with abdominal distension	Presence of features of a surgical cause
Presence of point of tenderness	
Presence of a palpable mass	
Signs suggestive of peritonitis	

Points to be Noted in Taking the History

1. Onset of pain and progression.
2. Location of pain. Presence or absence of radiation of pain.
3. Character of pain.
4. Any interference of normal activity.
5. Presence of associated symptoms viz. anorexia, nausea, vomiting, diarrhoea, constipation.
6. Presence of systemic symptoms viz. fever, headache, chills and rigor.
7. Presence extra abdominal symptoms viz. burning micturation, dysuria, chest pain, difficulty in breathing, dyspnea.

Physical Examination

A thorough general examination should be done keeping in mind the following in particular:

1. *Appearance:* Whether the child looks well or ill.
2. *Decubitus:* Is the child in a particular position to get relief of pain?
3. *Examination of vitals:* Pulse, blood pressure (to assess hemodynamic status), respiratory rate and temperature.
4. Examination of oral cavity and tongue, skin for purpuric spots.
5. Pallor, jaundice.
6. Edema.

Rectal Examination

A rectal examination should be done in children with abdominal pain and suspicion of intussusception. A dark ring around the rectal mucosa may be an early sign of lead poisoning.

Systemic Examination

The priority system for examination is the abdomen. The abdomen should be examined for distension, tenderness, organomegaly, abnormal mass and bowel sounds.

The respiratory, cardiovascular and neurological systems should be examined to exclude extra abdominal causes of acute pain abdomen.

Laboratory Investigations

The investigations should be picked up on the basis of the findings of clinical findings. The list includes the following:

1. Complete blood count: The following findings help in diagnosis:
   - *Microcytic hypochromic anemia:* May indicate peptic ulcer disease, inflammatory bowel disease.
   - *Basophilic stippling:* Lead poisoning.
   - *Polymorpho leucocytosis:* Urinary tract infection and infection of GIT.
   - *Eosinophilia:* Parasitic infections.
2. Urine analysis:
   - Routine examination and culture.
   - Watson-Schwartz test for porphobilinogen.
3. Stool examination for :
   - Routine examination, parasites and ova.
   - Tests for occult blood.
4. Biochemical test viz. serum amylase and lipase in case of diseases of pancreas.
5. Plain X-ray abdomen (in erect posture) which will help to rule out:
   - Intestinal obstruction.
   - Gall stones and renal calculi.
6. Barium study will help to confirm diagnosis of:
   - Malrotation.
   - Intestinal tuberculosis.
7. Ultrasonography, an non-invasive test, can help diagnosis of:
   - Choledochal cyst.
   - Gall stones.
   - Renal calculi.
   - Retro peritoneal mass.
   - Hydronephrosis.
8. Endoscopy is indicated only in patients with significant pain in whom a mucosal abnormality of upper or lower gut is suspected. It is usually not necessary in acute pain abdomen.

Recurrent Abdominal Pain

Recurrent abdominal pain (RAP) is a frequent and troublesome complaint in childhood and adolescence. It is probably the most common form of pain complain of children below 15 years age. It has been reported to occur in 10% to 15% of children between the ages of 4–16 years. The male to female ratio is 1: 2. The term recurrent abdominal pain was first coined by the British pediatrician John Apley in 1958.

The child is said to be suffering from RAP when there are at least 3 bouts of significant abdominal pain occurring over 3 months, the severe phase lasting at least 3 minutes occurring usually in children above 3 years of age.

'Significant pain' is usually a subjective decision. Generally, any abdominal pain that disturbs the daily routine of the child like studies, schooling, eating, sleep etc. can be considered as significant pain.

Causes of Recurrent Abdominal Pain

- **Dysfunctional**
- **Psychogenic**
- **Organic**

Infective

- Parasitic: Giardiasis, Amebiasis and Helminthiasis.
- Bacterial: Tuberculosis, Clostridium difficile, Yersinia, Campylobacter.
- Virus: CMV gastritis.

Inflammatory

- Gastroesophageal reflux disease (GERD), NSAID ulcer, Peptic ulcer, H. pylori, Gastritis, Eosinophilic gastroenteritis, Henoch-Schönlein purpura (HSP).
- Inflammatory Bowel Disease: Ulcerative colitis, Crohn's disease.
- Colitis: Lymphocytic, Collagenous.

Obstructive

- Malrotation with or without volvulus.
- Intussusception with lead point.
- Tuberculosis.
- Post surgical adhesions.
- Small bowel lymphoma.
- Crohn's disease.
- Eosinophilic GE.
- Angioneurotic edema.

Contd.

Contd.

- Malabsorption: Lactose, carbohydrate intolerance, celiac disease.

Motility

- Constipation gastroparesis, pseudobstruction, biliary dyskinesia.

Gynecologic

- Dysmenorrhea, tubo-ovarian mass.

Systemic

- Renal disease, chronic pancreatitis, chronic hepatitis, chronic cholecystitis.

Neurological

- Abdominal migraine, epilepsy, porphyria, psychiatric disorders.

Others

- Musculoskeletal, drugs, food allergies etc.

Clinical Manifestations

Children who have recurrent abdominal pain tend to exhibit one of the three clinical presentations: (i) Isolated paroxysmal abdominal pain, (ii) Abdominal pain associated with symptoms of dyspepsia (epigastric pain, nausea, vomiting, regurgitation, early satiety, bloating or belching and, in the presence of negative evaluation and no response to acid-blocking medication), and (iii) Abdominal pain associated with altered bowel movement with diarrhea, constipation or sensation of incomplete evacuation of bowel.

Steps of Evaluation

Once history suggests the possibility of recurrent abdominal pain, the *first step* is to rule out two situations: acute abdomen and malingering. Malingering is a situation where the child feels no pain at all but nevertheless complains of abdominal pain either for seeking attention or to avoid unpleasant tasks like exams, homework etc. The *next step* in evaluation of a child with recurrent abdominal is to determine the type of RAP.

Types of RAP

Recurrent abdominal pain may be of three types: Organic, psychogenic and dysfunctional.

Organic Pain

Around 15% of the recurrent abdominal pain is due to an organic cause. More than 80% of abdominal pain from organic causes, present as acute abdominal pain, or as recurrent pain which do not fit into the pattern of RAP syndrome. Some examples of organic recurrent abdominal pain which may be misdiagnosed easily as non-organic are:

1. *Sub Acute Appendicitis:* While controversy exists if appendicitis can be sub acute or chronic, it is well established that acute appendicitis if missed or inadequately treated can go on for a smoldering inflammation of the appendix which presents as recurrent abdominal pain. The typical right iliac fossa tenderness may be easily missed unless carefully looked for.
2. *Gastritis/Duodenitis:* Can be missed unless the child is subjected to an upper GI endoscopy.
3. *Constipation:* This is a fairly common cause of RAP often missed since the doctor doesn't elicit the history nor are the parents usually aware of the bowel habits of the children beyond the age of 2-3 years. This is an easily treatable and curable condition which should be picked up at the first consult itself.
4. *Helicobacter Pylori Infection:* Its role in causing RAP is still controversial but enough evidence exists that RAP with significant epigastric tenderness is often due to H. pylori infection. This organic cause can be easily missed unless an endoscopy and antral biopsy is done.
5. *Gastroesophageal Reflux:* This is not an uncommon phenomenon in children and the gold standard for diagnosis being 24 hours pH monitoring. It is not surprising that the diagnosis is often missed or over/underdiagnosed.
6. *Pin Worms and Giardiasis* are common gastro-intestinal infections where child can present with RAP.
7. *Malrotation of Gut* is a congenital anomaly of the small intestine which may be missed as a cause of RAP.
8. Hydronephrosis.

There are several other organic causes like gallbladder stones, peptic ulcer disease, etc. which can also present as RAP. But all of them have distinct clinical features and specific tests for diagnosis which makes it unlikely that they will be missed in a routine work up for RAP. The red flag signs that could reflect an organic disease of isolated paroxysmal RAP include the following:

Red Flag Signs

1. Pain awakening the child at night.
2. Pain further away from the umbilicus.

3. Presence of fever, jaundice, abdominal distension, dysuria, bilious vomiting, weight loss, growth deceleration, arthralgia, rash.
4. Positive family history of peptic ulcer and irritable bowel syndrome (IBS).
5. Blood in stools (Guaiac-positive).
6. Changes in bowel function.
7. Intermittent fecal incontinence.
8. Anemia.
9. Dysuria.
10. Elevated erythrocyte sedimentation rate.

Psychogenic Pain

Around 10% of RAP syndrome have a clearly recognizable psychiatric basis and need active psychiatric therapy. Besides abdominal pain, these children also have other behavioural disorders and a close connection to some precipitating events which make clinical diagnosis easy. These include school phobia, psychosis secondary to intra family problems and tragedies, depression, complaint modeling etc. In these situations the psychiatric component overshadows the problem of RAP.

Dysfunctional Pain

This constitutes the bulk (75%) of RAP seen in clinical practice wherein children complain of significant abdominal pain occurring over several weeks or months and clinical exam/all investigations fail to reveal an organic component. These children have normal behaviour pattern and are often quite intelligent. They do not have any significant psychiatric problem and no obvious precipitating factors besides routine stresses of childhood like exams, peer pressure, home work etc.

Pathogenesis of Dysfunctional Pain

Every body's intestines have variable number of non-propulsive spasmodic contractions whose number/amplitude is never severe enough to be felt by the individual as pain. In children with dysfunctional pain, these contractions are more severe, more sustained, and more frequent and hence felt as recurrent abdominal pain. This is the somatic component of dysfunctional pain. For reasons poorly understood, these contractions are more during periods of stress explaining the increased frequency of RAP nearer exams and other routine stresses of childhood. Dysfunctional abdominal pain is also sometimes called irritable bowel syndrome, to emphasize the role of spasmodic intestinal contraction creating the pain. However, now clear understanding exists of the connection between IBS of childhood and IBS of adults which presents as recurrent diarrhoea/constipation.

Characteristics of Dysfunctional Pain

1. Age commonly affected is 4–13 years with predominance in girls after 9 years age.
2. Symptoms are nonspecific.
3. The pain is usually described as a dull ache (may be colicky) in the periumbilical region or mid epigastrium that rarely radiates to other sites.
4. There is no consistent duration, frequency and periodicity, usually unrelated to food, bowel habit or other habits.
5. The pain is usually brief (< 1 hour) with fairly asymptomatic pain free interval inbetween, which ranges from days to weeks and improvement during weekends and school vacations.
6. The pain does not awaken the child from sleep or interfere with pleasurable activities.
7. Associated symptoms like headache, nausea, limb tingling, sleep difficulties and enuresis is common.
8. Growth and development are normal.

An Approach to a Case of RAP

While clinical examination should give a very good clue as to which of the above 3 groups of RAP we are dealing with, all RAP cases require a basic workup to rule out organic causes. All cases require:

- CBC, urine RE, stool exam, Mantoux test.
- CXR.
- LFT.
- Serum urea and creatinine.
- Serum amylase and lipase.

Most cases will require:

- USG (Abdomen).
- Barium swallow, meal, follow-through.

Selected cases will require:

- Upper GI endoscopy.
- Antral/Duodenal biopsy/H. pylori studies.

The positive yield from scopies (which is an invasive procedure) will improve if it is restricted to children with food related pain, epigastric pain, and epigastric tenderness.

When significant pain persists (all investigations are negative) and an organic cause is still suspected it may be worthwhile to arrange for screening for:

- Porphyria.
- Henoch-Schönlein purpura.
- Lead poisoning.
- Meckel's screening.

Management

Psychogenic Pain

The treatment of psychogenic pain requires psychiatric evaluation and treatment.

Organic Pain

Organic RAP resulting from specific organic causes require specific therapy.

Dysfunctional Pain

The child's complaint should be considered seriously and a careful history and thorough physical examination should be done in all cases. This reassures the parents and at times has an early therapeutic effect. The basic investigations should be done. Then the parents as well as the older child are to be assured that there is no serious underlying disorder and at the same time it should be informed that the pain is not imaginary. However, the parents should be instructed to avoid reinforcing the symptoms showing excessive concern. The child should be encouraged to participate in regular activities like school attendance and healthy exercises.

The child should be followed up. Successful management depends on close follow-up. It is more important when the family is not completely satisfied with the consultation and advice. It is also possible that an organic problem may not be apparent in the initial visit, but with time, the symptom complex may become more typical.

Pharmacologic therapy with antispasmodic, anticholinergic, antidepressant agents have not proved to be effective in children with dysfunctional RAP. However, medications sometimes may have a transient placebo effect. Biofeedback and relaxation technique have been useful in some children with functional pain.

Referral to a pediatric gastroenterologist or pediatric surgeon may be necessary in some cases to provide reassurance to both the parents and the clinician that nothing has been missed.

A full balanced diet should be advised for the child. Iron supplementation should be advised to prevent or treat deficiency anemia. The child should be also advised anthelmentics at 6 months interval.

Prognosis

With proper approaches and support from the physician, most children with dysfunctional RAP improve resulting in reduction or elimination of abdominal symptoms. But some children continue to have abdominal or other pain syndrome into adulthood. They become adults with functional disorders although nature of symptoms may change.

Helminthiasis

The helminthes of importance to human beings are divided into three main groups: nematodes or round worms, the cystodes or tapeworms, and the trematodes or flukes. Only the commonly encountered helminthic diseases have been described in this chapter viz. infestation with nematodes and cystodes.

NEMATODES OR ROUND WORMS

The most common round worm infestations include: Ascariasis, Enterobiasis, Trichuriasis, Hookworm and Filariasis.

ASCARIASIS

Ascariasis is widely distributed throughout the tropics and extends to the temperate zones as far north and south as latitude 40 degrees. Children between 1 and 10 years age is more infected by ascariasis than older children.

Etiology

Ascariasis is produced by the largest round worm ascariasis lumbricoides. It normally lives in the lumen of the host's small intestine. The mature female worm measures 20–35 cm in length and 3–6 mm in the greatest diameter and the male is about one fifth smaller. Both sexes have a triangular mouth surrounded by three fleshy lips. Both taper to a sharp posterior end, with the male curved ventrally at the posterior end. The female lays approximately 200,000 eggs each day which gets fertilized in presence of a male worm. The fertilized eggs are passed in the patient's feces in the one cell stage.

Pathology

The fertile eggs are able to survive practically all external conditions except heat and extreme desiccation. When deposited in a suitably moist medium in warm weather, the eggs embryonate within 9 days or more and contains a motile first stage larva. A week later, the eggs become infective. These eggs remain infective and viable for months to several years. The children take them into the mouth on contaminated fingers or play objects or as a result of eating dirt.

When the infective eggs are swallowed and reach the duodenum they hatch and the escaping larva enter the intestinal wall. The larvae penetrate into the mesenteric lymphatics or venules, and commonly migrating through the liver are carried to the lungs. After growth and one molt in the lungs, the third stage larvae reach the epiglottis from where it is swallowed and reaches the small intestine where they grow into adult worms. Between 60–75 days after the eggs are swallowed, the mature worms mate and the female worm starts laying eggs.

An acute cellular infiltration occurs in the immediate vicinity of the larvae. Large number of larvae migrating through the lungs produces Loeffler syndrome or atypical pneumonia. If the adult worms get irritated owing to digestive disturbances or fever, they may pass down the bowel to be spontaneously evacuated or they may enter the stomach to be vomited, or escapes through the nares. They may block the appendix, perforate the intestinal wall, block the common bile duct, migrate into the parenchyma of the liver or reach the pleural cavity.

Clinical Manifestations

The most common complaint of children is intestinal colic. However, intestinal infection with ascaris may be asymptomatic, or there may be such manifestations like nausea and vomiting, anorexia, loss of weight, insomnia, and low grade fever.

Children with heavy infestation may present with vomiting, abdominal distension and cramps. Worms may be passed in stool and vomitus. A large mass of worm may cause intestinal obstruction. Worms may migrate into the biliary and pancreatic ducts causing cholecystitis and pancreatitis. It is not clear whether ascariasis effects growth and development. However, some believe that children with recurrent heavy infection are at risk of protein energy malnutrition.

During the development in the lungs the larvae may cause an atypical pneumonia. There may be manifestations of asthma, urticaria and eosinophilia as a result of ascaris allergy. Loeffler syndrome, characterized by transitory symptoms such as cough and dyspnea, pulmonary infiltrates and blood eosinophilia with larvae in sputum is a common manifestation of pulmonary ascariasis.

Laboratory Diagnosis

Laboratory diagnosis may be described under two heads: direct and indirect evidences.

Direct evidence includes demonstration of adult worms in stool or vomitus and demonstration of ova in stool by microscopical examination of a saline emulsion of stool specimen. Sometimes barium study of the gastrointestinal tract for other purposes demonstrates worms. *Indirect evidence* includes eosinophilia in the early stages of invasion.

Treatment

Several chemotherapeutic agents are available for treatment of intestinal infestation but no effective agent is available to treat pulmonary phase of the infection. The treatment options for gastrointestinal ascariasis available include albendazole (200 mg per oral below 2 years, 400 mg per oral once above 2 years), mebendazole, used only above 2 years age (100 mg twice daily × 3 days) and pyrantel pamoate (11 mg/kg/dose, maximum 1 gm one dose).

For intestinal or biliary obstruction, piperizine citrate is the drug of choice. It is given in a dose of 150 mg/kg orally initially followed by six doses of 65 mg/kg at 12 hours interval per oral. It is given in the syrup form through a nasogastric tube. It causes neuromuscular paralysis of the parasite and rapid expulsion of the worms. Severe intestinal obstruction by ascaris may require surgery.

Prevention

The long-term measures include improvement of sanitary conditions and sewage facilities and health education.

Short-term measure includes anthelmintic therapy every 6 months which can be implemented in one of the three following ways:

1. Universal treatment to all individual in highly endemic areas.

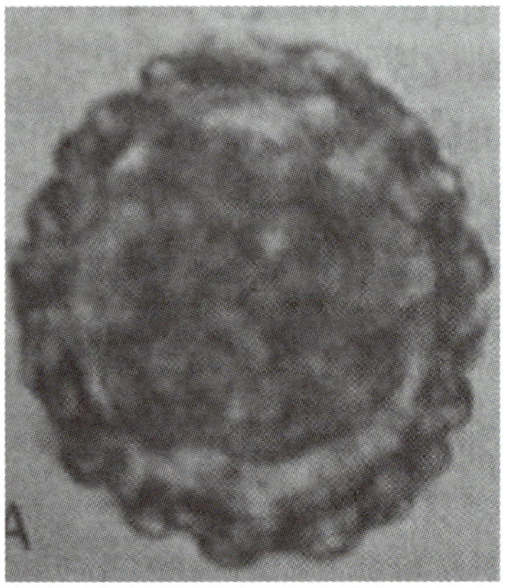

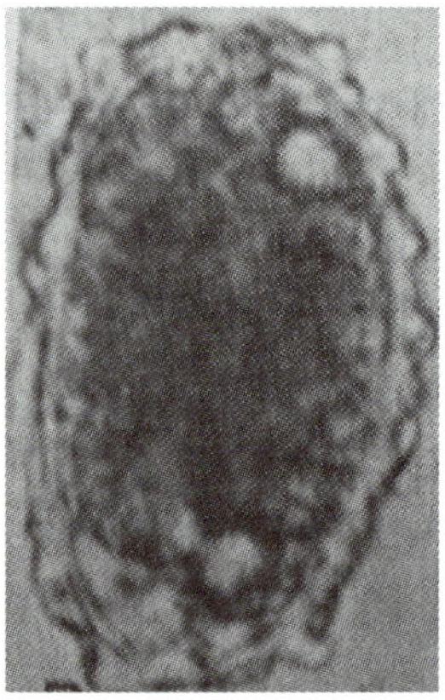

Fertilized **Unfertilized**

Ova of ascaris lumbricoides

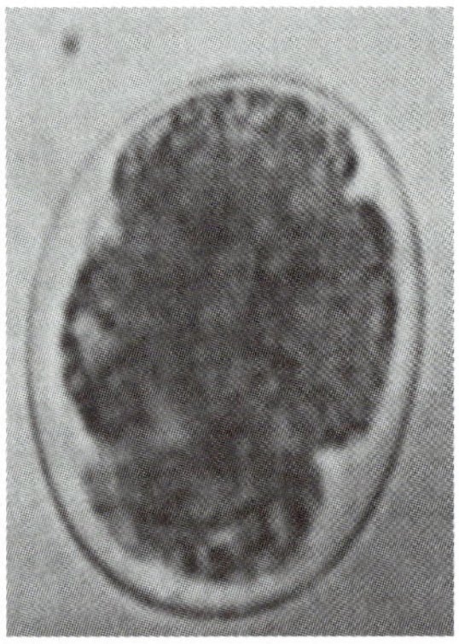

Ova of hookworm

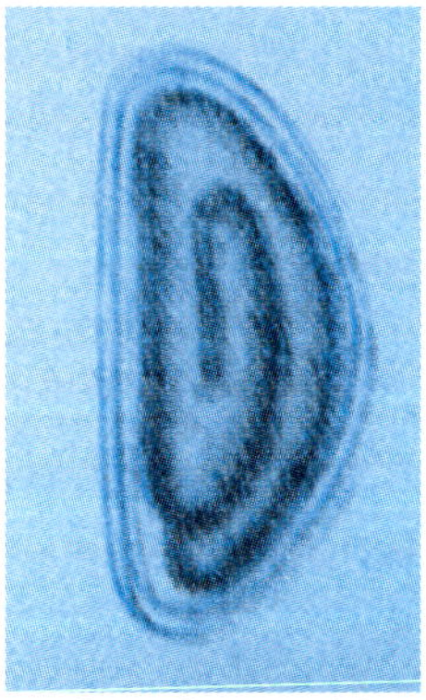

Ova of enterobius vermicularis

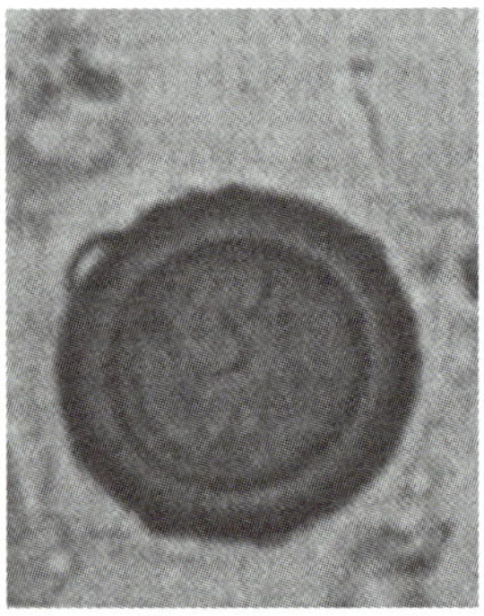

Ova of T. solium or T. saginata

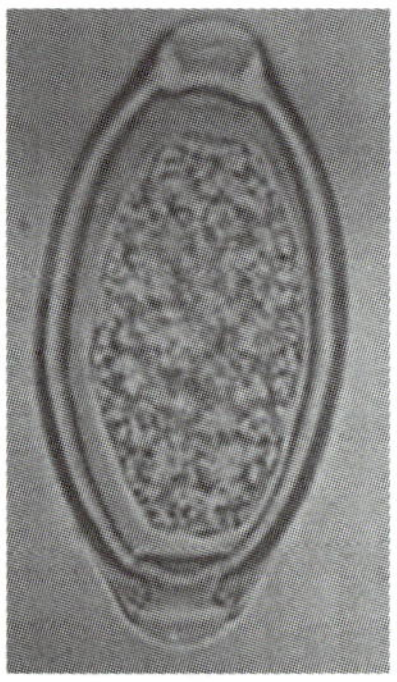

Ova of trichuris trichiura

Fig. 10.1: Ova of different nematodes

2. Offering treatment to target groups with high frequency of infection, e.g., preschool children.
3. Offering individual treatment based on intensity of recent or past infection.

ENTEROBIASIS

Enterobiasis or pinworm infection has a worldwide distribution. It occurs in all age groups irrespective of socioeconomic status. The prevalence of infection is highest in children from 5–14 years. Infection is common in areas where children live, play and sleep close together, thus facilitating egg transmission. Autoinoculation can occur in individuals who have the habit of putting the fingers in their mouth.

Etiology

Enterobiasis is caused by enterobius vermicularis. It is a nematode, 1 cm in length, white and threadlike. It typically inhabits the cecum, appendix and the adjacent areas of the ileum and ascending colon. The gravid female worms migrate at night to the perianal and perineal regions where they deposit eggs. Human infection occurs by ingestion of embryonated eggs that are carried on finger nails, clothing, bedding or house dust. The eggs embryonate within 6 hours of laying and larvae mature to form adult worms in 36–53 days after ingestion.

Clinical Manifestations

The most common complaints include nocturnal itching of the perianal and perineal regions and restless sleep. Rarely there may be development of perianal granuloma containing live or dead worms which may require surgical excision.

Aberrant migration to ectopic sites occasionally may lead to appendicitis, salpingitis, peritonitis, hepatitis and ulcerative lesions in the small and large intestine.

Laboratory Diagnosis

Enterobiasis is essentially a clinical diagnosis. Nocturnal perianal pruritus in children strongly suggests the diagnosis. Routine stool sample examination rarely demonstrates the ova.

Microscopic examination of adhesive cellophane tape pressed against the perianal region early in the morning frequently demonstrates eggs.

Worms can be demonstrated in the perianal region.

Treatment

Several anthelmintic drugs are used to treat enterobiasis. The drug should be administered to the infected individual and their family members. The drugs used are a single dose of Mebendazole (100 mg per oral, above 2 years old), single oral dose of Albendazole (200 mg per oral below 2 years, 400 mg per oral for above 2 years) repeated after 2 weeks or a single oral dose of pyarental pamoate (11 mg/kg/dose, maximum 1 gm).

Prevention

Repeated treatment every 3–4 months may be required in circumstances with repeated exposure such as institutionalized children. There is no evidence that personal cleanliness has a role in control of enterobiasis.

HOOKWORMS

(Ancylostoma Duodenale and Necator Americanus)

Hookworm infection is widely distributed in all tropical and subtropical countries. It occurs mostly in areas with high humidity because adequate soil moisture, warmth and shade are required for the development of the ova in soil. It is more common in rural areas where sanitation is inadequate or where human feces are used as fertilizers. China and India has the highest prevalence.

Etiology

Two species of hookworms infect human–Ancylostoma duodenale and Necator americanus.

The infective larval stage of both the hookworms lives in a developmentally arrested state in warm, moist soil. The larvae infect men either by penetrating through the skin (both species) or when they are ingested (Ancylostoma duodenale). After penetrating through the skin, the larvae travel through the venous circulation and lungs and are swallowed. When orally ingested they either travel through the venous circulation or remain in the gastrointestinal tract. In the small intestine they undergo two molts to become adult sexually mature male and female worms. The adult worms are around 5–13 mm in length. They are armed with teeth (A. duodenale) or cutting plates by which they attach to the mucosa and sub mucosa of the small intestine.

The hookworms can remain in the small intestine for 1–5 years where they mate and produce eggs. Eggs that are passed out and deposited on the soil with adequate moisture develop into first stage larvae and hatch. Over the ensuing several days, under appropriate conditions, the larvae molt twice to the infective stage. They migrate vertically in the soil until they either infect a new host or die after exhausting their lipid metabolic reserves.

Pathogenesis

Human hookworm infection result in blood loss. The adult worms adhere tenaciously into the mucosa and submucosa of the proximal small intestine. Each adult A. duodenale causes loss of an estimated 0.2 ml of blood/ 24 hours. Blood loss is less for N. americanus. Mild infection causes *hookworm infection* with very little blood loss and no anemia. Moderate to severe infection results in *hookworm disease* characterized by sufficient blood loss to develop iron deficiency anemia. With pre-existing dietary deficiency there may be hypoalbuminemia and consequent edema and anasarca.

Clinical Features

Ancylostoma dermatitis or ground itch occurs at the site of entry. It is characterized by vesciculation and edema. The skin lesion precedes general symptoms by 2–4 months and generally disappears by 7–14 days. *Creeping eruptions* on the skin may be sometimes seen in N. americanus infection when the larvae creep through the skin. Bronchitis and bronchopneumonia may occur when the larvae break through the pulmonary capillaries and enter the alveoli. There may be laryngotracheo-bronchitis and pharyngitis. At this stage there may be marked eosinophilia.

Intestinal hookworm infection may be asymptomatic or there may be pain, anorexia and diarrhea. The major clinical manifestations are related to blood loss. With heavy infection the child suffer from anemia and signs of protein energy malnutrition. Children with chronic hookworm disease acquire a yellow green color of the skin which is called chlorosis.

An infantile form of ancylostomiasis has been described. It results from heavy infection and is characterized by diarrhoea, melena, failure to thrive and profound anemia with significantly high mortality.

Diagnosis

Confirmation of diagnosis is possible by direct examination of stool and identification of the eggs. Quantitative estimation may be done to assess the degree of infection. The eggs of both species are morphologically indistinguishable. Species identification can be done by examination of the third stage larvae. Newer methods of diagnosis using polymerase chain reaction are under development.

Treatment

The goals of therapy are removal of adult worms from the intestine and appropriate nutritional supplement for children with hookworm disease.

Albendazole (200 mg per oral below 2 years, 400 mg per oral one dose above 2 years) and mebendazole (100 mg twice daily × 3 days or 500 mg single doses, contraindicated below 2 years age) are effective in eliminating hookworms from the intestine. Pyrantel pamoate (11 mg/kg once, maximum 1 gm × 3 days) is an effective alternative. Iron salt preparation should be given to treat iron deficiency anemia.

Prevention

In highly endemic areas, in addition to use of anthelmintic every 6 months, improved sanitation, health education, avoidance of human feces as fertilizer and improvement of socioeconomic condition are critical for reducing endemicity. Work is in progress to use vaccines in humans against hookworm infection, prepared by genetic engineering of the hookworm antigen.

TRICHURIASIS

Trichuriasis has a worldwide distribution. It is especially common in the rural community with inadequate sanitary facilities and soil contaminated with human or animal feces. The highest rate of infection occurs among children between 5 and 15 years. Infection develops after ingesting embryonated eggs by direct contamination of hands, food (raw fruits and vegetables) or drink. Transmission can also occur indirectly through flies or other insects.

Etiology

Trichuriasis is caused by the nematode Trichuris trichiura. The adult worm resembles a whip, the anterior three fifth is very thin and hair like and the posterior two-fifth is thick and stout resembling the handle of the whip. The male worm measures 3–4 cm and the female 4–5 cm. An adult worm sucks approximately 0.005 ml of blood / worm/24 hours. The principal host of T. trichiura is humans. Humans acquire the infection by ingestion of embryonated eggs. The larvae escape from the shell in the upper intestine and penetrate the intestinal villi. The worms move towards the cecum. They inhabit the cecum with the anterior whip like portion remaining within the superficial mucosa and the short posterior end free in the lumen. The female worms start deposition of eggs in 1–3 months. They produce 5000 to 20,000 eggs/24 hours. After excretion in the feces, embryonic development occurs in 2–4 weeks with optimal temperature and soil conditions.

Clinical Features

Trichuriasis is mostly asymptomatic with low worm load. There may be complaints of right lower quadrant or periumbilical abdominal pain.

In children with heavy infection clinical manifestations include chronic dysentery, rectal prolapse, anemia, and failure to thrive as well as developmental and cognitive deficits.

Diagnosis

Diagnosis is by demonstration of the characteristic ova in fecal smears. The trichuris egg is barrel shaped with a mucus plug at both ends. It is brown in colour (bile stained), has a double shell, the outer one is bile stained.

Treatment

Mebendazole (100 mg twice daily per oral × 3 days or single dose 500 mg per oral) is safe and effective but contraindicated below 2 years age. Albendazole (200 mg per oral for below 2 years, 400 mg per oral once for above 2 years age) is an alternative. In heavy infections it may have to be administered for 3 days.

Prevention

Trichuriasis can be prevented by personal hygiene, improved sanitary conditions, and eliminating the use of human feces as fertilizer.

TAENIASIS

Taeniasis has a worldwide geographical distribution. Prevalence in young children depends on the cultural practice of how well meat is cooked and how much is served to children.

Etiology

Taeniasis is caused by the cestodes T. saginata (beef tapeworm) and T. solium (pork tape worm). The adult worms of both live in the human small intestine (upper jejunum). The intermediate host harbours the larval stage.

The length of the adult worm is about 2–3 metres (T. solium) and 5–10 metres (T. saginata). The intermediate host in case of the former is a pig whereas in the latter it is a cow or buffalo. Hence they are also called pork tapeworm and beef tape worm respectively. The body of the adult worm is a connected series of hundreds or thousands of flattened segments, called proglottids, the most anterior end of which is called the scolex. The scolex of T. solium measures 1 mm in diameter is globular in shape and has 4 circular suckers and a rostellum with a double row of alternating large and small hooklets. The scolex of T. saginata is large, quadrate, with suckers but without a rostellum and hooks. The scolex anchors the parasite to the bowel walls. New segments arise at the caudal end of the scolex and after 2–3 months the terminal segments mature and become gravid. The gravid terminal segments contain 50,000 to 1,00,000 eggs. The eggs or the intact segments are passed in the stool.

Clinical Features

Taeniasis is usually asymptomatic except for non-specific abdominal symptoms. The proglottids passed in the stool are visually striking and sometimes cause a strong emotional reaction in older children and parents. The proglottids are motile and may cause anal pruritus. The adult worm may rarely cause intestinal obstruction, cholangitis and appendicitis.

Diagnosis

As proglottids are passed in stool, visual examination for gravid proglottids in the stool is a sensitive test for diagnosis of both the taenia infection. The eggs are often absent and it is also difficult to distinguish between the eggs of the two tape worms. If the worm is completely expelled, the scolex of each species is diagnostic.

Treatment

Praziquantel (5–10 mg/kg per oral once) is an effective drug for both types of tapeworm infection. Praziquantel tend to cause parasite death as well as resorption unless purged. An alternative drug is niclosamide (50 mg/kg/ per oral once).

Prevention

Improved sanitation can interrupt transmission by preventing infection in livestock. Prolonged freezing or thorough cooking of pork and beef kills the parasite and thus can prevent human infection.

CYSTICERCOSIS

Cysticercosis is caused by infection with the intermediate stage of T. solium with development of cysticerci in the tissues in the same way as in the pig. It preferentially invades the CNS and causes neurocysticercosis.

Humans acquire the intermediate forms by ingestion of food or water contaminated with eggs of T. solium. Cysticercosis, may, therefore develop even in individuals who do not eat pork. Individuals infected with T. solium also can infect themselves with the eggs by fecal-oral route. Auto infection may also result from reverse peristalsis of the intestine whereby the gravid segments are thrown back to the stomach, equivalent to swallowing of eggs.

In the small intestine, the egg releases an oncosphere that crosses the gut wall and is carried by circulation to all parts of the body. Wherever the eggs lodge there is formation of a cyst which contains some fluid and a protoscolex. The common sites for cysticercosis are brain, muscles and connective tissue. Neurocysticercosis is the most common and serious parasitic infection of the central nervous system.

While they remain alive and intact, the cystic stage does not provoke a strong immunologic response. Most cysts remain viable for 5–10 years and then begin to degenerate, followed by a vigorous host response. The natural history of the cysts is to resolve by complete resorption or calcification.

Clinical Manifestations

Neurocysticercosis can be classified as parenchymal, intraventricular, meningeal, spinal, and ocular on the basis of the anatomical location. The clinical features differ according to the type.

In *parenchymal neurocysticercosis*, the most common presentation is a seizure which is generalized in 80% cases but may begin as a simple or complex partial seizure. With a heavy initial infection, the child may present with a stroke due to cerebral infarction as a result of obstruction of small terminal arteries or vasculitis or as fulminant encephalitis. Extensive involvement of the frontal lobe may give rise to symptoms of intellectual deterioration with dementia or Parkinsonism. *Intraventricular type* is associated with hydrocephalus and acute, subacute or intermittent signs of increased intracranial pressure.

Meningeal cysticercosis is associated with signs of meningeal irritation and increased intracranial pressure. *Spinal type* presents with evidence of spinal cord compression, transverse myelitis, or meningitis. *Ocular neurocysticercosis* cause decreased acuity of vision due to cysticerci floating in the vitreous or retinal detachment or iridocyclitis.

Outside the nervous system, cysts can be palpated under the skin. Heavy infection in skeletal and cardiac muscles can result in myositis or carditis.

Diagnosis

The most useful diagnostic study for parenchymal neurocysticercosis is a CT scan. An MRI is better to detect intraventricular cysts as well as those in the spinal cord. It can delineate parasite membranes and the differences in signal intensity between the fluids and the tissues of the cysticercus. The protoscolex may even be visible within the cyst by MRI which is a pathognomonic sign of cysticercosis.

Proglottids (segments) or eggs are found in stool in 25% cases of neurocysticercosis.

Serological diagnosis using the enzyme linked immunotransfer blot (EITB) is available. Patients with many parenchymal cysts almost always have a positive serum EITB test.

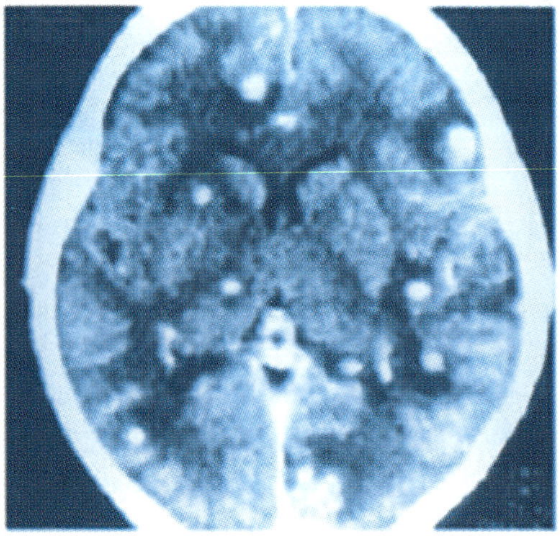

Fig. 10.2: A CT scan showing multiple neurocysticercosis

Treatment

Most treatment options of neurocysticercosis still remain controversial. Treatment may be medical or surgical.

Children with seizures, no hydrocephalous and only calcified, inactive lesions on CT require only anti-convulsant therapy. Parenchymal inflammation demonstrated by CT or MRI can be controlled using standard anticonvulsants.

Active parenchymal lesions usually resolve spontaneously. However, it has been shown that treatment with anti-cysticercal drugs is associated with fewer residual seizures on long-term follow-up.

The two effective drugs available are albendazole (15 mg/kg/day, maximum 800 mg/day two times daily, per oral for 28 days) and praziquantel (50–100 mg/kg/day 3 times daily, per oral for 30 days). Albendazole is found to be more effective than praziquantel. Many experts do not treat because administration of these drugs can cause worsening of the symptoms as the host responds to the dying parasite with increased inflammation. Corticosteroids (Prednisolone 1–2 mg/kg/day) for 2–3 days before and during drug therapy can ameliorate these effects. Antiparasitic therapy may also convert quiescent parenchymal lesion to active lesions or may worsen ventricular, spinal or ocular disease.

Surgical treatment is limited to placement of shunts, and removal of large and mobile cysts. Medical therapy in a child with evidence of hydrocephalous should always be preceded by a shunt as also in ventricular and spinal disease. Ocular cysticercosis needs surgery and in most cases enucleation is required.

HYMENOLEPIS

Hymenolepis is an infection with the dwarf tapeworm, hymenolepis nana. It is a prevalent disease in developing countries. It rarely causes overt disease. Although the intermediate stage develops in different hosts like rodents, fleas and ticks, the whole life cycle can be completed in human.

Diagnosis is made on the basis of presence of eggs in stool.

H. nana infection responds to Praziquantal (25 mg/kg per oral one dose) or Niclosamide (1gm per oral for children < 17 kg and 1.5 grams for 17 kg and above).

ECHINOCOCCOSIS/HYDATID DISEASE

Hydatid disease has a worldwide distribution although it is more common in the temperate climates.

Etiopathogenesis

It is caused by echinococcus granulosus, a tape worm also called dog tape worm. Man harbours the larval form.

The adult worm is harboured by the canine animals commonly the dog.

The adult worm measures around 3–6 mm in length. It comprises a scolex and a strobila of 3 or 4 segments. The first segment is immature, the second one is mature and the third one and fourth one (if present) is gravid. The terminal segment is the biggest, measuring 2–3 mm in length and 0.6 mm in breadth. The scolex bears 4 suckers and a rostellum with two circular rows of hooks. The eggs resembles other eggs of Taenia, contains a hexacanth embryo with 3 pairs of hooks.

The adult worms which lives in the small intestine of the definitive hosts viz. the dog or other canines like fox, jackals and wolves discharge eggs with the feces which contaminate the soil, water and the coats of the animals.

Humans are infected by ingesting food or water contaminated with eggs or by direct contact with infected animals usually a dog. In the duodenum, the embryos are hatched out. The embryos bore their way through the intestinal wall and are carried by vascular or lymphatic systems to the liver, lungs and less commonly to other tissues. Wherever the embryo settles it forms a hydatid cyst.

Two major echinococcus species are responsible for distinct clinical presentations. E. granulosus causes unilocular or cystic hydatid disease and the E. multilocularis which causes alveolar hydatid disease.

In areas where E. granulosus is endemic, the parasite is often acquired in childhood, but liver cysts require many years to become large enough to be detected or cause symptoms. In children, lungs appear to be the most common site. Cysts can develop in bone, the genitourinary system, bowels, subcutaneous tissue and brain. In E. multilocularis infection, there is formation of multiple cysts with more vigorous host reaction.

Epidemiology

Transmission of E. granulosus to human is common wherever animals are herded by humans with help of dogs. Transmission of E. multilocularis occurs primarily in temperate climate. It is, however, uncommon.

Clinical Manifestations

With a cyst in the lung, the child may present with cough, chest pain and hemoptysis. The cyst in the liver is asymptomatic in majority of cases and resolves spontaneously. It is a common cause of symptom less hepatomegaly. Some may have non-specific symptoms followed by increased abdominal girth, a palpable mass, vomiting or abdominal pain. There may be anaphylactic reaction if there is spillage of cyst fluid during surgery. Jaundice due to cystic hydatid disease is rare. The proliferating mass may compromise hepatic tissue or the biliary system and cause obstructive jaundice and hepatic failure. Bone cysts can cause pathological fracture. Cyst in the genitourinary system can produce hematuria.

Laboratory Diagnosis

A plain X-ray PA view chest can at times show a typical lung cyst.

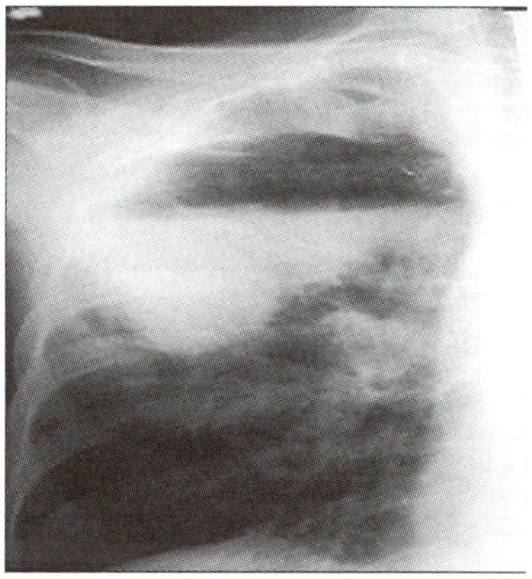

Fig. 10.3: (a) X-ray PA view chest showing a hydatid cyst

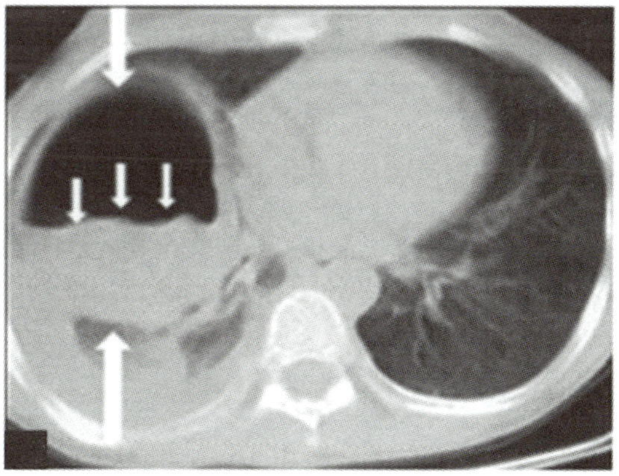

Fig. 10.3: (b) CT showing the water lily sign

Ultra sonography is a very useful tool for diagnosis of hydatid cyst. Presence of internal membranes and floating echogenic cyst material (hydatid sand) strongly suggests hydatid disease. CT findings are similar.

Protoscolices may be found in the sputum if a lung cyst ruptures.

Serological tests can be helpful but the false negative rate may be as high as 50% in hydatid disease of the lungs and in presence of young, intact liver cysts.

Treatment

Treatment is essentially surgical. The present preferred therapy for simple and easily accessible cysts however is USG or CT guided percutaneous aspiration, instillation of hypertonic saline or another scolicidal agent and reaspiration after 15 minutes (PAIR). The risk of spillage with PAIR is minimal. The risk of anaphylaxis is decreased by prophylactic medical therapy beginning before PAIR and continuing for a month thereafter. PAIR is contraindicated in bile stained cysts wherein risk of biliary complications is high.

Medical therapy alone may be attempted in patients where surgery and PAIR is contraindicated. The drug of choice is albendazole in a dose of 15 mg/kg/day in two divided doses (maximum 800 mg) for 2 weeks repeated for 3–12 courses with 15 days drug free interval inbetween two courses. The response to medical therapy is monitored by serial USG. Successful therapy is indicated by change in shape of cyst from spherical to elliptical or flat, progressive increase in echogenecity and separation of membranes from the capsule which is described as "water lily sign". CT findings are same. Albendazole therapy is safe. Common side effects include elevated transaminases and abdominal pain. Rarely there may be headache, abdominal distension or alopecia.

Prognosis

Prognosis is good if the age of the cyst is < 2 years, internal complexity of the cyst is low and size is small. Response to treatment is poor in bone cyst. Even after surgical removal, mortality is very high, within 10 years, in the alveolar type.

Prevention

Measures should be taken to interrupt transmission which includes thorough hand washing, avoiding contact with dogs in endemic areas, using boiled or filtered water, proper disposal of animal carcasses and meat inspection and proper disposal of refuse from slaughter houses.

The other measures include control and treatment of wild dogs and regular praziquantel treatment to pet and working dogs in endemic area.

FILARIASIS

Filariasis is a disease affecting the lymphatics. It results from infection with filarial worms viz. Wuchereria bancrofti, brugia malayi, loa loa and onchocerca volvulus. Lymphatic filariasis is caused by the former two and is common in our country. It is distributed along the sea coast and along the big rivers except Indus. It has also been reported from Rajasthan, Punjab, Uttar Pradesh and Delhi.

The Lymphatic Filariasis Worms and the Life Cycle

Wuchereria bancrofti, brugia malayi are threadlike nematodes that causes similar infections with similar clinical manifestations. The mosquito vector introduces the infective larvae into humans during a blood meal. The larval forms develop into adult worms over a period of 4–6 months. The worms reside in the afferent lymphatic vessels. Sexually mature adult female worms release large number of microfilariae that circulate in the blood stream. The mosquitoes, during a blood meal ingest the microfilariae which molt to form infective larvae over a period of 10 to 14 days and the life cycle is completed.

Clinical Manifestations

The early symptoms and signs include episodic fever, headache, myalgia, lymphangitis, of an extremity and lymphadenitis especially of the inguinal and axillary areas that last a few days to several weeks. The symptoms and signs of acute infection are most frequently observed in young persons. The chronic lymphatic filariasis which is characterized by hydrocele and elephantiasis, occurs mostly in adults 30 years of age or older. It is a result of anatomic and functional obstruction to lymph flow. Elephantiasis may involve one or more limbs, the scrotum, the breasts, or the vulva.

Tropical pulmonary eosinophilia can occur with microfilariae in the lungs and lymph nodes. It is seen mostly in men of 20–30 years of age but may occasionally occur in children. The clinical manifestations include paroxysmal nocturnal cough with dyspnea, fever, weight loss and fatigue. Hepatosplenomegaly and generalized lymphadenopathy are often seen in children. On auscultation of the chest there are rales and rhonchi.

Laboratory Diagnosis

Demonstration of microfilariae in the blood is confirmatory. The blood sample should be collected between 10 pm and 2 am.

The diagnosis of tropical pulmonary eosinophilia is suggested by residence in a filarial endemic area, eosinophilia (> 2,000/micro litre), increased serum IgE (> 1000 IU/mL) and high titres of antimicrofilarial antibodies in absence of microfilaria in blood. An X-ray PA view chest may show diffuse miliary mottling, increased bronchovascular markings, discrete opacities in the middle and basal regions of the lung or occasionally even a normal lung field.

Treatment

No antifilarial drug has been shown to modify the course of acute lymphangitis and acute lymphadenitis. Diethylcarbamazine may be given to asymptomatic patients with microfilaria in blood. It lowers the intensity of parasitemia and also kills a proportion of adult worms. Treatment with diethylcarbamazine is associated with complications like pruritus, fever, bodyache, hypertension and even death especially with high microfilarial levels. Hence the dose is increased gradually as 1 mg/kg per oral as a single dose on day 1; 1 mg/kg 3 times daily on day 2; 1–2 mg 3 times daily on day 3; and 6 mg/kg/day on days 4 to 15.

Tropical pulmonary eosinophilia responds to administration of diethylcarbamazine, 5 mg/kg/day per oral for 10 days. A second course may be required if there is a recurrence of symptoms.

Viral Hepatitis

Viral hepatitis is a major health problem in developing and developed countries. The term viral hepatitis is used to describe infection of the liver caused by hepatotropic viruses. These viruses are designated hepatitis A, B, C, D, E and G viruses. They are a heterogeneous group causing clinically similar illnesses except for hepatitis G virus which is, as yet, known to cause mild or no disease.

HBV is a DNA virus. HAV, HCV, HDV, HEV, and HGV are RNA viruses. HAV and HEV are not known to cause chronic illness, whereas HBV, HCV and HDV cause chronic infection and subsequent high morbidity and mortality. HGV can cause chronic infection with little morbidity or mortality.

Table 10.8 : Basic features of the six hepatotropic viruses

Features	*HAV*	*HBV*	*HCV*	*HDV*	*HEV*	*HGV*
1. **Nucleic acid**	RNA	DNA	RNA	RNA	RNA	RNA
2. **Incubation days**	30	100-120	7-9	2-4	40	Un-known
3. **Transmission**						
Percutaneous	Rare	Common	Common	Common	No	Common
Fecal-oral	Common	No	No	No	Common	No
Sexual	Rare	Common	Rare	Rare	Rare	Rare
Transplacental	No	Common	Rare	No	No	Rare
4. **Chronic infection**	No	Yes	Yes	Yes	No	Yes
5. **Fulminant disease**	Rare	Yes	Rare	Yes	Rare	No

Acute Viral Hepatitis

Acute viral hepatitis refers to an inflammatory disorder of the liver which is usually associated with complete clinical and histological recovery within a period of 4–6 weeks.

Acute viral hepatitis is a major public health problem in developing as well as developed countries. Among the six hepatotrophic viruses, HAV, HBV, HCV, HDV and HEV cause similar acute illness. HGV appears to cause no or mild disease. The existence of HBF virus is reported but not yet proved. In children, acute hepatitis is most commonly caused by HAV and HEV viruses. Hepatitis B infection rarely causes acute hepatitis in children. HDV, which occurs only in the presence of HBV, can cause disease in only a very small percentage of children.

Epidemiology

Hepatitis A infection has a worldwide distribution but more common in developing countries where the prevalence rate approaches 100% in children under 5 years age. Most infections in children, younger than 5 years of age, are asymptomatic or have mild with non-specific manifestations. HAV infection confers life long immunity.

Hepatitis B infection also has a worldwide distribution with high prevalence rate in the sub-Saharan Africa, China, and the Amazon basin, parts of middle-east and Pacific islands. Acute hepatitis, due to HBV infection, may be considered in children, receiving repeated blood transfusions (blood disorder), on hemodialysis and in adolescents (IV drug users, sexually promiscuous); and also in institutionalized mentally handicapped children. It is usually asymptomatic. If symptomatic, then the presentation may be with prominent extra hepatic manifestations, a serum sickness like prodromal picture with fever, arthralgia, skin lesions (purpura, maculopapular rashes and urticaria) and others like MPGN and aplastic anemia. The prodrome is usually prolonged. Jaundice appears in 25% infected children, 8 weeks after exposure and lasts for 4 weeks. Fulminant hepatitis may occur especially when associated with HDV co-infection.

Epidemiological Features of Hepatitis A and Hepatitis B

Features	*Hepatitis A*	*Hepatitis B*
1. Incubation period	15–45 days	60–160 days.
2. Onset	Abrupt	gradual
3. Season	Autumn and winter	Year round
4. Transmission	Feco–oral	Sexual, pricks
5. Age	children and young adult	All age groups
6. Fulminant hepatitis	0.1%	0.1–1 %
7. Chronicity	None	Neonates (90%) Older child (1–10%)
8. Carrier	None	1–30%
9. Immunity	Life long	None
10. Case fatality	0.1–2.7%	1–3 %

Hepatitis C infection is of worldwide distribution. It is commonly transmitted through blood transfusion, sexual transmission (multiple partners), and illegal drug use, with exposure to blood or blood products from HCV infected persons. Perinatal transmission has been described but is uncommon except when the mother is HIV infected or has high titre of HCV RNA. The mean incubation period of post transfusion acute HCV infection is 7–8 weeks, with a range of 2–26 weeks. Acute disease caused by hepatitis C infection tends to be mild and insidious in onset. The clinical pattern is similar to that of infection with other hepatitis viruses. It is, however, the most common cause of chronic liver disease.

Hepatitis D infection cannot produce infection without concurrent HBV infection. It can cause a co-infection with HBV or can infect a person who is already infected with HBV (super infection). Tramission usually occurs by intrafamilial or intimate contact. The developing countries are the areas of high prevalence. The incubation period of HDV super infection is about 2–8 weeks; with co-infection it is same as HBV infection. The symptoms of HDV infection are similar. With co-infection, acute hepatitis is much more severe than HBV infection alone but the risk of developing chronic hepatitis is low. With super infection, acute illness is rare but risk of fulminant hepatitis is high and chronic hepatitis is common.

Hepatitis E infection is reported from Indian subcontinent, the Middle East, South East Asia and Mexico. It occurs in an epidemic form. The route of infection, incubation period as well as clinical illness and course is similar to HAV infection but is often very severe and effects older children, above 15 years of age. The incidence of liver failure is higher (1–2 %) in comparison to HAV infection (0.1%) as well as the fatality rate which may go upto 4% in comparison to 2.7 % in HAV infection. Infection with HEV does not confer life long immunity.

Hepatitis G infection has been reported in children. It has a worldwide distribution. It is common in blood donors and injection drug users. Co-infection with chronic hepatitis B and C in adults have been reported. It is not yet clear whether HGV is a pathogen.

Pathology

The pathological changes in liver are similar in all the types of acute hepatitis. There is acute inflammation of the liver characterized by hepatocellular necrosis and infiltration of portal tracts with leucocytes and histiocytes. The sinusoids show infiltration with mononuclear cells, polymorphs and eosinophils. Hepatocytes show eosinophilic change (acidophil bodies). The surviving hepatocytes retain the glycogen. The reticulin framework is well preserved. The inflammatory cells disappear as the patient recovers. In cases with fulminant hepatitis, there is massive hepatocellular necrosis and the liver becomes shrunken which is a bad prognostic sign.

Clinical Manifestation

Whatever the virus, the clinical presentation of acute hepatitis can be divided into 4 phases: Incubation period, preicteric, icteric and convalescent phases. The incubation period differs according to the infecting virus.

Preicteric phase is characterized by nonspecific symptoms for 4–5 days before appearance of jaundice. Fever with signs of mild upper respiratory tract infection, mild headache, malaise and chills are present at the onset. Anorexia is an early symptom followed by nausea and vomiting. Upper abdominal pain is a frequent complaint. Constipation is common.

Icteric phase continues usually for 2–4 weeks with gradually increasing jaundice during the first weeks followed by gradual diminution. When jaundice appears, other prodromal symptoms abate except for anorexia. Urine is high colored and stools may be pale. There may be distressing pruritus. Tender hepatomegaly is present; splenomegaly may be present in around 15% cases.

Convalescence phase: Most children recover completely and resume normal activity within 2–3 weeks. However, the child may complain of malaise and fatigue for 1–2 months following complete resolution of the jaundice. Recovery is the rule in acute hepatitis except for HCV and at times HBV infection.

Atypical Presentation of Acute Hepatitis

Anicteric hepatitis: It is more common in infants and young children. The symptoms include anorexia, diarrhea, vomiting. Jaundice is absent. They may excrete the virus in the stool for many months and constitute a potential source of infection to others.

Complications

Hepatitis with predominant cholestasis: It is characterized principally by obstruction and dilatation of the bile canaliculi with little evidence of hepatocellular necrosis. The clinical manifestations include jaundice with pruritus, high colored urine and pale stools and an enlarged, non tender liver. Laboratory examination shows presence of bilirubin in urine, decreased fecal urobilinogen, increased serum alkaline phosphatase and 5, nucleotidase and slight increase in transaminases.

Chronic hepatitis: Occasionally in a patient with acute hepatitis, an elevation of serum indirect bilirubin or serum transaminases may persist for months without either clinical disease or pathologic changes on liver biopsy. It is common with HBV and HCV infection.

Relapsing hepatitis: Occasionally, there may be a relapse, after 3–90 days after the initial attack. The clinical manifestations and biochemical alterations resemble the original attack and the virus may be detected in the stools. It may last for several months but eventually, recovery is the rule.

Laboratory Diagnosis

Serology: Interpretation of Serological Markers

Hepatitis A: IgM anti-HAV is diagnostic of acute infection. It may be present upto 6 months. IgG anti-HAV appears after 6 months and persists for life and offer protection.

Hepatitis B: Following exposure to the virus, the first serological marker to appear is HbsAg, by 6 weeks. It usually disappears by 2–3 months of the onset of symptoms. Persistence for more than 6 months implies a carrier state. Anti-HBs appears a short period after the disappearance of HbsAg. This is called the window period, which can be diagnosed by demonstration of increased IgM-anti-HBc.

The second antigen to appear is HBeAg, immediately after HbsAg. Its presence indicates active intrahepatic viral replication and the presence in the blood DNA polymerase, HBV DNA and virion reflecting high infectivity. It disappears before HbsAg, coinciding with the fall of transaminases. It is followed by appearance of Anti-HBe. Its testing is indicated only in chronic infection and carriers.

IgM anti-HBc, the antibody of HBcAg appears in blood, 1–2 weeks after the appearance of HbsAg. It is the first antibody to appear. After 6 months, IgM anti-HBc is replaced by IgG anti-HBc. Thus the presence of former indicate recent infection and the presence of the latter a past infection.

The presence of anti-HBs without any other serological markers indicates immunity following vaccination.

HBV DNA is also a marker of viral replication and infectivity. The serum level helps to assess the progress of patients with chronic hepatitis under anti-viral chemotherapy.

Table 10.9 : Interpretation of serological markers in hepatitis B infection

HbsAg	*HBeAg*	*Anti-HBe*	*Anti-HBc*	*Anti-HBs*	*Significance*
+ ve	+ve	- ve	IgM	- ve	Acute HB, highly infectious
+ve	+ve	- ve	IgG	- ve	Chronic carrier state, highly infectious
+ve	- ve	-ve/ +ve	IgG	-ve	Chronic carrier, less infectious
-ve	-ve	-ve/+ve	IgM	-ve	Window period, infectious
-ve	-ve	-ve/ +ve	- ve	+ve	Immunity following HB vaccination
-ve	-ve	-ve	IgG	+ve	Immunity following natural infection

Hepatitis C: Detection of HCV infection is based on detection of antibodies to HCV antigens or testing directly for viral RNA or DNA. Anti-HCV antibody is not a protective antibody. Hence does not confer immunity.

Hepatitis D: The diagnosis is made by detecting IgM antibody to HDV. The antibodies to HDV develop about 2–4 weeks after co-infection and about 10 weeks after super infection.

Hepatitis E: IgM anti HEV is diagnostic of acute infection. Antibody appears after one week of illness. IgG anti HEV indicates resolved infection and disappears by 9–12 months.

Hepatitis G: The only diagnostic test available is PCR assays to detect HGV RNA.

Liver Function Test

Serum Transaminases, Serum Protein and Fractions

Serum ALT (alanine transaminase) is almost always raised in acute hepatitis; it is most specific of liver damage. Peak levels may vary between 400–4000 IU or more (upto 10,000 IU), but the levels do not correlate well with degree of liver damage. Levels subside with resolution of acute phase. In chronic hepatitis, levels are seldom more than 2–3 times normal, but are persistently raised.

A falling serum ALT with rises in serum bilirubin, often >20 mg/dl and fall in serum albumin, is a very grave sign–indicates fulminant progression, clinically altered sensorium, deepening jaundice, coagulopathy, ascites, rapidly shrinking liver size are danger signs.

Serum Bilirubin

Mostly, total serum bilirubin levels are equally divided between direct and indirect fractions. In acute hepatitis, rise may be very mild, may range from 5–20 mg/dl. Levels >20 mg/dl indicate fulminant hepatitis.

Serum Alkaline Phosphatase, GGT and 5, Nucleotidase

Levels are usually raised in acute hepatitis; reflect bile duct damage.

Prothrombin Time (PT)

It should be checked in all cases of hepatitis. It helps to differentiate between cholestatic jaundice and hepatocellular jaundice. It is of high prognostic value especially in acute hepatocellular disease. A prothrombin time more than 5–6 seconds prolonged indicates the possibility of fulminant hepatitis in patients with acute viral hepatitis. However, a prolonged PT is not specific of liver disease as it may be seen in coagulation disorders, and ingestion of drugs that affect the prothrombin complex.

International Normalization Ratio (INR)

The INR standardizes the prothrombin time for different thromboplastin agents thus providing a universal standard. Liver biopsy is contraindicated if INR > 1.3. An INR more than 1.5 is abnormal and indicate fulminant hepatic failure. The INR is calculated as follows: INR = T/C × ISI of thromboplastin (T = test, C=control, ISI = international sensitization index).

Urine Examination for Bile Salts and Pigments

Urobilinogen is increased (above 1: 20) in the pre icteric phase. It helps in early diagnosis of acute viral hepatitis before appearance of jaundice. In the icteric phase there is decrease in the urobilinogen content. There is a gradual rise in bilirubin and disappearance of urobilinogen followed by reappearance of urobilinogen in the convalescent phase indicating recovery.

Treatment

Treatment is supportive. It is aimed at supporting the child during the interval required for his own immunologic defenses to control the invading virus. The precipitating factors of hepatic encephalopathy (viz. excessive physical activity, dehydration, constipation, excessive protein intake, hepatotoxic drugs etc.) should be taken care of. *The parents should be reassured about the benign and self-limiting nature of the disease and the favorable outcome in case of HAV and HEV infections.*

Indications for Hospitalization

The indications for hospitalization include persistent vomiting, persistent fever, deepening jaundice, altered sensorium, bleeding tendency, G.I. bleed, presence of edema and ascites, decreasing liver span, prolonged prothrombin time.

Supportive Treatment

1. *Rest:* A previously healthy child should be advised periodic rest periods during the day rather than continuous bed rest. Physical activities should be held within limits of fatigue. Strict bed rest does not appear to produce more rapid recovery. They should not be allowed to go out and play. This is enforced till the patient is free from jaundice.

2. *Diet:* Regeneration of damaged liver requires an adequate supply of protein and calories. Hence maintenance of a reasonable state of nutrition during illness appears to be beneficial. After the initial period of anorexia has passed, a diet providing adequate calories for age and 1.5 to 2.5 gm/kg/day of protein with sufficient salt should be provided. Restriction of fat intake is not necessary and can be allowed as much as the child desires. Frequent feedings in small amounts are helpful in achieving adequate dietary intake.
3. Hydration should be maintained by plenty of oral fluids. When there is dehydration or excessive vomiting intravenous infusion of 10% dextrose with saline, ringers lactate or normal saline should be given.
4. The patient should have daily bowel movements. Stool softeners may be advised in presence of constipation.
5. Drugs should be avoided as far as possible. The parents should be advised not to use herbal or indigenous medicines for treatment. It is better to avoid *antipyretics* for fever especially paracetamol. Hydrotherapy i.e. sponging the whole body with warm water is the best treatment. Persistent vomiting is a danger sign. It may herald the onset of fulminant hepatitis. Such patients should be hospitalized and treated with IV fluids and monitored closely. It is better to avoid *antiemetics*.
6. Daily monitoring should be done in hospitalized patients to detect early signs of encephalopathy. The span of the liver should be measured daily because a decreasing span is a bad prognostic sign. A base line LFT and prothrombin time may be done. HbsAg should be done in all patients, even in clinically suspected HAV infection, because if the patient is already a carrier, the prognosis could be bad.

Signs of Recovery

The signs of recovery include improvement of general well-being, no vomiting or nausea, improvement of appetite, and decreasing jaundice.

The child may be allowed to go to school when there is no clinical jaundice. It is not necessary to wait till the serum bilirubin becomes normal (i.e. < 1 mg %).

Follow-up

The patient should be reviewed 3–4 weeks after discharge and if necessary at monthly intervals for 3 months. Special attention should be paid to the recurrence of jaundice and to the size of the liver and spleen. Tests should include serum bilirubin, ALT, HBV and HCV markers if initially positive.

Chronic Viral Hepatitis

Definition

Chronic viral hepatitis is defined as symptomatic, biochemical or serologic evidence of continuing or relapsing hepatic disease for more than 6 months with histologically documented inflammation and necrosis.

Etiopathogenesis

In children, chronic hepatitis is rare and is usually caused by hepatitis B, C and D viruses. Chronicity is inversely related with age–lower the age of acquisition, higher the chances of chronicity. The major concerns of chronic liver disease are the increased risks of progressing to cirrhosis and hepatocellular carcinoma.

HDV is an incomplete virus by itself; it needs a concurrent (co-infection) or preexisting (superinfection) HBV infection to produce infection. HDV superinfection causes chronic hepatitis more commonly than co-infection. Children are infected with these viruses and develop chronic hepatitis under special circumstances like:

- Perinatal transmission from an infected or carrier mother (HBV and HCV).
- Through blood and blood products (HBV, HCV, HDV).
- Through illicit use of IV drugs and unsafe sexual practices–HBV, HCV (rare) and HDV.
- Individuals with impaired immunity, e.g., children with Down's syndrome, leukemia, chronic hemodialysis.

Clinical Manifestations

Clinical features of chronic hepatitis are extremely variable and are not predictive of the outcome. The patient may present as:

Asymptomatic healthy carriers: They harbor the virus, but suffer little or no adverse effects; detected incidentally.

In some, persistently elevated serum transaminases are the only sign. Fluctuating levels of transaminases are very characteristic of chronic HCV infection.

The most common *symptom* is fatigue; less commonly malaise, anorexia. Occasional bouts of mild jaundice may occur. There may be presence of stigmata of chronic liver disease like palmar erythema, spider angiomas etc.

The extra hepatic manifestations of chronic HCV infection include cutaneous vasculitis, peripheral neuropathy, cerebritis, membranoproliferative glomerulonephritis and nephrotic syndrome.

Serology

1. *Hepatitis B:* Presence of serum markers
   a. HBs Ag, Anti-HBc, HBeAg and HBV DNA indicate chronic HBV infection with high infectivity.
   b. HbsAg, Anti-HBc and Anti-HBe indicate chronic infection with low infectivity or a healthy carrier.
2. *Hepatitis C:* Presence of serum markers
   a. Anti-HCV indicate chronic infection.
3. *Hepatitis D:* Presence of serum markers
   a. IgG and IgM anti-HDV indicates chronic infection.

Treatment

Hepatitis B

The current modalities of treatment for hepatitis B have better effect when the patient is highly infective. Recombinant interferon ∝ 2b—is a protein which occurs naturally also in our bodies; its function is to fight viruses by boosting the immune system. It is given in a dose of 5-10 million units/m^2 IM, thrice a week for 4-6 months. Long-term eradication rates reach 25-40%. Therapy is monitored by repeated estimation of HBeAg or HBV DNA and presence of HbsAg. Lamivudine–is an antiviral drug which is given orally. It is an inactive prodrug, converted intracellulary into active phosphorylated form which is a potent inhibitor of HBV reverse transcriptase. It is given in the dose of 3 mg/kg/day for 1 year. Successful therapy would mean HBeAg seroconversion and undetectable serum HBV DNA. Liver transplantation–for end stage liver failure (fulminant hepatitis).

Annual surveillance for development of hepatocellular carcinoma should be done by USG and serum alpha feto-protein estimation in all cases of chronic hepatitis B infection.

Hepatitis C

The treatment of hepatitis C includes monotherapy with Interferon (IFN), 3 million units/m^2, thrice a week for 6-12 months which has shown sustained response in 10-15% patients. Studies are on in children of combined therapy of IFN and ribavirin.

Prevention

Vaccines are available to prevent hepatitis A and hepatitis B infection. No vaccines are available against other hepatitis as yet.

General measures for hepatitis A include isolation of infected child for 1 week after onset of jaundice, strict hand washing, and proper disposal of feces and use of sanitary latrines.

Preventive measures for hepatitis B and C include proper screening of blood and blood products, advice regarding safe sexual practices, screening of all pregnant women and proper sterilization of surgical instruments.

Wilson Disease

Wilson disease is an autosomal recessive disorder characterized by degenerative changes in the brain, liver disease and Kayser-Fleischer rings in the cornea. It is an important cause of chronic liver disease and fulminant hepatitis in children. Specific treatment is available. It is fatal if untreated. In order to inherit it, both of the parents of an individual must carry an affected gene. Most cases have no family history of the condition. People with only one abnormal gene are called carriers (heterozygotes). Carriers may have mild, but medically insignificant, abnormalities of copper metabolism.

Etiopathogenesis

The abnormal gene for Wilson disease is on chromosome 13 with the locus at q14 - q21. The gene encodes amino acid structural motifs consistent with a role in copper transport. Mutations that completely destroy the gene function are associated with onset of symptoms as early as 2 - 3 years of age. Milder mutations can be associated with an onset of disease symptoms as late as 50 years of age.

The average intake of copper in breastfed babies is 50 microgram/kg/day. In older children it is 1 mg/kg/day. Of this 50% is not absorbed and passed in stool and 30% is lost through skin. The remaining 20% is absorbed within enterocytes by metallothionein (a sulphur rich copper binding protein). Fetal and neonatal liver normally contains relatively high concentrations of copper and metallothionein. Absence of this protein causes accumulation of copper within the enterocytes, failure of absorption and systemic copper deficiency.

The mechanism responsible for copper homeostasis in older children reaches maturity by 2 years of age. Therefore, the Wilsonian trait may be expressed after this time, but clinical manifestations of Wilson disease do not occur before 5 years age.

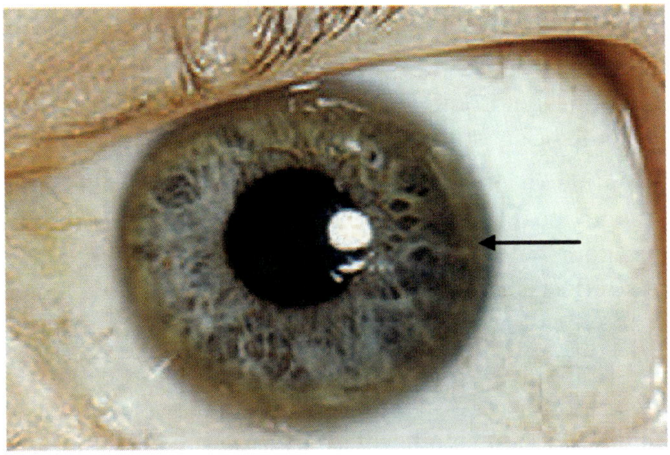

Fig. 10.4: Showing Kayser-Fleischer ring

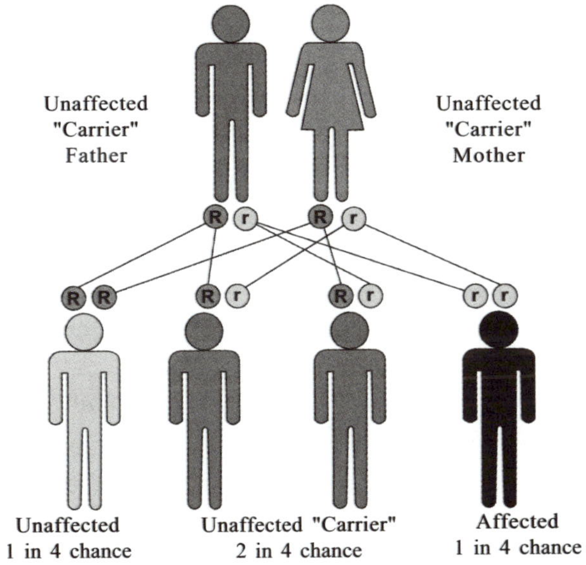

Fig. 10.5: Inheritance pattern of Wilson disease

Defective mobilization of copper from lysosomes in liver cells for excretion into bile is the basic defect for the multiorgan damage in Wilson disease. Excessive accumulation of copper in the liver lead to escape of copper from the overloaded liver to the circulation in a non-ceruloplasmin bound form. The free copper accumulates and damages the other organs, particularly the brain and kidneys and in the cornea to form the Kayser-Fleischer rings (KF rings). The underlying mechanism of liver damage is presumably oxidant injury to the hepatocyte mitochondria, which is the target organ in copper induced toxicity. Lipid peroxidation of the mitochondria resulting from copper overload leads to functional alteration.

The parents of patient with Wilson disease are heterozygotes. Clinical disease does not occur but they may have low serum ceruloplasmin, borderline normal urinary copper and elevated urinary copper on D-penicillamine challenge. There may be mild elevation of liver copper (100 - 250 microgram/gm of dry liver tissue). The risk to siblings is as follows: 25% will suffer from Wilson disease, 50% will be unaffected carriers and 25% normal.

Clinical Manifestations

The clinical manifestation depends of the age of onset. The child presents mainly with symptoms of liver disease and neuropsychiatric manifestations. In younger children, hepatic involvement is the predominant manifestation whereas beyond 20 years of age neuropsychiatric disorders predominate.

The hepatic manifestations include asymptomatic hepatomegaly (with or without splenomegaly), fulminant hepatic failure, subacute or chronic hepatitis and cirrhosis. The child may present with portal hypertension, ascites, variceal bleeding or other effects of hepatic dysfunction viz. delayed puberty, amenorrhea or coagulation defect.

The neuropsychiatric disorders develop gradually or precipitously. They are characterized by deterioration in school performance or behavioural changes, intention tremor, dysarthria and dystonia.

The Kayser-Fleischer ring may not be present in young patients with liver disease but are always present in patients with neurologic disease.

Some children may present with an acute hemolytic episode as an initial manifestation. This form is usually fatal without transplant. Such acute hemolysis is possibly related to the release of large amount of copper from damaged hepatocyte.

The child may present with Fanconi syndrome and progressive renal failure.

Unusual manifestations include arthritis and hypoparathyroidism.

Diagnosis

Wilson disease should be clinically suspected in children and teenagers with the following features:

1. Unexplained acute or chronic liver disease.
2. Neurologic symptoms of unknown cause.
3. Acute hemolysis.
4. Psychiatric illness and behavioural changes.
5. Fanconi syndrome or unexplained bone disease.

Laboratory Investigations

1. Estimation of serum ceruloplasmin level is the best screening test. Most patients with Wilson disease have a low level.
2. Serum copper level may be elevated in the early stages. Urinary copper excretion (normally < 40 micro gram/day) is increased to greater than 100 microgram/day or often upto 1000 microgram or more/day.

   In equivocal cases, estimation of urinary copper estimation after a 1 gm oral dose of D-penicillamine is helpful. The excretion increases to 1200 - 2000 microgram/day.
3. Liver biopsy helps in examination of the histology of liver and for estimation of hepatic copper content (normally < 10 microgram/gram dry weight). In Wilson disease, the hepatic copper content exceeds 250 micro gram/gm dry weight.

Treatment

The modalities of treatment include chelation therapy and supportive therapy and gene therapy.

Chelation Therapy: Chelation therapy helps in rapid excretion of excess deposition of copper. It is currently best managed by oral administration of the copper chelating agent D-penicillamine (Beta Beta dimethylcysteine) in a dose of 20 mg/kg/day, one hour before or 2 hours after meals as it is best absorbed in empty stomach. The maximum dose should not exceed 1 gm/day. However if there is no improvement, the dose may be increased to 1.5 to 2 gms/day. It usually takes about 6 months to reduce copper to subtoxic levels. The drug has to be continued. If treatment is discontinued the patient may deteriorate within 18 - 24 months.

The response to therapy is indicated by marked increase of urinary copper excretion and slow clinical improvement. With continued administration of D-penicillamine urinary copper levels become normal with marked improvement of hepatic and neurologic function and disappearance of KF rings.

Monitoring during the first two months of therapy include WBC count and platelet count twice weekly then monthly upto 6 months, then less frequently. Proteinuria should also be checked.

Toxic effects of D-penicillamine are uncommon but can be significant in 5 - 10% of patients. It consists of urticaria, agranulocytosis, aplastic anemia and lymphadenopathy. These are usually resolved by stopping therapy and restarting with slowly increasing doses along with prednisolone which is gradually withdrawn after about 2 weeks. D-penicillamine may also cause SLE and nephrotic syndrome. In the event of serious side effects, it should be substituted by trientine.

Trientine (triethylene tetramine dihydrochloride) is a second line drug. The dose is 0.5 - 2 gram/day (20 mg/kg one hour before food or two hours after food). Early toxic effects include aplastic anemia and proteinuria. Later it may cause SLE, Goodpasture's syndrome and sideroblastic anemia.

Zinc is another drug use for chelation of copper. It induces metallothionein synthesis in the absorptive cells of the intestinal villi that helps in copper trapping. As these cells slough into the intestinal lumen, the copper trapped in the cells are lost in the stools. Zinc can also stimulate metallothionein synthesis in liver, which will detoxify the remaining copper. However, zinc is slow in action and takes much longer to achieve a negative copper balance. Hence it is not an ideal agent for initial therapy in symptomatic patients. After initial treatment with D-penicillamine, zinc can be used for maintenance therapy. Combination of penicillamine and zinc can be used. If both drugs are used together, there can be an additive effect as both drugs work in different mechanism. It may also help to produce an optimum response without using toxic levels of penicillamine.

Zinc acetate salts are preferred as the incidence of gastritis is less. The dose is elemental zinc 25 mg thrice daily. The only side effect of zinc is gastritis which is however much less with acetate compounds.

Supportive Treatment

1. Restriction of copper intake to less than 1 mg/day. Foods such as liver, shell fish, dried fish, nuts and chocolates should be avoided. A vegetarian diet is better. Copper and brass utensils should not be used for cooking.
2. Additional amount of Vitamin B_6 should be supplemented as penicillamine is an antimetabolite of Vitamin B_6.

3. Liver transplant may be required in fulminant Wilson disease and patients with end stage liver disease.

Gene Therapy

Gene therapy is done by introduction of a normal allele of Wilson disease into the liver hepatocytes of a patient with homozygous inheritance.

Prognosis

Untreated disease is rapidly progressive and fatal. It is excellent in patients with good compliance with therapy even with cirrhosis or chronic hepatitis at diagnosis. Patients with neuropsychiatric symptoms may take months to years for recovery. In chronic hepatitis, the response to therapy is poor. Liver transplant may be life saving in such cases.

Liver Failure

Definition

Liver failure is defined as a clinical syndrome resulting from massive necrosis of hepatocytes or from functional impairment of hepatocytes with coagulopathy and encephalopathy, in a child who does not have a preexisting liver disease.

Acute liver failure is the term used to describe the disorder in which the severe impairment of liver function (INR = / > 1.5 with encephalopathy or INR = / > 2 with or without encephalopathy) is associated with hepatocellular necrosis, occurs in a child with no recognized chronic liver disease within 8 weeks of the initial symptoms.

If the features of acute liver failure occur within 4 weeks of onset of symptoms, it is termed as *fulminant liver failure* and when it occurs within one week of onset it is termed as *hyperacute liver failure*. When features of acute liver failure occurs gradually over a period of 4 weeks to 6 months after onset of symptoms, it is called *subacute liver failure*. It is associated with persistent icterus, ascites, and / or encephalopathy. If the signs of hepatic failure occur after 6 months of the onset of hepatic illness it is described as *chronic liver failure*. In children, liver failure is usually acute or fulminant.

The above definition of acute / fulminant liver failure may not be always applicable in children because metabolic disorders like Wilson's disease, Galactosemia etc., which are chronic liver diseases, may present for the first time with acute liver failure. In neonates, acute liver failure is usually due to an inborn error of metabolism or an intra-uterine insult which is again a pre existing condition. Moreover, the early stages of hepatic encephalopathy are difficult to assess in children, and in infants it may not be apparent until the terminal stages.

The pediatric acute hepatic failure study group (PALFSG), therefore, has proposed the following criteria:

- No history of known liver disease.
- Presence of biochemical evidence of liver injury.
- Coagulopathy not corrected by Vitamin K administration.
- INR> 1.5 if the patient has encephalopathy or > 2 if patient does not have encephalopathy.

It needs mention that whatever may be the type of liver failure, the etiology, clinical presentation and management is same.

Etiology

The common causes of liver failure are given in the following table. In India hepatitis A alone or in combination with hepatitis E is the most common cause in older children. In infants, the common causes are usually metabolic disorders and non-hepatotropic viral infections.

Table 10.10 : Causes of liver failure

	Infants	*Older children*
Metabolic disorders	e.g. Galactosemia, fructose intolerance, tyrosinemia, hemochromatosis	e.g. Wilson's disease.
Infections	Hepatitis B, adeno, parvo, herpes viruses, sepsis	Hepatitis A, B and E viruses, parvo and adeno-viruses.
Drugs	Valproate, INH, paracetamol	Valproate, phenytoin, paracetamol, INH.
Others	Severe asphyxia, neonatal hepatitis etc.	Autoimmune disease, Budd-Chiari syndrome etc.

Pathology

There is patchy or confluent massive necrosis of hepatocytes, multilobular or bridging necrosis associated with collapse of reticulin framework with little or no regeneration. Sometimes microvesicular fatty infiltration of hepatocytes is observed in Reye's syndrome and tetracycline toxicity. Acetaminophen toxicity and circulatory collapse is associated with centrilobular damage.

Pathogenesis

The exact mechanism leading to liver failure as a result of the different causes is not clearly known.

Massive necrosis of hepatocytes in viral hepatitis may be due to both a direct cytotoxic effect of the virus and an immune response to the viral antigen.

Drugs like acetaminophen and INH produces hepatotoxic metabolites which causes liver injury. Fulminant liver failure may follow depletion of intracellular substances, particularly glutathione, involved in detoxification.

Whatever may be the initial cause of liver injury, the factors contributing to liver failure may be impaired hepatocytes regeneration, altered parenchymal perfusion, endotoxemia and decreased hepatic reticuloendothelial function.

The pathogenesis of hepatic encephalopathy may relate to increased serum levels of ammonia, false neurotransmitters, amines, increased gamma amino butyric acid receptor activity or increased circulating levels of endogenous benzodiazepine like compounds. Decreased hepatic clearance of these substances may produce marked central nervous system dysfunction.

Clinical Manifestation

In infants, acute liver failure may complicate a previously known acute liver disease or it can be the presenting feature of the liver disease. An older child is usually healthy and often do not have a history of pre existing liver disease.

Fever, anorexia, pain abdomen, vomiting, progressive jaundice and fetor hepaticus are common presenting features. A hemorrhagic diathesis and ascites may develop. A rapidly decreasing liver size in absence of clinical improvement is an ominous sign.

Red Flag Signs

Clinical	*Laboratory*
Persistent jaundice	PT > 5 secs difference in spite of Vitamin K.
Deepening jaundice	Persistent hypoglycemia.
Relapse of jaundice	Low serum albumin.
Shrinking liver size	Raised SGPT > 3000 IU/dl.
Ascites	Serum bilirubin > 20 mg/dl.
Spontaneous bleeds	

Complications

The complications include the following:

1. Encephalopathy.
2. Coagulopathy and hemorrhage.
3. Hypoglycemia.
4. Cerebral edema.
5. Renal dysfunction.
6. Infection.

Laboratory Diagnosis

The *investigations* in a child with liver failure are directed towards guiding management, and for determining the etiology.

For guiding management:

i. Liver function test (S. bilirubin and fractions, S. protein and fractions, ALT, GGT, LDH, prothrombin time).
ii. Urea, creatinine.
iii. Electrolytes Na, K, Ca.
iv. APTT in the event of DIC.
v. Glucose, ammonia.
vi. CBC, blood culture, urine culture, chest X-ray to exclude infection.
vii. USG abdomen to study the size of liver and status of bile canaliculi.

For etiological diagnosis:

i. Viral markers viz. anti-HAV IgM, anti-HEV IgM, HbsAg.
ii. Copper studies for Wilson's disease viz. serum copper, ceruloplasmin, 24 hours urinary copper.
iii. For inborn errors of metabolism viz. urinary organic acids, reducing sugar, urinary and plasma amino acids.
iv. Viral markers for chronic active hepatitis.

Treatment

There is no specific therapy. Treatment is essentially directed towards hepatic support and prevention and treatment of complications while awaiting recovery.

Management should be ideally done in an ICU set up with intensive monitoring. The frequency of monitoring will depend on the grade of hepatic encephalopathy ranging from daily in grade I and II to 4–6 hourly in grade III and IV.

A central venous catheter for assessment of CVP and volume status and an indwelling arterial line for continuous measurement of blood pressure and for biochemical and acid base monitoring are essential.

A nasogastric tube should be passed to detect upper GI bleeding and the urinary bladder catheterized for strict urine output record to help in evaluation of fluid status and renal function.

Monitoring

The following clinical parameters are to be monitored:

a. Heart rate, respiratory rate, temperature 4 hourly.
b. Blood pressure and CVP 4 hourly.
c. Neurological/coma grading 12 hourly.
d. Physical examination to detect complications.

The following laboratory parameters are to be monitored:

a. Blood glucose 2–4 hourly.
b. Electrolytes Na and K 12 hourly.
c. ABG, blood urea, serum creatinine 12 hourly.
d. Prothrombin time 12 hourly.

Supportive Treatment

The supportive treatment includes general measures and prevention and treatment of complication.

General Measures

Fluid and Electrolyte Balance

The aim of fluid balance is to maintain urine output, to correct or prevent hypoglycemia, to maintain serum potassium concentration while preventing cerebral edema. Maintenance fluid consists of 10% dextrose in N/5 normal saline. Fluid intake should be 75% of normal maintenance requirements. Sodium intake of 0.5–1 mEq/kg/day is adequate. Potassium requirement may be high, 3– 6 mEq/kg/day depending on the serum concentration.

Nutrition

The aim of nutrition therapy is to maintain blood glucose > 75 mg/dl. This can be achieved by provision of sufficient carbohydrates. Protein intake should be around 1–2 gm/kg/day. 30% calories from fat.

Other Therapy

Vitamin K in the doses of 2.5 mg (< 6 months), 5 mg (6 months–2 years) and 10 mg (more than 2 years). It should be given I.V.

Prevention and Treatment of Complications

Hypoglycemia

Severe hypoglycemia (< 40 mg/dl) develops in majority of cases. Frequent bedside monitoring and I.V. administration of 10–50% dextrose (1 ml/kg) are required to prevent this complication.

Coagulopathy

Administration of Vitamin K parenterally assures the sufficiency of the Vitamin K dependent clotting factors. Thrombocytopenia is less a problem in children. Platelet count however, should be maintained above 50,000/micro litre.

Mild to moderate coagulopathy (Prothrombin time < 30 seconds) requires no therapy. Marked coagulopathy (Prothrombin time > 40 seconds) should be corrected with FFP, 10 ml/kg every 6 hours or continuous infusion at the rate of 3–5 ml/kg/hour.

It should be noted that prothrombin time is the most sensitive measure of hepatic synthesis of clotting factors. Prolongation often precedes other clinical evidence of encephalopathy. It is also a guide to the urgency of liver transplant.

Gastrointestinal Hemorrhage

Gastrointestinal hemorrhage may be life threatening. It may be due to stress ulceration or gastritis. Ranitidine, 2–3 mg/kg 8 hourly IV or omeprazole 10–20 mg/kg/day and sucralfate (250–500 mg 4–6 hourly) through nasogastric tube may be given to reduce GI bleeding. GI hemorrhage may respond to cold saline washes.

Encephalopathy

The precipitating factors of encephalopathy include constipation, infection, dehydration and electrolyte imbalance, hypovolemia and gastrointestinal hemorrhage.

The *clinical features* of hepatic encephalopathy depend on the grade as follows:

Grade	*Clinical features*
I	Mild drowsiness, impaired cognition, concentration, psychomotor functions, altered sleep awake cycle.
II	More drowsy, confused, inappropriate behaviour, mood swings, but capable of conversation.
III	Marked drowsiness but arousable, unresponsive to verbal commands, delirious, hyper reflexia, positive Babinski sign.
IV	Unconscious, decerebrate or decorticate rigidity, response to pain present (IV A) or absent (IV B).

The precipitating factors should be identified and corrected. Ammonia lowering therapy includes:

1. *Restriction of dietary protein*: No restriction of protein is required in Grade I and II while in Grade III and IV protein is restricted to 20 gms/day. It is advisable to give vegetable proteins which are source of branched chain amino acid.
2. Enema/bowel washes two times a day.
3. Lactulose, 0.5 ml/kg/dose orally every 6 hours titrated to produce 2–3 semi-loose stools daily. Lactulose, a non-absorbable disaccharide, is metabolized to organic acids by colonic bacteria. It probably lowers blood ammonia levels by decreasing microbial ammonia production and through trapping of ammonia in acidic intestinal contents.
4. Oral administration of a non-absorbable antibiotic may reduce enteric bacteria responsible for ammonia production.
5. Flumazenil, a benzodiazepine antagonist may reverse early hepatic encephalopathy.
6. Lornithine aspartate, zinc supplementation and anti-oxidant therapy are some new modalities tried.

Cerebral Edema

It is a major cause of death in patient with hepatic encephalopathy due to liver failure. Every effort should be made to prevent cerebral edema because current treatment available is inadequate.

1. Place head in neutral position with head end raised to 30–45% from bed.
2. Fluid restriction to 75% of maintenance.
3. Minimal handling of the patient.
4. Mannitol, 0.5 gm/kg IV infusion every 4–6 hours for 7–8 doses, help to control acute increase in intra-cranial pressure and may reverse acute neurological damage.
5. Elective hyperventilation should be performed in cases with coma Grade III and more or if cerebral edema is suspected. Hyperventilation prevents or postpones development of cerebral edema and intracranial hypertension.
6. Maintenance of cerebral perfusion by administration of blood products and ionotropic drugs. The aim is to maintain ICP below 20 mm Hg and cerebral perfusion above 50 mm Hg.
7. Convulsion should be treated promptly with phenytoin (10 mg/kg IV) or phenobarbitone (10–15 mg/kg IV). Persistent convulsion may respond to thiopentone infusion.

Renal Dysfunction

Renal insufficiency complicates the course of hepatic failure in around 75% of cases. The aim of management is to maintain the circulating volume and ensure a urine output of more than 0.5 ml/kg/hour.

An intake output chart should be maintained to diagnose renal failure at the earliest. Established renal failure requires dialysis or hemofiltration.

Sepsis

The signs of sepsis include subtle signs like tachycardia or a core toe temperature gradient <2°C, fall in blood pressure or urine output, hypoglycemia, and hypothermia, deterioration of mental state, convulsion and acidosis.

The common organisms causing an infection are staphylococcus, gram negative bacteria and occasionally fungus.

Broad spectrum antibiotics like IV Cloxacillin/Ampicillin combined with IV Cefotaxime/Ceftazidime are choice drugs. Anti-fungal and metronidazole may be added if there is no response in 48–72 hours. There is no role of prophylactic antibiotics.

Specific Therapy

1. N acetyl cystine, 140 mg/kg initially followed by 70 mg/kg 4 hourly should be started within 24 hours of ingestion of paracetamol and continued until liver failure has resolved.
2. Therapy for inborn errors of metabolism.

Hepatic Support

Various measures have been used to support the liver awaiting regeneration. They are:

1. Double volume exchange transfusion, plasmapheresis.
2. Charcoal hemoperfusion, extracorporeal perfusion.

These therapeutic maneuvers used to remove potential neuroactive toxins have shown to be useful in providing support during liver regeneration or while awaiting a donor. None have been shown to have benefit with regard to survival.

Liver Transplantation

Liver transplant, where available should be considered in all children with Grade III and IV encephalopathy. It is appropriate for all except those with multi-systemic disorders, uncontrolled sepsis etc.

Auxiliary liver transplantation has proved to be useful in children with acute liver failure. Here a part of the native liver is removed and replaced with either the respective right or left lobe of a reduced graft.

Prognosis

The overall mortality exceeds 70%. With intensive medical treatment, a survival rate of 50–60% may occur with hepatic failure complicating acetaminophen overdose and with fulminant HAV or HBV infection. Recovery can be expected in only 10–20% of patients with liver failure by the other viruses or an acute onset Wilson's disease. In general, the poor prognostic factors include:

1. Jaundice for more than 7 days before onset of encephalopathy.
2. Prothrombin time more than 50 seconds.
3. Serum bilirubin level more than 17.5 mg/dl.

Survival of 50–75% can be achieved in patients with poor prognostic factors after orthotropic liver transplantation.

The patients who recover from acute liver failure with supportive treatment only, do not usually experience chronic liver disease.

Portal Hypertension

The normal portal venous pressure is approximately 7 mm Hg. Portal hypertension is defined as elevation of portal pressure above 7–10 mm Hg or intra-splenic pressure above 17 mm Hg or wedged hepatic venous pressure (WHVP) more than 4 mm Hg above the inferior vena caval pressure. It is a major cause of morbidity and mortality in children with liver disease.

Classification

Portal hypertension may be classified as follows:

1. Pre or extrahepatic.
2. Intrahepatic
   a. Presinusoidal
   b. Sinusoidal
   c. Postsinusoidal
3. Post hepatic.
4. Hyperkinetic.

Pre or Extrahepatic Portal Hypertension (EHPHT)

Extrahepatic portal obstruction is an important cause of portal hypertension during childhood. The obstruction can occur at any level of the portal vein. In extrahepatic portal hypertension the block in the portal vein occurs before the blood reaches the liver. The liver function is normal and the wedged hepatic venous pressure is normal.

Etiology

The main causes of extrahepatic portal obstruction include developmental defects like portal vein cavernoma, umbilical sepsis, intraluminal trauma by catheterization of the portal vein in the newborn, intra-abdominal sepsis, blunt abdominal trauma damaging the portal vein, thrombocytosis and pancreatitis. However, in around 50% cases of EHPHT etiology cannot be found.

Causes of Extrahepatic Portal Hypertension

1. Developmental defects: Portal vein cavernoma
2. Umbilical sepsis
3. Post catheterization intraluminal trauma in newborn
4. Intra-abdominal sepsis
5. Blunt abdominal trauma
6. Thrombocytosis
7. Pancreatitis
8. Idiopathic

Umbilical sepsis is the most important cause of portal hypertension in developing countries. In intraluminal trauma, the wall of the portal vein is damaged by catheterization for exchange transfusion or infusion of sodium bicarbonate. Intra-abdominal sepsis like acute appendicitis or peritonitis can cause local phlebitis and the infected thrombus may ascend in the portal venous radicals to reach the main portal vein. Blunt abdominal trauma may damage the portal vein and cause thrombosis. Postoperative causes like thrombocytosis after splenectomy, difficult surgery like that for biliary strictures, cause portal vein thrombosis. Idiopathic EHPHT may sometimes be associated with autoimmune disorders like rheumatoid arthritis, hypothyroidism etc.

Intrahepatic Portal Hypertension

Intrahepatic portal hypertension may be of three types, in relation to the hepatic sinusoids: Presinusoidal, sinusoidal and post sinusoidal.

The basic differences between the three types are that the liver functions and the wedged hepatic venous pressure (WHVP) are normal in presinusoidal type. In the other two types the liver functions as well as the WHVP are abnormal.

A catheter is passed through the inferior or superior vena cava into a hepatic venous radicle until it can go no further. The pressure here measures the sinusoidal or the WHVP. Normally the inferior vena caval pressure is about 2 mm Hg. In sinusoidal and post sinusoidal portal hypertension, the WHVP is 4 mm Hg more than the inferior vena cava pressure and in cirrhosis the usual value is around 20 mm Hg.

Intrahepatic Presinusoidal Type

The common causes of presinusoidal portal hypertension include chronic active hepatitis, congenital hepatic fibrosis, infiltration of the portal zones with hemopoetic tissues in Hodgkin's disease and chronic myeloid leukemia, sarcoidosis, primary biliary cirrhosis, tropical splenomegaly, hypervitaminosis A, prolonged use of drugs like methotrexate, azathioprine and 6 mercaptopurine, hepatic cysts and neoplasm.

Intrahepatic Sinusoidal Portal Hypertension

The causes of intrahepatic sinusoidal portal hypertension are cirrhosis due to hepatitis B and C, metabolic disorders like Wilson's disease and alpha 1 antitrypsin deficiency, glycogen storage disease type IV, cholestatic disorders like neonatal hepatitis and extrahepatic biliary atresia, hepatotoxic drugs like methotrexate, and parenteral nutrition.

Intrahepatic Postsinusoidal Portal Hypertension

This includes the condition called veno-occlusive disease. It is characterized by nonthrombotic occlusion of the portal vein by connective tissue and collagen of the terminal hepatic venous radicles, without associated abnormalities of the hepatic veins or inferior vena cava. It may progress to extensive perivenular fibrosis, central to central bridging and eventually cirrhosis.

It is the most common cause of hepatic vein obstruction. This disorder usually occurs after total body irradiation with or without cytotoxic drug therapy that is commonly used before bone marrow transfusion. It can also occur after ingestion of herbal remedies containing pyrrolizidine alkaloids, which are sometimes taken as medicinal teas.

Common Causes of Intrahepatic Portal Hypertension

Pre sinusoidal	*Sinusoidal*	*Post sinusoidal*
Chronic active hepatitis Cong. hepatic fibrosis Hodgkin's disease CML Sarcoidosis Primary biliary cirrhosis Tropical splenomegaly	Cirrhosis Metabolic disorders viz. Wilson"s disease Alpha 1 antitrypsin deficiency Glycogen storage disease type IV	Veno occlusive disease (VOD) Ingestion of herbal remedies viz. pyrrolizidine alkaloids
Hypervitaminosis A Hepatic cyst & neoplasm Drugs: Methotrexate, azathioprine, 6MP	Neonatal hepatitis EHBA Parenteral nutrition Drug: Methotrexate	

Post Hepatic Portal Hypertension

This includes the condition called Budd-Chiari syndrome. It is characterized by thrombosis of the hepatic veins anywhere between the efferent hepatic veins and the entry of inferior vena cava into the right atrium. In most cases, no cause can be found but thrombosis can complicate neoplasms, collagen vascular disease, infection and trauma.

Hyperkinetic Portal Hypertension

This is caused by intrahepatic or extrahepatic arterio-venous fistula resulting from trauma. It may be seen with Osler-Rendu-Weber syndrome (hereditary hemorrhagic telangiectasia) and hypersplenism.

Clinical Manifestations

The clinical presentations of portal hypertension include upper gastrointestinal bleeding, hepatomegaly, splenomegaly, ascites and hepatic encephalopathy.

Bleeding from upper gastrointestinal tract is the most common presentation of portal hypertension. Regardless of the underlying cause, children with portal hypertension most commonly present with recurrent bouts of life threatening hemorrhage, as a result of bleeding from esophageal varices, in the form of hematemesis and melena.

In patients with portal obstruction but normal liver function, the bleeding is usually massive but the patient does not develop hepatic encephalopathy as the liver function is normal and bleeding stops spontaneously. In patients with intrahepatic disease, the combination of portal hypertension and poor liver function with coagulopathy can make bleeding much more difficult to control. Bleeding in intrahepatic portal hypertension can precipitate hepatic encephalopathy. This is not true with extrahepatic portal hypertension.

Splenomegaly is the most frequent sign of portal hypertension in children. It is usually moderately enlarged. Massive splenomegaly is rare. In late stages, some patients may present with features of hypersplenism. In extrahepatic portal hypertension the previously palpable spleen may temporarily reduce in size after a bout of bleeding.

The combination of gastrointestinal bleeding and splenomegaly is pathognomonic of portal hypertension until proved otherwise.

Hepatomegaly is a feature of early disease. Subsequently, the liver shrinks and there may be disproportionate enlargement of the left lobe. In patients with underlying hepatic disease physical examination may show presence of jaundice, and stigmata of cirrhosis viz. palmer erythema and vascular telangiectasia.

Ascites is frequently seen in sinusoidal and post sinusoidal portal hypertension. It is usually absent in extrahepatic and presinusoidal portal hypertension.

Cutaneous vascular signs like dilated veins over the abdominal wall around the umbilicus and caput medusa (prominent collateral vessels in the periumbilical region) is found in sinusoidal portal hypertension. A continuous murmur from low to high pitch may be heard between the umbilicus and the lower sternum (Cruveilhier-Baumgarten murmur) is pathognomonic of intrahepatic portal hypertension. These signs are not seen in extrahepatic portal hypertension.

Hepatic encephalopathy develops in patients with sinusoidal portal hypertension and portosystemic shunts.

The clinical presentations of *veno-occlusive disease* include sudden onset abdominal distension and pain due to hepatomegaly in a child between the age group of 1–6 years. Ascites is present in 70% cases. Around 30% of the cases develop cirrhosis and portal hypertension.

Budd-Chiari syndrome may be acute or chronic. Acute type is characterized by severe abdominal pain with vomiting, marked hepatomegaly, mild jaundice and rapid onset of ascites. The patient may progress to hepatic failure. In the chronic type, the patient develops massive ascites, hepatomegaly and upper gastrointestinal bleed with cutaneous vascular signs of inferior vena caval obstruction viz. dilated veins over the abdomen and back, with flow from below upwards.

Laboratory Diagnosis

Ultrasonography

The classic finding in portal hypertension is an increase diameter of portal vein > 17 mm. In normal patients, the portal vein increases in diameter during inspiration. The absence of this is suggestive of portal hypertension. There is presence of vascular collaterals in a thickened omentum and splenomegaly.

In extrahepatic portal hypertension, a hyperechogenic area, where multiple tortuous structures are seen, replaces the bifurcation of the portal vein.

In Budd-Chiari syndrome, abnormal hepatic veins are seen.

In cirrhosis, increased echogenecity of the liver and ascites can be seen.

Ultrasonography with Doppler Study

Doppler study can assess the blood flow within the portal vein. In severe portal hypertension there is reversal of blood flow. It also helps in assessment of the patency of the inferior vena cava and the size of splenic vein and superior mesenteric vein, when a portosystemic shunt is considered.

Endoscopy

Demonstration of esophageal varices by endoscopy clinches the diagnosis of portal hypertension.

Barium Studies

Barium swallow esophagus can demonstrate esophageal varices. Barium meal upper GIT can demonstrate gastric as well as duodenal varices. However with the advent of endoscopy, barium studies are rarely used now.

Treatment

Assessment of Degree of Blood Loss

Assessment of degree of blood loss is the first step in management. This can be done by the following methods:

1. Presence of disproportionate tachycardia (pulse rate > 150 / minute) which suggests a loss of about 20% blood volume.
2. **Tilt test:** The basal blood pressure and pulse rate are measured. The head end of the patient is then tilted or raised to 45%. If pulse rate rises by more

than 20-minute or if the diastolic pressure falls by more than 10 mm of mercury, the patient has suffered about 25% blood loss.

3. **Capillary refill time:** In a normal child if the nail bed is compressed and the pressure is released, the blood column comes back almost immediately. If it takes more than 5 seconds to come back it indicates that the patient has suffered 25% blood loss.
4. If the patient is in shock, the loss is around 40%.

Initial Stabilization

1. All patients with evidence of 20–25% blood loss should be given oxygen inhalation through a face mask or nasal cannula to maintain an oxygen saturation of 95% or more.
2. Patient in shock should be treated with intravenous crystalloids like normal saline or Ringers lactate. If an intravenous route is not available, the intraosseous route can be used for fluid administration.
3. A Ryles tube should be passed and gastric lavage given with normal saline at room temperature. Iced or chilled normal saline does not stop bleeding but may cause central hypothermia particularly in infant and young child. The tube should be kept in situ for continuous aspiration. It will help to know if bleeding is continuing or not. After bleeding has stopped, nasogastric aspiration should be continued every half an hour to detect recurrence of bleeding, till the patient is hemodynamically stable. Once the patient is stable aspiration should be done hourly for the next 24 hours.
4. Injection Vitamin K 5 mg should be given in case of hepatocellular failure and cholestatic jaundice.
5. Ideally, investigation of the cause of bleeding should begin after adequate resuscitation. However, if bleeding is torrential, diagnostic and therapeutic measures should be started simultaneously even in an unstable patient.

Monitoring

1. Vitals viz. pulse, respiration, blood pressure and sensorium. Pulse rate should be maintained below 100/minute and systolic blood pressure > 100 mm Hg.
2. Fluid intake/input and urine output chart should be maintained. If the patient is in shock, bladder should be catheterized to monitor urine output.
3. Monitoring of the central venous pressure helps to guide replacement therapy.

Management of Esophageal Variceal Bleed

Upper gastrointestinal bleed, due to ruptured esophageal varices, is an important cause of morbidity and mortality in children with portal hypertension. The treatment of choice is endoscopic sclerotherapy or endoscopic variceal ligation. A number of drugs however have been found to be useful in initial management.

The drugs to control bleeding include vasopressin, somatostatin, octreotide, metoclopramide.

Vasopressin is the drug used for treatment of variceal bleed for quite some time. Vasopressin acts by vasoconstriction of splanchnic vessels and thereby decreases the blood supply to the portal vein and the varices. It also constricts the lower end of esophageal sphincter. It is used in the dose of 0.33 units/kg in 20 minutes followed by an intravenous infusion of 0.33 units/kg/hour. If vasopressin fails to control bleeding within 4–6 hours or if bleeding recurs when it is withdrawn, it should be discontinued and some other drugs should be used. The side effects include myocardial infarction, ventricular fibrillation, cerebral hemorrhage, respiratory arrest, bowel ischemia and necrosis.

Somatostatin has a very short half-life. There are no sufficient placebo controlled trials in children. *Octreotide* is a synthetic analogue of somatostatin with a much longer half-life. It may be used with a loading dose 1 microgram /kg as an intravenous infusion over 30 minutes followed by 0.5 microgram/kg/hour. Both these drugs suppress gastrointestinal motility and secretion and cause flatulence, nausea and malabsorption. In high doses they may cause ischemia of the bowel. Both these drugs can be used freely only after further evaluation in children.

Metoclopramide is a powerful prokinetic and antiemetic drug. It can control hematemesis by constricting the lower esophageal sphincter thus cutting of the blood supply to the varices. The dose is 5–10 mg slow intravenous, may be repeated every 6 hours. It is found to be a useful drug in controlling the initial hemorrhage especially in extrahepatic portal hypertension. The main advantage of this drug is its low cost and easy availability.

Mechanical Methods to Control Bleeding

The Sengstaken-Blakemore tube and the Linton-Nachlas are designed to stop bleeding mechanically by balloons that compress esophageal and gastric varices. The former has three lumens, one each for gastric and esophageal balloons and one for aspiration. It is passed through the nose into the stomach and the gastric balloon is inflated with 75–100 ml of air and pulled against the gastro-esophageal junction. This compresses the gastroesophageal junction. If bleeding is not controlled, the esophageal balloon is then inflated to compress the esophageal varices. This tube is effective in controlling hemorrhage but it is associated with high incidence of recurrence of bleeding when the tube is removed. The latter tube is a single balloon triple lumen tube. It is more effective for control of bleeding from gastric varices.

Endoscopic Sclerotherapy (EST) and Endoscopic Variceal Ligation (EVL)

Endoscopic sclerotherapy is the treatment of choice for esophageal varices. It can be done as an emergency or as an elective procedure. EST acts by producing intimitis, followed by thrombosis and fibrosis of the vessels. EST is initially given at weekly intervals followed by monthly doses till sclerosis is complete. Followup EST is done at 6 months. If it is satisfactory then it is continued at yearly intervals. The complications of EST include esophageal ulceration and stricture, bronchoesophageal fistula, thoracic duct damage, cerebral abscess and paraplegia. There may be transient bacteremia. So prophylactic antibiotics should be given to children with congenital or acquired heart disease.

Endoscopic variceal ligation is a more popular method than EST at present because it is an effective method while complications are rare. The procedure is repeated as for EST.

Transjugular Intrahepatic Portosystemic Shunt (TIPS)

TIPS is a percutaneous technique that creates a shunt in the liver between the portal and the hepatic veins. It is used to treat variceal bleeding secondary to portal hypertension. The indications include refractory variceal bleeds, refractory ascites and hepatorenal syndrome.

Prevention of Variceal Bleed

Prevention may be primary, i.e., to prevent the first bleed which can be done by using propranolol in the dose of 1–2 mg/kg. It helps by lowering the venous flow and the portal venous pressure by decreasing the heart rate by 25% and blood pressure by 15 mmHg. It also causes splanchnic vasoconstriction and thereby decreases the portal blood flow.

Secondary prevention of bleeding is done after controlling the acute variceal bleed. This can be done by EST or EVL at 2–3 weeks interval or by surgical treatment. Surgical treatment is rarely necessary after the advent of endoscopic treatment. It may be indicated in varices due to extrahepatic portal hypertension when there are no facilities for endoscopic treatment, when EST fails to control varices, hypersplenism, and a child with a very rare blood group so that it is difficult to get blood in case of emergency.

Approach to Ascites

Ascites is an accumulation of serous fluid within the peritoneal cavity. The classical signs of ascites include uniform distension of abdomen or fullness of flanks, umbilical herniation in case of severe ascites, flank dullness, shifting dullness, fluid thrill and puddle sign. Very small amounts of fluid can be detected by ultrasound examination of the abdomen. The course, prognosis, and treatment of ascites depend entirely on the cause. Patients with any type of ascites are at an increased risk of spontaneous bacterial peritonitis.

Effects of Ascites

a. The body is unable to utilize the molecules like albumin and clotting factors that accumulates in the peritoneal cavity. Moreover, the child becomes anorexic and dyspneic as ascites increases. This effects nutrition and growth.

b. Ascites is a good culture medium for bacteria and hence spontaneous bacterial peritonitis is always a threat.

c. The disturbances in homeostasis aggravate sodium and fluid retention, which may precipitate hepato-renal syndrome in presence of liver disease.

Pathogenesis

The exchange of fluid between blood and the tissue spaces is controlled by the balance between 2 factors: (1) The capillary blood pressure, which forces fluid into the tissue spaces; and (2) The osmotic pressure of the plasma proteins which retains fluid within the vascular compartment. Imbalance between the two factors results in ascites.

The mechanisms for the accumulation of fluid in the peritoneal cavity are complex. Three pathways probably play a major role: hypoalbuminemia and reduced plasma osmotic pressure, renal retention of sodium and water, and increased hepatic lymph formation.

Hypoalbuminemia and Reduced Plasma Osmotic Pressure

Hypoalbuminemia can result from reduced synthesis (e.g. liver disease) and increased loss (e.g. nephrotic syndrome) resulting in reduction of plasma osmotic pressure. In face of portal hypertension this favours extravasation of fluid into the peritoneal cavity.

Renal Retention of Sodium and Water

During development of ascites, there is retension of sodium in spite of high total body sodium. Two theories have been propounded in this aspect: under fill theory and the over fill theory. According to the *under fill theory*, as a result of sequestration of fluid in the peritoneal cavity there is reduced effective circulating volume. This stimulates the juxtaglomerular cells to release renin. Renin converts angiotensin to angiotensin 1 which is converted to angiotensin 2 in the lungs by angiotensin converting enzyme. Angiotensin 2 releases aldosterone from zona glomerulus of the adrenal cortex. This increases the reabsorption of sodium and water and excretion of potassium from the distal convoluted tubules of the kidney thus contributing to formation of ascites. In case of cirrhosis of liver, the damaged liver is unable to metabolize ADH and aldosterone. This increases the blood levels of both and aggravates ascites.

Moreover, hypovolemia causes the release of ADH and contributes to ascites. Both these factors cause retention of sodium and water.

According to *the over fill theory* sodium and water retention is a primary response (for obscure reasons) with expansion of blood volume. Hypervolemia results in overflow from the congested portal system to the peritoneal cavity.

According to the *Nitric oxide theory (peripheral arterial vasodilatation theory)* when the portal pressure is above a critical threshold, nitric oxide levels increase leading to peripheral arterial vasodilatation resulting in decreased effective blood flow and increased sodium and water retention.

Increased Hepatic Lymph Formation

In case of cirrhosis, the hepatic architecture is distorted by fibrosis and nodule formation which compress the sinusoids. The increased sinusoidal pressure and the hepatic venous obstruction stimulate hepatic lymph production, which drains into the peritoneal cavity aggravating ascites. There is also decreased resorption of lymph from peritoneal surface and seepage from the splanchnic bed. The ascitic fluid often passes through the transdiaphrgmatic lymphatics into the pleural cavities, particularly on the right, to cause hydrothorax.

Etiology

Causes in Newborn

The causes of ascites in newborn may be associated with or without hydrops as follows:

1. **Associated with hydrops**
   a. *Cardiac causes:* Congenital heart block, Ebstein's anomaly, hypoplastic left heart syndrome.
   b. *Hematological disorders:* Homozygous alpha thalassemia, isoimmune hemolytic anemia.
   c. *Chromosomal anomalies* e.g. Turner's syndrome, Down's syndrome, Edwards syndrome, Patau syndrome.
   d. *Infections:* TORCH infection, congenital syphilis.
   e. *Renal causes:* Congenital nephrotic syndrome, posterior urethral valve.
   f. *G.I. and hepatic causes:* Intestinal atresia, neonatal hemochromatosis.
   g. *Malignant disease:* Wilms' tumour, neuroblastoma.
2. **Not associated with hydrops**
   a. Chylous ascites.
   b. Biliary ascites.
   c. Urinary ascites.
3. **Unknown cause.**

Causes in Older Children

The causes in older children may be enumerated as follows:

1. Liver disease
   i. Decompensated cirrhosis
   ii. Subacute hepatic failure
   iii. Veno-occlusive disease
   iv. Budd-Chiari syndrome

2. Peritoneal diseases
   i. Tuberculous peritonitis.
   ii. Bacterial peritonitis.
3. Renal causes
   i. Nephrotic syndrome.
4. Cardiac causes
   i. Cardiomyopathy.
   ii. Constrictive pericarditis.
5. Hypoalbuminemia
   i. Protein-losing enteropathy.
6. Endocrine causes
   i. Myxoedema.
7. Ovarian causes
   i. Meigs' syndrome.
   ii. Struma ovarii.
8. Miscellaneous
   i. Pancreatic ascites.
   ii. Filariasis.
   iii. Chylous ascites.
   iv. Polyserositis.
   v. Lymphatic obstruction.

Causes of Transudative Ascites

- Cirrhosis.
- Chronic congestive heart failure.
- Constrictive pericarditis.
- Nephrotic syndrome.
- Protein loosing enteropathy.

Causes of Exudative Ascites

- Tubercular peritonitis.
- Acute bacterial peritonitis.
- Pancreatitis.
- Malignant ascites.
- Myxedema.
- Budd-Chiari syndrome.
- Vasculitis.

Clinical Manifestations

Symptoms

Mild ascites is asymptomatic. As ascites increase, there may be sense of fullness of abdomen and abdominal discomfort. Massive ascites may cause respiratory distress, anorexia and nausea.

Signs

In *moderate* degree of ascites, the flanks are full. The umbilicus is everted with a horizontal slit. The distance between the pubic symphysis and the umbilicus seems to be decreased. In *massive ascites*, the abdomen is uniformly distended. The skin over the abdomen becomes shiny. There may be umbilical, femoral; and inguinal hernias due to increased intra-abdominal pressure. Scrotal edema is common.

The specific signs of fluid in the peritoneal cavity depend on the amount of fluid. Mild ascites can be detected by puddle sign and USG examination of the abdomen. In moderate ascites there is presence of shifting dullness but no fluid thrill. In massive ascites there is presence of fluid thrill and respiratory embarrassment.

Flank dullness is the most sensitive sign of ascites. Puddle sign helps to demonstrate minimal ascites (300–400 ml fluid). Fluid thrill is a late sign of massive ascites under tension and it is the most specific sign of ascites.

Grade	*Severity*	*Signs*
I	Mild	Puddle sign + ve USG examination
II	Moderate	Shifting dullness + ve No fluid thrill
III	Severe	Fluid thrill + ve Respiratory embarrassment

Complications

The complications which may occur with ascites may be as follows:

1. Spontaneous bacterial peritonitis.
2. Hydrothorax.
3. Gastroesophageal reflux.
4. Atelectasis of the lung due to elevation of the diaphragm.

Laboratory Diagnosis

1. **Ascitic fluid analysis:** Ascitic fluid is collected by abdominal paracentesis. 10–20 ml of fluid should be withdrawn for diagnostic studies. The ascitic fluid analysis includes examination of the gross appearance, chemical examination, cell count, serum ascites albumin gradient (SAAG), culture and cytology.

a. *Gross appearance:* Normally the peritoneal fluid is transparent or slightly yellow. It may be red in presence of red cells with a count more than 10,000/cu mm, milky if it is lipid laden, dark brown in presence of bilirubin, black or tea colored in pancreatic ascites, cloudy when the absolute neutrophil count is over 5,000/cu mm.

b. *Chemical examination:* Includes estimation of protein, amylase, adenosine deaminase (ADA), bilirubin, triglycerides and LDH (>225 IU/l). A protein level of > 3 gms/dl indicates exudative ascites. However, the concept of an exudative and transudative ascites has become obsolete now because it cannot differentiate ascites with and without portal hypertension. Amylase is increased in pancreatic ascites. ADA is increased in tubercular ascites (>60 u/l). A bilirubin level > 6 mg /dl indicates biliary or upper gut perforation. In Chylous ascites triglyceride level is very high (> 1000 mg/dl). An increased level of LDH (>225 mu/l) is often helpful in distinguishing spontaneous bacterial peritonitis from gut perforation. The above mentioned tests should be done only when indicated and not routinely.

c. *Cell count:* The upper limit of white cell count is 500 WBC per/dl with predominance of lymphocytes. The upper limit of polymorphs is 250 cells/dl. A cell count > 500 WBCs/dl suggest peritonitis. Predominance of polymorphs indicates likelihood of bacterial peritonitis whereas those of lymphocytes suggest tubercular peritonitis.

d. SAAG or the serum ascites albumin gradient is calculated by subtracting the ascitic fluid albumin level from serum albumin level. It is a superior method for categorizing ascites. Classifying ascitic fluid into transudate and exudate is not accurate and moreover it cannot differentiate ascites with or without portal hypertension. If the SAAG value is > 1.1 gm/dl, the ascites is due to portal hypertension. However, it cannot tell the etiology of portal hypertension. If the SAAG value is < 1.1 gm/dl, the ascites is due to some cause other than portal hypertension. The test is accurate irrespective of ascitic fluid infection, diuresis, therapeutic paracentesis, albumin infusion and etiology of liver disease.

Table 10.11 : Causes of ascites by SAAG

High gradient (> 1.1 gm/ dl)	*Low gradient (< 1.1 gm/dl)*
Cirrhosis	Tubercular peritonitis
Hepatitis	Nephrotic syndrome
Fulminant hepatic failure	Pancreatic ascites
Cardiac ascites	Bowel obstruction/ infarction
Budd-Chiari syndrome	Post operative lymphatic leak
Veno occlusive disease	Serositis in collagen disease

e. *Gram stain and culture:* Should be done on ascitic fluid for bacteria, mycobacteria and fungi in the appropriate clinical setting.

f. *Cytology* for malignant cells has an accuracy of 50–80%.

2. **Radioimaging:** *Ultrasonography* is sensitive as it can detect as little as 100 ml fluid. In minimal ascites, with the patient supine, fluid is detected in the flanks, more in the right flank. Very small collections are seen around the liver, in the pelvis and in the Morrison's pouch. A *CT scan* also can detect small collection (100 ml). It can also differentiate hemoperitoneum from other types of ascites.

3. **Peritoneal biopsy and peritoneoscopy:** Peritoneal biopsy is required if ascites is caused by a peritoneal disease. An unexplained ascites may require peritoneoscopy. It helps in inspection of the peritoneal cavity.

Management

The aim of therapy is to relieve ascites and treat the cause. The SAAG is helpful to therapeutic decision making. The treatment modalities will be depending on the type of ascites whether it is low albumin gradient or high albumin gradient. The etiology of ascites should be determined and appropriate treatment should be started.

Indications for Hospitalization

Children with ascites can be managed on an outpatient basis if compliance to therapy and regular follow up can be ensured. Hospitalization is necessary in the following circumstances:

1. No response to outpatient management for 4–6 weeks.
2. Tense (grade III) ascites.
3. Spontaneous bacterial peritonitis.

4. Presence of diuretic induced complications such as hyponatremia (Na < 125 mEq/L), hypokalemia (K<3 mEq/L), hepatic encephalopathy, refractory ascites etc.

Low Albumin Gradient Ascites

Treatment depends on the etiology of ascites. As these patients do not have portal hypertension, they do not respond to salt and water restriction and diuretics.

High Albumin Gradient Ascites

This type of ascites has portal hypertension. The plan of management is as follows:

1. *Bed rest* is essential because it give rest to the organs like liver in cirrhosis as it reduces the metabolites that have to be handled by the liver. It also increases the plasma volume and thereby increases renal perfusion.
2. *Salt restriction:* A negative sodium balance can be attained by restricting oral intake of salt to 2–3 grams/day or 2 mEq/kg/day in adolescents and 1 gm/day in younger children. For this no added salt should be allowed and salty snacks should be avoided.
3. *Fluid restriction:* Usually no fluid restriction is necessary unless there is hyponatremia (Na < 120 mEq/L). In such situation fluid should be restricted to 75% of the maintenance amount.
4. *Diet* should contain atleast 150% of the normal recommended calories out of which 15% should be from protein, 30–35% from fat and the rest from carbohydrates.
5. *Diuretics:* It is the mainstay of treatment and should be used liberally but carefully. In ascites associated with peripheral edema, diuretics should be prescribed in doses which will result in weight loss of less than 0.9 kg/day and in cases with only ascites the target of weight loss should be less than 0.5 kg/day. All diuretics should be given in a single dose to maximize compliance. Which diuretic to use?
   a. Potassium sparing diuretics to start with. *Spironolactone* in the doses of 1 mg/kg/day (in infant and young children) with increase in daily dose by 1 mg / kg/day upto a maximum dose of 6 mg/kg/day. In older children and adolescents, the dose is 100–200 mg/day which can be increased by 100 mg/day upto a maximum of 600 mg/day. *Amiloride* in the dose of 10 mg/day may be used in place of spironolactone.
   b. Loop diuretic such as frusemide is indicated in patients who respond partially to spironolactone. The starting dose is 1–2 mg/kg which can be increased by 1 mg/kg/day upto a maximum of 6 mg/kg/day.
   c. A combination of spironolactone and frusemide is found to be very effective.
   d. Hydrochlorothiazide is indicated when diuresis is inadequate on high doses of two diuretics. The dose is 2–3 mg/kg/day. It should be used along with spironolactone.
   e. The diuretics for treatment of ascites should be continued till ascites is relieved. When used for prevention it may have to be continued for months to years.
6. *Therapeutic paracentesis* decreases the systemic venous congestion, increases renal blood flow and glomerular filtration rate resulting in diuresis. It is indicated in cases with tense ascites, intractable ascites not responding to usual treatment and to release intra-abdominal pressure in Grade II and III ascites. A volume of upto 100 ml/kg can be safely tapped at any time. A large volume should be tapped in one sitting rather than frequent taps.

Monitoring During Diuretic Therapy

Patients on diuretic therapy should be monitored for too rapid fluid mobilization and for diuretic induced complications.

- The patient should be assessed 1 week after starting therapy and every two weeks thereafter.
- One should confirm strict adherence to salt restriction, bed rest and diuretics as prescribed.
- Measurement of abdominal girth and weight.
- Look for signs like edema, grade of ascites and subtle signs of SBP.
- A weight loss of more than 1% per day or 4–6%/week of the previous weight indicate too rapid mobilization of fluid and sodium which will require reduction of dose of diuretics and evaluation of renal function.

Management of Refractory Ascites

Refractory ascites is defined as ascites not responding

to salt restriction and high dose of diuretics. The treatment includes the following modalities:

1. *Repeated therapeutic paracentesis.*
2. *Peritoneal venous shunt* is a device which mechanically transfuses the ascitic fluid to the superior vena cava by a long perforated plastic tube, thereby producing a sustained expansion of the circulating blood volume.
3. *TIPSS (Transjugular intrahepatic portosystemic shunt)* is a technique where a stent is placed between the hepatic vein and the portal vein within the liver to provide portosystemic shunt to reduce portal pressure.
4. *Ascites ultrafiltration and reinfusion* is a technique where the ascitic fluid is removed via a peritoneal dialysis catheter with the help of a automated ultrafiltration apparatus. The concentrate after filtration contains 2–4 times more protein and the fluid is infused intravenously to the patient.
5. Orthotropic liver transplant.

Acute Pancreatitis

Acute pancreatitis is the most common disease of the pancreas in children. The common causes of acute pancreatitis include blunt abdominal injuries, viral illness, multisystem disease, congenital anomalies, drugs and biliary microlithiasis; the most common being trauma, drugs and viral infections.

Table 10.12 : Etiology of acute pancreatitis

Idiopathic
Trauma
Blunt injury, burns, child abuses, surgical trauma.
Drugs
Acetaminophen overdose, Erythromycin, Furosemide, Thiazides, Tetracycline, Sulphonamides, Pentamidine, Valproic acid, Enalapril, L-aspariginase, Vincristine, 6, Mercaptopurine, Venom (spider, scorpion).
Infections
Virus: Coxsakie B, EB virus, Hepatitis A, B, Influenza A and B, Measles, Mumps, Rubella, Varicella.
Parasite: Ascariasis, Malaria.
Others: Leptospirosis, Mycoplasma, Reye's syndrome.

Contd.

Contd.

Systemic disease
Collagen vascular disease, Diabetes mellitus, HUS, Hyperlipidemia type I and IV, V, SLE, Kawasaki disease, Malnutrition, Alpha 1 anti-trypsin deficiency, Brain tumours, Peptic ulcer, Hyperparathyroidism, Organic acidemia, Transplant– bone marrow, liver, heart etc.
Congenital abnormalities
Cholelithiasis, microlithiasis and choledocholithiasis, Pancreatic duct abnormalities, Duplication cysts, Spincter of Oddi dysfunction, Tumor, ERCP complication.

Pathogenesis

The exact pathogenesis is still not clearly defined. Several theories have been proposed. A recent theory suggests that following an insult, there is release of cytokines and subsequent depletion of antioxidants which leads to pancreastasis and activation of pancreatic proenzymes leading to auto digestion.

Histopathologically, there is interstitial edema initially followed by localized and confluent necrosis, blood vessel disruption leading to hemorrhage, and an inflammatory response in the peritoneum.

Clinical Manifestations

In *uncomplicated acute pancreatitis*, the patient presents with abdominal pain, persistent vomiting and fever. The pain is epigastric and continuous. The child assumes a typical position with hips and knees flexed, sitting upright or lying on the side. The child is very uncomfortable and irritable and appears acutely ill. The abdomen may be distended and tender and a mass may be palpable. The pain increases in intensity for 24–48 hours. During this time vomiting may increase and there may be dehydration which may necessitate hospitalization and I.V. fluid and electrolyte therapy. The child recovers and prognosis is excellent.

Severe acute pancreatitis is rare in children. It is a life threatening condition. The patient is acutely ill with severe nausea, vomiting and abdominal pain. There is high fever, jaundice, ascites and pleural effusion. The child may go to shock. A bluish discoloration may be seen around the umbilicus (Cullen sign) or in the flanks (Grey Turner sign). The mortality rate is around 50% and is a result of multiorgan failure (renal failure, DIC, ARDS, massive GI bleed, infection).

Laboratory Diagnosis

There is no single laboratory test for diagnosis of acute pancreatitis. Further, the available tests are non-specific and may be sometimes misleading. So it needs careful interpretation.

Serum amylase and lipase levels are the most commonly used tests. The serum amylase level is elevated for upto 4 days. However, serum amylase may be elevated in variety of other conditions without pancreatitis such as mumps, other viral parotitis, intestinal obstruction, peritonitis, appendicitis etc. Elevation of salivary amylase may mislead the diagnosis in a child with abdominal pain. Separation of amylase isoenzyme into salivary and pancreatic fractions is helpful in such a situation. Serum lipase is more specific for acute pancreatitis. The serum lipase remains elevated for 8–14 days longer than serum amylase. Serum lipase is elevated even when serum amylase may be normal in the initial stages.

The other abnormalities observed in acute pancreatitis include leucocytosis, hyperglycemia, glycosuria, hypocalcemia, hyperbilirubinemia, elevated gamma glutamyl transpeptidase. There may be hemoconcentration and coagulopathy.

Ultrasound and CT examination has a major role in diagnosis and follow-up of cases of acute pancreatitis. Findings may include pancreatic enlargement, hypoechoic, sonoluscent edematous pancreas, fluid collection and abscesses. However, in atleast 20% cases pancreatic imaging may be normal in the initial stages.

Endoscopic retrograde cholangiopancreatography (ERCP) or magnetic resonance cholangiopancreatography (MRCP) are essential investigations for recurrent pancreatitis, dysfunction of sphincter of Oddi and disease associated with gallbladder pathology. Endoscopic USG helps to visualize the pancreaticobiliary system.

A **chest X-ray** may demonstrate non-specific findings like atelectasis, basilar infiltrates, elevation of the hemidiaphragm, left sided (rarely right sided) pleural effusion, pericardial effusion and pulmonary edema.

A **plain X-ray of abdomen** may reveal dilatation of the transverse colon (cut off sign), small bowel ileus, pancreatic calcification (if recurrent), a pseudocyst, ascites, and pancreatic extra luminal gas bubbles.

Treatment

In uncomplicated acute pancreatitis the child should be advised nil orally and nasogastric suction when there is vomiting. Fluid and electrolyte imbalance should be restored and the balance maintained with IV fluid. Refeeding may be commenced when clinical symptoms are resolved and serum amylase is falling. The response to treatment is usually complete over 2–5 days.

Children with severe acute pancreatitis require total parenteral nutrition, prophylactic antibiotics to prevent infected pancreatic necrosis, gastric acid suppression with H_2 blockers, and peritoneal lavage to reduce secondary infection and rarely surgical drainage of necrotic material or abscesses. Endoscopic treatment is indicated when the cause is an anatomic abnormality such as strictures and calculus.

Prognosis

Children with uncomplicated acute pancreatitis recover over a period of 2–5 days. When pancreatitis is associated with trauma or systemic disease, the prognosis is related to the associated medical problems. Regarding severe pancreatitis, data in children is limited but suggests a mortality of around 50%.

Suggested Reading

1. National child survival and safe motherhood programme. Integrated skills course for physicians. Acute respiratory infections, diarrhoeal diseases and essential newborn care. MCH division. Department of Family Welfare, Ministry of Health and Family Welfare, Government of India.
2. IAP Text Book of Pediatrics. First edition. 1999. Published by Jaypee Brothers Medical Publishers (P) Ltd. New Delhi.
3. Indian Pediatrics, Vol. 37, 2000.
4. Pediatric Gastroenterology and Hepatology. A. Riyaz, 2nd edition, Paras Publishing, Hyderabad.
5. Practical Pediatric Gastroenterology, JA Walker, Smith J R, 1st edition, 1993.
6. Recent Advances in Pediatrics, Special Vol. 6 on Gastroenterology, Hepatology and Nutrition. Edited by Suraj Gupte, Published by Jaypee Brothers, New Delhi.
7. Paul N. Thiessen, Recurrent Abdominal Pain. Pediatrics Vol. 14, No. 3, 2003.
8. The liver and biliary system in infants and children. Edited by R.K.Chandra. Published by Churchill Livingstone, Great Britain.
9. Nelson's Textbook of Pediatrics, 16th, 17th and 18th editions, Saunders.
10. Parasitology by K.D. Chatterjee, 12th edition, 1980. Published by Chatterjee Medical Publishers, Kolkata.

11

Infectious Diseases

OUTLINES

Typhoid Fever

Etiology

Enteric fever or typhoid fever is an acute systemic febrile illness found exclusively in human beings. It is caused by salmonella typhi as well as para typhi A, B and C.

Epidemiology

The incidence, mode of transmission and consequences of typhoid fever differ significantly in developed and developing countries. The incidence has markedly decreased in developed countries whereas it is increasing in developing countries with increase number of cases occurring below 5 years with emergence of multi-drug resistant strains.

Ingestion of food contaminated with human feces is the most common mode of transmission. Water borne outbreaks due to poor sanitation and direct fecal oral spread due to poor personal hygiene of food handlers are encountered in developing countries. In developed countries it is usually caused by international travel. It may also result from consumption of food handled and contaminated by individuals who are chronic carriers.

Congenital transmission can occur by transplacental infection from a bacteremic mother to her fetus. Intrapartum transmission is also possible by fecal-oral route from a carrier mother.

Pathology

The morphological changes include hyperplasia of Peyer's patches with necrosis and sloughing of the overlying epithelium in the small intestine producing ulcers which may bleed. The ulcers heal without scarring. The inflammatory lesions occasionally penetrate the muscularis and serosa of the intestine and produce perforation. The mesenteric lymph nodes, liver and spleen are hyperemic and generally reveal areas of focal necrosis. Proliferation of the mono nuclear cells may be seen in the bone marrow in association with areas of focal necrosis. There is also inflammation of the gallbladder and bronchial mucosa. Inflammation may also be observed in the form of localized abscesses, pneumonia, septic arthritis, osteomyelitis, pyelonephritis, endophthalmitis and meningitis. It needs mention that the morphological changes are less prominent in younger children than in older children and adults.

Pathogenesis

After oral ingestion, the bacteria invade through Peyer's patches. Organisms are transported to the intestinal lymph nodes where multiplication takes place in the mono nuclear cells. The monocytes, unable to destroy the bacilli carry the organism to the mesenteric lymph nodes. Organisms then reach the blood stream through the thoracic duct causing a transient bacteremia. This marks the onset of fever. The circulating organisms then reach the RE cells in the liver, spleen and bone marrow and may seed other organs. After proliferation in the RE system, bacteremia recurs. This heralds the onset of the disease. The gallbladder is particularly susceptible to infection. Local multiplication of the organism in the walls of the gallbladder produces large numbers of salmonellae, which reach the intestine through bile.

Several virulence factors possessed by the salmonella seem to be important in the pathogenesis. A high inoculum size reduces the gastric acidity facilitating survival of the organism. The surface Vi capsular antigen found in S typhi interferes with phagocytosis. The ability of the organism to survive within macrophages is an important virulence trait. The circulating endotoxin which is a lipopolysaccharide component of the bacterial cell wall is thought to be responsible for the prolonged fever and toxic symptoms of enteric fever. There is a reduction in the number of T lymphocytes in patients who are critically ill with typhoid fever resulting in lowered cell mediated immunity. The carriers, on the other hand show impaired cellular activity to S. typhi antigens. The carriers pass into their intestine a large number of bacilli which are excreted in the stool without entering the epithelium of the host.

Clinical Manifestations

The clinical manifestations of typhoid fever differ according to age. The incubation period is usually 7–14 days, but it may range from 3 to 30 days.

Neonates

Enteric fever during pregnancy can cause abortion, preterm delivery and vertical transmission and intrapartum transmission. The neonatal disease usually begins within 3 days of delivery. Vomiting, diarrhea and abdominal distension are common. Temperature is variable but may be as high as 40.5°C. Seizure may occur. Hepatomegaly, jaundice and weight loss may be marked.

Infants and Young Children (< 5 years)

The disease is mild at presentation characterized by mild fever and malaise, often misinterpreted as a viral illness. Diarrhea is more common leading to a diagnosis of acute gastroenteritis. Recently multi-drug resistant typhoid is seen more commonly in this age group.

School Children and Adolescents

This is the most common age group of children to suffer from typhoid fever. The clinical picture evolves in around three weeks with different symptoms and signs.

First week illness: The onset is insidious with fever, malaise, anorexia, myalgia, headache and abdominal pain which develop over 2–3 days. Initially there may be loose motions of pea soup consistency but later constipation is the prominent symptom. There may be cough and epistaxis. Severe lethargy may develop in some children. Fever increases in a step ladder pattern, becomes continuous and high within one week; often may reach as high as 40°C.

Second and third week illness: High fever is sustained. Fatigue, anorexia, cough and abdominal symptoms increase in severity. The child appears acutely ill, disoriented and lethargic. Delirium and stupor may be observed. The physical findings on examination include hepatosplenomegaly and distension of abdomen with diffuse tenderness, rhonchi and scattered rales on auscultation of chest. Relative bradycardia disproportionate to high fever is uncommon in children.

In about 50% cases, rose spots appear on about 7th–10th day. It is a macular or maculopapular rash, usually discrete, erythematous and 1–5 mm in diameter. The lesions are slightly raised and blanch on pressure. They appear in crops of 10–15 lesions on the lower chest and abdomen and last for 2–3 days. They leave a brownish discoloration of skin on healing. Culture of the lesions has a 60% yield of salmonella organism.

Complications

Most complications occur after the first week of disease. Nausea and vomiting, if occurring in the second or third week suggests a complication. The following complications can occur in typhoid fever. However, permanent sequalae are rare.

1. *Severe intestinal hemorrhage and intestinal perforation:* Hemorrhage usually precedes perforation. It is manifested by decrease in temperature and blood pressure and increase in the pulse rate. Perforations may be of pin point size to as large as several centimeters. It is seen typically in the distal ileum. The characteristic manifestations include marked increase in abdominal pain, tenderness, vomiting and signs of peritonitis.
2. Hepatitis, cholecystitis and pancreatitis.
3. Pneumonia due to secondary infection is common.
4. Toxic myocarditis (manifested by arrhythmias, sino-atrial block or shock), endocarditis.
5. Neurologic complications include acute cerebellar ataxia, aphasia, deafness, psychosis, peripheral and optic neuritis, meningitis.
6. Pyelonephritis, nephrotic syndrome.
7. Bone marrow necrosis.
8. Osteomyelitis and septic arthritis, more common in children with hemoglobinopathies.

Multi-Drug Resistant Typhoid Fever (MDRTF)

Definition

Epidemiologically, in MDRTF salmonella typhi strain is resistant to any two known antibiotics usually effective against typhoid fever viz. Chloramphenicol, Ampicillin, Amoxicillin and Cotrimoxazole.

Clinical Presentations

MDRTF is more common in children below 5 years age. It has been reported in children below 2 years also. There is a history of protracted illness (7–10 days) characterized by fever of varying degrees and toxemia. There is frequent occurrence of high fever with chill.

Extra abdominal features are more common. These consist of:

a. Cough and respiratory distress. It is the most common presentation.
b. Cardiovascular complications follow next. It comprises toxic myocarditis, arrhythmias.
c. Neurological disorders viz. seizure, focal deficits, acute cerebellar ataxia and acute flaccid paralysis.
d. Hepatitis.
e. Abscess formation in brain, bone, liver, spleen and lymph nodes.
f. Abdominal features include diarrhea, constipation, abdominal distension, paralytic ileus, GI hemorrhage and perforation.

Laboratory Diagnosis

1. **Cultures:** Blood culture is the confirmatory test. It is positive in 40–60% of patients in the first week.

Stool and urine culture become positive after the 1st week. The stool culture is also occasionally positive during the incubation period. Bone marrow culture is the most sensitive method for diagnosis (positivity is 85–90%) and often yield positive results during later stages when blood culture is negative. It is less influenced by prior antibiotic therapy.

2. **Widal test** measures the antibodies against O and H antigens of S. typhi. Because of many false positive and false negative results, diagnosis of typhoid fever by Widal test alone is prone to error. It is positive usually after 7–10 days of onset of fever. Elevation of antibody against O antigen indicates acute infection and has a better diagnostic value. A four-fold rise of titre in a nonimmune individual is considered diagnostic. If a child had suffered from typhoid fever or had immunization against typhoid, the H titre rises rapidly with non-typhoid fevers but the O titre does not rise. For practical purposes and for optimal result Widal test should be done after 7 days of fever by the tube method and level of O and H antibody titre of 1: 160 should be taken as cut off value for diagnosis.
3. **Other serologic tests:** A dot enzyme immunoassay that detects IgG and IgM antibodies distinct from the somatic (O), flagellar (H) or capsular (Vi) antigen of salmonella typhi is available as *Typhidot.* The sensitivity and specificity of this test has been reported to vary from 70–100% and 43–90%. The detection of IgM reveals acute typhoid in early phase of infection, while the detection of both IgM and IgG suggest acute typhoid in middle phase. However in areas of high endemicity, as IgG will already be high it cannot differentiate between the acute and convalescent phase. To overcome this problem, the original test is modified by inactivating the total IgG in the serum samples. The *Typhidot M* test detects only the IgM antibodies of salmonella typhi and has been reported to be slightly more specific.
4. **Blood, urine, stool examination:** For practical purposes the CBC is unremarkable in enteric fever. *Leukocyte count* is normal or low in relation to fever and toxicity. Leucopenia, usually not less than 2500 cells/cumm is often found after the first or second week of illness. If there is a pyogenic complication the count may be as high as 20–25 thousand cells/cumm. Initially there is moderate neutropenia followed by relative lymphocytosis. Eosinopenia often absolute may be present in 70–80% cases. *Thrombocytopenia* may be striking in the second week of illness and persist for as long as 1 week. A normocytic normochromic anemia often develops due to intestinal blood loss or bone marrow suppression.

   Liver function tests including AST (SGPT): LDH ratio: The LFT is deranged. An AST: LDH ratio < 4 differentiates typhoid hepatitis and viral hepatitis.

   Proteinuria is common.

   Stool contains blood/RBCs and WBCs.
5. *Other laboratory tests* when indicated may be done are:
   a. X-ray PA view chest in presence of respiratory difficulty.
   b. ECG in suspected myocarditis.
   c. USG abdomen to exclude intestinal complications.
   d. Bone marrow examination in presence of signs of bone marrow suppression.

Treatment

Most typhoid cases can be treated at home with oral antibiotics and good nursing. Severe cases with persistent vomiting, inability to take oral feeds, severe diarrhoea, abdominal distension, need admission and administration of parenteral antibiotics.

Antimicrobial Therapy

Chloramphenicol (50 mg/kg/day 6 hourly PO) has been the standard treatment of typhoid fever in children. Other drugs used are Ampicillin (200 mg/kg/day 6 hourly PO), Amoxycillin (100 mg/kg/day 6 hourly PO) and Cotrimoxazole (trimethoprim 6–8 mg/kg/day 12 hourly PO). Most antibiotic regimens are associated with a recurrence risk of 5–20%.

Resistant strains of S. typhi are usually susceptible to 3rd generation cephalosporins. Quinolones are efficacious but not approved for children below 18 years and may be used only in cases resistant to all other recommended antibiotics.

The antibiotics recommended are as follows:

Antibiotic therapy for hospital admitted cases are:

1. Ceftriaxone 50–75 mg/kg/day IV 12 hourly for 24–48 hours followed by oral Cefixime 15–20 mg/kg/day 12 hourly.
2. Ceftriaxone 50–75 mg/kg/day 12 hourly.

3. Ciprofloxacin 10 mg/kg/day IV for 24 to 48 hours then orally 15 mg/kg/day 12 hourly.
4. Ofloxacin 10 mg/kg/day IV for 24–48 hours then orally 15 mg/kg/day 12 hourly.

Antibiotic therapy for ambulatory (OPD cases) include:

1. Cefixime 20 mg/kg/day 12 hourly.
2. Ciprofloxacin 15 mg/kg/day 12 hourly.
3. Ofloxacin 15 mg/kg/day 12 hourly.
4. Azithromycin 20 mg/kg/day 12 hourly.

Duration of Antibiotic Therapy

Most children become afebrile by 5–7 days. The antibiotic should be continued for 5–7 days after fever subsides or 10 days whichever is later.

Supportive Therapy

Control of temperature: Paracetamol 10–15 mg/kg/dose 4–6 hourly when axillary temperature is 101°F (axillary) or more. When temperature is > 104°F paracetamol should be given. If temperature does not come down after 45 minutes, it should be followed by tepid sponging of whole body for 20–30 minutes. This is helpful in bringing down the temperature. Other antipyretics should be avoided. Antipyretics should be used judiciously because they may cause precipitous fall in temperature.

Diet and fluid intake: The intake of calories, protein, iron and vitamins should be adequate for normal daily requirement. Diet should not be withheld because intestinal ulcers heal better in presence of food in the gut. Parenteral nutrition may be required in very sick children and in those with abdominal complications. Fluid intake and urine output should be maintained.

Nursing care: Frequent cleaning of oral cavity with antiseptic wash lotions, and appropriate care of the unconscious patient.

Dexamethasone, transfusion and surgical repair may be required in some cases. A short course of Dexamethasone (3 mg/kg IV for the initial dose followed by 1 mg/kg/dose IV 6 hourly for 2 days) should be given to patients presenting in shock, stupor or coma.

Transfusion and surgical repair for complications e.g. intestinal hemorrhage and perforation may be required. Platelet transfusion may be indicated for severe thrombocytopenia.

Relapse Typhoid Fever

5–10% of cases have a relapse 1–2 weeks after completion of therapy. It usually follows a milder course and responds to the initial antibiotic. A blood culture may be required if not done earlier and treatment started according to the sensitivity.

Prevention

The most effective way is routine immunization of the child. An unimmunized child should be given typhoid vaccine 3 months after recovery. In endemic areas improved sanitation and clean running water are essential to control. Personal hygienic measures, hand washing and attention to clean food preparation practices are important.

Carriers should be prevented to work in food or water processing activities if personal hygienic measures cannot be maintained. Chances of becoming carriers in children are low.

Malaria

Malaria is the most common parasitic disease of man. The word malaria comes from the Italian word 'mal air' and literally means bad air. The Italian writers thought that malaria was caused by offensive vapours from the marshes. Charles Louis Alphonse Laveran, a French army surgeon first claimed that malaria was caused by a parasite. In 1880, he examined fresh blood and identified parasites in the red blood cells. The parasitic stage in the mosquito was first reported by the Scottish physician, Ronald Ross in 1897. He identified the anopheles mosquito as the vector of human malaria and finally demonstrated plasmodium falciparum sporogony in anopheles mosquito. Both Laveran and Ross received Nobel prizes for their respective discoveries.

Etiology

Malaria is caused by intracellular plasmodium protozoa. Four species of plasmodium cause malaria in humans. They are P. falciparum, P. vivax, P. malariae and P. ovale. It is usually transmitted to humans by the bite of a female anopheles mosquito. The other modes of transmission are transfusion (whole blood, packed cells, platelets, leucocytes), organ transplant, by use of contaminated needles and vertical transmission from mother to fetus. Occasionally, malaria infection is caused by more than one species of plasmodium. In such mixed infections, one species may be temporarily suppressed by the other species. Thus, in a mixed infection of P. falciparum and P. vivax, the primary attack is due to P.

falciparum, but relapses occurring subsequently are produced by P. vivax.

Epidemiology

Malaria is a worldwide problem with much more importance in the developing world. Most malarial deaths occur in infants and children and are a result of plasmodium falciparum infection. Transmission of malaria has been eliminated in most parts of North America including the USA, Europe and the Caribbean, Australia, Chile, Israel, Japan, Korea, Lebanon, China and Taiwan.

Malaria is one of the major public health problems in India. Around 50% of the total malaria cases reported is due to P. falciparum. One of the reasons attributed to rise in proportion of P. Falciparum cases is resistance to Chloroquine, which was used for a long time as the first line of treatment of malaria cases. P. Falciparum infections are known to lead to severe malaria, if timely treatment with effective drugs is not administered.

Pathogenesis

Plasmodium species has a complex life cycle that enables them to survive in different cellular environments in the human host (asexual cycle) and the vector mosquito (sexual cycle).

The asexual cycle consist of two phases: exoerythrocytic phase, which occurs in the liver and erythrocytic phase which occurs in the red cells.

The *exoerythrocytic phase* begins with inoculation of sporozoites into the blood stream by a female anopheles mosquito. Within minutes, the sporozoites enter the hepatocytes of liver where they develop and multiply asexually forming schizonts which are filled with merozoites. After 1–2 weeks, the hepatocytes rupture and release thousands of merozoites into the circulation. The tissue schizonts of P. falciparum and P. malariae rupture once and none persists in the liver. There are two types of tissue schizonts for P. ovale and P. vivax. The primary type ruptures in 6–9 days while the secondary type remains dormant in the liver cells for weeks, months or even years before releasing merozoites and thereby causing relapse of infection.

The *erythrocytic phase* begins when the merozoites penetrate the red cells in the circulation. Once inside the erythrocytes, the parasite transforms into the ring form, which then enlarges to become a trophozoite. These two latter forms can be identified with Giemsa stain on blood smear. The trophozoite multiplies asexually to produce a number of erythrocytic merozoites. The merozoites are released into the blood stream when the red cell membrane ruptures. Over time some of these merozoites develop into male and female gametocytes and circulate in the blood.

Sexual Cycle

The gametocytes are ingested by the female anopheles mosquito during a blood meal. The male and female gametocytes fuse to form a zygote in the stomach cavity of the mosquito which develops into an oocyst beneath the outer membrane of the mid gut. A few thousand sporozoites develop within the mature oocyst. The oocyst burst and releases the sporozoites into the body cavity of the insect host. Most of the sporozoites migrate to the salivary glands of the mosquito and are inoculated into a new host with the next blood meal.

Pathophysiology

The pathophysiology of malaria results from destruction of erythrocytes, liberation of parasite and erythrocyte material into circulation and the host reaction to events. Four important pathologic processes have been described in patients with malaria:

1. *Fever:* Occurs as a result of rupture of erythrocytes and release of merozoites into circulation.
2. *Anemia:* Is caused by hemolysis, sequestration of erythrocytes in spleen and other organs, and bone marrow depression.
3. *Immunopathologic events:* Documented in malaria include:
   a. Hypergammaglobulinemia and formation of immune complexes.
   b. Immunodepression.
   c. Release of cytokines viz. Tumour necrosis factor (TNF).
4. Tissue anoxia: In falciparum malaria, two phenomena are noted in the pathogenesis of tissue anoxia:
   a. Cytoadherence of infected erythrocytes to the vascular endothelium leading to obstruction of blood flow and capillary damage with resultant vascular leak of protein and fluid, edema and tissue anoxia in the vital organs viz. brain, heart, lung, kidney and intestine.
   b. Sequestration of P. falciparum infected erythrocytes in the microcirculation of the vital organs which interferes with the microcirculatory flow and host tissue metabolism.

Clinical Epidemiology

There is a relationship between age and clinical presentation of severe malaria at different levels of malaria transmission.

In *hyper endemic areas* (spleen or parasite rate 50–75% and adult spleen rate is high), young infants (0 to 3 months) infrequently develop severe malaria as a result of passive transfer of maternal immunity and the high Hb F content of the infants' erythrocytes. These factors retard parasite development. Children between 3 months to 2–5 years have little specific immunity to malaria species and can suffer yearly attacks and potentially fatal disease.

In *holoendemic areas* (spleen or parasite rate over 75% and adult spleen rate is low), the main clinical impact of falciparum malaria is to cause severe anemia in the 1 to 3 years age group. With less intense, more variable or unstable transmission, the age range affected by severe disease extends to older children and cerebral malaria becomes a prominent manifestation of severe disease.

In *hypo endemic* areas (spleen rate or parasite rate 0–10%), the prominent manifestation is cerebral malaria and severe anemia. Acute renal failure is common after 5 years of age.

Presence of HbS in erythrocytes resists growth of malarial parasites. Erythrocytes containing HbF and ovalocytes are resistant to P. falciparum infection.

Clinical Manifestations

The incubation period of malaria infection is different for the different species viz. P. falciparum, 9–14 days; P. vivax, 12–17 days; P. malariae, 18–40 days; P. ovale, 16–18 days. The incubation period may be prolonged in patients with partial immunity or with inadequate chemoprophylaxis. It can be as long as 6–12 months in P. vivax.

The most severe form of malaria is caused by P. falciparum. It is associated with a high mortality if appropriate therapy is not instituted promptly. Hence the diagnosis of P. falciparum malaria is a medical emergency. P. vivax malaria is generally less severe but it causes relapse if radical treatment is not given. Relapse is common within 6 months after an acute attack but may occur as long as 5 years after the initial attack. P. malariae is the mildest infection. But it can cause chronic ill health in addition to febrile illness. P. ovale malaria is the least common type. It is commonly found in conjunction with P. falciparum malaria.

Clinically malaria may be (a) uncomplicated and (b) severe. In children, the classical features of malarial paroxysm, as seen typically in adults, are not common. Moreover, the clinical presentation differs according to the immune status of the child.

Uncomplicated Malaria

In non-immune children older than 2 months of age, fever is the characteristic clinical feature of malaria. Fever may vary widely from low grade to a temperature greater than 104°F. Fever is usually persistent but may be intermittent. The child usually complain of associated symptoms like headache, myalgia, anorexia, nausea. The child may present with febrile convulsion. Occasionally, gastrointestinal symptoms (vomiting and diarrhea) and respiratory symptoms (cough, increased respiratory rate, crepitations and rhonchi) may predominate.

Slight enlargement and tenderness of liver are found more consistently than splenomegaly. Spleen may be enlarged and tender especially if the illness has been present for a number of days or if the child has been exposed previously to malaria. Rupture of the spleen has been described in P. vivax infection but is a rare complication.

In children from highly endemic area, after a primary infection, parasitemia is minimal and symptoms are mild which include restlessness, anorexia, pallor, sweating and occasional fever. After some time, the inherited immunity declines and attacks become more severe.

The partially immune children, on marginal diet develop loss of weight, anemia, edema or frank Kwashiorkor and are not completely cured until malaria is treated. However, with a good diet, the effects of malaria are not marked.

Severe Malaria

Severe malaria is more likely during the first attack of malaria than in the subsequent attacks and in partially immune malnourished children from the endemic zone who are continuously exposed to malarial infection without any protection.

The WHO technical meeting in 1988 defined the following criteria for severe malaria. The patient who is clinically unwell, one or more of the following features qualify for the definition of severe malaria.

1. Cerebral malaria.
2. Severe normocytic normochromic anemia (Hb < 5 gm/dl with parasitemia > 10,000/ micro litre.
3. Renal failure (urine output < 12 ml/kg/day + creatinine > 265 micro mol/litre (> 3 mg / dl).
4. Pulmonary edema.

5. Hypoglycemia defined as whole blood glucose < 2.2 mmol/litre(< 40 mg/dl).
6. Circulatory collapse or shock – Hypotension (systolic pressure < 50 mm Hg in children aged 1–5 years and < 70 mm above 5 years) with cold clammy skin or core skin temperature difference > 10°C.
7. Spontaneous bleeding from gums, nose, GIT etc and /or laboratory evidence of DIC.
8. Repeated generalized convulsion – more than 2 convulsions in 24 hours despite cooling.
9. Acidemia (arterial pH < 7.25) or acidosis (plasma bicarbonate < 15 mmol/L).
10. Macroscopic hemoglobinuria (not drug induced).

Complications of Malaria

The complications of malaria may occur early in the course of the disease or may be late. The early complications include cerebral malaria, black water fever, renal failure, pulmonary edema, hypoglycemia, DIC, splenic rupture, algid malaria.

The late complications include septicemia and nephrotic syndrome. Septicemia is often caused by salmonella species, and may follow an attack of malaria, especially among patients with anemia. A small proportion of P. malariae infection is followed by an immune complex mediated nephritis and usually presents as nephrotic syndrome. This frequently progresses to end stage renal failure.

Cerebral Malaria

Cerebral malaria is the most common form of severe malaria. It is associated with a fatality rate of 20–40% but rarely causes long-term sequalae if it is treated appropriately. Although cerebral malaria due to P. falciparum infection is well documented, some reports mention P. vivax as a causative agent also. Cerebral malaria is more likely in patients with parasitemia greater than 5%. Onset may be insidious or rapid. It may be associated with very high fever but presence of fever is not a must for diagnosis of cerebral malaria. Presence of any manifestation of cerebral dysfunction in a case of malaria should be taken as an evidence of cerebral malaria. These manifestations of cerebral dysfunction include:

1. *Severe headache and drowsiness, confusion delirium, impaired consciousness, deep coma.* Loss of consciousness can occur very rapidly and some children are already in deep coma by the time they reach hospital.
2. *Abnormal neurological signs:* Localizing neurological signs are found infrequently. In severe cases there may be increased muscle tone, contracted or unequal pupils, hemiplegia, absent or exaggerated deep tendon reflexes, positive Babinski sign, opistotonus and decerebrate rigidity. Papilledema is rare but retinal hemorrhages are sometimes seen. CSF analysis reveals increased pressure and protein with minimal or no pleocytosis and a normal glucose concentration.
3. *Focal or generalized convulsion:* Sometimes high fever alone, without any cerebral pathology may produce febrile convulsion and some impairment of consciousness. If the post ictal unconsciousness persists for more than 30 minutes, such cases should be diagnosed as cerebral malaria.

Black Water Fever

Black water fever is a clinical syndrome characterized by severe hemolysis, hemoglobinuria and renal failure. It is usually transient. Acute renal failure, as a result of acute tubular necrosis, may develop in severe cases.

Chloroquine Resistant Falciparum Malaria

Chloroquine resistance should be assumed if:

1. Clinically the patient with slide positive falciparum infection does not respond within 72 hours.
2. If the parasite count does not drop rapidly (within 24–48 hours) and become negative after 4 days of treatment with adequate dose of chloroquine.
3. The national malaria treatment guidelines recommend that change of drug in case of resistance should be considered when treatment failure with chloroquine exceeds 10% in a minimum sample of 30 cases. In such situation a switch over to ACT should be considered.

Diagnosis of Malaria

There are no clinical features diagnostic of uncomplicated malaria. Malaria should be considered in differential diagnosis of any febrile child resident in a malaria endemic area or in a child who has been a recent visitor to such an area, even if chemoprophylaxis has been taken. Similarly, cerebral malaria must be considered in any child who presents with convulsion or develops impairment of consciousness which persists for more than 30 minutes. A diagnosis of clinical malaria appears justified if fever subsided rapidly in 24–48 hours of administration of an adequately dosed antimalarial.

Laboratory Diagnosis

Detection of Malaria Parasite in Peripheral Blood Smear

The diagnosis of malaria is established by detection of malaria parasite in a thick or thin film but it is not without fallacies. In *non-immune children*, symptoms may occur when parasitemia is only at a low level. This is also true in children who are on chemoprophylaxis or who have been already administered an antimalarial drug few hours before examination of the blood film. So a careful search for parasites is necessary preferably on more than one blood film before a diagnosis is excluded. In contrast, in *endemic areas*, many asymptomatic children have parasitemia which demonstrates the presence of infection but it does not determine disease.

Some degree of normocytic anemia, thrombocytopenia, and a polymorphonuclear leucocytosis are frequently found.

Preparation of the Blood Film

Steps

1. Swabbing of the skin of the ball of the ring or middle finger or great toe (in case of infants) with ether or alcohol.
2. When clean and dry, the skin is pricked with a triangular, cutting Hagedorn needle.
3. For the thick smear, a large drop of fresh blood is touched by a clean slide. The blood drop on the slide is then evenly spread with a corner of another slide to form a round or square smear about 1 cm in diameter and of thickness such that one is just able to read print through it. The film should be dried but not fixed. The smear is then stained with two stage Field's stain or Giemsa stain.
4. To make a thin film, a small drop of fresh blood is put on the slide. The slide is then laid on an even surface and the blood drop is touched by the edge of a second slide held at an angle so that the blood will spread along the line where the slide touches. A gentle rapid push of the second slide along the surface of the first will spread the blood into an even, thin film. Before staining, the thin film should be dried and fixed by covering it with a few drops of absolute methyl alcohol. The thick and thin films can be prepared in the same slide and stained with Giemsa stain.
5. The thick film examination is a time saving method which reveals even slight infections, since one microscopic field of a thick film is equivalent to about 30 fields of a thin film. The thin film allows for identification of the malaria species as well as determination of the percentage of infected erythrocytes.
6. Standard practice requires that a thick film be examined for at least 5 minutes while a thin film must be examined for 15–20 minutes before a negative report can be issued.
7. Although P. falciparum is most likely to be identified from blood just after a febrile paroxysm, the timing of the smears is less important than their being obtained several times a day over a period of 3 sucessessive days. A single negative smear does not exclude malaria. It may be necessary to repeat the smears as often as 4–6 hourly to make a diagnosis.

Antigen Detection Methods

These are simple, rapid, highly specific, but costly test for diagnosis of malaria. It is based on antibody detection of two malaria specific antigens in blood samples; histidine rich protein 2 (Pf HRP2) and parasite lactate dehydrogenase (Pf LDH). They are specific of P. falciparum malaria. The tests based on color reactions, provide a diagnostic sensitivity similar to trained microscopist. Pf LDH is cleared rapidly from blood and the test becomes negative within days of treatment. PfHRP2 is cleared very slowly from the blood, and may remain positive for upto 1 month particularly if the parasitemia was high. The disadvantage of this test is that it may show false positive result in endemic areas and in patients with persistent gamaetocytemia. It is a very useful test in the diagnosis of malaria in:

1. Severely ill patients who have received previous antimalarial treatment where parasitemia has cleared but the Pf HRP 2 will remain strongly positive; and
2. When there is mixed infection with P. vivax and P. falciparum where the former was not evident microscopically.

Treatment

Uncomplicated Malaria (P. Vivax, P. Ovale, P. Malariae Infection)

Oral Chloroquine is the drug of choice. It is given in a dose of 25 mg/kg body weight divided over three days, i.e., 10 mg/kg on day 1, 10 mg/kg on day 2 and 5 mg/kg on day 3 followed by Primaquine 0.25 mg base/kg/day as a single dose for 14 days to prevent relapse.

In cases where parasitological diagnosis is not possible due to non-availability of either timely microscopy or

RDT, suspected malaria cases should be treated with full course of Chloroquine till the results of microscopy are received. Once the parasitological diagnosis is available, appropriate treatment as per the species, is to be administered.

Children with 14 days regimen should be under close supervision to detect any complication. Patients should be instructed to report back in case of hematuria or high colored urine/cyanosis or blue coloration of lips and primaquine should be stopped in such cases. Care should be taken in patients with anemia.

If vomiting prevents oral chloroquine administration, it can be given by nasogastric tube. Sudden death has been attributed to parenteral administration. Hence, it is better avoided. Oral chloroquine should never be given in empty stomach and during high fever. It can cause cramps, nausea and vomiting. The temperature should be brought down. If vomiting occurs within 45 minutes of a dose of chloroquine, that particular dose is to be repeated after taking care of vomiting by using an antiemetic.

As primaquine can cause hemolytic anemia in children with G6PD deficiency, they should be preferably screened for the same prior to starting therapy. A known case of G6PD deficiency should not be given primaquine. As infants are relatively G6PD deficient, it is not recommended in this age group. In a case of borderline G6PD deficiency, once weekly dose of primaquine 0.6 to 0.8 mg/kg can be given for 6 weeks.

Clinical and blood smear response should be carefully monitored after chloroquine therapy. Patients need monitoring for possible recrudescence which may occur upto 90 or more days after therapy in case of low grade resistant malaria.

Uncomplicated P. Falciparum Malaria

According to the National Malaria Treatment Guidelines, the present recommendation for treatment of P. falciparum malaria is ACT – SP. The ACT – SP includes combination of oral Artesunate (4 mg/kg body weight daily for 3 days) combined with oral sulphadoxine (25 mg/kg body weight) + pyrimethamine (1.25 mg/kg body weight) for 3 days.

P. falciparum infection does not have relapse because gametocytes in the blood disappear soon after destruction of the asexual precursors by antimalarial drug but reinfection can occur. Gametocytes however, can be destroyed by a single dose of Primaquine (0.75 mg/kg) to prevent onward transmission of infection.

In view of the growing resistance to pyrimethamine and sulphadoxine, the present recommendation for treatment of uncomplicated P. Falciparum malaria in the north-eastern region is ACT–AL. The ACT–AL includes combination of Artemether + Lumafantrine. The dosage schedule is given in the schedule of treatment recommended by NVBDCP in the table below:

NVBDCP Guidelines for Treatment of Malaria and North-Eastern States, India

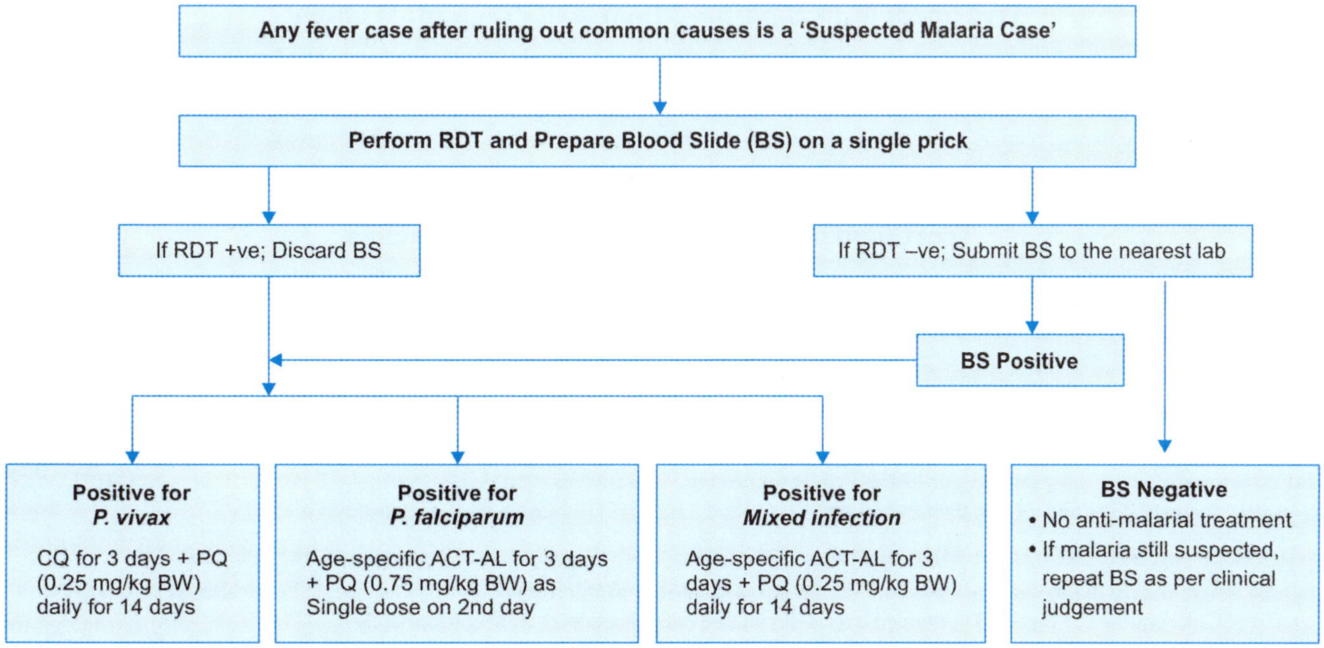

Dosage Chart for Treatment of *P. vivax* Malaria

Age (Yrs)	*Day 1*		*Day 2*		*Day 3*		*Day 4 to 14*
	CQ (250 mg)	*PQ (2.5 mg)*	*CQ (250 mg)*	*PQ (2.5 mg)*	*CQ (250 mg)*	*PQ (2.5 mg)*	*PQ (2.5 mg)*
<1	1/2	0	1/2	0	1/4	0	0
1 - <5	1	1	1	1	1/2	1	1
5 - <9	2	2	2	2	1	2	2
9 - <15	3	4	3	4	1½	4	4
15 and above	4	6	4	6	2	6	6
Pregnancy	4	0	4	0	2	0	0

CQ: Chloroquine (250 mg = 150 mg base); **PQ:** Primaquine – administer under supervision; to be taken after meals; **PQ** contraindicated for pregnant females, infants and G6PD cases (PQ to be stopped if patient develops dark coloured urine, yellow conjunctiva, bluish discolouration of lips; to contact health facility immediately.

Dosage Chart for Treatment of *P. Falciparum* Malaria

Co-formulated tablet ACT-AL	*6 months to <3 years (5 - <15 kg)*	*3 to <9 years (15 - <25 kg)*	*9 to <14 years (25 - <35 kg)*	*≥ 14 years (≥35 kg)*
Total Dose of Artemether + Lumefantrinefor 3 days	20 mg + 120 mg BD for 3 days	40 mg + 240 mg BD for 3 days	60 mg + 360 mg BD for 3 days	80 mg + 480 mg BD
No. of tablets per Pack Colour code	6 Yellow	12 Green	18 Red	24 White
Dosage1 Tab BD for 3 days	2 Tab BD for 3 days	3 Tab BD for 3 days	4 Tab BD for 3 days	
Primaquine (single dose)	0.75 mg/kg BW on day 2	0.75 mg/kg BW on day 2	0.75 mg/kg BW on day 2	0.75 mg/kg BW on day 2

ACT-AL not recommended in 1st trimester of pregnancy and for children <6 months; **ACT-AL** to be taken with high fat food OR milk; PQ to be taken after meals.

Treatment of *Falsiparum* Malaria in Pregnant Women

Uncomplicated P. falciparum malaria should be treated with:
- 1st Trimester: **Quinine** salt 10 mg/kg 3 times a day for 7 days.

Quinine may induce hypoglycemia; hence pregnant women should eat regularly while on Quinine treatment.
- 2nd and 3rd Trimester: **ACT-AL** as per schedule.

Treatment of Severe and Complicated Malaria

Initial parenteral treatment for at least 48 hours: CHOOSE ONE of following two options	**Follow-up treatment, when patient can take orally**
Inj Quinine: 20 mg salt/kg BW as loading dose on admission followed by maintenance dose of 10 mg/kg BW 8 hourly in 5% Dextrose/Dextrose Saline; IV infusion rate should not exceed 5 mg/kg BW per hour.	**Quinine** 10 mg/kg BW TDS **with** doxycycline (3 mg/kg BW OD) **or** clindamycin (10 mg/kg BW BD) in pregnant women and children <8 years of age, to complete 7 days of treatment.
Inj Artesunate: 2.4 mg/kg BW I.V. or I.M. given on admission (time=0), then at 12 hrs and 24 hrs, then once a day.	Full course of Age-specific ACT-AL for 3 days + PQ (0.75 mg/kg BW) as single dose on second day.

OD: Once a day; **BD**: Twice Daily; **TDS**: Three times a day; **BW:** Body Weight; **I.V.:** Intravenous; **I.M.:** Intramuscular.

In case where timely diagnosis is not possible due to non-availability of microscopy or RDT, suspected case should be treated with full course of Chloroquine (25 mg/kg BW divided over 3 days); and once diagnosed, treat appropriately.

Severe/Complicated P. Falciparum Malaria

Fever without a focus in any child who has left a P. falciparum endemic area within the incubation period of 9–14 days and is non-immune should be considered a medical emergency. A thick and thin smear should be immediately obtained and, if positive, the child should be hospitalized and treatment started. If blood films are negative, they should be repeated every 4–6 hours or an antigen card test should be ordered. If the child is severely ill, anti-malarial therapy should be initiated immediately.

Indications of Admission to ICU

The indications for admission to a pediatric ICU are as follows:

1. Patients who cannot retain oral fluids and medication due to vomiting.
2. Presence of neurologic dysfunction, pulmonary edema, renal failure.
3. Peripheral asexual parasitemia more than 5%.

Monitoring

The child should be monitored for the following:

1. Blood pressure for hypotension, temperature and respiration.
2. Clinical signs of dehydration.
3. Urine output and fluid intake.
4. State of consciousness by modified GCS.
5. Biochemical parameters viz. blood glucose, serum sodium, potassium, serum creatinine, urea, hemoglobin, ABG.

Supportive Treatment in Severe Falciparum Malaria

Cerebral malaria is the most common type of severe falciparum malaria. Usually a child present with altered sensorium. Anemia, hypoglycemia, seizures, disturbed fluid and electrolyte balance, and acidosis are usually present. Correction of these complications is equally important as the specific drug therapy for survival.

1. All cases should be attended to maintenance of airway, breathing and circulation. An IV cannula should be fixed.
2. The blood glucose should be checked with dextrosticks and treatment of hypoglycemia instituted. Even if dextrosticks are not available, treatment for hypoglycemia with 2 ml/kg 10% dextrose should be given as a bolus. The blood glucose should be monitored and maintained. There is hypoglycemia in severe malaria and administration quinine also causes hypoglycemia. Quinine should be prepared in 5% dextrose solution.
3. Hydration should be maintained with judicious administration of fluid and electrolytes. If the child presents in shock it should be treated with fluid bolus and vasoactive drugs when necessary.
4. If possible ABG should be checked. If a clinical sign of acidosis (e.g. acidotic breathing) is present it should be treated with correction of dehydration and sodibicarb.
5. Anemia is a common complication of P. falciparum malaria. Hemoglobin should be checked in all cases. Anemia should be treated with cell transfusion to maintain Hb% above 7 gm% and Hct above 20%.
6. Convulsion in cerebral malaria should be treated with anticonvulscents like diazepam, lorazepam and phenytoin.
7. Treatment of fever with paracetamol 15–20 mg/kg/dose 4–6 hourly, with or without tepid sponging.
8. There is no role of steroids and mannitol. Steroids are shown to be harmful and mannitol without benefit.
9. Exchange transfusion may be helpful in life threatening P. falciparum infection with parasitemia more than 5%.
10. Dialysis may be necessary in treatment of renal failure. The child is benefited with an early dialysis.

Specific Drug Therapy

Severe malaria is a medical emergency. Parenteral artemisinin derivatives or quinine should be used as specific therapy.

Artemisinin derivatives have a high killing rate (reduces parasite number 10,000 fold per cycle whereas other anti-malarials reduces 100 to 1000 fold per cycle). A rapid elimination rate, less serious side effects, and relatively low level of resistance are also important characteristics. The artemisinin derivatives include artesunate, artemether and arteether (not recommended in children). Among the three, artesunate is the most widely used.

Artesunate: 2.4 mg/kg body weight IV or IM given on admission, then at 12 h and 24 h and then once a day or *Artemether:* 3.2 mg/kg body weight IM given on admission and then 1.6 mg/kg body weight per day. It is advisable to switch over to oral therapy as soon as the child is able to take orally. For IV administration, the total dose should be diluted to 3-5 ml with 5% dextrose and given as a bolus.

After parenteral artemisinin therapy, patients will receive a full course of oral ACT for 3 days.

Quinine dihydrochloride: 20 mg/kg body weight on admission (IV infusion) followed by maintenance dose of 10 mg/kg body weight/dose 8 hourly. The infusion rate should not exceed 5 mg salt/kg body weight per hour. It is advisable to switch over to oral quinine sulphate (30 mg/kg/day) as soon as the child is conscious and can take orally. The loading dose of quinine i.e. 20 mg /kg body weight on admission may not be given if the patient has already received quinine or if the clinician feels inappropriate).

Those patients who receive parenteral quinine therapy should receive oral quinine 10 mg/kg body weight three times a day for 7 days (including the days when parenteral quinine was administered) plus doxycycline 3 mg/kg body weight once a day or clindamycin 10 mg/kg body weight 12 hourly for 7 days (Doxycycline is contraindicated in children under 8 years of age).

Prevention

Malaria can be prevented by chemoprophylaxis and personal prophylaxis.

Chemoprophylaxis

Chemoprophylaxis should be administered only in selective groups in high *P. falciparum* endemic areas like military personal in night patrol duties. It is not practised in children because of the adverse effects of the drugs.

Personal Prophylaxis

Use of personal protection measures should be encouraged for pregnant women and children as well as vulnerable populations including travellers for longer stay.

1. The children should be kept indoors from dusk to dawn. Sleeping indoors under mosquito nets should be encouraged. Use of insecticide treated bed nets (ITN) / long lasting insecticidal nets (LLIN) have shown to be effective.
2. Use of mosquito repellants and mosquito proofing of houses may be practised.

Kala Azar

Kala azar or visceral leishmaniasis is a disease which results from infection with L. donovani characterized by a long incubation period and a chronic course, remittant fever, hepatosplenomegaly and leucopenia.

Epidemiology

Kala azar is endemic in many places in India, China, Africa, Southern Europe, South America and Russia. In India, it was especially common in Assam and Bengal along the coasts of the Ganges and Brahmaputra. It was also endemic in Bihar, Orissa, Tamilnadu and eastern parts of Uttar Pradesh. In India, the disease is commonly seen in older children and young adults; it commonly occurred in epidemics but has practically disappeared.

About the Parasite

The parasite is named after its discoverers, Leishman (from London) and Donovan (from Tamilnadu), both of whom reported simultaneously in 1903.

Life Cycle

In the Indian disease, the reservoir is man. In man it exists in the non-flagellete form as small oval bodies between 2–5 microns in length and containing a large laterally placed nucleus to which the small rod shaped kinetoplast is turned end on.

The vector is a female sand fly of species phlebotomus, which becomes infected by sucking blood containing parasites from an infected human or animal reservoir. In the insect, the parasite rapidly develops into the flagellate leptomonad form/promastigote form which multiplies in great numbers and eventually blocks the pharynx and buccal cavity. The fully developed promastigote forms are long slender spindle shaped bodies, 15–20 microns in length and 1–2 microns in breath with a central nucleus. The kinetoplast lies transversely near the anterior end with an eosinophilic granule in front. The flagellum may be of the same length as the body even longer.

When the blocked insects attempts to feed, the parasites escape into the wound and enter the tissues where they are taken up by the fixed and mobile macrophages in which they are transformed into leishmania forms/ amastigote form. They multiply by fission and the host cells eventually ruptures, liberating the organisms which then infect other cells in which the cycle is repeated. They are carried by the blood macrophages to all tissues of the body, where the invasion of the reticuloendothelial cells is continued.

Transmission by phlebotomus spp. in this way is probably the only natural way. Occasionally the infection may be transmitted in transfused blood.

Clinical Manifestations

The incubation period generally varies from 3–6 months but it may exceed 1–2 years. The onset of the disease may be acute or more frequently insidious.

Fever is often an early symptom. It may be continuous or remittent type to start with becoming intermittent at a later stage. In 20% cases the fever shows a double rise in 24 hours. There is no associated malaise or apathy and the patient may be unaware of the fever. The patient has a good appetite. In a fully developed case emaciation and anemia become noticeable. Jaundice sometimes occurs, but usually not before the third month of the overt disease.

The most striking feature is the enlarging spleen, which grows in size rapidly and over the weeks and months may fill the left side of the abdomen upto the pelvis. The organ is firm and non tender except when perisplenic or capsular lesions develop. The liver is also enlarged but not as large as the spleen. Generalized lymphadenopathy may be observed but is more common in the African type.

The skin over the entire body becomes dry and rough and is often pigmented particularly over the face, malar prominences, temples, and sometimes around the mouth. The hair becomes brittle and fall out with patches of alopecia. In African kala azar, warty eruption on the skin and mucocutaneous lesion may appear. Diarrhoea is common and is probably arising from infiltration and proliferation of macrophages in the gut walls.

If untreated, 75–95% of the patients die within a period of 2 years. Death in kala azar is always due to some complications viz. shigiella dysentery, pneumonia, pulmonary tuberculosis, malaria and cancrum oris.

Laboratory Diagnosis

1. Identification of Parasite by Microscopic Examination of a Stained Film

Commonly smears are studied from peripheral blood and bone marrow material. Splenic puncture is sometimes done as an alternative and is said to be more sensitive when the parasites are scanty. Smears are stained by Leishman or Giemsa's stain. The parasites are difficult to find in peripheral blood but are plentiful in the bone marrow and spleen. They are seen as the amastigote form (LD bodies) mostly within the cytoplasm of the macrophages, but may be found free also.

2. Blood Culture

Blood culture is indicated when organisms are not seen in tissue or peripheral blood. The blood culture is done in NNN medium at 22°C and incubated for 1–4 weeks. On culture, the organisms reveal as the promastigote forms. The disadvantage of this method is that it takes about a month to give the diagnosis.

3. Indirect Evidences of Diagnosis

a. *Serological tests:* These tests are dependent on the increase in protein content especially the gamma globulin level. They are not specific and may be positive in other conditions also.

   i. *Formol gel test* is carried out by adding one drop of commercial formalin in one ml of serum in a small glass tube. The mixture is shaken and left at room temperature. A positive result is indicated by jellification of milk white opacity like the white of a hard boiled egg in 2–20 minutes. This test is not positive till the disease is of atleast 3 months duration.

   ii. *Antimony test:* A positive test is indicated by the formation of a profuse flocculent precipitate when a 4% solution of urea stibamine in distilled water comes in contact with whole serum or serum diluted 1 in 10. This test is less reliable than the former.

   iii. *Complement fixation test:* This test is of distinct advantage in the early diagnosis of the disease. It becomes positive within 3 weeks of the infection. The test is, however, also positive in leprosy, pulmonary tuberculosis and tropical eosinophilia. The test is carried out with an antigen prepared from Kedrowsky's acid fast bacillus.

b. *Blood count:* There is leucopenia with marked reduction of polymorphonuclear leucocytes and relative increase of the lymphocytes and monocytes. The initial total count which may be around 3000/cumm progressively decrease to as low as 1000/cumm with progression of the disease. There is anemia.

Treatment

The specific chemotherapeutic drugs include the antimony compounds and synthetic non-metallic compound. The pentavalent antimony compounds are the drug of choice and include urea stibamine, sodium stibogluconate. *Urea stibamine* was the widely used drug in India. This drug causes painful damage to muscles and other tissues and is therefore given only intravenously. Very rarely, a condition resembling shock accompanied by high fever may develop after the fifth or sixth injection of the antimony compounds. General treatment including adrenaline and blood volume adjustment is all that is needed for management of the condition. WHO recommends *Sodium stibogluconate.* It is given in the dose of 20 mg/kg/day for 20 days preferably 28 days and even upto 40 days in areas with high resistance.

Cases which are refractory to treatment with antimony compounds may respond to higher or more prolonged doses. Alternatively, *Pentamidine isethionate* may be used in the doses of 3–4 mg/kg body weight deep intramuscularly for 10–12 days. *Hydroxystilbamidine* isethionate is said to be more effective and less toxic. It is given intravenously in the doses 3 mg/kg body weight daily for 7–10 days. If necessary the dosage schedule may be repeated after 10–14 days. The diamidine drugs are toxic. Hypoglycemia is common which can be prevented by encouraging glucose drinks. Hypoglycemia should be treated. A few cases of myelitis have been reported following administration of Hydroxystilbamidine. Skin rashes may develop which can be taken care of by use of antihistaminics.

Cases refractory may respond to *amphotericin B.* The dose is 0.25 mg–1.0 mg/kg body weight given very slowly mixed with 5% dextrose in a concentration not more than 0.1 mg per 1 ml. The treatment is given every alternate day for 3–8 weeks. The drug is toxic. If proteinuria develops or if the blood urea begins to rise administration should be stopped. Occasionally in a very refractory case splenectomy may be effective.

Prevention

In India, for attack on the parasite, control measures should centre on treatment of cases as the reservoir of infection. Measures against sand fly control and personal prophylaxis viz. use of mosquito nets and periodic fumigation are also important.

Tuberculosis

Tuberculosis appears to be a disease as old as history of human race. Bones of prehistoric man dating back to 8000 BC have shown typical changes of tuberculosis. The Rigveda has described tuberculosis as *Yakshma* as early as 2000 BC. Tuberculosis stands as the prototype of infections which exists in man most often without causing significant disease and yet capable of producing both acute and chronic disease patterns of sufficient seriousness to be one of the leading causes of death.

History

In 1882, Sir Robert Koch demonstrated that tuberculosis is caused by the acid fast bacillus. The generic name Mycobacterium was proposed by Lehmann and Newman in 1896. Subsequently, Smith showed that the disease can be produced in man by bovine and human tubercle bacilli. In 1890, Koch discovered tuberculin. Albert Calmette and Camille Guerin subsequently developed Bacillus Calmette Guerin (BCG) vaccine on the basis of theory of allergy evolved by Koch. BCG vaccine was first used in 1921 as a preventive tool. In early years treatment of tuberculosis consisted of rest, nutrition and fresh air. With the discovery of streptomycin in 1921, followed by isoniazid and para amino salicylic acid, effective chemotherapy treatment started. With the discoveries of drugs like Rifampicin, ethambutol and pyrizinamide in early seventies, long-term therapy has been replaced by short course chemotherapy of 6–9 months.

Epidemiology

Childhood tuberculosis is a very small and constantly decreasing problem in developed countries, seen only in a few high risk groups of children like children of migrant workers from countries with high prevalence. On the other hand, the incidence in the developing countries is relatively high and increasing, mainly due to excess incidence of infectious tuberculosis due to HIV infection.

Transmission

Transmission is from person to person, usually by airborne mucus droplet particles that contain M. tuberculosis. Transmission can also occur by direct contact with an infected discharge or fomites.

The chances of transmission to children increases when the adult patient has:

1. AFB positive sputum.
2. An extensive upper lobe infiltrate or cavity.

3. Copious production of thin sputum; and
4. Severe and forceful cough.

Most adults no longer transmit the organism within several days to 2 weeks after beginning adequate chemotherapy.

Young children with pulmonary tuberculosis rarely infect other children or adults. This is because, in children, bacilli are sparse, cough is often absent or lacks the tussive force required to suspend the particles of the correct size.

Older children and adolescents with post primary tuberculosis can transmit the organism.

Pyramid of Childhood Tuberculosis

Patients with tuberculosis in pediatric age group can be placed in three categories:

Group I

Constitute 6–10% of total pediatric admissions. They suffer from serious tubercular disease like meningitis, miliary tuberculosis, disseminated tuberculosis or severe complicated intrathoracic disease. They constitute the apex of the pyramid.

Group II

Consists of cases of tuberculosis with mild to moderate disease. Only a few of them have characteristic symptoms of tuberculosis. Majority present with nonspecific symptoms and remain undiagnosed. If diagnosed they are inadequately treated.

Group III

This group forms the base of the pyramid. These children are either asymptomatic or have nonspecific symptoms. They are usually undiagnosed and hence untreated. They constitute the reservoir of primary infection from which various post primary complications develop. These children are also forerunners of a large percentage of chronic pulmonary tuberculosis in adults.

Tuberculous Infection and Disease

Tuberculosis has two stages. First is the stage of infection. *Tuberculous infection* is defined as the entry of tubercle bacilli into the body but there is no clinical, radiological or bacteriological evidence of the lesion. In immunocompetent children, the response to the initial infection with M. tuberculosis usually provides protection against reinfection when a new exposure occurs. Untreated infants with tuberculous infection have upto 40% chance of developing disease with a high risk of progression. The greatest risk for progression occurs in the first 2 years after infection.

Tubercular disease, on the other hand, is the condition which after entry of bacilli, is characterized by symptoms, clinical and/or radiological evidence of tubercular lesion and isolation of mycobacterium tuberculosis from sputum or from gastric aspirate.

In adults, there is a vast difference between infection and disease. The total population may have infection but disease may be present in around 2–10% of those infected. In other words, infection remains dormant in the majority of the infected adults, though there is chance of reactivation into disease in near future, particularly in the underprivileged population.

In the children, on the other hand, apparently silent infection may result in dangerous or fatal disease like miliary tuberculosis, meningitis, or disseminated disease, especially during infancy and early childhood. This shows the difficulty of separating infection from disease in children.

Differences Between Childhood and Adult Tuberculosis

Childhood tuberculosis differs from adult tuberculosis in various aspects. It is essential to note the differences from the point of view of diagnosis and management. The differences are shown in a tabular form below:

Table 11.1 : The differences between childhood and adult tuberculosis

Parameters	*Childhood tuberculosis*	*Adult tuberculosis*
1. Type	Primary	Post primary
2. Route of infection	Inhalation, ingestion micro inoculation	Reinfection or reactivation of an old focus
3. Bacterial load	Low	High
4. Infectivity	Low or absent (unless main lesion communicate with bronchus)	High
5. Delayed hypersensitivity	Takes 6–12 weeks to develop	Already present
6. Lesion	Primary focus, lymphangitis, and regional lymphadenitis	Only in lung parenchyma with cavitation. No lymphadenopathy
7. Healing	By calcification	By fibrosis
8. Hematogenous spread	Very common	Uncommon
9. Prevention by BCG	Prevent hematogenous spread	None

Clinical Forms of Childhood Tuberculosis

Tuberculosis can involve practically any organ or tissue of the body. Intrathoracic tuberculous infection accounts for atleast 90% of recognized tuberculous disease in children.

Clinical Forms of Intrathoracic Tuberculosis

1. Asymptomatic mantoux positive.
2. Symptomatic mantoux positive.
3. Pulmonary primary complex (PPC)
   a. Nodal
   b. Parenchymal
   c. Nodal + parenchymal.
4. Progressive primary disease (PPD) which may present with features of:
   a. Consolidation
   b. Consolidation and collapse
   c. Significant pleural effusion
   d. Bronchopneumonia.
5. Miliary tuberculosis.
6. Tuberculosis of tracheobronchial lymph nodes.
7. Bronchiectasis.
8. Pericardial effusion.

Clinical Forms of Extrathoracic Tuberculosis

1. Tuberculosis of tonsils and cervical lymph glands.
2. Abdominal tuberculosis.
3. Tuberculosis of central nervous system: meningitis, tuberculoma.
4. Tuberculosis of skin.
5. Tuberculosis of bone and joints.
6. Tuberculosis of genitourinary tract.
7. Tuberculosis of eye: Phlyctenular conjunctivitis, chorioretinitis.
8. Tuberculosis of middle ear.

PULMONARY TUBERCULOSIS

Lungs are the common site for tuberculous disease in children. Both the lung parenchyma and the lymph nodes are involved to various degrees. The clinical manifestation largely depends on the extent of infection in the lung parenchyma or in the lymph nodes.

PULMONARY PRIMARY COMPLEX (PPC)

Pathophysiology

Primary infection with M. tuberculosis in children usually occurs following inhalation of viable microorganisms. Although all parts of the lung are apparently at equal risk, the usual sites of primary tuberculous implantation in lungs are the lower segments of middle lobe and upper segments of lower lobe. Lesions are more common in the right lung because of greater volume and the right bronchus being more vertical, short and wide. Seventy percent of primary pulmonary focus is subpleural because sluggish air current in the peripheral parts of the lung allow the bacilli to thrive longer there. In 80% cases there is one primary focus.

With the introduction of infection, initially there is polymorphonuclear response which is later replaced by macrophage / mononuclear response. The mycobacteria are phagocytosed by macrophages. They continue to multiply intracellulary. In about 2–4 weeks time there is development of cell mediated immune response after which the lesion undergo caseous necrosis in the central part and bacillary multiplication decreases. The area of necrosis is surrounded by macrophages, lymphocytes, giant cells and collagen fibres forming a granuloma, called tubercle. Some tubercle bacilli traverse into the regional lymph nodes via the lymphatics and cause an inflammatory response in the glands. The common group affected is the mediastinal glands. The right paratracheal glands may be involved frequently even with a left sided parenchymal focus. This is because the lymphatic drainage of the lungs occurs predominantly from left to right. The cervical glands may also be involved because they have communications with the paratracheal lymph nodes and also drain the apical pleura. The primary focus, the draining lymphatics and involved lymph glands are collectively called the *pulmonary primary complex*.

Natural History of Untreated Primary Infection

About 4–8 weeks after infection the body becomes sensitized to tubercular protein. This is manifested by a positive Mantoux test. With high degree of hypersensitivity, there may be fever, phlyctenular conjunctivitis and erythema nodosum (more commonly seen in temperate region where tuberculosis is uncommon).

The sequence of events that follows thereafter depends on the immune response of the host. The risk factors of complications include age below 1 year and adolescents, poor nutritional status and occurrence of intercurrent infections viz. whooping cough, measles. The outcome may be described under the following heads:

Primary Focus

If the host resistance is good, the inflammatory exudate around the primary focus is absorbed and the caseous area inspissated. Healing occurs by fibrosis and calcification. When cell mediated response of the host is weak, the bacilli continue to multiply and the inflammatory process extends to the contiguous areas. The focus enlarges steadily and develops a large caseous centre. The central portion then liquefies and empty into an adjacent bronchus leaving a soft walled cavity. The bacilli may spread into other parts of the lung or the entire lung. This may lead to consolidation of an area of the lung or to bronchopneumonia. Such an extensive pulmonary infiltration is termed as *progressive primary disease.* The focus may enlarge, cause adhesions with the pleura or rupture into the pleural space causing effusion.

Lymphadenitis

The enlarged lymph nodes may compress the neighbouring airway. An incomplete obstruction leads to a ball valve effect resulting in emphysema distal to obstruction. A complete obstruction of the bronchus leads to atelectasis. The enlarged paratracheal glands can cause pressure over the trachea and cause stridor and respiratory distress. Sub carinal glands may impinge on the esophagus and cause dysphagia. They may also rupture into the pericardial sac and cause pericardial effusion. A caseated gland may erode through the wall of the bronchus leading to endobronchial tuberculosis. Discharge of the caseated material with mycobacterium into the lumen may lead to bronchial dissemination.

Hematogenous Dissemination

Hematogenous dissemination occurs when the bacilli find their way into the blood stream when a caseous focus erodes through the wall of a blood vessel in the lung, resulting in foci of infection in various organs. If the host immune response is good, then these foci are contained and the disease does not occur. Lowering of host immunity any time may lead to activation of these metastatic foci and development of the disease. The risk factors include young infants, severe malnutrition and immunodeficiency including HIV infection.

With poor immune response, tubercular meningitis and miliary tuberculosis are most likely to occur in the second six months of acquiring the infection. Bone and joint lesion (usually single) occur from towards the end of the first year to the third year after infection. Skin and renal tuberculosis occur later. Renal tuberculosis is rare before 10 years of age and occurs 5–7 years after primary infection.

Post Primary Pulmonary Tuberculosis

Post primary pulmonary tuberculosis which results from endogenous reactivation of foci of infection is uncommon in children but may be seen in adolescents. The common site for this type of tubercular disease is the apex of the lung (Puhl's lesion). Regional lymph glands are usually not involved in this type of tuberculosis.

Clinical Spectrum of PPC

Most children suffer from pulmonary primary complex. Pulmonary primary complex may be asymptomatic or symptomatic. It may be picked up accidentally during evaluation of intercurrent infection.

Asymptomatic Pulmonary Primary Complex

The child has a positive tuberculin test with no clinical manifestations or radiological signs.

Symptomatic Pulmonary Complex

A history of contact may be present. The symptoms and physical signs are much less considering the extent of radiographic changes often seen. Infants are more likely to experience symptoms. They may present with vague systemic symptoms like fever, night sweats, anorexia, and failure to gain weight or weight loss. Non-productive cough and mild dyspnea are common symptoms. Signs are even less striking.

The child has a positive tuberculin test with radiological signs of primary tuberculosis which may be nodal, parenchymal or combination of both. Radiological findings may also consist of one or more calcified foci in the lung parenchyma or calcified lymph glands, hilar or tracheobronchial. Such findings indicate a healed state even in presence of a positive tuberculin test. However, these children should be kept under observation for detection of exacerbation, especially during adolescence.

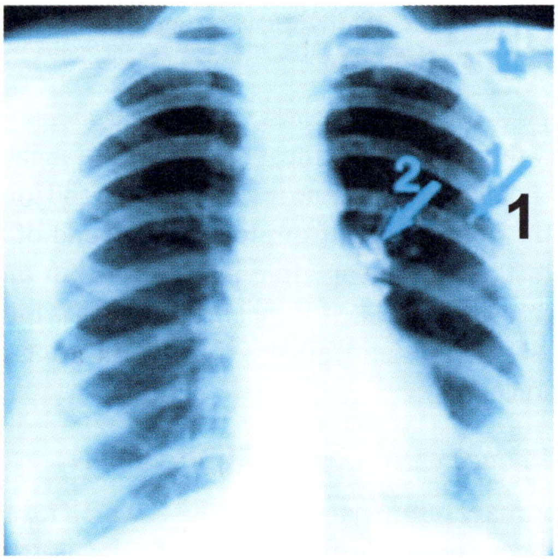

Fig. 11.1: X-ray showing (1) Ghon's focus and (2) Hilar glands

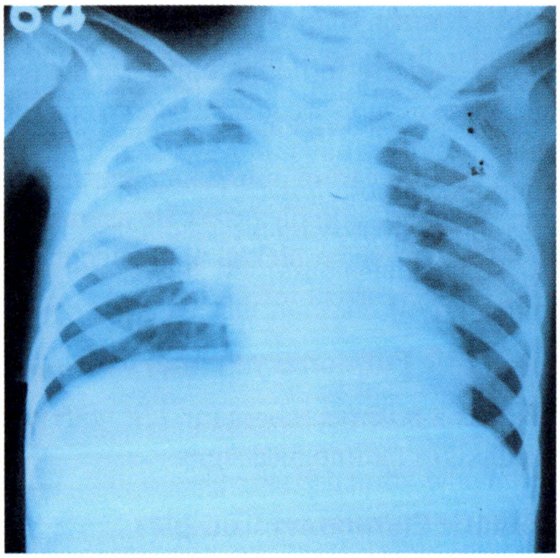

Fig. 11.2: X-ray showing primary progressive disease (consolidation, collapse and mediastinal glands)

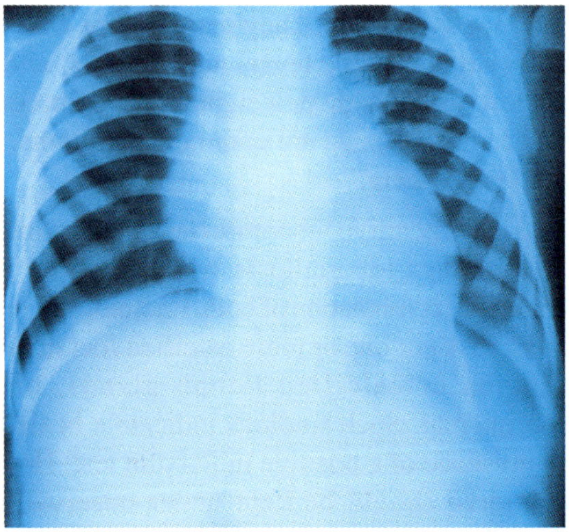

Fig. 11.3: X-ray showing hilar lymph glands (left)

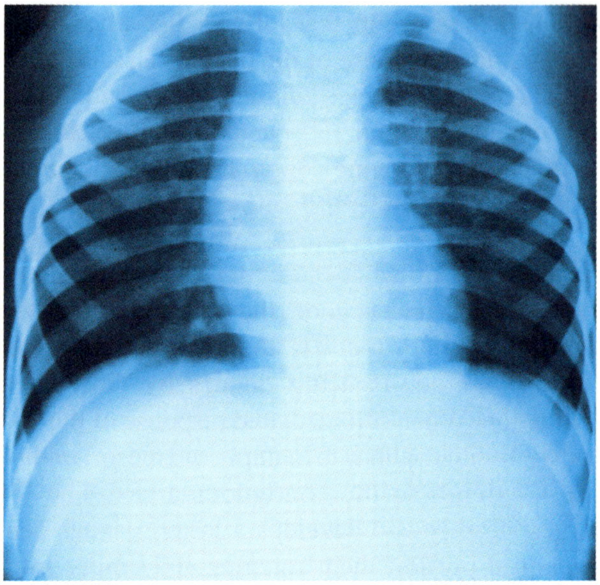

Fig. 11.4: X-ray showing calcified hilar lymph glands (left)

PROGRESSIVE PRIMARY DISEASE

A child with progressive primary disease presents with high fever, cough, hemoptysis, weight loss and night sweats. The signs depend on the extent of involvement. There may be signs of consolidation, collapse or cavitation.

A child with endobronchial tuberculosis may present with high fever, troublesome cough with or without expectoration, dyspnea, wheezing and cyanosis. The possibility of endobronchial tuberculosis should be always kept in mind in a wheezing child below 2 years age, especially if there is poor response to bronchodilators. The signs depend on the lesions present viz. emphysema, consolidation and collapse.

MILIARY TUBERCULOSIS

Miliary tuberculosis is the most clinically significant form of disseminated tuberculosis. It occurs when massive numbers of tubercle bacilli are released into the blood stream causing disease in two or more organs. Miliary tuberculosis usually complicates the primary infection and occurs within 2–6 months of the initial infection.

This form of disease is most common in infants and young children but may occur in adolescents as well; as a result of breakdown of a previously healed primary pulmonary lesion.

Clinical Manifestations

The clinical manifestations of miliary tuberculosis depend

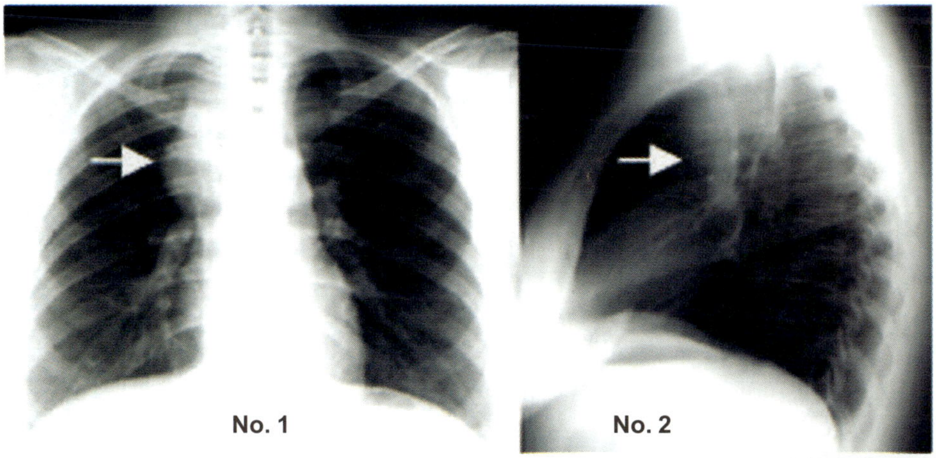

Fig. 11.5: X-ray showing hilar glands (No.1) and middle lobe collapse (No. 2)

on the load of organism and the organ they lodge in. The common organs involved are the lungs, liver, spleen and bone marrow.

The onset of disease may be abrupt and the child may become gravely ill in several days. More often however, the onset is insidious with nonspecific symptoms viz. fever, anorexia and weight loss. Fever tends to run an irregular course frequently with peaks as high as 40°C (104°F). Physical signs are absent at this stage. Choroid tubercles may be an early manifestation and may be detected by fundoscopy. Spleen may be enlarged and there may be abdominal distension. These findings with high fever and absence of respiratory signs may suggest the diagnosis of typhoid fever. In course of several weeks, in around 50%cases, there is development of generalized lymphadenopathy and hepatosplenomegaly. In this stage, fever becomes higher and more sustained but respiratory symptoms are absent or minimal. The chest radiograph is also normal. Localized signs do not appear until the last week or so of the illness in the untreated patient. The child develops cough, dyspnea and wheeze. Fine rales may be heard all over the chest.

The chest radiograph shows multiple tubercles which are usually smaller than 2–3 mm in diameter when first visible. The smaller lesions may coalesce to form larger lesions and sometimes extensive infiltrates. They give a mottled appearance to lung which is frequently described as resembling snow flakes.

If left untreated, the pulmonary disease progresses, and the child may present with pneumothorax and pneumomediastinum resulting in respiratory distress and hypoxia.

Chronic or recurrent headache in an advanced case of miliary tuberculosis indicates presence of meningitis

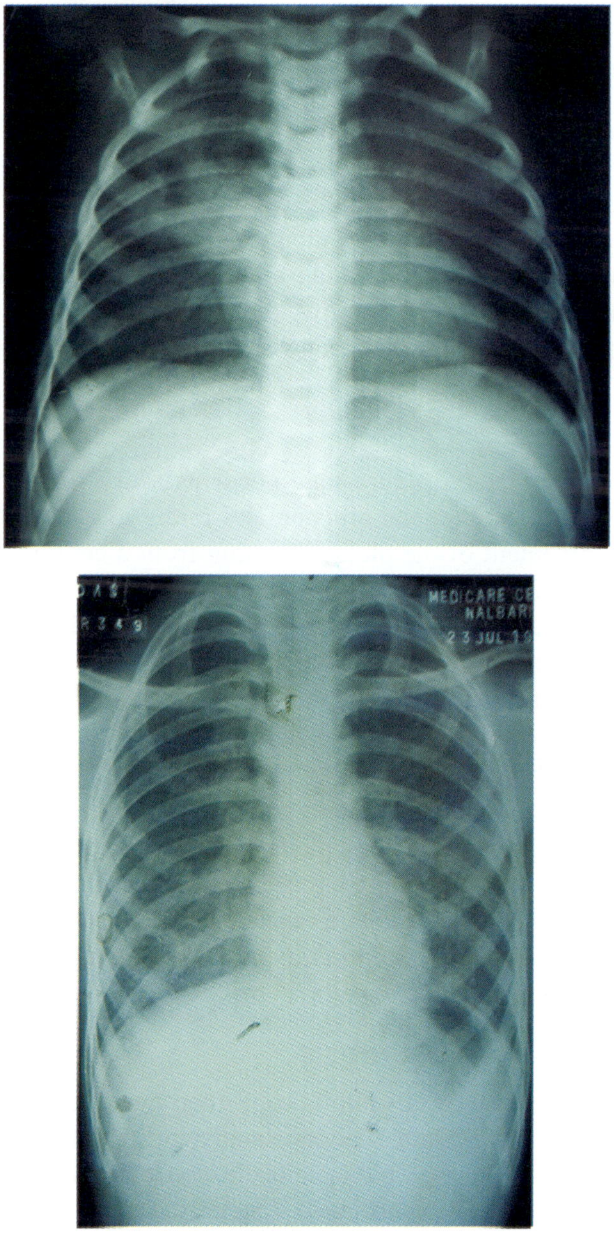

Fig. 11.6: X-rays showing miliary motting with hilar adenopathy

whereas abdominal pain or tenderness is a sign of tubercular peritonitis.

Diagnosis

A high index of suspicion on the part of the treating physician is often required for an early diagnosis. The child may present as a case of pyrexia of unknown origin. The most important clue is usually a history of recent exposure to an adult with infectious tuberculosis. The tuberculin test is negative in about 40% cases. An X-ray chest shows miliary mottling. Sputum or gastric aspirate cultures have a low sensitivity. Biopsy of the liver or bone marrow with appropriate bacteriologic and histologic examination more often yields an early diagnosis.

Course and Prognosis

In untreated cases, death usually occurs within 4–6 weeks. With early diagnosis and adequate treatment recovery is possible in majority of cases and prognosis is excellent. However resolution is slow even with proper therapy. Fever takes around 2–3 weeks to show a decline after initiation of therapy. The chest radiographic abnormalities may take many months to resolve.

PLEURAL EFFUSION

Involvement of pleura may occur as a dry fibrinous pleurisy, as a serous effusion and rarely as a necrotic involvement of the pleura resulting from a contiguous caseous focus in the lung. Tuberculous effusion is infrequent in children below 6 years age and rare in children below 2 years age. Effusions are usually unilateral but may be bilateral.

Clinical Manifestations

Tuberculous pleurisy usually has a sudden onset with low to high grade fever, chest pain on deep inspiration on the affected side, and shortness of breath. Clinical signs are absent in small effusions. Even with large effusions, often the radiographic abnormality is more extensive than symptoms and signs.

Laboratory Diagnosis

The presence of effusion is confirmed by a radiograph and etiology is established by examination of pleural fluid and pleural biopsy. The colour of the fluid is usually yellow and occasionally blood tinged. The specific gravity is 1.012 to 1.025. The protein level is high (2–4 gms/dl) and glucose level is usually normal (20–40 mg/dl). Cytological examination shows a total cell count ranging from several hundreds to several thousands per cubic millimeter. There is predominance of polymorphonuclear cells in the early stage followed by high percentage of lymphocytes. Acid fast stain of pleural fluid is rarely positive. Culture of the fluid for AFB is positive in less than 30% cases but AFB yield from acid fast stain or culture of pleural biopsy material is more. The tuberculin test is positive in about 70–80% cases. The adenosine deaminase (ADA) level > 60 units/L is diagnostic.

When to Suspect Pulmonary Tuberculosis?

The diagnosis of tuberculosis in children rests largely on the result of clinical history, family contact history, tuberculin skin test, X-ray examination and examination of gastric aspirate for AFB.

There are no definite clinical features to suggest active tuberculosis. The following clinical setting may help one to suspect.

1. Fever and/or Cough

Fever of recent onset lasting for > 2 weeks should arouse suspicion of tuberculosis. It is important to document fever to avoid erroneous reporting by parents. Fever can be of any type and the often described evening rise of temperature is not specific to tuberculosis.

Cough can be dry or moist and may be severe. As cough and fever are otherwise also common, it is the unabated persistence of these symptoms for over 2 weeks which makes tuberculosis more likely.

Recurrent symptoms with normal intervening period are less likely to be due to tuberculosis and more likely to be asthma. Cough persisting beyond 2 weeks, particularly as an only symptom in an otherwise healthy child can be due to viral infection and is often not due to tuberculosis. Such children, therefore, do not always warrant extensive investigations.

2. Unexplained Weight Loss

Recent unexplained loss of weight is an important pointer to the suspicion of tuberculosis. Unexplained poor weight gain in infancy is relevant. However, it is not so in older children as several other conditions also can lead to poor weight gain or weight loss. Loss of weight is defined as a loss of more than 5% of the highest weight recorded in the past three months.

3. History of Contact

History of exposure to an infectious TB patient (smear positive) should always prompt detailed examination for presence of the disease. However, in a symptomatic child, contact with a person with any form of active tuberculosis within last two years may be significant as many a times there can be a coexisting pulmonary involvement which went unrecognized due to lack of chest symptoms.

4. Risk Factors

Diagnosis is also more likely in a symptomatic child in presence of risk factors such as recent history of measles or whooping cough and immunocompromised state including steroid therapy. In our country tuberculosis remains an important cause of persistent pneumonia not responding to antibiotic therapy.

5. Significant Superficial Lymphadenopathy

Significant superficial lymphadenopathy must be specially looked for, as it may often coexist. Inguinal lymph glands > 1.5 cm and other superficial (cervical and axillary) glands > 1 cm size or any gland of >2 cm size is considered as significant enlargement. In 40–50% of patients superficial lymphadenopathy is present and hence should be looked for.

6. Failure of Therapeutic Response

Failure of therapeutic response to an appropriate and adequate trial with a broad spectrum antibiotic (e.g., Amoxicillin 40 – 50 mg/kg/day 8 hourly for 7 – 10 days) in a symptomatic child supports the probability of tuberculosis. Therapeutic trial with anti-tubercular drugs is not recommended. All attempts must be made to diagnose tuberculosis by proper investigations.

Laboratory Tests

Diagnosis of tuberculosis can never be reliably made on clinical features alone. The subject with above mentioned clinical features – in isolation or in combination is only a suspect. Further investigations are always necessary to establish the diagnosis. The laboratory tests include bacteriology, radiology and tuberculin skin test (TST).

Bacteriology

Demonstration of AFB from anybody fluid or tissue is confirmatory of tuberculosis. Such a proof is often lacking in childhood tuberculosis because of difficulty in collection of sputum and due to paucibacillary primary disease in children. However, studies do report that the yield of a positive test in advanced cases may be as high as in adults. Therefore, every attempt must be made to bacteriologically prove the diagnosis in every case of suspected tuberculosis.

Sputum smear examination is the primary investigation of choice if sputum specimen is available from the child. If sputum smear is positive, patient is diagnosed as smear positive pulmonary TB and should be initiated on anti-tuberculous treatment.

If sputum smear is negative or not available, then the patient is prescribed a course of antibiotics for duration of seven days. Care should to be taken to use antibiotics which do not have anti-TB activity. Fluoroquinolones should not be used as antibiotics at this point in time. In case the symptoms continue unabated despite antibiotics, then chest X-ray and Tuberculin skin test (TST/Mantoux test) should be done. However, in a sick looking or distressed child with persistent symptoms of >2 weeks duration, chest X-ray and TST test should be performed immediately along with other workup for non-TB infections.

Even where the chest X-ray is highly suggestive of tuberculosis (showing Hilar/paratracheal lymphadenitis with or without parenchymal lesion, Miliary TB, fibro cavitary pneumonia) and TST is positive, an attempt should be made for establishing bacteriological diagnosis using alternative specimens like Gastric Lavage (GL)/ Induced sputum (IS) or Bronchoalveolar lavage (BAL) depending on the facilities available. Given that the sensitivity of TST is not 100%, in any case with highly suggestive radiology, one must attempt bacteriological diagnosis (as mentioned above) even if the TST is negative. Based on the bacteriological results, case may be labelled as smear positive or negative TB and treated appropriately.

In a pediatric pulmonary tuberculosis suspect who has persistent symptoms and/or non-specific radiological shadows but efforts for a bacteriological diagnosis have failed, further investigative scheme is broadly divided into three possible situations:

1. If both TST and X-ray findings are negative, then tuberculosis is highly unlikely and an alternative diagnosis should be looked for.
2. In situations where the CXR has persistence of non-specific shadows despite a course of antibiotics,

alternative samples, viz. Gastric aspirate/Induced sputum/BAL, should be sent to establish bacteriological diagnosis irrespective of the TST positivity. In case the alternative sample is AFB positive, then classify and treat as smear positive case. In case these samples are negative, then an alternative diagnosis should be diligently looked for. If no alternative diagnosis is established, the case may be classified and treated as smear negative TB.

3. If only TST is positive and X-ray chest is not suggestive, then look for tuberculosis at an extra-pulmonary site or an alternative diagnosis. Cases with persistent symptoms with TST positive but no evidence at pulmonary/extrapulmonary site thus far, often need expert help and detailed investigations like CT chest, etc.

Bacteriological investigations using following alternative specimens can be attempted:

1. *Early morning gastric aspirate* is a preferred specimen for most young children with suspected TB for detecting AFB or isolating Mycobacterium tuberculosis.
2. *Sputum collection* is possible in older children with extensive and cavitary disease, particularly if the patient has a wet cough.
3. *Induction of sputum by 3% nebulized hypertonic saline* can be tried in other children. The patient is pre-treated with nebulized bronchodilators like salbutamol prior to induction. Following saline nebulisation, chest physiotherapy is done to loosen up the secretion and the samples are collected from the throat or nasopharynx using a collector attached to a suction at one end and a catheter/tube to the other. The suction catheter provokes cough and the secretions brought up are collected via suction.
4. *Bronchial washings/bronchoalveolar lavage (BAL)* can also be used as a diagnostic tool though the availability is limited. Bronchoscopy and BAL is often needed for evaluating cases of persistent pneumonia.
5. *FNAC lymph node:* Sometimes, there may be a co-existent peripheral lymphadenopathy, which is easily accessible and the aspirates from these can be used for bacteriological/cytological diagnosis.

Experience shows that one needs to collect at least two samples of whatever type of the respiratory specimens one decides to choose to get the optimal yield. If the facilities are limited, these tests may be prioritized and at least be done in all children with wet cough or children who have definite parenchymal lesion on chest X-ray.

The bacteriological examination can be done by the following methods:

(a) *Ziel-Neilson (ZN) stain and culture:* ZN stain can reveal AFB only if sample contains > 10,000 bacilli per ml.

(b) *Culture methods* such as LJ medium, Radiometric (Bactec) and Non-radiometric (MGIT) can be used for confirming diagnosis in paucibacillary state. The newer methods are capable of giving faster results and may be used if available. Mycobacterial culture and drug sensitivity assumes special significance in case of suspected drug resistance and should be attempted in cases needing retreatment (particularly the defaulters and failures but preferably in all cases).

Radiology

Chest X-ray: There are no pathognomonic radiological signs of tuberculosis. In relevant clinical setting, certain radiological lesions may strongly suggest tuberculosis and they include miliary, hilar or paratracheal lymphadenopathy with or without parenchymal involvement, pleural effusion and fibrocaseous cavitary lesions.

Rarely chest X-ray may be normal. Such cases should be referred to an appropriate centre for further detailed investigations, if the clinical suspicion and epidemiological risk (e.g. close contact of an infectious case, etc.) is high.

In clinical practice, non-resolving shadows in a chest X-ray, despite adequate antibiotic therapy in a symptomatic child, raises the possibility of tuberculosis. However, it is worth mentioning that all persistent radiological lesions are not necessarily due to tuberculosis.

Asymptomatic patients may have persistent shadows due to parenchymal scarring, pleural thickening, and healed fibro-atelectatic changes. On the other hand, a child with bronchiectasis or an interstitial lung disease may have presence of non-resolving shadows with persistent symptoms.

Ultrasonography of chest is helpful to assess pleural fluid collection; although decubitus chest X-ray film may also reveal similar information.

CT scan is rarely necessary and is not cost and radiation effective. Chest CT scan, however, may offer an opportunity for CT guided biopsy for tissue diagnosis.

Tuberculin Skin Test (TST)

The standard tuberculin skin test, recommended for use is the Mantoux's test. Commercially available tuberculins in the country are of the strength of 1, 2 and 5 Tuberculin Unit (TU) PPD (RT23 equivalent).

It is important to raise a wheal of about 6 mm after the intra-dermal injection and the test is read 48-72 hours after an injection. Ballpoint or palpatory methods are used to read the induration.

The width of reaction (induration) in the horizontal plane is noted for interpretation. Mantoux test or PPD skin test is considered positive if the induration is 10 mm or more. This cut off was recommended using a 1 TU PPD RT23. It is recommended that the 10 mm cut off may be continued to be used for strength of PPD only up to 5TU. However, 2TU PPD RT23 is considered to be the most suitable strength. In no case strength higher than 5 TU should be used.

It needs mention that the degree of reaction (including necrosis and ulceration), may not necessarily differentiate infected from diseased. In addition, a negative tuberculin test does not necessarily exclude tubercular infection. Prior BCG vaccine has minimal influence on PPD reaction.

If the patient returns for reading beyond 72 hours but by 7th day, a positive test can still be read. If the tuberculin test is negative but there is a strong clinical suspicion, the test may be repeated. Repeat tuberculin skin test, when required, should preferably be done on the other forearm.

The tuberculin test may be false negative within 6 – 8 weeks of infection, in miliary tuberculosis and tubercular meningitis, severe protein energy malnutrition, in presence of viral infections (e.g., measles, mumps, chickenpox,

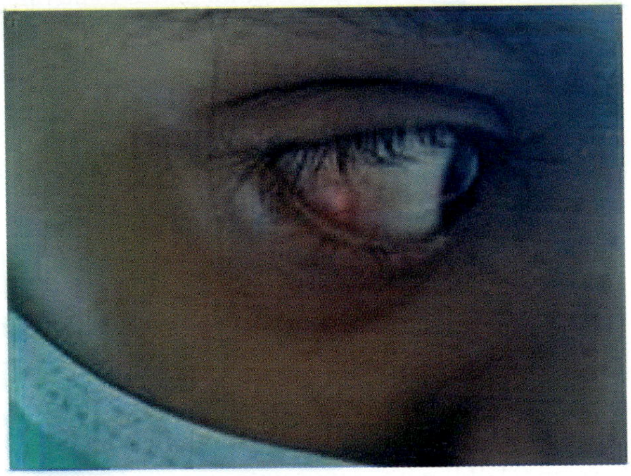

Fig. 11.7 : Phlyctenular conjunctivitis

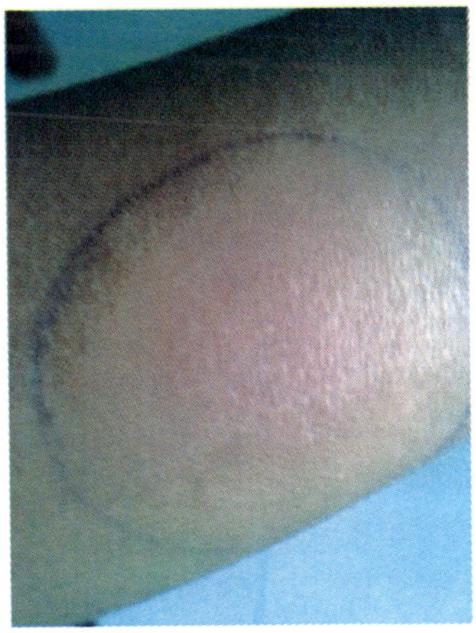

Fig. 11.8 : Positive tuberculin test

HIV infection) or bacterial infections (e.g., leprosy, brucellosis), faulty technique and errors in reading and if the child is on steroid therapy or other immunosuppressive drugs.

It may be false positive in infections with non-tuberculous mycobacteria, recent BCG vaccination, faulty technique and erroneous reading.

Tuberculin test is a manifestation of hypersensitivity. The other hypersensitive manifestations of primary tuberculosis include phlyctenular conjunctivitis and pleural effusion.

Status of Other Tests in Vogue for Diagnosing Active Tuberculosis in Children

1. *BCG Test*: BCG test is not recommended in diagnosis of tuberculosis.
2. *Serodiagnostic Tests*: As mycobacterial antigens overlap in different stages of infection and disease, there are no specific antigens that can confirm natural infection or active disease. These tests are not recommended for use.
3. *Interferon Gamma Release Assays (IGRAs)*: These new generation tests measure the production of interferon gamma by the peripheral mononuclear cells. These tests have been developed to identify the patients with TB disease or latent infection. These tests are skin tests which do not require repeat visit by the patient for reading purposes. However, these expensive tests do not differentiate the TB infection from disease. The exact advantage of these tests in high burden situation is still not clear. Hence, these are not recommended for use in the diagnostic algorithm for tuberculosis in India.

4. *PCR Tests and Gene Expert*: The in house nucleic acid amplification tests (NAAT) and several commercial tests have poor sensitivity for diagnosing TB in smear negative samples. These tests are, therefore, not recommended for the diagnosis of childhood TB. However, Hemi nested, cartridge based real time PCR marketed as Xpert MTB/RIF™ is now endorsed by WHO for use, where available, particularly in previously treated cases or cases who are contacts of chronic/MDR TB adults. The test has ability to detect MTB as well as rifampicin resistance in a matter of hours.

SUPERFICIAL TUBERCULAR LYMPHADENITIS

Superficial tubercular lymphadenitis, often referred to as scrofula, is one of the most common forms of extra-pulmonary tuberculosis. It may be localized to one region depending upon the site of the primary focus or may be generalized following hematogenous dissemination, particularly in children immunocompromised by HIV infection and AIDS.

Tuberculous lymphadenitis most often involves the cervical lymph glands. The tonsillar, anterior cervical, submandibular and supraclavicular lymph glands are involved. It is thought to have its origin in the lymphatic spread from a pulmonary primary focus via the hilar and paratracheal glands. However, in a minority of cases it may originate from a primary focus in the tonsils or some other point in the oropharynx or tissues of the head and neck. Infected lymph glands in the inguinal, epitrochlear or axillary regions results from regional lymphadenitis associated with tuberculosis of skin or skeletal system.

Etiology

Earlier scrofula was usually caused by drinking unpasteurized cow's milk containing Mycobacterium bovis. In areas where milk is pasteurized and M. bovis is under control, M. tuberculosis is the common responsible organism. In developed countries where incidence of tuberculosis is low, Mycobacterium avium intracellulare is reported to be the common organism.

Pathogenesis

There is tubercle formation and lymphoid hyperplasia which may be followed by caseation and necrosis. Usually more than one lymph gland is involved, although one may be more involved than the other. Periadenitis and spread of inflammation causes adjacent nodes to adhere to one another. Abscess formation as a result of necrosis and involvement of overlying skin may lead to sinus formation. If left untreated, there is gradual healing of the glands over a period of many months with scar formation and calcification in some.

Clinical Manifestations

Superficial tubercular lymphadenitis can occur soon after the primary infection or much later. Most cases occur within 6–9 months of the initial infection.

The common presentation is with enlargement of one or a group of glands, sometimes accidentally noticed in a healthy child. The enlarged gland is firm, painless, not attached to the skin or underlying structures. Small glands can be palpated down the line of lymph drainage. The primary node, where the infection starts, remains the largest in the chain of the glands. In general, the younger the child larger the glands. Left without treatment, the firm glands tend to soften and become matted within six months of first appearance. Occasionally, the nodes seem to regress and resolve completely, but remain palpable though very small in size.

Sometimes in a child, usually above the age of 10 years, the onset may be rapid. The palpable glands is associated with constitutional symptoms and high fever (40°C). The glands are swollen and tense but not tender as in case of streptococcal infection.

A child may even present with a hard swelling due to calcification of the infected glands. Calcification may indicate the infection of some years duration.

In general, the changes in the superficial tuberculous glands may be divided into several stages ranging from enlarged, discrete, firm and mobile nodes to advancing nodal or perinodal involvement, to sinus tract formation.

Differential Diagnosis

Many other conditions may be confused with tubercular lymphadenitis. These include pyogenic infection (Group A streptococcus and staphylococcus aureus), acute lymphoblastic leukemia, lymphoma (Nonhodgkin and Hodgkin's), infectious mononucleosis, HIV infection/AIDS, fungal infection (Histoplasmosis, Coccidiodomycosis), Toxoplasmosis, Brucellosis, Sarcoidosis and atypical mycobacterial lymphadenitis.

Acute pyogenic lymphadenitis is characterized by enlargement of lymph glands with signs of inflammation and constitutional symptoms. Response to appropriate and adequate antibiotic therapy (Amoxicillin 30–40 mg/kg/day 8 hrly × 10 days) is dramatic.

Slow, painless enlargement of cervical lymph glands unilateral or bilateral without any preceding illness raises the possibility of leukemia and lymphoma. There are associated features like fever, anemia, bleeding manifestations and hepatosplenomegaly in leukemia and Nonhodgkin lymphoma and the child is ill. The glands in Hodgkin's disease are typically enlarged, discreet with rubbery consistency and the child is not so ill. Bone marrow examination and lymph gland histology is confirmatory.

Infectious mononucleosis presents with constitutional symptoms and generalized lymphadenopathy. Paul Bunnel test is confirmatory.

Nontubercular mycobacterial lymphadenitis is characterized by solitary, unilateral involvement of the submandibular, preauricular and submental glands. There are no constitutional symptoms and no history of contact. Chest X-ray is usually normal and the tuberculin test is negative or weakly positive.

Laboratory Diagnosis

1. Fine Needle Aspiration Cytology (FNAC)

It is a very useful method for diagnosis of tubercular lymphadenitis. FNAC has now replaced routine lymph gland biopsy. FNAC should be done always before starting therapy because prior antituberculous therapy results in definite change in histopathological picture. A lymph gland biopsy is indicated when the FNAC is inconclusive. The different histopathological findings on FNAC may be as follows:

a. *Definite tuberculous lymphadenitis is* characterized by caseation with central necrosis along with granulomatous changes. AFB is visible in a few cases. Presence of pus cells and acute inflammatory cells with AFB visible in a lymph gland histopathology specimen indicates tubercular lymphadenitis.

b. *Granulomatous lymphadenitis* is characterized by only granulomatous changes with giant cells with absence of caseation necrosis.

c. *Reactive lymphadenitis* is characterized by presence of nonspecific cellular changes of chronic inflammation.

2. Chest Radiograph

The most common abnormal finding is presence of primary pulmonary tuberculosis. X-ray abnormality may be present in around 60% cases.

3. Tuberculin Test

Tuberculin test is positive in around 40–80% cases only.

NEUROTUBERCULOSIS

Neurotuberculosis or tuberculosis of the central nervous system is the most serious form of tuberculosis in children and is fatal without treatment. The most frequent forms of neurotuberculosis are tubercular meningitis and tuberculoma. Considering all age groups, tubercular meningitis is a more frequent form of neurotuberculosis than brain tuberculoma. Neurotuberculosis in BCG vaccinated children present as a modified clinical entity which may have a normal CSF but a positive PCR for tuberculosis and/or tubercular antigen by ELISA.

Most tubercular infections of central nervous system are caused by M. tuberculosis. It is believed that the tubercular bacilli reach the central nervous system by the hematogenous route secondary to disease elsewhere in the body. There is formation of a focus (Rich's focus) which may be situated in the meninges, the subpial or subependymal surface of the brain or the spinal cord. Rupture of a focus into the subarchnoid space or into the ventricular system results in meningitis. With a sizable inoculation of organisms or in the absence of adequate cell mediated immunity, the parenchymal cerebral tubercular focus may develop into a tuberculoma or a tubercular brain abscess.

TUBERCULAR MENINGITIS

Tubercular meningitis is the most common form of neurotuberculosis in children. It is the most serious complication of childhood tuberculosis with high mortality and morbidity. Tubercular meningitis complicates about 0.3% of untreated tubercular infections in children. Tubercular meningitis usually occurs within 3–6 months of the primary infection and accompanies in about 50% of cases of miliary tuberculosis.

Pathogenesis

During the lymphohematogenous spread of primary infection, there is formation of metastatic caseous lesion in the cerebral cortex or meninges. This lesion increases in size and discharges small numbers of tubercle bacilli into the subarchnoid space or ventricular system. There is formation of a gelatinous exudate which infiltrates the blood vessels of the cortex and meninges producing inflammation, obstruction and subsequent infarction of cerebral cortex. The site of greatest involvement is the brainstem with associated dysfunction of III, VI and VII cranial nerves. The exudate also interferes with the normal flow of the cerebrospinal fluid in and out of the ventricular system at the level of the basilar cisterns resulting in communicating hydrocephalous.

Clinical Manifestations

Tubercular meningitis is common in children between the age group of 6 months and 6 years. The most common age group is 9 months to 3 years. A prior history of tuberculosis is obtained in approximately 50% of children suffering from tubercular meningitis.

The onset and progression of tubercular meningitis may be rapid or gradual. Rapid progression is seen more often in infants and young children, who may experience symptoms only several days before the onset of acute hydrocephalous, seizures and cerebral edema. More commonly, the progression is gradual over several weeks and can be divided into three stages as follows:

First Stage or Prodromal Stage lasts for 1–2 weeks and is characterized by non-specific symptoms viz. fever, headache, malaise, irritability and drowsiness. There may be sleep disturbances, lack of interest in play, altered behavior, stagnation or loss of developmental milestone in infants. The young children (below 3 years of age) often cannot localize the symptoms. In them fatigue and altered behavior may be subtle signs.

Second Stage or Stage of Meningeal Irritation is characterized by moderate to high fever, increased headache and vomiting. The child develops apathy; lies curled up in the bed and resent handling. The common features are presence of signs of meningeal irritation (viz. neck rigidity, Kernig and Brudzinski), focal or generalized seizures, cranial nerve palsies, hypertonia, focal neurological deficits and signs of raised intracranial pressure (vomiting, papilledema on fundoscopy). The acceleration of the clinical illness correlates with the development of hydrocephalous, increased intracranial pressure and vasculitis.

Some children have signs of encephalitis instead of signs of meningeal irritation. These include disorientation, movement disorders or speech impairment.

Third Stage or Stage of Local or Diffuse Cerebral Involvement is marked by coma, neurological deficits like hemiplegia or paraplegia, hypertension, decerebrate rigidity, deterioration of vital signs and death.

Diagnosis

A high index of clinical suspicion is necessary to diagnose tubercular meningitis. Often the key to diagnosis is a history of exposure to an adult with infectious tuberculosis. Tubercular meningitis can be diagnosed in a child who develops basilar meningitis with hydrocephalous, cranial nerve palsy or stroke with no other apparent cause. Evidence of tuberculosis occurring elsewhere in the body is an important diagnostic clue and should be looked for.

Laboratory Investigations

1. Examination of Cerebrospinal Fluid

The most important laboratory test for the diagnosis of tubercular meningitis is examination and culture of the cerebrospinal fluid.

The CSF is usually under pressure (30–40 cm H_2O). The CSF may be clear or opalescent. On standing, a pellicle or a cobweb coagulum may form in the centre of the tube. The coagulum is composed of cells, tubercle bacilli enmeshed in fibrin. The CSF may be hemorrhagic or xanthochromic. Xanthochromia results from high protein content which may results from spinal meningitis (with increased protein and cells) or Froin syndrome (with marked increased protein and no increase in cells).

The protein level is elevated above 40 mg/dl and is often more than 100 mg/dl. The glucose level is usually reduced to about two third of the blood sugar.

On cytological examination, the leukocyte count is in the range of 10–500/mm^3. Polymorphonuclear leucocytes may be present initially, but later lymphocytes predominate.

A definitive diagnosis depends on the detection of the tubercle bacilli in the CSF. This can be done either by smear examination or bacterial culture. The smear is made from the sediment after centrifuging the CSF or teasing the cobweb and stained with Ziel-Neilson stain. Culture in a traditional media like Lowenstein Jensen media requires 6–8 weeks before any growth is detected. The use of the BACTEC system detects the growth of AFB in 8–14 days. The bacterial yield in smear and culture of CSF is variable. The yield can be increased by taking a larger volume of CSF (5–10 ml), repeated examination for several days and examination of smear for atleast 30 minutes.

2. **Neuroimaging**
    a. An X-ray of skull may show signs of raised intracranial tension.
    b. Computed tomography (CT) and magnetic resonance imaging (MRI) of the brain are useful in diagnosis. A contrast enhanced MRI is superior to CT in detecting meningeal granuloma and delineating infarcts. For routine management of cases, a contrast enhanced CT is sufficient.

    A CT or MRI may be normal in the early stages. As the disease progresses, thick basilar exudates which appear as intensely enhancing areas in the basal cisterns and sylvian fissures with communicating type of hydrocephalous and signs of cerebral edema or focal infarcts in thalamus, basal ganglia and internal capsule are common findings. Multiple, small, silent tuberculomas, occurring most often in the cerebral cortex and thalamic region, may be seen in small infants when TBM is a part of miliary tuberculosis. Findings in late disease include atrophy, meningeal calcification and focal infarcts.

3. **Biochemical Markers in CSF**

    Many biochemical markers have been used for early diagnosis of tubercular meningitis. They are detection of indolic acid, tuberculostearic acid, bromide partition test and adenosine deaminase (ADA) assay. Among these, ADA assay is presently increasingly used. The significant level of ADA in CSF for diagnosis of TBM is more than 10 U/L. It has been shown to be specific and sensitive.

4. **Immunodiagnosis**

    The tubercular antigen has been detected by ELISA, latex particle agglutination and radio immunoassays. These tests appear to be rapid, sensitive and specific but need validation in large number of patients before it can be used routinely.

5. **Polymerase Chain Reaction (PCR)**

    This test has been found to be highly sensitive and specific in the diagnosis of tubercular meningitis. The expense involved in the test is its main disadvantage.

6. **Electrophysiological Studies**

    Among the two electrophysiological studies viz. electroencephalogram (EEG) and brainstem evoked response (BAER), the latter is useful for early detection of hearing impairment which is a common sequelae of TBM.

TUBERCULOMA

Tuberculoma is another form of tuberculosis of the central nervous system. Clinically it usually presents as a space occupying lesion. It primarily occurs in young children in conjunction with tubercular meningitis or independently. In children they are often located in the infratentorial region in the cerebellum, temporal lobe, brainstem and spinal cord. Tuberculomas are most often singular but may be multiple.

Clinical Manifestations

In single tuberculomas, the clinical manifestations are similar to other space occupying lesions viz. features of raised intracranial pressure, focal or generalized seizures and focal deficits. The child may present with cerebellar manifestations and multiple cranial nerve palsy. The constitutional symptoms are absent. With multiple lesions, constitutional symptoms are present and the incidence of signs of intracranial pressure is higher.

Laboratory Diagnosis

The CSF examination is unremarkable except an elevated protein levels. The tuberculin test is reactive. Chest X-ray is normal in single lesion but shows hilar lymphadenopathy in patients with multiple lesions.

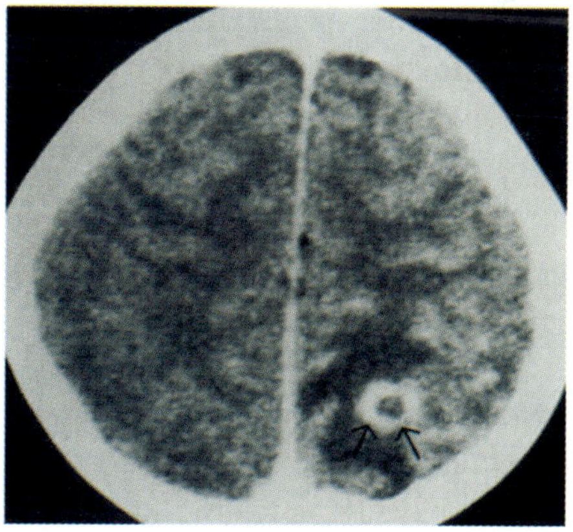

Fig. 11.9: CT scan brain showing a tuberculoma

In the CT and MRI of brain, the tuberculomas are mostly located in the posterior fossa. They are discrete lesions with irregular borders and surrounding edema. The "target sign" with a central calcification or nidus surrounded by a ring that enhances on contrast administration is considered pathognomonic of a tuberculoma. Differentiating tuberculomas from neurocysticercosis is important. Neurocysticercosis is smaller in size, more common in the gray-white junction.

INTRA-ABDOMINAL TUBERCULOSIS

Tuberculosis of the oral cavity or pharynx, esophagus is uncommon in children. They are usually associated with extensive lesions in the lungs but may occur in the absence of pulmonary disease by spread from the mediastinal or peritoneal lymph glands.

The prevalence of abdominal tuberculosis in pediatric age group has been reported as 0.8% by Indian workers.

Etiopathogenesis

In India, all the reported cases of abdominal tuberculosis in children are caused by the human strain of M. tuberculosis. Boiling of milk, pasteurization and eradication of infected cattle may be factors responsible for the decreasing incidence of M. bovis.

Abdominal tuberculosis in children can occur in three forms: intestinal, peritoneal and glandular. Morphologically, the intestinal lesions are classified into ulceroconstrictive, which is seen in the small bowel and hypertrophic seen in the ileocecal region. The infection may be primary and the source of infection may be swallowed infected sputum or secondary to lymphohematogenous spread. In both primary and secondary lesions, the mesenteric and at times the retroperitoneal lymph glands are involved. In primary infections, the intestinal lesion is overshadowed by glandular involvement. The common sites of intestinal involvement are the jejunum, ileum near Peyer's patches and the appendix.

Tuberculous peritonitis may be a part of a generalized hematogenous infection or more frequently results from rupture of a caseous mesenteric lymph gland or by extension from an ulcerative intestinal lesion or from contiguous extension from adjacent organs. Peritoneal tuberculosis can have three forms viz. ascitic, fibrinous or plastic and the caseous or ulcerative forms. However, all these processes are frequently present in a single case with no sharp distinction. In children, the involvement of peritoneum and lymph nodes are more common than intestinal tuberculosis.

Tuberculosis of the liver and spleen is usually a part of generalized miliary tuberculosis.

Clinical Manifestations

Children above the age of 5 years are affected more frequently. It is particularly more common in children with malnutrition and in those who come from rural and low socioeconomic background.

Abdominal tuberculosis is usually a disease of insidious onset but it may also have an acute onset. Constitutional symptoms like fever, night sweats, weight loss etc. may or may not be present. Three clinical categories of abdominal tuberculosis have been described but with overlapping of symptoms and signs.

Intestinal Tuberculosis

The clinical features of intestinal tuberculosis may be those of ileocolitis with tenesmus and diarrhoea with bleeding, and alternate diarrhoea and constipation. Abdominal distension and tenderness may be present. Tuberculosis may be suspected from the chronic nature of the illness or from the presence of tubercular infection elsewhere in the body, especially in the lungs.

The child may present with recurrent attacks of subacute intestinal obstruction which often resolves to conservative treatment. The child may also present with abdominal pain, distension and a doughy feeling on palpation of the abdomen. The doughy feeling results due to adherent intestinal loops and the omentum. Often a lump is palpable, usually in the right iliac fossa which consists of variable portions of terminal ileum, cecum, omentum and lymph nodes at the ileocecal angle.

Peritoneal Tuberculosis

In presence of ascites, the abdomen is distended and there are signs of fluid in the peritoneal cavity viz. shifting dullness or fluid thrill according to the amount of fluid. Children presenting with ascites are usually severely malnourished and anemic. The child may present with an asymptomatic lump due to loculated ascites.

Lymph Node Tuberculosis

When the involvement is predominantly glandular, the child usually presents with a lump and /or signs of intestinal obstruction due to kinks and adhesions. Rarely, there may be signs of obstruction of bile duct, pancreatic duct, duodenum, inferior vena cava and ureter by enlarged lymph nodes.

Others

Uncommonly the presentation may be that of acute

abdomen as a result of rupture of caseous lymph nodes, gastrointestinal perforation, tuberculous peritonitis or rarely acute appendicitis. Another uncommon presentation of abdominal tuberculosis is with pyrexia of unknown origin. Involvement of uterus or fallopian tubes in female adolescents may present with menstrual irregularities or infertility.

Laboratory Diagnosis

For definite diagnosis, characteristic histological findings in presence of suggestive clinical features are adequate in endemic areas. Abdominal tuberculosis is a paucibacillary disease and microbiological proof is not always possible. Caseation is the histological marker for abdominal tuberculosis. However, granuloma with caseation may be present in the lymph nodes and absent in intestinal lesions. Moreover, non-caseating granuloma may be seen due to a good host defence or low virulence of the organism. Tissue specimens for histological examination may be obtained by one of the following techniques:

1. Ultrasound or CT guided fine needle aspiration cytology (FNAC) from an abdominal mass.
2. Endoscopic guided FNAC for submucosal lesions.
3. Culture of biopsy tissue for AFB.
4. Ascitic fluid examination: The ascitic fluid in abdominal tuberculosis looks clear or straw colored with a glucose concentration less than 30 mg/dl, protein content more than 2.5 gram/dl and white cell count greater 100/ mm^3. The serum to ascites fluid albumin (SAAG) ratio less than 1.1 gm/dl is a better guide to diagnosis than ascitic fluid protein alone. Ascitic fluid smear and culture for AFB is confirmative. The yield of organism is high if atleast 1 litre of ascitic fluid can be concentrated by centrifugation. Determination of ascitic fluid enzyme adenosine deaminase activity is a major advance in diagnosis. The test is highly sensitive as well as specific. The normal level of adenosine deaminase in ascitic fluid is less than 40 U/L; between 40 and 60 U/L it is indeterminate. A level above 60 U/ L is diagnostic.

Investigations which provide supportive evidence are as follows:

1. Tuberculin test may be positive in around 50% cases.
2. *Serologic tests (ELIZA test):* A positive test has 80% sensitivity and 80–90% specificity in serodiagnosis of abdominal tuberculosis.
3. *Radiology:* The radiological tests include a chest X-ray, plain X-ray abdomen, barium enema, barium meal study and abdominal ultrasound and CT scan study as and when indicated.

   A positive chest X-ray is seen in a very small number of cases. A plain X-ray of abdomen may show mottled calcification in the mesenteric lymph nodes. The findings in barium study include filling defects in cecum and small intestine, strictures in small intestine, increased or decreased intestinal transit time and hypersegmentation or thickened mucosal folds. The characteristic sonographic and CT features are mesenteric thickness, mesenteric lymphadenopathy and ascites.
4. Endoscopy of the upper and lower GI tract with biopsy from ulcer margins can give a rapid diagnosis.
5. Laparoscopy with directed biopsy is currently the best way to make a rapid specific diagnosis. It is preferred over blind percutaneous peritoneal biopsy.

TREATMENT OF CHILDHOOD TUBERCULOSIS

The first drug found to be effective in tuberculosis was streptomycin which when used alone was found to become resistant in 3 months. It was used around the year 1940. The next two drugs discovered were para amino salicylic acid in 1949 and isoniazid in 1952. Use of the three drugs in combination helped in prevention of resistance. However, this combination of drugs was to be given for 18–24 months.

Discovery of newer and more potent drugs, viz. Rifampicin, Pyrazinamide, Ethambutol led to the use of shorter regimens. Use of a combination of streptomycin, rifampicin and isoniazid reduced the period of treatment to 9 months. With addition of pyrizinamide the period of treatment was further shortened to 6 months.

Previous Drug Regimens

Earlier intermittent therapy was not recommended in children as compliance was found to be generally poor and hence an increased risk of drug resistance. A standard WHO clinical categorization and suggested clinical conditions of tuberculosis in children followed in TB clinic in AIIMS is given below.

Table 11. 2 : Standard WHO clinical categories and suggested clinical conditions of tuberculosis in children (TB clinic AIIMS)

Category	*As suggested by WHO*	*Suggested conditions*	*Suggested regimens*
I	New Sputum positive Pulmonary TB	PPD, TBL, Pleural effusion, abdominal TB, osteoarticular TB, genitourinary TB, CNS TB	2HRZE, 4HR Or 2HRZ, 4HR
II	Relapse, treatment failure, Return after adult default (Interrupted treatment)	Relapse, Treatment failure, Interrupted treatment	2SHRZE, 1HRZE, 7HRE
III	Sputum negative Pulmonary with limited parenchymal involvement, extrapulmonary TB (with less severe forms)	Single lymph node, small pleural effusion, PPC, skin TB	2HRZ, 4HR

PPC - Pulmonary primary complex, PPD - Progressive primary disease, TBL - Tubercular lymphadenitis, CNS - Central nervous system, TB -Tuberculosis.

H = Isoniazid, R = Rifampicin, Z = Pyrazinamide, E = Ethambutol, S = Streptomycin.

According to this recommendation all drugs should be administered in a single daily dose on an empty stomach. The drugs are safe if used in the recommended doses. Vitamin B6 is not necessary in children taking isoniazid.

Indications of Steroid (Prednisolone)

- Neurotuberculosis.
- Miliary tuberculosis.
- Pleural effusion, ascites.
- Endobronchial tuberculosis, segmental lesions.
- Genitourinary tuberculosis, sinus formation.

Dosage schedule: 1–2 mg/kg/day single dose 4–8 weeks (8–12 weeks in neurotuberculosis).

Management of Hepatotoxicity after Antituberculosis Treatment

The clinical features of hepatoxicity in a child on antituberculosis drugs include jaundice and hepatomegaly. The child should be advised laboratory test for liver function and the hepatotoxic drugs viz. HRZ should be temporarily stopped. The child should be started on streptomycin and ethambutol. When the SGPT enzyme returns to normal which takes about 2–4 weeks, isoniazid (H) is restarted and the three drugs should be continued. After one week, rifampicin (R) is restarted and streptomycin and ethambutol is stopped. Pyrizinamide (Z) should be started after another one week if stoppage was required in the intensive phase.

Recommendation on Treatment of Pediatric Tuberculosis under RNTCP (2012)

It has been recommended that all pediatric TB patients should be registered under RNTCP and treated with intermittent short course chemotherapy given under direct observation (DOTS).

Intermittent versus Daily Regimen

According to the recent recommendation (RNTCP), the intermittent therapy will remain the mainstay of treating pediatric patients. However, among seriously ill admitted children or those with severe disseminated disease/neurotuberculosis, the likelihood of vomiting or non-tolerance of oral drugs is high in the initial phase. Such, select group of seriously ill admitted patients should be given daily supervised therapy during their stay in the hospital using daily drug dosages. After discharge they will be taken on thrice weekly DOT regimen.

The anti-tuberculous drugs to be used for the daily regimen and their daily doses are:

- Rifampicin 10-12 mg/kg (max 600 mg/day).
- Isoniazid 10 mg/kg (max 300 mg/day).
- Ethambutol 20-25 mg/kg (max 1500 mg/day).
- PZA 30-35 mg/kg (max 2000 mg/day); and
- Streptomycin 15 mg/kg (max 1gm/day).

New Case Definitions of Pediatric TB (RNTCP)

The following are the new case definitions for pediatric TB patients:

1. *Failure to respond*: A case of pediatric TB who fails to have bacteriological conversion to negative status or fails to respond clinically/or deteriorates after 12 weeks of compliant intensive phase shall be deemed to have failed response provided alternative diagnosis/reasons for non-response have been ruled out.
2. *Relapse*: A case of pediatric TB declared cured/ completed therapy in past and has clinical or bacteriological evidence of recurrence.
3. *Treatment after default*: A case of pediatric TB who has taken treatment for at least 4 weeks and comes after interruption of treatment for 2 months or more and has active disease (clinical or bacteriological).
4. *Others:* All types of retreatment cases where bacteriological evidence could not be demonstrated but decision to treat again was taken on clinical grounds would continue to be recorded and reported as "OTHERS" for surveillance purposes.

Diagnosis of Extrapulmonary Tuberculosis (RNTCP)

TB Lymphadenitis

This is most common form of extra pulmonary tuberculosis. Clinical correlate of diagnosis includes progressive enlargement of lymph node for more than 2 weeks, firm, minimally tender or not tender, sometimes fluctuating, may be matted and may have chronic sinus formation.

Fine needle aspiration cytology (FNAC) is usually adequate for accurate diagnosis and it correlates well with biopsy in > 90% of cases. Histopathology typically shows necrosis and epitheloid granuloma. It is important to look for AFB in FNAC specimen and it may be positive in 20-70% of patients. When FNAC is inconclusive, biopsy is necessary for confirmation of diagnosis.

It needs mention that in children, lymphadenopathy is common due to recurrent tonsillitis and URTIs as well. Such reactive lymphadenitis may clinically mimic tuberculosis but does not warrant anti-TB drugs. Persistent lymphadenopathy of significant size (say more than 2 cm in the neck) should however, be investigated. TST is mostly positive in a significant proportion, but isolated skin test positivity is not enough to establish a diagnosis of TB. Hence anti-tuberculous drugs should not be given unless the diagnosis of TB is confirmed by FNAC or histopathology.

Pleural Effusion

If chest X-ray is suggestive of pleural effusion, pleural aspiration should always be performed for biochemical, cytological and smear examination by ZN stain to confirm the diagnosis.

Typically, a tubercular effusion fluid is straw coloured, has large numbers of cells (in hundreds; predominantly mononuclear), with high proteins (>3 g/dL). Adenosine Deaminase (ADA) levels over 60 IU/L may be suggestive of tuberculous pleural effusion but is not diagnostic of tuberculosis. Pleural biopsy may be performed, where available, particularly when the fluid aspirate findings are inconclusive. It should be noted that pus, if aspirated, is very rarely due to tuberculosis.

Tubercular Meningitis (TBM)

Children with TBM present with a rather longer (>1 week) duration of fever, with vague CNS symptoms such as behaviour changes, irritability, drowsiness, headache, vomiting and seizures.

Physical examination reveals typically global encephalopathy with focal deficits, hydrocephalus and movement disorder.

Risk factors for TBM include age < 5 years, contact with an adult suffering from tuberculosis, PEM grade III and IV and HIV infection.

CSF examination typically shows a clear to opalescent CSF, usually does not show very high cell count (below 500 cells/mm^3) with lymphocytosis. Biochemical investigations reveal increased proteins and mild reduction in glucose. The typical CSF picture may, however, not always be seen. Furthermore, the typical CSF picture described above can also be mimicked by partially treated pyogenic meningitis. In such a situation, reassessing after 48-72 hours of treatment with a fresh set of broad spectrum potent antibiotics to evaluate improvement in clinical status as well as in CSF can be useful.

Besides routine CSF examination, CSF ADA is high in TBM. Various studies have a cut-off point between 7 and 11.3 IU/L for diagnosis. This may offer supportive evidence in favour of TBM but should not be taken in isolation. CSF antigen and PCR tests are neither routinely available nor reproducible. They are, therefore, not recommended. CSF antibody tests have poor sensitivity and specificity and hence are not useful.

TST, chest skiagrams and bacteriological examination should be done to establish the diagnosis by collecting more supportive evidence. Bacteriological diagnosis from appropriate samples including CSF is diagnostic. Many a time concomitant TB lesions elsewhere in the body (say, pulmonary) coexist and can clinch the diagnosis. Mycobacterial culture from CSF should also be attempted but CSF culture has poor sensitivity (16%) though specificity is high (90%).

Neuroimaging (CT scan) is an important diagnostic modality. It may reveal one or more of the following findings: basal meningeal enhancement; hydrocephalus with or without periventricular ooze, Tuberculoma(s), or infarcts may be seen in different areas, especially in basal ganglia. Normal CT scan does not rule out TBM and in case of strong clinical suspicion of diagnosis, a repeat follow-up CT scan after few days may show newly developing lesions.

Tuberculoma

Often seen in older children, it may present as a focal seizure in supratentorial cortical lesion or with symptoms and signs of raised intracranial tension with multiple localizing signs and hydrocephalus in posterior fossa lesion. It may sometimes also be seen as a part of tubercular meningitis. Differentiation from other ring lesions, especially neurocysticercosis (NCC) is difficult in cortical lesion. A ring enhancing lesion is not pathognomonic of tuberculoma. A larger lesion > 20 mm, disc lesion or ring lesion with thicker rim with central nodule favours tuberculoma while multiple, smaller, thin rim with epicentric nodule favour NCC. MR spectroscopy may help in diagnosis of tuberculoma.

Abdominal Tuberculosis

It may present as localized disease such as mesenteric lymphadenopathy, intestinal disease, peritoneal involvement or systemic disseminated disease presenting as hepatosplenomegaly. Large matted lymph node mass may be clinically evident and ultrasound guided biopsy may help in confirming the diagnosis.

There are no standard guidelines for sonography diagnosis of abdominal tuberculosis. However, corroborative evidence includes: echogenic thickened mesentery with lymph nodes > 15 mm in size; dilated and matted bowel loops; thickened omentum, and ascites. None of these findings, however, is specific to tuberculosis alone.

Barium follow-through examination may be suggestive of intestinal disease but is not confirmatory.

Exudative peritoneal disease presents as ascites that is often clinically evident. The ascitic tap should always be done in such situations and the fluid tapped is an exudate, typically showing lymphocytic predominant cellular response with high proteins (>3 g/dL).

Treatment Regimens

There will be only two treatment categories – one for treating 'new' cases and another for treating 'previously treated cases'. The treatment regimens are summarized in the Table 11.3.

Table 11.3 : Showing treatment categories and regimens for childhood tuberculosis

Category of treatment	*Type of patients*	*Treatment Regimen*	
		Intensive phase	Continuation phase
New cases	• New smear positive pulmonary tuberculosis (PTB) • New smear negative PTB • New extra pulmonary TB	2 H_3 R_3 Z_3 E_3 *	4 H_3 R_3*
Previously treated cases	• Relapse, failure to respond or treatment after default • Re-treatment Others	2 $S_3H_3R_3Z_3E_3$* + 1 H_3 R_3 Z_3 E_3*	5 H_3 R_3 E_3*

H=Isoniazid, R= Rifampicin, Z= Pyrazinamide, E= Ethambutol, S= Streptomycin

* The number before the letters refers to the number of months of treatment. The subscript after the letters refers to the number of doses per week.

- Pulmonary tuberculosis (PTB) refers to disease involving lung parenchyma.
- Extra pulmonary TB refers to disease involving sites other than lung parenchyma. If both pulmonary and extra pulmonary sites are affected, it will be considered as pulmonary for registration purposes. Extra Pulmonary TB involving several sites should be defined by most severe site.
- *Smear positive:* Any sample (sputum, induced sputum, gastric lavage, bronchoalveolar lavage) positive for acid fast bacilli.
- *New Case:* A patient who has had no previous ATT or had for less than 4 weeks.
- *Relapse:* Patient declared cured/completed therapy in past and has evidence of recurrence.
- *Treatment after Default:* A patient who has taken treatment for at least 4 weeks and comes after interruption of treatment for 2 months and has active disease.
- *Failure to respond:* A case of pediatric TB who fails to have bacteriological conversion to negative status or fails to respond clinically/or deteriorates after 12 weeks of compliant intensive phase shall be deemed to have failed response provided alternative diagnosis/reasons for non-response have been ruled out.
- *Others:* Cases who are smear negative or extra pulmonary but considered to have relapse, failure to respond or treatment after default or any other case which do not fit the above definitions.
- In patients with TB meningitis on Category I treatment, the four drugs used during the intensive phase can either be HRZE or HRZS. The present evidence suggests that Ethambutol can be used in children.
- Under Revised National Tuberculosis Program (RNTCP), all patients shall be covered under directly observed intermittent (thrice weekly) therapy. The supervised therapy is considered as the most optimal treatment and is followed under RNTCP. It is important to ensure completion of treatment in every case put on treatment to prevent emergence of resistance, particularly to Rifampicin. In the rare circumstances where a patient is given daily therapy, observation and completion of therapy remains as important. It is the duty of the prescriber to ensure appropriate and complete treatment in all cases.

Extending Intensive and Continuation Phase

1. Children who show poor or no response at 8 weeks of intensive phase should be given benefit of extension of intensive phase for one more month.
2. In patients with TB meningitis, spinal TB, miliary/disseminated TB and osteoarticular TB, the continuation phase shall be extended by 3 months making the total duration of treatment to a total of 9 months. A further extension may be done for 3 more months in continuation phase (making the total duration of treatment to 12 months) on a case to case basis in case of delayed response and as per the discretion of the treating physician/pediatrician.

Drug Dosage

There will be six weight bands and three generic patient-wise boxes will be used in combination to treat patients in the six weight bands. These products are supplied under RNTCP.

To ensure that every child gets correct dosages, weighing of the patient in minimal clothing (as appropriate) using accurate weighing scales is essential.

Chemoprophylaxis

INH is the drug used for chemoprophylaxis. The dose is 10 mg/kg administered daily for 6 months.

Preventive therapy should be provided to:

1. All asymptomatic contacts (under 6 years of age) of a smear positive case, after ruling out active disease and irrespective of their BCG or nutritional status.
2. Chemoprophylaxis is also recommended for all HIV infected children who either had a known exposure to an infectious TB case or are Tuberculin skin test (TST) positive (>/=5 mm induration) but have no active TB disease.
3. All TST positive children who are receiving immunosuppressive therapy (e.g., Children with Nephrotic syndrome, acute leukemia, etc.).
4. A child born to mother who was diagnosed to have TB in pregnancy should receive prophylaxis for 6 months, provided congenital TB has been ruled out. BCG vaccination can be given at birth even if INH chemoprophylaxis is planned.

CONGENITAL TUBERCULOSIS

In spite of tuberculosis being so common, congenital tuberculosis is rare. However, with increase in cases of multidrug resistant tuberculosis and HIV there is an increase in incidence of tuberculosis in the women of child bearing age and in the babies born to them.

Pathophysiology

Congenital tuberculosis is acquired transplacentally when the tubercular bacilli gains access by the umbilical vein or by aspiration of the amniotic fluid either in utero or during the passage through the birth canal. Rarely, the infection can occur in the neonatal period by inhalation or ingestion of infected droplet from the mother or an open case in the family.

Transplacental infection usually occurs in late pregnancy. The primary focus is formed in the liver with involvement of the periportal lymph glands. The tubercle bacilli reach the liver via the umbilical vein. The bacilli may pass through the liver resulting in a hematogenous spread to form multiple foci in different organs.

A caseous lesion in the placenta may rupture into the amniotic cavity. If the baby swallows the infected amniotic fluid, multiple foci forms in the lungs, gut and the middle ear with enlargement of the mediastinal, mesenteric lymph glands or both. Middle ear involvement leads to multiple perforations in the tympanic membrane and otorrhea.

Clinical Manifestations

The symptoms and signs may be present at birth but more commonly begin by second or third week of life. The symptoms include respiratory distress, fever, poor feeding, lethargy or irritability, seizures, failure to gain weight and draining from ear. There is hepatomegaly and/or splenomegaly, lymphadenopathy, jaundice. The most common presenting features however are hepatosplenomegaly, respiratory distress, fever, growth failure and generalized lymphadenopathy.

The clinical presentation of congenital tuberculosis is similar to that caused by bacterial sepsis or congenital intrauterine infection**.** The important clue to diagnosis is presence of a maternal or family history of tuberculosis and absence of response to adequate antibiotic therapy or evaluation for congenital infections is unrevealing.

Laboratory Diagnosis

1. The tuberculin test is negative initially, but may become positive in 1–3 months.
2. The X-ray of chest often reveals hilar and mediastinal lymphadenopathy with parenchymal infiltrates.
3. Direct acid fast stains of gastric aspirate, ear discharge, tracheal or nasopharyngeal aspirates. The positive gastric aspirate yield is very high.
4. Examination of cerebrospinal fluid including culture. The culture yield is however very poor.
5. Bone marrow aspiration cytology, biopsy of lymph glands, liver biopsy are the other diagnostic modalities which may be considered.

Prognosis

The mortality rate of congenital tuberculosis is very high because of delayed diagnosis. Complete recovery is possible with early diagnosis and adequate chemotherapy.

Treatment

The consensus statement of Indian Academy of Pediatrics recommends treatment with INH (5 mg/kg/day) rifampicin (10 mg/kg/day) and pyrizinamide (30 mg/kg/day) for 2 months followed by INH and rifampicin for 7 months.

Management of a Neonate Born to a Mother with Tuberculosis

Separation of the baby from mother is not considered mandatory once antituberculous therapy is started in the mother. Breastfeeding should be continued. Prophylactic INH (5 mg/kg/day) is recommended after ruling out congenital tuberculosis. INH therapy should be continued in the infant atleast until the mother has been shown to be noninfectious (culture negative) for 3 months. The infant should receive INH for a total of 6 to 9 months. Vaccination with BCG appears to decrease the risk of tuberculosis in exposed infants, but the effect is variable.

Separation of the baby from the mother should be advised in the following circumstances: (1) The mother is ill enough to require hospitalization (2) If she has been or is expected to be non-adherent to treatment or (3) if she is infected with a drug resistant strain of M. tuberculosis.

MULTI DRUG RESISTANT TUBERCULOSIS

Multi drug resistant tuberculosis (MDR) is rare in children. It should be considered when child has a contact with MDR tuberculosis or there is failure of response to adequate treatment for 8–12 weeks. Before considering the diagnosis of MDR TB in children, diagnosis of tuberculosis itself should be reviewed. The diagnosis of multi drug resistance should be confirmed by bacteriological study and the patient should be treated in a referral centre.

Treatment

In MDR TB, 3 sensitive drugs should be given for 2 years after culture is negative in both HIV positive and negative patient. In patients with only INH resistant and HIV negative status, the patient should be treated with Rifampicin, pyrizinamide and ethambutol for 12 months whereas in HIV positive cases, the same drugs should be given for 18 months or 12 months after culture is negative. In case of isolated rifampicin resistance and HIV negative status, the patient should be treated with INH, pyrizinamide, and ethambutol for 18–24 months whereas HIV positive cases, the same drugs should be given for 18–24 months or 12 months after culture is negative.

HIV AND TUBERCULOSIS

Tuberculosis is one of the most common opportunistic infection in HIV infected children especially in high prevalent areas. HIV infection increases the susceptibility to primary and post primary tuberculosis as well as drug resistant tuberculosis.

Clinical Manifestations

The clinical presentation is usually with unusual features and extrapulmonary disease is more common. Careful history with emphasis on a history of contact with a person with infectious tuberculosis is important for diagnosis. In HIV positive but immunocompetent patients, clinical manifestations are similar to those seen in general population. In HIV positive and immunosuppressed, tuberculosis is extensive. Progressive depletion and dysfunction of CD 4 cells with defects in the function of macrophages and monocytes associated with HIV infection is responsible for the development of extensive tuberculosis. Extensive tuberculosis includes miliary tuberculosis, presence of hepatosplenomegaly, lymphadenopathy, tuberculous meningitis and genito-urinary tuberculosis.

Laboratory Diagnosis

1. Tuberculin test is considered positive if the induration is 5 mm or more.
2. The chest radiograph may show the features of (i) confluent, patchy consolidation involving more than half of the lung, (ii) massive hilar/paratracheal lymphadenopathy, (iii) dense lobar/segmental collapse.
3. Isolation of acid fast bacilli from gastric lavage, bronchoalveolar lavage or sputum and stained with Zeil-Neilson or Auramine-Rhodamine stain.
4. Culture of the specimens in radiometric blood culture media for antibiotic susceptibility. For extrapulmonary tuberculosis, tissue samples should be stained and cultured in the same way.
5. The PCR test for sputum, pleural fluid and cerebrospinal fluid can help in diagnosis.

Treatment

Antituberculous Drugs

Tuberculosis with HIV infection is treated with a 4 drug regimen consisting of isoniazid, rifampicin, pyrizinamide, and ethambutol or streptomycin for a period of 6–12 months for pulmonary tuberculosis and for a minimum of 12 months in extrapulmonary disease. Directly observed therapy (DOT) is recommended for the initial months. Children with tuberculin test positive but without any other manifestations of active disease should receive isoniazid and rifampicin for 12 months. When MDR TB is suspected, 6–7 drugs should be started till the sensitivity report is available. Besides the first line drugs such as INH and pyrizinamide, the second line drugs include ofloxacin, ethionamide, cycloserine, capreomycin and PAS. The minimum duration of treatment in cases with MDR TB is 12–15 months.

The drugs dosage of the antituberculous drugs:

a. *INH:* 10–20 mg/kg/day in single or two divided doses (maximum dose 300 mg/day).
b. *Rifampicin:* 10–20 mg/kg/day in single or two divided doses (maximum dose 600 mg/day).
c. *Pyrizinamide:* 30 mg/kg/day in single or two divided doses.
d. *Ethambutol:* 15 mg/kg/day as a single dose.
e. *Streptomycin:* 20–30 mg/kg/day IM in two divided doses.

Anti-retroviral Drugs

WHO recommends that in a patient with CD4 count less than 200, anti-retroviral drugs should be started two weeks to two months after starting of anti-tuberculous drugs. If the CD4 count is higher, such patients can wait until the induction phase of anti-tuberculous therapy is complete.

Amebiasis

Amebiasis is the condition of harboring the protozoon Entamoeba histolytica. The organism may live for a long time in the lumen of the large intestine as a commensal, without invading the intestinal wall. When invasion occurs, lesions are developed in the mucosa which may give rise to clinical conditions viz. amebic colitis or to extra-intestinal lesions. Human infection is prevalent worldwide, occurring specially in unhygienic conditions and warm climate.

Etiology

There are two morphologically distinct species of entamoeba that commonly infect humans. Entamoeba histolytica is the pathogenic species which causes symptomatic disease. Entamoeba dispar is associated with an asymptomatic carrier state. Infection is established by ingestion of parasite cysts. The cysts are resistant to environmental conditions such as low temperature and the concentration of chlorine commonly used in water purification.

Pathogenesis

On ingestion, the cyst which is resistant to gastric acidity and digestive enzymes, encyst in the small intestine to form eight trophozoites. These are large, actively motile organisms that colonize the lumen of the large intestine and may invade the mucosal lining under conditions that are currently unknown. They attach to the colonic mucosa by a galactose-specific lectin-receptor. The trophozoites do not transmit infection because they degenerate rapidly outside the body or in the low pH environment of the stomach.

Once attached to the colonic mucosa, amebas release a cysteine rich proteinase that allows for penetration through the epithelial layer. Once E. histolytica trophozoites invade the intestinal mucosa, they produce tissue destruction by cytolysis. The organisms multiply and spread laterally underneath the intestinal epithelium to produce flask shaped ulcers. These lesions are commonly seen in the cecum, transverse colon, and sigmoid colon. The ameba may produce similar lytic lesions if they reach the liver.

Clinical Manifestations

The clinical presentations of amebiasis include asymptomatic cyst passers, amebic colitis, amebic dysentery, ameboma and extra-intestinal disease viz. amebic hepatitis and liver abscess which may spread to the brain and lungs. Severe disease is more common in young children, malnourished and children on corticosteroids.

Asymptomatic amebiasis has the potential to become invasive and thus should be treated.

Intestinal amebiasis usually occurs after two weeks of infection or may be delayed for months. The onset is gradual with colicky abdominal pain and frequent bowel movements (6–8 times/day). Generalized constitutional symptoms and signs are characteristically absent although fever may occur in 30% of cases. Amebic infections can occur at any age but the incidence is high in the age group of 1–5 years. Severe infection in infants and young children tend to be rapidly progressive with frequent extra-intestinal involvement and high mortality rates. *Amebic colitis* is characterized by some looseness of stool and mild diarrhoea which eventually subsides, but tends to recur at intervals. Some cases pass on to *invasive amebic colitis* with passage of blood stained mucus motions with offensive smell. Occasionally, amebic dysentery is associated with sudden onset of fever, chills and severe diarrhoea which may result in dehydration and electrolyte imbalance. This is usually associated with malnutrition, debilitating conditions and concurrent infection. Uncommonly, a chronic form develops, which can mimic chronic inflammatory bowel disease. It is characterized by bouts of abdominal pain and bloody diarrhoea, often recurring over several years. Hence chronic amebic dysentery should be excluded before starting steroid therapy for inflammatory bowel disease.

Complications

Complications can occur in few patients. These include ameboma, toxic megacolon, local hemorrhage or perforation and extra intestinal extension. The *ameboma* is formed by extension of infection in the gut wall and contiguous tissue. It is felt as a mass through the abdominal wall, usually in the region of the cecum and sigmoid colon. It is tender when palpated per rectum.

The most common extra intestinal extension is amebic liver abscess but there is usually no clear history of intestinal disease. The child presents with fever, pain and distension of abdomen. The liver is enlarged soft and tender. An abscess may rupture into the peritoneal cavity or pleural cavity. The child then has signs of peritonitis and pleural effusion respectively. Laboratory examination findings are mild leucocytosis, moderate anemia, high ESR and nonspecific elevation of enzymes (particularly alkaline phosphatase). Stool examination is negative in more than 50% cases of documented amebic liver abscess. In most cases, the abscess can be localized and size delineated with a USG, CT, MRI or an isotope scan.

Laboratory Diagnosis

Diagnosis is based on detection of organisms in stool samples, smears obtained by sigmoidoscopy, tissue biopsy and liver abscess aspirate.

Stool samples should be fresh and examined within 30 minutes of passage and looked for motile trophozoites containing erythrocytes. Examination of 3 fresh stool samples by an experienced pathologist has 90% sensitivity. E. histolytica is distinguished from E. dispar on microscopy, from presence of phagocytosed RBCs. Patients with invasive colitis also have a stool occult blood test positive.

Table 11.4 : Macroscopic and microscopic differences between stools of amebic and bacillary dysentery

Findings	*Amebic dysentery*	*Bacillary dysentery*
Macroscopic		
Number	6 – 8 motions/day	> 10 motions/day
Amount	Relatively copious	Small
Odour	Offensive	Odourless
Colour	Dark red	Bright red
Nature	Blood and mucus mixed with feces	Blood mucus no feces
Reaction	Acid	Alkaline
Microscopic		
RBC	In clumps, reddish yellow in color	Discrete/ rouleaux Bright red in color
Pus cells	Scanty	Numerous
Macrophages	Very few	Numerous contain RBCs
Parasite	Trophozoites of E. histolytica	Nil
Bacteria	Nil	Many motile bacteria
CL crystals	Present	Nil

Sigmoidoscopy and biopsy should be performed when the stool sample results are negative and there is a strong suspicion of amebiasis.

Serologic tests viz. indirect hemagglutination test is positive in 95% of patients with symptomatic disease of more than 7 days duration and most asymptomatic carriers of pathogenic E. histolytica. E. dispar does not elicit a humoral response. The test can be done in both stool and serum. However these tests are not routinely available.

Treatment

The principle of treatment is destruction and elimination of E. histolytica in the intestine and the tissues. Two types of drugs are available. Iodoquinol and diloxanide furoate are primarily luminal amebecides. Metronidazole, chloroquine and dehydroemetine are drugs effective in the treatment of invasive amebiasis.

All children with E. histolytica trophozoites or cysts in stool whether symptomatic or not should be treated. *Metronidazole* (30–50 mg/kg/day in 3 doses per oral for 10 days; maximum dose 500–750 mg/dose) is the drug of choice for invasive amebiasis of the intestine, liver or other organs. *Diloxanide furoate* (20 mg/kg/day 3 doses per oral per day for 10 days) is also a safe drug in intestinal amebiasis, but should not be used in children below 2 years. Aspiration may be necessary in case of large abscess if rupture is imminent or if the patient shows poor response 4–6 days after administration of amebecidal drugs. *Dehydroemetine*, in fulminating cases and *chloroquine* in cases of liver abscess was used earlier.

Stool examination should be repeated every 2 weeks until the result is negative after the completion of antiamebic therapy to confirm cure.

Prevention

Control of amebiasis can be achieved by adopting proper sanitary measures to avoid feco-oral contact. Regular screening of food handlers and thorough investigation of diarrheal outbreaks may identify the source of infection. There is no drug or vaccine for prevention.

Giardiasis

Giardiasis is a protozoal infection caused by the Giardia intestinalis/lamblia. The organism was first seen by Leewenhoek in 1681 while examining his own stool. Infection results in a wide variety of manifestations ranging from asymptomatic colonization to acute or chronic diarrhoea and malabsorption.

Epidemiology

Giardiasis is endemic in the areas of the world with poor levels of sanitation. It is also a cause of morbidity in the developed countries where they are associated with urban child care centres, residential centres for mentally handicapped and water borne and food borne outbreaks. Infection is more prevalent in children than in adults. The major reservoir and vehicle for spread of Giardia appears to be water contaminated with Giardia cysts, but food borne transmission also occurs. Person to person spread also occurs particularly in areas of low hygiene standards, frequent fecal-oral contact and overcrowding. Humoral immunodeficiency predisposes to chronic symptomatic Giardia infection. Human milk contains glycoconjugates and secretary IgA antibodies that may provide protection to babies on breastfeeding.

Etiology

Giardia intestinalis exists in two forms – the trophozoite and the cyst. It habitats the duodenum and the upper part of jejunum. The body of the trophozoite is tear drop shaped measuring 10–20 µm in length and 5–15 µm in breath. It contains two oval nuclei anteriorly, a ventral disk, a curved median body posteriorly and four pairs of flagella. The fully formed cyst is oval in shape and measures 12 µm in length and 7 µm in breadth. There are four nuclei. The remains of the flagella and the margins of the disk may be seen inside the cytoplasm.

Pathogenesis

Infection in man is brought about by ingestion of as few as 10–100 cysts. Within 30 minutes of ingestion, the cyst hatches out two trophozoites which then multiply in enormous numbers and colonize in the duodenum. To avoid the high acidity of duodenum, the trophozoites often localizes in the biliary tract. With the help of the disc, the trophozoite attaches itself on to the convex surface of the epithelial cells in the intestine and may cause disturbance of intestinal function leading to malabsorption of fat. Consequently there is persistent looseness of bowels and mild steatorrhoea. The parasite is also capable of producing harm by its toxic effects (allergy), traumatic and irritative effect as well as spoliative action i.e. by diverting the nutrients.

As the trophozoites get detached and pass down the intestinal tract, they encyst to form oval cysts. The cysts are passed in stool and they may remain viable in water as long as 2 months. Their viability is often not affected by the usual concentration of chlorine used to purify water for drinking. Boiling is effective for inactivating cysts.

Clinical Manifestations

The incubation period of Giardia infection usually is 1–2 weeks but may be longer. An infected child may present with clinical presentations varying from asymptomatic cyst passers to acute and chronic diarrhoea. There is usually no extra intestinal spread, but occasionally trophozoites may migrate into the bile or pancreatic ducts.

Symptomatic infections occur more frequently in children than in adults. Majority of cases present with acute diarrhoea associated with nausea and anorexia with or without fever. In a small percentage of cases, there may be an intermittent or protracted course characterized by diarrhoea, abdominal distension and cramps, bloating, malaise, flatulence, nausea, anorexia and weight loss.

Initially, the stools may be profuse and watery and later become greasy and foul smelling and float in water. Abnormal stool may alternate with periods of constipation and normal bowel movements.

Laboratory Diagnosis

A definitive diagnosis can be made by examination of a stool specimen or duodenal aspirate for trophozoite, cyst or giardia antigen.

Examination of Stool

The examination can be done on direct smear or after concentration of stool specimen. The stool specimen should be examined within 1 hour of passage. If examination is delayed, the specimen should be preserved in vials containing polyvinyl alcohol or 10% formalin. Both trophozoites and cysts should be looked for. However, the trophozoites are unstable and cysts stable outside the GI tract. Direct examination of three stool specimens will yield more than 90% diagnosis while one examination 70%. The child should not take any medication for 48–72 hours before collection of stool specimen.

Duodenal Aspiration and Biopsy

Aspiration or biopsy of the duodenum or upper jejunum is indicated in patients when Giardiasis is suspected but stool examination yields a negative result. In a fresh specimen, the trophozoites can be identified in a direct wet mount. The biopsy specimen can be used to make touch preparations and tissue sections for identification of Giardia as well as to visualize histological changes.

Radiological and Blood Studies

Contrast studies of the small intestine may show irregular thickening of the mucosal folds. Blood cell counts are normal.

Serological Tests

Use of polyclonal and monoclonal antibodies against Giardia organism specific antigen in immunofluorescent assays has been tried in an effort to improve diagnosis. For environmental monitoring, polymerase chain reaction (PCR) and gene probe based detection system specific for Giardia have been used. These are tools for research purposes.

Treatment

All symptomatic cases should be treated with oral antimicrobials. The asymptomatic cyst passers do not require treatment except under the following circumstances: (a) for outbreak control, (b) for prevention of household transmission by toddlers to pregnant women and patients with cystic fibrosis and hypergammaglobulinemia, (c) malabsorption which hampers absorption of antibiotic therapy.

Table 11.5 : Antimicrobials for treatment of giardiasis

Agent	*Dose*
Albendazole	400 mg once a day for 5 days per oral
Metronidazole	20 mg/kg /day in 3 divided doses for 5 days per oral (maximum 750 mg/day)
Furazolidone	6 mg/kg/day divided into 4 doses for 10 days per oral (maximum 400 mg/day)
Tinidazole	50 mg/kg once (maximum 2 gm) per oral
Quinacrine	6 mg/kg /day divided into 3 doses per oral (maximum 300 mg/day)

Metronidazole is the widely prescribed drug for giardiasis. Albendazole appears to be as effective as metronidazole with fewer side effects among children above 2 years. It is a broad spectrum anthelmentic making it also useful in multiple parasitic infestations. Furazolidone is less effective than metronidazole. Refractory cases are treated with a combination of metronidazole and quinacrine.

Prevention

Strict hand washing by infected persons and person at risk after contact with feces. Purification of public water supply by chlorination, sedimentation and filtration. Avoidance of swimming during episodes of diarrhoea by adults as well as children.

Travelers to endemic areas should avoid uncooked food.

Purification of drinking water by a filter with a pore size of 1 µm or less or by brisk boiling of water for atleast 20 minutes. Treatment of water with chlorine or iodine is less effective.

Diphtheria

Diphtheria is an acute toxic infection caused by corynebacterium diphtheriae and characterized by a membranous exudate at the site of infection which is followed by distant toxic effects.

Etiology

Corynebacterium diphtheriae is a gram positive bacillus. It is an aerobic, noncapsulated, non spore forming, mostly motile organism which appears segmented or clubbed. It grows in Loeffler's and tellurite medium and ferments glucose. There are three main strains viz. gravis, intermedius and mitis, each capable of causing diphtheria. They are differentiated by colonial morphology, hemolysis and fermentation reactions. Gravis and intermedius groups are most virulent and grow well on human tissue while the mitis strains multiply less readily and remain more superficial. All the strains produce an exotoxin which is responsible for the majority of the serious complications. The toxin can be demonstrated in vitro by the agar immuno precipitin technique (Elek test), by polymerase chain reaction or by the in vivo toxin neutralization test in guinea pigs.

Diphtheroids are organisms morphologically similar to diphtheria bacilli. They include Hoffman's bacillus frequently recovered from ear, nose and less often from the throat and corynebacterium xerosis obtained from the conjunctiva. These may cause confusion in bacteriological diagnosis.

Epidemiology

The incidence of diphtheria has decreased worldwide after introduction of active immunization. The disease is rare under 6 months age and above 15 years age. The most common age group is 2–10 years. The disease can occur in adults who lack natural exposure and in those who have low rates of booster vaccinations. The disease is spread by droplet infection from carriers and cases, the latter being the most dangerous source. Anterior nasal diphtheria, which causes little ill health, but copious nasal discharge, is highly infectious.

Pathogenesis

The organisms multiply locally at the site of infection which may be the skin or the respiratory mucous membrane. They are non-invasive. Multiplication of the organisms leads to production of the 62–kd polypeptide exotoxin which inhibits protein synthesis and cause local tissue necrosis. The constitutional symptoms arise from absorption of the toxin. The necrosis is deeper and the toxin is absorbed much more readily from the fauces and nasopharynx than from the nose or larynx where there is little soft tissue between mucous membrane and cartilage.

Within a few days of the respiratory infection there is formation of a gray brown colored pseudomembrane. It consists of a dense necrotic coagulum of organisms, epithelial cells, fibrin, leucocytes and erythrocytes. The Corynebacteria are present at the margin of the membrane. The membrane can be removed with difficulty leaving behind a bleeding submucosa. The membrane may extend down the respiratory tract to the trachea and major bronchi where it is less adherent than in the fauces. The membrane is false in that it consist of invaded and necrotic layers of the mucosa and is not an exudate superimposed on an intact surface.

The paralysis of the palate and hypopharynx is an early local effect of the toxin. Toxin absorption can lead to necrosis of kidney tubules, thrombocytopenia, cardiomyopathy and demyelination of nerves. The latter two complications can occur 2–10 weeks after mucocutaneous infection. Hence the pathophysiology is also suspected to be immunologically mediated.

Clinical Manifestations

The incubation period is commonly between 2 and 5 days with extremes of 1–10 days.

The fauces are most often the site of infection and is usually associated with severe toxemia. The diphtheritic membrane can be found in the nose, nasopharynx, fauces or larynx. Infection in other sites is rare.

The acute stage of all types covers the first week where the most prominent symptoms are due to the local lesion. Thereafter, in more severe infections, the local symptoms fade and the illness is dominated by cardiovascular and still later by neurologic symptoms.

Clinical classification of diphtheria is an anatomical one including the following types:

Faucial Diphtheria

This is the most common type. The onset of disease is insidious with lassitude, mild headache, malaise and sore throat. The temperature seldom rises above 101°F (38.40°F). However, sore throat may not be a marked symptom in many children.

The membrane which is characteristic of the disease may not be present at the onset and in the mildest form where the fauces may be only injected. Typically, the membrane begins on one or both of the tonsils and may spread on to the pillars of the fauces, uvula and the palate and become extensive within 24 hours. The membrane may be thin or thick, greyish, or creamy or dirty grey in color. In early stages, it may glisten. It can be removed with difficulty usually leaving a bleeding surface. In most cases, there is an area of inflammation visible as a hyperemic zone surrounding the membrane separating it from the pale edematous fauces. There is often a characteristic fetor. There is also some degree of cervical lymphadenitis which is slightly tender. In many cases, a serous or blood stained nasal discharge appears in later stages. Vomiting, pallor, drowsiness, tachycardia are signs of early toxicity.

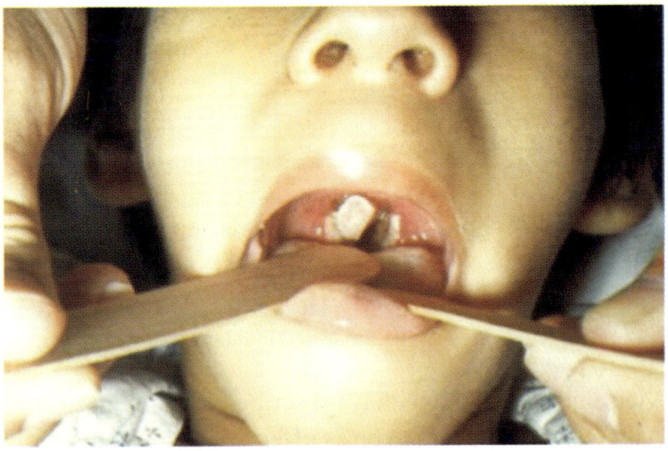

Fig. 11.10: Diphtheria membrane in the throat

Posterior Nasal (Nasopharyngeal) Diphtheria

This type is similar in all respects to faucial diphtheria with which it is generally associated. The membrane is formed in the nasopharynx hidden behind the palate and therefore not easily visible on ordinary throat inspection.

Anterior Nasal Diphtheria

This type is seldom serious to the patient but highly

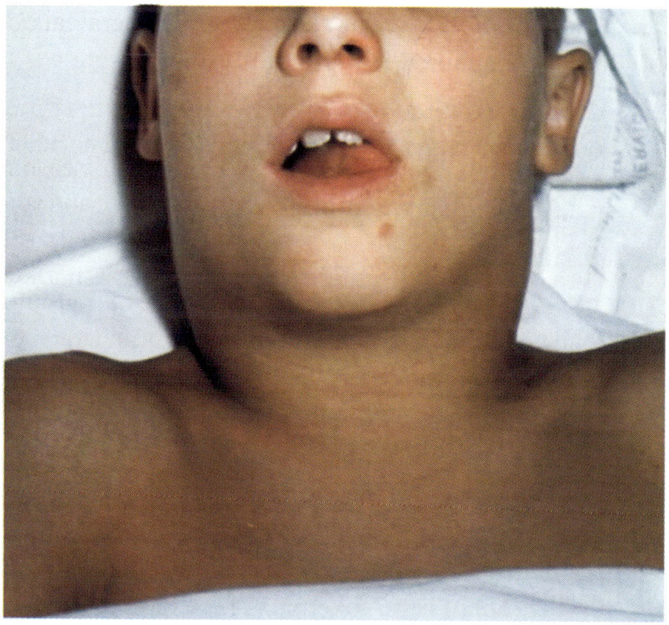

Fig. 11.11: Bull's neck due to enlarged lymph glands

infectious; hence of considerable epidemiological importance. The onset is insidious with symptoms like minimal fever and malaise. There is profuse, thin, blood stained, serous nasal discharge together with small ulcers or crusted sores appearing at the anterior nares, and extending on to the upper lip and cheeks. The membrane is confined to the front of the nose, usually the nasal septum. Undiagnosed, the nasal discharge may persist for weeks. Following treatment, the discharge ceases rapidly.

Laryngeal Diphtheria

Laryngeal diphtheria is characterized by progressive laryngeal obstruction with relatively less toxemia unless associated with faucial diphtheria. The membrane may spread down the trachea into the major bronchi.

Early in the illness, there are periodic attacks of laryngeal spasm with resulting acute laryngeal obstruction. Any one of these attacks may prove to be fatal. Later the symptoms of croup viz. hoarse voice, inspiratory stridor and cough appear. These symptoms increase until there are signs of airway obstruction viz. chest indrawing, restlessness, pallor, cyanosis and asphyxia. In rare instances, membranous casts are coughed out giving relief of symptoms.

Other Sites

Skin, conjunctiva, middle ear, genital mucosa and umbilicus in the newborn are rare sites of diphtheria infection.

Complications

The chief complications are cardiovascular and neurological. The complications are related to the virulence of the infecting strain, the amount of membrane (hence the toxin) formation and the time interval between onset and administration of antitoxin. The more the exotoxin formed sooner the onset of complications. The diphtheria antitoxin can neutralize the circulating toxin only. Once the toxin is fixed to the cardiac muscles or peripheral nerves it is not affected by administration of antitoxin.

Cardiovascular Complications

Some degree of myocarditis is present in all cases of faucial diphtheria where there is membrane formation. Severe myocarditis with circulatory failure is the commonest cause of death. Cardiovascular symptoms may appear at any time between the 3rd day and 21st day of onset depending on the severity of the attack. The early signs are vomiting, pallor and tachycardia followed by symptoms and signs of congestive cardiac failure. Heart block of all degrees can occur in severe cases of myocarditis. Recovery from myocarditis is usually complete in almost all cases. However in severe cases it may take over 3 months.

Neurological Complications

The paralytic complications develop in a constant order with the palate being first affected.

Palatal palsy commonly occurs between the 3rd and 6th weeks. It may be evident as early as 7th day. It is characterized by nasal quality of voice or nasal regurgitation of fluids. On examination palatal movement is seen to be decreased or absent. The paralysis is due to local action of toxin on the nerve endings. If palatal palsy develops in the second week of illness, the patient is expected to suffer from extensive paralysis. Conversely if palatal palsy develops late, in the 5th or 6th week, it is likely to be the sole neurological manifestation. Palatal palsy and eye palsies usually recover in 1–3 weeks.

Eye palsies follow palatal palsy. It is manifested by blurred vision due to weakness of accommodation. External rectus muscle is sometimes involved.

Peripheral neuritis of the limbs and trunk occurs from the 4th week onwards. It is fairly symmetrical and may be extensive. Sensory symptoms are usually absent but sensory ataxia is found in cases that develop neuritis late. The degree of peripheral neuritis depends on the amount of toxin fixed in the peripheral nerves before administration of antitoxin.

Respiratory failure as a result of diaphragmatic paralysis, pharyngeal paralysis or both usually occurs after the 6th week. If recovery occurs, it may take 6 months or more.

Hemiplegia due to cerebral embolism from an intra cardiac thrombus is a rare complication.

Other Complications

There may be albuminuria, casts and red cells in urine. In cases of laryngeal diphtheria, there may be bronchitis, bronchopneumonia and atelectasis. In faucial diphtheria, there may be mixed infection with diphtheria and hemolytic streptococci, characterized by an atypical membrane, painful lymphadenitis and usually marked toxemia.

Differential Diagnosis

The differential diagnosis is different for each clinical type.

Anterior Nasal Diphtheria

A foreign body in the nose can give rise to profuse, foul smelling purulent nasal discharge. Examination with a nasal speculum will reveal the membrane and hence the cause. Examination of a swab from the discharge will confirm the diagnosis.

Faucial Diphtheria

Faucial diphtheria needs differentiation from a number of conditions as mentioned below:

a. *Streptococcal tonsillitis:* In streptococcal tonsillitis, the exudate is yellow, usually patchy and can be easily removed. It is confined to the tonsils. The rest of the throat is erythematous. The tonsillar glands are tender. Temperature is usually above 102°C.
b. *Quinsy:* Causes unilateral faucial edema with acute pain and tenderness. It is seldom accompanied by membrane formation.
c. *Vincent's angina:* The lesion is ulcerative rather than membranous. The onset is insidious. There may be a greyish exudate.
d. *Infectious mononucleosis:* It is the common infection to cause real difficulty in diagnosis. There may be formation of a greyish membrane and edema identical to diphtheria. The other evidence viz. generalized lymphadenopathy, splenomegaly and abnormal mononuclear cells in the peripheral blood helps in diagnosis. Paul Bunnel test is positive.
e. *Acute leukemia and agranulocytosis* may be complicated with a membrane in the throat. The other specific features *viz.* pallor, bleeding tendency, hepatosplenomegaly and blood examination will help in diagnosis.
f. *Oral thrush* is characterized by presence of multiple small white patches on the buccal mucosa and tongue. They can be removed with difficulty leaving behind a red area. Lack of constitutional symptoms is characteristic.
g. *Herpes zoster of the palate:* There may be an extensive unilateral membrane with discrete herpetic lesions in the buccal mucosa or in the external auditory meatus. There is no toxemia. There is hyperacusis, deafness or earache on the affected side. These may be the initial symptoms.

Laryngeal Diphtheria

The differential diagnosis of laryngeal diphtheria includes the following conditions which are discussed in different chapters. They are:

a. Croup.
b. Retropharyngeal abscess.
c. Foreign body.
d. Angioneurotic edema of larynx, papilloma larynx and congenital laryngeal stridor.
e. Epiglotitis.

Laboratory Diagnosis

The diagnosis is confirmed by culture of a portion of the membrane with underlying exudate. The culture isolates should be identified to the species level, toxigenicity and antimicrobial sensitivity. Evaluation of a direct smear using Gram stain or specific fluorescent antibody is unreliable.

Treatment

The treatment of diphtheria may be supportive and specific.

Supportive Therapy

(a) *Isolation:* All children suffering from diphtheria should be isolated till 3 negative nose and throat swab cultures are obtained after treatment.

(b) *Rest:* All cases of diphtheria should be kept in bed for a minimum of 2–3 weeks as there is risk of myocarditis. In presence of myocarditis, mobilization is advised when clinical and ECG evidence of myocarditis has subsided. The patient is best managed in the supine position except when there is heart failure when child may be comfortable in the propped up position. There is some evidence that Carnitine in a dose of 100 mg/kg/day in 2 divided doses for 4 days prevent myocarditis.

(c) Maintenance of nutrition and hydration.

(d) Laryngeal obstruction may necessitate tracheostomy to establish airway.

(e) Treatment of myocarditis includes use of digoxin, appropriate antiarrhythmic drugs, ACE inhibitors and diuretics.

(f) Acute polyneuropathy needs supportive care such as nasogastric feeding, mechanical ventilation.

(g) The child should be immunized after complete recovery because there is no permanent protection after an attack of diphtheria.

Specific Therapy

Diphtheria antitoxin is the mainstay of treatment. The dose required is dependent of the type of disease, its duration and extent of the membrane. It is unrelated to the age of the patient. WHO/UNICEF recommends the following dosage schedule of Diphtheria antitoxin. A repeat dose is usually not necessary if a correct assessment is originally made. However a further dose can be safely given after 2–3 days if the membrane continues to spread.

Table 11.6 : WHO / UNICEF Dosage Schedule

Type of diphtheria	*Total dose in units*
Nasal	10,000 – 20,000
Laryngeal/Pharyngeal	20,000 – 40,000
Tonsillar	20,000 – 30,000
Combined types/delayed diagnosis	40,000 – 60,000
Severe disease*	80,000 – 100,000
Carrier/Contact	Not required

*Defined as extensive disease/more than 3 days duration/neck edema/tachycardia/collapse/breathlessness.

Points to be Noted

1. Treatment with antitoxin should be started immediately when diphtheria is suspected in an unimmunized child or if there is severe disease, without waiting for the smear results. In an immunized child or in mild disease or where the diagnosis is doubtful, treatment may be deferred till the smear results are available. It is important that the patient should receive the first dose not later than the third day of the disease.
2. Before giving anti-diphtheric serum (ADS), a history regarding previous serum injection and possible allergy should be obtained. If this is negative, 0.2 ml of undiluted serum is injected subcutaneously. If there is no reaction after an hour, then the whole dose can be safely administered.
3. In any patient with a hypersensitive reaction, the need for anti-diphtheric serum should be reassessed. If necessary, desensitization should be done. Pretreatment with antihistamines and prednisolone is recommended.
4. In severe cases, 50,000 units intramuscularly can serve as a test dose before giving 100,000 units intravenously. Intravenous administration should be done very slowly to avoid complications. If the patient is shown to be sensitive, therapy should be begun with a small dose which is gradually increased every 20–30 minutes provided there is no reaction.
5. Epinephrine (1: 1000 dilutions) solution and Inj hydrocortisone should be immediately available in a syringe whenever ADS is administered.

Antimicrobial therapy is indicated to halt toxin production, treat localized infection and prevent transmission of the organism. Penicillin and erythromycin are the recommended drugs. Appropriate therapy is as follows: Erythromycin, 40–50 mg/kg body weight (maximum 2 gms/day) 6 hourly per oral or IV Or, Aqueous penicillin G, 1–1.5 lakh units/kg/day IV or IM, 6 hourly or, Procaine penicillin 25,000–50,000 units/kg/day 12 hourly. The microbial therapy should be continued for 14 days.

Eradication of organism should be established by at least two successive negative cultures from the nose and throat obtained 24 hours apart after completion of therapy. Treatment with erythromycin should be repeated if the culture is positive. Antimicrobial therapy is not a substitute for antitoxin therapy.

Prevention

All suspected cases of diphtheria should be reported to the local and state health departments. The subsequent investigation is aimed at prevention of the disease in the contacts, determining the source and carriers to halt spread to unexposed individuals.

The asymptomatic case contacts should be closely monitored for illness through the 7 days incubation period. Cultures of throat, nose and any skin lesion should be taken. Regardless of immunization status antimicrobial therapy should be given using erythromycin (40–50 mg/kg/day, max 2 gm/day, per oral 6 hourly × 7 days), or a single dose of benzathine penicillin G (6 lacs units IM < 30 kg and 12 lacs units IM => 30 kg weight). The efficacy of antimicrobial therapy in contacts is presumed but not proved.

Active immunization of children is possible with the use of DPT (Triple) vaccine. It should be advised at 6 weeks of age. It is given as 3 primary doses at 4 weeks interval followed by booster doses at 16–18 months and 4–5 years age.

In case of dropout from the immunization schedule, the child should be given the booster doses appropriate for the age. If the child has not completed the primary three doses or is found to be of doubtful immunization status he/she should be immunized with age appropriate schedule.

Asymptomatic carriers are put on antimicrobial therapy as mentioned in case of contacts. They are placed in isolation until atleast two subsequent cultures are found negative when taken 24 hours apart after completion of antimicrobial therapy. A course of erythromycin should be repeated if the cultures are positive. No antitoxin is recommended in carriers or contacts even if they are unimmunized.

Pertussis

It is an acute infectious disease characterized by attacks of coughing commonly followed by an inspiratory whoop. Hence the name whooping cough.

Etiology

The causative organism is *Bordetella Pertussis.* It is a small slender gram negative rod. Two other organisms have been identified in a number of outbreaks. One is *Bordetella parapertussis,* which is morphologically identical but showing cultural and serological differences. Infection with parapertussis probably accounts for the occasional rare attack of pertussis. An occasional attack may be caused by another organism, *B. bronchiseptica.*

It should be noted that paroxysmal cough can occur during infection with certain respiratory virus viz. adenovirus or parainfluenza virus. However, these illnesses tend to be of much shorter duration than pertussis.

Epidemiology

The disease has a worldwide distribution. It is more prevalent and tends to be more severe in cold climates. It is endemic year round. The incidence has come down with active immunization. Ninety percent of cases occur in children under 5 years of age. No age is however immune. There is little or no passive protection of the newborn infant. Infection in the first six months of life is particularly serious. Infection is followed by life long immunity. Illness in the elderly may be due to waning of this protection. Two attacks in childhood are probably always due to separate infection with B. pertussis and B. parapertussis.

It is a highly infectious disease. Spread take place through droplets. The disease is at its most infectious state in the first week or two when diagnosis is difficult on clinical grounds. The mild case missed is often responsible for the spread of the disease. Infectivity falls sharply once the paroxysmal phase develops. However, organisms have been isolated as late as 8 weeks in severe cases. The organisms do not become invasive and have never been isolated from outside the respiratory tract.

Pathology

There is inflammation of the respiratory mucous membranes from the trachea to the bronchioles accompanied by infiltration with polymorphonuclear and mononuclear cells and production of mucus. Initially thin, the mucus becomes progressively more viscid until plugs are formed which consist of sticky mucus and cellular debris. This irritant material precipitates coughing. Temporary relief follows the bringing up of the mucus plugs. However, bringing up is usually moving of plugs from one bronchiole to another. The whoop is caused by a long drawn inspiration through a larynx narrowed by a combination of spasm and mucus. Obstruction of bronchi and bronchioles leads to areas of atelectasis and emphysema. Pneumonia can occur as a result of secondary bacterial infection.

Clinical Manifestations

It is a disease of insidious onset with an incubation period of 7–10 days. Most attacks of pertussis can be divided into two stages: catarrhal stage and paroxysmal stage.

The *catarrhal stage* starts insidiously with fever, coryza and dry cough resembling a severe cold. After 3–4 days, fever remains, the cough increases occurring in bouts, more at night, followed by vomiting. On examination, there is evidence of mild upper respiratory inflammation. There may be signs of bronchospasm although auscultation of chest may be normal throughout the disease. The temperature may be upto 101°F (38.3°C).

The *paroxysmal stage* usually develops insidiously after 4–8 days after the onset of the illness. In some patients, the onset may be with cough which rapidly becomes paroxysmal without the preceding catarrhal stage. As the character of the cough changes from simple to spasmodic one, the temperature falls to normal.

The fully developed paroxysmal stage in an unimmunized child consists of a toneless inspiration followed by short sharp coughs with open mouth and protruding tongue. This long expiratory coughing phase is continued until the face becomes congested, the superficial veins engorged and the eyes fill with tears. The eyeballs may protrude and skin becomes bathed with sweat, mucus running from the nose and mouth until sometimes a sticky plug of mucus is coughed up. In a severe attack, cyanosis and respiratory distress follow. Relief eventually comes from a long inspiration which is accompanied by the whoop. In very young infants, the whoop is often absent. Vomiting during or after the spasm is usual. When several coughing bouts follow one after another in succession, the child becomes exhausted.

The coughing bouts may be spontaneous or provoked by a stimulus viz. eating, excitement or examination of the throat. The number of paroxysm in moderately severe cases may be upto 15–20/day while in severe cases it may be upto 40/day. Examination of the respiratory system immediately after the coughing attack may reveal scattered rhonchi or signs of atelectasis which often disappear after a few hours. In between paroxysms most patients are afebrile and feel well with examination of the respiratory system unrewarding. Presence of subconjunctival hemorrhage and ulceration of frenum linguae are suggestive findings of pertussis.

The course of the illness is variable. The spasms reach their height within a week. Thereafter decrease rapidly or may persist for even 6–10 weeks.

Complications

Mechanical complications occur during the paroxysmal stage due to increased pressure and include epistaxis, subconjunctival hemorrhage, petechiae, retinal detachment, hernia and rectal prolapse.

Gastrointestinal complications include vomiting, malnutrition and dehydration.

Respiratory complications include pneumonia, apnoeic attacks, emphysema, spontaneous pneumothorax, subcutaneous emphysema and lighting up of a latent primary tuberculous infection.

Neurological complications include generalized convulsion, post whooping cough encephalopathy.

Laboratory Diagnosis

In catarrhal stage the diagnosis can be suspected if there is a history of contact with a known case within 15 days. In the paroxysmal stage diagnosis is essentially clinical on the basis of clinical symptoms and signs.

Two laboratory tests can be helpful in doubtful cases: (a) Culture of the organism in the first two weeks (b) Examination of nasal swab taken immediately after a cough. As the organism is slow growing, reports are available after 4–5 days by which time a clinical diagnosis becomes evident. A negative culture never excludes the diagnosis. The indirect evidence include a total WBC count which is usually 15,000 to 25, 000/cumm but may go upto 1,00,000/cumm out of which 50% or more are lymphocytes. The ESR is normal in uncomplicated cases.

An X-ray chest should be done in all cases except the mildest cases, after convalescence is well established, to exclude residual atelectasis. Mantoux testing is indicated if recovery is slow.

Treatment

Supportive Treatment

Supportive treatment is the mainstay of management. Isolation of patient should be advised for 3 weeks from the onset of the paroxysms. Contacts need not be quarantined or kept away from school.

The child should be advised to play quietly, avoid excitement and should be advised small frequent meals. Severe cases may require nasogastric feeding. More severe cases need admission to hospital where oxygen and a suction apparatus should be available.

Cough mixtures are not effective for control of cough. For patients with severe spasm, maintenance of a warm humid atmosphere is helpful. For a nervous child whose spasms are easily provoked, small regular doses of phenobarbitone are helpful. Heavy sedation should be avoided as it carries the risk of atelectasis. An antiemetic before each feed may help to reduce vomiting.

Persistent atelectasis responds to vigorous physiotherapy. Bronchoscopy may be sometimes necessary. The hemorrhagic complications do not require treatment except reassurance to the parents.

During an apnoeic attack secretions are removed from the pharynx with the right index finger while the back is percussed with the left hand. Pharyngeal suction may be required to remove secretions. Oxygen is administered once the airway is cleared. Artificial respiration may be required.

Convulsions are treated with anticonvulscents in the usual line.

Specific Treatment

There is no specific treatment of pertussis. Antibiotics viz. tetracycline/erythromycin started early in the catarrhal stage may lessen the duration and severity of the attack. This is very useful in an infant with a history of contact. In such cases the drug should be started with the first sign of upper respiratory infection and continued for 2 weeks.

Prevention

Active immunization with DPT vaccine is effective.

Tetanus

Tetanus is an infectious disease characterized by paroxysms of muscle spasms superimposed on a generalized tonic rigidity, most consistently affecting the masseters and the trunk muscles.

Etiology and Epidemiology

Tetanus is caused by bacillus Clostridium tetani which is a slender, spore bearing, anaerobic rod. They are present in human and animal feces and are widely distributed in dust and soil. Tetanus follows injury in majority of cases. Puncture wounds viz. by a nail or rose thorn, are more favorable for the germination of the spores than superficial scratches. The risk of tetanus increases with severe injury with a wound with debris because tissue necrosis provides a suitable culture medium for the bacilli. Outbreaks have also occurred in hospitals from contamination of gauze, catgut and other surgical materials.

Pathology

The organism enters through the skin. Secondary bacterial infection in a tetanus contaminated wound increases the risk of clinical tetanus because it causes increased tissue destruction.

Cl. tetani produces an exotoxin which has an affinity for nerve tissue. The toxin travels along the peripheral nerves to the central nervous system and also in the blood stream. The action of the toxin on the neuromuscular end plates results in the tonic rigidity. Reflex spasms, on the other hand, are caused by the toxin increasing the excitability of the anterior horn cells in the spinal cord. Once the toxin is fixed in the nerve cells it can no longer be neutralized by antitoxin. Secondary effects of tetanus include myocarditis, pneumonia and vertebral fractures.

No immunity develops following an attack of tetanus because the fatal dose is very small to be antigenically active.

Clinical Manifestations

The incubation period is commonly 2–21 days. Longer the incubation period better is the prognosis. Fatal attacks with long incubation period may be due to the reason that the spores remain dormant until tissue destruction, sepsis, surgical manipulation etc change the environment into a suitable one for their germination.

Most cases of tetanus pass through three clinical stages– prodromal stage, stage of tonic rigidity and stage of reflex spasms.

The *prodromal symptoms* consist of fleeting back pain, progressive difficulty in swallowing, which may precede 24 hours before the onset of spasm.

The first indication of tonic rigidity is *trismus* i.e. painless spasm of the masseters. It may be the first symptom. It begins with slight stiffness in the jaw increasing till the teeth are firmly clenched and the mouth cannot be opened at all. Involvement of facial muscles leads to production of *risus sardonicus* which cause a grin due to retraction of the angles of the mouth. At the same time the abdominal recti become stiff which steadily increases to produce a board like but painless rigidity. Trismus due to local cause can be differentiated from trismus due to tetanus by the presence of abdominal rigidity. In a severe case the rigidity reaches maximum in 48 hours producing head retraction and opisthotonus. In a mild attack, it may take upto 7 days to develop to such an extent. Tonic rigidity is much less marked in the limbs than in the trunk. In some cases, local rigidity develops around the site of the wound. It may be severe and may precede trismus by a few days. In such cases the ultimate attack is usually mild.

Reflex spasms appear within a few hours of tonic rigidity in the severe cases or may be delayed up to 5 days. In mild cases no spasms occur. Spasms may be spontaneous or precipitated by extraneous stimuli viz. noise. At the onset they are usually brief, but gradually increase in severity, duration and frequency as the disease develops. Occasionally the first spasm is severe and may even prove fatal. Spasms may persist for 2–3 weeks or occasionally longer. They become intensely painful. A typical spasm is characterized by sudden increase in muscle tone with clenching of the jaw, increase in head retraction and opisthotonus combined with extension of the limbs. A severe spasm may cause laryngeal obstruction and may stop respiration. The patient becomes cyanosed.

The tendon reflexes in tetanus are usually exaggerated. The disease is essentially afebrile. There may be a terminal hyperpyrexia. A mild rise in temperature of 37.3°C (99°F) is not unusual. A more marked rise of temperature indicates secondary infection viz. pneumonia. The mind remains clear. The CSF is normal.

Course

In most severe cases, the first reflex spasm may prove fatal, death taking place on the 2nd or 3rd day. In severe cases tonic rigidity may persist for upto three months. In moderate cases reflex spasm persist for 7–10 days; complete recovery taking around 6 weeks.

Complications

The most important complications are related to the respiratory system. These include asphyxia, collapse consolidation, insidious underventilation due to tonic chest wall rigidity, and acute underventilation due to laryngeal spasm or respiratory arrest during a spasm. In addition there may be retention of urine or obstinate constipation. Severe spasms may cause laceration of the tongue and compression fracture of the vertebrae. Myocarditis may occur.

Differential Diagnosis

The local common causes of trismus viz. quinsy and dental abscess are painful and have fever. Mumps can also cause trismus; the presence of other signs can differentiate it.

The spasm present in strychnine poisoning resembles tetanus but there is no tonic rigidity; the muscles become quite flaccid between the spasms.

Neonatal Tetanus

Neonatal tetanus typically manifests within 3–12 days of birth. It starts with progressive difficulty in feeding (sucking and swallowing) with associated hunger and crying. The full blown picture is characterized by paralysis or diminished movements, stiffness to touch, and muscles spasm with or without opisthotonus. The umbilical cord stump may hold remnants of dirt, dung etc or it may appear clean.

Localized Tetanus

Localized tetanus is characterized by painful spasms of the muscles adjacent to the wound site. It may precede generalized spasms of tetanus.

Laboratory Diagnosis

Diagnosis of tetanus is essentially clinical. The typical setting is an unimmunized child (and/or mother) who was injured or born within the preceding two weeks and who presents with trismus, other rigid muscles, and a clear sensorium.

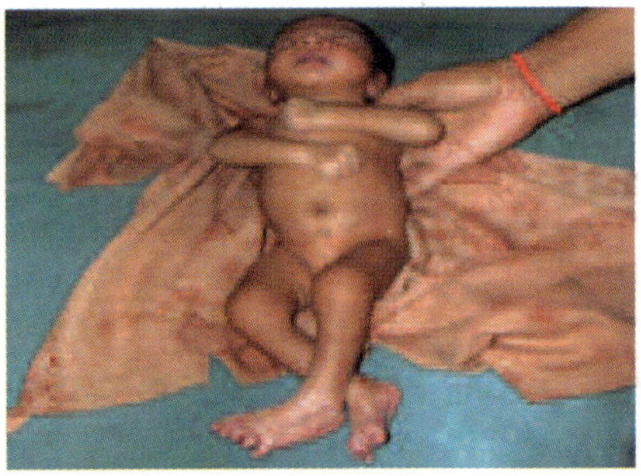

A. Trismus

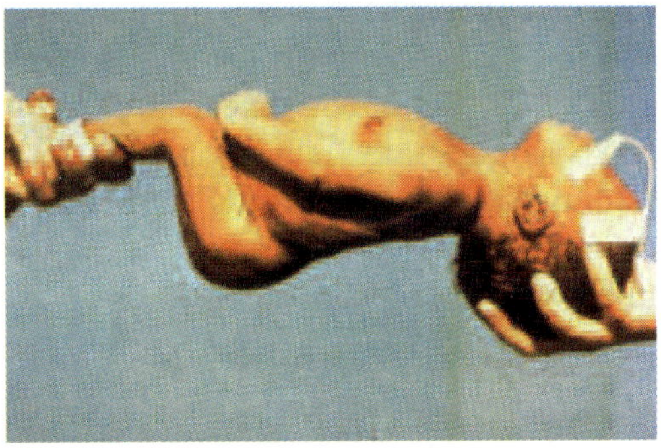

B. Opisthotonus

Fig. 11.12A and B: Showing neonatal tetanus

Routine laboratory examination is usually normal. There may be leucocytosis as a result of secondary infection of the wound or may be stress induced from sustained muscle spasm. The CSF is normal but pressure may be increased due to intense muscular contraction. C. tetani is visible on gram stain of wound material in about one third of cases.

Treatment

The treatment of tetanus includes toxin neutralization, eradication of C. tetani, wound management, symptomatic treatment of seizures and respiratory problems and supportive treatment.

Toxin neutralization is done by administration of Tetanus immunoglobin (TIG). It should be given as soon as possible because once the toxin has begun its axonal ascent to the spinal cord it cannot be neutralized. A single intramuscular dose of 500 units of TIG is sufficient to neutralize systemic tetanus toxin. Local infiltration of TIG into the wound is now considered unnecessary.

Penicillin G (100,000 units/kg/day IV 4–6 hourly for 10–14 days) remains the antibiotic of choice. Erythromycin (30–40 mg/kg orally 8 hourly) and tetracycline (for children 8 years or older) are alternatives for penicillin sensitive patients.

Diazepam is useful for control of seizures as well as a muscle relaxant. The initial dose is 0.1–0.2 mg/kg every 3–6 hourly subsequently titrated to control the muscle spasm. It should be continued for 2–6 weeks. Midazolum (0.1–0.3 mg/kg/day) can also be used.

In generalized tetanus, the best survival rates are achieved with neuromuscular blocking agents such as vecuronium and pancuronium. They produce general flaccid paralysis which is then managed by mechanical ventilation.

Supportive care should be provided in a quiet, dark room because tetanic spasm may be triggered by minor stimuli. It is preferable to do endotracheal intubation before laryngeal spasms develop. If intubation is not possible, a tracheostomy kit should be ready at hand. An early tracheostosmy is preferable in a severe case not managed by pharmacologically induced paralysis.

The cardiorespiartory status should be monitored. Frequent suctioning, maintenance of fluid and electrolytes and nutrition is important. Care of the oral cavity, bladder and bowel should be done as in case of an unconscious patient.

Complications

Respiratory complications include aspiration pneumonia, pneumothorax and mediastinal emphysema following mechanical ventilation. Seizures may result, in lacerations in the tongue or mouth, in intramuscular hematomas and rhabdomyolysis with myoglobinuria and renal failure. It may also result in long bone and spinal fractures. The involvement of the autonomic nervous system manifests with cardiac arrhythmia, unstable blood pressure and a labile temperature.

Prognosis

A favourable prognosis is associated with a long incubation period, absence of fever and with localized disease. An unfavorable prognosis is associated with young age, with a week or less period between the injury and onset of trismus and generalized muscle spasm. Most fatalities occur within the first week of illness. The case fatality reported in generalized tetanus is between 5% and 35%. That in neonatal tetanus it may be as low as 10% with intensive treatment or more than 75% without intensive treatment.

Prevention

Active immunization is done by DPT vaccine and tetanus toxoid. DPT vaccine should be started at 6 weeks age with three primary doses at 4 weeks interval with boosters at 16–18 months and 4–5 years age. This should be followed by tetanus toxoid at 10 and 15 years age and subsequently every 10 years. An unimmunized older child above 5 years age can be given two primary doses at 4–6 weeks interval followed by a third dose 6 months to 1 year after the second dose.

A child who recovers from tetanus should be immunized at discharge with a full course depending on the age as there is no long-term protection.

Poliomyelitis

Poliomyelitis is an acute infectious disease characterized by local or widespread muscular paralysis due to destruction of anterior horn cells in the spinal cord or the corresponding cells in the medulla.

Etiology

The polio viruses are RNA viruses belonging to the picornaviridae family, in the genus enterovirus. It is commonly a harmless inhabitant of the nasopharynx and intestinal tract. Three types of viruses are identified: Type I (Brunhilda) which is the most virulent, carries the highest incidence of paralysis and is responsible for most polio epidemics; type II (Lansing) and type III (Leon) which has the greatest propensity for vaccine associated paralytic poliomyelitis (VAPP). All three has been responsible for paralytic attacks in the human. They are serologically distinct and one type does not confer protection against the natural disease caused by the other types. The Coxsakie and ECHO group of viruses is sometimes associated with an illness clinically indistinguishable from paralytic poliomyelitis.

Epidemiology

The disease has a preference for the young but no age is immune. The largest number of cases occurs in the second and third year of life. Mortality and degree of disability are greater after the age of puberty. It is most common during the summer months. Sporadic cases can occur throughout the year. Man is the only reservoir of infection and the infection is spread from person to person. Fecal-oral transmission is most common route of infection in areas where sanitation is poor. The virus continues to be excreted in stool for 6–8 weeks after infection.

Pathogenesis

The polio virus infects cells by adsorbing to specific genetically determined receptors, including polio virus receptor (PVR). The virus penetrates the cell and is then uncoated and releases the RNA. The RNA is translated to produce proteins responsible for replication of the RNA, shut off host cell protein synthesis and synthesis of structural elements that compose the capsid. Mature virus particles are produced in 6–8 hours and are released into the environment by disruption of the cell.

In the contact host, polio virus enters through the gastro-intestinal tract. The primary site of replication may be the M cells lining the mucosa of the small intestine. The regional lymph nodes are infected and primary viremia occurs after 2–3 days. The virus seeds the reticuloendothelial system, the brown fat deposits, and skeletal muscles. With the first appearance of non-CNS symptoms, a secondary viremia probably occurs as a result of enormous viral replication. The exact mechanism of entry into the CNS is not known. The virus probably gains access to the CNS along the peripheral nerves. Once entry is gained, the virus may traverse neural pathways and multiple sites within the CNS may be affected. A mixed perineuronal inflammatory reaction with both polymorphonuclear leucocytes and lymphocytes occurs and is associated with extensive neuronal destruction. The poliovirus primarily infects motor neurone cells in the spinal cord (the anterior horn cells) and the medulla oblongata (the cranial nerve nuclei). Involvement of the intermediate and the dorsal horn and dorsal root ganglia in the spinal cord cause the typical hyperesthesia and the myalgias that are seen in acute poliomyelitis. Other neurons affected are the nuclei in the roof and vermis of the cerebellum, the substantia niagra and occasionally the red nucleus in the pons and variable involvement of the thalamic, hypothalamic, pallidal nuclei and the motor cortex.

Infants acquire transplacental immunity from their mother which disappears at a variable rate during the first 6 months of life. Natural infection results in type specific humoral and local active immunity which may be life long. An infection with other serotypes is possible. After exposure, poliovirus neutralizing antibodies develop within several days as a result of replication of the virus in the M cells in the intestinal tract and deep lymphatic tissues. These IgG antibodies protects against CNS infection. Local mucosal immunity is conferred mainly by secretory IgA which protects against subsequent reinfection of the GI tract.

Tonsillectomy and intramuscular injections may enhance the risk of acquisition of bulbar and local paralysis respectively. Increased physical activity and fatigue during the early phase of illness are factors leading to an increased risk of paralytic disease.

Clinical Manifestations

The incubation period of polio virus infection is 8–12 days, with a range of 5–35 days. The most common type of infection is the *silent infection* in which the children are asymptomatic. By 5 years nearly 70% and by 10 years 90–95% children get exposed to all the three polio viruses. A silent infection can be detected only by laboratory isolation of the virus in stool and examining the blood for antibody titre.

Clinical poliomyelitis is recognized in three forms: abortive, pre-paralytic/non-paralytic and paralytic poliomyelitis.

Abortive Poliomyelitis

Abortive poliomyelitis occurs in about 5% of children exposed to polio virus. The children present with influenza like viral illness, an acute gastrointestinal illness or an acute upper respiratory tract infection like illness. The child can be suspected to have a polio infection in presence of a history of contact during an epidemic of polio infection. The symptoms and signs subside by 24–48 hours without any residual affect and the spinal fluid is normal.

Pre-paralytic/Non-paralytic Poliomyelitis

In the pre-paralytic form there is fever which may last for 1–3 days. It may sometimes extend upto 7–13 days. Neurological signs viz. positive head lag (tripod sign), nuchal rigidity are present. There is local or generalized pain, rigidity and muscle tightness. Large muscles of the lower limbs are more affected. The deep tendon reflexes may be exaggerated. Recovery is rapid with no paralysis. The diagnosis of poliomyelitis can be confirmed by laboratory diagnosis.

Paralytic Poliomyelitis

On the basis of the portion of the CNS most severely affected three types of paralytic poliomyelitis have been recognized: (1) The spinal form where the paralysis may be confined to the muscles innervated by the spinal cord, (2) The bulbar or bulbospinal form where affected muscles are those innervated by the bulbar nuclei either exclusively or in addition to spinal paralysis, and (3) The rare form of polio encephalitis.

Spinal Poliomyelitis: The onset and course of paralysis are variable and age related. When a history of intramuscular injection precedes paralysis, patient may present with fever and paralysis of the part (provocative paralysis). Older children may have a single phase in which the prodromal symptoms and paralysis occur in a continuous fashion.

Infants and young children most frequently manifest a biphasic course. The patient appears to recover and feel better for 2–5 days after the abortive phase. Then there is an exacerbation of the previous systemic symptoms associated with severe muscle pain with sensory and motor phenomena viz. paresthesia, hyperesthesia, fasciculations and spasms. Within 1–2 days, asymmetric flaccid paralysis occurs. The distribution of paralysis is characteristically spotty involving single, multiple or groups of muscles. The most common is involvement of one leg followed by involvement of one arm. The proximal areas of the extremities tend to be involved to a greater extent than the distal parts. The paralysis reaches its height within 24 hours from the onset. Progression of paralysis rarely occurs beyond 2–3 days.

On physical examination muscles are tender, there is presence of nuchal rigidity or stiffness, and deep tendon reflexes are initially hyperactive and later absent or diminished. There may be weakness of the muscles of the abdomen, diaphragm, neck, trunk and thorax. Sensation is intact. The degree and duration of muscle pain are variable. Some patients have none while others complain for days and weeks. In some patients there is spasm and increased muscle tone with transient increase in deep tendon reflexes whereas in others flaccid paralysis can occur abruptly. Once the temperature returns to normal no further paralysis is noted in most patients.

Improvement of paralysis starts in the first few days or weeks but is usually evident within 6 months and continues for as long as 18 months. Lack of improvement from paralysis within the early weeks is an indicator of permanent paralysis. Atrophy of the muscles of the affected limb, failure of growth and deformity is common especially in the growing child.

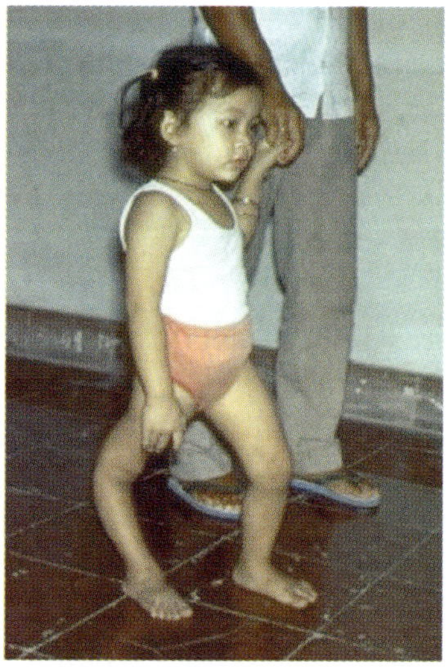

Fig. 11.13: A child with atrophy of muscles and deformity after paralytic poliomyelitis

Bulbar Poliomyelitis: Bulbar form of poliomyelitis can occur as a separate clinical entity with dominance of clinical manifestation by dysfunction of cranial nerves and medullary centres or as a culmination of ascending paralysis from initial involvement of the lower extremities. Pure bulbar poliomyelitis involves paralysis of the motor cranial nerve nuclei with or without involvement of the vital centres. Bulbo spinal poliomyelitis with respiratory insufficiency affects the respiratory muscles.

The clinical findings of bulbar poliomyelitis include: (1) Nasal twang to the voice or cry caused by pharyngeal and palatal weakness; (2) Inability to swallow;

(3) Accumulated pharyngeal secretions; (4) Absence of effective coughing; (5) Nasal regurgitation of fluids, (6) Deviation of uvula, palate or tongue; (7) Paralysis of one or both vocal cords causing hoarseness of voice, aphonia and asphyxia needing emergency tracheostomy; (8) Involvement of vital centres manifested by irregularities of rate, rhythm and depth of respiration; hypertension, hypotension and shock, arrhythmias and rapid changes of body temperature and color; (9) The rope sign characterized by an acute angulation between the chin and larynx is caused by weakness of the hyoid muscles.

The clinical features of involvement of respiratory muscles include (1) Anxious expression; (2) Inability to speak without frequent pauses, resulting in short, jerky, breathless sentences; (3) Increased respiratory rate; (4) Movement of alae nasi and of the accessory muscles of respiration; (5) Inability to cough or sniff with full depth; (6) Paradoxical abdominal movements; (7) Immobility of intercostal muscles.

The course of bulbar form varies from complete recovery to death due to extensive involvement of the vital centres.

Polio Encephalitis: It is a rare form of poliomyelitis with severe involvement of the higher centres of the brain. The manifestations are similar to encephalitis of any cause. It can be attributed to polio viruses by specific viral diagnosis or if accompanied by flaccid paralysis.

Diagnosis

The clinical features to suspect poliomyelitis include nonspecific febrile illness, aseptic meningitis or paralytic disease in an unimmunized or incompletely immunized child. The combination of fever, headache, neck and back pain, asymmetric flaccid paralysis without sensory loss and pleocytosis in CSF does not regularly occur in any other disease.

Vaccine associated paralytic poliomyelitis (VAPP) should be considered in any child with paralytic disease occurring 7–14 days or more after receiving oral polio vaccine. It should be considered in any child with paralytic disease in countries or regions where wild type polio virus has been eradicated and OPV has been administered to the child or a contact.

Laboratory Diagnosis

Isolation of Polio Virus in Stool

Laboratory diagnosis for confirmation can be done by isolation of polio virus in stool and specific identification of wild type and vaccine type strains by DNA sequence studies. For the purpose, 2 stool specimens of minimum 8–10 grams weight (size of an adult thumb) should be collected 24–48 hours apart and within 14 days of onset of paralysis. The specimen should be sent at a temperature below 8°C to one of the WHO certified laboratory for analysis. Polio virus can be isolated from 80–90% acutely ill patients. The yield decreases to less than 20% within 3–4 weeks.

Examination of CSF

Examination of CSF is normal during the period of minor illness but demonstrates pleocytosis between 20–300 cells/cumm with CNS involvement. Initially there is polymorpho leucocytosis shifting to mononuclear cells soon afterdwards. The CSF values return to normal by second week of major illness. The CSF protein rises to between 50–100 mg/dl by the second week of illness. In polio encephalitis the CSF may remain normal or show minor changes.

Serology

Serology will demonstrate seroconversion or a 4-fold or greater rise of antibody titre during the acute phase of illness and 3–6 weeks later.

Differential Diagnosis

Poliomyelitis is one of the many causes of acute flaccid paralysis in children. The diseases mainly confused are Guillain-Barré syndrome, transverse myelitis and traumatic paralysis due to sciatic nerve injury and non-polio enterovirus infection.

There are many other causes of acute flaccid paralysis viz. neuropathies (post diphtheric, Cl. botulinum infection, and tick bite paralysis), myasthenia gravis, polymyositis, viral myositis, hypokalemic periodic paralysis, Rabies, varicella zoster infection, epidural abscess and spinal cord compression. In most cases the typical clinical features are sufficient to differentiate the various diseases.

Guillain-Barré Syndrome

This acquired demyelinating disease of the peripheral nervous system is a common cause of acute flaccid paralysis in children. It is common in children above 2 years of age. There is a preceding history of a respiratory tract infection, GI syndrome, surgery or immunization, 1–4 weeks (average 2 weeks) before the onset of symptoms. The identified agents include EB virus, cytomegalo virus, herpes virus, mycoplasma, campylobacter jejuni.

There is symmetrical weakness evolving rapidly over a period of days or weeks (<4 weeks) then plateauing. Paralysis starts in the distal part of lower limb and then ascends. It is more severe in the proximal muscles. Initially there is hyporeflexia followed by areflexia. There is transient involvement of bladder and bowel. There may be involvement of cranial nerves and presence of autonomic disturbances with sinus tachycardia, fluctuating blood pressure, facial flushing etc. CSF examination after 1 week shows CSF protein upto 200 mg, WBC < 50 cells /cumm, PMN not > 2/cumm. Nerve conduction velocity done after 3 weeks is normal.

Transverse Myelitis

It is an immune mediated disease due to a viral insult. It is common in the age group 4 years and above. Fever may be present before the onset of acute flaccid paralysis but rarely during onset. The child complains of backache followed by symmetrical paralysis of the lower limbs, depressed or absent DTR. There is early onset of bladder and bowel dysfunction and profound anesthesia to all kinds of sensation. Flaccidity usually changes to spasticity after several weeks and areflexia replaced by hyper reflexia. CSF WBC count is normal, protein raised or normal. MRI shows swelling and hyperintensity of cord onT2 weighted images.

Traumatic Paralysis

There is a history of injury to sciatic nerve by intramuscular injection in gluteal region. Onset of paralysis is within 1 hour to 5 days after injection. There is associated pain in the region of trauma or along the affected limb. Muscle tone is decreased or absent. Muscle power at hip and knee is normal. Child walks with foot drop. The knee jerk is present, ankle jerk is absent. Atrophy may appear 40 to 60 days later (difference between calf and thigh circumferences does not exceed 0.5–1.5 cm). CSF analysis is normal.

Non-polio Enterovirus Infection

A number of non-polio enteroviruses are known to cause acute flaccid paralysis. Coxsakie A and B, echo and enterovirus types 70 and 71 have been associated with polio like illness. Unlike poliomyelitis, most cases show complete recovery within 60 days of onset.

Treatment

There is no specific anti-viral drug to treat polio virus infection. Treatment is essentially supportive. Intramuscular injections and surgical procedures should be avoided during the acute phase of illness especially in the first week because these may result in progression of the disease.

Abortive and Non-paralytic Poliomyelitis

It can be treated at home. The modalities of treatment are similar in abortive and non-paralytic forms.

Bed rest should be advised until the child's temperature is normal. Exertion should be avoided for the ensuing 2 weeks. A careful neurological and musculoskeletal examination should be done after 2 months to detect minor residual effects.

Analgesics combined with the application of hot packs for 15–30 minutes every 2–4 hours are effective for relief of discomfort of muscle tightness, and spasm of neck, trunk and extremities. This should be followed by gentle physical therapy. A firm bed is desirable and a foot board should be used to keep the feet in right angles to the legs. A nutritious and attractive diet should be served.

Paralytic Poliomyelitis

Most cases would require hospitalization for monitoring bulbar and respiratory paralysis.

Complete bed rest should be advised for 2–3 weeks. The affected limbs should be placed in the neutral position to give comfort and avoid excessive skeletal deformity. The neutral position for the lower limbs would be with feet at right angles to the legs, knees slightly flexed and hips and spine straight. The position may be achieved with sand bags or light splints and use of boards to make a firm bed. Active and passive movements are indicated as soon as there is relief of pain.

Moist hot packs and analgesics can be used to relieve muscle spasm and pain. Sedatives or opiates should not be used in cases with impairment of ventilation or impending respiratory failure.

There may be bladder paralysis which rarely lasts for more than a few days. One of the following procedures may be used for evacuation: (1) Manual expression; (2) Psychological effect of running water; (3) Parasympathetic stimulant drugs; (4) Aseptic bladder catherization. Constipation is common and fecal impaction should be avoided with the help of purgatives/enemas.

The child is usually anorexic. So the diet should be nutritious as well as appealing. An adequate fluid intake should be advised.

Bulbar Poliomyelitis

The management of bulbar poliomyelitis includes maintenance of airway, prevention of aspiration of secretions viz. saliva, food or vomitus and close monitoring for early signs of respiratory failure.

The patient should be nursed with foot end of the bed elevated 20–25 degrees in prone position with face turned to one side for gravity drainage. Patients with paralysis of muscles of respiration or difficulty in swallowing should be nursed in semi prone or lateral position. Oral and pharyngeal aspiration should be done with aspirators with semi rigid or rigid tips. Soft, flexible catheter may be used for nasopharyngeal aspiration.

Oral or tube feeding may incite vomiting during the first few days. Fluid and electrolyte balance should be maintained with intravenous infusion.

The child should be monitored for early signs of respiratory failure (anxious look, restlessness and fatigue) and hypertension. Tracheostomy is indicated in patients with pure bulbar, bulbospinal and spinal respiratory muscles paralysis because these patients are unable to cough. Mechanical ventilators are often indicated.

Prognosis

Abortive and non-paralytic forms have a uniformly good outcome. In the paralytic form maximum paralysis occurs 2–3 days after the onset of the paralytic phase of the illness. This is followed by stabilization and gradual return of muscle function. The recovery phase usually lasts for about 6 months. Paralysis persisting beyond that is permanent. The outcome of paralytic disease is determined by the degree and severity of CNS involvement. Mortality is high in bulbar poliomyelitis and low in spinal form.

Prevention

The only method of effective prevention of poliomyelitis is vaccination. Two vaccines are available viz. inactivated polio vaccine (IPV) and the live attenuated oral polio vaccine (OPV). Both the vaccines have established efficacy in preventing polio virus infection and paralytic poliomyelitis. Both vaccines induce production of antibodies against the three strains of polio virus. IPV produces higher serum IgA antibody titre. OPV also induces significantly greater mucosal IgA immunity in the oropharynx and the gastrointestinal tract that limits replication of wild polio virus at these sites. Vaccination by oral polio vaccine limits transmission of wild polio virus by fecal spread. IPV has no adverse effects whereas OPV can cause VAPP in those vaccinated and their contacts, the overall risk of which is 1 case/6.2 million doses.

According to the national immunization schedule, all children in India should receive polio drops at birth, 6 weeks, 10 weeks, 14 weeks age followed by booster dose at 16–18 months. The Indian Academy of Pediatrics recommends additional doses at 9 months and a second booster at 4–5 years ages. The vaccine confers 95% immunity and is virtually without any side effects.

Measles

Measles is a highly infectious disease characterized by respiratory catarrah, Koplik's spot on the buccal mucosa and maculopapular rash.

Etiology

Measles is caused by the measles virus which is able to survive only for a few days in room temperature but for long periods in low temperature. It is an RNA virus of genus morbillivirus belonging to paramyxoviridae family. Man is the only reservoir.

Epidemiology

Measles is a disease of worldwide distribution. Both sexes are equally susceptible. The disease is rare in the first 6 months of life due to passive protection received from the mother. A diagnosis of measles under the age of 6 months is always a suspect unless the mother has never suffered from measles infection. Measles in pregnancy tends to cause abortion or premature birth. The preterm infant is usually born with congenital measles. Measles in early pregnancy carries a slight risk of fetal damage.

Spread of the disease takes place by direct contact or by droplet infection. The virus enters through the intact conjunctiva and the respiratory tract. Patients are at their most infectious state during the prodromal period before the development of the rash.

The infective phase however is usually 4 days before and 5 days after the appearance of rash. The disease is common in preschool children and occur in all seasons; more common during winter and spring.

Pathology

The Koplik's spot on the buccal mucosa consist of minute areas of endothelial proliferation which break down into shallow ulcers at the base of which are cells which are undergoing active mitosis. The characteristic lesion of measles, which appears in the pharyngeal and bronchial mucosa, is the large multinucleated giant cells with associated general mucosal inflammation. Giant cells are also found in the tonsils, lymph nodes, spleen and appendix. Fatal cases show interstitial pneumonia. Secondary bacterial pneumonia is common.

Clinical Manifestations

The incubation period varies between 8–12 days. The onset of illness is rapid with fever, malaise and irritability. There is coryza, dry cough, watery eyes and running nose. Croup is not uncommon and diarrhoea also frequent. This is called the *catarrhal stage*. After around three days the temperature may fall and the child improve to deteriorate again with appearance of the rash.

Koplik's spot usually appear two days before the appearance of the rash. They consist of small irregular spots of bright red color with a minute bluish-white speck. They appear in clusters and are most numerous on the inner aspects of the cheek opposite the molar teeth and near the gum margin. Sometimes they are so numerous as to cover nearly the whole buccal mucous membrane. Koplik's spots are pathognomonic of measles. They are present for 48 hours before the rash and for few hours after it begins to appear.

The *measles rash* appears on the third or fourth day of illness although it is sometimes delayed as long as 6–7 days. It is usually accompanied by a sharp rise of temperature, increased respiratory rate and widespread crepitations audible throughout the lungs. The appearance and distribution of the rash is typical. It is first seen on the forehead, behind the ears and along the hair margin at the back of the neck. Within 12–48 hours it spreads rapidly over the face, neck, trunk and limbs. The individual lesions are at first discrete dusky pink macules; they rapidly enlarge in size to become maculopapular. Many of the lesions coalesce giving the typical blotchy appearance in which large areas of skin are covered by patches of rash with an irregular outline. Petechial hemorrhages into the rash are common and are not of grave importance as they merely indicate a heavy rash. Itching is rare.

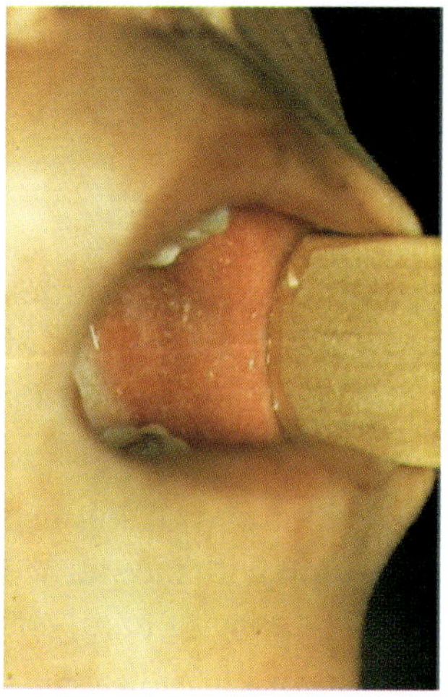

Fig. 11.14: Koplik's spots

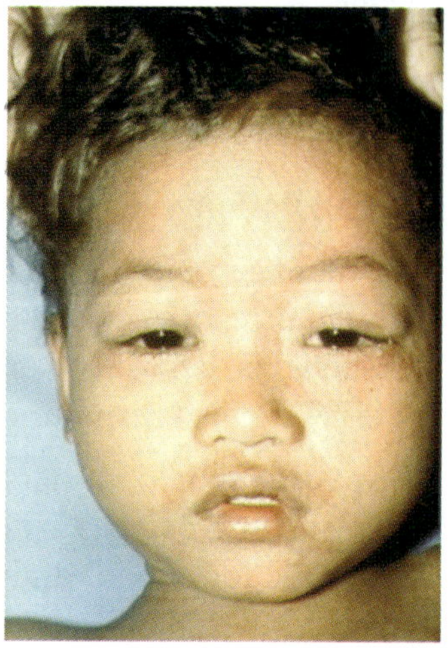

Fig. 11.15: Measles rash and conjunctivitis

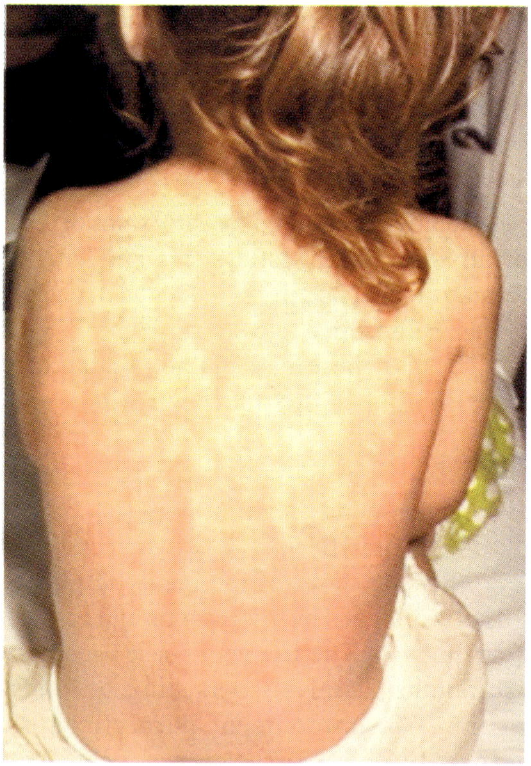

Fig. 11.16: Maculopapular rash over the trunk

The eruption fades in the order of its appearance, usually disappearing from the face after 2–3 days. It leaves behind a brownish staining due to extravasation of plasma. In heavy or hemorrhagic rashes the staining may persist for a fortnight. With the disappearance of the rash a fine, branny desquamation develops but this is much less constant than the staining and is confined to the areas where the rash has been profuse.

With the development of the rash, the temperature may continue to rise but falls by rapid lysis once the rash starts to fade. Thereafter convalescence is rapid in the absence of complications.

Milder attacks of measles may occur with rash appearing with a febrile cold but with relatively less constitutional disturbance. Abortive attacks can occur with no rash but with only Koplik's spots. Hemorrhagic measles is a severe and frequently fatal form characterized by hyperpyrexia, delirium, hemorrhage into skin and mucous membrane of mouth and intestinal tract.

Complications

The chief complications of measles are otitis media, pneumonia and encephalitis.

Otitis media, catarrhal or suppurative, often starts about fifth day and is a common cause of temperature failing to settle as the rash subsides.

Pneumonia: Measles virus can cause interstitial pneumonia (giant cell pneumonia) in the prodromal phase. Bacterial pneumonia can occur when the rash is at its height or within the next few days. The bacteria implicated are Group A streptococcus, S. pneumoniae, H. influenzae type B and staphylococcus. Measles pneumonia in HIV infected patients is often fatal and is not always accompanied by rash.

Neurologic complications are common in measles than in any other exanthematous disease. The incidence of encephalomyelitis is 1–2/1000. Symptoms appear 5–10 days after the onset. In a few instances, encephalitic involvement may occur in the pre eruptic period. On the other hand, subacute sclerosing panencephalitis (SSPE) is a progressive fatal neurologic disease, due to measles virus, seen mainly in late childhood. The etiology of measles encephalitis remains controversial. It has been suggested that direct viral invasion may be the cause for encephalitis early in the course of the disease although measles virus has not been isolated from brain tissue. Encephalitis that occurs later is predominantly demyelinating and may reflect an immunological process.

Measles encephalitis is usually of sudden onset. The patient is on way to convalescence when one of the following neurological features appears: retention of urine, drowsiness, irritability, convulsion, vomiting or severe headache. Fever may recur. Signs of meningeal irritation may or may not be present. The CSF usually shows rise of protein but the cells may be within normal limit or show a moderate increase upto 500 per cu mm.

Subacute sclerosing panencephalitis is a rare condition in which behavioral disturbances and convulsions are followed by development of involuntary movements, ataxia, mental deterioration and death within a few months. Boys are affected 3 times more than girls. The onset is usually some months or years of an attack of measles.

Other central nervous system complications viz. Guillain-Barré syndrome, hemiplegia, retrobulbar neuritis can occur rarely.

Exacerbation of an existing tuberculous focus is one of the potential dangers of measles. This possibility should be always considered when convalescence is slow and a child fails to thrive. There may be temporary loss of hypersensitivity to tuberculin. A negative Mantoux test upto 6 weeks after measles does not exclude tuberculosis.

Myocarditis is an infrequent serious complication but transient ECG changes are relatively common.

Diagnosis

The diagnosis of measles is essentially clinical. The development of a maculopapular rash on the third or fourth day of a coryzal illness with Koplik's spot in the mouth is pathognomonic. However in the eruptive stage, measles rash may be confused with those of Rubella, roseola infantum, other viral infections (echo, adeno and coxsakie viruses), rickettsial diseases, meningococcemia, infectious mononucleosis, serum sickness and drug rash. The rashes of rubella, other viruses, and roseola infantum are less striking, appear after the fever subsides, more in the trunk and are transient. The rash in rickettsial diseases rarely invades the face. In acute meningococcemia the rash is characteristically petechial and purpuric. Infectious mononucleosis may have a rash but is associated with generalized lymphadenopathy, atypical lymphocytes and a positive Paul Bunnel test. The absence of history of administration of drugs usually serves to exclude serum sickness and drug rash. Serum rashes are usually itchy and frequently show an urticarial element.

Treatment

Measles is a self limiting disease. In majority of patients symptomatic therapy is all that is required.

The patient should be nursed in bed until the rash has faded and the temperature has been normal for 48 hours. Isolation within the family is usually unnecessary as other susceptibles would have been infected before the diagnosis is made. However, limitation of visitors to the household is highly desirable to prevent secondary bacterial infection. There is no need of diet restriction in children who retains appetite. An adequate fluid intake should be advised. The mouth and teeth should be cleaned regularly. A regular bath is important. The bed clothes should be changed every day.

In presence of photophobia due to severe conjunctivitis, the child should be nursed in a dark room. Steam inhalation or humidification relieves laryngitis and cough. Simple cough linctus should be prescribed for an irritating cough. Paracetamol can alleviate mild to moderate fever. If temperature rises to 104°F (40°C) it should be lowered by tepid sponging and paracetamol. Bacterial complications should be treated with appropriate antibiotics. Good supportive care is necessary for encephalitis.

Low Vitamin A level can lead to higher rates of complications and death in measles. Synergy of measles and Vitamin A deficiency has additive effect on epithelia and immune system. Measles itself may lead to severe acute depletion of Vitamin A and precipitate keratomalacia and blindness. Two doses of Vitamin A should be administered in all cases of measles immediately on diagnosis and on next day.

Course

The uncomplicated case of measles is non infectious 5 days after the appearance of the rash and recovers within 15 days of onset. Considerable weight loss may occur in the severe attack but convalescence is rapid.

Prevention

Active immunization with measles vaccine is widely practised. One dose is given at 9 completed months age (270+ days). A second dose is recommended at 12 to 15 months which may be in the form of MMR / Measles vaccine. Measles vaccine can be given to a child below 6 months age within 3 days of exposure to prevent measles. These children however, should have a repeat dose at 9 months. The vaccine given below 6 months does not give full protection.

Post exposure prophylaxis can be done by passive immunization to susceptible contacts with immunoglobin (0.25 ml/kg IM, maximum 15 ml). It is effective for prevention and attenuation of measles if given within 6 days of exposure. Immunocompromised children should receive immunoglobulin (0.5 ml/kg IM; maximum 15 ml) regardless of the immunization status.

Rubella

Rubella is a mild infectious, viral disease characterized by a long incubation period followed by a short invasive period with rash and lymphadenopathy.

Etiology and Epidemiology

The rubella virus is a RNA virus of genus Rubivirus in the family Togaviridae. Rubella infection in early pregnancy may cause the congenital rubella syndrome which affects virtually all organ systems. Infection is spread by oral droplet or transplacentally to fetus. It has a worldwide distribution affecting both sexes equally. The incidence is greatest in spring and early summer. The peak incidence is among children between 5–14 years but is often seen in adolescents and young adults. Life long immunity is usual after rubella infection. During clinical illness, the virus has been recovered from the nasopharynx 7 days before exanthema and 7–8 days after its disappearance.

Pathogenesis

The pathogenesis of rubella is not well understood. An immune process has been suggested. The risk of congenital defects and disease is greatest with primary maternal infection during the first trimester. Incidence of congenital defects is around 90% when the mothers acquire infection before 11th week of pregnancy. It diminishes to about 10-20% by the end of first trimester. Maternal infection after 16th week of pregnancy poses a low risk of congenital defects although infection of fetus can occur.

Clinical Manifestations

The incubation period is 14–21 days. Prodromal symptoms are often absent in children; the rash being the first evidence of the disease. In some children and in most adults, however, a mild and brief prodromal illness for 1–3 days precedes the rash. There is mild fever, sore throat, headache and conjunctivitis. Approximately two thirds of infections are subclinical. There is tender enlargement of the posterior cervical lymph glands which may be the most common and may be the sole pre-eruptive sign. The lymphadenopathy is evident atleast 24 hours before the rash appears and remains for one week or more. In 20% cases an enanthem appears before the appearance of the skin rash. It consists of discrete rose colored spots on the soft palate that may coalesce into red blush and extend over the fauces.

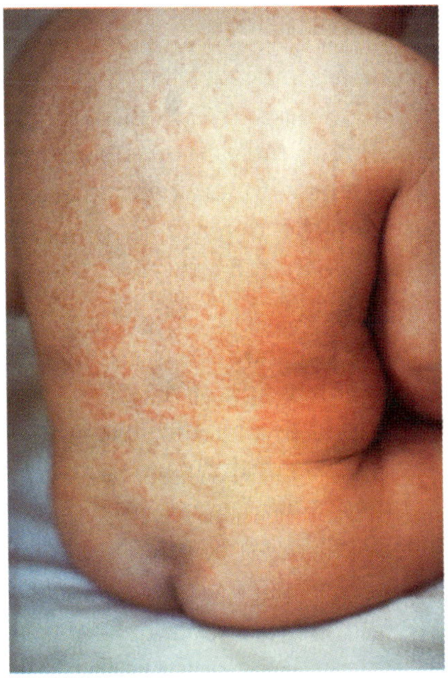

Fig. 11.17: Rash in rubella

The rash appears in the face first and spreads rapidly over the entire body usually within 24 hours. Its evolution is so rapid that the rash may be fading on the face by the time it appears on the trunk. The rash is maculopapular and discrete, may be confluent particularly in the face. In the trunk it may be pinpoint. Mild itching may be present. The eruption usually clears by third day. Desquamation is minimal. Rubella can occur without rash also. Fever may be low grade or absent during the rash.

In the older girls, polyarthritis may occur with pain, swelling, tenderness, and effusion but usually without any residual effect. The small joints of the hand are affected most frequently but any joint may be involved. It occurs on the third to seventh day with a return of fever. Arthritis usually persists for several days to two weeks but may persist for months.

CONGENITAL RUBELLA SYNDROME

Congenital rubella syndrome affects virtually all organ systems. Rubella embryopathy is either due to inhibition of cell growth or to cellular necrosis. The most common manifestation is intrauterine growth retardation. The other common findings include: eye defects (cataract, glaucoma, and retinopathy), heart lesions (patent ductus arteriosus, ventricular septal defect, and pulmonary stenosis), cerebral defects (mental retardation, meningoencephalitis), sensori neural deafness, thrombocytopenic purpura, hepatosplenomegaly, and skeletal abnormalities.

Ninety percent of the infected infants have neutralizing IgM antibodies. The virus can be readily isolated from the throat, urine or rectum of infants infected in utero. Virus excretion may last upto 12 months.

Laboratory Diagnosis

Diagnosis of rubella is essentially clinical. It may be confirmed by serology or virus culture. Detection of IgM antibodies in the first few days of illness is considered diagnostic. Detection of IgM antibodies in the newborn is useful in diagnosis of congenital rubella syndrome. Seroconversion or 4 fold rise of IgG titre is diagnostic. Rubella virus can be cultured from the nasopharynx and blood.

Differential Diagnosis

The conditions for differential diagnosis are same as that of measles.

Complications

Complications are rare in childhood. Encephalitis similar to that of measles can occur; but is uncommon. Symptoms in survivors resolve within 1–3 weeks without sequelae.

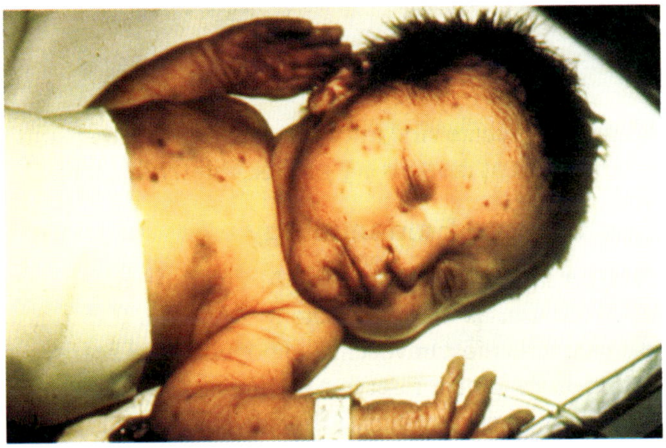

Fig. 11.18: Congenital rubella syndrome

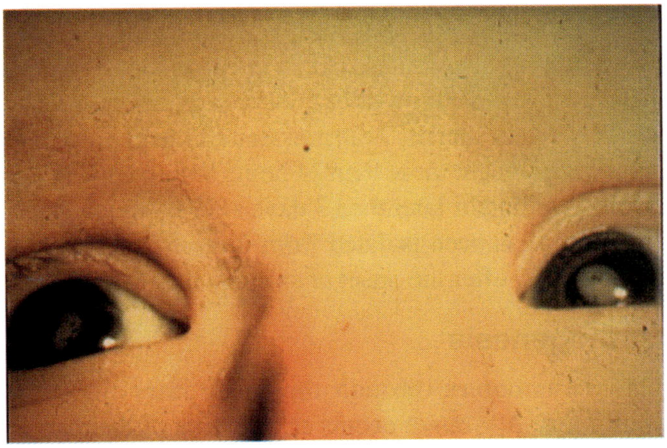

Fig. 11.19: Congenital cataract

Treatment

Treatment is symptomatic with rest in bed during the febrile period. There is no specific anti viral therapy. Antipyretic drugs may be necessary for fever.

The patient can be regarded as non-infectious once the rash has faded. No quarantine is necessary for the contacts.

Course

Rapid, uneventful recovery is the rule. Immunity is permanent. The incidence of reinfection on exposure to wild virus is 3–10% among those with a history of previous rubella infection and 14–18% among those immunized with vaccine. Reinfection may lead only to a booster immune response or to clinical rubella. The significance of rubella infection is controversial.

Prevention

Active immunization is recommended with 2 doses of MMR (Measles, Mumps and Rubella) vaccine. The first dose should be given at 12–15 months age followed by the second dose at 5 years age.

Mumps

Mumps is an acute viral infection characterized by painful enlargement of the salivary glands, chiefly the parotids.

Etiology and Epidemiology

The mumps virus is an RNA virus of the genus paramyxovirus in the family paramyxoviridae. The disease is endemic in most unvaccinated population. The virus is spread from human reservoir by direct contact, airborne droplets, fomites contaminated by saliva, and possibly urine. Epidemics occur at all seasons but are slightly more common in late winter and spring. It is common in children younger than 15 years of age.

The virus has been isolated from saliva as long as 6 days before and upto 9 days after the appearance of swelling of the salivary glands. Transmission of the disease does not seem to occur more than 24 hours before appearance of the swelling or later than 3 days after it has subsided. The virus has been isolated from urine from the 1st to the 14th day after the onset of salivary gland swelling.

Pathogenesis

The virus enters through the respiratory tract and multiplies. A viremia occurs at the onset of the disease with localization in glandular and nervous tissue.

Clinical Manifestations

The incubation period is 18–21 days with probable extremes of 14–30 days. The common presentation of mumps is swelling of the salivary glands. However, the patient may present with any complication as the sole manifestation of the disease in about 10% cases. Subclinical attacks are not uncommon and seen in 30–40%.

In the common form of the disease, swelling of one parotid gland may be the first sign of the disease. This may be associated with mild fever and constitutional symptoms which commonly precede the gland swelling by 1–2 days. There may be earache or pain in the region of the masseter muscle or shivering with slight sore throat may be premonitory symptoms.

The parotid swelling is at first unilateral. It increases for 2–3 days forming an ill defined elastic swelling which is much more clearly seen than felt. The lobe of the ear is pushed upwards and forwards. The swelling fills the space between the posterior border of the mandible and the mastoid. The swelling is limited above by the zygoma. Rarely the skin over the gland is reddened or edematous. The other parotid swelling starts after a day or two. The swelling gradually subsides within 3–7 days. May occasionally lasts longer. The other salivary glands may be involved. The swollen glands are uncomfortable rather than painful. The thought or sight of food may cause increased pain due to salivary secretion. Trismus may occur. The lacrimal glands are rarely involved. There may be moderate enlargement of cervical lymph nodes. The orifices of the salivary ducts particularly the Stensen's duct are often swollen and red in the early stages.

Mild pyrexia, 101°F–102°F (38.3°C–38.9°C) may accompany the onset and persist for 1–2 days but many attacks remain afebrile throughout especially in young children. One attack usually confers life long immunity.

Complications

The viremia of mumps may give rise to a wide variety of glandular or neurological complications. Of the glandular complications, orchitis is by far the most common followed by oophoritis and pancreatitis. Rarely the thyroid, breast and Bartholin's gland may be involved. The neurological manifestations include aseptic meningitis and meningoencephalomyelitis.

Orchitis occurs in 20–30% of post pubertal males. It appears 7–14 days after the onset. In some instances orchitis precedes the swelling of the salivary glands. In the majority of cases it is unilateral. It subsides spontaneously within a week. Some degree of testicular atrophy may follow but loss of libido or sterility as may be a rare sequelae of bilateral involvement.

Oophoritis is a much less frequent complication in post-pubertal females. There is no evidence of impairment of fertility.

Pancreatitis, mild or subclinical is common. Severe pancreatitis is rare. It may be unassociated with salivary gland manifestations. The child may present with epigastric pain and tenderness with fever, chills vomiting and prostration. An elevated serum amylase level may be present in mumps with or without pancreatitis. Symptoms most often appear on the 3rd to 5th day and subside rapidly in 3–4 days in most cases.

Thyroiditis is uncommon in children. It occurs one week after the onset of parotitis. Antithyroid antibodies subsequently develop.

The most frequent neurological complication is **aseptic meningitis** which may be the sole manifestation of mumps infection or it may precede or follow the parotitis by a few days. Recovery takes place within 1–7 days in the majority of cases. **Meningoencephalomyelitis** is rare. It may appear in the second week. The pathogenesis may be either a primary infection of the neurons or post infectious encephalitis with demyelination.

Nerve deafness is rare but a serious complication because it is usually permanent and complete but unilateral. **Optic neuritis** may occur as a part of post mumps encephalopathy. Rarely there may be facial palsy due to facial nerve neuritis.

Myocarditis is infrequent but ECG evidence of temporary damage to heart has been demonstrated.

Acute benign arthritis may arise in the 2nd or 3rd week. It is usually monoarticular affecting a large joint accompanied by fever and raised ESR. It does not respond to salicylates, may respond to other NSAIDs or steroid. Usually there is rapid spontaneous recovery within 2 weeks. However symptoms may last for a few days to 3 months.

Laboratory Diagnosis

The typical case in which swelling of one parotid gland is followed by the other presents no diagnostic difficulty. In cases with unilateral parotitis or presentation with a complication, history of contact with mumps approximately 3 weeks previously is of great help but laboratory confirmation is necessary. Serum amylase level is a useful test to employ. The rise tends to parallel the parotid swelling and then return to normal within 2 weeks.

Microbiologic diagnosis is by serology or viral culture. Enzyme immunoassay for mumps IgG and IgM antibodies are most commonly used for diagnosis. A four-fold rise in antibody is diagnostic. The IgM antibodies are detectable in the first few days of illness and are considered diagnostic. They may remain elevated from weeks to months. The IgG antibodies appear later and are a useful indicator of a previous attack. Mumps virus can be cultured from the saliva, urine, brain and other infected tissues.

Differential Diagnosis

The conditions for differential diagnosis include other viral parotitis (viz. influenza, parainfluenza type 1 and 3, cytomegalo, coxsakie viruses and HIV), acute suppurative parotitis, recurrent parotitis of unknown cause or due to salivary calculus, and preauricular or anterior cervical lymphadenitis. The diagnosis of suppurative parotitis is established by watching pus at the duct orifice on massaging the gland. Preauricular or anterior cervical lymph glands can be differentiated by the well defined borders of the lymph nodes and a location that is completely posterior to the angle of the mandible. Recurrent nature in parotitis of unknown etiology excludes mumps.

Treatment

Isolation is recommended for 7 days from appearance of gland swelling. Contacts need not be quarantined.

The patient should be nursed in bed till the glands are subsiding. Patients with myocarditis should rest until the ECG returns to normal.

There is no specific treatment for mumps and most patients do not require even symptomatic relief. The diet should be adjusted to the patient's ability to chew. Orchitis should be treated with local support and bed rest. The patient should be reassured that they neither be impotent nor sterile as a result of orchitis. Mumps arthritis may respond to a 2-week course of NSAID or corticosteroids. Neurological complications are also treated symptomatically.

Prevention

Active immunization with 2 doses of MMR vaccine is the present recommendation.

Varicella

Chickenpox or varicella is an acute and highly infectious disease characterized by a vesicular rash which tends to appear in successive crops. Although often it is a mild illness in childhood, chickenpox can cause substantial morbidity and mortality.

Etiology

Varicella-zoster virus is a neurotropic human herpes virus. It causes primary, latent and recurrent infections. The primary infection is manifested as varicella or chickenpox. Reactivation of a latent infection causes herpes zoster. Chickenpox during pregnancy can be severe in the mother and can cause a rare but distinct intrauterine syndrome. Chickenpox in the newborn can be severe and life threatening.

Epidemiology

Varicella is a universal communicable disease of childhood. Most children are infected by 15 years of age. The incidence has decreased in countries with moderate to high levels of vaccine coverage after the introduction of varicella vaccine in 1995. Varicella is a more serious disease with higher rates of complications and mortality in the infant, adults and the immunocompromised.

The disease is spread mainly by droplet and direct contact but it can be spread by fomites. Patients with varicella are contagious from 24–48 hours before the rash appears and until vesicles are crusted, usually 3–7 days after the onset of rash. The crusts are not infectious.

Herpes zoster is uncommon in children. The lifetime risk of herpes zoster for individual with a history of varicella is 10–15% and 75% of cases occurring after 45 years of age. Herpes zoster is a milder disease in children and is less frequently associated with post herpetic neuralgia. It may be recurrent and severe in children on immunosuppressive therapy and in those with HIV infection.

Varicella can occur in immunized children; called break through varicella, is usually very mild. It may be progressive particularly in immunosuppressed children.

Pathogenesis

Primary infection results from the inoculation of the virus in the respiratory mucosa. The virus multiplies during the incubation period in the respiratory tract. This is followed by a brief subclinical viremia. Widespread cutaneous lesions occur during a second viremic phase. The infectious virus is carried in the blood by mononuclear cells generating new crops of vesicles for 3–7 days. The virus is also transported back to the respiratory mucosa during the late incubation period permitting spread to susceptible contacts before the appearance of rash. Host immune responses limit the viral replication and facilitate recovery from infection. Failure of immune response, especially cell mediated immune responses, in immunocompromised child results in continued viral replication with resultant injury to the lungs, liver, brain and other organs.

Varicella-zoster establishes latent infection in sensory ganglia cells in all individuals who experience primary infection. Subsequent reactivation of latent virus causes herpes zoster characterized by a vesicular rash of dermatomal distribution.

The skin lesions in varicella and herpes zoster are identical in histopathology. The infectious varicella-zoster virus is present in both. Varicella produces humoral and cell mediated immunity that is highly protective against symptomatic re-infection.

Clinical Manifestations

The incubation period of varicella infection is 11 to 21 days. The illness usually begins 14–16 days after exposure.

Prodromal symptoms may be present particularly in older children. Fever, malaise, anorexia, headache and occasionally mild abdominal pain may occur 24–48 hours before the appearance of rash. The temperature is usually moderate degree. Occasionally the onset may be with vomiting, convulsion and high fever. Fever and other systemic symptoms persist during the first 2–4 days after the onset of the rash.

The eruption of chickenpox appears first on the trunk but soon spreads to the face, scalp and proximal parts of the limb. The distribution of the rash is predominantly centripetal. The initial lesions in the skin consist of intensely pruritic erythematous macules that evolve through the papular stage to form clear fluid filled vesicles. Clouding and umbilication of the lesions begin in 24–48 hours. While the initial lesions are crusting, new crops form on the trunk and then in the extremities. The simultaneous presence of lesions in various stages of evolution viz. papules, vesicles, pustules and scabs, is characteristic of varicella. Ulcerative lesions involving the oropharynx and vagina are also common. Many children have vesicular lesions on the eyelids and

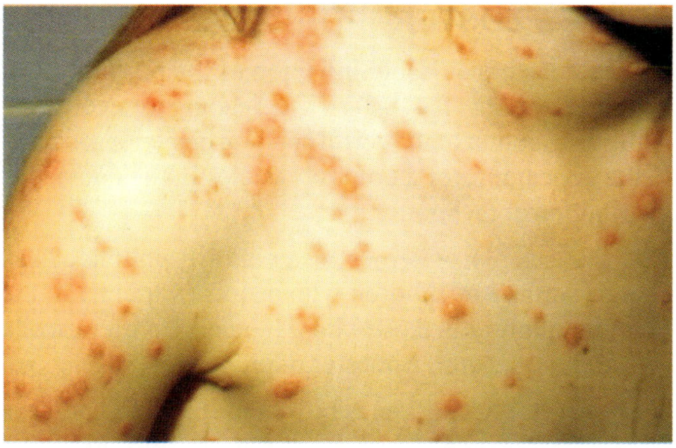

Fig. 11.20: Rash of varicella in different stages

conjunctiva. Corneal involvement and serious ocular disease is rare. Hypopigmentation or hyper pigmentation of lesion sites persists days to weeks in some children.

Complications are more common in immunocompromised children. The main complications include secondary bacterial infection of the skin lesions, pneumonia, and encephalopathy. Mild thrombocytopenia and bleeding tendency may occur. Rare complications include nephritis, myocarditis, pericarditis, pancreatitis and orchitis.

Differential Diagnosis

Papulovesicular urticaria occasionally causes confusion in diagnosis. The skin lesions in this condition are smaller, seldom involve the face and frequently occur in clusters on the legs. If vesicles are present they are pin point size. The lesions of insect bites are similar to papular urticaria.

CONGENITAL VARICELLA SYNDROME

When pregnant woman contracts varicella zoster infection about 25% of fetuses gets infected but all fetuses are not clinically affected. Upto 2% of fetuses whose mother has varicella in the first 20 weeks of pregnancy may demonstrate varicella embryopathy. Fetuses infected at 6–12 weeks of gestation appear to have maximum abnormality with limb development. Fetuses infected at 16–20 weeks may have eye and brain involvement. In addition, damage to the sympathetic nerve fibres in the cervical and lumbosacral cord may lead to divergent effects viz. Horner's syndrome and dysfunction of the urethral or anal sphincters.

Most of the stigmata can be attributed to virus induced injury to the nervous system. Histologic examination of the brain demonstrates necrotizing cerebral lesions involving the leptomeninges, the cortex and the adjacent white matter. The stigmata involve mainly the skin, extremities, eyes and brain. The stigmata include the following:

a. Damage to sensory nerves resulting in cicatricial skin lesion, hypopigmentation.
b. Damage to optic stalk and lens vesicle resulting in micropthalmia, cataracts, chorioretinitis and optic atrophy.
c. Damage to brain due to encephalitis resulting in microcephaly, hydrocephaly, calcification and aplasia.
d. Damage to cervical or lumbosacral cord resulting in hypoplasia of an extremity, motor and sensory deficits, absent tendon reflexes, anisocoria, Horner's syndrome and anal/urinary sphincter dysfunction.

Diagnosis of congenital varicella syndrome is based essentially on history of chickenpox during pregnancy combined with presence of stigmata in the fetus. The usefulness of laboratory tests for patient management and counseling has not been properly defined. Viral DNA can be detected in tissue samples by PCR. Some infants have varicella-zoster specific IgM antibody detectable in the cord blood sample. The titre however, drops quickly. The virus cannot be cultured from the affected newborn. Chorionic villous sampling and fetal blood samples for detection of viral DNA, virus or antibody has been used for diagnosis of fetal infection.

The damage caused by fetal varicella-zoster infection does not progress postpartum which indicates that there is no persistent viral replication. Therefore antiviral treatment of infants with congenital varicella syndrome is not indicated. It is uncertain whether administration of varicella-zoster immunoglobulin to the susceptible mother exposed to chickenpox modifies infection in the fetus. Similarly safety and efficacy for the fetus is not known in case acyclovir treatment is given to the mother with severe varicella.

NEONATAL CHICKENPOX

The risk to the newborn developing neonatal varicella is dependent on the amount of maternal anti varicella-zoster antibody that the fetus has acquired transplacentally before birth. The newborn frequently suffers from severe varicella when delivered within 1 week before or after onset of maternal varicella. If there was an interval of 1 week or more, it is likely that the newborn has acquired sufficient transplacental antibody to ameliorate neonatal

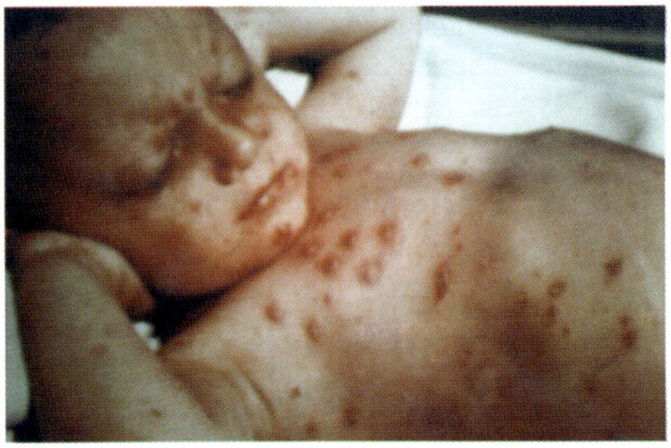

Fig. 11.21: Neonatal chickenpox

infection. Neonates can suffer from community acquired varicella infection in the postpartum period when delivered to woman who is susceptible to varicella-zoster virus. Complications however decline rapidly in the weeks after birth.

BREAKTHROUGH VARICELLA

Breakthrough disease is varicella in a child vaccinated more than 42 days before rash onset. Rash occurring within the first 2 weeks of vaccination is most commonly due to wild virus. Rash occurring 2–6 weeks after vaccination could be due to either the wild or vaccine strains.

The rash in breakthrough disease is frequently atypical, predominantly maculopapular. Vesicles are uncommon. The illness is commonly mild with fewer than 50 skin lesions and little or no fever.

The children with breakthrough disease should be considered potentially infectious and excluded from school until lesions have crusted or until no lesions are occurring.

PROGRESSIVE VARICELLA

It is a dreaded complication of primary varicella-zoster virus infection characterized by visceral organ involvement, coagulopathy, severe hemorrhage, and continued lesion development.

The risk of progressive varicella is highest in children with congenital cellular immune deficiency disorders and in those with malignancy particularly if chemotherapy is given during the incubation period and the absolute lymphocytic count is < 500 cells/cumm. The children are at risk of progressive varicella after organ transplant, when on high dose oral steroids and inhaled corticosteroids. However, children on long term, low dose systemic corticosteroids are not considered to be at higher risk.

HERPES ZOSTER

Herpes zoster is an acute infection of the posterior root ganglion by varicella-zoster virus, leading to severe pain in the distribution of the corresponding posterior root, and to the appearance of a crop of vesicles in the cutaneous distribution of the root.

An increased risk of herpes zoster in early childhood has been described in children who acquire varicella in the first year of life or in those whose mothers have a varicella infection in the third trimester of pregnancy.

Herpes zoster in children is however, mild and course is brief. Localized pain, hyperesthesia, pruritus and fever are infrequent. The rash is mild. Symptoms of acute neuritis are minimal. Complete resolution occurs within 1–2 weeks. Post herpetic neuralgia is unusual in children.

Herpes zoster may be more severe in immunocompromised children. Manifestations then are similar to those seen in adults. Onset is with fever which may persist for 2–4 days. There is pain which may be intense at the site where later the rash appears by 3rd or 4th day of the illness. The rash appears as patchy erythema upon which appear vesicles filled with clear fluid. The vesicles dry up and shrink progressively to form a scab from the 5th to 10th day. The scab finally drops leaving scars. These scars may be anesthetic to touch, pain and temperature. Immunocompromised children may also experience disseminated cutaneous disease that mimics varicella with pneumonia, hepatitis, encephalitis and DIC. Children with HIV infection, severely immunocompromised, may have unusual, chronic or relapsing cutaneous disease, retinitis or central nervous system disease without rash.

Laboratory Diagnosis

The diagnosis of varicella is essentially clinical. With the typical features it causes no difficulty. Rapid laboratory diagnosis is often important in high risk patient. Varicella-zoster virus can be identified quickly by direct fluorescence assay of cells from cutaneous lesions and by polymerase chain reaction testing. The infectious virus can be recovered by using tissue culture methods. The IgG antibody tests are useful for diagnosis as well as to determine the immune status of an individual. A four-fold rise is confirmatory of acute infection.

Treatment

Varicella

The disease is self-limiting and majority of the patients require no treatment. The patient should be isolated until all the skin lesions are dry, usually a period of 10–14 days. Skin irritation can be treated with liberal application of calamine lotion and anti-histamines like promethazine (dose 0.5–2 mg/kg/day per oral 6–8 hourly).

Treatment of varicella in children and adolescents with acyclovir is acceptable in view of its demonstrated efficacy and safety profile. However, the American Academy of Pediatrics does not recommend its use in uncomplicated varicella in the otherwise healthy child because of the marginal benefit, the cost of the drug, and the low risk of complications. Therefore acyclovir is indicated in children 12 months or older in age with:

1. Chronic cutaneous lesions or pulmonary disorders.
2. Children on short-term, intermittent or aerosolized corticosteroids.
3. Children on long-term salicylate therapy.
4. Presence of disseminated varicella including pneumonia, severe hepatitis, thrombocytopenia or encephalitis.

To be effective, treatment should be initiated preferably within 24 hours of onset of exanthema. Oral therapy with acyclovir in a dose of 20 mg/kg/dose (maximum 800 mg/dose) 6 hourly should be continued for 5 days. In disseminated infections, immediate therapy should be started with intravenous acyclovir in a dose of 10 mg/kg/dose 8 hourly and continued for 7 days or until no new lesions have appeared for 48 hours.

Neonatal Varicella

Newborns whose mothers develop varicella 5 days before or 2 days after delivery should receive 1 vial (125 units IM) of varicella-zoster immunoglobulin. Every preterm infant born to mother with active chickenpox at delivery (even if present > 1 week) should receive immunoglobulin.

Perinatally acquired varicella is life threatening and should be treated with acyclovir 10 mg/kg/dose IV 8 hourly for 5 days.

Herpes Zoster

In otherwise healthy children, treatment with antiviral drugs may not be always necessary. Some advocate administration oral acyclovir (10 mg/kg/dose in divided doses; maximum 800 mg/ dose for 5 days) to shorten the duration of the disease.

Immunocompromised children with herpes zoster should receive IV acyclovir 10 mg/kg/dose 8 hourly for 5 days. With uncomplicated herpes zoster, oral acyclovir is sufficient.

Prevention

Varicella-zoster infection is difficult to prevent because the infection is contagious for 24-48 hours before the rash appears. Active immunization is recommended with varicella vaccine to all children at the age of 15 months or above. Children between 15 months and 12 years receive a single dose. Above 12 years age 2 doses are required at 4 weeks apart.

The vaccine given to normal children within 3–5 days of exposure is effective in preventing or modifying varicella. It is recommended for post exposure use for outbreak control. Post exposure prophylaxis is also possible with administration of herpes zoster immunoglobulin. It is recommended for immunocompromised children in a dose of 125 units/10 kg (maximum 625 units) intramuscularly as soon as possible but within 96 hours after exposure. Newborns whose mother develops varicella 5 days before to 2 days after delivery should receive 125 units of herpes zoster immunoglobulin.

Japanese Encephalitis

Japanese encephalitis (JE) is a mosquito borne disease of humans, horses, swines and other domestic animal. The JE virus was first isolated by Japanese workers in 1934. The virus was initially called Japanese B encephalitis virus in order to distinguish it from an unusual epidemic of von Economo (type A) encephalitis that occurred in Japan in 1920s.

Epidemiology

The principal vectors of zoonotic and human JE from Taiwan to India are Culex tritaeniorhynchus and Culex vishnui. Seasonal rains are accompanied by increases in mosquito population and increased transmission. Pigs are amplifying host.

Etiology

The JE virus is a positive-sense single stranded RNA virus. It is a member of the family Flaviviridae.

Clinical Manifestations

The incubation period varies from 4–14 days. The clinical manifestation progresses through 3 stages: prodromal stage, encephalitis stage, late stage.

Prodromal Stage

This phase is characterized by high grade fever with or without rigors, headache, malaise, nausea, abdominal pain and vomiting, sensory changes including psychotic episodes. A definitive clinical diagnosis is usually not possible at this stage.

Encephalitis Stage

This phase is marked by CNS symptoms starting from 3–5 days of onset. The manifestations include altered sensorium, generalized tonic clonic seizures, less frequently intention tremor and cog wheel type rigidity of the muscles. Rapidly changing CNS signs (e.g. hyper reflexia followed by hypo reflexia or changing planter response) is a characteristic sign. The sensory status of the patient may vary from confusion, disorientation, delirium or somnolence, progressing to coma. There may be features of raised intracranial pressure like oculocephalic reflex, acute onset hemiparesis with hypertonia and decorticate and decerebrate rigidity. The extra CNS features in JE include gastric hemorrhage in absence of coagulation abnormalities and pulmonary edema. Death usually occurs due to neurological illness within 7–10 days of onset.

Late Stage

It is the stage of recovery or neurological sequelae. Children, who survive, slowly regain neurological function over several weeks. About one third cases recover normal neurological function. Residual impairment includes speech defects, aphasia, paresis and intellectual deficits. Localized paresis is more common and upper limb is commonly involved. There may be complications like pneumonia, urinary tract infection and stasis ulcers during the recovery period.

Atypical Presentations

A child with JE may present with a brief period of altered sensorium, a short duration of altered behaviour, and an acute flaccid paralysis like illness as the initial presenting feature.

Laboratory Diagnosis

CSF analysis: Increase of cells (100–1000 WBC/cumm), initially polymorphonuclear leucocytosis but in a few days becomes predominantly lymphocytic.

Neuroimaging: A CT scan and MRI may be useful in distinguishing JE from herpes encephalitis. The MRI is more sensitive than CT scan. The T2 weighted images on the MRI shows extensive hyperintense lesions of the thalamus, cerebrum, and cerebellum. In herpes encephalitis the lesions are mainly frontotemporal. The EEG changes are generalized and nonspecific viz. diffuse theta and delta waves, burst suppression, epileptiform activity, and alpha coma. In herpes encephalitis it is localized.

Serology: The etiologic diagnosis of JE is established by testing an acute phase serum collected early in illness for the presence of virus specific IgM antibodies or, alternatively, demonstrating a four-fold or greater increase in IgG antibody titres by testing paired acute and convalescent sera. The virus can be identified by PCR. Isolation of virus or demonstration of viral antigen or genomic sequences in blood are used for research purposes and has no role in routine diagnosis of JE.

Diagnosis

1. Patient from endemic area with history of exposure to night biting mosquitoes, during transmission season.
2. Clinical features and CSF analysis for diagnosis of encephalitis.
3. Acute phase serum for virus specific IgM antibodies.
4. A four-fold or greater increase in IgG antibody titre by testing paired acute and convalescent sera.
5. Identification of virus by PCR.

Prognosis

Patient fatality is 24–42%. Fatality is highest in children aged 5–9 years. Frequency of sequelae is 5–70%. Sequelae are directly related to the age of the patient and to the severity of the disease. It is most common in children younger than 10 years. The more common sequelae are mental retardation, severe emotional instability, personality changes, motor abnormalities and speech disturbances.

Treatment

There is no specific treatment for JE. Supportive treatment is the mainstay.

Supportive Treatment

Resuscitation includes normalization of circulation and respiration which includes ABC of resuscitation and maintenance of adequate oxygenation. Temperature should be maintained. High fever should be controlled with paracetamol. Hypothermia should be prevented.

Monitoring parameters should include GCS, fluid intake and urine output, seizures, oxygen saturation, ABG, serum sodium, blood glucose.

Fluid, electrolytes and blood sugar should be maintained. No fluid restriction is advised unless there is evidence of SIADH.

If there are signs of *raised intracranial pressure* like bradycardia, shallow respiration, headache, squint, vomiting, hemiplegia etc., child should be kept in supine position with head elevated at 30°C. Drugs used are Frusemide in the dose of 1 mg/kg/dose IV or mannitol. Mild hyperventilation is helpful because it reduces cerebral blood flow through vasoconstriction of the cerebral blood vessels. There is no role of steroids in raised ICT or prevention of mortality and morbidity.

Mannitol is useful in treatment of acute intracranial hypertension. It is an osmotic diuretic and promotes a shift of fluid from intracellular to intravascular space. It is less beneficial in severe disruption of blood brain barrier. It may enter the CNS and draw fluid into the brain. If mannitol creates a hyperosmolar circulatory state, renal failure and hemolysis may ensue. Frusemide is safer but a less effective alternative. Usually the combination of both is prescribed.

Intubation and mechanical ventilation may be required if there is brain stem involvement, Glasgow coma scale < 8, cardiac or respiratory signs suggestive of raised ICT and uncontrolled seizures.

Care of the comatose patient to prevent aspiration, bed sores, nosocomial infection, malnutrition and contractures should be given.

Seizures lasting for >10 minutes should be treated aggressively. Seizures lasting >30 minutes is status and seizure lasting >60 minutes despite anticonvulscent therapy are called refractory seizures. The drugs effective for seizures are: diazepam lorazepam, phenytoin, phenobarbitone. In status and refractory cases phenobarbitone and phenytoin are used as first line drugs followed by IV midazolum and valproic acid. In refractory cases repeated doses of phenobarbitone may be used to achieve high levels (50–100 mg/dl). In addition a midazolum drip may be used followed by a pentobarbital coma.

Extrapyramidal symptoms such as tremors, rigidity, spasticity, hemiballismus, dystonia etc can be controlled with haloperidol, diazepam, chloral hydrate etc.

Specific Therapy

There is no specific antiviral drug available yet. Monoclonal antibodies and recombinant interferon alpha has been used in experimental studies. They do not have established role in management in JE.

Prevention

Vaccination of humans is the method of choice for prevention of Japanese encephalitis. At present the cell culture derived *JE vaccine*, a vaccine based on a stable neuroattenuated strain of JE virus is licensed in India. The dose is 0.5 ml for all ages. Initial studies demonstrated an efficacy of 80% with single dose and 98% with 2 doses. Recent studies have shown efficacies of 98.5% at 12–15 months and 96.2% at 5 years with a single dose of the vaccine. Along with infants, all susceptible children upto the age of 15 years should be administered catch up vaccination. The vaccine can be safely co-administered with measles vaccine at 9 months age. Recent recommendation of routine vaccination includes 1 dose at 9 months age and a second dose at 16 to 24 months age.

Other measures include reduction of exposure to mosquitoes by avoiding evening outdoor exposure, using repellants, covering the body with clothing and using mosquito nets, insecticide application from portable sprayers, helicopters and light aircrafts.

Pigs are the major amplifying hosts. Piggeries should be built away from the townships. Vaccination in pigs decreases viral amplification but annual immunization of pigs should be done. Birds also transmit the disease but migration of bird population cannot be regulated. Hence control of reservoirs is not easy.

Rabies

Rabies is a viral infection of the central nervous system usually transmitted by contamination of a wound with saliva from a rabid animal. The disease is virtually 100% fatal once symptoms develop. However, it can be prevented by post exposure prophylaxis.

Etiology

Rabies virus belongs to the family Rhabdoviridae and classified under genus Lyssavirus. The viral particles resemble striated bullets, 75–80 nm in diameter and 130–380 nm in length. They have a lipid containing envelope with a helical nucleocapsid containing one molecule of negative sense single stranded RNA genome. The envelope contains a glycoprotein that elicits neutralizing antibodies and act as a protective antigen in animal experiments. Recent investigations viz. monoclonal antibody analysis, reverse transcriptase followed by polymerase chain reaction has revealed considerable antigenic variation of the virus. The result has been identification of variant strains, rabies related viruses, and antigenic differences among the true rabies viruses.

Epidemiology

Rabies infection occurs in warm blooded animals. Two patterns are recognizable: one which occurs in wildlife maintained by mammals like wolves, mongoose, fox, jackals and bats, and an urban type in which the dog alone is responsible, although during an epidemic other domestic animals viz. cats and cattle may be affected. Rodents, rats, mice, rabbits and other mammals are not infected.

Human rabies occurs routinely in India, South-East Asia and Africa. Children are particularly at risk for rabies exposure and infection because of their short stature, fearlessness of animals, and inability to protect themselves. Human rabies is a rare disease in countries where domestic animals are routinely vaccinated and animal control efforts have been successful.

Rabies infection in animals causes encephalitis followed by spread of virus down nerves away from the brain. The virus multiplies in many organs. Multiplication in the salivary glands is most important for transmission. It should be noted that not all animals have virus in their saliva and even when it is present, the quantity is variable. The viral shedding in saliva of dogs occurs for only 3–6 days before visible symptoms begin. The incubation period for rabies in dogs is 14–180 days. Rabies transmission from a dog appearing normal for 10 or more days after a biting incident has not been reported. Less than half of untreated bites by rabid animals results in rabies. The variability of virus in saliva explains the low transmissibility.

Non-bite exposures can also result in transmission of rabies. Scratches by claws of rabid animals are dangerous because animals lick their claws. Saliva applied to mucosal surfaces e.g. conjunctiva may be infectious. Bat excreta contain enough viruses to pose a danger of rabies either by inhalation or physical contact. Transmission can occur by corneal transplant from patients with undiagnosed rabies encephalitis to healthy recipients. It is advisable to exclude donors dead of unexplained neurologic disease. Human to human transmission is possible.

Humans infected with rabies are infectious for about 1 week before onset of symptoms and can continue to be infectious for upto 5 weeks.

Pathogenesis

After inoculation with contaminated saliva from the bite or scratch, the virus infects and multiplies in the striated muscles cells, to which it attaches via several receptors, probably including nicotinic acetylcholine receptor. After the multiplication, the virus has to overcome two barriers before it causes the disease. It is hypothesized that antibody, interferon, and other host factors act on the virus as it leaves the muscles. If these factors are insufficiently protective, the virus eventually attaches to the nerve. At this stage development of rabies becomes inevitable. However, electron microscopy studies shows that another barrier exist that is passing from the first infected neuron to the other neurons.

It should be noted that the exact means by which the rabies virus travels from the wound to the brain is still ill understood.

Pathology

Rabies virus causes neuronal destruction in the brainstem and medulla. The hippocampus, thalamus, and basal ganglia show neuronal destruction and glial infiltrates. The most severe disease is evident in the pons and the floor of the fourth ventricle. The cerebral cortex is usually normal. In presence of severe anoxia before death, excess of CSF, petechial hemorrhage of the pia, archnoid and injection of its vessels may be found on autopsy. Histological examination reveals cellular infiltration of the perivascular lymph spaces and Negri bodies within the cytoplasm of the nerve cells and their process. The Negri body consists of clumped viral nucleocapsid. They are globular or ovoid structures of variable diameter (0.5–25 microns), especially seen in the purkinjee cells of the cerebellum and the hippocampus. Absence of Negri bodies does not exclude rabies because fluorescent antibody stains of brain section or smears may be positive in their absence.

Clinical Manifestations

The incubation period is extremely variable in human rabies. Usually it is 20–180 days. Incubation period as short as 9 days following severe exposure and as long as

7 years, confirmed by strain identification have been reported. The incubation period tends to be shorter in children.

The disease starts with a prodromal phase which lasts for 2–10 days. It is characterized by pain, pruritus or paresthesia at the site of the wound, non-specific symptoms like fever, malaise, headache, anorexia and vomiting. The patient may also have apprehension, anxiety agitation or depression.

The next phase of the disease is characterized by a stage of excitement or paralysis and may last from 2–21 days. In the type characterized by excitement, the patient is restless, excited and turns furious. The pathognomonic sign is hydrophobia. It is characterized by sudden spasm of the muscles of the mouth, pharynx and larynx and sometimes the respiratory muscles during attempts to swallow liquids, including saliva. Eventually, a psychological component exacerbates the spasm, and even the site of water evokes terror. The voice is altered. Frothy saliva collects in the throat and mouth and is flung off the lips during the attacks which may be characterized by profound terror. Hydrophobia appears to be an exaggerated respiratory tract protective reflex, perhaps mediated by neuronal dysfunction in the brainstem. Aerophobia may be present. It is elicited by fanning a current of air across the face which causes violent spasm of the pharyngeal and neck muscles. It is considered by some as pathognomonic of rabies. Lastly, there may be opistotonus and general respiratory spasm. In the interval, the mind is clear and patient remains in bed in a quiet state. If the patient does not die from cardiorespiratory failure during the acute phase and survives long enough paralysis develops and ultimately dies in coma. Rabies after bat bites may present with ascending symmetric flaccid paralysis.

Diagnosis

A clinical diagnosis should be suspected in patients with a history of an animal bite or proximity to bats associated with wounds with paresthesia or dysesthesia surrounding the wound site, signs of CNS involvement, hydrophobia and/or aerophobia.

Laboratory diagnosis includes demonstration of virus by fluorescent antibody stain or reverse-transcriptase polymerase chain reaction (RT–PCR) in smears of corneal epithelial cells or sections of skin from the neck to the hair line. The virus can also be isolated in saliva. Serologic diagnosis is also possible in patients who survive beyond the acute stage. Neutralizing antibodies may be more than 100 IU/ml in both serum and CSF.

Autopsy examination of the brain of patients will show Negri bodies and positive fluorescent antibody test or positive RT–PCR test for rabies.

Treatment

There is no specific treatment for rabies. Therapies with interferon, high dose rabies immunoglobulin and antiviral drugs have been tried but were successful only in prolongation of clinical course.

Prevention

Pre-Exposure Immunization

Primary prevention of rabies infection includes routine vaccination of all domestic animals and avoiding contact with potentially rabid animals. The children should be taught to avoid wild animals, stray animals and animals with strange behavior. Pre-exposure prophylactic vaccine should be advised to all high risk persons such as veterinarians, laboratory workers, and travelers to rabies-enzootic areas. For pre- exposure immunization, a three dose vaccination schedule on days 0, 7 and 28 days should be advised. A booster dose is given after 1 year of primary vaccination and every 5 years thereafter.

Post Exposure Prevention

Post exposure prevention aims at reducing the risk of infection and includes local wound care, passive immunization with human rabies immunoglobulin and active immunization with antirabies vaccine. Local wound care is designed to remove or kill the virus by mechanical and virucidal action. Passive immunization provides immediate blockage of attachment of virus to the nerve endings and active immunization replaces the fading passive immunity. Human exposure to a potentially rabid animal is considered to be present if the person (1) bitten or scratched by a potentially rabid animal, (2) has a contamination of a scratch, abrasion or open wound with potentially infectious material viz. saliva or CNS tissue from a potentially rabid animal.

Local Wound Care

Local wound care consists of immediate thorough cleansing of the wound with soap and water. Vigorous cleaning has shown to be effective in preventing infection. Wounds should be irrigated for atleast 10 minutes preferably with a virucidal agent like povidone iodine. Catheter should be used to irrigate punctured wound.

Passive Immunization

Passive immunization is possible with Human rabies immunoglobulin (HRIG). The dose is 20 IU/kg which should be thoroughly infiltrated into and around the wound. If an amount is left out it should be administered IM. Equine immunoglobulin is available and can be used in a similar way in a dose of 40 IU/kg. The immunoglobulin should be given within 7 days but preferably together with the first dose of the vaccine on the day of exposure. There is no use of giving HRIG after 7 days of starting the vaccine.

Post Exposure Vaccination

For previously unvaccinated children, the schedule of post exposure vaccination is 5 doses given intramuscular in the deltoid or anterolateral aspect of the thigh on days 0, 3, 7, 14 and 28. The dose is same as in adults. Immune response to post exposure schedule takes around 14 days. For effective prophylaxis to rabies, it is mandatory to provide passive as well as active immunization. No failure has been reported after combined use of HRIG and vaccine.

For re-exposure, the recent recommendation of WHO for previously vaccinated children is two vaccine doses given at 0 and 3 days at any time of re-exposure. There is no need for giving HRIG.

HIV Infection and HIV Disease

Acquired Immunodeficiency Syndrome (AIDS) or HIV disease is a serious disorder of the immune system in which the body's normal defences against infection is broken down, leaving it vulnerable to a host of life threatening infections/conditions including unusual malignancies.

AIDS was first detected in June 1981 in the USA. Since then it has been reported from all the continents. The causative organism human immunodeficiency virus (HIV) was independently identified by a team of French scientists led by Dr. Luc Montagnier of Pasteur Institute and American scientists lead by Dr. Robert C. Gallo of National Cancer Institute in 1983.

The Problem

About 95% of all HIV/AIDS infected people are living in the developing countries. Although HIV/AIDS can affect all age groups, about a half of new infections occur in young adults below 25 years of age. Both sexes are equally affected.

In India, HIV infection was first detected in the commercial sex workers in Tamilnadu in 1986. Since then there has been a steady increase in the number of AIDS cases.

Mortality from AIDS has however, presently fallen markedly due to large use of the new anti-retroviral drugs which control viral loads, improve quality of life and prolong duration. Although these drugs may reduce transmission, there is no evidence that they can cure people of HIV/AIDS infection.

The Agent

The HIV virus is a lenti virus, belonging to class retroviruses and family Lentiviridae. They have a unique enzyme, reverse transcriptase, which copies the viral ribonucleic acid (RNA) into deoxyribonucleic acid (DNA), which eventually disintegrates into host cell chromosome. Hence, the HIV virus persists within cells for years and cannot be eradicated from the host cells by the retroviral drugs.

There are two types of HIV viruses viz. HIV 1 and HIV 2. The latter (HIV 2) is prevalent in Western and Southern Africa. It is a rare cause of infection in children.

Reservoir of Infection

People harbouring HIV in their body are the reservoir of infection. They may be asymptomatic healthy carriers or full blown AIDS cases. In the developed countries, 50% of the infected people are likely to develop AIDS within 10 years after being first infected. In developing countries, the interval between infection and disease is probably shorter.

Source of Infection

Infected blood, semen, vaginal fluids are the prime sources of infection. Infected breast milk is a source of infection for transmission from mother to child. Saliva and tears are not considered to be epidemiologically important sources of infection.

Modes of Transmission

Ninety percent of the children living with HIV are infected through mother-to-child transmission during pregnancy, around the time of birth or through breastfeeding.

Table 11.7: Estimated risk and timing of parent to child transmission (PTCT) in the absence of interventions

Timing of HIV infection	*Children at risk*
During pregnancy	5–10%
During labour and delivery	10–15%
During breastfeeding	5–20%

Source: De Cook KM, *et al.* JAMA 2000; 283(9):1175-82.

Other routes of transmission include:

1. Transfusion with blood products from HIV-infected donor.
2. Injections with contaminated needles.
3. Sexual transmission either through sexual abuse or among children/adolescents with early sexual contact.

Routes of Transmission of HIV

Transmission of HIV can occur by the following routes:

1. **Blood and blood products:** Responsible for 3-6% Pediatric AIDS cases.
2. **Unprotected sexual contact:** Through vaginal and seminal fluid.
3. Use of unsterilized syringes, needles and other instruments.
4. **Parent to child transmission:** Primary route of transmission in children (13-50%).

Pathogenesis

The incubation period is 2 weeks – 6 weeks (longest 36 weeks).

The portal of entry of the virus may be the mucosa or blood vessels. When mucosa is the portal of entry, the first cells to be infected are the dendritic cells. These antigen presenting cells transport the HIV virus to lymphoid tissue. When blood vessels are the portal of entry, the virus, through gp120, targets the CD4 cells which reach the lymphoid tissue.

Humoral immunity is intact during the asymptomatic stage of HIV infection. Specific antibodies are produced against viral proteins, but the antibodies are not protective, and are not able to interfere with cell to cell transmission and infectivity of virus on account of constant variation of virus due to mutation in the same patient.

Progression of HIV infection from asymptomatic to symptomatic stage and then AIDS involves shift of the Th 1 type of response (CMI responses) to Th2 responses (humoral immune responses). The shift in immune response is associated with shift in cytokine profile also. Cytokine induced immune dysregulation is a central component in progression to AIDS. This change in profile results in inability of host macrophages to get rid of opportunistic pathogens resulting in opportunistic infections and neoplasms.

Kinetics of Humoral Immune Response

The entry of the virus into the body leads to a transient period of plasma viremia and p24 antigenemia. The levels of these however, come down with concomitant body immune response. Humoral response is evidenced by formation of antibodies of different classes. The antibodies appear in blood within 2–8 weeks but usually become detectable after 3–12 weeks with the assays presently available. The period following entry of HIV into the body and the appearance of detectable levels of antibodies with the available tests is called "window period". During this period the individual is infected, infectious but nonreactive with the antibody detection tests.

The anti-HIV antibodies may be IgA, IgM and IgG. Detection of IgM is valuable for identifying early seroconversion particularly following needle stick injury and infection in newborn. IgA is the predominant immunoglobulin in seromucus secretions (saliva, colostrum, genitourinary secretions). Since IgA does not cross the placenta, detection of anti HIV IgA in a newborn is diagnostic of congenital HIV infection. Among the three immunoglobulins, IgG response is consistent and better understood. Moreover, sensitivity of ELISA and Western blot to detect IgA and IgM is low.

HIV Disease (AIDS)

It is the advanced stage of HIV infection characterized by decrease in all virology markers in peripheral blood, severe immune deficiency, clinical symptoms, increased susceptibility to opportunistic infection and malignancies. These act as surrogate clinical indicators of AIDS. Survival after diagnosis of AIDS is short (1–2 years on average).

How Pediatric HIV Differs From Adult HIV?

1. There is a much more rapid rate of disease progression. The average time to an AIDS diagnosis after HIV infection is 8–17 months in children.
2. Normal T cell counts are significantly higher in children of less than 6 years and can fluctuate greatly. Thus

it is difficult to determine when opportunistic infections might occur and to determine whether or not ART (antiretroviral therapy) is yielding the desired effect.

3. HIV infected children have higher viral load, possibly due to high T-cell count.
4. There is an increased incidence of recurrent invasive bacterial infections in children.
5. In children opportunistic infections often represent as primary disease with more aggressive course with lack of immunity due to prior infection. But in adults, majority of opportunistic infections are reactivation of latent infections.
6. In most children, B-cell activation occurs early in the infection as evidenced by hypergammaglobulinemia (>1.750 g/L) with high levels of anti HIV-1 antibody.
7. CNS involvement is more common in pediatric patients.

Clinical Manifestations

An infant or child up to 12 years is suspected of having AIDS when presenting with at least two major and two minor signs in the absence of known causes of immune suppression.

Major Signs

a. Loss of weight or FTT (failure to thrive) which is not known to be due to other medical causes.
b. Chronic diarrhea (intermittent or continuous) > 1month duration.
c. Prolong fever (intermittent or continuous) > 1 month duration.

Minor Signs

a. Repeated common infections (e.g., Pneumonia, otitis, pharyngitis).
b. Generalized lymphadenopathy.
c. Oropharyngeal candidiasis.
d. Persistent cough for > 1 month.
e. Disseminated maculopapular dermatitis.

In case of children above 12 years of age, AIDS is suspected when they present with:

1. a. Significant weight loss (10% of body weight) within last one month or cachexia not known to be due to a condition other than HIV infection.
   b. Chronic diarrhea (intermittent or continuous) >1 month duration; or
   c. Prolong fever (intermittent or continuous) >1 month duration.
2. Tuberculosis: Extensive pulmonary tuberculosis, disseminated, miliary, or extra pulmonary tuberculosis.
3. Neurological impairment preventing independent daily activities, not known to be due to the conditions unrelated to HIV infection.
4. Candidiasis of the oesophagus.
5. Clinically diagnosed life-threatening or recurrent episodes of pneumonia, with or without etiological confirmation.
6. Kaposi sarcoma.
7. Other conditions, viz.
   - Cryptococci meningitis.
   - Neuro toxoplasmosis.
   - CMV retinitis.
   - Recurrent and multi dermatome herpes zoster.
   - Disseminated molluscum.

The presence of generalized Kaposi sarcoma or Cryptococcus meningitis is sufficient by themselves for the diagnosis of AIDS.

Paediatric HIV Classification System (1994, CDC Revised Classification)

This classification is useful to predict the severity and prognosis. It is based on two parameters:

1. Clinical status.
2. Degree of immunologic impairment.

Clinical Status

Category N

Asymptomatic, i.e., children who have no signs or symptoms considered to be the result of HIV infection or who have only one of the conditions listed in Category A.

Category A

Mildly symptomatic, i.e., children with 2 or more of the following conditions but with none of the conditions listed in Category B and C.

Showing degree of immunological impairment			
Category	*< 12 months CD_4 cells/ micro litre (%)*	*1 – 5 years CD_4 cells/ micro litre (%)*	*6 years and more CD_4 cells/micro litre*
No evidence of immune suppression	=/> 1500 (>25%)	=/> 1000 (=/> 25%)	= /< 500 (= /> 25%)
Moderate immune suppression	750 – 1499 (15 – 24%)	500 – 999 (15 – 24%)	200 – 490 (15 – 24%)
Severe suppression	< 750 (<15%)	<500 (<15%)	< 200 (< 15%)

They are lymphadenopathy (>0.5 cm at more than 2 sites; bilateral in one site), hepatomegaly, splenomegaly, dermatitis, parotitis, recurrent or persistent upper respiratory infection; sinusitis or otitis media.

Category B

Moderately symptomatic, i.e., Children who have symptomatic conditions other than those listed in Category A and C that are attributable to HIV infection. They are children with oropharyngeal thrush persisting for >2 months, recurrent or chronic diarrhea persisting >1 month, hepatitis, recurrent herpes simplex stomatitis or HSV esophagitis or pneumonitis, disseminated varicella (i.e., with visceral involvement), cardiomegaly or nephropathy.

Category C

Severe symptoms, i.e., children with two serious bacterial infections (e.g., Sepsis, meningitis, pneumonia) in a 2 years period, esophageal or lower respiratory tract candidiasis, cryptococcosis, cryptosporidiosis (>1 month duration), encephalopathy, malignancies, disseminated myco-bacterial infection, Pneumocystis carinii pneumonia (PCP), cerebral toxoplasmosis (onset after 1 month of age) and severe weight loss.

Immunological Impairment

The degree of immunological impairment is shown by the CD4 cell count as shown in the table above.

Laboratory Diagnosis

HIV Testing

At least 2 different antigens or principles based on rapid/ ELISA tests are positive in symptomatic HIV patients. Most ELISA kits presently available are 100% sensitive and specific and therefore considered to be the best to diagnose HIV infection in children more than 18 months of age. Latest ELISA test is rapid test, gives results in 10 minutes, 100% sensitive and 99% specific.

Immune status is tested by CD_4, CD_8 cell counts, and CD_4/CD_8 ratio. In case of infant of HIV infected mother, it should be performed at 1 and 3 months. If HIV infected or status unclear, 3 monthly from 6 months of age then 4-6 weekly, if the CD_4 count declines rapidly. Plasma viral loads by RNA-PCR should be done whenever possible.

Other Tests

- Full blood counts, liver and renal function tests.
- Tuberculin test.
- Chest X-ray.
- Investigations for opportunistic infections, e.g., bronchoalveolar lavage for PCP, isolation of Mycobacterium Avian from blood.
- Diagnosis of HIV infection during window period: It can be done by P-24 antigen assay, Viral culture and PCR.

Treatment

The goal of treatment of HIV in children is to:

1. Achieve normal growth and development.
2. Avoid opportunistic infection.
3. Avoid organ dysfunctions due to HIV.
4. Maintain a healthy and normal lifestyle as much as possible.

When to Start Therapy?

Treatment should be started before substantial immunodeficiency ensues. The principle is "Hit the virus early and hit it hard". The indications of therapy are as follows:

(A) In children < 12 months of age

Clinical category	*CD_4 cells*	*Plasma HIV RNA copy number*	*Recommendations*
Symptomatic	< 25%	Any value	Treat category (A, B or C)
Asymptomatic	>25%	Any value	Consider (clinical) category N

(B) In children > 12 months

Clinical category	*CD_4 cells*	*Plasma HIV RNA copy number*	*Recommendations*
AIDS	<15%	Any value	Treat category C
Mild moderate Cat A or B	15–25%	>100000 copies/ml	Consider treatment
Asymptomatic Cat N	>25%	< 100000 copies/ml	Defer therapy and monitor

Which Agents to Start With?

Single agents are no longer recommended. Combination therapy is shown to be far better as synergistic action at different sites means lower dose and lesser side effects and delay in emergence of resistance.

Antiretroviral Drugs

1. *Nucleoside Reverse Transcriptase Inhibitors (NRTI):* Zidovudine, Stavudine, Lamivudine, Didanosine, Zalcitabine, Abacavir.
2. *Non-Nucleoside RTI (NNRTI):* Nevirapine, Efavirenz.
3. *Protease Inhibitors (PI):* Saquinavir, Ritonavir, Nelfinavir, Amprenavir, Indinavir.

The reverse transcriptase inhibitors (NRTIs, NNRTIs) suppress HIV replication by competitive inhibition of viral reverse transcriptase. PIs prevent the late stages of viral replication by interfering with the formation of structural proteins of the virion core.

Adverse Effects of ART

1. *NRTI:* Hepatitis, fatty liver, lactic acidosis, pancreatitis, myopathy, peripheral neuropathy, cardiomyopathy, bone marrow suppression.
2. *NNRTI:* Rash, granulocytopenia, hepatotoxicity, psychosis.
3. *PI:* Hyperglycemia, lipodystrophy, hyperlipidemia, osteoporosis, diabetes, increased bleeding tendencies.

Highly Active Antiretroviral Therapy (HAART)

HAART (Highly active antiretroviral therapy) is the internationally recommended therapy. It consists of:

1. Combination therapy including 3 drugs.
2. A combination of Two NRTI + one P I or Two NRTI + Two NNRTI or Two NRTI + Hydroxyurea.

Principles of Treatment with ART

1. To interrupt destruction of the immune system and progression to AIDS.
2. To prevent emergence of ARV drug resistant mutants.
3. Maximal viral suppression by targeting at different points of the viral cycle and stages of cell activation.
4. Adherence to the complex drug regimens.

Goals of ART

1. Reduction in viral load to undetectable levels (<50 copies/ml) for as long as possible.
2. Achievement of immune status that is quantitative and qualitative.
3. Drugs must have least possible side effects so that their adherence is not a major problem.

How Long to Give ART?

The WHO consolidated guidelines on the use of ARV drugs for treating and preventing HIV infection were updated in 2013 and again in 2016. WHO now recommends lifelong antiretroviral therapy (ART) for everyone from the time when any adult (including pregnant and breastfeeding women) or child is first diagnosed with HIV infection.

Monitoring of ART

1. Minimum two CD_4 counts and two HIV RNA viral loads should be obtained prior to initiation of therapy.
2. HIV RNA levels should be measured at 4 weeks and 3–4 months after initiation of ART, because initial virologic response of at least 5 fold reductions in viral load should be achieved within 4 weeks of initiation of ART. Maximum response to therapy (<50 copies/ml) usually occurs within 12–16 weeks.
3. CD_4 count should be monitored every 3–4 months.
4. In developing countries, where viral load and CD_4 counts are not routinely available, clinical parameters such as weight, absolute lymphocyte count will give some indication of treatment response and disease progression.
5. Potential drug toxicity should be monitored for the first 8–12 weeks.

Future Therapies

Alpha interferon, although a drug with antiviral activity, it has not been proven to have a role as an anti-retroviral agent. TIBO is another promising new drug which has been shown to be five times more potent than zidovudine.

A combination of anti-retroviral agents, immunotherapy and gene therapy is being increasingly considered as the best hope for the persons with HIV/AIDS.

Followup of a Child on ART

1. History and physical examination: 3 monthly.
2. Systemic review: 3 monthly.
3. Developmental assessment should be done 3 monthly in children below 1 year, 6 monthly in children between 1 and 6 years and annually above 6 year olds.
4. Chest radiography: Annually.
5. Laboratory test: CBC, CD_4, CD_4 / CD_8, Liver and Kidney function tests should be performed 3 monthly.
6. Mantoux test: Annually.
7. Examination of eyes, cardiovascular system, CT/MRI annually.

Prophylaxis for Opportunistic Infections (OI)

A. Pneumocystis Pneumonia (PCP)

PCP is the most common opportunistic infection in HIV infected children and occurs in the first year of life. The drug used is trimethoprim and sulphamethoxazole in the doses 150 mg/750 mg/square metre body surface once daily. All HIV infected children and children with unconfirmed infection should be started on PCP prophylaxis from 6 weeks of age.

B. Serious Bacterial Infections

The child should be put on 150 mg (trimethoprim), 750 mg (sulphamethoxazole) / metre square body surface once daily. In children with hypogammaglobinaemia, IVIg 400 mg/kg/month should be given. IVIg is also considered in HIV infected child with history of > 2 invasive bacterial infections in 1 year.

C. Mycobacterium Tuberculosis Infection

For prevention of tuberculosis the child should be on INH 5 mg/kg once daily for 12 months, when Tuberculin test > 5 mm, and who had previously not received ATT, when there is a recent history of contact with an infectious patient suffering from open tuberculosis or if there is history of prior untreated or inadequately treated infection.

D. Disseminated Mycobacterium Avian Intracellular Infection (MAC)

Indications of Therapy:

i. <12 months of age, CD_4 count <750.

ii. 1–2 years, CD_4 count < 500.

iii. 2–6 years, CD_4 < 75.

iv. >6 years, CD_4 count <50.

Drugs: Clarithromycin or Azithromycin.

Primary prophylaxis against OIs may be discontinued if there is sustained (>6 months) immune reconstruction with HAART.

Supportive Care

Nutrition: The aim of nutrition rehabilitation is to preserve the body weight. Most children require 200 kcal/kg and 4 g/kg of protein. Calorie intake should be increased if there is fever or weight loss. The child should be offered small frequent feeds. Attention should be given to food hygiene and proper hand washing. The diet should be nutrient dense. Iron deficiency anemia should be treated with high iron containing food, supplements of iron, folic acid and vitamin B_{12}.

Diarrhoea: It should be treated according to the cause. The child should be investigated for malabsorption.

PARENT TO CHILD TRANSMISSION

The HIV infected adult male can transmit the infection to women and thus HIV infection becomes a serious threat to children of such parents. In India, sexual route is the most common route of transmission of HIV. After implementation of effective blood safety programme, parent to child transmission (PTCT) has emerged as the second important cause of infection. It is the most important cause of HIV infection in children.

In the developing countries like India, most of the mothers are getting infection from their husbands through the sexual route, i.e., fathers are equally responsible for the transmission of HIV to their children. Hence, in order to ensure that mothers alone should not be blamed for mother to child transmission (MTCT), MTCT has been renamed as PTCT (Parent to child transmission) in India.

Timing of Vertical Transmission

Vertical transmission can occur during pregnancy, labour and delivery as well breastfeeding. The incidence of the different routes is as follows:

1. Intrauterine: 30 – 40%.
2. Intrapartum: 60 – 70%.
3. Postpartum: 29% when mothers acquire HIV infection postnatally.

Postulated Mechanisms of PTCT

Parent to child transmission of HIV virus can occur by the following mechanisms:

1. Transplacental micro-transfusion, especially during late pregnancy.
2. Exposure of the baby's mucocutaneous surface to maternal blood and cervical secretions of the mother during delivery.
3. Virus transmission through breast milk.

Prevention of Parent to Child Transmission (PPTCT)

India has launched the PPTCT programme to monitor and to take measures to prevent perinatal transmission. PTCT blockage involves 4 strategies:

1. Primary prevention of HIV infection among the child bearing age parents and prevention of unwanted pregnancy among HIV positive females.
2. Measures to decrease viral load in HIV infected mothers by administration of anti-retroviral therapy (ART).
3. Measures to decrease exposure of baby to maternal fluids by promotion of delivery by elective LSCS.
4. Measures to decrease chances of HIV in an exposed baby by administration of ART to the baby.

Interventions

All the components of the PPTCT programme must be adequately emphasized for achieving the primary goal of reducing overall maternal and infant morbidity and mortality. The components of the PPTCT programme include:

- Information, education, counselling.
- Condom promotion.
- VCTC (Voluntary counselling and testing centre) for HIV/AIDS.
- Treatment of STDs in mother.
- Good antenatal care.
- Prevention of transmission with anti-retroviral therapy (ART).
- Safe delivery practices.
- Counselling and support for safe infant feeding practices; and
- Community action in order to make the programme successful and safeguard future generation.

Components of Care of HIV-exposed Infant/Child

1. Immediate care at birth.
2. Infant feeding.
3. ARV prophylaxis.
4. Cotrimoxazole prophylaxis (CPT).
5. Immunization and Vitamin A supplementation.
6. Growth monitoring and development assessment.
7. Early infant diagnosis.
8. Followup.

Immediate Care at Birth

The immediate care of the newborn infant at birth should follow standard neonatal care guidelines including resuscitation guidelines. However, the following should be adhered to:

- Follow universal precautions.
- Do not milk the cord.
- The cord should be clamped soon after birth.
- Cover the cord with gloved hand and gauze before cutting to avoid blood splattering.
- Initiate breastfeeding within the first hour of birth in accordance with the preferred and informed choice of the mother.

Infant Feeding

The 2016 WHO Recommendations on HIV and Infant Feeding

- Mothers living with HIV should breastfeed for at least 12 months and may continue breastfeeding for up to 24 months or longer (similar to the general population) while being fully supported for ART adherence.
- Mothers living with HIV and health care workers can be reassured that ART reduces the risk of postnatal HIV transmission in the context of mixed feeding. Although exclusive breastfeeding is recommended, practising mixed feeding is not a reason to stop breastfeeding in the presence of ARV drugs.

- Mothers living with HIV and health care workers can be reassured that shorter duration of breastfeeding of less than 12 months are better than never initiating breastfeeding at all.
- If infants and young children are known to be living with HIV, mothers are strongly encouraged to exclusively breastfeed for the first six months of life and continue breastfeeding in accordance with the recommendations for the general population: that is, up to two years or beyond.
- Women who are HIV negative or of unknown status should exclusively breastfeed for the first six months, and continue breastfeeding until 24 months or beyond because of the many benefits for both mother and child.
- All infants should be started on complementary foods from six months of age.

ARV Prophylaxis

ARV prophylaxis to the infant must be given in accordance with the current National PPTCT Guidelines. For all the exposed infants syrup Nevirapine (NVP) has to be given for 6 weeks and these children has to be linked to the Early Infant Diagnosis (EID) programme. The ART provision shall depend on the result of EID.

All Infants born to women who are receiving ART / maternal triple ARV prophylaxis/who present directly-in-labour and receive intra partum ARV prophylaxis should be started on daily NVP prophylaxis at birth and continue for a minimum of 6 weeks (i.e., till the first immunization visit for the infant).This regardless of whether the infant is exclusively breastfed or receives replacement feeding it helps in reducing the risk of postpartum HIV transmission.

In situations where infants are born to women who present directly-in-labour and receive intrapartum ARV prophylaxis, the daily NVP prophylaxis for the infant should not be stopped at 6 weeks. These infants should be continued on NVP prophylaxis until the mother is initiated on ART/ARV prophylaxis and complete a minimum of six weeks of therapy.

Daily Dose of Infant NVP Prophylaxis

(Considering the content of 10 mg Nevirapine in 1 ml suspension)

- Birth weight < 2000 gm: 2 mg/kg once daily 0.2 ml/kg once daily
- Birth weight 2000 – 2500 gm: 10 mg once daily/1 ml once daily
- Birth weight more than 2500 gm: 15 mg once daily/1.5 ml once daily

Preventive Therapy (CPT)

Cotrimoxazole Preventive Therapy (CPT) protects the infant from Pneumocystis jiroveci pneumonia (PCP), toxoplasmosis and other bacterial diseases. It is the standard component of HIV care to reduce the morbidity and mortality of children less than five years of age.

Ideally all exposed infants should be advised pneumocystis carinii pneumonia (PCP) prophylaxis from 6 weeks age with Cotrimoxazole till 5 years or until perinatal HIV infection is excluded. The recommended dose is 5 mg/kg/day of TMP once daily.

Children with the history of severe adverse reaction (grade 4 reaction) to Cotrimoxazole or other sulpha drugs and children with G6PD (glucose-6-phosphate dehydrogenase deficiency) should not be initiated on CPT. The alternative drug is Dapsone 2 mg/kg once daily (not to exceed 100 mg/day) orally. Aerosolised pentamidine administered via respigard II inhaler in the dose of 300 mg once a month is another alternative for children > 5 years.

In addition, it is worth considering additional 6–9 months chemoprophylaxis against tuberculosis, to be started as two drug INH and RMP regimen at birth, in view of the high prevalence of tuberculosis and its coexistence with HIV infection, especially in developing countries.

Immunization and Vitamin A Supplementation

HIV-exposed/infected children should be immunized according to the National Immunization schedule. However, live vaccines should be avoided in all severely immune compromised infants (CD_4 %< 25% or WHO stage 3 and 4). Live vaccines should be avoided in symptomatic children till such a time when their CD_4 count improves as a response to ART.

Vitamin A supplementation should be as per the national immunization schedule.

Growth Monitoring and Development Assessment

Growth monitoring should be done using growth charts in all HIV exposed infants and children as per scheduled visits. If the child's growth curve is falling down, flattening or faltering, reinforce nutrition and work up for urgent assessment for nutrition status, HIV related features and also screen for treatable causes, e.g., nutritional deficiency, chronic infections such as respiratory, gastrointestinal, urinary tract infection and TB. For children on ART with growth flattering or decline look for treatment failure.

Developmental Assessment: All children require a routine screening of development milestone to detect delays or regression of milestones. Remembering the Red flag signs help (See Table 11.8). Early detection of developmental aberration allows for early interventions which is a key to successful management.

Delayed development or loss of milestones after attaining them (Regression of Milestones), may be the first sign of HIV infection suggesting HIV encephalopathy, if other common causes are ruled out. Even in these circumstances, early identification of developmental delay and neurologic abnormalities, confirmation of HIV and initiation of ART can facilitate intervention and suitable remedial actions. Therefore it is crucial to assess the development in an HIV-exposed/HIV-infected infant and child.

Table 11.8: Showing the developmental red flag signs

Age	*Red flag sign*
4 – 6 months	Poor head control, Failure to smile
By 5 months	Failure to reach for objects
6 – 12 months	No sounds or babbling
By 10 months	Inability to localize sounds
12 – 24 months	Lack of consonant production
Prior to 18 months	Presence of hand dominance (indicates contralateral weakness)
By 16 months	No imitation of speech and activities
Any age	Loss of previously attained milestones

(Baylor College of Medicine's HIV Curriculum for the Health Professional, 2006)

Early Infant Diagnosis

Maternal HIV antibody transferred passively during pregnancy can persist for as long as 18 months in children born to HIV-infected mothers. Hence, positive HIV antibody test does not necessarily indicate HIV infection in the infant/child. In children who are breastfed, since they have ongoing risk for HIV transmission, HIV infection can only be excluded after 6 weeks of complete cessation of breastfeeding.

In the current Early Infant Diagnosis (EID) program, virologic tests, i.e., HIV-1 DNA PCR by Dried Blood Spot (DBS) and on Whole Blood Sample (WBS) are being done for infants and children below 18 months of age, as per the algorithm. Antibody tests, using rapid test method can be used for children > 18 months of age for diagnosis of HIV infection as in adults.

Followup of HIV Exposed Infants and Children

In view of ARV prophylaxis to all exposed babies for at least 6 weeks of age, the first followup visit should be at 2 weeks of age. During the first followup visit at 2 weeks of life, child should be looked for any adverse reaction to NVP.

The subsequent visits should be according to the immunization schedule starting at 6 weeks of age. The road to health card for HIV-exposed children will include information on maternal HIV status, Cotrimoxazole prophylaxis, infant HIV diagnosis and infant feeding information.

The exposed infants and children should be followed up at ICTCs at 6, 10, 14 weeks of age and then at 6, 9, 12 and 18 months of age. If they test positive by DBS-DNA PCR test done at ICTC, they should be referred to ART centre for confirmation of the diagnosis by WBS-DNA PCR.

Activities at Each Followup Visit

Activities at each followup visit Birth 6 weeks, 10 weeks, 14 weeks, 6 months, 9 months, 12 months, 18 months.

- *Cotrimoxazole prophylaxis therapy (CPT):* Start from 6 weeks (or first immunisation visit) for all HIV-exposed infants and children.
- Continue CPT for those tested to be HIV infected beyond 6 weeks. Stop cotrimoxazole: For those tested to be HIV un-infected. Stop at 6 weeks of life or after at least 6 weeks of ART to mother whichever is later.
- Counselling for infant feeding.
- Growth monitoring and developmental assessment.
- Immunisation and Vitamin A supplements as per national and state immunization protocol.
- Clinical assessment HIV testing.
- *Counselling and Psychosocial support:* At every visit, give information and talk to the mother or caregiver on common HIV related conditions, opportunistic infection, availability of Early Infant Diagnosis (EID), psychosocial concerns, reinforce the importance of co-trimoxazole prophylaxis, infant feeding and nutrition, and the importance of followup and adherence to ARV prophylaxis/ART.

Appropriate counselling is ultimately the responsibility of the team providing care to the HIV exposed infant and child.

Dengue Fever and Dengue Hemorrhagic Fever

Dengue fever is an acute febrile illness caused by several arthropod-borne viruses and characterized by biphasic fever, myalgia, arthralgia, rash, leucopenia, and lymphadenopathy. Dengue hemorrhagic fever is a febrile disease caused by dengue viruses. It is characterized by abnormalities in hemostasis and by leakage of fluid and protein from capillaries, which in severe cases results in shock (dengue shock syndrome).

The criteria for diagnosis proposed by the WHO for *dengue hemorrhagic fever* are fever, minor or major hemorrhagic manifestations, thrombocytopenia (=/< 100,000/cumm) and objective evidence of increased capillary permeability (hematocrit increased = / > 20%), pleural effusion (by chest X-ray) or hypoalbuminemia.

The criteria for diagnosis of *dengue shock syndrome* (DSS) include those for dengue hemorrhagic fever as well as hypotension or narrow pulse pressure (= / < 20 mm Hg).

Etiology

There are at least four distinct types of dengue viruses, members of the family Flaviviridae. In addition three other arthropod-borne (arboviruses) viruses cause similar or identical febrile illness.

Epidemiology

Dengue viruses are transmitted by mosquitoes. Aedes aegypti, a daytime biting mosquito is the principal vector. All four types of the virus have been recovered from it. Dengue outbreaks in urban areas infested by Aedes aegypti may be explosive involving upto 70-80% of the population. Spread of an epidemic occurs mainly through viremic human beings. In areas where dengue is endemic, the adults become immune. Children and susceptible foreigners may be the only persons to acquire the disease.

Dengue hemorrhagic fever occurs where multiple types of dengue virus are simultaneously or sequentially transmitted. It is currently endemic in tropical America and Asia. It is largely due to the warm environmental temperature, practice of water storage and availability of outdoor breeding sites for Aedes aegypti. Under these circumstances infection with all types of dengue viruses is common. Second infection with heterologus types is frequent. Dengue like diseases can occur as epidemics. The common such diseases occurring in India are Chikungunya caused by the virus of the same name and West Nile virus.

Pathogenesis

The pathogenesis of dengue hemorrhagic fever is not well understood. Epidemiological studies suggest it is usually associated with second infection with dengue virus types 1-4. Early in the acute stage of secondary dengue infection, there is rapid activation of the complement system. Shortly before or during shock, blood levels of soluble tumor necrosis factor receptors, interferon gamma, and interleukin 2 are elevated. C1q, C3, C4, C5-8 and C3 proactivators are depressed.

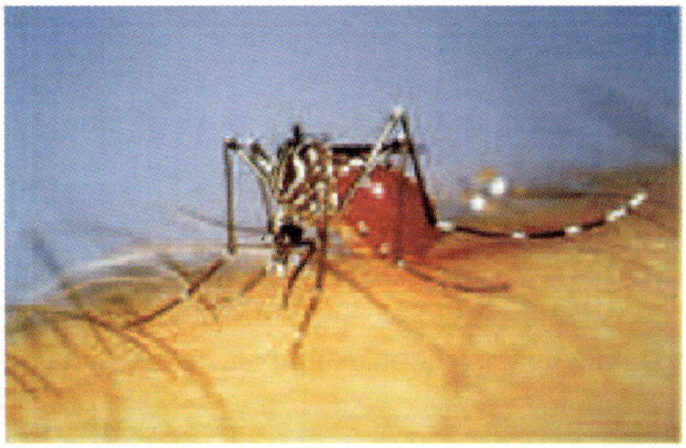

Fig. 11.22: Aedes aegypti mosquito

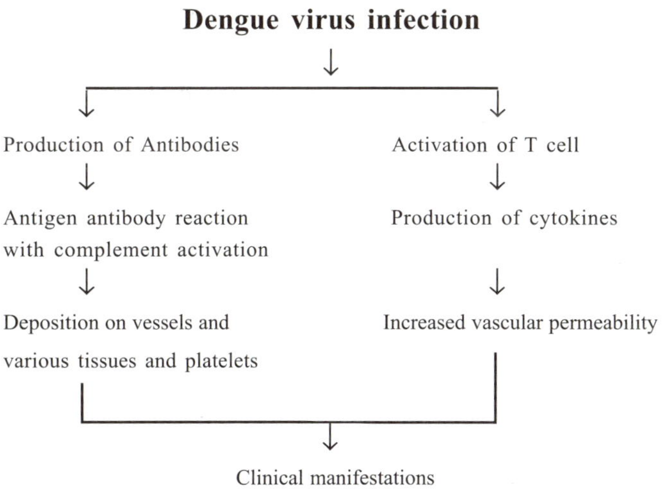

Fig. 11.23: Pathogenesis of dengue hemorrhagic fever

These factors may interact at the endothelial cell to produce increased vascular permeability through the nitric oxide final pathway. The blood clotting and fibrinolytic systems are activated and the levels of factor XII are depressed. The mechanism of bleeding in dengue hemorrhagic fever is not clear. A mild degree of DIC, liver damage, and thrombocytopenia may operate synergistically. Capillary damage allows fluid electrolytes, small proteins and in some instances red cells to leak into the extra vascular spaces. The internal redistribution of fluid, together with deficits caused by fasting, vomiting, results in hemoconcentration, hypovolemia, increased cardiac work, tissue hypoxia, metabolic acidosis and hyponatremia.

Clinical Phases

There is a history of living in or travel to a dengue endemic area. The incubation period is 1-7 days. After the incubation period, the illness begins abruptly and is followed by the three phases viz. febrile, critical and recovery.

Febrile Phase

Patients typically develop high-grade fever of sudden onset. This acute febrile phase usually lasts 2-7 days and is often accompanied by facial flushing, skin erythema, generalized body ache, myalgia, arthralgia and headache. Some patients may have sore throat, injected pharynx and conjunctival injection. Anorexia, nausea and vomiting are common.

It can be difficult to distinguish dengue clinically from non-dengue febrile diseases in the early febrile phase. A positive tourniquet test in this phase increases the probability of dengue. The earliest abnormality in the complete blood count is a progressive decrease in total white cell count, which should alert the physician to a high probability of dengue.

These clinical features are indistinguishable between severe and non-severe dengue cases. Therefore monitoring for warning signs and other clinical parameters is crucial to recognizing progression to the critical phase.

The warning signs include abdominal pain or tenderness, persistent vomiting, clinical fluid accumulation, mucosal bleed, lethargy, restlessness, liver enlargement >2 cm, increase in HCT concurrent with rapid decrease in platelet count.

Critical Phase

Usually on days 3-7 of illness, there is defervescence and the temperature drops to 37.5-38°C or less and remains below this level. The beginning of the critical phase is marked by an increase in capillary permeability in parallel with increasing hematocrit levels. The period of clinically significant plasma leakage usually lasts 24-48 hours. At this point, patients without an increase in capillary permeability will improve, while those with increased capillary permeability may become worse as a result of lost plasma volume.

Those who improve after defervescence are said to have non-severe dengue. However, some patients progress to the critical phase of plasma leakage without defervescence.

Those who deteriorate will manifest with warning signs. This is called dengue with warning signs. Cases of dengue with warning signs will probably recover with early intravenous rehydration. Some cases will deteriorate to severe dengue.

Recovery Phase

If the patient survives the 24-48 hours critical phase, a gradual reabsorption of extra vascular compartment fluid takes place in the following 48-72 hours. General well-being improves, appetite returns, gastrointestinal symptoms abate, hemodynamic status stabilizes and diuresis ensues. Some patients may have a rash of "isles of white in the sea of red". Some may experience generalized pruritus. Bradycardia is common during this stage.

The hematocrit stabilizes or may be lower due to the dilutional effect of reabsorbed fluid. White blood cell count usually starts to rise soon after defervescence but the recovery of platelet count is typically later than that of white blood cell count.

Clinical Problems During Different Phases

1. *Febrile phase:* Dehydration, high fever may cause neurological disturbances and febrile seizures in young children.
2. *Critical phase:* Shock from plasma leakage, severe hemorrhage, organ function impairment.
3. *Recovery phase:* Hypervolemia, pulmonary edema or congestive heart failure (only if intravenous fluid therapy has been excessive and/or has extended into this period).

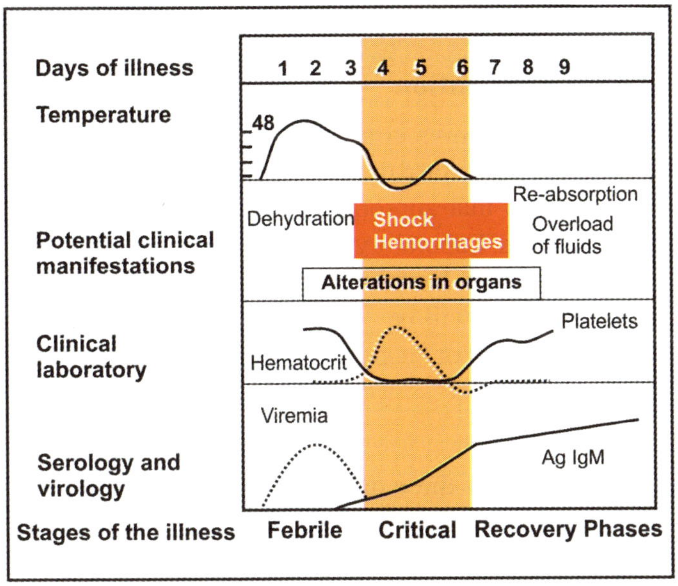

Fig. 11.24: Showing the phases of dengue illness

Severe Dengue

Severe dengue should be considered if the patient is from an area of dengue risk presenting with fever of 2-7 days plus any of the following features:

1. Evidence of plasma leakage, such as high or progressively rising hematocrit; pleural effusion or ascites; circulatory compromise or shock (tachycardia, cold and clammy extremities, capillary refill time greater than three seconds, weak or undetectable pulse, narrow pulse pressure or, in late shock, unrecordable blood pressure).
2. Significant bleeding.
3. Altered level of consciousness (lethargy or restlessness, coma), convulsions.
4. Severe gastrointestinal involvement (persistent vomiting, increasing or intense abdominal pain, jaundice).
5. Severe organ impairment viz. acute liver failure (AST or ALT =/> 1000), acute renal failure, encephalopathy or encephalitis, cardiomyopathy or other unusual manifestations (See Table 11.9).

Laboratory Diagnosis

For Confirmations of Clinical Diagnosis

Dengue virus infection produces a broad spectrum of symptoms, many of which are non-specific. Thus, a diagnosis based only on clinical symptoms is unreliable. Early laboratory confirmation of clinical diagnosis may be valuable because some patients progress over a short period from mild to severe disease and sometimes to death.

Before day 5 of illness, during the febrile period, dengue infection may be diagnosed by virus isolation in cell culture, by detection of viral RNA by nucleic acid amplification tests (NAAT), or by detection of viral antigens by ELISA or Haemagglutination Inhibition (HI) test.

The isolation and identification of dengue viruses in cell cultures usually takes several days. Nucleic acid detection assays may identify dengue viral RNA within 24-48 hours. However, these tests require expensive equipment and reagents and must be performed by experienced technicians. Dengue serologic tests are available. Specimen transport is not a problem as immunoglobulins are stable at tropical room temperatures. Results of rapid tests may be available within less than one hour. A four-fold or greater increase in antibody levels measured by IgG ELISA or by haemagglutination inhibition (HI) test in paired sera indicates an acute or recent flavivirus

Table 11.9: Suggested dengue case classification and levels of severity (2010)

Probable dengue	*Warning signs (requiring strict observation and medical intervention)*	*Severe dengue*
Live in or travel to dengue endemic area Fever and 2 of the following criteria: • Nausea, vomiting • Rash • Aches and pains • Tourniquet test positive • Leucopenia • Any warning sign • Laboratory confirmed dengue (important when no sign of plasma leakage)	• Abdominal pain or tenderness • Persistent vomiting • Clinical fluid accumulation • Mucosal bleed • Lethargy, restlessness • Liver enlargement >2 cm • Laboratory: Increase in HCT concurrent with rapid decrease in platelet count	Severe plasma leakage leading to: • Shock (DSS) • Fluid accumulation with respiratory distress • Severe bleeding as evaluated by clinician • Severe organ involvement Liver: AST or ALT >/=1000 CNS: Impaired consciousness Heart and other organs involvement

infection. The interpretation of dengue diagnostic tests is as shown below:

Highly suggestive	*Confirmed*
One of the following: 1. IgM + ve in a single serum sample 2. IgG + ve in a single serum sample with a HI titre of 1280 or greater	One of the following: 1. PCR + ve 2. Virus culture + ve 3. IgM seroconversion in paired sera 4. IgG seroconversion in paired sera or four fold IgG titer increase in paired sera

Other Investigations

1. A full blood count should be done at the first visit. A hematocrit test in the early febrile phase establishes the patient's own baseline hematocrit. A decreasing white blood cell count makes dengue very likely. A rapid decrease in platelet count in parallel with a rising hematocrit compared to the baseline is suggestive of progress to the plasma leakage/critical phase of the disease.
2. Additional tests should be considered as and when indicated. These should include tests of liver function, glucose, serum electrolytes, urea and creatinine, bicarbonate or lactate, cardiac enzymes, ECG and urine specific gravity.

Management

Disease Notification

In dengue-endemic countries, cases of suspected, probable and confirmed dengue should be notified as soon as possible so that appropriate public health measures can be initiated. Laboratory confirmation is not necessary before notification. In non-endemic countries, usually only confirmed cases will be notified. Suggested criteria for early notification of suspected cases are:

1. The patient lives in or has travelled to a dengue endemic area.
2. Has fever for three days or more.
3. Has low or decreasing white cell counts, and/or has thrombocytopenia ± positive tourniquet test.

Treatment

Depending on the clinical manifestations and other circumstances, patients with Dengue fever may be sent home, those with Dengue hemorrhagic fever be referred for in-hospital management, while those with Dengue shock syndrome may require emergency treatment and urgent referral to a higher centre.

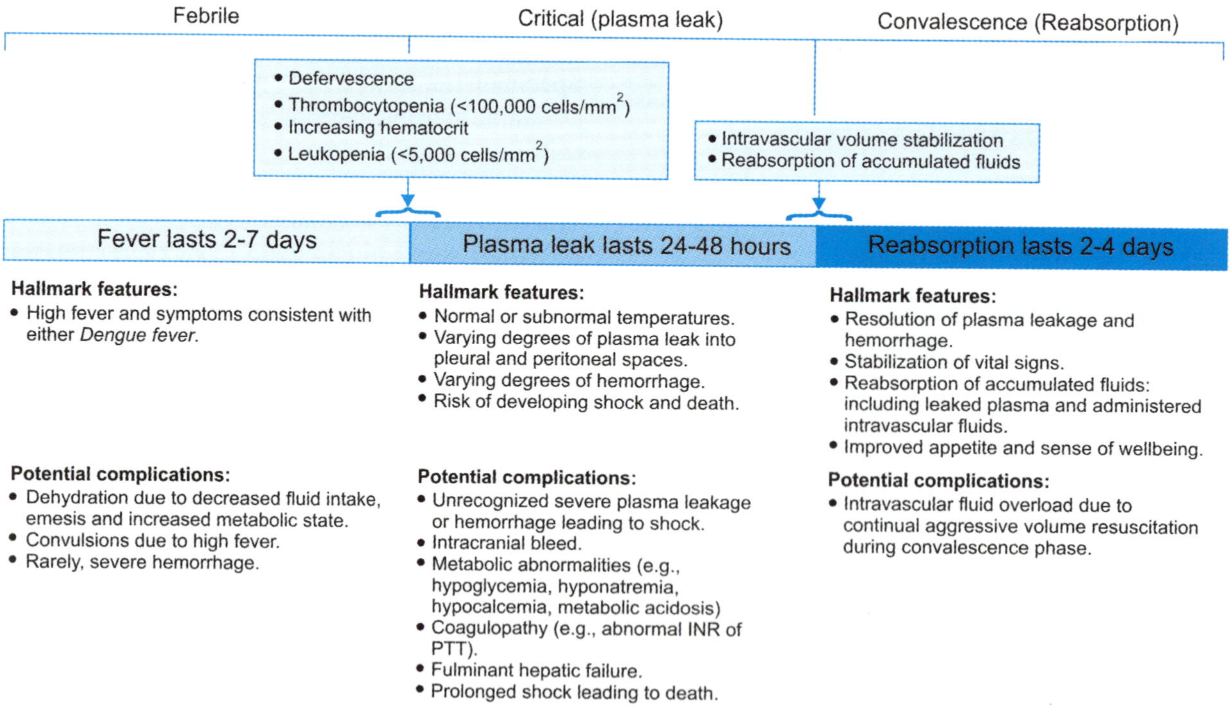

Fig. 11.25: Showing the hallmark features and potential complications in different phases

Dengue Fever

These patients are able to tolerate adequate volumes of oral fluids and pass urine atleast once every 6 hours. They do not show any of the warning signs, particularly when fever subsides.

Ambulatory patients should be reviewed daily for signs of disease progression, viz. decreasing white blood cell count, defervescence and presence of warning signs until they are out of the critical period. They can be sent home after being advised to return to the hospital immediately if they develop any of the warning signs and to adhere to the following measures:

- Oral intake of oral rehydration solution (WHO ORS), fruit juice and other fluids containing electrolytes and sugar to replace losses from fever and vomiting. (Caution: Fluids containing sugar/glucose may exacerbate hyperglycemia of physiological stress from Dengue).
- Paracetamol (10 mg/kg/dose) should be advised for fever (101°F or more) if the patient is uncomfortable. The interval of Paracetamol dosing should not be less than six hours. Tepid sponge if the patient still has high fever. *No acetylsalicylic acid (aspirin), ibuprofen or other non-steroidal anti-inflammatory agents (NSAIDs)* should be used for fever, as these drugs may aggravate gastritis or bleeding. Acetylsalicylic acid (aspirin) may be associated with Reye's syndrome.
- Care givers should be instructed that the patient should be brought to hospital immediately if any of the following occur: no clinical improvement, deterioration around the time of defervescence, severe abdominal pain, persistent vomiting, cold and clammy extremities, lethargy or irritability/restlessness, bleeding (e.g., black stools or coffee ground vomiting), not passing urine for more than 6 hours.
- Patients who are sent home should be monitored daily by health care providers for temperature pattern, volume of fluid intake and losses, urine output (volume and frequency), warning signs, signs of plasma leakage and bleeding, hematocrit, and white blood cell and platelet counts.

Patients with Warning Signs

These patients may need to be admitted to a secondary health care centre for close observation, particularly as they approach the critical phase. These include the following:

(a) Patients with warning signs.

(b) Those with co-existing conditions that may make dengue or its management more complicated (such as infancy, renal failure, chronic hemolytic diseases).

(c) Those with certain social circumstances (e.g., living far from a health facility without reliable means of transport).

If the patient has dengue with warning signs, the action plan should be as follows:

- Obtain a reference hematocrit before fluid therapy. Give only isotonic solutions such as 0.9% saline or Ringer's lactate.
- Start with 5-7 ml/kg/hour for 1-2 hours, then reduce to 3-5 ml/kg/hour for 2-4 hours, and then reduce to 2-3 ml/kg/hour or less according to the clinical response.
- Reassess the clinical status and repeat the hematocrit. If the hematocrit remains the same or rises only minimally, continue with the same rate (2-3 ml/kg/hour) for another 2-4 hours. If the vital signs are worsening and hematocrit is rising rapidly, increase the rate to 5-10 ml/kg/hour for 1-2 hours. Reassess the clinical status, repeat the hematocrit and review fluid infusion rates accordingly.
- Give the minimum intravenous fluid volume required to maintain good perfusion and urine output of about 0.5 ml/kg/hr.
- Intravenous fluids are usually needed for only 24-48 hours. Reduce intravenous fluids gradually when urine output and/or oral fluid intake is/are adequate, or hematocrit is decreasing below the baseline value in a stable patient.
- Patients with warning signs should be monitored until the period of risk is over. A detailed fluid balance chart should be maintained. Parameters that should be monitored include:
  1. Vital signs and peripheral perfusion (1-4 hourly until the patient is out of the critical phase).
  2. Urine output (4-6 hourly).
  3. Hematocrit (before and after fluid replacement, then 6-12 hourly).
  4. Blood glucose and other organ functions (such as renal profile, liver profile, coagulation profile) as indicated.

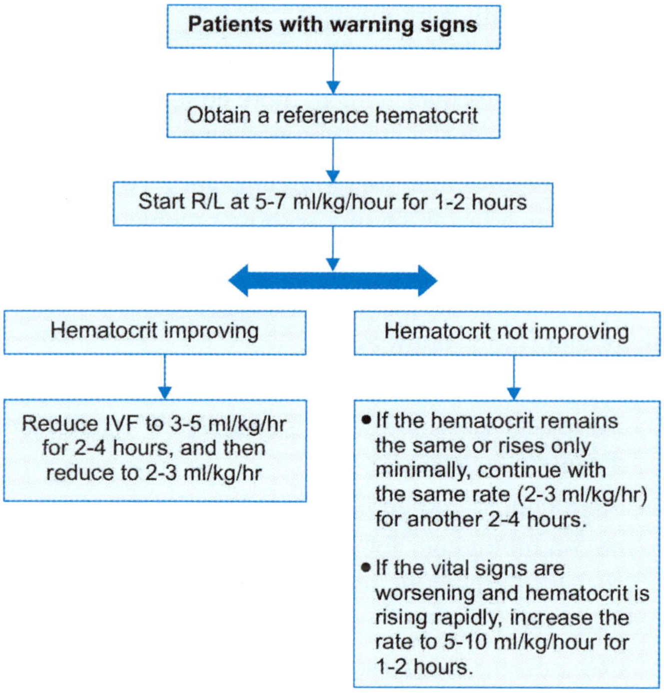

Fig. 11.26: Algorithm showing the management of dengue with warning signs

Severe Dengue (Dengue Hemorrhagic Fever, Dengue Shock Syndrome)

These patients require emergency treatment and urgent referral when they are in the critical phase of disease, i.e., when they have:

1. Dengue shock and/or fluid accumulation with respiratory distress.
2. Severe hemorrhage.
3. Severe organ impairment (hepatic damage, renal impairment, cardiomyopathy, encephalopathy or encephalitis).

All patients with severe dengue should be admitted to a hospital with access to intensive care facilities and blood transfusion.

Interventions

Judicious intravenous fluid resuscitation is the essential and usually the sole intervention required. The crystalloid solution used should be isotonic and the volume just sufficient to maintain an effective circulation during the period of plasma leakage.

Plasma losses should be replaced immediately and rapidly with isotonic crystalloid solution or, in the case of hypotensive shock, colloid solutions. If possible, hematocrit levels should be obtained before and after fluid resuscitation. For overweight or obese patients, the ideal body weight should be used for calculating fluid infusion rates.

Blood group determination and cross match should be done for all shock patients. Blood transfusion should be given only in cases with suspected/severe bleeding.

Goals of Fluid Resuscitation

1. Improving central and peripheral circulation (decreasing tachycardia, improving blood pressure and pulse volume, warm and pink extremities, and capillary refill time <2 seconds); and
2. Improving end-organ perfusion, i.e., stable conscious level (more alert or less restless), urine output > 0.5 ml/kg/hour decreasing metabolic acidosis.

Fluid Management in Cases with Compensated Shock

In cases where there is bleeding tendency, thrombocytopenia with rise of hematocrit but vital signs are stable fluid management is as follows:

Start intravenous fluid with a bolus 5-10 ml/kg of crystalloid (Sodium chloride/Ringers lactate) in 1 hour.

Reassess vital signs, capillary refill time, hematocrit, urine output. The next steps will on the situations as follows:

1. If condition of the child improves, intravenous fluids should be gradually reduced to 5-7 ml/kg/hour for 1–2 hours, then 3–5 ml/kg/hour for 2–4 hours, then 2–3 ml/kg/hour and then further depending on the hemodynamic status, which can be maintained upto 24–48 hours.
2. If vital signs are still unstable, check the hematocrit. If the hematocrit increases or is still high (>50%), repeat a second bolus of crystalloid solution at 10–20 ml/kg/hour for 1 hour.
3. After the second bolus, if there is improvement:
   (a) Reduce the rate to 7–10 ml/kg for 1–2 hours and then continue to reduce similarly as cited above.
   (b) If the hematocrit decreases (<40%) it indicates bleeding. It is an indication for blood cross match and transfusion.
   (c) Further boluses of crystalloid or colloid solutions may be needed to be given during the next 24–48 hours.

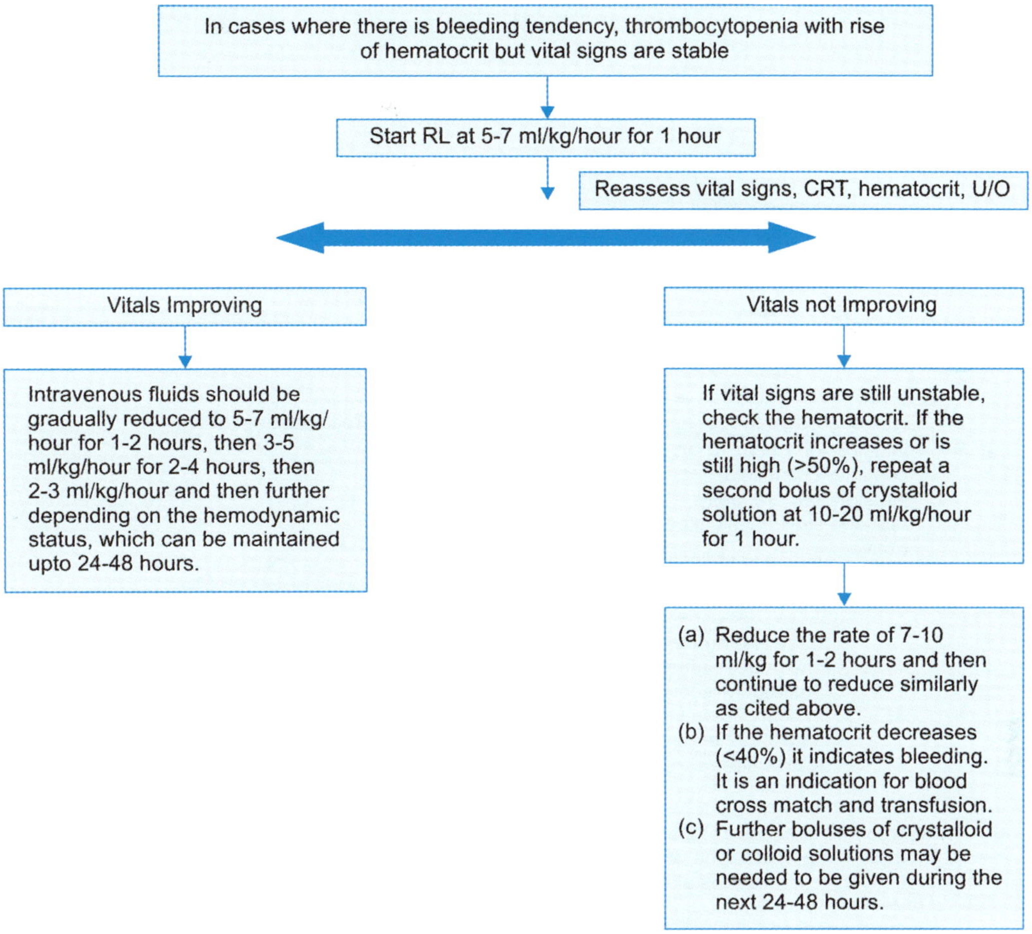

Fig. 11.27: Algorithm showing management of dengue with bleeding tendency

Treatment of Hypotensive Shock

The action plan for such patients is as follows:

1. Check the hematocrit before starting infusion. Initiate IV fluid resuscitation with crystalloid/colloid (if available) at 20 ml/kg as bolus over 15 minutes, to bring patient out of shock as early as possible.

   If the patient condition improves, give a crystalloid/colloid infusion for 1 hour. Then continue crystalloid infusion and gradually reduced similarly as cited above.

2. If the vital signs are still unstable (i.e., shock persists) recheck hematocrit.
   (a) If the base line hematocrit was low or post infusion hematocrit is low (<40%) it indicates bleeding and indicates need for blood transfusion as soon as possible.
   (b) If the hematocrit is high compared to the baseline hematocrit, change intravenous fluids to colloid solution at the rate of 10–20 ml/kg/hour for 1–2 hours; then change back to crystalloid and then reduce the rate of infusion similarly as cited above.

If the condition is unstable even after the second bolus. Repeat hematocrit after the second bolus.

(i) If the hematocrit decreases compared to the previous value (<40%), this indicates bleeding and need for blood transfusion.

(ii) If the hematocrit increases compared to the previous value or remains high (>50%) continue colloid solution at the rate of 10–20 ml/kg over 1 hour as the third bolus. After this dose, reduce the rate to 7–10 ml/kg/hour then change back to crystalloid and gradually reduce the rate of administration as cited earlier when patient's condition improves. These patients may need further bolus infusion titrated to the clinical response.

If the hematocrit decreases compared to the previous value (<40%), this indicates bleeding and the need to transfuse blood as soon as possible.

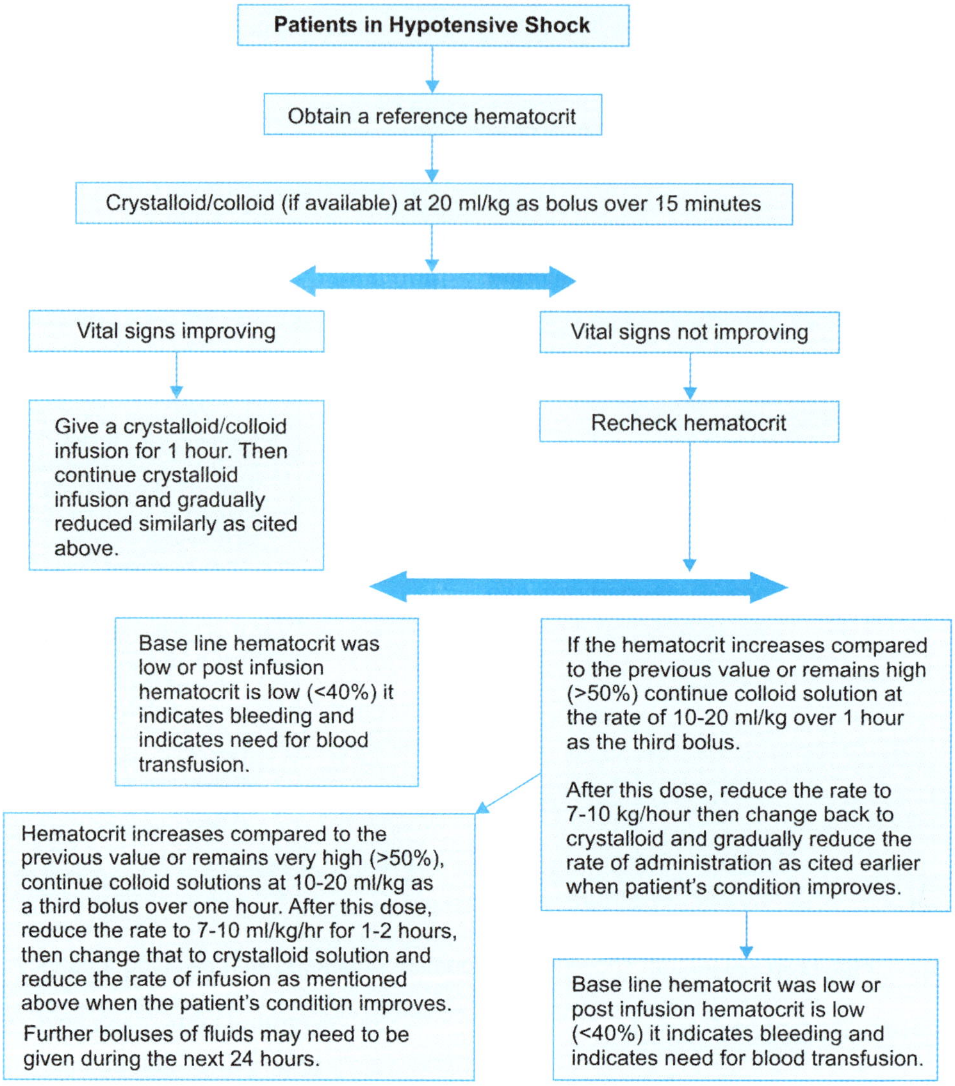

Fig. 11.28: Algorithm showing treatment of hypotensive shock

If the hematocrit increases compared to the previous value or remains very high (>50%), continue colloid solutions at 10-20 ml/kg as a third bolus over one hour. After this dose, reduce the rate to 7-10 ml/kg/hr for 1-2 hours, then change back to crystalloid solution and reduce the rate of infusion as mentioned above when the patient's condition improves.

Further boluses of fluids may need to be given during the next 24 hours. The rate and volume of each bolus infusion should be titrated to the clinical response**.**

Monitoring

Patients with severe dengue should be admitted to the high-dependency or intensive care area. Patients with dengue shock should be frequently monitored until the danger period is over.

1. A detailed fluid balance of all input and output should be maintained.
2. Parameters that should be monitored include vital signs and peripheral perfusion (every 15-30 minutes until the patient is out of shock, then 1-2 hourly). In general, the higher the fluid infusion rate, the more frequently the patient should be monitored and reviewed in order to avoid fluid overload while ensuring adequate volume replacement.
3. If resources are available, a patient with severe dengue should have an arterial line placed as soon as practical. The reason for this is that in shock states, estimation of blood pressure using a cuff is commonly inaccurate. The use of an indwelling arterial catheter allows for continuous and reproducible blood pressure

measurements and frequent blood sampling on which decisions regarding therapy can be based.

4. Monitoring of ECG and pulse oximetry should be available in the intensive care unit.
5. Urine output should be checked regularly (hourly till the patient is out of shock, then 1-2 hourly). A continuous bladder catheter enables close monitoring of urine output. An acceptable urine output would be =/> 0.5 ml/kg/hour.
6. Hematocrit should be monitored (before and after fluid boluses until stable, then 4-6 hourly).
7. Monitoring of arterial or venous blood gases, lactate, total carbon dioxide/bicarbonate (every 30 minutes to one hour until stable, then as indicated).
8. Blood glucose (before fluid resuscitation and repeat as indicated).
9. Other organ functions (such as renal profile, liver profile, coagulation profile, before resuscitation and as indicated).

Treatment of Hemorrhagic Complications

1. Mucosal bleeding in a stable patient or who remains stable with fluid resuscitation/replacement should be considered as minor. The bleeding usually improves rapidly during the recovery phase.
2. In patients with profound thrombocytopenia, strict bed rest and protection from trauma should be advised to reduce the risk of bleeding. No intramuscular injections should be given to avoid hematoma. Prophylactic platelet transfusions for severe thrombocytopenia in otherwise hemodynamically stable patients have not been shown to be effective and are not necessary.
3. If major bleeding occurs it is usually from the gastrointestinal tract, and/or vagina in adolescent females. Blood transfusion is life-saving and should be given as soon as severe bleeding is suspected or recognized. However, blood transfusion must be given with care because of the risk of fluid overload. Consider repeating the blood transfusion if there is further blood loss or no appropriate rise in hematocrit after blood transfusion.
4. The action plan for the treatment of hemorrhagic complications is as follows: Give 5-10 ml/kg of fresh-packed red cells or 10-20 ml/kg of fresh whole blood at an appropriate rate and observe the clinical response. It is important that fresh whole blood or fresh red cells are given.

Treatment of Other Complications

The treatment of other complications, viz. overhydration and ARDS, hypo and hyperglycemia, fluid and electrolyte and acid base disturbances should be done in the usual line.

Supportive Care and Adjuvant Therapy

Supportive care and adjuvant therapy may be necessary in severe dengue. This may include:

- Renal replacement therapy, with a preference to continuous veno-venous hemodialysis (CVVH), since peritoneal dialysis has a risk of bleeding.
- Vasopressor and inotropic therapies as temporary measures to prevent life threatening hypotension in dengue shock and during induction for intubation, while correction of intravascular volume is being vigorously carried out.
- Further treatment of organ impairment, such as severe hepatic involvement or encephalopathy or encephalitis.
- Treatment of cardiac abnormalities, such as conduction abnormalities that may occur usually not requiring interventions.
- There is little or no evidence in favour of use of steroids and intravenous immunoglobulins, or of recombinant Activated Factor VII.

Criteria for Discharge of Patients

- Absence of fever for at least 24 hours without the use of anti-fever therapy.
- Return of appetite.
- Visible clinical improvement.
- Good urine output.
- Minimum of 2/3 days after recovery from shock.
- No respiratory distress from pleural effusion or ascites.
- Platelet count > 50,000/cum.

Prognosis

Primary infections with dengue fever are usually self-limiting and benign. Dengue hemorrhagic fever with shock can have a mortality upto 40-50%. Survival is directly related to early and aggressive supportive treatment.

Prevention

Preventive measures primarily consist of avoiding mosquito bites by using mosquito nets, insecticides, and repellants, destroying mosquito (A. aegypti) breeding sites with malathion spray. Several vaccines are under development. However, the possibility exists that dengue vaccination may sensitize a recipient so that ensuing dengue infection could result in hemorrhagic fever.

Syphilis

Syphilis is a systemic communicable infection, once a very common disease is now exceedingly rare in developed countries. It is, however, still common in many parts of the developing world including India.

Etiology

It is caused by Treponema pallidum, a spirochete belonging to the family Spirochaetaceae.

Epidemiology

Two forms of syphilis are encountered in children: congenital and acquired. Congenital syphilis results from transplacental transmission of spirochetes. Transmission can occur at any stage of pregnancy. Pregnant women with primary and secondary syphilis and spirochetemia are more likely to transmit infection to fetus than are women with latent infection. The incidence of congenital infection in the offspring of untreated infected women remains highest during the first 4 years after acquisition of infection.

Acquired syphilis is transmitted almost exclusively by sexual contact. Less frequently it may be transmitted by transfusion of contaminated blood or direct contact with infected tissues.

Congenital Syphilis

Fetal or perinatal death occurs in around 40% affected infants. The survivors may not develop frank signs of the disease for weeks or even months. Syphilis is not a common cause of early abortion.

The manifestations of congenital syphilis have traditionally been divided into early and late.

Early Manifestations

The early manifestations appear during the first two years of life as a result of transplacental spirochetemia and are analogous to secondary stage of acquired syphilis. There is no lesion in congenital syphilis corresponding to primary stage of acquired syphilis. Approximately 60% of infected infants are asymptomatic at birth and are identified by routine perinatal screening. If the screened infants are left untreated, symptoms and signs develop within weeks or months.

The early manifestations result from multisystem involvement and are varied. These include variety of rashes, severe rhinitis (snuffles), moist lesions at the mucocutaneous junctions of mouth, anus and genitalia, painful pseudo paralysis of limbs and enlargement of liver, spleen and lymph nodes.

The *rash* may be scant or diffuse. It is reddish or maculopapular, sometimes bullous lesions, followed by desquamation involving the palms and soles ("washerwoman's skin"). The nails may be ridged and syphilitic paronychia may occur from finger sucking. The rash may disappear spontaneously but may recur a few weeks or months later. No permanent stigma remains from skin eruptions even if not treated.

Snuffles are one of the most characteristic manifestations. It is due to osteitis and osteochondritis of the nasal bones and cartilages. There is nasal obstruction with a purulent and blood stained discharge. The nasal discharge commonly excoriates the upper lip living fine scars. When the nasal osteitis heals, the collapse of the nasal bridge remains as the pathognomonic "saddle nose". A permanent stigma of the disease.

The *mucocutaneous lesions* about the mouth, anus and genitalia are moist and irritating. They produce fissures which heal with permanent scars ("rhagades") especially around the corners of the mouth and chin.

A painful *pseudo paresis* (Parrot's paralysis) may occur in one or more limbs due to bone changes resulting from osteochondritis and periostitis. This is a common presentation.

Rubbery discrete lymph node enlargement is common, and involvement of epitrochlear gland is especially characteristic. So also is hepato splenomegaly with jaundice.

Edema may be seen in severe cases, owing to hypoproteinaemia and sometimes to renal involvement (syphilitic nephrotic syndrome / nephritis). Coomb's negative hemolytic anemia is characteristic.

General features which may be present include failure to thrive, fever and increased susceptibility to bacterial infection.

Obvious *clinical signs of meningeal involvement* are uncommon. However, in many cases the CSF shows an increase cell count and protein, and positive serological tests. Therefore the CSF should be examined in all cases because acute meningovascular syphilis in early infancy has severe sequalae which include mental retardation, hydrocephalous and convulsions.

Radiological changes in the skeleton include multiple sites of osteochondritis (moth eaten appearance with separation of epiphyses) at the elbows, wrists, ankles and knees and periostitis (periosteal elevation) of several long bones and occasionally of skull bones.

Course of Early Syphilis

Untreated, early syphilis frequently subsides spontaneously, but T. pallidum persist in the tissues. The infant soon becomes noncontagious but the child may bear stigma of early syphilis viz. flat bridge of the nose, cranial bossing (Olympian brow), unilateral or bilateral thickening of the sternoclavicular portion of the clavicle, and rhagades. Other changes which were initiated early but take time to appear include the changes in the permanent teeth. Each permanent incisor may become notched (Hutchinson teeth) and the cusps of the first molar surface may appear squeezed (mulberry molar). Defects in enamel formation lead to repeated caries and eventual tooth destruction. The deciduous teeth are normal.

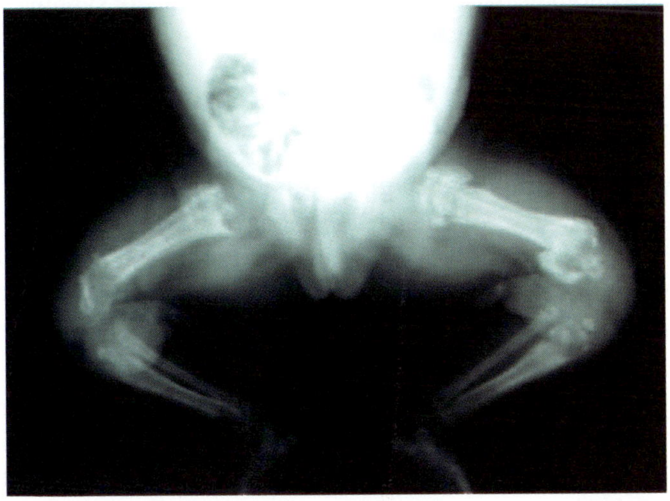

Fig. 11.29: Figure showing skeletal changes in congenital syphilis (osteochondritis, periostitis with periosteal elevation in long bones)

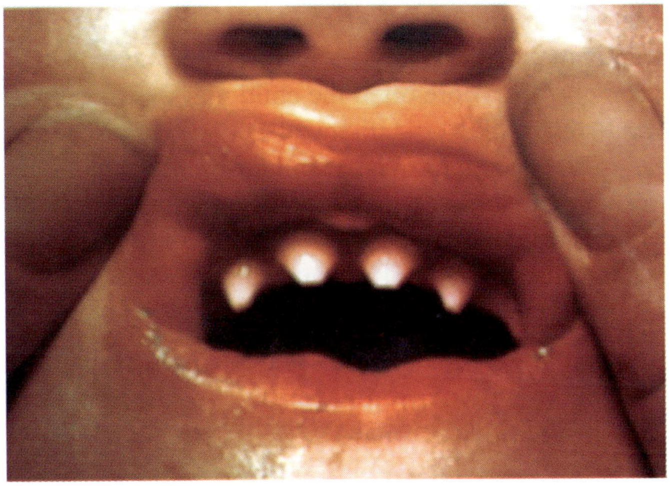

Fig. 11.30: Figure showing Hutchinson's teeth

Late Manifestations

The late manifestations include those signs which appear only after infancy. These signs may help diagnosis in children with no history early manifestation of infancy.

The classic *Hutchinson's triad* of late congenital syphilis consists of nerve deafness, interstitial keratitis and Hutchinson incisors. Nerve deafness due to involvement of the eighth nerve may be unilateral or bilateral and can appear at any age. Initially it presents as vertigo and high tone deafness and progresses to permanent deafness. Interstitial keratitis represents a hypersensitivity phenomenon. It may be unilateral or bilateral with symptoms viz. intense photophobia and lacrimation, followed within weeks or months by corneal opacification and complete blindness. The less common late ocular manifestations are choroiditis, retinitis, vascular occlusions and optic atrophy.

The *skeletal changes* include persistent or recurrent periostitis which causes thickening of the bone is best seen in the tibia where there is anterior curving of the shaft (Saber shin). Dactylitis may occur as a late manifestation. There may be unilateral or bilateral synovitis involving the joints of lower extremities (usually the knee) which presents as painless joint swelling with sterile synovial fluid (Clutton joint). Spontaneous recovery occurs after a period of several weeks. Gummas of the bones of the nose or palate may lead to destruction of the nasal bridge or to perforation of the palate.

A *latent meningovascular syphilitic infection* may abruptly manifest in prepubertal children by hemiplegia or convulsions. More often the child may present with mental retardation or anti-social behaviour. Juvenile paresis, an uncommon latent meningovascular infection, may present during adolescence with behavioural changes, focal seizure or loss of intellectual function. Juvenile tabes with involvement of the spinal cord and cardiovascular involvement with aortitis is extremely rare.

Paroxysmal hemoglobinuria is a rare late manifestation which is precipitated by exposure to cold and is a hypersensitivity phenomenon.

Laboratory Diagnosis

T. pallidum cannot be *cultured*. However, direct examination of the organism can be done by two methods: dark field microscopy and fluorescent microscopy. Dark field microscopy examination of scrapings from moist cutaneous and mucocutaneous lesions in early congenital syphilis is both sensitive and specific. Live organisms can be recognized by their cockscrew morphology and flexing hairpin motility. Fluorescent microscopy requires staining of the specimen with fluorescein labeled T. pallidum globulin and a fluorescent microscope. This method is not available in clinical practice.

Serologic Testing

Serologic testing is particularly helpful when the patient does not have any clinical lesions that can be microscopically evaluated or when antibiotic therapy has reduced the sensitivity of microscopy. There are two types of serologic essays: nonspecific non-treponemal assays and specific treponemal assays.

The two *non-treponemal tests* most widely used are the Venereal Disease Research Laboratory test (VDRL) and the rapid plasma reagin test (RPR). These tests are relatively inexpensive, easy to perform and sensitive making them useful for screening purposes. As they can be quantitated, they can be used to monitor response to therapy. Certain conditions such as autoimmune diseases may give false positive results in serum but not in CSF. However, false positive results are less common because of the introduction of purified cardiolipin-lecithin-cholesterol antigen. The serum usually becomes non-reactive in the nontreponemal tests within 1 year of adequate therapy of primary syphilis and within 2 years of secondary syphilis.

The specific *treponemal tests* which are often used include fluorescent treponemal antibody absorption test (FTA–ABS), T. pallidum immobilization test (TPI), the microhemagglutination assay for antibodies to T. pallidum (MHA–TP), and the hemagglutination treponemal test for syphilis (HATTS). These tests are very sensitive and specific but are relatively expensive, difficult to perform. Treponemal antibody titers become positive soon after initial infection and usually remain positive for life, even with adequate therapy. These antibody titers do not correlate with disease activity and are not quantified. They are useful for diagnosis of a first episode of syphilis and for distinguishing false positive results of nontreponemal antibody tests. They are of limited usefulness in the evaluation of response to therapy and possible reinfection.

Tests for IgM antibodies and PCR have been developed. These tests are relatively insensitive and are generally not available.

Gross and Microscopic Examination of the Placenta

Gross and microscopic examination of the placenta can be useful in diagnosis of congenital syphilis. The placenta is disproportionately large. Characteristic histological features include focal proliferative villitis, endovascular and perivascular arteritis and focal or diffuse immaturity of placental villi.

Diagnosis

The diagnosis of congenital syphilis depends on clinical judgement and appropriate use and evaluation of microscopic, serologic, radiologic and sometimes epidemiologic data. However, serologic testing for syphilis is the mainstay of screening and diagnosis.

Evaluation of the Newborn Born to a Seropositive Mother

A syphilitic mother can give birth to a clinically normal infant but the serological tests will be positive because of the presence of maternal IgG antibodies transferred from the mother across the placenta. Such passively acquired antibody is suggested by a raised neonatal titer less than four-fold compared to the maternal titer. This can be verified by the gradual decline in antibody titer in the infant, usually becoming undetectable by 3–6 months age.

If the maternal treatment was adequate and given at one month or before one month of delivery, a positive VDRL test represents passively acquired antibody and the infant does not require treatment at delivery. Follow-up serology should be advised till nontreponemal serology (VDRL) is negative. If the mother's evaluation is incomplete, these infants must be assumed to be infected and treated.

Infants symptomatic at birth should be thoroughly evaluated and treated. Asymptomatic infants considered at risk of congenital syphilis because of maternal seropositivity should be evaluated. A VDRL titer four-fold greater than the mother's titer indicates an infection in the infant.

Diagnosis of neurosyphilis is difficult because of the poor sensitivity of the CSF VDRL and lack of CSF changes in the newborn period. It is now accepted that all infants with presumptive diagnosis of congenital syphilis should be treated with regimens effective for neurosyphilis because it cannot be properly excluded.

Treatment

Penicillin remains the drug of choice because T. pallidum is extremely sensitive to penicillin and there is no evidence of emerging penicillin resistance. Even in patients allergic to penicillin, desensitization followed by standard penicillin therapy is considered the most reliable strategy.

Current recommendations include regimens of aqueous penicillin G (100,000–150,000 units / kg / day in two divided doses at 12 hourly interval IV for the first week of life and 8 hourly thereafter) or procaine penicillin G, (50,000 units/kg IM once daily) for 10 days. Both penicillin regimens are recognized as adequate therapy. However, higher concentration of penicillin is achieved in the CSF with IV aqueous penicillin than with IM procaine penicillin.

Treated infants should be followed up serologically to confirm decreasing nontreponemal antibody titers. Reversion to negative requires some months. Radiographic skeletal changes, especially those of the periosteum, may not disappear for a long time.

An acute febrile reaction, the Jarisch-Herxheimer reaction, with exacerbation of lesions can occur in 15–20% cases treated with penicillin. It is not an indication for discontinuation of penicillin therapy.

Acquired Syphilis

Infants, children and adolescents may acquire the infection from an adult.

Clinical Manifestations

The clinical manifestation depends on the stage of the disease. The *primary stage* is characterized by a chancre and adjacent regional lymphadenitis. The chancre is a painless papule which appears at the site of inoculation after 2–6 weeks of contact. The papule soon develops into a clean, painless ulcer with raised borders. The chancre contains viable T. pallidum and is highly contagious. Usually seen on the genitals but may be seen in other areas (anus, face, lips, mouth etc) depending on the site of initial inoculation. The chancre heals spontaneously within 4–6 weeks leaving a thin scar. It should be noted that a detectable chancre is not common in children. The condition comes to medical attention only when manifestations of secondary stage appear.

If untreated, the patient develops manifestations of secondary syphilis 2–10 weeks after the chancre heals. The manifestations of *secondary syphilis* include a rash, condylomata, flu like illness, and generalized lymphadenopathy. The rash is nonpruritic maculopapular or sometimes pustular which can cover the whole body including the palms and soles. The condylomata occur in the moist areas around the anus and vagina. They are grey white to erythematous wart like plaques. A flu like illness with low grade fever, headache, malaise, anorexia, weight loss, sore throat myalgia and arthralgia is often present. Around 30% cases may present with asymptomatic meningitis with CSF pleocytosis and elevated protein level. Secondary infection becomes latent within 1–2 months after the onset of rash. Relapses with secondary manifestation can be seen during the first year of latency. This is followed by the tertiary stage which may be asymptomatic or symptomatic. The symptoms of tertiary stage include neurologic, cardiovascular and gummatous lesions.

Laboratory Diagnosis

Same as in congenital syphilis. The diagnosis of neurosyphilis in acquired syphilis is made by demonstrating pleocytosis and increased protein in CSF and a positive CSF VDRL along with neurological symptom.

Treatment

Primary, secondary and early latent syphilis can be treated with a single dose of benzathene penicillin G (50,000 units/kg deep IM; maximum upto 2.4 million units). Non-pregnant penicillin sensitive women and penicillin sensitive patients without neurosyphilis can be treated with Doxycycline (100 mg per oral12 hourly for 2 weeks) or Tetracycline (500 mg 6 hourly per oral for 2 weeks).

All HIV infected persons should have a CSF analysis before starting treatment as they are prone to develop neurosyphilis. The CDC guidelines recommend the same treatment schedule as for the non-HIV infected patients.

Leptospirosis

Leptospirosis, an infectious disease that affects humans and animals is considered the most common zoonosis in the world. The disease was first described in 1812, among Napoleon's troops and was known as bilious typhoid in Europe throughout the 19th century. In 1986, Adolph Weil described the clinical manifestations as severe jaundice, fever and hemorrhage with renal involvement and hence later known as Weil's disease.

Etiology

Leptospirosis is caused by spirochetes of genus Leptospira. They are finely coiled, thin, and long with a terminal hook at one or both ends. They can be visualized by dark field microscopy and by silver staining. They are slow growing organisms and can be cultured in liquid media. Although all serotypes are potentially pathogenic to human, most human infections seem to be due to L. icterohemorhagica, L. canicola and L. pomona.

Epidemiology

Leptospirosis occurs worldwide but more common in the tropical and subtropical developing countries. The rat is the principal source of human infection although leptospires can infect many species of animals including pets and livestock. The majority of human infection results from occupational exposure to water or soil contaminated with rat urine. In western countries, the major animal reservoir is dog and contact with spirochetes is often associated with recreational activities that result in contact with contaminated soil or water. Transmission *via* animal bites and directly from person to person, is rare but has been reported.

Pathogenesis

Leptospires enter humans through abrasions and cuts in the skin or through mucous membranes. After entry they circulate in the blood stream and spread to all the organs in the body. The primary lesion caused by leptospires is damage to the endothelial lining of the small blood vessels resulting in ischemic damage to the liver, kidneys, meninges and muscles.

Two phases of the disease has been described: septicemic phase and immune phase. The *septicemic phase* begins after an incubation period of 7–12 days. In this phase leptospires can be isolated from blood, CSF and other tissues. This phase lasts for 2–7 days to be followed by a brief period of well being followed by the *symptomatic or immune phase*. This phase is associated with appearance of circulating antibody, the disappearance of organisms from blood and CSF, and localization of leptospires in the tissues resulting in localized symptoms and signs. This phase may last for several weeks.

Clinical Manifestations

Most of the cases of human leptospirosis are subclinical or very mild. Symptomatic infection may present as an acute febrile illness with non-specific clinical features in 70% cases, as aseptic meningitis in 20% and as hepatorenal dysfunction in 10%.

In general, leptospirosis occurs as two recognizable syndromes: anicteric leptospirosis and icteric leptospirosis. In both types onset is sudden and the illness tends to follow a biphasic course: a septicemic phase and immune phase.

Anicteric Leptospirosis

The *septicemic phase* is typically characterized by sudden onset of fever, shaking chills, lethargy, severe headache malaise, nausea, vomiting and severe myalgia.

The important physical findings include severe muscle tenderness especially involving the lower limb muscles, lumbosacral region and abdomen, conjunctival suffusion with photophobia and orbital pain, generalized lymphadenopathy and hepatosplenomegaly.

Some patients have bradycardia and hypotension but circulatory collapse is uncommon. During this phase leptospires can be isolated from the blood, CSF as well as urine.

The *immune phase* starts after a brief asymptomatic period. It is characterized by recurrence of fever, a transient truncal rash lasting for less than 24 hours, aseptic meningitis, and unilateral or bilateral self limiting uveitis. Although abnormal CSF findings can be found in 80% cases frank signs of meningitis can be found in only 50% cases. The CSF findings include modest rise of pressure, increase in total cells (not > 500 cells/mm^3) with initial increase in polymorphonuclear leucocytes followed by increase in mononuclear cells, normal or slightly elevated protein and normal glucose. Symptoms of CNS involvement resolve spontaneously within about a week with almost no mortality.

The leptospires, in this phase is present in the urine only.

Icteric Leptospirosis (Weil Syndrome)

Icteric leptospirosis is a severe form and occurs in less than 10% cases. It is less common in children.

The *septicemic phase* is characterized by the same manifestations as in the anicteric type.

The *immune phase* is characterized by liver and renal dysfunction. In fulminating cases there may be hemorrhagic phenomena and cardiovascular collapse.

Features of hepatic dysfunction include hepatomegaly and pain in the right upper abdomen, hyperbilirubinemia (direct and indirect) and modest elevation of enzyme. The liver function returns to normal after recovery.

Renal involvement is common. Acute renal failure is the principal cause of death. Features include oliguria, anuria, and hematuria. All patients have findings on urine analysis (viz. hematuria, proteinuria and casts) and azotemia.

ECG findings of myocarditis are present but congestive cardiac failure is uncommon.

Hemorrhagic manifestations are rare but when present include epistaxis, hemoptysis and GI and adrenal hemorrhage. Transient thrombocytopenia may occur.

Laboratory Diagnosis

The diagnosis is established by serologic tests and by isolation of the organism from blood, CSF and urine.

Serologic tests are the frequently used diagnostic tests. The reference serological test is the microscopic agglutination test. This test is read by dark field microscopy for agglutination and titers are determined. A four-fold or greater rise in titer in paired acute and convalescent sera confirms the diagnosis. Agglutinins usually appear by the 12th day of illness and reach a maximum titer by the third week. Low titers may persist for years. ELISA methods, including an IgM specific dot–ELISA test have also been developed.

Identification of the leptospires in infected tissue and body fluids can be done by Warthin-Starry silver staining, immunofluorescent and immunohistochemical methods as well as by phase-contrast or dark field microscopy. These are insensitive methods.

Leptospires can be easily cultured on commercially available media containing rabbit or bovine serum albumin and long chain fatty acids. Leptospires can be recovered from blood (in the first week), CSF (during the first 10 days) and from urine (after the second week). The number of leptospires is small and their growth rate is slow; hence prolonged incubation is required. Cultures may not become positive for 2–4 months.

Diagnosis

Leptospirosis should be considered in the differential diagnosis of any acute febrile illness when there is history of direct contact with animals or with soil or water contaminated with animal urine and the onset is abrupt with chills, severe myalgia, conjunctival suffusion, headache, and nausea and vomiting.

Treatment

Initiation of treatment within 7 days of onset probably shortens the clinical course and decreases the severity of the infection. The two drugs commonly used are Penicillin G (6–8 million units/m^2/day in divided doses IV 4 hourly for 7 days) is the drug of choice. In penicillin sensitive cases and children over 8 years, tetracycline (10–20 mg/kg/day in divided doses 6 hourly per oral/IV is an alternative).

Suggested Reading

1. Pediatric Infectious Diseases. Editors D.Engelhard, M.I. Marks, D.Branski, 1st edition, 1993, Reprints 1997. Published by S. Karger, AG, and P.O. Box No. CH – 4009, Basel (Switzerland).
2. Manson's Tropical Diseases, edited by Gordon C. Cook and Alimuddin Zumla, 21st edition 2003.
3. Diseases of children in tropics and subtropics edited by DB Jelliffe and J.P. Stanfield. Third ELBS edition, 1978, Great Britain.
4. Nelson Textbook of Pediatrics, 10th edition, 1975. Published by W.B. Saunders Company, Philadelphia.
5. Nelson Textbook of Pediatrics, 17th edition, 2004. Published by Saunders, Philadelphia.
6. Practical Pediatric Problems, 6th edition, 1986. Published by PG Publishing Pvt. Ltd., 304 Orchard Road, Singapore.
7. Price's Textbook of the Practice of Medicine. Edited by Sir Ronald Bodley Scoot. Eleventh ELBS edition, 1973, Great Britain.
8. Essentials of Tuberculosis in Children, 3rd edition, 2006. Published by Jaypee Brothers Medical Publishers (P) Ltd., New Delhi-110002.
9. RTI Facts. IAP Action Plan 2006. IAP consensus guidelines on rational management of respiratory tract infections in children.
10. Consensus statement of Childhood Tuberculosis. Working group on Tuberculosis, Indian Academy of Pediatrics (IAP). Indian Pediatrics 2010, vol 47, Pages 41–55.
11. Dengue guidelines: Treatment, prevention and control (WHO 2009).
12. Textbook of Pediatric Infectious Diseases. Feigin, Cherry, Demmler-Harrison, Kaplan, 6th edition, 2009. Reprinted in India 2011, Saunders.

12

Nephrology

OUTLINES

Proteinuria

Proteinuria may be present in normal children. Albumin represents the largest fraction (< 30 mg/24 hours). The remainder of normal urinary protein is Tamm–Horsfall protein, a mucoprotein of unknown function produced in the distal tubule.

In normal infants and children, the concentration of protein in urine is less than 20 mg/dl. The volume of urine depends on fluid intake and on the concentrating ability of the kidney. Accordingly, when a given quantity of protein is excreted per unit time, the urine protein concentration will vary with the dilution of the urine. For this reason, if proteinuria in excess of 20–30 mg/dl is detected, the total quantity of protein excreted over 24 hours should be measured. The upper limit of normal protein excretion in healthy children is 150 mg/24 hours.

Definition

The term proteinuria should apply only when the total daily excretion of protein excretion exceeds 150 mg. More specifically, normal protein excretion in children is less than or equal to 4 mg/sq m/hour. Abnormal proteinuria is defined as urinary protein excretion between 4–40 mg/sq m/hour. Nephrotic range of proteinuria is defined as more than 40 mg/sq m/hour.

Determination of urine protein/creatinine (Upr mg/dl/Ucr mg/dl) ratio on a random urine sample is an alternative to quantitative estimation of protein in urine. A ratio less than 0.5 in children younger than 2 years of age and less than 0.2 in children 2 years or older suggest normal protein excretion. A ratio greater than 3 suggests nephrotic range proteinuria. Upr/Ucr ratios have been shown to have a high correlation with 24 hours protein excretion. It can be used when 24 hours urine collection is not practical.

Classification

Proteinuria may be transient or persistent.

In *transient proteinuria*, the excessive protein excretion is apparently not the result of a diseased state. It is never associated with edema. The proteinuria does not exceed 2 + on the dipstick and is less than 1 gm/24 hr. The mechanism of transient proteinuria is not known. Febrile proteinuria is considered benign if it resolves when the fever subsides. Benign exercise induced proteinuria resolves after 48 hours of rest. A child with transient proteinuria does not need evaluation.

Proteinuria is said to be *persistent* when it is present on 4 separate occasions. If persistent proteinuria is present in both supine and upright position it is called fixed proteinuria. It may be caused by either glomerular or tubular disorders.

Glomerular and Tubular Proteinuria

Proteinuria following glomerular disorders is a result of increased permeability of glomerular capillary wall. Glomerular proteinuria may range from less than 1 gm to more than 30 grams/24 hours. It may be selective i.e. loss of plasma protein of molecular weight upto and including albumin or nonselective i.e. loss of albumin as well as larger molecular proteins e.g. IgG. Glomerular proteinuria should be suspected in any patient with proteinuria > 1 gm/24 hours or is associated with hypertension, hematuria, or renal dysfunction.

Proteinuria following tubular disorders is a result of injury to proximal tubules which result in diminished reabsorptive capacity and the loss of low molecular weight proteins in urine. Tubular proteinuria is low grade fixed proteinuria usually <1 gram/24 hours. It may be associated with other defects of proximal tubular function such as glycosuria, phosphaturia, aminoaciduria etc. Tubular proteinuria is rarely a diagnostic problem because the underlying disease is usually detected before the proteinuria.

Causes of Proteinuria

Transient Proteinuria

1. Fever > 38.3°C (101°F)
2. Exercise
3. Dehydration
4. Exposure to cold
5. Seizure
6. Congestive cardiac failure
7. Stress

Persistent Proteinuria

1. Glomerular causes
   a. Acute post infectious glomerulonephritis
   b. Focal segmental glomerulosclerosis
   c. Mesangial proliferative glomerulonephritis
   d. Membranous nephropathy
   e. Membrano proliferative glomerulonephritis
   f. Lupus nephritis
   g. IgA nephropathy
   h. Henoch-Schönlein purpura nephritis
   i. Amyloidosis
   j. Diabetic nephropathy
   k. Sickle cell nephropathy
   l. Alport's syndrome
2. Tubular diseases
   a. Hereditary
      i. Proximal renal tubular acidosis
      ii. Cystinosis
      iii. Wilson's disease
      iv. Galactosemia
      v. Lowe syndrome
   b. Acquired
      i. Interstitial nephritis
      ii. Acute tubular necrosis
      iii. Heavy metal poisoning (mercury, lead, copper, chromium, cadmium, gold)
      iv. Antibiotics

Laboratory Evaluation of a Case Presenting with Persistent Fixed Proteinuria

A *detailed history* with particular importance to presence of hematuria, edema, urinary symptoms like dysuria, frequency, and intake of medicines and family history of renal disease should be taken. The important *physical examinations* include confirmation of edema, accurate measurement of blood pressure, and assessment of hearing and ophthalmologic examination. The *laboratory evaluation* should include the following investigations: urine analysis and culture, 24 hours urinary protein and creatinine, serum creatinine, serum protein and fractions and serum cholesterol, serum C 3 level, hepatitis B surface antigen and a renal USG. Renal biopsy is indicated when there is increasing proteinuria in excess of 1 gram/24 hours and/or development of hematuria, hypertension or renal dysfunction.

Hematuria

Hematuria is defined as the presence of atleast 5 red blood cells per high power field in the sediment of a 10 ml centrifuged fresh specimen of urine. However, when the hematuria is of clinical importance, many times this number of RBCs is usually seen.

Types of Hematuria

Hematuria may be gross or macroscopic when the urine has a reddish or brown colour due to the presence of RBCs, free hemoglobin as a result of hemolysis of excreted RBCs.

The term microscopic hematuria is used when the colour of the urine is normal and hematuria is detected only by microscopic examination or dipstick. Only microscopic hematuria does not necessarily represent a disorder of the kidney or urinary tract. Microscopic hematuria may occur following strenuous exercise and with a variety of intercurrent unrelated conditions viz. viral or bacterial respiratory tract infection, any febrile disorder, gastroenteritis with dehydration, contamination by red blood cells from external genitalia e.g. a meatal ulcer or menstrual blood.

If proteinuria is also present, the hematuria is usually clinically important and probably has a renal source. If casts are present, the source of hematuria must be the kidney. The association of both proteinuria and tubular casts with hematuria is evidence that the hematuria is most likely the result of a glomerular disorder.

Source of Bleeding

Blood appearing at the beginning of the urinary stream indicates a lower urinary tract cause while uniform staining throughout the stream points to a cause higher up. Terminal hematuria is typical of severe bladder irritation by stone or by infection. Upper urinary tract sources of hematuria originate from the nephron (i.e. glomerulus, convoluted/collecting tubules and interstitium). Lower urinary tract sources originate from the pelvicalyceal system, ureter, bladder or urethra.

Brown or tea coloured urine is more likely to be of renal source. Bright red urine with or without clots suggest an extra renal or lower urinary tract source of bleeding.

Glomerulus and Extraglomerulus Hematuria

Hematuria from within the glomerulus is frequently associated with brown, or cola coloured urine, proteinuria > 100 mg/dl, RBC cast and deformed RBC in urine. Hematuria originating from the tubules may be associated with the presence of leucocytes or epithelial casts.

Lower urinary tract bleeding is associated with gross hematuria, terminal hematuria, blood clots, minimal proteinuria (i.e. < 100 mg/dl) and normal urinary RBC morphology.

Causes of Red Coloured Urine Without RBCs

Red coloured urine without RBCs may be heme positive or heme negative. Heme positive urine without RBCs is caused by the presence of hemoglobin or myoglobin. Hemoglobinuria without hematuria may occur in the presence of hemolytic anemia and myoglobinuria without hematuria occurs in presence of rhabdomyolysis. Rhabdomyolysis may occur secondary to viral disease, crush injury, severe electrolyte abnormalities (hypernatremia, hypophosphatemia), hypotension, disseminated intravascular coagulation and prolonged seizure.

Heme negative red coloured urine without RBCs may appear red, cola coloured or burgundy which may result from ingestion of drugs or food dyes. Dark brown or black coloured urine may result from various urinary metabolites.

The drugs responsible are rifampicin, phenolphthalein, pyridium, salicylates, ibubrufen, metronidazole, nitrofurantoin, phenothiazines, chloroquine, sulphasalazine, desferrioxamine. The metabolites include homogentisic acid, melanin, methemoglobin, porphyrin, urates.

Common Causes of Hematuria in Children

1. Urinary tract infection viz. pyelonephritis, cystitis, urethritis.
2. Meatal stenosis.
3. Perineal irritation.
4. Trauma.
5. Urolithiasis.
6. Crystalluria viz. calcium, oxalate, uric acid.
7. Coagulopathy.
8. Tumours viz. Wilms', rhabdomyosarcoma.
9. Glomerular causes: IgA nephropathy, Non-MCNS, Alport syndrome, post infectious glomerulonephritis, Henoch-Schönlein purpura (HSP), Hemolytic uremic syndrome (HUS), Sickle cell glomerulopathy, and systemic lupus erythematosus (SLE).
10. Congenital abnormalities viz. hydronephrosis, polycystic kidneys.

The most common cause of gross hematuria is urinary tract infection. Less than 10% have evidences of glomerulonephritis. Recurrent episodes of gross hematuria suggest IgA nephropathy, Alport syndrome, Hypercalciuria/Urolithiasis and thin glomerular basement membrane disease. In a child with gross hematuria, the entity urethrorrhagia should be excluded. Urethrorrhagia refers to urethral bleeding in absence of urine, associated with dysuria and blood spots on underwear after voiding. This condition, which often occurs in pre-pubertal boys at intervals of several months for several years, is a benign condition with a self limiting course.

Clinical Evaluation

Patients with hematuria usually present with associated features suggestive of specific disorders related to upper or lower urinary tract, glomerular or extraglomerular. Tea or cola coloured urine with facial/body edema, hypertension and oliguria suggest glomerular disease. High fever and loin pain suggest an upper urinary tract and frequency, dysuria suggest a lower urinary tract infection. Renal colic suggests nephrolithiasis. Hematuria with a recent history of upper respiratory, skin or gastrointestinal infection suggest post infectious glomerulonephritis, HUS or HSP. Presence of joint pain or rash point towards SLE or HSP.

Physical findings can be pointers to a specific disease. For example presence of edema, hypertension, and signs of heart failure suggest acute glomerulonephritis. Abdominal masses may be caused by posterior urethral valves, hydronephrosis, and polycystic kidneys. Presence of anatomic abnormalities of the external genitalia may be associated with renal disease.

Laboratory Diagnosis

A Child with Asymptomatic Isolated Microscopic Hematuria

Asymptomatic patients with isolated microscopic hematuria should not undergo laboratory evaluation until atleast 2 additional urine specimens collected over 2 weeks period demonstrate an abnormal number of RBCs. If a child is found to have persistent asymptomatic hematuria of greater than 2 weeks duration the following laboratory investigation should be done step by step:

1. *Urine culture:* If urine culture is negative then the following should be done.
2. Urine for calcium and creatinine.
3. A sickle cell screen.
4. USG of kidney, ureter and urinary bladder (KUB) to rule out structural lesion.
5. Serum creatinine and electrolytes if the initial studies are normal.

Children with persistent asymptomatic isolated hematuria and normal laboratory evaluation should have their serum creatinine values checked annually and blood pressure and urine checked every 3 months until hematuria resolves. The diagnoses to be considered in such cases include resolving post infectious glomerulonephritis, IgA nephropathy, thin basement membrane disease, heavy exercise or trauma.

A Child with Glomerular Hematuria

A child with clinical features of glomerular disease should be subjected to the following lab investigations:

1. Urine for routine examination.
2. Complete blood count with differential count.
3. 24 hours urine total protein, and creatinine clearance.
4. Serum protein and fractions, serum cholesterol.
5. Serum C_3 level.
6. ASO/Anti-DNase B titre.
7. Anti nuclear antibody titre.
8. Throat/skin culture if indicated.

A Child with Extraglomerular Hematuria

The child with no clinical features of glomerular disease should have a urine culture done as the first step. If the urine culture is negative then the following initial investigations should be done as the next step:

1. Urine calcium and creatinine.
2. Sickle cell screen.
3. Ultrasound of kidney, ureter and bladder.
4. Urinalysis of parents and siblings.
5. Serum electrolytes, creatinine and calcium.
6. MCU, Renal scan, cystogram if there is hydronephrosis/pyelocaliectasis on USG.
7. 24 hours urinary calcium, creatinine, uric acid, oxalate if there is crystalluria, urolithiasis, or nephrocalcinosis.

Acute Glomerulonephritis (AGN)

Acute glomerulonephritis includes a number of distinct entities where in some, the glomerulus is primarily affected while in others, renal involvement is only one manifestation of a systemic disorder. It is characterized by a relatively abrupt onset of variable degrees of hematuria, edema, hypertension, oliguria along with diminished GFR, fluid and salt retension and circulatory congestion.

Etiology of Glomerulonephritis

Post streptococcal
a. Acute post streptococcal glomerulonephritis.
Non-post streptococcal
a. Acute glomerulonephritis due to other bacterial infection viz. Gr. C beta hemolytic streptococci, Streptococcus pneumoniae, Staphylococci, Klebsiella pneumonae, Meningococci, Salmonella.
b. AGN due to viral infection viz. Measles, Varicella, Mumps, Hepatitis B and C, cytomegalovirus, infectious mononucleosis and HIV.
c. AGN due to spirochetes: Leptospirosis, Treponema pallidum.
d. AGN due to parasites: P. falciparum, Toxoplasmosis.
e. Secondary to SLE, Infective endocarditis, Infected shunts for hydrocephalus, Henoch-Schönlein purpura, HUS.
f. Acute exacerbation of chronic renal failure.

Common Clinical and Laboratory Abnormalities of AGN

The clinical and laboratory abnormalities of the various types of acute glomerulonephritides may range from minimal to severe. The features include:

Clinical

1. Oliguria with urine volume less than 180/sqm/24 hours.
2. Edema, usually minimal, seldom massive.
3. Hematuria with urine color smoky, brownish red to tea colored.
4. Hypertension and circulatory congestion, common to most forms of AGN.

Laboratory

1. Urine examination: Characteristically contains:
   a. Proteinuria which varies from moderate to nephrotic range.
   b. Red blood cells, WBC and mixed granular and RBC casts.
2. Azotemia, elevated S. creatinine, phosphorous and uric acid, depressed serum calcium.
3. Mild normochromic anemia.
4. Electrolytes acid base disturbances viz hyperkalemia, hyponatremia and acidosis.

Features to Suggest AGN Due to Causes Other than APSGN

1. Presence of varying degrees of nonspecific general symptomatology.
2. Presence of clinical features of the primary disease viz. arthritis, rash, purpura, hepatomegaly.
3. Normal C_3 level.

Features to Suggest Acute Exacerbation of Chronic Glomerulonephritis

1. Presence of prior history of renal symptoms viz. hypertension, urinary abnormalities.
2. Onset of AGN after a short latent period of 1–4 days.
3. Presence of stunting, severe anemia at the onset.
4. Presence of azotemia disproportionate to clinical findings.
5. A nephrotic presentation of AGN with C_3 levels failing to return to normal by 4–6 weeks.

Acute Post Streptococcal Glomerulonephritis (APSGN)

APSGN is an acute, specific, self-limiting glomerulonephritis which follows a pharyngeal or cutaneous infection (Impetigo) with a nephritogenic strain of Group A beta hemolytic streptococci. It is the most common form of acute glomerulonephritis in children. It is characterized by sudden onset of gross hematuria, edema, hypertension and renal insufficiency.

Etiology

The precipitating event is a streptococcal infection of the upper respiratory tract or the skin. The overall attack rate of nephritis in patients with either pharyngitis or impetigo is 10–15%. Subclinical episodes occur 4–10 times more frequently than overt clinical disease. Microscopic hematuria is the most common abnormal urinary finding in asymptomatic contacts.

The clinical presentation of nephritis is the same following infection at either sites but there are a number of differences including the serotype and antibody response. Only certain serotypes of Gr. A beta hemolytic streptococci characterized by either M or T antigen, cause APSGN. The factors that allow only certain strains of streptococci to be nephritogenic are unclear. The most common pharyngeal and skin streptococci are M types 12 and 49 respectively. The serum antibodies to streptococcal diphosphopyridine nucleotidase (DPNase) and to a lesser extent to streptococcal deoxyribonucleic B (anti-DNase B) and anti-streptolysin O (ASO) are usually present in nephritis after pharyngeal infection. In nephritis following skin infection, a significant increase of anti-DNase B or antihyaluronidase response is seen. Accordingly, the anti-DPNase test is confirmatory for pharyngeal infection while anti-DNase B tests for skin infection.

Epidemiology

Although the clinical presentation is same, there are number of differences in the epidemiology between APSGN following pharyngitis and impetigo.

Table 12.1 : The epidemiological differences

Features	*APSGN following pharyngitis*	*APSGN following impetigo*
1. Climate	Temperate or cold climates	Tropical or hot climate
2. Season	Winter and spring	Late summer, early fall
3. Age	5–15 years	3–5 years
4. Sex	M: F = 2:1	Equal
5. Latent period	9–11 days	3 weeks or longer.

Pathogenesis

The morphologic findings and a depression in the serum complement (C_3) level strongly suggest that post streptococcal glomerulonephritis is mediated by immune complexes. However, the exact mechanism by which nephritogenic streptococci induce complex formation is yet to be determined. It is likely that the immune complexes are formed in situ. Nephritogenic antigens derived from streptococci may bind directly to sub-epithelial glomerular sites. Antibodies formed against these antigens combine and result in an inflammatory response, leading to activation of complement (both classical and alternative pathway), infiltration of neutrophils, and proliferation of glomerular cells and expansion of mesangial matrix.

Pathology

As in most forms of AGN, the kidneys are bilaterally enlarged.

On *light microscopy*, all glomeruli appear enlarged and relatively blood less and show diffuse mesangial cell proliferation with an increase in mesangial matrix. There is infiltration of polymorphonuclear leucocytes in the glomeruli in the early stages. In severe cases crescents and interstitial inflammation may be seen.

Immunofluorescence microscopy shows deposits of immunoglobulin and complement on the glomerular basement membrane (GBM) and in the mesangium.

On *electron microscopy*, electron dense deposits are seen on the epithelial side of the GBM.

Clinical Manifestations

The common age group is between 5–15 years in case of throat infection and 3–5 years in case of impetigo. It is rare below the age of 3 years. In most cases, the clinical pattern is fairly characteristic. The cardinal features are abrupt onset of edema, hematuria and oliguria which occurs after a latent period of around 2 weeks (in case of pharyngitis) and around 3 weeks (in case of impetigo). Development of features of AGN within 1–4 days of onset of streptococcal infection suggests a pre-existing glomerulonephritis.

Edema starts in the face, particularly in the periorbital area, more prominent in the morning hours. It is followed by edema of the ankle. As edema is dependent it is shifting in nature. It is minimal and hence turgid.

Hematuria: Microscopic hematuria is present in all children and presents with a smoky colored urine. Gross hematuria with tea or red colored urine may be present in 30–50% cases. Gross hematuria usually clears within 7 days but microscopic hematuria may persist upto 4–8 weeks.

Oliguria: There is abrupt onset of decreased urinary output which gradually increases by 4–10 days

General symptoms, which are less common, include irritability, general malaise, low grade fever and flank or midline abdominal pain.

Other features may include:

Acute hypertension with symptoms viz. headache, vomiting, somnolence. Hypertension may be mild to severe, often with a biphasic character. The first phase lasts for the initial 3–5 days and is of severe degree followed by a brief period of 2–5 days when pressure elevation is less marked. This is followed by a less severe but more persistent blood pressure elevation which may last for an additional period of 1–2 weeks. Persistent hypertension beyond 3–4 weeks usually indicates chronic disease or rapidly progressive AGN. To identify presence of hypertension early, blood pressure should be measured every 4–6 hours.

Features of circulatory congestion, characterized by cough, dyspnea and orthopnoea with pulmonary rales in the bases is apparent in majority of cases. The child may present with features of pulmonary edema and left ventricular failure (tachypnoea, tachycardia, gallop, rales and wheeze). However, in presence of previously normal cardiac condition, cardiac failure and pulmonary edema are unusual.

Hypertensive encephalopathy has been reported in around 5% hospitalized cases. Hypertension is severe and is accompanied by one or more signs of CNS dysfunction viz. headache, vomiting, diplopia, confusion, seizures, drowsiness and coma. Hypertensive encephalopathy appears to occur in the child who has minimal edema.

Atypical Presentations

Less commonly, the child may present with the following atypical features:

Seizures due to hypertensive encephalopathy or **acute pulmonary edema** with cardiac failure. These may direct attention away from the correct diagnosis. The urinary abnormalities are minimal or absent. Presence of a history of a prior streptococcal infection, a positive family history and a depressed C_3 level is usually sufficient to suggest the diagnosis.

Features of nephrotic syndrome, clinical and laboratory but with a preceding history of streptococcal infection and the presence of hypertension, circulatory overload and characteristic laboratory data.

APSGN may occur in a **sub clinical form** among children with streptococcal infection. Urinary findings and depressed C_3 levels confirms diagnosis.

Complications

The major life threatening problems are encountered during the initial 1–2 weeks. They include:

(a) Acute renal insufficiency.

(b) Circulatory congestion with pulmonary edema and LVF.

(c) Acute hypertension with hypertensive encephalopathy.

Laboratory Diagnosis

In majority of cases a *routine examination of urine* clinches the diagnosis. Urinalysis demonstrates reduction of volume, a smoky, cola or red color, high specific gravity, mild to moderate proteinuria and RBC, polymorphonuclear leucocytes, RBC cast on microscopy.

Hb% and PBS for cell morphology shows a mild normochromic anemia as a result of hemodilution and low grade hemolysis.

The following investigations may be required in cases with atypical presentation or when recovery takes more than 2 weeks:

1. Serum C_3 level. It is usually reduced in the acute phase and returns to normal 6–8 weeks after onset.
2. Evidence of streptococcal infection include elevated anti DPNase and ASO titre (elevated after pharyngitis) and elevated DNase B (elevated after impetigo).
3. Blood urea and serum creatinine is raised in presence of acute renal insufficiency.
4. An X-ray PA view chest may help in case of pulmonary edema.
5. Renal biopsy: The indications of renal biopsy are as follows:
   (a) Presence of acute renal failure and nephrotic like presentation.
   (b) Absence of evidence of streptococcal infection or normal complement levels.
   (c) When hematuria and proteinuria, diminished renal function and/or low C_3 level persist for more than 2 months.

Treatment

Treatment of APSGN is essentially symptomatic.

Reassurance: Since the attacks of gross hematuria are self limiting and the course is benign, the condition should be discussed and parents reassured.

Bed rest: Bed rest should be advised only during the acute phase when there is gross hematuria and hypertension. The blood pressure should be monitored 4–6 hourly in the initial days for early detection of hypertension.

Fluids: Fluid restriction is necessary and is advised as follows:

(a) *Day I:* Only insensible loss (i.e. 300 ml/sq m/day).

(b) *Day II onwards:* Insensible water loss + last 24 hours urine output + fluid loss in diarrhea and vomiting if any.

(c) Fluid restriction is withheld when urine output is more than 1 ml/kg/hour.

Diet: Carbohydrates and fats are freely allowed to meet the daily calorie requirement. Protein, 1.5 gms/kg/day should be allowed. The amount may be reduced to 0.7 gm/kg/day if blood urea is elevated and oliguria is present. Sodium should be restricted to 1.5 gms/sqm/day in presence of edema and hypertension. Potassium rich food should be withheld till oliguria is present. The *diet of the child* can consist of rice, milk, salt less roti, sugar, sweet biscuits, potato and all vegetables. Potassium rich fruits and fruit juices should be avoided during the oliguric phase.

Treatment of Residual Streptococcal Infection

Antibiotic therapy does not affect the natural course of the disease. It helps to limit the spread of nephritogenic organism. Any one of the following regimens may be used.

(a) Oral phenoxymethyl penicillin 250 mg 8 hourly × 10 days.

(b) Oral Amoxycillin 30–40 mg/kg/day in divided doses 8 hourly × 10 days.

(c) One dose of Benzathene penicillin, 6 lacs (below 27 kg body wt.) 12 lacs (above 27 kg body weight) deep I.M. after negative skin test with benzyl penicillin.

Treatment of Hypertension

Mild to moderate hypertension should be treated with bed rest, fluid and salt restriction and an oral antihypertensive, nifedepine (dose 0.25 mg/kg/ day in 3 divided doses.

Severe hypertension (Systolic blood pressure > 180 mmHg and diastolic pressure > 110 mm Hg) without signs of hypertensive encephalopathy should be treated with nifedepine 0.25–0.5 mg/kg sublingually (onset of action 5–30 minutes) followed by per oral nifedepine. Antihypertensive drugs should be gradually tapered after blood pressure comes down below 95th percentile for age and height.

Treatment of Hypertensive Encephalopathy

Hypertensive encephalopathy warrant emergency treatment. A rapidly acting drug like Diazoxide (5–10 mg/kg rapid IV) is the choice. If not available can be treated with sublingual nifedepine. Approximately one third of the desired reduction of blood pressure should be achieved within 6 hours. A further 1/3rd over the next 12 – 24 hours and the rest 1/3rd in next 1–2 days. The target blood pressure level is 95th percentile value for age and height. Oral medication should be started when the crisis is under control. Frusemide, 1–2 mg/kg I.V. should be given as a stat dose. Seizures should be treated with an anticonvulsant viz. dizepam 0.3 to 0.5 mg/kg/dose.

Treatment of Circulatory Congestion and Pulmonary Edema and Left Ventricular Failure

Treatment modalities depend on the degree of cardiopulmonary symptoms:

(a) Salt and fluid restriction.

(b) Frusemide (1–2 mg/ kg), blood less phlebotomy, letting out of 300 ml of blood, peritoneal dialysis in succession, if the child has pulmonary edema and LVF.

Clinical Course and Prognosis

The clinical course of APSGN is characterized by subsidence of the acute process within 1–2 weeks. Microscopic hematuria can persist upto 6 months and mild proteinuria upto 1 year and apparent resolution of the disease takes 6 to 12 months. Presence of hematuria and proteinuria alone or in combination beyond this period and persistent hypertension beyond 3 weeks needs further evaluation. The eventual recovery in APSGN is 95%. Mortality in the acute phase can result from complications viz. acute renal failure, hypertension and cardiac failure which can be prevented by appropriate management.

Criteria for Discharge

The child can be discharged from the hospital when there is:

(a) General well-being.

(b) Edema subsides, blood pressure becomes normal.

(c) Urine volume and colour is normal. There is no macroscopic hematuria.

(d) Urine analysis is normal. Microscopic hematuria and/ or proteinuria may be present.

(e) Blood urea and serum creatinine if elevated earlier has come to normal.

Follow-up

A plan of follow-up of the child should be clearly outlined and discussed with the parents. Blood pressure measurement and urine examination should be done at 4 weeks interval for the first 6 months, then at an interval of 3 months until there is persistent absence of proteinuria and hematuria for 1 year. After that urine analysis once a year appears sufficient.

Nephrotic Syndrome

Nephrotic syndrome is an arbitrarily defined clinical state characterized by proteinuria (40 mg/m^2/hour or more) and hypoalbuminemia (less than 2 gms/dl), usually accompanied by massive edema and hypercholesterolemia with generalized hyperlipidemia and sometimes accompanied by hypertension, hematuria and reduced glomerular filtration rate.

Etiology

There is a primary glomerular abnormality in around 95% cases of nephrotic syndrome. In the remainder, the disorder results from glomerular involvement as a part of systemic diseases. Nephrotic syndrome associated with primary glomerular disease is termed as primary nephrotic syndrome. When it occurs as a part of a recognized systemic disease or results from some evident cause, it is termed secondary nephrotic syndrome. Rarely the disorder may be congenital. In 85% of children with primary glomerular abnormality histology shows insignificant glomerular abnormalities on light microscopy, hence termed as minimal change nephrotic syndrome (MCNS) and good response to steroid therapy with a good outcome, whereas others have several distinct glomerular lesions and termed as non-minimal change nephrotic syndrome (Non-MCNS) with no response to steroid therapy, progressive renal damage and poor outcome.

Classification

A. Primary Nephrotic Syndrome

1. Corticosteroid responsive
   i. Minimal change nephrotic syndrome (MCNS).
2. Corticosteroid non-responsive (Non MCNS)
   i. Focal Segmental glomerulosclerosis.
   ii. Mesengioproliferative glomerulonephritis.
   iii. Membranoproliferative glomerulonephritis.
   iv. Membranous glomerulopathy.

B. Secondary Nephrotic Syndrome

In children secondary nephrotic is most often associated with:

1. Systemic lupus erythematosus.
2. Anaphylactoid purpura.
3. Sickle cell disease.

Other rare causes:

1. Renal vein thrombosis.
2. Amyloidosis.
3. Diabetes mellitus.
4. Syphilis.
5. Plasmodium malariae infection.
6. Reaction to bee sting, drugs and heavy metals.

The common drugs and heavy metals include penicillamine, Captopril, NSAIDs, methimazole, lithium, and phenytoin and mercury compounds.

C. Congenital Nephrotic Syndrome

1. Finish type.
2. Due to congenital infections viz. Syphilis, Toxoplasmosis, Cytomegalovirus, Rubella, HIV, Hepatitis B.

Diagnostic Features of Secondary Nephrotic Syndrome

1. Age of onset more than 8 years.
2. Presence of hypertension, hematuria, renal dysfunction.
3. Extra renal features:
   (a) Butterfly rash in SLE.
   (b) Purpura in anaphylactoid purpura.
   (c) Arthralgia in collagen diseases.

Diagnostic Features of Congenital Nephrotic Syndrome

1. Age of onset within first 3 months age.
2. Most common type is Finnish type presenting with:
   (a) Massive proteinuria (detectable in utero by increased alpha feto protein).
   (b) Massive edema.
   (c) Large placenta.
   (d) Prematurity, respiratory distress and separation of cranial sutures.
   (e) Natural history is persistent edema, recurrent infection, progressive renal failure and death by the age of 5 years.
   (f) No response to corticosteroids and immunosuppressive agents.

   ACE inhibitors, indomethacin, and unilateral nephrectomy help decrease proteinuria and ameliorate the nephrotic state. The child ultimately needs chronic dialysis and kidney transplant.
3. Nephrotic syndrome as a result of intrauterine infections presents with similar features but is less severe and may improve or resolve with treatment of the underlying cause.
4. Depressed serum complement (C_3) levels.

Common congenital infections include TORCH and syphilis. Hepatitis B and HIV has also been reported.

MINIMAL CHANGE NEPHROTIC SYNDROME (MCNS)

Approximately 90% of children with nephrotic syndrome suffer from minimal change nephrotic syndrome.

Pathophysiology

The underlying abnormality in nephrotic syndrome is an increase in permeability in the glomerular capillary wall, which leads to massive proteinuria and hypoalbuminemia. The cause of increased permeability is not well understood. The current hypothesis regarding minimal change disease cites the possibility that T-cell activation leads to production of a cytokine, which may affect the filtration of proteins by the glomerular capillaries, by interfering with the polyanionic charge or through some other undefined mechanism.

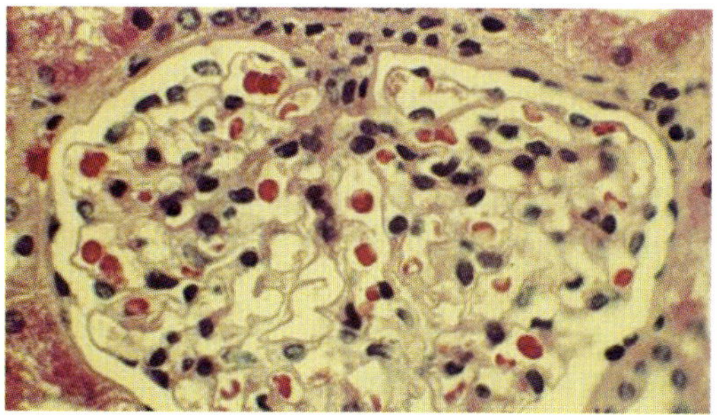

Fig. 12.1: MCNS: Light microscopy (no change)

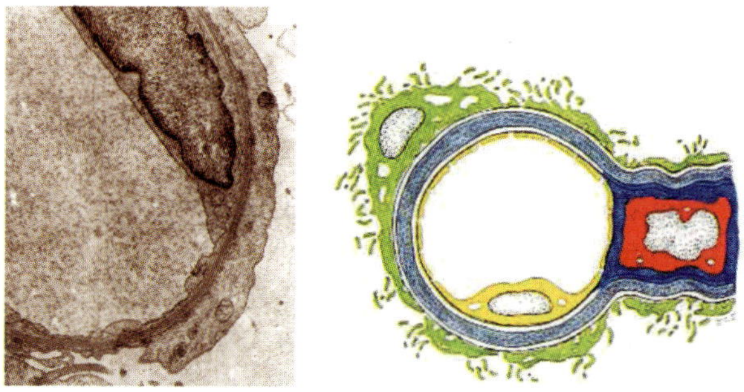

Fig. 12.2: MCNS: Electron microscopy

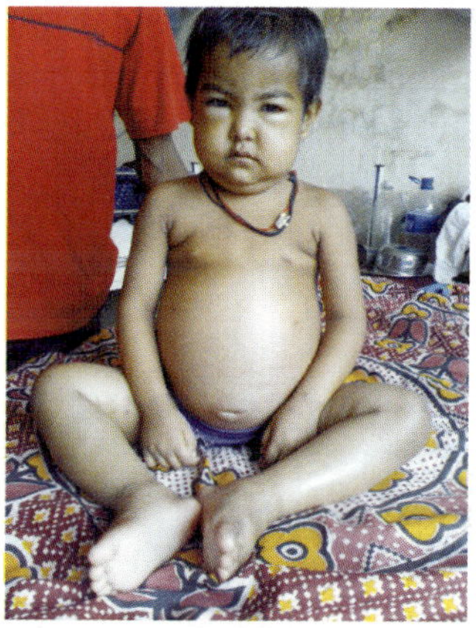

(a) With generalized edema

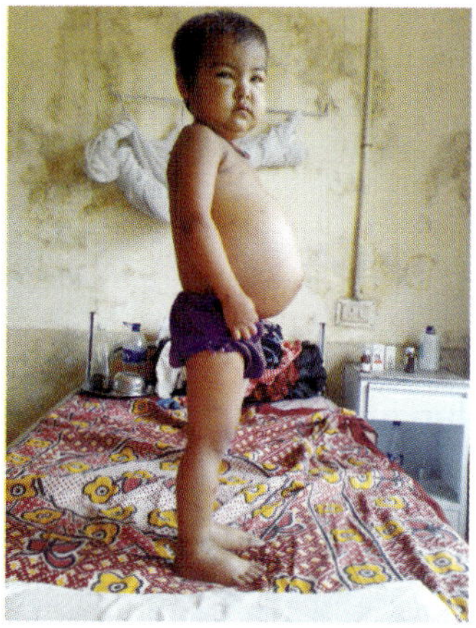

(b) With massive ascites

Fig. 12.3: A child with nephrotic syndrome

Pathology

On light microscopy, the glomeruli appear normal or show minimal increase in mesangial cells and matrix. Findings on immunofluorescence are typically negative. Electron microscopy reveals effacement of the epithelial foot process.

Clinical Manifestations

Minimal change nephrotic syndrome (MCNS) affects more males with a male-female ratio 2:1. It is most commonly seen between the age group 2–8 years. The child usually presents with edema of gradual onset which develops over the course of several weeks. The edema characteristically is first noted around the eyes, which decreases through the day, and in the lower extremities. With time, the edema becomes generalized, with development of ascites, pleural effusion and genital edema. The urine volume decreases and urine is high colored. Transient hematuria may be present but gross hematuria is uncommon. Transient hypertension may be present in 5–10% cases. The child usually does not appear ill even in presence of generalized edema but may sometimes complain of lethargy, anorexia and weight gain. Sometimes an initial episode appears to be precipitated by a respiratory viral infection.

Differentiating Features of MCNS and Non-MCNS

Features	*MCNS*	*Non-MCNS*
1. Age of onset	2–8 years	<1 year and > 10 years
2. Clinical presentation	Gross edema, Transient hematuria Hypertension	Gross hematuria, persistent hypertension, azotemia
3. Proteinuria	Highly selective proteinuria, normal C_3 level	Poorly selective proteinuria, low C_3 level
4. Histology	Negative morphological findings	Positive morphological findings
5. Response to steroid	Responsive	Non-responsive
6. Course	High tendency to relapse	Downhill

Untreated patients with MCNS tend to have a prolonged course characterized by recurrent episodes. In some instances remission may occur spontaneously or after an intercurrent illness such as measles.

Occasionally, generalized edema may develop abruptly and may be associated with gross hematuria and oliguria. These cases require detailed investigations including renal biopsy before starting treatment.

Laboratory Diagnosis

The laboratory tests may be divided as follows:

(a) Tests for confirmation of clinical diagnosis include:
   i. Urinalysis.
   ii. Serum protein and fractions, serum cholesterol.
   iii. Serum C_3 level.
   iv. Renal biopsy.

(b) Tests for assessment of renal function:
   i. Serum urea and serum creatinine.
   ii. Serum electrolytes viz. sodium, potassium, calcium.

(c) Tests for excluding infection and anemia:
   i. Total WBC count, differential leucocytic count, hemoglobin.
   ii. Mantoux test to exclude tuberculosis.
   iii. X-ray PA view chest.
   iv. Urine culture, blood culture when indicated.

The characteristic findings on *urinalysis* are as follows: Urine volume, colour, specific gravity is normal. The volume may be reduced, urine high coloured and specific gravity high in cases with massive edema. There is 2 + or more proteinuria (in excess of > 40 mg/m^2/hour), RBCs in 20% cases, plenty of WBCs and hyaline cast. WBCs in urine do not indicate an infection unless there are relevant symptoms of urinary tract infection.

Massive proteinuria is accompanied by reduction of total serum protein with albumin level < 2.5 gm/dl and elevation of alpha 2 globulins. The cholesterol (> 250 mg/dl) and triglyceride levels are elevated. Generalized massive edema is associated with a serum albumin level of < 1.5 gms/dl and cholesterol level of > 500 mg/dl. There is an inverse relation between serum albumin and serum cholesterol. The serum C_3 level is normal.

Kidney biopsy is not required for confirmation of diagnosis in most children. It is indicated only in children with features that make minimal change disease less likely viz. (i) Persistent hematuria, (ii) Persistent hypertension, (iii) Renal insufficiency, (iv) Hypocomplementemia, (v) Age <1 year or > 8 years.

There may be increase in both *serum urea and serum creatinine*, especially in cases of massive edema as a result of diminished renal perfusion consequent to contraction of intravascular volume.

All cases of nephrotic syndrome should undergo the investigations to exclude an infective focus before steroid therapy is started.

It needs mention that a case of relapse, occurring in a previously diagnosed case, on regular follow-up, may require only the investigations to exclude infection and for assessment of renal function.

Management

The first step in management is to identify whether the child is suffering from MCNS or Non-MCNS. In case of presence of features of Non-MCNS, renal biopsy should be carried out before starting treatment.

Corticosteroids remain the mainstay in the treatment of minimal change nephrotic syndrome for the initial episode as well as relapses. The aim is to induce remission of proteinuria and to maintain the remission over a length of time. If clinical and laboratory evaluation confirms the diagnosis, the first step would be to initiate steroid therapy following ISKDC (International Study of Kidney Diseases in Children) regimen for 8 weeks or IAP regimen for 12 weeks. Most children respond within 4 weeks/6 weeks of continuous therapy.

The initiation of daily treatment with steroids for either the first attack or relapse however, can be delayed for a week or so because of the following reasons:

a. Spontaneous remission can occur particularly if the episode has been precipitated by an intercurrent infection.
b. To detect latent infections like tuberculosis and UTI, in presence of which steroid therapy should not be started.
c. To treat massive edema and ascites if present, before starting steroid therapy. Steroid therapy in such children will aggravate sodium and water retension.

Principles of Treatment

1. Treatment of edema.
2. Detection and treatment of infection.
3. Dietary management.
4. Steroid regimen.
5. General care.

Treatment of Edema

The treatment depends on the severity of edema. A child with massive edema has intravascular contraction and hypovolemia. The child should be examined for signs of hypovolemia. Aggressive diuretic therapy in presence of hypovolemia can lead to shock.

Mild edema can be treated with salt restriction alone. The usual amount of salt in cooking is allowed but salty snacks should be temporarily withheld. No fluid restriction should be advised. The child can drink as much as he desires. Diuresis starts within 48–72 hours of starting steroid therapy.

Moderate to severe edema: Children with severe symptomatic edema, including ascites, pleural effusion and genital edema should be hospitalized.

The patient should be advised *no added salt diet*. Fluid restriction should be advised when there is hyponatremia. The water intake may be limited to replacement of insensible loss plus urine output minus a planned weight loss. The target weight loss is 1% body weight loss/day. A swollen scrotum should be elevated with pillows to enhance the removal of fluid by gravity.

Oral diuretics, Frusemide 1–3 mg/kg/dose should be started in 2–3 divided doses. The dose may be increased to 4–8 mg/dose depending on the response. Oral doses are preferred due to sustained diuresis. Onset of action is within 30 minutes, peak diuresis occurs at 2 hours and action lasts for 6–8 hours. In children requiring higher doses (> 4 mg/kg) and prolonged frusemide (> 7 days), spironolactone, 2–3 mg/kg/day in a single dose needs to be added.

In severely edematous children with very low sodium, diuresis can be augmented by IV/oral administration of chlorothiazide (10 mg/kg/dose every 12 hours) or metolazone (0.1 mg/kg/dose twice daily) in addition to IV or oral frusemide (1–2 mg/kg/dose 12 hourly).

In intractable edema, diuresis can be induced by IV frusemide bolus in the dose of 1–3 mg/kg/dose 8–12 hourly. The bolus doses should be given very slowly over 10–15 minutes not exceeding a rate of 4 mg/minute. Patient who shows diuresis with IV bolus doses can be put on IV frusemide infusion as it is safer and more effective than IV bolus doses. An IV infusion should be given @ 0.1 to 1 mg/kg/hour after an initial bolus dose. Onset of action of IV therapy is within 5 minutes. It should be noted that those who fail to respond to IV bolus are also less likely to respond to IV infusion.

In an occasional case with severe edema with serum albumin level below 1 gm/dl associated with hypovolemia, diuretics are ineffective unless blood volume is expanded. In such cases, IV infusion of 20% salt free albumin, 0.5 gm/kg body weight is administered slowly over 60 to 90 minutes with a dose of IV frusemide, 1–2 mg/kg/dose administered towards the end of infusion. The resulting increase in diuresis is usually transient. Hence, infusion of albumin should be multiple and preferably given on alternate days.

Head out water immersion therapy is an effective method for diuresis in children with generalized edema with severe ascites. The child is immersed in a drum of water with the head out. The procedure leads to movement of edema fluid from the interstitial space to the intravascular space. Expansion of the intravascular space cause stretching of the atrial wall and release of atrial natriuretic peptides, which inhibit sodium and water reabsorption from the medullary collecting duct. This therapy can be advised in an older child for 2–4 hours each day for a few days.

Detection and Treatment of Infection

Infections remain the most common cause of morbidity and hospital admission and the chief cause of mortality in nephrotic syndrome. A child with anasarca and already on immunosuppressive therapy is more susceptible to bacterial infection. Peritonitis and cellulitis are the most common infections. Empyema, bone and joint infection, septicemia and tuberculosis are also frequent. Streptococcus pneumoniae is the most common pathogen. Infection due to gram negative organisms like E. coli and H. influenzae has also been reported.

The signs of infection may be masked. A child even with anasarca usually looks well and is active. If such a child looks ill or complains of vague abdominal pain, headache or vomiting, infection should be suspected. Such a child should be admitted to a hospital and appropriate investigations carried to rule out infection.

Peritonitis is mostly seen in children with relapse and ascites. The onset is acute with mild abdominal pain and low grade fever. The usual causative organisms is S. pneumoniae. Peritonitis is confirmed on examination of peritoneal fluid. The fluid appears hazy or frankly turbid with presence of neutrophils and organisms on gram stain. Peritoneal fluid culture is usually negative. A polymorphonuclear leucocytosis is present and blood culture is often positive. Hence an ascitic fluid examination should be ordered even in a child with ascites and presence of vague abdominal pain. Peritonitis should be treated with parenteral antibiotics for 7–10 days.

Cellulitis: Cellulitis is also common in children with generalized edema. At times it can progress to septicemia and shock. The focus of infection may be a venepuncture site, a minor trauma or a spontaneous break in the edematous skin. Cellulitis should be treated with suitable parenteral antibiotics covering both gram positive and gram negative bacteria.

Other infections: viz. urinary tract infection is common when associated with anomalies of the urinary tract. Bone and joint infection, empyema and meningitis although not common should be kept in mind in a sick edematous child. The child may present with only mild headache and vomiting (meningitis) pain in limb and limp (bone and joint infection), cough with breathing difficulty (pneumonia and empyema). Every child should have a Mantoux test and an X-ray chest done to exclude tuberculosis.

Common pathogens: The common pathogens causing infection in a nephrotic child are S. pneumoniae, Staphylococcus, H.influenzae, E. coli and Klebsiella.

Treatment: Even if the infection appears localized, it should be treated with parenteral antibiotics. A blood culture should be sent and a third generation cephalosporin (or Ampicillin) and an aminoglycoside should be started. Antibiotic may be changed after the results of culture and sensitivity are obtained.

Prophylactic antibiotic should not be used routinely.

Dietary Management

In minimal change nephrotic syndrome, the child should be advised a high protein diet with supplements of vitamin and micronutrients. A high protein diet increases serum albumin and also urinary excretion of protein. However, in MCNS, proteinuria is resolved in 10 – 14 days with corticosteroids and a high protein diet helps in restoration of body protein. Salt and fat should be restricted during daily administration of prednisolone to the decrease tendency to hypertension and obesity respectively.

In patients with non-MCNS, dietary protein should be restricted to 1.5 gms/kg/day of first class protein with an aim to reduce proteinuria. In steroid resistant cases with persistent proteinuria, calcium and Vitamin D supplements are required. Potassium supplements should be advised to replenish diuretic induced potassium losses.

Steroid Regimen for Initial Episode

ISKDC regimen: Prednisolone 2 mg/kg/day (60 mg/sq m/day) in 2–3 divided doses for 4 weeks followed by 1.5 mg/kg/day (40 mg/sq m/day) as a single morning dose on alternate days for 4 weeks after which it is discontinued. Tailing off the steroid is not necessary. The prednisolone dose should be given in full stomach to avoid gastritis.

A steroid regimen of 6 weeks daily therapy followed by 6 weeks of alternate day therapy with the same dose of prednisolone as in ISKDC regimen has been suggested. There is good evidence that an initial 6 weeks course of daily steroid treatment may lead to lower relapse rate, although the frequency of steroid induced side effects is higher. It has also been suggested that children in their first episode should be treated for at least 3 months of alternate day therapy with tapering doses of prednisolone.

The optimum duration of steroid treatment for the initial episode is still under investigation.

Definitions and Terminologies to Describe Response to steroids in patients with MCNS

Urinary remission: Protein trace or nil urine for 3 consecutive days within 7 days.

Complete remission: Serum albumin 3.5 gms/dl or more.

Relapse: Urine protein (1 + or more) on 3 consecutive days on 3 separate days within 7 days.

Infrequent relapse: Less than 2 relapse within 6 months of initial response.

Frequent relapse: 2 or more relapses within 6 months of initial response.

Steroid dependence: Relapse while on alternate day steroid therapy or within 28 days of stopping prednisolone therapy.

Steroid resistance: Continue to have proteinuria (2+ or more) after 8 weeks of daily steroid therapy.

Treatment of Relapse

Of the children who respond to prednisolone in the initial episode, 25–40% has infrequent, 40% has frequent relapses and the remainder show steroid dependence. A relapse may be precipitated by an infection and proteinuria may resolve with treatment of infection. So the standard treatment can be deferred for some days and the child can be observed for a spontaneous remission. If the child has an infection related proteinuria during alternate day therapy, the dose of alternate day steroid should be doubled for a week or two. Such brief episodes of mild proteinuria (< 2 +) which resolves spontaneously may not be regarded as a relapse.

An *infrequent relapse* is treated with prednisolone 2 mg/kg/day in 2–3 divided doses till urine is protein free for 3 consecutive days or for 14 days. Thereafter prednisolone is given as 1.5 mg/kg/day in single morning dose on alternate days for 4 weeks and stopped abruptly. The same regimen should be used to treat each relapse.

A *frequent relapse* or steroid dependence should be treated in a similar manner as infrequent relapse for induction of remission. The prednisolone is then tapered gradually to maintain the patient in remission on an alternate day dose of 0.5 mg/kg/day or lower for 9–12 months.

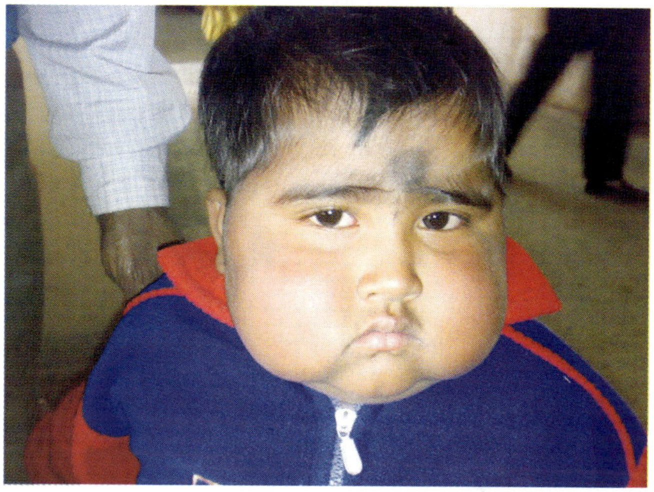

Fig. 12.4: Cushingoid facies in steroid toxicity

Patients with frequent relapse who show persistence or development of signs of steroid toxicity such as Cushingoid features (obesity, hirsutism, striae), hypertension, impaired glucose tolerance, posterior subscapular lenticular opacities, emotional problems and growth retardation, needs institution of steroid sparing agents. Serious complications of steroid therapy should not be allowed to develop.

Steroid Sparing Agents

The widely used steroid sparing agents include cyclophosphamide and cyclosporine A. Newer additions to the list are tacrolimus and mycophenolate. Steroid sparing agents are indicated in patients with signs of steroid toxicity and if the prednisolone threshold to maintain remission is higher than 0.5 mg/kg/day on alternate days. At present, cyclophosphamide is the most widely used agent.

Cyclophosphamide may induce long lasting remission or rarely permanent remission in children. It should be started after induction of remission with the standard regimen of prednisolone. The results are better in older children and in those frequent relapsers without steroid dependence. Alopecia, hemorrhagic cystitis and gonadal toxicity are uncommon side effects. A standard course with a cumulative dose of 168 mg/kg is reasonably safe. However, the interval between two courses of cyclophosphamide should be one year. Hemorrhagic cystitis can be prevented by maintaining a high urine flow rate. Cyclophosphamide is given as a 8-12-week course at a dosage 2-3 mg/kg/day as a single dose along with prednisolone 1–1.5 mg/kg/day as a single dose on alternate days. The TLC should be monitored every 2 weeks. If the count falls below 4000/cumm, the drug is withheld till the count reach normal values.

Cyclosporine A is recommended in children who continue to show steroid dependence or frequent relapse despite a course of cyclophosphamide. The dose is 3–5 mg/kg/day 12 hourly. It is preferably combined with alternate day prednisolone for 12 to 20 weeks. Cyclosporine A is continued for 1 year.

Tacrolimus (0.15 mg/kg/day 12 hourly) is also effective in maintaining prolonged remission and is useful as a steroid sparing agent. *Mycophenolate* (dose 20–25 mg/kg in two divided doses), may maintain remission in children with steroid dependent or frequently relapse nephrotic syndrome. However, further trials are required to recommend routine use of this drug.

It needs mention that, most of the patients who respond to cyclosporine A, tacrolimus and mycophenolate therapy, tend to relapse when medication is discontinued.

Steroid Dependence

These children require continued daily administration of prednisolone for maintenance of remission. Some of these patients may be managed with relatively higher doses of prednisolone given on alternate days and continued for 9–12 months or longer provided there are no side effects. Patients who develop serious steroid toxicities should be treated with steroid sparing agents.

MCNS with Initial Steroid Resistance

Eighty to ninety percent of children will respond to a steroid regimen (urine trace or negative for protein for 3 consecutive days) by two weeks. Majority of children will do so within the first 4 weeks of treatment. Children who continue to have proteinuria (2+ or more) after 8 weeks of daily steroid therapy are considered as steroid resistant. A diagnostic renal biopsy should be performed in these cases. Steroid resistant nephrotic syndrome is usually FSGS (80%), MCNS (20%) and rarely mesangio-proliferative. The following treatment modalities can be used in cases with resistance.

(i) A 12 weeks course of cyclophosphamide (2–3 mg/kg/day, single dose). Alternate day steroid therapy (prednisolone 1.5 mg/kg/day) is often continued during the course of cyclophosphamide administration. During cyclophosphamide therapy, the white cell count must be monitored weekly, and the drug withheld if the count fall below 4000/cumm.

(ii) Pulse therapy with bolus doses of methyl prednisolone 30 mg/kg body weight (upto maximum 1000 mg) 3–6 intravenous injections on alternate days followed by tapering doses of oral prednisolone on alternate days starting at 1.5 mg/kg for 4–12 months. Dexamethasone can be used in place of methyl prednisolone. It is less expensive and easily available. The dose is 4–5 mg/kg. Schedule is same as that of methyl prednisolone. Despite the large doses side effects of pulse therapy is not very significant. Patients should be monitored for hypertension and infection and treated promptly.

(iii) Cyclosporine A along with alternate day steroid is a useful regimen. It should be continued for 1–2 years. Most patients who respond do so within 3 months of therapy.

(iv) Angiotensin converting enzyme (ACE) inhibitors and angiotensin II blockers may be helpful as an adjunct therapy to reduce proteinuria in steroid resistance cases.

MCNS with Late Steroid Resistance

Three to 5% cases of children with frequent relapse or steroid dependence eventually cease to respond to steroids. Kidney biopsy should be done to study the renal histology. The patients who show changes of MCNS respond to cyclophosphamide and later may become steroid responsive. A small percentage develops focal segmental glomerulosclerosis (FSGS). These cases have an unfavorable outcome.

General Care

1. The parents should be made aware of the disease in detail. They should be talked about the treatment regimens, the nature of response and side effects of the drugs used, the course of the disease and the outcome.
2. During the stay at the hospital, they should be taught how to test urine for protein and keep record of the urine tests and drug intake.
3. During the remission period, the child should be treated as a normal child, should go to school. The family

should be given constant reassurance and guidance and impressed on the compliance of treatment and routine follow-up.

4. All children above 2 years should receive pneumococcal and varicella vaccine. Administration of live vaccines should be withheld until steroid therapy has been discontinued for atleast 4–12 weeks. If a child is continuously on immunosuppressant, the siblings should not receive OPV. IPV can be given instead.

Complications

The complications in nephrotic syndrome include infections, hypovolemia, thromboembolism and hyperlipidemia.

Infections and Hypovolemia

Infections are the chief cause of mortality in children suffering from nephrotic syndrome. They are more common in children with generalized edema who are on immunosuppressive therapy. Peritonitis and cellulitis are most common. Bone and joint infection, empyema, sepsis and tuberculosis are frequent. A child should be investigated to exclude infection before starting a steroid regimen.

Children with generalized edema often shows signs of *hypovolemia* characterized by cold periphery, collapsed neck veins, hypotension, oliguria, prolonged capillary refill time, and a raised hematocrit, raised blood urea and low urine sodium content. These abnormalities can be rapidly corrected by infusion of saline, plasma or albumin. Rarely there may be development of acute tubular necrosis usually in presence of sepsis. A careful clinical and laboratory evaluation should be done and volume deficit should be corrected in case of hypovolemia.

Thromboembolism

Thromboembolism is uncommon in children. The predisposing factors including hemoconcentration from hypovolemia, increase in blood viscosity and fibrinogen level, low antithrombin III and protein S activity etc have been suggested. Thromboembolism can be prevented by avoiding dehydration, prompt treatment of infection, judicious use of diuretics and avoiding deep vein puncture. Thrombotic complications are initially treated with heparin and maintained with Warfarin for 6 months or longer.

Hyperlipidemia

Hyperlipidemia in nephrotic syndrome may contribute in the development of glomerulosclerosis and progressive renal injury. In steroid responsive cases, the raised lipids fall after remission. High levels may persist in patients with continued heavy proteinuria. All components of the lipid profile is raised except HDL which decrease or remains normal. There is an increased LDL/HDL cholesterol ratio.

The treatment of hyperlipidemia includes nonpharmacological as well as pharmacological treatment. In severe and persistent cases, diet should contain less than 30 % fat with equal amounts of polyunsaturated and saturated fatty acids and low cholesterol (< 250 mg/day). If dietary modification is not effective, drugs like use of HMG – CoA reductase inhibitors (lovastatin, simvastatin, atrovastatin) may be tried. Use of these medications is not well-defined. The treatment of hyperlipidemia is still unsatisfactory.

NON-MINIMAL CHANGE NEPHROTIC SYNDROME (NON-MCNS)

The non-minimal change nephrotic syndrome includes conditions with significant glomerular histological lesions such as focal segmental glomerulosclerosis (FSGS), mesangioproliferative glomerulonephritis (MesPGN), membranoproliferative glomerulonephritis (MPGN) and membranous nephropathy (MGN). These conditions presents with the features of non-MCNS. Most of these histological types are resistant to steroids and response to other modalities of treatment and outcome are different. Except FSGS the other types are not common in children.

Focal Segmental Glomerulosclerosis (FSGS)

FSGS constitutes about 30–35% children with non-MCNS. It is the most common type of progressive glomerular disease in children. Most patients with FSGS have either initial or late steroid resistance. The response to treatment with cyclophosphamide is unpredictable. More aggressive treatment modalities have been found to be beneficial in a significant number of cases. The treatment modalities include:

(a) Pulse methyl prednisolone, 30 mg/kg (maximum 1 gm) three times a week for 2 weeks, once a week for 8 weeks, once in 2 weeks for another 8 weeks, and thereafter once a month for 6–12 months. Two weeks after starting the treatment, prednisolone is administered at the dose of 2 mg/kg/body weight on alternate days with reduction of dose gradually for a period of 12 months. Cyclophosphamide (2–3 mg/kg) is also given for 12 weeks as a part of this protocol. With this regimen, sustained remission has been shown in 60% patients.

(b) Cyclosporine (150–200 mg/kg) with concurrent use of alternate day prednisolone (30 mg/kg) is also shown to cause partial or complete remission in 30–50% cases.

(c) Cyclophosphamide (500–750 mg/m^2) given once a month for 6 months along with oral prednisolone has shown variable benefit.

The overall prognosis of FSGS is unsatisfactory. Forty to 50% patients with steroid resistance progress to end stage renal disease within 10–15 years.

Supportive Care in Non-Minimal Change Nephrotic Syndrome

Edema should be controlled with moderate salt restriction and diuretics. No other dietary restriction is necessary. Hypertension should be kept controlled. Schooling should be continued and physical activity should be encouraged. Prevention and early treatment of infection and avoidance of nephrotoxic agents are important measures.

In cases with heavy proteinuria not responding to treatment, ACE inhibitors (Enalapril) and angiotensin receptor antagonists (Losartan) are effective in reducing the amount of filtered protein. Enalapril can be administered in the dose of 0.2–0.5 mg/kg/day in two divided doses. It reduces proteinuria by 30–40%, increase serum albumin and reduce serum cholesterol levels. Long-term therapy with Enalapril is safe. Combination of Enalapril with Losartan may enhance the anti-proteinuric effect.

Course and Prognosis

The *majority* of children with MCNS have repeated relapse which generally decrease and stop by 14–20 years age and sometimes earlier. They fully recover without any residual effect. Children with younger age at onset usually have a lengthy relapsing course. However, it is not possible to predict when the relapses would cease. The steroid responsive disease never develops chronic renal failure. Children with steroid resistant disease develop progressive renal insufficiency and ultimately end stage renal failure.

Hemolytic Uremic Syndrome

The hemolytic uremic syndrome (HUS) is an acute disorder characterized by renal failure with or without oligoanuria, microangiopathic hemolytic anemia, and thrombocytopenia. It is the most common cause of acute renal failure in young children. Two broad subgroups have been described. The first is commonly seen in infants and is associated with a diarrheal prodrome. This is called D + HUS. The second form is not associated with antecedent diarrhea and is called D-HUS, is rare in children. D-HUS is a heterogenous group and can be familial, drug induced or recurrent. Clinical and laboratory features are similar to D+HUS.

Etiology

The etiology is unknown. Inciting and precipitating factors have been recognized. An acute enteritis with diarrhea caused by verocytotoxin producing Escherichia coli 0157: H 7 precedes 80% or more of cases of HUS in developed countries. In the developing countries, the common organism is Shiegella dysentriae type 1 that produces shiga toxin 1. HUS is associated, less often, with other bacterial (viz. Salmonella, Campylobacter, S. pneumoniae) and viral (viz. coxsackie, echo, influenza, varicella, HIV, Ebstein-Barr) infections.

Pathogenesis

The primary event is capillary and arteriolar endothelial injury in the kidney which leads to localized clotting. The microangiopathic anemia results from mechanical damage to the red blood cells as they pass through the damaged microvasculature. Thrombocytopenia is caused by intra-renal platelet adhesion or destruction.

Pathology

Light microscopy shows thickening of the capillary walls, narrowing of the capillary lumens and widening of the mesangium in the glomerulus. Electron microscopy shows sub-endothelial and mesangial deposition of a granular and amorphous material of unknown origin. The glomerular capillaries are seen filled with fibrin thrombi and there may be cortical necrosis. Severely involved glomeruli may show partial or total sclerosis.

Clinical Manifestations

Children below 5 years are mostly affected. The onset may be preceded by an episode of dysentery or acute gastroenteritis. Less often an upper respiratory infection may precede the onset of HUS. The dysentery caused by Shiegella is usually severe and continue well beyond the development of HUS. When the prodrome is acute gastroenteritis it may be mild to severe, and subside by the time HUS develops.

HUS presents with sudden onset of pallor, irritability, drowsiness, lethargy, convulsion and oliguria which usually occurs 5–10 days after the initial respiratory or gastro-intestinal illness. In those with a prolonged history of oliguria or anuria, complications of acute renal failure may be present. Physical examination may reveal presence of irritability, dehydration, edema, petechiae, hypertension and hepatosplenomegaly.

D-HUS is mostly seen in older children. The onset is insidious. There may be heavy proteinuria, gross hematuria and severe hypertension.

Laboratory Diagnosis

The peripheral blood smear shows features of hemolytic anemia viz. broken and deformed RBCs. The platelet counts are almost invariably decreased but return to normal in 2–3 weeks. In the post dysenteric form there is a polymorphonuclear leucocytosis. Fibrinogen levels are normal. The serum potassium is low initially as a result of gastrointestinal losses. Urine examination shows red cells and occasional casts.

Treatment

There is no specific treatment. Supportive treatment is the mainstay. Meticulous attention to fluid and electrolytes, control of hypertension, nutrition and early institution of dialysis has brought down the mortality significantly. Interference with oral feeding in cases of prolonged diarrhea/dysentery can lead to severe PEM and may require parenteral nutrition.

Acute Renal Failure

Acute renal failure is a clinical syndrome resulting from an acute reduction in or cessation of renal function. It is characterized by anuria or oliguria (urine volume < 0.5 ml/kg/hour), electrolyte and acid base disturbance (notably hyperkalemia and metabolic acidosis), and impaired excretion of substances such as creatinine, urea and phosphate.

Reduction in urine volume however, is not an essential feature of acute renal failure, and the other features can be present in presence of a normal or slightly reduced urine volume. This condition is called non-oliguric renal failure which is specially seen in acute renal failure in association with nephrotoxic drugs.

Table 12.2 : Causes of renal failure

Prerenal causes
Acute gastroenteritis, blood loss, shock
Fulminant hepatitis
Reye's syndrome
Congestive heart failure
Hepato-renal syndrome, and
Drugs (ACE inhibitors, NSAIDs)
Renal causes
Renal vein thrombosis and renal arterial obstruction
Hemolytic uremic syndrome
Henoch-Schönlein syndrome
Polyarteritis
Acute glomerulonephritis
Acute interstitial nephritis
Acute tubular necrosis
Intravascular hemolysis
Sepsis
Nephrotoxic agents
Snake bite
Falciparum malaria
Leptospirosis
Post renal
Obstructive uropathy as a result of bilateral obstruction of pelvi ureteric junction and ureters, bladder outlet and urethra by calculi and blood clots and pus debris.

Etiology

Acute renal failure is conventionally classified into three types: pre renal, intrinsic renal and post renal depending on where the principal disturbance lies. The causes are as follows:

Pre renal causes include acute gastroenteritis, blood loss, shock, fulminant hepatitis, Reye's syndrome, congestive cardiac failure, hepatorenal syndrome and drugs like ACE inhibitors, NSAIDs.

Renal causes include renal vein thrombosis and renal arterial obstruction, hemolytic uremic syndrome, Henoch-Schönlein syndrome, polyarteritis, acute glomerulone-phritis, acute interstitial nephritis and acute tubular necrosis as a result of prolongation of pre renal failure, intravascular hemolysis, sepsis, nephrotoxic agents, snake bite, falciparum malaria, leptospirosis.

Post renal causes include obstructive uropathy as a result of bilateral obstruction of pelvi ureteric junction and ureters, bladder outlet and urethra by calculi, blood clots and pus debris.

The most common causes in childhood are renal hypoperfusion due to acute gastroenteritis with dehydration and shock, hemolytic uremic syndrome, acute glomerulonephritis and interstitial nephritis, congenital developmental anomalies of the kidney and urinary tract, septicemia, acute tubular necrosis. Malaria, leptospirosis, snake bite and intravascular hemolysis in G6PD deficient subjects are common in different parts of India. ARF in ICUs is associated with extensive trauma, burns and sepsis and multi organ failure.

The common nephrotoxic drugs which causes ARF are aminoglycoside, amphotericin B, cisplatin, ifosphamide, radio contrast media, fluorinated anesthetic agents (methoxyflurane).

Table 12.3 : Common causes of acute renal failure

Acute gastroenteritis with dehydration and shock
Hemolytic uremic syndrome
Acute glomerulonephritis
Interstitial nephritis
Congenital developmental anomalies of the kidney and urinary tract
Septicemia
Acute tubular necrosis
Severe malaria

Pathogenesis

Pre renal failure: Reduction in effective circulating arterial volume leads to inadequate renal perfusion and a resultant decreased glomerular filtration rate. Evidence of kidney damage is absent. If the underlying cause of kidney hypoperfusion is corrected promptly, renal function returns to normal. If hypoperfusion is sustained, intrinsic renal parenchyma damage may develop.

Intrinsic renal failure is characterized by kidney parenchymal injury which may be predominantly in the tubules or in the glomerulus with resultant hypoperfusion or ischemia. In classic acute intrinsic renal failure resulting from tubular damage, the course may be divided into 3 stages: anuric or oliguric, diuretic and convalescent. The management of these stages is different. In children this sequence is however not clear cut.

Post renal failure results from obstruction of urine flow at some point in the pelvicalyceal collecting system or in the ureter.

Biochemical Alterations

The biochemical alterations in acute renal failure include hyperkalemia, sodium and water overload, metabolic acidosis and elevation of BUN, plasma creatinine and uric acid levels.

Hyperkalemia in acute renal failure develops because of decreased renal excretion of potassium. It may also result from a hyper catabolic state like trauma, hemolysis, infection or hypoxia. Presence of acidosis results in increase plasma potassium as a result of intracellular shift of H ion in exchange of potassium. The cardio toxic effects of hyperkalemia result from a decreased ratio of cellular to extracellular potassium.

Sodium and water overload usually occurs during oliguric phase (reduced excretion of urine) and may lead to interstitial and pulmonary edema, pleural effusion, hypertension and circulatory congestion. Hyponatremia in acute renal failure is the result of dilution of body fluids as a consequence of excessive intake of water relative to that of sodium.

Metabolic acidosis with or without increased H^+ ion concentration (acidemia) is common in acute renal failure. It reflects impaired ability of the kidney to eliminate acid as well as increased catabolic production of acids.

Blood urea nitrogen, plasma creatinine and uric acid concentrations are elevated as a result of reduced excretion.

Clinical Manifestations

The clinical features include (a) manifestations of the precipitating cause and (b) features related more specifically to acute renal failure.

The clinical presentation of acute renal failure is often overshadowed by manifestations of the precipitating cause. Features that suggest the underlying cause may be as follows:

Table 12.4 : Features that suggest the underlying cause

Underlying cause	*Features*
1. Acute tubular necrosis	History of fluid or blood loss with severe dehydration or shock.
2. Acute glomerulonephritis	Edema, hematuria and hypertension.

Contd.

Contd.

3. Hemolytic uremic syndrome	Dysentery, pallor and petechiae.
4. Acute intravascular hemolysis	Sudden passage of dark red urine, pallor and jaundice.
5. Obstructive uropathy	History of interrupted urinary stream, a palpable bladder or kidney, anuria.

The clinical features related more specifically to acute renal failure include decreased urinary output (oliguria to anuria), peripheral or pulmonary edema, altered sensorium and convulsion due to advanced uremia or hypertensive encephalopathy, cardiac arrhythmia and deep and rapid breathing (Kussmaul's respiration) due to metabolic acidosis.

ARF may be occasionally superimposed on chronic renal disease. In such cases chronic renal disease is indicated by the presence of features like failure to thrive, signs of rickets, retinopathy, hypocalcemia, hypophosphatemia and small contracted kidneys.

Investigations and Management

Acute renal failure is an emergency situation where proper and timely management is life saving. The metabolic consequences of acute renal failure is life threatening. Hence immediate attention should be directed towards detection and management of the complications that may be present when the child is first seen. Hence investigation and management of acute renal failure go simultaneously.

When acute renal failure is suspected in a child the initial evaluation of the patient should lay emphasis on the following points:

1. History and physical findings of dehydration, shock, fluid overload and signs of congestive cardiac failure.
2. Pattern of breathing e.g. presence of Kussmaul's respiration indicating acidosis.
3. Evidence of encephalopathy, pericarditis.
4. A palpable kidney and urinary bladder.
5. Presence of pallor and its degree.

Post Evaluation Plan of Management

The post evaluation management depends on the situation with which the child presents:

1. In presence of dehydration or overhydration, one should establish ARF with challenge test:
   (a) If the child passes urine after challenge test, it indicates absence of renal failure.
   (b) If the child does not pass urine after the test, diagnosis of intrinsic renal failure is established. The child should undergo laboratory investigation, supportive treatment, dialysis as indicated.
2. Presence of signs of pericarditis, encephalopathy, and Kussmaul's respiration indicates established renal failure. A child presenting with such features should undergo:
   (a) Laboratory investigation, supportive treatment, dialysis as indicated.
3. Presence of a palpable kidney, urinary bladder indicates obstructive uropathy. The obstruction should be removed. If the child still does not pass urine the child should be subjected to:
   (a) Laboratory investigation to confirm presence of complication and institution of supportive treatment, dialysis as indicated.
   (b) The child should also undergo investigation and treatment of the cause after recovery from renal failure.

The Challenge Test

In a child with oliguria/anuria:

(a) With signs of dehydration, intravascular volume expansion should be done by IV administration of 20–30 ml/kg of isotonic saline /Ringers lactate over 45 to 60 minutes. If urine volume increases but signs of hypovolemia persist then infusion may be continued. If urine output is <1 ml/kg/hour after 2 hours and there is no sign of hypovolemia, frusemide 2-3 mg/kg/dose IV @ 4 mg/min should be given. If there is no urine output in the following hour, one should treat as intrinsic renal failure.

(b) With signs of overhydration or no signs of dehydration, frusemide 2–3 mg/kg/dose should be given @ 4 mg/minute. If there is no increase in urine output in the following 1 hour the child should be treated as intrinsic renal failure.

(c) With post renal cause, if possible the obstruction should be removed with emergency surgical intervention. If there is no improvement of urine output after removal of obstruction, the child should be treated as a case of intrinsic renal failure.

After establishment of intrinsic renal failure, the child should be subjected to investigations. The investigations in acute renal failure may be grouped as:

1. Immediate investigations which should include:
   i. Urinalysis.
   ii. Estimation of blood urea, serum creatinine.
   iii. Electrolytes: Sodium, potassium, calcium, bicarbonate.
   iv. X-ray PA view chest and ECG.
2. Further investigations are necessary to determine the cause. These are not done in all cases. They should be picked up as and when necessary:
   i. Peripheral blood smears in hemolytic uremic syndrome, and for malaria parasite.
   ii. C_3 level, ASO titre in acute glomerulonephritis.
   iii. Total leucocytic count, differential leucocytic count, platelet count.
   iv. Urine and blood culture for septicemia.
   v. X-ray: Plain picture abdomen, wrist and hand, knee in acute on chronic renal failure.
   vi. Ultrasonography of KUB region for structural abnormalities of kidney and ureter, calculi and renal size.
   vii. Micturiting cystourethrogram (MCU), DTPA/DMSA scan for obstructive lesions and parenchymal disease of kidney respectively.
   viii. Kidney biopsy should be planned in (a) case of unremitting ARF lasting longer than 2–3 weeks, (b) patients in whom etiology is not identified, and (c) suspected drug induced ARF in a patient receiving a nephrotoxic drug (cyclosporine in post renal transplant).

Urinalysis

A carefully done urinalysis helps to a great extent to differentiate between the various causes of acute renal failure.

Urinary findings	*Cause*
1. Scanty urinary findings	Pre renal and post renal acute failure, Hemolytic uremic syndrome
2. Protein, granular cast, epithelial cells	Acute tubular necrosis
3. Protein, RBC and RBC cast	Acute parenchymal disease
4. Protein, eosinophils	Acute interstitial nephritis

Management

The management of intrinsic renal failure includes:

(a) Management of immediate complications.

(b) Supportive care.

Complications: The complications of acute intrinsic renal failure include:

1. Hyperkalemia, hyponatremia, hypocalcaemia.
2. Pulmonary edema and heart failure.
3. Metabolic acidosis.
4. Hypertension.
5. Anemia.
6. Gastrointestinal bleed.

Management of Immediate Complications

1. Hyperkalemia

Table 12.5: Differentiation between pre renal (functional) oliguria and acute tubular necrosis

	Parameters	*Functional oliguria*	*Acute tubular necrosis*
1.	Urinary sodium (meq/ L)	Less than 20	More than 50
2.	Urine: plasma creatinine ratio	More than 40	Less than 20
3.	Urine: plasma osmolality	More than 2	Less than 1.5
4.	Urine: plasma urea ratio	More than 10	Less than 10
5.	Renal failure index*	Less than 1	More than 1
6.	Challenge test	Positive	Negative

* Renal failure index: Urinary Na/Urinary creatinine.

(a) The child with oliguria/anuria should not receive any potassium containing food, fluid or medicine until adequate renal function is reestablished.

(b) Serum potassium level should be measured every 12–24 hour and an ECG obtained if necessary. If serum potassium level rise upto 5.5 mEq/litre, measures to deplete body potassium should be initiated with sodium polystyrene sulphonate resin, 1 gm/ kg orally suspended in 2 ml /kg 70% sorbitol. It can also be given per rectally suspended in 20% sorbitol 10 ml/kg. Resin therapy is repeated 2 hourly. One gram resin/kg body weight reduces serum potassium by 1 mEq/L.

(c) If the serum potassium rises above 7 mEq/litre, the following emergency measures are to be started, awaiting dialysis, in addition to resins and given sequentially:

i. 10% calcium gluconate 1.0 ml/kg IV over 3 - 5 minutes.

ii. 7.5% sodium bicarbonate 1 - 2 mEq/kg IV over 5 - 10 minutes.

iii. 50% glucose (1 ml/kg) with regular insulin (0.1 unit/kg IV over 1 hour).

iv. Salbutamol 5-8 microgram/kg IV or by inhalation.

It should be noted that the duration of action of these measures is only a few hours. Persistent hyperkalemia, especially in patients requiring emergency measures should be treated with dialysis.

2. *Acidosis:* Mild to moderate acidosis does not require any treatment. Severe acidosis (pH < 7.1, serum bicarbonate < 8 mEq/litre) should be managed immediately by partial correction (i.e. enough to raise pH to 7.2 and serum bicarbonate level to 12 mEq/litre) on the basis of the formula:

   mEq of sodium bicarbonate = 0.3 × wt (in kg) × (12 – serum bicarb level).

   The remainder correction should be done only after normalization of serum calcium and phosphorous and is done by oral sodium bicarbonate tablet or sodium citrate solution. When a facility for blood gas measurement is not available the bicarbonate correction can be done with 7.5% sodium bicarbonate, 3 mEq /kg given slow IV.

3. *Pulmonary edema and heart failure, hypertension:* Can be managed in the same line as discussed earlier in the chapter of APSGN.

4. *Hypocalcaemia:* Hypocalcaemia without tetany should be treated by giving oral antacid containing calcium carbonate, 15 ml 4 times daily with meals and at bedtime. Tetany should be treated with IV 10% calcium gluconate under ECG monitoring The dose of 10% calcium gluconate is 1.0 ml/kg IV over 3–5 minutes .

5. *Hyponatremia:* Should be treated with fluid restriction. If there is sensorial alteration or seizures, the serum sodium is < 120 mEq/l, it should be elevated to 125 mEq/l with IV infusion of 3% sodium chloride. The dose is 6–12 ml/kg over 30–90 minutes. The amount to be infused can also be calculated on the basis of the formula:

   mEq of NaCl required = 0.6 × wt (kg) × (125–serum sodium).

6. *Anemia* of ARF is generally mild (Hb 9–10 gm%), normocytic normochromic and primarily results from volume expansion (hemodilution). Children with HUS, SLE, active bleeding or prolonged ARF may require transfusion. Transfusion of packed red cells is indicated if the Hb level goes below 7 gm%. In hypervolumic patients, transfusion carries the risk of further volume expansion, which may precipitate hypertension, heart failure and pulmonary edema. Slow transfusion (in 4–6 hours) with packed red cells (10 ml/kg) diminishes the aggravation of hypervolemia and use of fresh, washed RBC minimizes the risk of hyperkalemia. If anemia is associated with severe hypervolemia and hyperkalemia, transfusion can be safely administered during dialysis.

7. *Gastrointestinal bleed:* Should be prevented by IV H_2 blockers (Ranitidine 2–3 mg/kg/day 12 hourly IV). In case of a bleed transfusion will be indicated according to the degree of bleed.

8. *Infection:* Should be prevented by maintaining asepsis during all procedures, monitoring IV lines, oral hygiene, avoidance of long-term catheterization of bladder. Frequent physical examination should be done for early detection of infection. In case infection is suspected, culture and sensitivity of appropriate specimen should be done and appropriate antibiotics should be administered.

Supportive Treatment

Oliguric phase:

The duration of oliguria may be for a few hours to several weeks. In uncomplicated acute tubular necrosis, it usually lasts for 5–10 days.

1. *Monitoring:* The following parameters are to be monitored:
   (a) Fluid intake and urine output.
   (b) Stool output and other fluid loss.
   (c) Daily body weight and a detailed physical examination twice daily.
   (d) Estimation of serum sodium and potassium daily.
   (e) Serum urea and serum creatinine daily.
2. *Fluid restriction*
   (a) *On day 1:* Insensible water loss i.e. 300–400 ml/sq m/day.
   (b) *From day 2:* Insensible water loss + 24 hours urine output + other extra loss e.g. loss through diarrhea and vomiting.

   Type of fluid: Insensible water loss should be replenished by 10% dextrose; urine output and other losses with 0.45% saline in 5% dextrose.
   (c) In presence of marked hypervolemia total fluid restriction should be advised. No replacement of insensible fluid loss and other losses needs to be to be done.
   (d) No fluid restriction is necessary for non-oliguric renal failure.
3. *Diet:* In most cases sodium, potassium and phosphorous should be restricted. The diet should be of high calorie content with protein of high biological value. 50–60 calories/kg/day should be advised for which sugar, honey, butter milk, milk, butter, ghee, and oil should be given in adequate amounts. 0.6–0.8 gm/kg/day of protein should be advised. A higher amount of protein (3–5 gms/kg/day) should be advised if the child is on dialysis. Milk and eggs are good sources. Eggs are preferred to restrict fluid intake. Vitamins and micronutrients should be given in adequate amounts. In critically ill patients, parenteral nutrition with essential amino acids should be considered.
4. *Indications for dialysis*
   (a) Volume overload with hypertension and/or pulmonary edema refractory to diuretic therapy.
   (b) Hyperkalemia with serum potassium > 7 mEq/L or between 6–6.5 mEq/L with ECG changes.
   (c) Severe metabolic acidosis (pH < 7.2) not responding to medical treatment.
   (d) Presence of neurologic symptoms viz. altered sensorium, seizures.
   (e) Blood urea nitrogen > 100–150 mg/dl.

Dialysis

The major dialysis modalities include peritoneal dialysis, hemodialysis and continuous hemofiltration. The former two are equally effective in the management of acute renal failure. *Peritoneal dialysis* is sufficient in most cases and is commonly used in children. It is easy to perform, requires minimal equipment and infrastructure. It is tolerated by critically ill children. It is technically feasible in the smallest infants.

Continuous arteriovenous hemofiltration (CAVH) is particularly useful for the management of overhydration complicating ARF, and in patients with major surgical procedures, burns, heart failure and septic shock. CAVH is best undertaken in units with expertise in extracorporeal dialysis.

Diuretic Phase

The diuretic phase is characterized by progressive increase of urine output which may reach as high as 2–3 liters per day. The blood urea and creatinine usually continue to rise to fall only after several days. During the diuretic phase complications such as infection, gastrointestinal bleed, convulsion and electrolyte abnormalities (e.g. hypokalemia) are frequent.

With glomerular disease, though the urine volume may be high, excessive loss of fluid and electrolytes do not occur because the tubules are able to exhibit homeostatic function. There is only excretion of excess fluid and electrolytes accumulated during the oliguric phase. On the other hand, when ARF is the consequence of tubular damage, an excessive diuresis can occur as tubular regeneration and function begins to return.

The child should be monitored for dehydration, infection, gastrointestinal bleeding and hypokalemia. The urine output should be replaced with 0.45 saline and potassium replaced if necessary.

Surgical Treatment

The children with a surgical cause leading to obstruction of renal tract and acute renal failure need urgent management to remove obstruction to urine flow. Definitive surgery should be performed after treatment of acute renal failure.

Outcome

In uncomplicated acute renal failure, oligoanuria may last for 7–10 days at the end of which the urine output may start and progressively increase. Such patients may require only a single dialysis. If acute renal failure is prolonged beyond 2–3 weeks, multiple dialysis may be required. In these cases, maintenance of nutrition and prevention of infections become crucial. Most patients die of infection and inanition before significant recovery of renal function can occur.

For a better outcome, urgent dialysis is indicated when the child presents with uremic complication. Early dialysis should be planned in cases with HUS and hypercatabolic states (e.g. infection, trauma).

The outcome also depends on the precipitating cause. The prognosis is good in acute tubular necrosis and intravascular hemolysis. In glomerular disease, the prognosis depends on the severity of renal injury. The factors associated with high mortality are sepsis, multiple organ failure, cardiac surgery and delayed referral.

Prevention

Most of the precipitating causes of acute renal failure are preventable. Preventive measures may be as follows:

1. Prompt fluid therapy for correction of dehydration in acute diarrhea.
2. Avoidance or judicious use of nephrotoxic drugs.
3. Careful prescription of antimalarial drugs.
4. Maintenance of hydration for patients undergoing diagnostic procedures with radio contrast media.

Chronic Renal Failure

Chronic renal failure (CRF) is defined as an irreversible deterioration of renal function. It gradually progresses to end stage renal disease which is characterized by decline of renal function to a degree when life cannot be sustained without renal replacement therapy either in the form of dialysis or renal transplant.

Etiology

In children, the causes of chronic renal failure may be congenital, acquired, inherited or metabolic renal disease. The causes may be different depending on age at presentation.

In children younger than 5 years the causes are:

1. *Congenital anomalies:* Renal hypoplasia, dysplasia, polycystic kidney disease.
2. *Obstructive uropathy:* Pelvi-ureteric or uretero-vesical junction obstruction, posterior urethral valve, calculi.
3. Renal cortical necrosis, infantile polycystic kidney disease, congenital nephrotic syndrome.

After 5 years of age, acquired diseases predominate. These include:

1. *Various forms of glomerulonephritis:* Idiopathic, SLE, anaphylactoid purpura, polyarteritis nodosa.
2. *Inherited disorders:* Nephronophthisis, Alport syndrome.
3. *Miscellaneous:* Amyloidosis, hemolytic uremic syndrome, bilateral Wilms' tumor.

Metabolic disorders viz. cystinoisis, hyperoxaluria and certain inherited disorders like polycystic disease of kidney can present with CRF at any age.

Clinical Manifestations

The clinical features include anorexia, failure to thrive, growth retardation, easy fatigability, anemia, hypertension and osteodystrophy. The late features with extreme reduction of GFR include left ventricular failure and pulmonary edema, pericarditis, and altered sensorium, severe acidosis and hyperkalemia.

The diagnosis of CRF should be considered if any one or more of the above manifestations are present without an obvious cause.

Laboratory Diagnosis

Laboratory investigations to confirm CRF:

1. Estimation of blood urea, creatinine; both are elevated. Hemoglobin is low. A peripheral blood smear shows normocytic normochromic anemia.
2. Measurement of GFR. It can determine degree of renal dysfunction.
3. Serum electrolytes viz. sodium and potassium. There may be hyperkalemia and hyponatremia if there is volume overload.

Laboratory investigations to find out the cause are to be done selectively depending on the clinical diagnosis. They are as follows:

1. Urinalysis: Glomerular diseases are suggested by proteinuria and hematuria and casts.

2. Serum protein and fractions low, serum cholesterol and triglycerides high in glomerular diseases.
3. Skeletal survey, serum calcium and phosphorous in presence of osteodystrophy.
4. Ultrasonography for examination of renal size, abnormalities, obstruction.
5. Radionuclide imaging to examine for renal scars. It is not helpful if GFR is below 20–30 ml/min/1.73 m^2.
6. Renal biopsy and histological examination in case of renal parenchymal disease.

Treatment

The aim of treatment is to maintain well-being and quality of life. Normal physical activity and schooling should be encouraged. Counseling of the family and emotional support to the child is important.

The treatment of CRF includes monitoring the progress, measures to retard progression of renal dysfunction and replacement therapy for diminished or absent renal function.

Monitoring

The management of CRF requires close monitoring of the clinical and laboratory status. The laboratory parameters for monitoring include hemoglobin level, serum electrolytes, blood urea nitrogen, serum creatinine, calcium, phosphorous, albumin and alkaline phosphatase. For early detection of osteodystrophy, periodic measurement of parathyroid hormone and X-ray of bones help. Echocardiography, done periodically can help in identifying left ventricular hypertrophy and cardiac dysfunction.

Measures to Retard Progression of CRF

The measures to retard progression of CRF include protein restriction, strict control of hypertension, use of angiotensin converting enzyme (ACE) inhibitors, and control of hyperlipidemia. Studies have shown that ACE inhibitors slow the progress of renal disease, an effect independent of control of hypertension. Control of hyperlipidemia is also shown to be helpful. However, a benefit of protein restriction in children is not proved.

Diet: Food should be tasty and attractive. The recommended calorie and protein intake appropriate for age and weight should be provided. The protein should be of high biological value that is metabolized primarily to usable amino acids rather than to nitrogenous wastes. The proteins of highest biological values include those in eggs and milk followed by meat, fish and foul. Dietary intake however should be adjusted according to response, preferably through a dietician. If oral intake remains inadequate supplemental feedings may be provided via nasogastric feeding. In infants, the calorie intake may be enhanced by addition of carbohydrates (polycose) and fat (medium chain triglyceride oil).

Children with CRF may become deficient in water soluble vitamins either because of inadequate intake or dialysis. Routine administration of vitamins supplements should include 1mg each of B_1, B_2 and folic acid, 10 mg each of pantothenic acid and pyridoxine, vitamin C 50 mg, B_{12} 5 mg and biotin 300 mg per day. Fat soluble vitamins, A, E and K are usually not required. Iron and zinc supplements should be added only when deficiency is confirmed.

Fluid and electrolytes: There is no need to restrict salt and water because children with CRF can maintain water and sodium balance until there is terminal renal failure. If there is no edema and hypertension, the usual salt intake should be allowed. If the blood pressure is high, salt intake should be restricted to 0.8 to 1 gm per day. Salt restriction and diuretics may be required in children with edema and heart failure. Fluid restriction is necessary when the child develops end stage renal disease and requires dialysis. Both hypo and hyperkalemia can occur in CRF. Hypokalemia can result from excessive use of diuretics. If serum potassium is less than 3 mEq/l, intake of potassium rich articles like citrus fruits, bananas, green vegetables should be advised. Hyperkalemia may be treated by restriction of potassium containing food articles and potassium exchange resins.

Hypertension: Sodium and water retension are the major causes of hypertension in CRF. Hence most cases of hypertension can be controlled by salt restriction and diuretics. Some patients may require antihypertensive. The commonly used antihypertensive drugs include ACE inhibitors, alpha and beta blockers and clonidine. Hypertensive emergency should be treated with sublingual nefidepine or IV nitroprusside or labetolol.

Anemia: Most patients need iron and folic acid supplements. Recombinant erythropoietin (EPO) can be given to patients predialysis or to those on dialysis. The dose is 50–150 units/kg weekly subcutaneously. The dose is tailored to achieve a hematocrit level (34–36%). During EPO therapy serum ferritin should be kept above 100 microgram/litre to ensure adequate iron supplies.

Packed cell transfusion (10 ml/kg) may be given when hemoglobin level is less than 6 gm% under careful monitoring. Leukocyte poor blood is preferred. A normal or near normal hematocrit improves appetite, increase energy and quality of life.

Metabolic acidosis: Mild acidosis may not require correction. A serum bicarbonate less than 15 mEq/l, can be treated with oral supplement of bicarbonate in the dose of 2–3 mEq/kg. The dose should be titrated to maintain serum bicarbonate level at around 20 mEq/l.

Hyperlipidemia: Many patients with CRF may have high cholesterol and triglycerides. Diet restriction and exercise are helpful in correction of lipid abnormalities to some extent. Lipid lowering drugs have limited role in children.

Infection: Urinary tract and respiratory tract infection are common in children with CRF. The symptoms may be mild or even absent. Antibiotics should be used with appropriate dosage modification. However, it is necessary to give a normal loading dose of the drug.

Growth: One of the significant long-term sequalae of CRF is short stature. Children who remain less than – 2 SD for height despite optimal medical treatment may benefit with pharmacologic doses of recombinant human growth hormone. Treatment should be started with 0.05 mg/kg/day subcutaneously, with periodic adjustment in the dose to achieve a goal of normal height velocity for age. The treatment should be continued until the patient (i) reaches the 50th percentile of mid parental height, (ii) achieves a final adult height, or (iii) undergoes renal transplant. Treatment with human growth hormone helps the majority of the patients to achieve a normal adult height.

Osteodystrophy: A spectrum of bone disorders is seen in children with CRF. It is most commonly caused by secondary hyperparathyroidism, the chief stimulus for which is hyperphosphatemia.

The clinical manifestations include muscle weakness, bone pain, and fractures with minor trauma. In growing children, rachitic changes, varus and valgus deformities of long bones, slipped capital femoral epiphysis may be seen. Laboratory studies may demonstrate a decreased serum calcium level, increased serum phosphorous level, increased alkaline phosphatase and a normal parathyroid level.

To prevent such bone disorders, the serum phosphate levels should be maintained as close to normal as possible. Children and adolescents should be advised a low phosphorous diet. The infants should be advised a low phosphorous formula. It is not possible to fully restrict phosphorous intake. So phosphate binders like calcium carbonate and calcium acetate are commonly used. The starting dose is 50–60 mg/kg/day of calcium (as carbonate or acetate). These should be prescribed with meals.

The therapy for renal osteodystrophy is administration of vitamin D. It is indicated in patients with (i) high parathyroid hormone levels greater than 3 times the normal, or (ii) persistent hypocalcaemia despite reduction of the serum phosphorous level below 6 mg/dL. Therapy can be initiated with calcitriol (1, 25 $(OH)_2 D_3$) 0.01 to 0.05 microgram/kg/day. The phosphate binders and vitamin D should be adjusted to maintain the intact parathyroid hormone level 2 – 3 times the upper limit of normal and the calcium and phosphorous levels within normal range for age.

Immunization: Data suggests that children with CRF respond suboptimally to vaccination. However, all children with CRF should receive all standard immunizations according to schedule. The live vaccines should be withheld in children under immunosuppressive drugs. The MMR and the varicella vaccine should be administered before renal transplant and all children should be advised influenza vaccine yearly.

Replacement Therapy for Diminished or Absent Renal Function

Patients with end stage renal disease, which is defined as decline in renal function to an extent that life threatening biochemical abnormalities persist despite optimal medical management, require renal replacement therapy in the form of maintenance dialysis or renal transplant.

Urinary Tract Infection

Urinary tract infection (UTI) in children is important not only because of the frequency of their occurrence but also because of their potential to cause lasting kidney disease. The incidence of urinary tract infection is highest during the early years, when the propensity to renal damage is also the greatest.

The renal cortex in the neonates and infant is functionally and structurally immature and in the growing stage. Hence infection of upper urinary tract carries the risk of severe damage and scarring. In the neonates and infants, who are the high risk group for damage, the signs and symptoms of urinary tract infection are non-specific, which usually does not point to the genitourinary system and unless specifically looked for, the diagnosis of UTI is missed.

UTI in children may be an indicator of an underlying abnormality of the genitourinary system. UTI related kidney damage is most often the result of unrecognized or inadequately managed infection during infancy or early childhood.

A very high index of suspicion of UTI should be maintained in any sick child and frequent urine cultures should be asked for especially during the high risk period.

For all practical purposes, UTI in children should be considered as upper UTI so that unnecessary damage to renal cortex is prevented.

Unless UTI is promptly and adequately treated, long term complications like renal scarring, chronic renal failure and end stage renal disease, hypertension and renal stones may develop in later life.

Epidemiology

Urinary tract infection is the third common bacterial infection in children after those of respiratory tract and gastrointestinal tract. The precise data on incidence and prevalence in developing countries is not available as most UTI remain unrecognized because of non-specific signs and symptoms. In western countries, UTI occurs in 3–5% of girls and 1% of boys. In both sexes, the first UTI occurs during the first year of life. UTIs are more common in uncircumcised boys. The male-female ratio varies with age. There is male preponderance during the first year of life. Beyond 1–2 years there is female preponderance. Obstructive lesions may be found in 10% of boys. 30–40% patients show vesicoureteric reflux. The risk factors associated with renal scarring include UTI in children less than 1 year old, delay in initiating antibacterial treatment, recurrent UTI and presence of moderate to severe vesicoureteric reflux.

Etiology

E.coli is the most common organism during a first symptomatic infection in all age groups. Nearly 70 – 80% of recurrent UTI are also caused by E.coli. In males older than 1 year proteus is as common as E.coli. It can be a causative organism in about one third of boys with cystitis. Other organisms like Klebsiella, Staphylococcus epidermidis and streptococcus fecalis may be occasionally responsible. Pseudomonus and proteus are associated with recurrent UTI, instrumentation and nosocomial infection. Candida infection is common in preterm infants. Viral infection, particularly adenovirus, may occur as a cause of cystitis.

Pathogenesis

In the neonatal period, the renal parenchymal infection is due to hematogenous spread. Beyond neonatal period, it is an ascending infection. Bacteria reach the urethra and bladder through the ascending route and ureter and kidney through vesicoureteral reflux. The source of bacteria is usually the bowel. In boys, bacteria under the prepuce reach the bladder by ascending the urethra. This explains why uncircumcised boys have more UTI.

The predisposing factors for UTI include a short urethra in the females which permits easy entry of bacteria into the bladder and uncircumcised boys in spite of a long urethra, probably due to bacterial colonization under the prepuce. Babies born to mothers with bacteriuria during pregnancy have a higher incidence of UTI as a result of development of rapid colonization by uropathogens. An increased predisposition to UTI is seen in presence of obstructive uropathy, urinary calculus, constipation, incomplete voiding with residual urine and thread worm infestation. Another important predisposing factor is therapy with broad spectrum antibiotics for minor infections. This may abolish the normal bacterial flora of the perineum and allow colonization by more virulent organism.

Classification

There are three basic forms of urinary tract infection: pyelonephritis, cystitis and asymptomatic bacteriuria. UTI may be simple, complicated and recurrent.

Pyelonephritis indicates involvement of the renal parenchyma. If there is no parenchymal involvement it is called pyelitis. Acute pyelonephritis may result in renal injury which is termed pyelonephritic scar.

Cystitis indicates involvement of bladder. It does not cause renal injury.

Asymptomatic bacteriuria refers to presence of significant bacteriuria on two or more specimens in a child with no symptoms. A colony count of $> 10^5$/ml of a single species in a mid stream catch of urine is called significant bacteriuria.

Simple UTI is characterized by low grade fever, dysuria, frequency, urgency and absence of symptoms of complicated UTI.

Complicated UTI is characterized by presence of fever > 39°C, systemic toxicity, persistent vomiting, dehydration, renal angle tenderness and raised creatinine.

Recurrent UTI is defined as the second attack of UTI.

Clinical Manifestations

The clinical features of UTI differ according to the age, the form and the presence or absence of anatomical abnormalities.

Newborn Period

In the newborn period, symptomatic UTI is generally a part of septicemia. They may present with non-specific features like jaundice, poor feeding, irritability and weight loss. Only failure to gain weight may be an early indication of UTI in this age group.

Age Group Between 1 Month and 3 Years

In children between the age group of one month and 3 years, failure to thrive is the leading feature. Some infants may present with non-specific features like jaundice, poor feeding, irritability and weight loss. A few may present with macroscopic hematuria without any signs and symptoms pointing to the urinary tract. The child may also present with fever, irritability, abdominal pain, vomiting, malodorous diapers and meningism. In infants, unexplained fever may be the only symptom of acute pyelonephritis.

Older Children

In older girls, reappearance of symptoms like enuresis may be a presenting feature. Older boys have fewer symptoms related to the urinary tract. May present with only macroscopic or microspic hematuria. However, older children with pyelonephritis may present with abdominal or flank pain, fever with chill and rigor, malaise, nausea, vomiting and occasionally diarrhoea. The symptoms of cystitis include dysuria, urgency, frequency, suprapubic pain, incontinence and malodorous urine. Fever is not a feature of cystitis.

Features Suggesting Underlying Structural Abnormality

In UTI complicated with congenital abnormality, the age of onset is early, starting during the first few months of life. In case of acquired obstruction, the onset may be at any age. In addition to the signs and symptoms of UTI, the following features will suggest an underlying structural abnormality:

(a) History of straining at micturition, dribbling, poor urinary stream, crying during micturition and intermittent voiding indicating an abnormality of the distal urinary tract.

(b) A distended bladder, palpable enlarged kidneys.

(c) Tight phimosis, vulval synechiae.

(d) Palpable fecal mass in colon.

(e) Patulous anus; neurological deficit in the lower limbs.

(f) Previous surgery of urinary tract, anorectal malformation or meningomyelocele.

Laboratory Diagnosis

The diagnosis of UTI is made on the basis of clinical features, microscopic examination of urine and urine culture. Clinical features can only suggest and supportive evidence can be obtained from microscopic examination of urine. The only valid criterion for diagnosis is demonstration of significant bacterial growth by urine culture.

Microscopic Examination of Urine

Urine analysis should be always performed on a freshly voided urine sample (preferably within 30 minutes) to avoid false positive and negative results. A microscopic examination of urine is especially helpful in making a tentative diagnosis of UTI in an acutely ill child awaiting results of culture and sensitivity.

Interpretation

1. The presence of > 5 leucocytes/high power field in centrifuged urine sample or > 10 leucocytes/cu mm in uncentrifuged urine may suggest urinary tract infection. Leucocytes may be also found with fever, dehydration, acute post streptococcal glomerulonephritis, and renal tuberculosis. However, absence of bacteria in urine in these conditions will help to exclude UTI.
2. Presence of 1 bacteria, on gram stain, in an uncentrifuged specimen of urine is shown to correlate well with a bacterial colony count of > 100,000/cu mm. A normal uncentrifuged specimen should have no organism per oil immersion field and not > 20 when centrifuged. In absence of facilities of bacterial culture, presence of bacteria permits a tentative diagnosis of UTI.

Nitrite Test and Leukocyte Esterase Test

A positive nitrite test is suggestive of significant bacteriuria. It is due to conversion of nitrate to nitrite by gram negative rods e.g. E. coli. A positive leukocyte esterase test results from the presence of white blood cells. By this test pyuria can be detected even if the urine sample contains damaged or lysed white cells. A combination of these two tests by dipsticks is reliable, but its sensitivity is low in infants who void frequently and have a less vigorous inflammatory response.

Urine Culture

Urine culture is the gold standard to diagnose urinary tract infection. Urine should be collected carefully, to prevent contamination by periurethral flora, in a sterile container. The routine procedure for collection is a clean catch, if possible a mid stream specimen. Washing the genitalia with soap and water can minimize contamination of periurethral and prepucial flora. Prompt plating of urine specimen, within an hour of collection, is important. The sample should be refrigerated at 4°C, if delay is anticipated. In the young infant supra pubic aspiration or urethral catheterization is the best way to collect the sample, as a clean catch specimen is difficult. Culture of urine enables to measure the number of colonies in a known volume of urine. The colony counts should be interpreted based on the method of collection.

Table 12.6 : Diagnostic colony counts for UTI

Method of collection	*Colony count*	*Probability of infection*
Suprapubic aspiration	Any number of pathogens	99%
Urethral	$> 5 \times 10^4$ CFU/mL	95%
Midstream	$> 10^5$ CFU/mL	90–95%

A urine culture should be repeated in case contamination is suspected, e.g. mixed growth of 2 or more pathogens, or growth of organisms that normally constitute the periurethral flora viz. the lactobacilli in healthy girls and enterococci in infants and toddlers.

Blood Examination

A blood culture should be done in neonates and infants and in older children with complicated UTI. The TLC and DLC show polymorphonuclear leucocytosis. There is raised ESR (> 30 mm at 1 hour) and CRP (> 20 mg/dl) in acute pyelonephritis.

Imaging Studies

A radiological evaluation is usually necessary in all children with symptomatic UTI in view of the high incidence of renal abnormalities associated with UTI. The indications of imaging studies are as follows:

1. All children below 5 years with symptomatic UTI. Above 5 years, females with UTI with fever and males with symptomatic UTI.
2. Any child with UTI and palpable bladder after voiding, renal mass, congenital skeletal abnormalities.
3. UTI with complications viz. metabolic acidosis, hypertension and acute renal failure.

The modes of radiological evaluation include:

1. Plain picture abdomen to exclude calculus.
2. USG of KUB region to evaluate kidney size and to demonstrate any dilatation of collecting system.
3. Micturating cystourethrogram (MCU)/Radio nuclide (Rn) MCU to demonstrate vesicourethral reflux (VUR) and diagnose posterior urethral valves (PUV). Rn MCU is a more convenient procedure in children and radiation exposure is 1/100 of conventional MCU.
4. Intravenous pyelography/Radionuclide (Rn) scans using DMSA and DTPA: Rn scan with 99 Tc di mercapto succinic acid (DMSA) is more sensitive in detection of renal cortical scars. Rn scan with 99 Tc di amino tetra ethyl penta acetic acid (DTPA) gives an excellent idea of the functional status of the kidneys. Radiation exposure in both procedures is much less. The importance of intravenous pyelography (IVP) has declined following the availability of radioisotope scans. However, an IVP may be performed to examine for renal scarring if facilities for Rn scan is not available.

Points to be Noted

1. Diagnostic procedures, except plain picture abdomen and ultrasound scan, should be delayed till 4–6 weeks, because functional defects caused by the episode of UTI may last till this period.
2. Children requiring imaging studies should be first subjected to the preliminary investigations viz. PP abdomen and USG. Further investigation will depend on the findings of these tests.

Treatment

For convenience of treatment UTI may be classified as follows:

1. Symptomatic (first) infection:
   (a) Uncomplicated infection.
   (b) Complicated infection.
2. Recurrent infection.
3. Asymptomatic bacteriuria.
4. UTI with VUR.

Symptomatic (First) Infection

In complicated UTI treatment should be aggressive. Newborn and infants should be hospitalized and treated with parenteral antibiotics. Older children with complicated UTI also need parenteral antibiotics initially for the first 48–72 hours. Antibiotic therapy should be started after obtaining a urine culture. The antibiotic may have to be changed later depending on the sensitivity pattern of the infecting organism. In addition, due attention should be paid to fluid, electrolytes, control of pyrexia and renal status. In older children, once the clinical condition improves and oral intake is satisfactory, antibiotics may be given orally.

Children with uncomplicated UTI are to be treated with oral antibiotics depending on the sensitivity pattern of the infecting organism.

Table 12.7 : Common antimicrobials for treatment of UTI

Medication	Doses
PARENTERAL	
Coamoxiclav	30–35 mg/kg amoxicillin 12 hourly IV
Gentamycin	5–6 mg/ kg/day 12 hourly
Amikacin	15–20 mg/kg/day 12 hourly
Cefotaxime	100–150 mg/kg/day 8 hourly
Ceftriaxone	75–100 mg/kg/day daily/ 12 hourly
ORAL	
Medication	*Doses*
Cephalexin	50–70 mg/kg/day 8 hourly
Co amoxyclav	30–35 mg/kg/day 8 hourly (Amoxycillin)
Cefixime	8–10 mg/kg/day 12 hourly
Ciprofloxacin	10–20 mg/kg/day 12 hourly
Cefaclor	40 mg/kg/day 8 hourly

Choice of Antimicrobials

For empirical parenteral therapy, a combination of ampicillin and gentamycin or a third generation cephalosporin (cefotaxime/ceftriaxone) is preferred. Once the child shows clinical improvement with resolution of fever and toxicity, antibiotics can be administered orally.

In young infants (< 3 months age) and children with positive blood culture parenteral antibiotics should be continued for the entire duration of treatment.

Oral amoxycillin, cotrimoxazole or cephalosporin is the preferred drug. Ciprofloxacin should not be used as first line drugs and reserved for serious infection. Nalidixic acid and nitrofurantoin should not be used to treat UTI because they do not achieve therapeutic concentration in renal parenchyma and blood stream.

Urine cultures need not be repeated after cessation of antibiotic therapy. If expected clinical response does not occur within 2 days, a repeat urine culture and an ultrasonography should be performed to exclude complicating factors.

Duration of Treatment

The usual duration of treatment is 10–14 days for infants and complicated UTI and 7–10 days for uncomplicated UTI. Short course treatment for 1–3 days is not recommended in children.

Following the treatment of UTI, prophylactic antibiotic should be initiated in children below 2 years and continued until appropriate imaging studies are completed.

Supportive Therapy

During an episode of acute UTI, it is important to maintain adequate hydration. A liberal intake of fluid also helps to alleviate dysuria. Antipyretics are used to relieve fever.

Evaluation After First UTI

The evaluation of the first UTI is done by imaging of the urinary tract to identify patients at risk of renal damage. It is recommended that all children *below 1 year age* should be screened by ultrasonography (USG), followed by MCU (micturating cystourethrogram) and DMSA (Dimercaptosuccinic acid) scintigraphy. In children *between 1 and 5 years age,* an USG and DMSA scan should be advised. If the USG or DMSA scan is abnormal an MCU should be advised. *Above 5 years,* if the USG is abnormal, an MCU and DMSA scan should be advised. No further tests required if the USG is normal.

The USG should be done soon after the diagnosis of UTI. The MCU is recommended 2–3 weeks later, while the DMSA scan is carried out 2–3 months after treatment. Patients showing hydronephrosis in the absence of VUR should be evaluated by diuretic renography using ^{99m}Tc-labeled diethylenetriamine-pentaacetic acid (DTPA) or mercaptoacetylglycine (MAG–3). These techniques provide quantitative assessment of renal function and drainage of the dilated collecting system.

All patients with recurrent UTI should be advised detailed evaluation with USG, DMSA and MCU.

Recurrent Infection

All recurrent infection should be treated as that of acute infections but should be followed by prophylaxis.

Table 12.8 : Antimicrobials for prophylaxis

Medication	*Dose (mg/kg/day)*	*Remarks*
Cotrimoxazole	1–2 (trimethoprim)	Avoid < 3 months age and G6PD deficiency
Nitrofurantoin	1–2	Avoid < 3 months age, G.I. upset
Cephalexin	10	Drug of choice in first 3–6 months age.

The suitable drug is given as a single dose at bed time for an initial period of 2–4 months. If a recurrence occurs shortly after stopping prophylaxis, a therapeutic course is given for 10 days followed by prophylaxis for 6 months. Some children may require prophylaxis for several years. Follow-up urine cultures should be done every 2–3 months during prophylaxis.

Children with more than one episode of UTI, irrespective of age, should be evaluated with an USG, MCU and DMSA scan. A patient showing hydronephrosis without VUR should be evaluated by DTPA scan for assessment of quantitative renal function and drainage of the dilated collecting system.

Measures to Reduce Recurrent UTI

1. General measures include regular bowel habit to avoid constipation, frequent complete bladder emptying and increasing fluid intake. Wiping in girls after defecation should be in an anterior to posterior direction to avoid periurethral soiling with fecal matter. Attention to undergarments and perineal hygiene including foreskin in boys should be advised.
2. Circumcision may be considered in boys with recurrent UTI.

Asymptomatic Bacteriuria

The frequency of asymptomatic bacteriuria is about 1% in girls and 0.5% in boys. About 80% children have recurrences. Absence of symptom and signs, normal ESR, CRP and an USG scan explains the benign nature. The causative organism isolated is E. coli which is a low virulent organism and lack the characteristics present in the invasive form that cause pyelonephritis. It has been suggested that presence of such organisms prevent colonization with more virulent organisms. Eradication of these organisms with antibiotics may lead to infection with more virulent organism. Asymptomatic bacteriuria hence does not require treatment. Bacteriuria may persist for many years but resolve with time.

UTI with Vesicourethral Reflux

The severity of VUR is graded from I to V, based on the appearance of the urinary tract on contrast MCU. The treatment options for VUR are continuous antibiotic prophylaxis or surgical repair. Therapeutic recommendations depend on the patient's age at diagnosis, grade of VUR, findings on renal imaging and occurrence of breakthrough infection on follow-up.

Most children are managed on long-term antibiotic prophylaxis while awaiting spontaneous resolution of VUR. The patient should be kept on close follow-up for occurrence of breakthrough UTI. A MCU is repeated every 12–18 months to evaluate resolution of reflux. A DMSA renal scan is repeated in patients having break through UTI to detect fresh renal scarring.

Table 12.9 : Management of vesico ureteric reflux

Grade of reflux	*Management*
Grades I and II	Antibiotic prophylaxis until 1 year old. Restart antibiotic prophylaxis if there is breakthrough febrile UTI.
Grade III to V	Antibiotic prophylaxis upto 5 years of age. Consider surgery if there is breakthrough febrile UTI. Beyond 5 years: Prophylaxis is continued if there is bowel bladder dysfunction.

The risk of recurrent UTI and renal scarring is low after 4–5 years of age. Hence it has been recommended that prophylaxis be discontinued in children beyond 5 years of age with normal bowel and urinary habits, even if mild to moderate reflux persists.

Long-Term Follow-Up

Children with renal scarring should be followed up through adulthood twice a year. Clinical assessment includes monitoring of physical growth and blood pressure. Investigations include urinalysis for proteinuria every 6 months, blood urea and serum creatinine every year. Urine should be promptly cultured in patients having signs of UTI. Renal growth should be monitored by yearly ultrasound scan.

Posterior Urethral Valve

Posterior urethral valve (PUV) is the most common cause of lower urinary tract obstruction in boys. The valves are located just distal to the verumontanum at the junction of the anterior and posterior urethra. There are three types:

Type I: It is the most common type. These valves are bilateral cusps with a slit like opening between the cusps and produce obstruction to flow of urine.

Type II: These valves spread proximally and do not produce obstruction to the flow of urine. They usually go undetected.

Type III: This type is less common consisting of a diaphragm with a central hole. They may get treated when retrograde catherization tear the valves.

Obstruction to flow of urine causes dilatation of posterior urethra and hypertrophy of bladder neck. The bladder wall thickens and there is trabeculation. There may be gross reflux into ureters with associated pyelonephritis and reflux nephropathy. The renal changes range from mild hydronephrosis to severe renal dysplasia. The degree of severity of renal changes probably depends on severity of obstruction and the time of its onset in fetal life.

Clinical Manifestations

Antenatal ultrasonography can detect a dilated urinary system with bilateral hydronephrosis, hydro ureter and a thick walled bladder. Renal dysplasia may be associated with oligohydramnios. Prenatally diagnosed posterior urethral valves, particularly when discovered in the second trimester, carry a poor prognosis than those detected after birth.

Infants, who do not undergo routine ultrasonography, generally present with dribbling of urine, pain (crying) during micturation, urinary tract infection or sepsis. The urine stream is weak and there is a palpably distended bladder. If the obstruction is severe and goes unrecognized during the neonatal period, infants may present in later life with failure to thrive due to uremia or sepsis caused by infection in the obstructed urinary tract. With lesser degree of obstruction, children present later in life with difficulty in achieving diurnal urinary continence or with recurrent urinary tract infection.

Laboratory Investigation

The diagnosis is confirmed by micturating cystourethrogram (MCU); findings of which include a dilated posterior urethra, poor flow into the distal urethra and abnormalities of the bladder viz. thickened wall and trabeculation. There may be vesico urethral reflux, bilateral hydroureter and hydronephrosis. After the diagnosis is established, renal function should be evaluated.

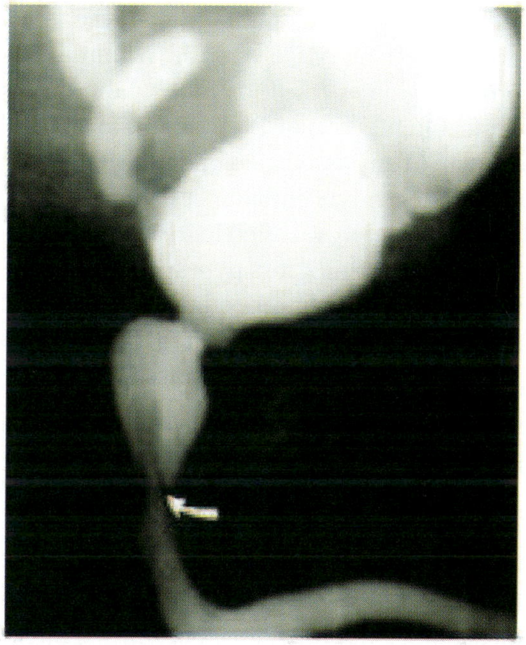

Fig. 12.5: Figure showing posterior urethral valve with dilated posterior urethra and dilated ureter (MCU)

Treatment

Antenatal treatment: Urinary tract obstruction in utero leads to decreased urinary output which can result in oligohydramnios. Amniotic fluid is also necessary for proper development of the lungs. Absence of amniotic fluid may lead to pulmonary hypoplasia also. It is important to identify fetus with good renal function. The predictors for good renal function in the fetus are sodium < 100 mEq/l, chloride < 90 mEq/l and osmolality below 200 mOsm/kg in three consecutive urine samples on three different days.

Vesicoamniotic shunt is the procedure used in antenatal treatment. It helps to overcome poor outcome, to gain time for prolonging pregnancy and protecting the developing kidney and lungs. The shunt procedure may reverse oligohydramnios, but does not influence the outcome and long term results of the patients with PUV. Fetal intervention has been attempted with variable results but is not regarded as a practical procedure.

Postnatal treatment: The favourable prognostic factors include a normal ultrasonography at 18 and 24 weeks of gestation, a serum creatinine level less than 0.8 to 1 mg/dL after bladder compression and visualization of corticomedullary junction on renal sonography.

If a male infant is born with suspected PUV, an MCU and drainage of the bladder should be done by catherization with a 6 F feeding tube. If catheterization is not possible, then a supra pubic puncture is made for drainage as well as MCU. If the infant is stable, endoscopic incision or resection of the valves is done at the earliest. Fulguration of PUV should be carried out after treatment of any associated infection and correction of fluid and electrolyte imbalance. Vesicostomy is a procedure occasionally resorted to in a very small infant when there is sepsis and gross pyuria or if the necessary expertise for the former procedures is not available locally. High urinary diversion viz. high loop ureterostomy is considered in the following situations:

- Very sick patients with gross pyuria and the trial of bladder drainage have not helped.
- Recurrent upper UTI.
- Increase upper tract dilatation in spite of adequate bladder drainage.

Once the general condition improves, further evaluation is carried out and the valves are fulgurated.

In upto 80% cases, PUV is associated with Vescicoureteric reflux with bilateral involvement in around 30%. High grade reflux is mostly associated with poor function of the kidneys. These patients require long-term monitoring for assessment of bladder function status. Bladder dysfunction is usually associated and should be investigated.

Renal Tubular Acidosis

Renal tubular acidosis (RTA) is a disease state characterized by a normal anion gap metabolic acidosis resulting from either impaired bicarbonate reabsorption or impaired urinary acid (hydrogen ion) excretion. The two common forms seen in children include distal RTA (type I) and proximal RTA (type II). A third form (type IV) characterized by hyperkalemia and hypoaldosteronism is rare in children. A mixed lesion i.e. those with elements of type I and type II RTA has been described. This type is primarily seen in patients with inherited carbonic anhydrase deficiency. The tubular defect may be primary or secondary, as a result of tubular damage due to a variety of congenital or acquired diseases or a part of a global tubular dysfunction (e.g. Fanconi syndrome).

Table 12.10 : Common causes of renal tubular acidosis

Distal (Type I RTA)

Primary: Genetic, sporadic.

Secondary: SLE, Sickle cell anemia, obstructive uropathy, reflux nephropathy, Amphotericin B and cisplatin toxicity.

Proximal (Type II RTA)

Primary: Genetic, sporadic.

Fanconi syndrome (multiple tubular dysfunctions)

Primary: Genetic, sporadic.

Secondary: Cystinosis, Wilson's disease, Lowe syndrome, Tyrosinemia, Galactosemia, Vitamin D dependent rickets, Amyloidosis, drugs (lead, aminoglycosides, cisplatin, ifosfamide).

Hyperkalemic (Type IV RTA)

Aldosterone deficiency without renal disease: Addison's disease, isolated aldosterone deficiency.

Aldosterone deficiency in chronic renal insufficiency: Interstitial nephritis, nephrocalcinosis, aldosterone resistance.

Distal (Type I) Renal Tubular Acidosis

Distal renal tubular acidosis results from impaired distal urinary acidification (hydrogen ion secretion). Because of impaired hydrogen ion secretion, urine pH cannot be reduced below 5.5, despite the presence of severe metabolic acidosis. Loss of sodium bicarbonate in urine results in hyperchloremia and hypokalemia. Hypercalciuria is usually present and may lead to nephrocalcinosis or nephrolithiasis. Chronic metabolic acidosis also impairs urinary citrate excretion. Low citrate in urine further increases the risk of calcium deposition in the tubules. Rickets is common due to mobilization of organic components from bone to serve as buffers to chronic acidosis.

Clinical Manifestation

The common presentation during infancy is growth failure. Additional symptoms include polyuria, dehydration, anorexia, vomiting, constipation and hypotonia and occasionally transient paralysis. Later, there may be manifestations of rachitic changes in the bones. Some patients have sensorineural deafness.

Laboratory Diagnosis

The blood pH is below 7.2 and bicarbonate below 15 mEq/L. Serum potassium levels may be normal or decreased and often below 2.5 mEq/L. Urine pH is more than 6 (distal RTA is virtually excluded if it is < 5.5) and there is bicarbonaturia. There is hypercalciuria and hypo citruria. Urinary ammonia excretion is low in spite of marked systemic acidosis. X-ray long bones show signs of rickets and in untreated cases nephrocalcinosis may be present.

Treatment

Correction of acidosis and hypokalemia is the mainstay. Correction of hypokalemia should be done before correction of acidosis with administration of 2–3 mEq/kg/day of potassium. Acidosis can be corrected by administration of alkali solution at an initial dose of 2–3 mEq/kg/day which may have to be increased upto 5 to 10 mEq/kg/day to maintain acid base status. A useful mixture is a solution of sodium and potassium citrate: 100 gm of each salt diluted in 1 liter of distilled water which provides approximately 2 mEq of citrate per milliliter. If there is severe rickets and osteopenia, small doses of Vitamin D may be administered.

With adequate correction of acidosis, the potassium requirement is decreased but in some patients, prolonged therapy may be required in some patients. The alkali requirements usually decrease after 5 years age. However, alkali therapy is usually life-long.

After treatment, the growth velocity markedly increases in infants within a few weeks while in older children it may take several months. A persistent hypercalciuria may need administration of thiazides.

Proximal (Type II) Renal Tubular Acidosis

Proximal RTA results from impaired reabsorption of bicarbonate in the proximal tubule. Isolated proximal RTA is rare. It more commonly occurs as a component of global proximal tubule dysfunction (Fanconi syndrome).

Clinical Manifestation

The common presenting features include failure to thrive, vomiting and muscle weakness. Rachitic deformities are rare in isolated type but common in Fanconi syndrome. Nephrocalcinosis is also uncommon.

Laboratory Diagnosis

The blood pH and bicarbonate levels are low and urine pH is relatively alkaline; may fall below 5.5 if the blood pH and bicarbonate levels are markedly decreased. Urinary calcium and citrate excretion is normal. Determination of fractional excretion of bicarbonate is confirmatory. After an infusion of bicarbonate to increase plasma levels to more than 22 mEq/L, more that 15% of filtered bicarbonate is excreted in urine. The difference between the urine and blood PCO_2 is more than 20 mm Hg.

Treatment

Correction of acidosis is the mainstay. It requires administration of sodi bicarb or sodium citrate solution, 5–10 mEq/kg/day as starting dose along with restriction of dietary sodium. Often larger doses are required. In mild proximal RTA, administration of potassium is not necessary. In severe proximal RTA, as seen in Fanconi syndrome, administration of potassium may be mandatory. In very severe forms, diuretic therapy appears to be most effective. Hydrochlorothiazide, 1.5 – 2 mg/kg /day initially, followed by a smaller dose after correction of acidosis, appears to be effective. Potassium supplements are obligatory to prevent secondary hypokalemia.

Fanconi Syndrome

It is a condition with global dysfunction of proximal tubules. It is characterized by glucosuria, phosphaturia and generalized aminoaciduria in addition to impaired absorption of water, bicarbonate, sodium, potassium and organic acids. Cystinosis is frequently an underlying cause in children.

Clinical manifestations include failure to thrive, polyuria, polydypsia, recurrent episodes of fever and dehydration. Vitamin D resistant rickets of varying severity is a striking feature.

Laboratory diagnosis includes presence of generalized aminoaciduria, glucosuria, mild proteinuria, uricosuria, excessive urinary loss of sodium, potassium and bicarbonate, hypophosphatemia and acidosis.

Treatment consists of appropriate treatment of the underlying condition. The patient may need fluid replacement with 0.9 percent saline with added potassium. Sodium, potassium, bicarbonate and phosphate should be supplemented. Adequate fluid intake is important during infancy. Rickets can be treated with phosphate neutral salts (1–3 grams daily), correction of acidosis and administration of moderate doses of vitamin D.

Hyperkalemic (Type IV RTA)

It is characterized by RTA, hyperkalemia and ability to appropriately acidify urine. The common associated clinical conditions are hyporeninemic hypoaldosteronism and chronic tubulointerstitial disease. Type IV RTA is rare in children.

Suggested Reading

1. Pediatric Nephrology, 4th edition, 2006 by R.N. Srivastava and Arvind Bagga. Jaypee Brothers, New Delhi.
2. Pediatric Kidney Diseases. Editor Chester M. Edelman vol I and II, 1st Edition 1978. Little Brown and Company.
3. Nelson Text Book of Pediatrics, 17th edition 2004 edited by Behrman, Kliegman and Jenson, Saunders.
4. Pediatric Nephrology edited by BR Nammalwar and M. Vijaykumar, 2nd edition, 1991. Alamu Printing Works, Madras.

13

Neurology

OUTLINES

Microcephaly

Microcephaly may be defined as head size below the 10th centile in relation to gestation in the newborn period, or two or more standard deviations below the mean for the age for older children.

Etiology

Microcephaly may be subdivided into two main groups: Primary (genetic) and secondary. Primary microcephaly follows a Mendelian pattern of inheritance and is not

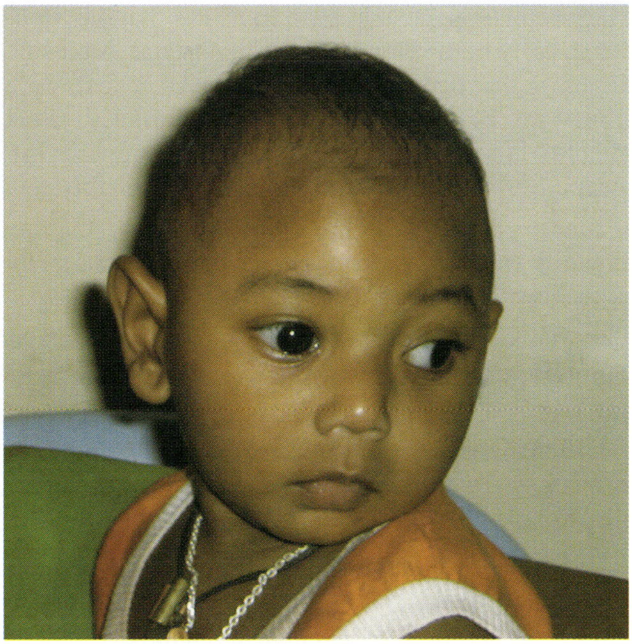

Fig. 13.1: A child with microcephaly

associated with any other malformations. It may be associated with a specific genetic syndrome. The affected infants are usually identified at birth because of a small head circumference. Secondary microcephaly results from a condition that may affect the fetus in utero or the infant during the period of rapid brain growth, particularly in the first two years of life. Microcephaly is usually associated with moderate to severe mental retardation.

Table 13.1: Common causes of microcephaly

Primary (Genetic)
Familial (autosomal recessive and autosomal dominant)
Syndromes: Down (21 trisomy), Edward (18 trisomy), Cri-du-chat
Secondary (Non-genetic)
Exposure to radiation
Congenital infections: Rubella, cytomegalovirus, Toxoplasmosis
Drugs: Fetal alcohol, fetal hydantoin
Meningitis, encephalitis
Hyperthermia
Hypoxic ischemic encephalopathy
Metabolic: Maternal diabetes mellitus, maternal hyperphenylalaninemia
Malnutrition

Diagnosis

A thorough history keeping in mind the causes of microcephaly will help in etiological diagnosis.

Every newborn should have the measurement of head circumference after 24 hours of birth and head circumference compared with the percentile chart. Microcephaly present at birth indicates that the process began early in the embryonic or fetal stage. An insult to the brain that occurs beyond the age of 2 years is less likely to produce severe microcephaly. Serial measurements of head circumference are more meaningful in case of mild degree of abnormality.

In case of a child with microcephaly, the head circumference measurement should be done in the siblings as well as the parents.

One should also look for facial dysmorphism to exclude chromosomal anomalies.

Laboratory investigations in a case of microcephaly is determined by history and physical examination.

A CT scan or MRI may be useful in identification of structural anomalies or intracerebral calcification.

A karyotype is obtained if a chromosomal anomaly is suspected or if the child has facial dysmorphism, short stature and additional congenital anomalies.

Additional studies include fasting plasma and urine amino acid analysis, serum ammonia, TORCH titers of mother and child and urine culture for cytomegalovirus.

If the cause cannot be identified, the mother's serum phenylalanine level should be determined. High serum phenylalanine levels in an asymptomatic mother can produce severe brain damage in an otherwise normal non-phenyl ketonuric infant.

Treatment

Genetic and family counseling is the mainstay of supportive treatment of a child with microcephaly. A good number of cases will have associated mental retardation. The children should be placed in an appropriate program that will provide maximum development.

Hydrocephalus

The term hydrocephalus means excess of cerebrospinal fluid. Two varieties of hydrocephalus are recognized: obstructive and communicating. *Obstructive hydrocephalus* is characterized by raised intracranial pressure as a result of an obstruction in some point between its formation in the choroid plexus and its exit from the fourth ventricle by the median and lateral apertures. In *communicating hydrocephalus*, there is no obstruction within or to the outflow from the ventricular system and the CSF freely reaches the spinal subarachnoid space and is found to be in increased pressure.

Table 13.2: Causes of hydrocephalus

Congenital

- Stenosis of cerebral aqueduct.
- Arnold-Chiari malformation type II (in which a tongue of cerebellum protrudes into the foramen magnum with obstruction to the outflow from the fourth ventricle).
- Dandy-Walker syndrome (cystic expansion of fourth ventricle as a result of developmental failure of the roof of the 4th ventricle).
- Malformation of vein of Galen.
- Intrauterine viral infection.

Acquired

- Obstruction to CSF flow due to adhesions following hemorrhage due to birth trauma.
- Adhesions following meningitis, arachnoiditis.
- Subarachnoid hemorrhage.
- Parasitic cysts and posterior fossa tumours.
- Superior sagittal sinus thrombosis.
- Leukemic infiltrates.

The most common cause of obstructive hydrocephalus is aqueductal stenosis or a lesion in the fourth ventricle such as posterior fossa tumours, Arnold-Chiari malformation and Dandy-Walker syndrome. An abnormally narrow aqueduct of Sylvius may be inherited in a small percentage of cases as a sex linked recessive trait. Aqueductal stenosis may also result from gliosis of the ependymal layer of the fourth ventricle following neonatal meningitis or subarachnoid hemorrhage in a preterm infant.

Communicating hydrocephalus most commonly follows subarachnoid hemorrhage as result of obliteration of cisterns and arachnoid villi by blood in the subarachnoid space and obstruction to CSF flow. Pneumococcal and tubercular meningitis have a propensity to produce a thick, tenacious exudate and obstruct the basal cisterns. Intrauterine infection destroys the CSF pathways and leukemic infiltrates may seed the subarachnoid space.

Clinical Manifestations

In an infant, the most prominent sign is an accelerated rate of increase of the head circumference. The normal average increase in the first 4 months after birth is 2 cm/month. If the increase is more than 1 cm in 2 weeks, it indicates an accelerated growth. In severe cases the anterior fontanel is wide open and bulging and the scalp veins are dilated. The forehead is broad and the eyes deviated downwards producing the setting sun sign (Fig. 13.2). The child may also have signs of pyramidal tract involvement particularly in the lower extremities as a result of stretching and disruption of the corticospinal fibres originating from the leg region of the motor cortex.

In the older child as the cranial sutures are partially closed the symptoms and signs may be more subtle. The child may present with lethargy, irritability, poor appetite and headache. There may be a gradual change in personality and deterioration of scholastic performances. Percussion of the head may produce a cracked pot or Macewen sign indicating separation of sutures. Papilledema, Abduscens/6th cranial nerve palsy, and signs of pyramidal tract involvement, particularly in the lower extremities, are apparent in most cases.

Some particular features may indicate the cause of hydrocephalus. A prominent occiput suggest Dandy-Walker syndrome. A cranial bruit is audible in association with malformation of the vein of Galen. Transillumination test of the skull is positive in Dandy-Walker syndrome or with massive dilatation of the ventricular system. Chorioretinitis suggest intrauterine infection due to toxoplasmosis.

Laboratory Investigations

A plain X-ray of the skull, in the older child, typically shows separation of the sutures, erosion of the posterior clinoid process, and thinning of inner table of skull and increase in the convolutional markings (beaten silver appearance) of the calvarium in long standing cases. A CT scan and/or MRI are the important studies to identify the specific cause of hydrocephalus.

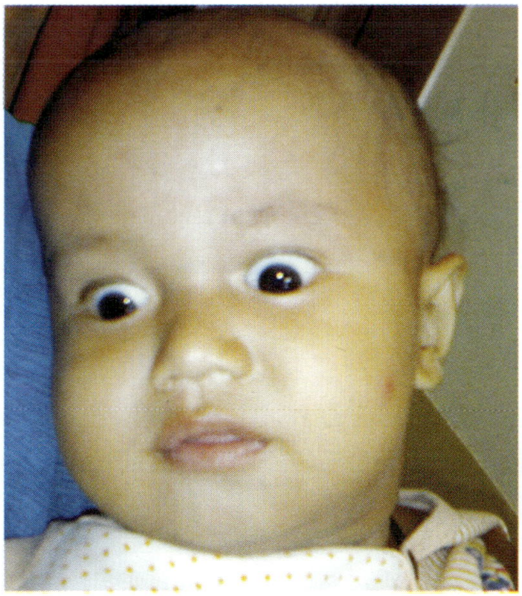

Fig. 13.2: Hydrocephalous with setting sun sign

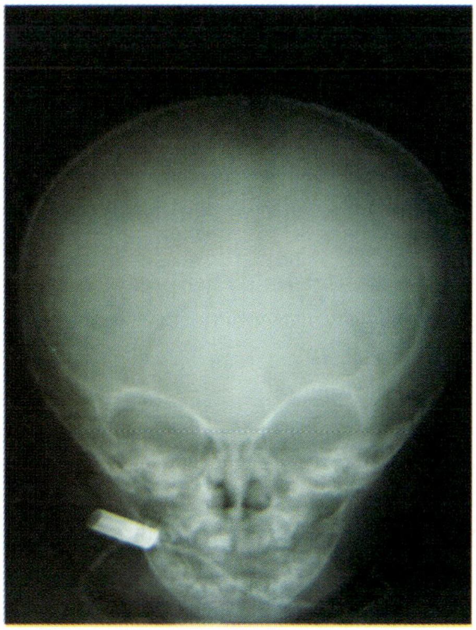

Fig. 13.3: AP view of skull showing thinning of cortex

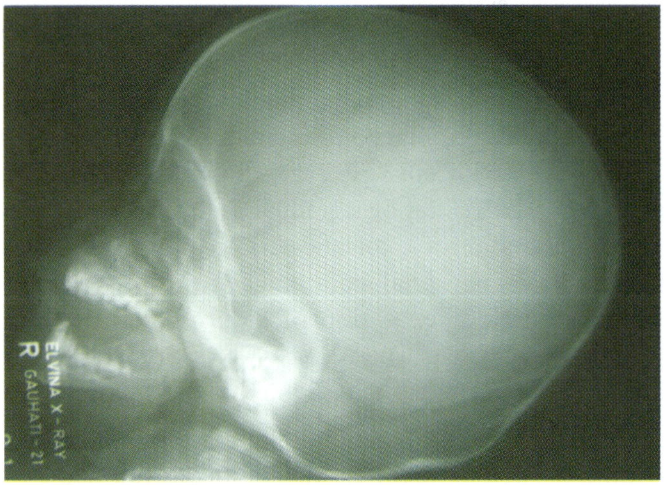

Fig. 13.4: Lateral view of skull showing thinning of the cortex, erosion of posterior clinoid process

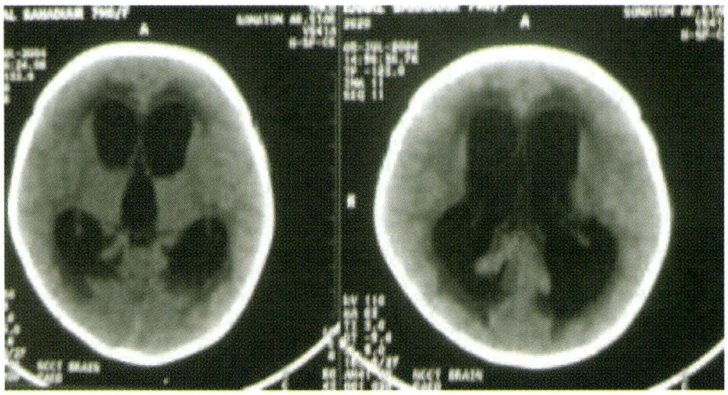

Fig. 13.5: CT scan showing hydrocephalus

Prognosis

Untreated cases of congenital hydrocephalus usually proves fatal during the first 4 years of life. Exceptionally, the disorder becomes arrested and a state of equilibrium is reached between formation and absorption of CSF. In patients who survive, mental deficiency, epilepsy and blindness are common. The prognosis of acquired hydrocephalus depends on its cause and how far it is amenable to treatment.

Treatment

Treatment depends on the cause. Medical therapy such as administration of acetazolamide and frusemide may provide temporarily relief by reducing the rate of CSF production but long-term results are disappointing. Most cases require a shunt particularly a ventriculoperitoneal shunt.

Craniosynostosis

Craniosynostosis is defined as premature closure of the cranial sutures. It may be classified as primary and secondary. *Primary* craniosynostosis refers to closure of one or more sutures due to abnormalities of the development of the skull. *Secondary* type results from failure of brain growth and expansion. The cause of primary type is not known in the majority of cases. However, genetic syndromes account for 10–20% of cases.

Majority of cases are evident at birth and are characterized by a skull deformity. Palpation of the sutures reveals a prominent bony ridge over the suture. The fusion of the suture may be confirmed by a plain skull X-ray or a bone scan which shows signs of raised intracranial pressure such as beaten silver appearance (Fig. 13.6). The most common form of craniosynostosis is scaphocephaly due to premature closure of the sagittal suture, produces a long and narrow skull. It is associated with a prominent occiput, a broad forehead and a small or absent anterior fontanel. The condition is sporadic and more common in males. It does not produce increased intracranial pressure or hydrocephalus and child is neurologically normal. Craniosynostosis may be isolated or associated with syndromes like Apert syndrome, Crouzon syndrome, Carpenter syndrome etc.

Treatment

Treatment is surgery. Craniectomy is mandatory to manage ICP. Premature fusion of only one suture rarely

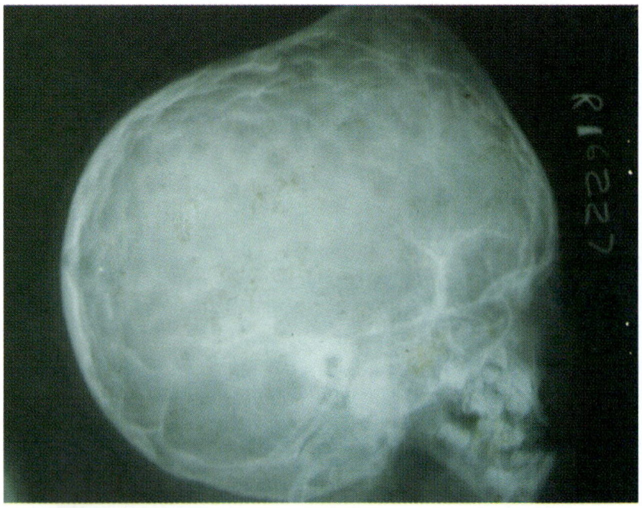

Fig. 13.6: Lateral view of skull with premature clossure of suture and beaten silver appearance in craniosynostosis

causes a neurological deficit. In such situation surgery is indicated to enhance the child's cosmetic appearance. Neurologic complications like hydrocephalus and increased ICP are more likely to occur when there is fusion of two or more sutures. In these cases operative intervention is essential.

Non-syndromic craniosynostosis may be surgically corrected with good outcome and relatively low morbidity and mortality.

Neural Tube Defects

The congenital malformations due to closure defects of the neural tube include anencephaly, encephalocele, spina bifida occulta, meningocele, meningomyelocele and dermal sinus.

Normal Formative Stages of the Nervous System

In human the first evidence of development of neural tissue occurs at about 20 days of gestation at which time the neural groove appears in the dorsal ectoderm of the embryo. Over the next few days this groove deepens, and the two margins of the groove become apposed and fuse. This fusion results in formation of the neural tube. The fusion begins near the centre of the embryo and progresses cephalad and caudad and by about 23 days gestation the neural tube is complete, except for an opening (neuropore) at each end. Failure of closure of the anterior neuropore results in anencephaly and encephalocele. Closure defect of the posterior neuropore leads to spina bifida and meningomyelocele.

Anencephaly

Anencephaly is a condition where there is absence of the membranous skull as well as the cerebral hemispheres.

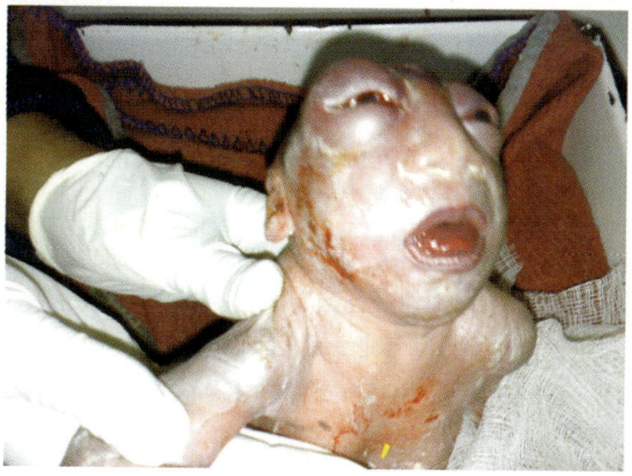

Fig. 13.7: Anencephaly

The brainstem and the basal nuclei may be well formed and are visible at the base of the skull. The infants are either stillborn or die within a few days of birth. The recurrence rate of neural tube defect in a mother giving birth to a baby with anencephaly is about 10% for each subsequent pregnancy.

An antenatal diagnosis can be made by ultrasound scan at 16–18 weeks. Increased level of alpha feto protein in amniotic fluid is helpful in utero diagnosis of the condition. The mother needs proper counseling for a subsequent pregnancy.

Encephalocele

An encephalocele consists of a herniation of brain and meninges through a defect in the skull, resulting in a sack like structure. When the defect contains only meninges it is called a cranial meningocele. About 75% of the encephaloceles occur in the occipital region; the remainder is parietal, frontal and nasopharyngeal.

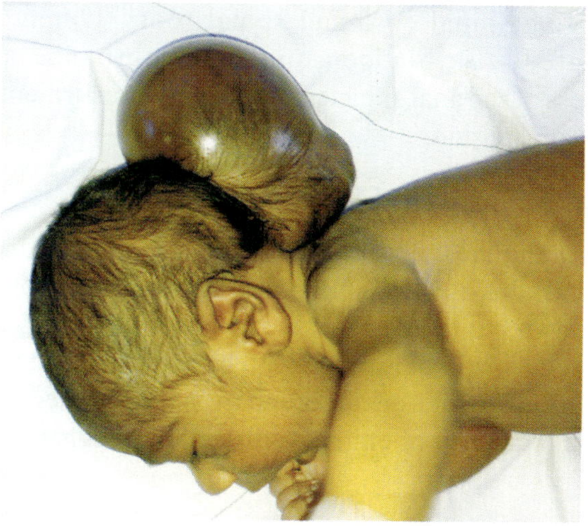

Fig. 13.8: Encephalocele in the occipital region

At birth, the encephalocele is an obvious swelling with a midline skull defect. It may be pedunculated or sessile. The nasopharyngeal encephalocele is not visible externally. The child may present with nasal airway obstruction or with cleft palate. Inspection of the nasal passage shows a smooth, round mass projecting downward. A frontal encephalocele may extend into the orbit and may present as proptosis of one eye.

An encephalocele may be clinically differentiated from a cranial meningocele by palpation and transillumination test. A transillumination test is positive in meningocele. A CT scan/MRI may show hydrocephalus in two third of patients with encephalocele.

Therapy consists of surgery. The associated hydrocephalus requires a shunt.

The prognosis is good in cranial meningocele with normal intellectual and motor function in 60% of the affected infants.

Spina Bifida Occulta

Spina bifida occulta consists of a defect of the vertebral arch with failure of the posterior fusion of the vertebral laminae and often with absence of the spinous process. The anomaly is most common at L5 and S1 levels but it may affect any portion of the vertebral column. The overlying skin and subcutaneous tissues may be normal, or there may be abnormalities such a tuft of hair, telangiectasia or a subcutaneous lipoma at the site. Spina bifida occulta may be an isolated insignificant finding detected on radiological examination of the spine. A small percentage of affected children, however, may have functionally significant developmental defects of the underlying spinal cord and spinal roots. It may be associated with bladder spincter disturbance and weakness of the anal spincter and sensory impairment in the perianal region.

Spina Bifida with Meningomyelocele

This is a midline defect of the skin, vertebral arches and the neural tube, usually in the lumbosacral region. Etiology is unknown but there appears to be an etiologic linkage with anencephaly. A women who have had a child with meningomyelocele or anencephaly has a higher than average incidence of either in subsequent pregnancy.

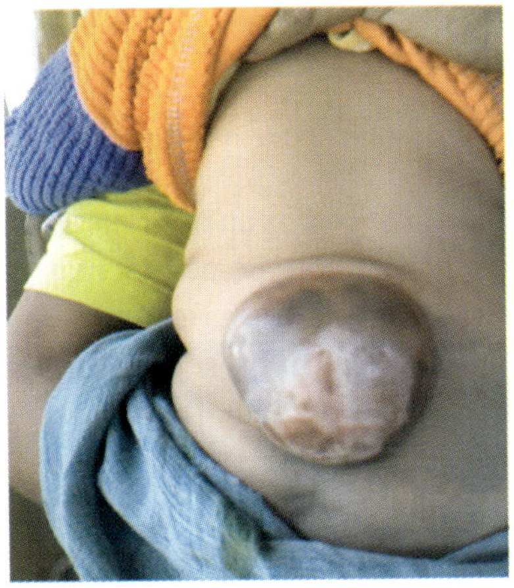

Fig. 13.9: Meningomyelocele in the back

A myelomeningocele is evident at birth as a skin defect over the back, bordered laterally by bony prominences of the unfused neural arches of the vertebrae. The defect is usually covered by a transparent membrane. Initially CSF leaks from this membrane but soon after birth, drying of the membrane tends to decrease its permeability. Meningomyelocele is associated with other developmental anomalies of neural tissue like Arnold-Chiari malformation (which consist of maldevelopment and downward displacement of the parts of cerebellum, 4th ventricle and medulla oblongata into the cervical spinal canal) and aqueductal stenosis. Both these abnormalities results in hydrocephalus in 90% cases.

There is usually presence of spinal cord dysfunction in an infant with meningomyelocele. Therefore, a neurological assessment should be carried out soon after birth to determine the upper level and its severity. The upper level of spinal cord dysfunction can be determined from the following:

1. Sensory level by observing the response to pinprick over legs and trunk. Functional integrity is present when the sensory stimulus leads to limb movements and to arousal and crying. However, stimulus induced limb movements without change in the infant's behaviour may be due to spinal reflexes which has no functional connection with higher centres.
2. Defective innervation of the bladder is indicated by urinary dribbling and that of perianal region by a patulous anal sphincter and lack of anal reflex.
3. The denervated limbs are flaccid and areflexic.
4. Presence of medullary and lower cranial nerve dysfunction, including difficulty in swallowing, stridor and atrophy of the tongue indicate presence of Arnold-Chiari malformation.

An organized plan for management by a specialized multi-disciplinary clinical group is essential. Optimal therapy of meningomyelocele consists of prompt surgical closure of the skin defect, preferably within 48 hours after birth inorder to prevent meningeal infection. The associated abnormalities like hydrocephalus, hip and foot deformities and urinary diversion operations for infants with bladder dysfunction should be simultaneously looked after.

Dermal Sinus

Dermal sinus is a small midline closure defect. It is of importance primarily because the sinus may be a route of entry of bacteria into the subarachnoid space leading to recurrent meningitis. The sinus is usually located in the lumbosacral area but may occur at any level of the spine or in the midline of the cranium.

Its point of entry in the skin is visible as a dimple often surrounded by a tuft of hair or by a small hemangioma. The sacral defects known as pilonidal sinus usually end blindly without communication with the subarachnoid space and hence not of significance. The sinus tracts above this level should be surgically explored and closed.

Approach to A Comatose Child

Altered states of consciousness may vary from mild impairment to deep unresponsiveness and can signal present or impending life threatening situations. The different states of altered level of consciousness include the following: *Confusion* (i.e. slowed, impaired cognitive abilities), *delirium* (succession of confused and unconnected ideas), *obtundation* (awake but not alert) *stupor* (aroused only with repeated, vigorous stimuli) and *coma*.

Coma is defined as a mental status where the patient is completely unarousable and does not respond to any form of stimuli.

Common Causes of Coma

1. *Infections:* Meningitis, encephalitis, septicemia and cerebral malaria.
2. *Mass lesion:* Bleed from ruptured arteriovenous malformations, cerebrovascular accident, trauma, intracranial tumor and abscess.
3. *Metabolic/toxic disorders:* Hepatic encephalopathy, diabetic ketoacidosis, inborn errors of metabolism, hypo and hypernatremia, severe dehydration, uremia, hypercapnia, drugs (morphine, antiepileptics, salicylates and organophosphorous).
4. *Non-metabolic encephalopathies:* Post status epilepticus, degenerative brain disorders, anoxia.

Pathophysiology

Coma results from lesions involving the cerebral cortex and/or brainstem. The common disorders that cause coma can be categorized into three broad groups:

1. Supratentorial lesion causing compression or displacement of the diencephalons or the brainstem.
2. Subtentorial lesion by damaging or compressing the reticular activating system (RAS).
3. Metabolic encephalopathies that affect the brain diffusely often the cortex as well as the brainstem.

Secondary injury to central nervous system can occur regardless of the primary neurologic injury. Ischemia may result from hypoxia, shock or local hypoperfusion resulting in death or severe and permanent CNS injury.

Clinical Diagnosis of Lesions Causing Coma

The clinical characteristics of coma depend on the type of lesion whether supratentorial, subtentorial or metabolic.

Supratentorial Lesions

Supratentorial lesions are characterized by asymmetric upper motor neuron type of focal neurological signs, signs of raised intracranial pressure and focal lesions in EEG and imaging studies.

Subtentorial Lesions

Subtentorial lesions are characterized by presence of abnormal oculocephalic (Doll's eye) reflex, abnormal Oculovestibular (calorie stimulation) reflex, respiratory abnormalities, cranial nerve palsy and features of focal lesions in EEG and imaging.

Metabolic Lesions

Metabolic lesions are characterized by generalized involvement, absence of focal signs; motor signs if present are symmetrical, abnormal movements and hyperventilation, spontaneous fluctuation in the level of consciousness, deep coma with preservation of pupillary light reflex, usually a hypotonic limp state. Sometimes hypertonia, decerebrate or decorticate rigidity may be observed in hypoglycemia, hepatic coma and short acting barbiturate induced coma. CT and MRI are normal. EEG is abnormal (slowing of background).

Initial Assessment and Immediate Intervention

Coma is a medical emergency. In the first encounter the comatose child needs a quick assessment and at the same time immediate intervention aimed at saving life. The initial rapid evaluation is critical in preventing secondary injury to the CNS and hence a systemic approach is required.

Table 13.3 : The seven questions for immediate assessment and management

Question	*Check*	*Action*
1. Airway clear?	ABG	Intubate if GCS < 8 or if there is pooling of secretion. Give oxygen
2. Seizure?	Blood glucose	10% glucose (5 ml/kg) IV, diazepam, oxygen
3. Major hemorrhage/ shock?	Maintain circulation	Bolus IV NS/ RL (20 ml/kg), vasopressors
4. Signs of craniofacial trauma?	CT scan	Neurological opinion
5. Neck broken?	Splint neck	X-ray neck
6. Signs of hyper-glycemia?	Check blood glucose, and urine ketones	Treat
7. Evidence of intoxication, drug overdose?	Examine pupil, ventilation	Treat

Assessment for the Cause

After immediate assessment and interventions one should start looking for the cause. This should be done by thorough history taking, physical examination and neurological examination along with some investigations.

History

A detail history should be taken from all possible sources e.g. parents, attendants, friends, observer, particularly giving stress on the following points: mode of onset, history of trauma, past history of epilepsy, heart disease, history of bite or sting-animal, snake, scorpion etc. History of ingestion of toxic substances, associated symptoms like fever, headache, viral prodrome, diarrhoea, vomiting, convulsion etc., and is the patient from a malaria pocket.

Physical Examination

A thorough clinical examination should include measurement of temperature, blood pressure, examination for jaundice, pallor, and pattern of respiration, signs of trauma, organomegaly, cardiac abnormality, any peculiar odour.

The presence of *Cushing's triad* (hypertension with widened systolic-diastolic gap, bradycardia and abnormal respiration) indicates increased intracranial pressure.

Examination of the Respiratory Pattern

The characteristic respiratory pattern indicating the causes are as follows:

Respiratory Pattern: Several characteristic patterns	
Hyperventilation	Metabolic acidosis or primary respiratory alkalosis
Hypoventilation	Metabolic alkalosis or respiratory acidosis
Cheyne-Stokes	Common in metabolic encephalopathy
Central neurogenic hyperventilation	Mid brain dysfunction
Apneustic	Anoxic encephalopathy or severe meningitis

Cheyne Stokes respiration is characterized by hyperapnea regularly alternating with apnea. It results from dysfunction deep in cerebral hemispheres or diencephalon.

Central neurogenic hyperventilation is characterized by regular rapid respirations despite normal oxygenation and low Pa CO_2.

Apneustic respiration is characterized by irregular, sporadic, respiration of varying amplitude. It results from pontine infarction.

Neurological Examination

The following neurological examinations should be done:

1. Level of consciousness.
2. Pupillary size and reflex.
3. Extra ocular movements.
4. Examination of the motor system.
5. Fundoscopy.

Level of Consciousness

An accurate assessment of level of consciousness is essential, with serially repeated evaluation to track trends. The assessment of level consciousness is done by using the Glasgow coma scale for children and AVPU scale.

Glasgow Coma Scale for Children

1. Eye opening (total points 4)		**2. Motor response (total points 6)**	
Spontaneous	4	Obeys command	6
To voice	3	Localizes pain	5
To pain	2	Withdraws	4
None	1	Flexion to pain	3
		Extension to pain	2
		None	1
3. Verbal response (Total points 5)			
Older children		*Infants and young children*	
Oriented	5	Appropriate words, smile, fixes and follows	5

Contd.

Contd.

Confused	4	Consolable crying	4
Inappropriate	3	Persistently irritable	3
Incomprehensible	2	Restless, agitated	2
None	1	None	1

The Glasgow coma scale (GCS) provides an accurate assessment of cerebral cortical function. The total score is 15. A decreasing score indicates increasing depression of cortical function. Patients with GCS score 8 or less require aggressive management, including mechanical ventilation and monitoring of intracranial pressure.

AVPU Scale

The Glasgow coma scale is accurate but lengthy. A valuable quick assessment tool is the AVPU scale: A = Awake and alert, V = Responsive to verbal stimuli, P = Responsive to pain stimuli and U = Unresponsive.

Pupillary Size and Reflexes

Reaction to light is the most important feature to distinguish between structural and metabolic causes. Preservation of pupillary light reflex indicates a metabolic cause. Change of pupillary reflex indicates a structural brain lesion.

Pupillary size and reflex	*Structural lesions*
Unilateral fixed dilated pupil	Mass lesion, uncal herniation with 3rd nerve palsy
Fixed dilated pupils	Transtentorial herniation: Pupils initially small, may become asymmetric with progressive herniation, then fixed and dilated
Mid position fixed pupil	Mid brain lesion
Pin point fixed pupils	Pontine lesion

Extra Ocular Movements

Defects in eye movements indicate a subtentorial lesion. The abnormalities in ocular movements include the following:

1. *Conjugate deviation of eyes at rest*
   - (a) *Cerebral lesion:* Look towards the side of lesion.
   - (b) *Brainstem lesion:* Look away from the side of lesion.
   - (c) *Upper mid brain lesion and hydrocephalus:* Downward deviation (setting sun sign).
2. *Oculocephalic reflex (Doll's eye response)*

The head is rotated from side to side with eyes held open.

- (a) *Intact brainstem:* Conjugate deviation of the eyes opposite to the direction of head turning.
- (b) *In brainstem lesion:* The eyes remain in the centre of the orbit regardless of any stimuli.

It is contraindicated if cervical spine injury is suspected.

3. *Oculovestibular reflex (Cold caloric stimulation)*
   - (a) Normally, cold water placed in the external ear elicits nystagmus with quick phase away from the side of stimulation and slow conjugate movement to the irrigated side. A normal response indicates a normal brainstem.
   - (b) This test is only indicated when Doll's eye response is absent. It is more sensitive. It is contraindicated in presence of perforation of tympanic membrane.

Examination of the Motor System

On assessment of muscle tone, strength and deep tendon reflexes, the following motor responses may be encountered:

(a) *Decorticate posturing*: Characterized by flexion of upper extremities and extension of lower limbs. It indicates cerebral cortex and subcortical white matter dysfunction, intact brainstem.

(b) *Decerebrate posturing:* Characterized by rigid extension of upper and lower extremities. It indicates brainstem dysfunction.

(c) *Flaccid posture:* With no response to painful stimuli indicates injury deep in the brainstem.

Other Neurological Examinations

1. Look for signs of head injury, e.g., local bruising, fracture and penetrating wounds, bleeding from nose, ears or any site.
2. If no neck injury (clinically and by X-ray) check for signs of meningeal irritation.

Fundoscopy

To look for retinal hemorrhage and papilledema (a late sign of raised ICP).

Investigations

Routine Investigations

- Complete blood count, PBS for MP, blood glucose.
- ABG, serum electrolytes sodium, potassium, calcium.
- LFT (SGPT), PT, APTT, INR, KFT (blood urea and serum creatinine).

- Routine examination of urine.
- X-ray chest and ECG.
- A lumbar puncture is often done in unexplained cases specially if there is fever.

Selective Investigation

- CSF analysis in suspected meningitis.
- CT scan, MRI, USG for suspected mass lesion, CNS infection.
- EEG for suspected encephalopathy and post ictal coma.
- Toxic screening for suspected toxic encephalopathy.
- Metabolic screening for suspected inborn errors of metabolism.

Management

The common goal in treatment is to prevent secondary injury by maintaining oxygen delivery to the brain. Hence ABC of resuscitation supersedes all other intervention.

After initial stabilization in the emergency room, the comatose child should be shifted to the ICU and managed as follows:

1. Supportive measures and monitoring.
2. Specific treatment.

Supportive Measures

1. Nursing care
    - Child should be nursed on a side.
    - Position should be regularly changed every 2 hourly.
    - Oral hygiene should be maintained by daily cleaning with an antiseptic solution.
    - Care of the skin with measures to prevent bed sores.
    - Care of the eyes to prevent drying by instilling lubricant eye drops.
    - Care of the bladder: Catheterization or condom drainage.
    - Care of the bowel.
    - Maintenance of nutrition preferably by NG feeding or parenteral nutrition.
2. Monitoring of vital signs and neurological parameters
    - Heart rate, respiratory rate, blood pressure, temperature.
    - Maintenance of fluid intake and urine output chart.
    - Frequent reevaluation of ABC and level of consciousness, intracranial pressure.
    - Early intubation and ventilation is necessary in a child with coma because children with coma but breathing on their own are at risk of hypoventilation, airway obstruction and aspiration. Moreover, infants have inherent airway laxicity and chances of airway obstruction from a large tongue. Hence life support should be started early and continued till the child is out of coma.
3. Treatment of complications, e.g., seizure, cerebral edema, peripheral circulatory collapse etc.

Specific Management

It depends on the cause of coma. Early institution of specific therapy is life saving.

Poor Prognostic Indicators

(a) Coma due to anoxia has the worst prognosis.

(b) Reye's syndrome.

(c) Children presenting with:

- Hypothermia.
- Shock.
- GCS < 6.
- Nonreacting pupils.
- Absent corneal reflex.
- Decerebrate or decorticate posturing.
- Apnea.
- Ataxic or gasping respiration.

Outcome of Coma

Children have better outcome than adults. However, outcome is related to many variables. They are as follows:

(a) *Duration of coma:* Longer duration worse prognosis.

(b) Intoxication carries good prognosis, anoxia carries bad prognosis.

(c) Complete recovery from traumatic coma of several days duration is possible in children.

(d) Some survivors however, are left in a vegetative state or with severe neuropsychiatric disabilities.

Febrile Seizure

Febrile seizures are one of the most common neurological problems in late infancy and early childhood. It is a condition responsible for generating tremendous fear and anxiety amongst the parents.

Definition

The 1980 consensus conference sponsored by the national institute of health, USA, defined a febrile seizure as an event occurring between 3 months and 5 years of age, associated with fever but without evidence of intracranial infections or defined causes. Seizures with fever in children who suffered a previous afebrile seizure were excluded. It is a widely accepted definition.

Characteristics of the Fever

- A rectal temperature of 38°C or more is usually accepted in the definition.
- A rapid increase in body temperature has been postulated as triggering the seizure.
- The suddenness in rise of temperature is thought to be more important than the height of temperature reached.
- On certain occasion, it is also noted that fever has been ushered in by the seizure. This is thought to be due to the fact that the seizure occurred when the child had a low grade fever and the fever rose to height only after the convulsion or may be parents became aware of the child's fever only after the seizure. This type of febrile seizure should be carefully assessed.
- The seizure usually occurs in the first few hours of onset of fever and within 24 hours in the majority of cases. Seizures after 24 hours are uncommon even if temperature remains high.
- The most common cause of fever is a viral illness (viral upper respiratory infection in 80% cases). Otitis media, urinary tract infection, GI infection, measles, malaria, DPT vaccination may be other causes.

Types of Seizure

It is customary to classify febrile seizure as simple or complex. 80–90% cases suffer from a *simple febrile seizure* which is characterized by:

(a) Generalized tonic clonic seizure, only tonic with the child becoming stiff and rigid with uprolling of eyeball or only clonic from the beginning in a neurologically normal child.
(b) Lasting for less than 15 minutes.
(c) Only one seizure in one episode of fever.
(d) Post ictal manifestations are virtually absent.

The rest may have a *complex febrile seizure* which is characterized by:

(a) Focal seizure.
(b) Lasting for more than 15 minutes.
(c) Multiple recurrences within 24 hours of onset of fever.
(d) Todd paralysis.

The above classification is debated for use because it has no prognostic value in terms of later recurrences or development of epilepsy.

Febrile seizure is now thought to constitute a heterogenous group with three subgroups:

(a) Children with a genetically determined susceptibility to febrile seizures. This forms the largest group.
(b) Children who have fever associated convulsion due to an unrecognized brain insult caused by the febrile disease.
(c) Children with fever triggered seizures which later unmasks into epilepsy.

Incidence

Febrile seizure is one of the most common pediatric emergencies. It occurs in about 3–5% of children below 5 years.

Age and Sex Incidence

90% of febrile seizures occur in children after 6 months of age and within 3 years; about 2% presenting in the younger age group and about 6% in older children. The peak incidence is at about 18–22 months. The incidence decreases by 6–8 years, after which such seizures are rare. Febrile seizures are common in boys but girls tend to have an early onset.

The Recurrence Rate

After a febrile fit, although children enjoy good health, they are prone to recurrence. The predictors of recurrence are:

(a) Age less than 18 months at the time of initial seizure.
(b) A low temperature threshold (< 40°C).
(c) Seizure occurring within 1 hour of onset of fever.
(d) Family history of febrile seizure in the first degree relative.

With no risk factor the recurrence rate is around 14%. With presence of 3 or more risk factors the incidence of recurrence increases to 63%. The younger age at onset is however, the only consistent predictor of risk of recurrence. A 50% recurrence rate in children with onset in the first year, and 28% when the onset was after 1 year has been reported.

Subsequent Epilepsy

The risk of development of epilepsy is about 4 times higher in children with febrile seizure than those without. The incidence of afebrile seizure or epilepsy following febrile seizure is around 2–4%. Three predictors have been identified which increase the risk of epilepsy in children who suffer from febrile seizure. They are:

(a) Family history of epilepsy in a first degree relative.
(b) Abnormal developmental or neurological status prior to onset.
(c) Complex febrile seizure with pre existing brain disease.

The most common type of epilepsy following febrile seizure is generalized tonic clonic epilepsy but any type can occur.

Clinical Manifestations

Febrile seizures are of sudden onset preceded by a brief febrile illness. Sometimes the initial symptom may be the seizure, the fever discovered after the seizure as it remained unnoticed by the parents. Irrespective of the seizure being simple or complex, the child appears well after the attack is over. In a few children there may be a post ictal phase characterized by drowsiness to sleep for varying duration.

The important physical findings are rise of temperature and occasional Todd's palsy. Other findings are related to the cause of fever, viz., cough, earache, vomiting, splenomegaly etc.

Diagnosis

The diagnosis of febrile seizure is made solely on clinical grounds. A CNS infection should be kept in mind, especially in an infant with the first febrile seizure. Presence of undue irritability, drowsiness or coma following the febrile seizure should lead one to investigate and exclude intracranial pathology viz. meningitis, cerebral malaria, encephalitis. During a recurrence also, a CNS infection should not be overlooked.

Investigations

1. Lumbar Puncture and CSF Analysis

Is indicated in:

(a) Infants under one year age on the slightest suspicion, because signs of meningitis may not be evident.
(b) Children who continue to be lethargic or drowsy or have signs of meningeal irritation on repeat examination after the seizure is over.
(c) Children with prior treatment with antibiotics which may mask the signs of meningitis.

2. Electroencephalogram (EEG)

An EEG is not an essential investigation as evidenced by the following facts about the status of EEG in febrile convulsion:

(a) EEG does not help as a guide to treatment or prognosis and is of limited value in evaluation of a child with febrile seizure.
(b) An EEG performed at the time of presentation or within the following month does not predict the risk of recurrence of febrile seizure or the development of future afebrile seizures.
(c) An abnormal EEG in febrile seizure should be regarded as an expression of a genetic predisposition to epilepsy and not an indication for the development of future epilepsy.

3. Neuroimaging

Should be advised in a child with complex febrile seizure with neurodevelopmental delay. Imaging in these cases may help in revealing structural abnormalities.

4. Blood Studies

Are not routinely required in evaluation of a febrile seizure. May be ordered, if required for diagnosis of cause of fever.

Treatment

The treatment of febrile seizure may be divided into:

(a) Treatment during interictal period.
(b) Treatment of the ongoing seizure.

Treatment During Interictal Period

In most children the febrile seizures are very brief and it is over by the time the child is with the doctor. However, they should be kept under observation for few hours for any recurrence.

The parents should be reassured and the benign nature of the event should be explained. They should be taught the simple way of administering per rectal diazepam.

At discharge the following advice should be given to be followed in the event of a recurrence:

i. To put the child in semiprone position to one side with head slightly lower than the trunk. Overcrowding should be avoided and room should be cool.

ii. To bring down the body temperature by tepid sponging but not to spill water over the face.

iii. Not to put anything inside the mouth.

iv. To administer per rectal diazepam if possible; and

v. To contact a doctor/shift to a hospital if the seizure does not stop within 5 minutes.

Treatment of an Ongoing Seizure

The child should be put in a semiprone position on one side with the head a little below the trunk. All clothes should be loosened. Crowding around the child prevented.

Clenching of teeth if present can be tackled by putting a gauge roll of appropriate size in between the teeth. A tongue depressor or any hard object should not be used because it may cause injury.

Oxygen inhalation should be started in case of a prolonged seizure.

Drugs

Diazepam is a useful drug for terminating seizures quickly but has a short anti-convulsant half life. The initial dose is 0.3–0.5 mg/kg (maximum 10 mg/dose, 30 mg/day) IV to be given very slowly, not faster than 1 mg/minute. If there is no response within 15–20 minutes the same dose is repeated. With partial response half the dose may be given. A third dose may be necessary sometimes. The dose of diazepam can be calculated by a simple formula viz. Age in years + 1= mg of diazepam. Alternatively 2 ml diazepam (10 mg) may be diluted with 8 ml normal saline and given slowly IV till seizure is terminated. Diazepam can also be given per rectally in the same dose, with the same effect. Diazepam is a respiratory depressant. However, with the recommended dose, when given very slowly IV, except for mild respiratory irregularity, no side effects have been observed.

Lorazepam (0.05 – 0.1 mg/kg/dose over 2 – 5 minutes IV or IM. May repeat dose after 10 – 15 minutes) or *Midazolam* (Intra nasal spray 0.2 mg/kg) can also be used.

If a child does not respond, a loading dose of *Phenytoin*, 15 mg/kg or *Phenobarbitone*, 15 mg/kg is usually sufficient to control the seizure. It should be followed by a maintenance dose 5 – 6 mg/kg/day for 48 – 72 hours. In case the child goes to febrile status, the child should be referred to a higher facility because it should be managed in the line of status epilepticus.

Prevention of Recurrence

To prevent recurrence of a febrile seizure, the following measures can be advised to the parents:

1. Lowering of Temperature

Lowering of temperature with Paracetamol 10–15 mg/kg/dose 4 hourly in order to keep the temperature below 38.5°C (101.3°F) with or without physical cooling for the first 24–48 hours when the risk of seizure is maximum. Thereafter paracetamol can be given 6 hourly when temperature is 38.9°C (102°F). Ibuprofen 5 mg/kg body weight/dose has also been tried. Aspirin should be avoided because of risk of precipitation of Reye's syndrome. It needs mention that use of antipyretics without anticonvulsants has been shown to be ineffective in prevention of recurrent febrile seizure.

Parents should be advised to keep the child in the coolest room of the house with minimum clothing.

Plenty of fluids should be advised to be given orally.

2. Anticonvulsant Drugs

Two modes of therapy are possible with anticonvulsant drugs for prevention of febrile seizure–intermittent and continuous.

The drugs currently in use for *intermittent prophylaxis* are oral and per rectal diazepam, and oral clobazam.

The recommended dose of per rectal diazepam is 0.5 mg/kg (5 mg for children < 3 years, 7.5 mg for children > 3 years) every 12 hours. The dose of oral diazepam is 0.6–0.8 mg/kg/dose every 8 hours. Oral diazepam is reported to be less effective than per rectal diazepam because of erratic absorption.

The recommended dose of clobazam is 5 mg/day upto 5 kg, 10 mg/day from 5–10 kg and 15 mg/day from 11–15 kg weight.

Prophylactic therapy should be continued for 48–72 hours from the onset of fever.

Intermittent therapy with phenobarbitone is not recommended because after a therapeutic dose it takes more than a week before a stable therapeutic level is established. By then fever would have subsided.

The potential drawbacks of intermittent prophylaxis are that the seizure, in many instances, can occur before the fever is noticed by the parents. Lethargy, drowsiness and ataxia are known side effects of diazepam and it can mask the evolving signs of CNS infection. Intermittent prophylaxis when child has fever as opposed to early treatment of seizures is still debatable. *Only indication of intermittent prophylaxis may be to advise for children of very anxious parents.*

The drugs effective for *continuous prophylaxis* are phenobarbitone and Sodium Valproate. Phenytoin and carbamazepine have not been shown to be effective in preventing recurrences. Continuous anti epileptic drug prophylaxis should not be advised because there are conflicting reports of prevention of recurrence by continuous AED therapy. Moreover both the drugs have serious side effects. Phenobarbitone is often associated with behaviour problem and cognitive dysfunction which are detrimental to normal development of the growing child. Adverse effects of sodium valproate are hepatotoxicity (especially below the age of 1 year), thrombocytopenia, pancreatitis etc. Further, continuous therapy for a prolonged period does not prevent development of subsequent epilepsy.

Therefore, it would be wise not to use such toxic drugs for prolonged period for prevention of a relatively benign, self limiting disorder. At present one should always say 'NO' to continuous prophylaxis in recurrent febrile seizures.

Parental Education

Parental education plays a very important role in management and prevention of febrile seizures. The steps include information to parents about the condition and discussion of therapeutic approach for prevention.

1. *Information:* The parents should be informed about the nature and course of the disease with importance on the following points:
   (a) It is a common, frightening but non-fatal, benign condition.
   (b) Subsequent neurological and mental development is normal.
   (c) There is a low possibility of subsequent epilepsy in a group of children with high risk factors.
   (d) To report immediately if the child with recurrent febrile seizure has an afebrile seizure.
2. Discussion of therapeutic approach for prevention:
   (a) Discussion on general measures.
   (b) Demonstration and training of rectal administration of diazepam.

Status Epilepticus

Definition

Status epilepticus is defined as a continuous seizure lasting for longer than 20 to 30 minutes or the occurrence of serial convulsions between which there is no return of consciousness.

It is believed that a seizure which lasts for more than 5 minutes should be treated with an anticonvulsant because they have the tendency to be a prolonged seizure. Therefore, practically any child brought to the physician convulsing should be considered as status epilepticus. There is also good evidence that early treatment with rectal diazepam or nasal midazolum may abort a potential status epilepticus.

Status epilepticus is often preceded by a cluster of seizures which culminate into status epilepticus. A seizure lasting for more than 30 minutes, can lead to a decompensated state which can result in irreversible brain damage.

Any type of seizure may evolve into status but GTCS predominates. In children major subtypes are:

(a) Prolonged febrile seizure–the most common type.
(b) Idiopathic status epilepticus.
(c) Symptomatic status epilepticus due to an underlying neurologic or metabolic cause.

Precipitating Factors

1. Febrile illness viz. viral sore throat or URTI.
2. Inadequate or irregular AED therapy.
3. Sudden discontinuation of AED.
4. Sleep deprivation, emotional upset.
5. Metabolic causes viz. hypoglycemia, hypocalcemia.
6. CNS infection.

Classification

SE is generally classified as convulsive and nonconvulsive. It may be classified also on the basis of the etiology.

Convulsive SE	*Nonconvulsive SE*
Generalised	Absence
Focal motor	Complex partial
Myoclonus	NCSE* with coma

*Nonconvulsive SE.

Convulsive Status Epilepticus

Generalised convulsive SE (GCSE) constitute majority of SE in children. It is characterized by tonic, clonic, tonic clonic seizure activity that involves all extremities. GCSE can be primary or secondary, which is difficult to distinguish with prolonged seizure. However, in secondary type, seizure begins focally but spread to involve the entire brain.

Focal motor SE is also called simple complex SE or epilepsy partialis continua. It is less common and frequently associated with a focal brain lesion. It is characterized by involvement of a single limb or side of the face.

Myoclonic SE is more common in comatose patients and is associated with anoxia or cardiac arrest. It is characterized by irregular, asynchronous, small amplitude repetitive jerking of the face or limbs.

Nonconvulsive Status Epilepticus (NCSE)

NCSE can occur in comatose or ambulatory patients. It is characterized by continuous, non-motor seizures which require confirmation by EEG.

Absence SE is the most common type seen in ambulatory children. It is characterized by altered consciousness and a generalized 3 Hz symmetric spike and wave pattern in EEG.

Complete partial SE in an ambulatory patient is marked by altered consciousness and focal activity on EEG, usually involving the temporal lobe.

NCSE with coma should be considered in any patient with prolonged obtundation after cessation of seizure or with coma of unclear etiology.

The diagnosis of NCSE in critically ill patients requires high degree of suspicion and is probably under recognized. NCSE is more common among younger children particularly those between 1 month and 1 year of age and it is frequently associated with structural lesions.

Table 13.4: Showing etiologic classification of Status Epilepticus

Etiology	*Definitions*
Idiopathic	SE without any pre-existing neurologic abnormality
Remote symptomatic	SE with known history of neurologic insult, viz. traumatic brain injury, stroke, static encephalopathy
Febrile	SE proved solely by fever without a history of afebrile seizure
Acute symptomatic	SE during an acute illness, viz. meningitis, hypoxia, hypoglycemia, hypocalcemia, hyponatremia
Progressive	SE in a patient with neuroencephalopathy, degeneration, malignancy, neurocutaneous syndromes

Stepwise Management

Management of the critically ill child with SE is directed towards (a) rapid cessation of seizure, (b) supportive care of associated systemic derangement or complication, (c) treatment of underlying condition, and (d) prevention of seizure recurrence.

Initial Stabilization

1. *Ensure airway patency and control*: The patient should be positioned so that ongoing seizure activity will not cause physical harm. Nothing should be placed into the patient's mouth due to risk of aspiration. Supplemental oxygen should be provided. In patients with hypoxia, hypoventilation or a Glasgow Coma Scale score < 8, rapid sequence endotracheal intubation should be considered for airway protection and respiratory support.
2. Ensure oxygenation.
3. *Reliable IV access* (preferably 2) should be established as soon as possible. If IV catheter placement is difficult or takes time, intraosseous catheter may be considered. Hypotension or dehydration should be treated with isotonic fluid resuscitation.
4. *Blood samples* to be sent for CBC, glucose, urea, electrolytes, serum calcium, drug levels, ABG.
5. *Serum glucose level check* should be promptly done to detect hypoglycemia. In the absence of rapid testing IV 10% dextrose bolus 5 ml/kg can be administered followed by 2/3rd maintenance of N/2 saline in 5% dextrose.

   In older children with nutritional deficiencies, Thiamine (50–100 mg IV) should be considered prior to dextrose administration. Serum electrolytes should be checked and replaced appropriately.

   Investigations to determine the cause should go on simultaneously together with treatment.
6. High dose antibiotics should be administered empirically to patients at risk of bacterial infection.

In patients with new onset SE and fever, empiric antibiotics and Acyclovir should be considered, if risk of bacterial or herpetic infection is suspected.

Supportive Care

Prolonged seizure activity is usually associated with metabolic acidosis, hyperthermia and hypertension.

Metabolic acidosis usually corrects spontaneously after cessation of seizure and adequate hydration.

Hyperthermia (>38.5°C) should be treated with surface and/or systemic cooling to achieve normothermia promptly. Precaution should be taken to prevent shivering associated with active cooling.

Hypertension may be present with ongoing seizure activity. It should not be treated unless it persists after seizure activity has stopped.

Laboratory Diagnosis

It needs emphasis that anti-convulsant therapy should not be delayed to facilitate diagnostic tests because swift cessation of seizure is crucial.

Every patient should have serum glucose and electrolytes tests.

Serum anti-convulsants levels should be measured in children on chronic therapy.

Further tests should go on simultaneously with anti-convulsant treatment. These include the following:

1. Blood and urine specimens for culture in febrile children.
2. Serum and urine toxicology screening tests when possible ingestion is suggested.
3. A CT scan after seizure has stopped to exclude mass intracranial lesions (viz. Tumour, abscess, hemorrhage) or cerebral edema.
4. Lumbar puncture is indicated in patients at risk of meningitis or in those with a new onset seizure disorder. It needs emphasis that it should be done only after the CT scan shows normal findings. Lumbar puncture is contraindicated in patients with evidence of increased intracranial pressure due to risk of downward herniation of brain.
5. Screening tests for inborn errors of metabolism viz. Serum ammonia, lactate, serum amino acid and urine organic acid should be checked in infants and children at risk for inborn errors of metabolism.

Treatment of Seizure

The goal of therapy should be cessation of seizure within 30 minutes of presentation. Administration of anticonvulsants should proceed along a defined timeline.

The steps of treatment of a seizure include:

(a) Administration of first line agent.
(b) Administration of second line agent; and
(c) Initiation of pharmacologic coma for treatment for refractory SE.

About the First Line Agents

Benzodiazepines: Commonly used benzodiazepines for SE includes diazepam, lorazepam and midazolam. Among the three, *Lorazepam* is the preferred first line agent, as it can be used as a first line medication in all types of SE. The peak effect of IV lorazepam occurs 15 minutes after dosing, and the duration of action is 3–6 hours. The dose is 0.05 – 0.1 mg/kg slow IV(Over 2–5 min), maximum 2 doses at 15 minutes interval.

Administration of *diazepam* per rectum is convenient in patients who receive prehospital care or those without established IV access. The bioavailability of rectal diazepam is 90%. The peak effect occurs after 1.5 hours after administration. The dose of rectal diazepam is 0.3 to 0.5 mg/kg. It should be diluted with 3 ml of normal saline and placed into the rectum by a syringe and a flexible tube. A repeat dose can be given after 10 minutes if required. As diazepam has a short half-life, a simultaneous dose of Phenytoin should be given.

Alternatively *midazolam* IM (0.1–0.15 mg/kg, max 0.5 mg/kg), buccal (0.3 mg/kg), intranasal (0.2–0.5 mg/kg) may be administered in patients without IV access. It should be noted that buccal administration of midazolam is easy and safe, and it may be more efficacious than PR diazepam. An appropriate dose of the IV preparation of midazolam is placed between the gum and cheek. Similarly, intra nasal midazolam has been shown to be safe and more efficacious than rectal diazepam.

About the Second Line Agents

Phenytoin is the preferred second line agent. If seizure persists after administration of the first line agent, Phenytoin should be given in the dose of 15 to 20 mg/kg over 15 to 20 minutes.

Valproate is the preferred second line agent in case of Absence seizure. It can be given in the dose of 25 – 35 mg/kg slow IV or Syrup valproate in 1:1 dilution per rectal by retention enema. Valproate has been added as an adjunctive therapy. Valproate may be particularly helpful in patients with Myoclonic SE and Lennox Gastaut syndrome.

Table 13.5: Showing the preferred first line and second line agents

Convulsive SE	*Nonconvulsive SE*
1st line	**1st line**
Lorazepam	Lorazepam
2nd line	**2nd line**
Phenytoin/Phosphenytoin	Phenytoin/Phosphenytoin
	Valproate (Absence seizure)

Refractory Status Epilepticus

SE of any type that fail to respond despite treatment with adequate doses of two anticonvulsants is termed as refractory SE.

A child with refractory SE is at ongoing risk for seizure induced cerebral injury and systemic complication. Whether convulsive or non-convulsive, refractory SE should be treated urgently. In such cases, irrespective of the medications used for induction of pharmacologic coma, the patient with refractory SE needs invasive blood pressure and central venous pressure monitoring to guide titration of ventilator, fluid and vasopressor support and to minimize systemic side effects of prolonged SE and high anticonvulsant doses.

Pharmacologic Coma

The child should be transferred to ICU as the child may need ventilatory support. Pharmacologic coma is typically continued for 24 hours after seizure control. Then tapering should be started. If seizures recur on a reduced dose of the medication, coma can be reinstated for an additional 24 hours. Recurrence after discontinuation of pharmacologic coma is a poor prognostic sign.

Three common therapies used to induce pharmacologic coma are midazolam, pentobarbital and propofol infusions. Benzodiazepine is targeted to seizure cessation, if there is no response, barbiturates are titrated to burst suppression.

(a) *Continuous Midazolam infusion*: It should be started with a loading dose of 0.2 mg/kg followed by 0.1 mg/kg/hour. The dose should be titrated every 15 minutes upwards by 0.05 mg/kg/hour till control. Maximum dose upto 1 mg/kg /hour can be safely used. This procedure has been shown to be effective in more than 85% cases.

The only adverse effect is transient, mild, hypotension which responds to moderate fluid resuscitation. In a small percentage of cases there can be breakthrough seizures and relapse of SE after discontinuation of midazolam.

(b) *Barbiturate coma*: Pentobarbital and Thiopental are the barbiturates in use. Pentobarbital is the most commonly used agent. The dose is usually titrated to burst suppression. The dose of Pentobarbital is 10 – 15 mg/kg IV initially then increase by 2 – 5 mg every 5 min to stop seizure followed by 1 – 3 mg/kg/hour.

Barbiturates suppress cerebral metabolism and may be beneficial for patients with increased ICP. Due to cardiovascular effects of high barbiturate doses fluid resuscitation and low dose vasopressor or inotropic support are frequently required. In addition, the adverse effects of high dose barbiturate includes hypothermia, ileus, and increased susceptibility to infection especially ventilator associated pneumonia. Due to long elimination half-life gradual tapering is usually not necessary.

(c) *Propofol* use for sustained sedation has been contraindicated in children due to the side effects.

Newer Agents

(d) *Ketamine* (1.5 mg/kg IV followed by 0.01– 0.05 mg/kg/hour infusion) can be used in prolonged refractory SE. It may increase ICP. Hence, should not be administered without excluding intracranial mass lesion by neuroimaging.

(e) *Topiramate* in high doses (25 mg/kg by nasogastric tube. Increase by 5 – 10 mg/kg/day) is efficacious for infantile spasm.

Anticonvulsant Therapy after Control of Status Epilepticus

Long-term anticonvulsant therapy should be maintained in children with history of recurrent or with a progressive neurological disorder before the onset of status epilepticus. For an initial attack of idiopathic status epilepticus, particularly that following a febrile seizure anticonvulsant therapy is maintained for 3 months and discontinued if the child remains asymptomatic.

Table 13.6: Suggested algorithm for goal directed treatment of Pediatric Status Epilepticus

Seizure duration	*Stage of SE*	*Location*	*Supportive care measures*	*Anticonvulsant therapy*
< 5 min	Prodromal	Prehospital	Support ABC Obtain IV access	Benzodiazepam (rectal, buccal or intranasal) IV administration of 1st line agent
5 – 10 min	Early	Emergency department	Check glucose and electrolytes Correct abnormalities Endotracheal intubation if: - inadequate airway protection - hypoventilation - hypoxia Begin investigation of cause and empiric therapy	Repeat IV dose of 1st line agent and/or start 2nd line agent Optimize 2nd line agent
10 – 30 min	Established	PICU	Consider EEG monitoring Provide airway, ventilatory and vasopressor support	Pharmacologic coma
>30 min	Refractory	Do	Invasive arterial BP and CVP monitoring Continuous EEG monitoring	Pharmacologic coma

Adapted from Kimberly D. Statler and Colin B. Van Orman. Status Epilepticus. Rogers' Text Book of Pediatric Intensive Care, 4th edition. Editor in Chief David G. Nichols. Lippincott Williams and Wilkins, Philadelphia.

Outcome

Cognitive and motor disabilities have been reported after status epilepticus. Risk of morbidity is more especially if SE is prolonged. Risk factors for poor outcome include age < 12 months, presence of neuroimaging abnormalities and acute symptomatic or progressive encephalopathy etiology.

Common Types of Epilepsy

COMMON TYPES OF CHILDHOOD EPILEPSY

Two unprovoked seizures greater than 24 hours apart suggest the presence of an epileptic disorder within the brain which will lead to future recurrence. The occurrence of a seizure without a provocative stimulus like fever is often considered a harbinger of epilepsy. However only 50% of these children go on to develop a second seizure. Therefore it is important to carefully evaluate to look for the cause of the seizures as well as the need for treatment with antiepileptic drugs. A simple classification of epilepsy in children is as follows:

International Classification of Epileptic Seizures

Generalized Seizures

- Generalized tonic clonic.
- Absence seizures.
- Infantile spasms.

Partial Seizures

- Simple partial (Consciousness retained).
- Complex partial (Consciousness impaired).

Unclassified Seizures

Source: Nelson Textbook of Pediatrics, 17th Edition.

GENERALIZED TONIC CLONIC SEIZURE (GTCS)

Generalized tonic clonic seizures are characterized by dramatic onset of unconsciousness and clonic movements of extremities, usually lasting for about 5–15 minutes or may be prolonged but not more than 30 minutes.

Classification

Generalized tonic clonic seizures (GTCS) may be classified into primary or idiopathic and secondary or symptomatic.

Primary or idiopathic GTCS constitutes about 7–27% of all seizure types in children. It involves the whole body from the onset. There is usually a positive family history. There is absence of any definable abnormalities. Seizures may show a marked diurnal pattern. Primary GTCS is generally precipitated by sleep deprivation, fatigue, and photosensitization. Response to AED therapy is excellent.

Secondary or Symptomatic GTCS is characterized by focal onset, subsequently becoming generalized. It is usually associated with a definable cause. Presence of aura is a characteristic feature. Most common aura is epigastric discomfort, headache and dizziness. There is prolonged weakness of an extremity following an attack. Incidence of status is about 5–6 times higher than that of primary type. Response to AED therapy and prognosis is not good. Requires poly therapy and may land up into intractable epilepsy.

Investigations

GTCS occurring in a neurologically normal child requires no investigation except an EEG.

Neuro imaging (CT or MRI) is required for:

(a) GTCS in infants and young children.

(b) Symptomatic or secondary GTCS.

(c) Distinguishing primary from secondary GTCS.

(d) Focal discharge in EEG.

Other investigations should be done according to the suspected cause on the basis of history and physical examination.

Treatment

Treatment includes treatment of an ongoing seizure and prevention of recurrence with long-term antiepileptic drug therapy.

Treatment of Ongoing Seizure

1. *Maintenance of ABC:* Lateral decubitus position, suctioning, oxygen administration when seizure is prolonged.
2. *Termination of Seizure:* Diazepam, 0.3 mg/kg/dose (max 10 mg) IV/PR, rate not exceeding 2 mg/min, may be repeated upto 3 doses at 10 to 15 minutes interval or lorazepam, 0.1 mg/kg/dose may be repeated once after 15 minutes. They usually respond to this regimen. If not should be treated along the line of status epilepticus.

Long-term Antiepileptic Drug (AED) Therapy for GTCS

The candidates for long-term antiepileptic therapy include those children with:

(a) Recurrent seizure (> 1 seizure).

(b) First seizure with presence of risk factors viz.

1. Symptomatic seizure (e.g. atrophy, inflammatory granuloma in CT).
2. Abnormal EEG.
3. Positive family history of epilepsy.

GTCS Which Do Not Require AED Prophylaxis

1. Single seizure in absence of the risk factors.
2. Symptomatic GTCS of acute onset, e.g., hypoglycemia, dyselectrolytemia, CNS infection.
3. GTCS with infrequent recurrences, i.e., widely spaced (several years). They should be kept under follow-up.

Selection of the Drug

Four drugs viz. Phenobarbitone, phenytoin, carbamazepine and valproic acid are commonly used for the treatment of GTCS. The rate of seizure control by these four drugs is more or less similar. Phenobarbitone is often associated with cognitive dysfunction and valproic acid is sometimes associated with severe hepato toxicity in infants which may be fatal. Among these carbamazepine and phenytoin are devoid of serious side effects. Phenytoin causes gum hyperplasia on prolonged use and may not be acceptable by adolescents. Thus in children with GTCS, carbamazepine and valproic acid are the preferred drugs. However, phenobarbitone is still a drug of choice in patients from poor socioeconomic class. It can be withdrawn if there is hyperactivity.

Stepwise AED Therapy Plan for a Newly Diagnosed Patient

Step 1

Identify and avoid precipitating factors, e.g., fever, sleep deprivation, fasting, photosensitivity.

Table 13.7 : Commonly used AEDs for chronic prophylaxis in GTCS

Drug	*Dose (mg/kg/day)*	*Therapeutic concentration (microgram/ml)*	*Time to steady state (days)*
Phenobarbitone	3–5 OD, bid	15–40	14–21
Phenytoin	5 OD, bid	10–20	7–10
Carbamazepine	10–30, bid, tid	6–12	3–4
Valproic acid	10–60, bid, tid	40–150	1–2

Step 2

Explain the parents the need for starting treatment, potential side effects and need for strict drug compliance. Explain that AED prophylaxis in GTCS has to be prolonged and uninterrupted. Interruption of treatment often results in recurrence of seizure, even a status, and further prolongs the duration of prophylactic treatment.

Step 3

Choose the appropriate drug (check economic status of parents). The appropriate AED should be started in the lowest dose. In case of recurrence of seizure, dose should be increased @ 25% of initial dose at an interval of 2–4 weeks according to the frequency of recurrences.

Step 4

If one drug fails to control the seizure, despite a trial for about 2–3 months in the maximum dose then one should consider the following:

(a) Reconsider the diagnosis of epilepsy.

(b) Check doses and compliance.

(c) Exclude triggering factors.

(d) Exclude structural lesion.

Step 5

If everything is in order a second drug has to be added. To add another first line AED; start in the lowest dose and increase to the optimal dose with 25% increment as in the case of the first AED. If seizure control is achieved, taper off the first drug @ 25% of the dose at an interval of 2 weeks and withdraw. The doses of the second AED taken alone should be adjusted to optimum.

Step 6

If seizure still recurs, a combination of two first line drug should be used. When a second drug is added one should be careful of drug interaction which may worsen the seizure control. Most cases of GTCS, however, can be controlled with one drug. It should be noted that seizure control can take time. Polytherapy is often associated with problems of seizure control and drug toxicity due to drug interaction and summation of toxicities.

Period of AED Therapy

If the child has responded to the antiepileptic drug therapy withdrawal should be planned if the child is seizure free for 2–3 years.

Withdrawal of AED

1. The period of tapering the dose is 3-6 months.
2. In case of polytherapy, the AED started first should be tapered and withdrawn first.
3. Tapering should be done @ 25% of the dose every 4 weeks. The lowest dose should be continued for 4 weeks followed by 4 weeks on alternate days and then stopped.

Follow-up

All patients on AED should be followed up regularly to avoid unwarranted manipulation of drug and dose. The patient is to be asked to visit regularly or whenever there is a recurrence or there is any side effect of the AED.

Initially, the patient should be asked to visit the epilepsy clinic 2–4 weekly depending on the seizure frequency. Subsequent visits should be at an interval of 3–6 months. At each follow-up record should be made about drug doses, compliance, and presence of side effects and recurrence of seizure.

Investigations During AED Prophylaxis

No baseline or subsequent investigations are recommended. Only during the first 3 months of AED prophylaxis, CBC should be done every month. Other investigation should be done if indicated clinically. AED blood levels should be done in case of (1) Seizures difficult to control in spite of adequate therapy (2) Unexplained drug toxicity; and (3) Suspected non-compliance.

The drug level can help to decide about increment of dose, decide about polytherapy and use of other methods of seizure control like surgery.

ABSENCE EPILEPSY

Absence seizures represent a form of epilepsy characterized primarily by negative clinical phenomena, i.e. loss or diminution of normal activity. Staring and transient loss of responsiveness are the most common manifestations, although subtle motor activity may occur, including eyelid fluttering or myoclonic jerks. Due to the brief and subtle nature of these episodes, absence epilepsy may go unrecognized for long periods of time or be mistakenly attributed to day-dreaming or attention deficit disorder.

Absence spells may last upto 10 seconds a piece and occur dozens of times daily. Patients have no recollection of events occurring during a seizure and will resume their previous activity without any postictal symptoms.

EEG classically shows intermittent runs of generalized, 3 cycle per second spike and wave activity which may be precipitated by hyperventilation.

A genetic basis for absence epilepsy has been postulated, since neuroimaging is typically normal and close relatives frequently demonstrate generalized epileptiform abnormalities on EEG. The specific mode of genetic transmission awaits precise elucidation.

Treatment

The aim of treatment should be complete resolution of the seizures and elimination of all spike wave pattern from the EEG.

Drugs

1. *Ethosuximide:* Should be started with 10 mg/kg/day in 2 divided doses and gradually increased at an interval of 8–10 days to 20–30 mg/kg/day. The therapeutic blood level range is 40–100 mcg/ml.
2. *Valproic acid:* Should be started with 10 mg/kg/day in 2–3 divided doses and slowly increased at an interval of 8–10 days until seizures are controlled. The maximum dose is 60 mg/kg body weight. The therapeutic blood level range is 5–120 mcg/ml. Valproate is the drug of choice where absence seizures are complicated by concurrent grand mal seizures.
3. Clonazepam is as effective as ethosuximide but side effects are more. Treatment is started with 0.05 to 0.2 mg/kg/day with a slow increment of 0.25 to 0.5 mg every 4–5 days to a maximum of 8 mg/day.

Duration of treatment: Seizure free interval of 3 years.

PARTIAL SEIZURES

Partial seizures form a sizable part of seizure disorders in children which merit detailed evaluation in order to help treatment and prognostication. Partial seizures may be classified as simple partial seizure where consciousness is maintained and complex partial seizures where conscious is impaired.

Simple Partial Seizures (SPS)

The most common symptom of SPS is *motor activity* characterized by asynchronous clonic tonic movements which tend to involve face, neck and extremities. Seizure movements consisting of head turning and conjugate eye movements are particularly common in SPS. *Automatism* does not occur with SPS, but some patients complain of aura (chest discomfort and headache) which may be the only manifestation of a seizure. However, children have difficulty in describing an aura and often may refer as "feeling funny" or "something crawling inside". The average duration of a seizure is 10–20 seconds. The most characteristic feature of SPS is that the patient remains conscious and may verbalize during the seizure and there is no post ictal phenomenon. The *EEG* may show spikes or sharp waves unilaterally or bilaterally or a multifocal spike pattern in patients with SPS.

Simple partial seizure may need differentiation from tics. Tics are characterized by movements which primarily involve the face and shoulder viz. shoulder shrugging, eye blinking, facial grimacing. Tics can be briefly suppressed whereas SPS cannot be controlled. EEG is normal in tics.

Complex Partial Seizure (CPS)

Complex partial seizure may present as an SPS with or without an aura, followed by unconsciousness. The onset may also coincide with an altered state of consciousness. Automatisms are common occurring in about 50–75% cases. Spreading of epileptiform discharge during CPS can result in secondary generalization with a tonic clonic convulsion. During the spread, contralateral turning of head, dystonic posturing, and tonic clonic movements of the extremities and face including eye blinking may be noted. The average duration of CPS is 1–2 minutes. It is much longer than an SPS or an absence seizure.

The *aura* in CPS consists of vague unpleasant feelings, epigastric discomfort or fear. It is seen in around 30% cases of SPS and CPS. The presence of an aura always indicates a focal onset of seizure. *Impaired consciousness* may be characterized by a brief blank stare, or sudden cessation or pause in activity. It is difficult to appreciate in infants and children and is usually overlooked by the parents as a normal phenomenon. Furthermore, the child is unable to describe the periods of impaired consciousness. Usually only an experienced observer or an abnormal EEG can identify such abnormal events. *Automatisms* develop after the loss of consciousness and may persist into the post ictal phase but they are not recalled by the child. The automatic behaviours observed in infants include lip smacking, chewing, swallowing and excessive salivation. They may be normal phenomenon in an infant. When prolonged and repetitive and associated with blank stare or with a lack of responsiveness, almost always indicate CPS in an infant. In older children, the automatic behaviour consist of semi-purposeful, incoordinated, unplanned gestures like picking and pulling at clothing or bed sheets, rubbing or caressing objects and walking and running in a non-directive, repetitive, and often fearful fashion. A common presentation in a child is a sudden psychic disturbance with a sensation of fear or strangeness and the child usually runs and clings to the mother which is followed by clonic movements.

Complex partial seizures are associated with interictal *EEG findings* viz. anterior temporal lobe sharp waves or focal spikes and multifocal spikes. Some children have interictal sharp waves or spikes originating from the frontal, parietal or occipital lobes. Approximately 20% infants and children with CPS have a normal routine interictal EEG. The techniques used to increase the identification of spikes and sharp waves in these cases include, sleep deprived EEG study, use of zygomatic leads, prolonged EEG recording or Video EEG study in hospitalized children weaned from anticonvulsants.

Radioimaging studies like CT scan and MRI (more useful) may identify a lesion in the temporal lobe which may include mesial temporal sclerosis, hamartoma, post encephalitic gliosis, subarachnoid cysts, infarction, arteriovenous malformations and slow growing glioma. A positron emission tomography (PET) is helpful in precisely localizing the focus with quantification of underlying physiological process.

Biochemical parameters viz. blood sugar, serum calcium, magnesium and sodium may help to eliminate metabolic triggering factors, when suspected.

Treatment of partial seizures consists of anticonvulsant therapy and surgery. Carbamazepine is an effective drug. Sodium valproate, clonazepam alone or in combination may be tried. In refractory complex partial seizures, Gabapentin can be used as an add on drug in children 12 years and older. Vigabatrin, another new drug, is useful as adjunctive therapy for poorly controlled seizures. Surgery should be considered for children with intractable seizures unresponsive to anticonvulsant therapy.

Benign Partial Epilepsy with Centrotemporal Spikes (BPEC)

BPEC, also called Rolandic Epilepsy is a common type of partial seizure in childhood with good prognosis. It occurs between the ages 9–10 years. The child is otherwise neurologically normal. There is often a family history of epilepsy. Approximately 20% children experience only one seizure episode and about 25% have multiple seizure clusters. About 75% seizures occur during sleep. The motor and somato sensory symptoms are usually confined to the face. They include excessive salivation, guttural noises, dysphagia, tonic contraction and paresthesia of the tongue, unilateral numbness of the cheek, clonic movements or paresthesia of the ipsilateral limb. Consciousness may be intact or impaired. The partial seizure may proceed to secondary generalization. The EEG finding is diagnostic and is characterized by a repetitive spike focus localized in centrotemporal or Rolandic area with normal background activity.

Carbamazepine is the drug of choice. It should be prescribed only for children who have frequent seizures. It should be continued for 2 years or until 14–16 years of age, when spontaneous remission of BPEC usually occurs.

Epilepsia Partialis Continua

It is characterized by focal seizures continuing for hours or days. Rasmussen encephalitis, a subacute encephalitis may be one cause. There may be a preceding history of non-specific febrile illness. The onset is usually before the age of 10 years. The seizure episode is usually left with sequelae like hemiplegia, aphasia and hemianopia. The EEG reveals diffuse paroxysmal activity with a slow background. The disease is progressive and usually lethal. It may become self limiting with significant neurologic deficits.

INFANTILE SPASM

Infantile spasm is a type of seizure characterized by brief symmetric contractions of neck, trunk and extremities. Seizures occur in clusters or volleys and may persist for minutes with brief intervals between each spasm. A cry may precede or follow an infantile spasm. The spasms occur during sleep or arousal. It has a tendency to develop while the patient is drowsy or immediately upon awakening. The EEG most commonly shows hypsarrhythmia or a modified hypsarrhythmia pattern.

Types of Spasm

There are three types of infantile spasm–flexor, extensor and mixed. *Flexor spasm* consists of sudden flexon of the neck, arms and legs on to the trunk. *Extensor spasm* produces extension of the trunk and extremities. The *mixed spasm* which consists of flexion in some volleys and extension in others is the most common type of infantile spasm.

Classification

Infantile spasms are classified into two groups: cryptogenic which constitute 10–20% and the rest symptomatic. The child with *cryptogenic infantile spasm* usually has an uneventful pregnancy and birth history. Developmental milestones are normal prior to the onset of seizures. The neurological examination and the CT scan is normal. Prognosis is good in the cryptogenic type.

The *symptomatic infantile spasm* is related to prenatal, perinatal and post natal factors, viz., HIE, congenital infections, inborn errors of metabolism, tuberous sclerosis, lissencephaly, and schizencephaly, prematurity, postnatal CNS infection, and head trauma. 80–90% of the symptomatic type has the risk of mental retardation. The underlying CNS disorder plays the major role in the neurologic outcome.

Pathogenesis

A recent hypothesis implicates corticotrophin-releasing hormone (CRH) in the pathogenesis of infantile spasm. Normally, CRH acts on the pituitary to enhance the release of ACTH. Glucocorticoids and ACTH suppress the metabolism and secretion of CRH by a feedback mechanism. It has been proposed that specific stresses or injury to the infant during the critical period of neurodevelopment causes over production of CRH resulting in neuronal hyper excitability and seizures. The number of CRH receptors reaches a maximum in the infant brain followed by spontaneous reduction with age. Perhaps this accounts for the eventual resolution of infantile spasm, even without treatment. Treatment with exogenous ACTH and glucocorticoids suppress synthesis of CRH. This explains their effectiveness in treatment of infantile spasm.

Treatment

ACTH is the preferred drug for the treatment of infantile spasm. A common dosage schedule is ACTH, 20 units daily IM for 2 weeks. If no response occurs dose is increased to 30 units IM daily for two weeks then 40 units IM daily for two weeks.

Prednisolone is equally effective. It is given as 2 mg/kg/day for two weeks. If seizures persist treatment time is extended by further 4 weeks.

Control can be expected in around 70% cases but one third of the patients relapse when ACTH or prednisolone is discontinued.

Acute Bacterial Meningitis

Meningitis is a common neurological disease in childhood. It is one of the acute emergencies in which a prompt diagnosis and treatment is necessary in order to avoid delay which may make a critical difference between full recovery and chronic disability or death.

Etiology

The etiology of acute bacterial meningitis relates to the age of the patient. During the *first two months of life*, the bacteria that cause meningitis in normal infants reflect the maternal flora and the environment to which the infant is exposed. The most common pathogens include gram negative enteric bacilli, Group B streptococci, and listeria monocytogenes. In addition, occasionally it may be due to H. influenzae B and the other pathogens more typically found in older children.

In children *between 2 months and 12 years of age,* bacterial meningitis is caused by S. pneumoniae, N. meningitides and H. influenzae B. Frequency of infection with H. influenzae B decreases beyond 5 years of age. Meningitis in infants *between 1 and 3 months* may be due to pathogens found in both neonates and older children.

Less common pathogens such as pseudomonas aeruginosa, staphylococcus aureus, and coagulase negative staphylococcus, salmonella and listeria monocytogenes cause meningitis in immunocompromised children.

Epidemiology

Ninetyfive percent of cases of acute bacterial meningitis occur between 1 month and 5 years of age. This is due to the attenuated immunologic response in this age group. All types of meningitis occur sporadically except meningococcal meningitis which may occur in epidemic form.

The *common risk factors* include poor socio economic condition, recent colonization with pathogenic bacteria, close contact with patients, overcrowding, splenic dysfunction, immunocompromised host, and communications (congenital or acquired) across the mucocutaneous barrier.

Pathogenesis

Organisms can gain entry into the meninges in a variety of ways viz. hematogenous dissemination of micro-organism from a distant site of infection; may follow bacterial invasion from a contiguous focus of infection such as paranasal sinusitis, otitis media, mastoiditis, orbital cellulitis and cranial or vertebral osteomyelitis, or may occur after introduction of bacteria via a penetrating cranial trauma, dermal sinus tracts and meningo-myelocele. Meningitis may occur during endocarditis, pneumonia or thrombophlebitis or associated with burns, indwelling catheters, or contaminated infusion equipment.

Bacterial meningitis, however, most commonly results from hematogenous dissemination of microorganisms from a distant site of infection. Bacterimia usually precedes or occur concomitantly. Bacterial colonization of the nasopharynx with a potentially pathogenic organism is the usual source of bacterimia. Prior or concomitant viral upper respiratory tract infection may enhance the pathogenecity of the bacteria producing meningitis.

In case of N. meningitides and H. influenzae type B, the organism attach to the mucosal epithelial receptors. After attachment to the epithelial cells, the bacteria breach the mucosa and enter the circulation. Bacteria gain entry into the CSF through the choroid plexus of the lateral ventricle and the meninges and then circulate to the extra cerebral CSF and subarachnoid space. As the CSF concentration of complement and antibody is inadequate and cannot contain bacterial proliferation, the organisms rapidly multiply. The presence of bacterial cell wall lipopolysaccharide of gram negative bacteria (H. influenzae type B and N. meningitides) and of pneumococcal cell wall components stimulates a marked inflammatory response with local production of tumor necrosis factor, interleukin-1, prostaglandin E and other cytokine inflammatory mediators. The subsequent inflammatory response is characterized by neutrophilic infiltration, increased vascular permeability, alterations of the blood brain barrier and vascular thrombosis. Excessive cytokine induced inflammation continues after the CSF has been sterilized and is thought to be responsible for the chronic inflammatory sequelae of pyogenic meningitis.

Pathology

Whatever the causative organism, the pathological changes in acute bacterial meningitis are similar. A *meningeal exudate* of varying thickness becomes rapidly diffused through the whole subarachnoid space of the brain and spinal cord. The exudate may be distributed around the cerebral veins, venous sinuses, convexity of the brain and cerebellum and the sulci and sylvian fissures, basal cistern and the spinal cord. There may be ventriculitis, subdural effusion and rarely empyema. Cerebral infarction may result from vascular occlusion due to inflammation, vasospasm and thrombosis. The infarct size ranges from microscopic to involvement of an entire hemisphere.

Inflammation of spinal nerves and roots produces the signs of meningeal irritation. Inflammation of the cranial nerves produces neuropathies. The common nerves affected are optic (2nd), occulomotor (3rd), facial (7th) and auditory (8th). The 3rd and the 6th nerve may be affected due to increased intracranial pressure. Third nerve palsy may be result of temporal lobe compression of the nerve during tentorial herniation. Sixth nerve palsy is a false localizing sign of increased intracranial pressure.

Increased ICP in bacterial meningitis may due to cell death (cytotoxic cerebral edema), cytokine induced increased capillary vascular permeability (vasogenic cerebral edema) and increased hydrostatic pressure as a result of obstructed reabsorption of CSF in the arachnoid villus or obstruction to flow from the ventricles (interstitial cerebral edema).

Communicating hydrocephalus can develop as an acute complication due to adhesive thickening of the arachnoid villi around the cisterns at the base of the brain. *Obstructive hydrocephalus* may develop after fibrosis and gliosis of the aqueduct of Sylvius or the foramina of Magendie and Luschka. There is also *damage to the cerebral cortex* due to focal or diffuse effects of vascular obstruction, hypoxia, cerebritis, toxic encephalopathy, elevated ICP, ventriculitis and transudation which results in clinical manifestations like impaired consciousness, seizures, cranial nerve deficits, motor and sensory deficits and later psychomotor retardation.

Clinical Manifestations

The clinical presentation of acute bacterial meningitis is related to the nonspecific findings associated with a systemic infection and to manifestations of meningeal irritation.

Early symptoms are often vague and younger the child more non-specific are the symptoms. The onset is commonly insidious with several days of fever, accompanied by upper respiratory tract or gastrointestinal symptoms, followed by nonspecific symptoms of CNS infection such as lethargy or drowsiness, irritability and refusal to feed.

Symptoms of increased intracranial pressure include headache, vomiting in older children and shrill cry, and tense, bulging fontanel in infants.

The onset may be sudden with rapidly progressive manifestations of shock, purpura, disseminated intravascular coagulation (DIC) and reduced level of consciousness. This is seen in cases of meningococcal meningitis.

The *signs of meningeal irritation* include pain in the back, nuchal rigidity, Kernig sign and Brudzinski sign. In young children, particularly those below 2 years age, these signs are consistently not present. In this age group, the *signs of increased ICP* are present which include a bulging fontanel, sutural diathesis, hypertension with bradycardia, apnea or hyperventilation and cranial nerve palsy viz. 6th and 3rd nerve palsy, decorticate or decerebrate rigidity, stupor, coma or signs of herniation.

Seizures (focal or generalized) occur in about 30% cases of acute bacterial meningitis. A high concentration of tumour necrosis factor has been associated with occurrence of seizure. The other causes include ceribritis, infarction and electrolyte disturbances. Generalized seizures that occur on presentation or within 4 days are of no prognostic significance. Seizures that persist beyond 4 days and are difficult to control may be associated with poor prognosis.

Papilledema is an uncommon finding but if present indicates subdural effusion or brain abscess.

Altered sensorium is common and is manifested by irritability, lethargy, stupor, obtundation and coma. It may result from increased ICP, cerebritis or hypotension.

Complications

Complications of acute bacterial meningitis can develop early in the course of illness or late or develop as a sequalae.

Table 13.8 : Complications and sequalae

1. Early complications
   - Subdural effusion
   - Ventriculitis
   - Motor deficits: Hemiparesis, quadriparesis
   - Cranial nerve palsy: Facial, occulomotor and optic nerves
   - Hydrocephalus
   - Hearing loss
   - Systemic: Peripheral circulatory failure, DIC, SIADH, arthritis
2. Late complications and sequalae
   - Mental retardation
   - Seizures
   - Sensorineural hearing loss
   - Behaviour problems
   - Motor deficits
   - Ataxia
   - Hydrocephalus

Laboratory Diagnosis

The diagnosis of acute bacterial meningitis is confirmed by analysis of the CSF which reveals microorganisms on gram stain and culture. However, isolation of causative organism from CSF culture requires a minimum of 24–48 hours and the results can be misleading if antimicrobials have been administered before collection of CSF. The outcome of acute bacterial meningitis depends on early and appropriate antimicrobial therapy. Hence, immediate diagnosis has to be made by physical, chemical and cytological examination and gram stain of CSF.

CSF Findings in Acute Bacterial Meningitis

On *physical examination* the CSF may be clear, hazy or turbid. Turbid CSF is present when the CSF total cell count is more than 200–400/cumm.

Chemical examination reveals increase in protein, reduction of CSF glucose as well as reduction of the CSF: blood glucose ratio which is normally about 66%. The blood sample for estimation of glucose should be taken before lumbar puncture in order to avoid the false increase due to the stress.

Cytological examination typically shows a polymorphonuclear leucocytosis with a total cell count usually more than 1000 / mm^3 and neutrophils constituting

75–95%. However, presence of 4 or more polymorphonuclear leucocytes (PMNL) in a neonate and more than a single PMNL in a child over 6 weeks is suggestive of acute bacterial meningitis.

A traumatic LP affects the interpretation of CSF leucocytes and protein but gram stain, culture and glucose level may not be influenced. In such cases one should rely on the bacterial diagnosis.

Variations of CSF Findings

A CSF total leukocyte count of less than 250/mm^3 may be present in 20% cases. In about 10–13% cases there may be predominately lymphocytosis. CSF lymphocytosis is common when the leukocyte count is less than 1000 cells / cumm. It may be seen in early stages of infection when it is also associated with milder biochemical alterations. In such cases, a repeat lumbar puncture after 24 hours commonly shows PMNL predominance. Prior antibiotic therapy may also lead to CSF lymphocytosis. A low CSF leukocyte count may also be associated with a poor outcome presumably reflecting an inadequate host response to infection.

Rapid Diagnostic Tests

The rapid diagnostic tests are helpful in patients in whom prior antimicrobial therapy may interfere bacterial culture. The tests are based on detection of antigen or antibody in various body fluids like CSF, serum and urine. It should be noted that a positive antigen test is usually meaningful but a negative test is unreliable to exclude diagnosis of meningitis. However, these tests are useful adjunct to CSF examination. Bacterial antigen can be detected by counter current immune electrophoresis (CIE), latex particle agglutination (LPA) and enzyme linked immunosorbent assay (ELISA). These tests are especially helpful in cases of partially treated meningitis and where gram stain does not reveal any organism.

Non-specific markers like raised C reactive protein, lactate dehydrogenase (LDH), and lactic acid in CSF indicate CSF inflammation, breakdown of blood brain barrier and qualify the type of inflammation. Among these tests, CSF LDH levels above 100 units/L is a reliable non-specific marker for diagnosis of acute bacterial meningitis.

Gram Stain

Gram stain is positive in around 70–90% patients with acute bacterial meningitis. Gram stain of buffy coat from blood or petechial lesion may help in early identification of organisms.

Blood Culture

Blood culture may help in isolation of the organism in patients with sterile CSF in around 80–90% of cases of acute bacterial meningitis in children.

Radiological Studies

Radiological studies useful in bacterial meningitis include ultrasonography (in infants with an open fontanel) and CT scan of skull. These investigations should be considered if response to therapy is not satisfactory or if complications are suspected. Complications should be suspected under the following circumstances:

1. Presence of signs of increased ICP, focal neurological deficits, increased head circumference.
2. Prolonged fever during therapy.

Differential Diagnosis

The common diseases which may present with symptoms and signs similar to acute bacterial meningitis include aseptic meningitis, tubercular meningitis and brain abscess. A careful examination of CSF, gram stain and CSF culture usually confirm the diagnosis. In doubtful cases and partially treated cases, tests for detection of bacterial antigen can help in establishing the diagnosis.

In cases of meningitis partially treated with oral or parenteral antibiotics, the CSF becomes rapidly sterile, particularly if the organism is S. pneumoniae or meningococcus but the CSF pleocytosis, elevated protein and low glucose still persist and indicate a diagnosis of acute bacterial meningitis. In such cases, CSF, blood and urine should be tested for bacterial antigen for confirmation of diagnosis.

Management

Acute bacterial meningitis is a medical emergency. The goal is to begin antibiotic therapy as early as possible within 60 minutes of patient's arrival in the emergency room. It is always advisable to start an empirical antibiotic if there is a strong clinical suspicion before a lumbar puncture even though it may reduce the chances of detecting the organism in CSF. The justification is that any delay in treatment may increase the possibility of permanent sequalae or death. The management may be broadly categorized into antibiotic therapy, adjunct therapy and supportive care.

All cases of meningitis should be admitted to hospital. On admission the patient should be evaluated for presence of signs of increased intracranial pressure or peripheral circulatory failure. Secondly, a lumbar puncture should be done and samples send for analysis. Sample of blood for culture and blood sugar should also be taken. In case lumbar puncture is contraindicated due to any reason, initial antibiotic therapy should be started before the spinal tap.

Antibiotic Therapy

The empirically chosen antibiotic should be one which (i) can achieve sufficient bactericidal concentration in CSF, (ii) provide coverage against the common pathogen, i.e., H. influenzae, S. pneumoniae and N. meningitidis.

The initial drug of choice is ceftriaxone (100 mg/kg/day in two divided doses) or cefotaxime (200 mg/kg/day in 6 hourly doses). These drugs achieve a high bactericidal concentration in CSF and rapidly sterilize the CSF. Alternatively, ampicillin (300 mg/kg/day 6 hourly) and chloramphenicol (100 mg/kg/day 6 hourly) can be used as initial therapy. In case of known resistance of S. pneumoniae to beta lactum drugs, recommended empirical antibiotic therapy is vancomycin (60 mg/kg/day 6 hourly) in combination with either ceftriaxone or cefotaxime. Higher doses of cefotaxime (250 – 300 mg/kg/day) may be used because it may help in overcoming some degree of cephalosporin resistance.

If a patient is immunocompromised and gram negative bacteria is suspected, the initial therapy might include ceftazidime and an aminoglycoside.

Subsequent antibiotic therapy should be guided by culture and sensitivity results.

Duration of Therapy

Ideally antibiotic therapy should be continued for atleast 5 days after the CSF becomes sterile. Empirically the duration of therapy depends on the presumed organism as identified by a positive gram stain/bacterial antigen as follows:

H. influenzae: 7–10 days.

N. meningitides: 7–10 days.

S. pneumoniae: 14 days.

Gram negative bacilli: 3 weeks.

Adjunct Therapy

The only adjunct therapy recommended is the use of intravenous dexamethasone, 0.15 mg/kg/dose given every 6 hours for two days in acute bacterial meningitis due to H. influenzae type B. Corticosteroids appear to have maximum benefit if given 1–2 hours before initiation of antibiotics. Studies show that the corticosteroid recipients had less fever, lower CSF protein and lactate levels, and a reduction of permanent auditory nerve damage than did placebo recipients. Dexamethasone has no role in a child with partially treated pyogenic meningitis.

Supportive Care

Complications are common in first 72 hours. The patient should be monitored for neurological and systemic complications.

Fluid should be restricted to 60–80% of normal maintenance until SIADH and raised ICP is excluded.

A child presenting with *septic shock* should be treated with fluid resuscitation and vasoactive drugs such as dopamine.

Patients with *raised ICP* should be treated as follows:

(a) Elevation of head end of the bed to 30°.

(b) Administration of mannitol (0.5–1 gm/kg) and frusemide (1 mg/kg).

(c) Endotracheal intubation and hyperventilation to maintain PCO_2 approximately at 25 mm Hg.

Seizures are treated with diazepam (0.1–0.2 mg/kg/dose) or lorazepam (0.05 mg/kg/dose) followed by a bolus dose of phenytoin (15–20 mg/kg) and maintained with a dose of 5 mg/kg/day. Phenytoin is preferred over phenobarbitone because it produces less CNS depression and allows assessment of sensorium.

Metabolic complications like hyponatremia, hypocalcaemia or hypoglycemia should be monitored and treated as and when necessary with specific therapy.

Prognosis

The mortality rate is around 16–27% in developing countries. Case fatality is reported to be much less, less than 10% in western countries. The highest mortality rate is observed in pneumococcal meningitis.

The poor prognostic clinical features include age <6 months, seizures occurring after 4th day into therapy, presence of focal neurological signs and / or coma at presentation, septic shock. The laboratory parameters with poor prognosis include TLC < 10,000/mm^3 or

> 20,000/mm^3, CSF cell count > 5000 / mm^3, CSF glucose < 20 mg/dl or protein > 500 mg / dl, more than 10^6 CFU of bacteria/ml in CSF, infection with E. coli, P. aeruginosa.

Severe neurodevelopmental sequelae may occur in 10–20% patients recovering from acute bacterial meningitis and as many as 50% may have subtle neurobehavioral morbidity. The common neurologic sequelae include hearing loss, mental retardation, seizures, and delay in acquisition of language, visual impairment and behavioural problems. Sensorineural hearing loss is the most common sequalae and occurs in as many as 30% of patients with pneumococcal, 10% with meningococcal and 5–20% in H. influenzae B meningitis. All patients with bacterial meningitis should undergo hearing assessment before or soon after discharge from hospital.

Prevention

Prevention of acute bacterial meningitis is possible by chemoprophylaxis and vaccination.

Chemoprophylaxis

Chemoprophylaxis helps in prevention of secondary cases. It is possible by rifampicin prophylaxis of the index case and close contacts for H. influenzae B infection. All household contacts of the index case should be administered. Rifampicin 20 mg/kg/day for 4 days when atleast one contact is less than 4 years of age irrespective of the immunization status. The index case should receive chemoprophylaxis at or near the completion of therapy.

In case of infection with N. meningitides, chemoprophylaxis is recommended for all close contacts regardless of age and immunization status. The drug used is rifampicin (10 mg/kg every 12 hours for 2 days). No prophylaxis is required for S. pneumoniae for normal hosts.

Vaccination

Three vaccines are available viz. Hib vaccine, meningococcal and pneumococcal vaccine. The Hib vaccine is recommended as routine immunization for children. Widespread use of this vaccine has significantly controlled Hib infection in western countries. In our country it is recommended as an additional vaccine. Meningococcal vaccine has been used for mass immunization to control outbreaks. The clinical efficacy of pneumococcal vaccine is yet to be established.

Brain Abscess

A brain abscess is a focal, suppurative infection within the brain parenchyma, typically surrounded by a vascularized capsule.

Epidemiology

Brain abscess can occur in children of any age but are most common in children between 4 and 8 years. Most brain abscesses are single but around 30% are multiple and may involve more than one lobe.

The predisposing conditions include otitis media, mastoiditis, paranasal sinusitis, pyogenic infection in any part of the body, congenital cyanotic heart disease (commonly tetralogy of Fallot), penetrating head injury or neurosurgical procedures (ventriculoperitoneal shunt operation), dental infection and immunodeficiency states (HIV infection). Upto one third of cases of brain abscess is associated with otitis media and mastoiditis.

Etiology

The common responsible bacteria are S. aureus, S. pneumoniae, S. viridens, and fusobacterium. Hematogenous spread accounts for around 25% of cases and it results in multiple abscesses. The etiological agent has a relation to the primary site of infection. For example, abscesses that develop as a complication of infective endocarditis is often due to S. viridens or staphylococcus, that due to lung infection are streptococci, staphylococci, bacteriodes or fusobacterium. Enterobacteriaceae and P. aeruginosa are causes of abscess associated with urinary sepsis. Abscess that follow head trauma and neurosurgical procedures are frequently due to staphylococcus, enterobacteriaceae and pseudomonas. Streptococci are the most common pathogens in causation of abscess in association with congenital cyanotic heart disease.

Pathogenesis

The intact brain parenchyma is relatively resistant to infection. The prerequisite for effective bacterial invasion include preexisting brain ischemia, necrosis or hypoxia.

The route of infection may be by (i) direct spread from a contiguous cranial site of infection such as paranasal sinuses (10%), ear, mastoid or dental infection (2%); or as (ii) a result of hematogenous spread from a remote site of infection (25%); or (iii) following head trauma or neurosurgical procedure. No apparent source of infection is detected in 25% of cases.

Once the infection is established, the brain abscess evolves through four stages. The *stage of early cerebritis* (1–3 days) is characterized by a perivascular infiltration of inflammatory cells which surrounds a central core of coagulative necrosis. In the *stage of late cerebritis* (days 4–9), there is enlargement of the necrotic centre with formation of pus which is surrounded at its border by macrophages and fibroblasts. A thin capsule of fibrous tissue develops gradually and the surrounding area of cerebral edema becomes more distinct. The third stage or *stage of early capsule formation* (days 10–13) is characterized by the formation of a capsule that is better developed on the cortical side rather than the ventricular side. This stage correlates with appearance of a ring enhancing capsule on neuroimaging. The final stage or *stage of late capsule formation* (day 14 and beyond) is defined by a well formed necrotic center surrounded by a dense collagenous capsule. The surrounding area of edema regresses but there is marked gliosis with development of large number of reactive astrocytes outside the capsule. The gliotic process may contribute to the development of seizures as a sequalae of brain abscess.

Clinical Manifestations

Although an infectious process, brain abscess typically presents as a space occupying lesion. The classic clinical triad of headache, fever and signs of focal neurologic deficits is present in less than 50% cases.

The onset of symptoms is variable ranging from hours to weeks or even months. The most common symptom is headache which is described as constant, dull, aching sensation either hemicranial or generalized, which progressively become more severe and refractory to therapy. Fever is not a constant feature and its absence does not exclude the diagnosis. There may be focal or generalized seizure. Focal neurological deficits including hemiparesis, aphasia, or visual field defects are a part of the initial presentation.

The *focal neurological signs* depend on the location of the abscess, the nature of the primary infection if present, and on the level of increased intracranial pressure (ICP). Hemiparesis is the most common localizing sign of a frontal lobe abscess. A temporal lobe abscess may present with dysphasia or an upper homonymous quadrantanopia. Nystagmus and ataxia are signs of cerebellar involvement. *Signs of raised ICP* viz. nausea, vomiting, papilledema and drowsiness or confusion can be the dominant presentation in some cases. *Signs of meningeal irritation* are present when there is a rupture of the abscess into the ventricle or the subarchnoid space.

Laboratory Diagnosis

Neuroimaging is diagnostic. An MRI is better than a CT scan to demonstrate an abscess in the early (cerebritis) stage and superior in identifying abscesses in the posterior fossa.

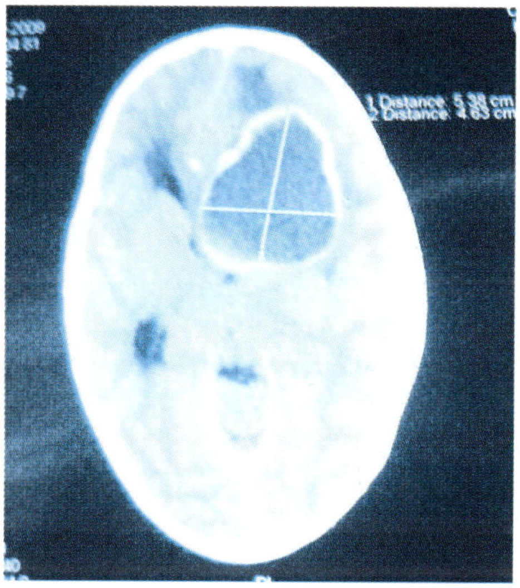

Fig. 13.10: CT scan showing cerebral abscess

A lumbar puncture should not be performed in a patient suspected to have a brain abscess or a subdural empyema. CSF analysis does not contribute to diagnosis or therapy and a lumbar puncture increases the risk of herniation. A microbiologic diagnosis is most accurately determined by gram stain and culture of abscess material obtained by stereotactic needle aspiration.

The indirect markers include a peripheral leucocytosis, elevated ESR and C reactive protein and positive blood culture.

Differential Diagnosis

The conditions that can present with headache, fever and focal neurological signs and seizure include subdural empyema, bacterial meningitis, viral meningoencephalitis, superior sagittal sinus thrombosis, and acute disseminated encephalomyelitis. When fever is absent, primary and metastatic brain tumours are the main differential diagnosis.

Treatment

Specific Therapy

The optimal therapy of brain abscess includes a combination of high dose parenteral antibiotics and neurosurgical drainage.

Empirical therapy for community acquired infection includes a third generation cephalosporin (e.g. cefotaxime, 200 mg / kg / day 6 hourly or ceftriaxone, 100 mg/kg/day 12 hourly) and metronidazole (30 mg/kg/day 6 hourly). In patients with history of penetrating head trauma or recent neurosurgical procedures, empirical treatment should include ceftazidime (150 mg/kg/day 8 hourly) and Vancomycin (60 mg/kg/day 6 hourly) to enhance coverage of pseudomonas and to cover staphylococcus respectively. Empirical antibiotic cover should be modified based on the results of Gram's stain and culture of the abscess contents. All patients should receive a minimum of 6–8 weeks of parenteral antibiotic therapy.

Excision of an abscess by craniotomy or craniectomy is generally reserved for multiloculated abscess or those in which stereotactic aspiration is unsuccessful.

Supportive Therapy

The patients should also receive prophylactic anticonvulsant because of high risk of seizures. Anticonvulsant therapy should be continued for atleast 3 months after resolution of the abscess. The decision for withdrawal is based on the EEG finding. If the EEG is abnormal, anticonvulsants should be continued. If the EEG is normal, the anticonvulsants should be gradually withdrawn, with close follow-up and repeat EEG after stopping the drug.

Follow-up

For documentation of resolution of the abscess, serial CT scan or MRI should be done on a monthly or twice monthly basis. More frequent follow-up may be required in patients who are receiving medical therapy alone. A small amount of enhancement may remain for months after the abscess has been completely treated.

Prognosis

The mortality from brain abscess has declined with the development of neuroimaging techniques, improved neurosurgical procedures for stereotactic aspiration and availability of potent antibiotics. However, significant sequelae which include seizures, persisting weakness, aphasia, or mental impairment may occur in survivors.

Subdural Effusion

Subdural effusion is characterized by collection of fluid in the subdural space. It may be associated with any of the bacterial meningitis but occurs most often following hemophilus influenzae meningitis. The peak incidence is at the age 4–6 months. The majority of subdural effusions are small collections and reabsorb spontaneously. The incidence of large collection, which cause significant increase in intracranial pressure and which require therapy, has become less with modern day therapy.

Pathogenesis

The pathogenesis of subdural effusion after meningitis is not completely understood. In the infant, the arachnoid membrane is a poor barrier to the spread of infection into the subdural space. Initially the fluid is an inflammatory exudate which is purulent and bacteria may be grown from it.

Several mechanisms appear to act to maintain and enlarge the fluid collection after the infection has been controlled. There may be rupture of the bridging veins due to expansion of the subdural space when the fluid becomes bloody. Transudation of fluid from inflamed capillaries may also be important because the protein composition of the subdural fluid is that of a transudate of plasma.

Clinical Manifestations

The symptoms are similar to those of meningitis like irritability, vomiting, convulsion and persistent drowsiness. The physical signs include persistent fever, a bulging fontanelle and abnormal enlargement of head and a positive transillumination test in a child suffering from bacterial meningitis and receiving treatment.

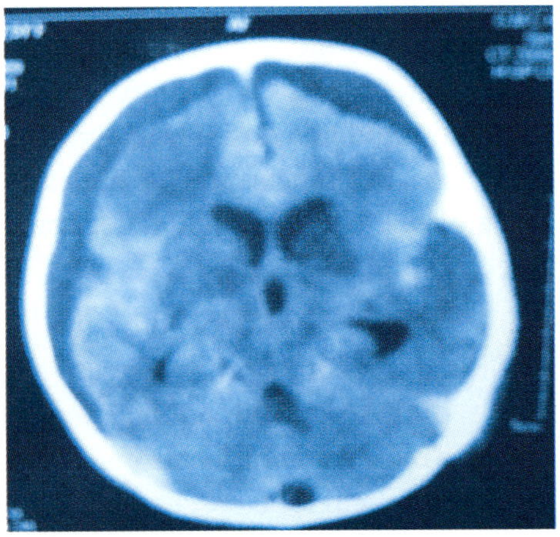

Fig. 13.11: CT scan showing fronto–parietal subdural effusion

The diagnosis may be confirmed by a CT scan or a bilateral subdural tap.

Treatment

Small effusions do not cause increased intracranial pressure, and subside spontaneously with treatment of meningitis. Large effusion should be prevented with repeated subdural taps at an interval of 24–48 hours in order to prevent brain damage by compression. Repeated taps are indicated in infants with bulging fontanelle or abnormal head enlargement. However, too many taps should be avoided as it may cause worsening of the condition by causing bleeding into the subdural space.

The subdural space needs surgical drainage via bilateral burr holes if large quantities of bloody fluid or fluid with high quantity of protein continue to accumulate after two weeks of repeated tapping.

Subdural and Epidural Empyema

It is characterized by collection of pus in subdural or epidural spaces. It is a condition which occur secondary to frontal sinusitis or to infections of the scalp and skull.

The purulent exudate acts as a space occupying lesion, compressing the underlying brain. In addition, there is thrombophlebitis of the cortical veins that pass through the infected subdural space. Interference with venous drainage leads to severe cerebral swelling.

The course is subacute, with fever, severe headache, lethargy, convulsion and hemiparesis in a child with a history of frontal sinusitis, scalp or skull infection. Papilledema is present and there is rapid progression to coma and tentorial herniation.

The diagnosis is confirmed by a CT/MRI scan.

Treatment consists of prompt surgical drainage followed by appropriate antibiotic therapy.

Acute Viral Meningitis

Acute viral meningitis is an acute inflammatory process involving the meninges and to a variable degree, brain tissue; hence also called viral meningoencephalitis.

Etiology

Enteroviruses (ECHO, coxsakie and adeno) account for 75–90% of acute viral meningitis. The other viruses include arboviruses (St. Louis and California encephalitis viruses), herpes simplex type 1 and type 2, mumps virus and varicella zoster virus. Meningoencephalitis is caused occasionally by rubella, rubeola, rabies and respiratory viruses.

Pathogenesis

There is neurologic damage which is caused either by direct invasion and destruction of neural tissues by actively multiplying viruses or by a host reaction to viral antigen. Most neuronal destruction is due to viral invasion. The host tissue response induces demyelination and vascular and perivascular destruction. The cerebral cortex, especially the temporal lobe is often severely affected by herpes simplex virus. The arboviruses tend to affect the entire brain and rabies virus has a predilection for the basal structures.

Pathology

There is meningeal congestion and mononuclear infiltration, perivascular cuffs of lymphocytes and plasma cells, some perivascular necrosis with myelin breakdown, and neuronal disruption in various stages.

Clinical Manifestations

The onset of illness is generally acute. The progression and severity of the disease depends on the degree of meningeal and parenchymal involvement, which in part is determined by the etiologic agent.

Some children may appear to be mildly affected initially, only to relapse into coma and die suddenly. In others, the illness is characterized by high fever, convulsions interspersed with bizarre movements and hallucinations alternating with brief periods of clarity, followed by complete recovery.

In general, there is a history of nonspecific febrile illness preceding the appearance of CNS symptoms and signs. The infant may present with lethargy and irritability. The older child complains of headache and hyperesthesia. Headache is most often frontal or generalized; frequently retrobulbar in adolescents and is accompanied with photophobia and pain on moving the eyes. There is also fever, malaise, nausea and vomiting, photophobia, and pain in the neck, back and legs, abdominal pain and/or diarrhoea. The temperature rises and there is mental dullness progressing to stupor with bizarre movements and convulsion. The seizures or focal neurological signs suggest involvement of brain parenchyma and do not occur in uncomplicated viral meningitis. There may be focal neurologic signs which may remain stationary, fluctuating or progressive. Loss of bowel and bladder control and unprovoked emotional outbursts may occur. In exanthematous infections, exanthems accompany or precede the CNS signs.

On examination nuchal rigidity is present in most cases but may be mild. Evidence of severe meningeal irritation, such as Kernig's and Brudzinski's signs are generally absent.

Laboratory Diagnosis

The most important laboratory test in the diagnosis of viral meningitis is examination of CSF. The typical profile is a cell count 25–500 cells / mm^3 with lymphocytic predominance, a normal or slightly elevated protein level and normal glucose level and a normal or mildly elevated opening CSF pressure. Organisms are absent on gram's stain, acid fast stains or India ink preparation.

However, initially there may be a polymorphonuclear leucocytosis changing to lymphocytic pre-dominance in 8–12 hours. The protein concentration may be very high if brain destruction is extensive as in cases of herpes simplex infection. There may be a substantial decrease in glucose concentration with certain viral infection like mumps virus, herpes simplex type 2, and varicella zoster virus.

The CSF should be cultured for viruses, bacteria, fungi and mycobacteria. The culture positivity is around 70% only, that too early in illness. Detection of viral DNA or RNA by polymerase chain reaction may be useful in the diagnosis of CNS infection caused by herpes simplex and enteroviruses respectively. PCR is claimed to be more sensitive than culture.

An EEG showing focal seizure and CT/MRI showing a focal lesion, especially involving the temporal lobes suggest herpes simplex infection. In other cases the EEG shows diffuse slow wave activity without focal changes and a CT/MRI show swelling of the brain parenchyma.

A chest X-ray and tuberculin test should be advised in all cases of aseptic meningitis to rule out tubercular meningitis in our country.

Treatment

In majority of cases treatment is symptomatic. Mild cases usually do not require hospitalization. They should be advised rest in a quiet room with reduction in room light and visitors. Acetaminophen (10–15 mg/kg/dose 4–6 hourly) is recommended for control of fever and pain and antiemetics for vomiting. Intravenous fluids are occasionally necessary because of poor intake. More severe cases require hospitalization and intensive care.

The severe cases should be monitored for development of complications like cerebral edema, convulsions, hyperpyrexia, disturbed fluid and electrolyte balance, aspiration, and cardiac or respiratory arrest of central origin and managed in usual lines.

In prolonged states of coma, parenteral nutrition is indicated. The serum sodium should be monitored for early detection of SIADH. A normal blood glucose, serum calcium and magnesium must be maintained to minimize the likelihood of convulsions. In case there is convulsion or cerebral edema, prompt treatment should be instituted.

The only drug treatment available is acyclovir. Oral or intravenous acyclovir may be of benefit in patients with herpes simplex virus and severe cases of enterovirus and varicella zoster infection. Intravenous acyclovir (30 mg/kg/day in 3 divided doses 8 hourly for 7 days) should be advised in all seriously ill cases. Oral acyclovir may be tried in less severely ill patients. The dose is 20 mg/kg 8 hourly for 7 days.

Prognosis

Most children recover completely from viral meningitis with the exception of herpes simplex meningitis which may either cause death or leave the survivors with severe sequelae. Mumps meningitis can cause deafness. Approximately 10% of children younger than 2 years of age with enteroviral infection suffer from an acute complication like seizures, increased intracranial pressure or coma. However, almost all have favourable long-term neurologic outcome.

Prevention

Vaccination is an effective method of preventing the development of neurological complications associated with viral infection. At present the available vaccines are against measles, mumps, rubella and varicella.

Encephalitis

Encephalitis is primarily an infection associated with inflammatory response limited largely to the brain parenchyma although there may be evidence of associated meningitis (meningoencephalitis) and, in some cases, involvement of the spinal cord or nerve roots (encephalomyelitis, encephalomyeloradiculitis).

It is one of the most serious infections of the central nervous system in children with high mortality, frequently with incapacitating sequelae in the survivors and virtually with no specific treatment.

Epidemiology

Host immune status is an important factor in the occurrence of viral infections. The most susceptible period of life is between the age group of 6 months and 5 years. The viruses causing encephalitis also show considerable geographic variation depending on the type of vector and climate. For example adeno and arbor viral infection are common in summer, enterovirus in summer and fall and lymphocytic choriomeningitis virus in winter. However, herpes viruses (herpes simplex type I and II), does not show significant seasonal variation.

Etiology

Large number of viruses causes encephalitis. Those documented to cause encephalitis in children include arbor viruses (e.g. Japanese encephalitis virus, St. Louis, California virus etc), herpes viruses (Herpes simplex type I and II), varicella zoster, cytomegalovirus, Epstein-Barr, enteroviruses (polio, coxsakie, echo), mixoviruses (influenza, parainfluenza, measles, mumps), adeno virus, rubella, rabies, and lymphocytic choriomeningitis virus.

A few viruses cause slowly progressive, encephalitis in children. The documented ones are measles, rubella and HIV.

Pathogenesis

There is a stage of primary replication followed by viremia and secondary replication. The *primary replication* of the virus commonly occurs in the mucous membrane and lymph nodes of the respiratory, gastrointestinal and genitourinary tract. It depends on the presence of suitable receptors on the host's cell membrane and the permissiveness of the host's cell.

The viruses are obligatory intracellular parasite. Following a viral infection of the body, the viruses adsorb into the host cell membrane and penetrate the cell. Inside there is uncoating of the virus, replication of nucleic acid and production of viral protein and production of mature viral particle or virion followed by viremia.

Viremia occurs in the susceptible host and the virus is disseminated to other organs and tissues in the body. The usual mode of spread is hematogenous route. The neural route of dissemination occurs in case of herpes and rabies virus infection. The virus infects the peripheral nerve endings, spread to the spinal cord and then infects other neurons and finally reaches the brain.

Secondary replication occurs in those tissues which intensifies the infection. The viral infection is associated with immune response. IgM antibodies usually appear within 2 weeks of infection. IgG antibodies usually appear within 2–6 weeks. Parallel to the humoral response, there is also development of cell mediated immunity. In certain viral infections the alternate common pathway is also activated. These immune responses are aimed at neutralization of the virus particles. Viral infection is also associated with production of interferon which inhibits virus multiplication.

Although these immune responses are helpful for the body, sometimes it may result in destruction of host's cells as a consequence of the intense reaction.

Pathology

On macroscopic examination, the brain may appear usually edematous but may be sometimes normal. On light microscopy, there is lymphocytic infiltration of the leptomeninges, mononuclear infiltration of brain parenchyma, perivascular cuffing, infarcts, and necrosis and microglial nodule. These changes may be focal or diffuse. Electron microscopy may show virus particle.

Clinical Manifestations

All types of encephalitis have the same clinical presentation irrespective of the causative agent. In majority of cases there is a phase of prodromal or antecedent illness followed by signs and symptoms of encephalitis.

The *antecedent illness* is characterized by features of a systemic viral infection such as fever, headache, vomiting, loose motions, myalgia, decreased appetite, conjunctivitis, rash, and photophobia. After an interval of 3–7 days (maximum 4 weeks) in most cases, the symptoms of cerebral involvement manifest. However, in about 2% cases, there may be no history of such antecedent illness.

The *stage of encephalitis* is usually of acute onset; sometimes insidious. There is high fever, may be hyperpyrexia, with chills, accompanied by symptoms and signs of diffuse or focal cerebral involvement.

The *features of diffuse cerebral involvement* include altered sensorium, convulsions, vomiting, headache, photophobia, abnormal movements, abnormal respiration, behaviour disturbances, and signs of raised intracranial pressure. There may be neck rigidity, altered tone and reflexes and loss of bowel and bladder control.

The most important feature of encephalitis, *altered sensorium* may be in the form of irritability, agitation, confusion, screaming spells, drowsiness, delirium, stupor and/or coma. Seizures are usually generalized. *Abnormal movements* may be present in the form of bizarre movements of the body, ataxia, tremor and decerebrate and dystonic postures. *Respiration* may be irregular and there may be hyperventilation. *Abnormal behaviour* is observed in the form of changes in mood, hallucinations, apathy, aggressiveness, emotional outbursts and staring spells.

The *signs of raised intracranial pressure* include rapid deterioration of consciousness, frequent seizures, bulging fontanelle, decerebration, pupillary abnormalities and papilledema. Neck stiffness is present in those cases with meningeal involvement. The tone and reflexes are variable. Plantar reflex is often extensor.

The *focal cerebral signs* depend on the site of involvement. HSV encephalitis is usually associated with focal neurological signs and features of *temporal lobe involvement* like visual and auditory hallucinations, abnormal behaviour and aphasia. *Brainstem involvement* causes bulbar and pseudo bulbar palsies. *Cerebellar involvement* which is usually seen with coxsakie virus infection is primarily manifested by ataxia, nystagmus and incoordination. *Hypothalamic involvement* is manifested by disturbances of abnormal temperature control and fluid and electrolyte disturbances.

Certain features can give a clue to the etiological diagnosis of encephalitis. These include exposure to ticks, mosquitoes and insects (arbovirus), preceding history of rash (measles, rubella, and varicella), presence of keratoconjunctivitis (adenovirus), history of parotitis and orchitis (mumps), presence of mucocutaneous lesions and aphasia (HSV) and history of dog bite (rabies).

Subsequent Course

The clinical course of encephalitis varies widely. Some cases present with mild symptoms, rapidly progresses to coma and death. Others present with marked sensorial changes and decerebration but recover within a short time with minimal sequelae while some patients continue to remain in coma for prolonged period and ultimately show remarkable recovery or develop sequalae.

Laboratory Diagnosis

Laboratory investigations are necessary to confirm the diagnosis of encephalitis as well as an etiological diagnosis. These include CSF analysis, virologic study, EEG, and neuroimaging.

CSF Analysis

A properly done CSF analysis is probably the most simple and useful laboratory investigation available in clinical setup. It should be done in every case of suspected encephalitis unless contraindicated by presence of raised ICP. It helps in confirmation of viral encephalitis as well as exclusion of bacterial meningitis.

The usual findings include a clear fluid, a normal glucose level, mildly elevated protein level and lymphocytic pleocytosis. In HSV encephalitis CSF may be hemorrhagic. The glucose level may be low in HSV and mumps encephalitis. The cell count, in majority of cases, is above 5 cells/micro litre and rarely exceeds 500 cells/micro litre. A count > 1000 cells/micro litre should raise the suspicion of a bacterial infection. Early in the course of illness there may be polymorphonuclear leucocytosis. In such a situation a repeat CSF after 24 – 48 hours will show a reversal of cellular response to a predominantly lymphocytic type.

CSF PCR shows a high sensitivity and specificity with HSV encephalitis. However, it should be noted that a negative HSV CSF PCR test in a patient with high likelihood of HSV encephalitis based on clinical and other laboratory investigations significantly reduces the likelihood of HSV encephalitis but does not exclude it. The positivity of CSF PCR is more if done after 72 hours and the positivity is decreased significantly after 7 days of antiviral therapy.

The sensitivity and specificity of CSF PCR tests for other viruses have not been definitely characterized.

Gram stain and culture is negative in cases of encephalitis.

Virologic Studies

The basic approach to serodiagnosis is to detect virus specific antibody (IgM and IgG) and antigen in different specimens like CSF, scrapings of mucocutaneous lesions, brain tissue, respiratory secretions, urine, feces, oral secretions, and whole blood. Recent infection is supported by detection of virus specific IgM antibodies or four-fold rise in IgG antibody titre. However, IgM antibodies appear within 2 weeks of onset of infection and IgG appear even later limiting the utility of early diagnosis. In HSV encephalitis, antibody detection may be helpful in cases which present after 1 week and in cases where CSF PCR is negative.

Neuroimaging (CT, MRI) and EEG

These tests help identify or exclude alternative diagnosis and assist differentiation of focal and diffuse encephalitic process. Focal findings in a case of encephalitis should always raise the possibility of HSV encephalitis. The focal findings include (1) areas of increased signal intensity in frontoparietal, cingulated or insular regions of the brain on MRI, (2) temporoparietal areas of slow absorption, mass effect and contrast enhancement on CT, and (3) periodic focal temporal lobe spikes on a background of slow or low amplitude activity on EEG. Some patients have a distinctive EEG pattern consisting of periodic, stereotyped, sharp-and-slow wave complexes originating from one or both temporal lobes and repeating at regular intervals of 2 to 3s. These periodic complexes are typically noted between the 2nd and 15th day of illness and are present in around two third of cases.

MRI is more sensitive than CT. 90% of CSF PCR positive cases will show abnormalities in the temporal lobe in comparison to only 30% in CT. EEG abnormalities occur in > 90% of PCR documented cases of HSV encephalitis.

The positivity of these tests is significantly less in other forms of encephalitis.

Brain Biopsy

Once considered the gold standard for diagnosis is now reserved for patients in whom CSF PCR studies fail to lead to a specific diagnosis, who have focal abnormalities in MRI and who continue to show progressive deterioration despite treatment with acyclovir and adequate supportive treatment.

Differential Diagnosis

The common differential diagnosis include meningitis (bacterial, tubercular and fungal), cerebral malaria, intracranial space occupying lesion, intracranial hemorrhage, Reye's syndrome, head injury. These conditions have specific features and can be differentiated by proper history, examination and laboratory investigations.

Treatment

Treatment of encephalitis is essentially symptomatic except in cases with HSV infection. Symptomatic treatment is targeted at supporting vital functions and treatment of complications. Vital functions should be monitored and supported when necessary. In the initial stages, many patients will require care in the ICU.

Treatment of Complications

Monitoring, clinical and biochemical parameters helps in early recognition and prompt treatment of complications. A base line clinical examination and biochemical tests should be done on admission. The *clinical parameters* for monitoring daily should include vitals, sensorium, presence of focal deficit, and fluid intake and urine output. The *biochemical parameters* like serum electrolytes, blood sugar, serum calcium and ABG should be done on admission. The electrolytes should be repeated daily when the patient is on intravenous fluid. ABG repeated daily or more frequently if situation demands. Serum calcium and blood sugar need to be repeated in presence of seizures.

The complications that need emergency treatment include cerebral edema, seizures, hyperpyrexia, SIADH, airway obstruction, and cardiorespiratory arrest.

Cerebral Edema

Development of cerebral edema and resulting increased intracranial pressure is the condition which needs urgent treatment. Monitoring of intracranial pressure is the best way to improve the outcome of treatment of raised ICP. The cerebral perfusion pressure should be maintained above 50 mm of Hg and the ICP at or below 15 mm of Hg.

The therapeutic measures commonly used to treat cerebral edema are as follows:

1. Raising the head end approximately to 30° or above the level of the heart.
2. Restriction of IV fluid to 2/3 of maintenance.
3. Intravenous infusion of mannitol (0.5–2 gms/kg over 20–30 minutes), can be repeated 3–4 times/day if necessary. It is most commonly used measure. However, the action of mannitol wanes after 72 hours because of rebound phenomena. Hence should not be used beyond 72 hours.
4. Administration of frusemide (1 mg/kg/dose IV). It can be given alone or in combination with mannitol which is shown to be more effective.
5. Hyperventilation is a quick and effective method for bringing down the ICP. It can be done manually with

bag and mask or endotracheal tube or using a ventillator, to maintain the $PaCO_2$ between 25–30 mm Hg.

6. If cerebral edema persists, reduction may be tried with administration of glycerol (0.5–1 ml/kg/dose 8 hourly).
7. In very severely ill cases, the methods used are removal of CSF through a ventricular catheter, barbiturate coma, use of hyperbaric oxygen and hypothermia.

Close monitoring of fluid and electrolyte levels, acid base status is essential during treatment of cerebral edema because measures to reduce ICP may lead to complications like dehydration, hyponatremia, hypokalemia with mannitol and frusemide. Hyperventilation, vigorously done can cause cardiac depression.

Seizures

Seizures should be treated promptly because it can cause structural neuronal damage. The cause of seizure may be multifactorial like toxic encephalitis, hypoxemia, vasculitis, electrolyte disturbance and hypocalcaemia.

An occasional seizure can be treated with intravenous diazepam (0.3 mg/kg/dose). Recurrent seizures should be treated with phenytoin (loading dose 15 mg/kg/dose) followed by maintenance dose of 5–6 mg/kg/day. If there is an accompanying biochemical anomaly, it should be treated simultaneously.

Hyperpyrexia

Presence of hyperpyrexia increases metabolic demand of the brain and chances of seizures. It should be treated with antipyretics, tepid sponging and ice bath.

Syndrome of Inappropriate ADH (SIADH)

SIADH lead to fluid retention and aggravation of cerebral edema. It is characterized by hyponatremia, weight gain and increase in urine osmolality. The treatment is restriction of fluid.

Airway Obstruction

Airway obstruction can result from accumulation of secretions, and/or vomitus in the throat especially in the patients in coma. This in turn can result in episodes of hypoxia, respiratory arrest and aspiration pneumonia. The patient in coma needs frequent suction of throat to prevent such complications.

Cardiorespiratory Arrest

Cardiorespiratory arrest can occur. Therefore, it is important to remain alert for the need of intubation and resuscitation. The patients with respiratory failure will need ventilatory support.

Specific Therapy

Acyclovir is of benefit in treatment of herpes simplex viral infection. It should be started empirically in patients with suspected viral encephalitis while awaiting viral diagnostic studies. Treatment should be discontinued in patients found not to have HSV encephalitis. Acyclovir (30 mg/kg/day) is given by I.V. infusion over a period of 1 hour in 3 equally divided doses for duration of 10 days.

Acyclovir is a purine analogue that inhibits virus replication by inhibiting viral DNA polymerase. The drug is safe and outcome is better if administered early. Patients with clinical features of HSV encephalitis (viz. focal neurological signs, hemorrhagic CSF, EEG and neuroimaging findings) should be treated with acyclovir even in absence of a serological diagnosis or virus isolation.

Vidarabine, a non-specific inhibitor of viral replication can be used if acyclovir therapy fails. It can be given by continuous infusion over 12 hours in the dose of 30 mg/kg/day for 10–14 days.

Spinal Paraplegia

The term paraplegia denotes partial or complete weakness of both legs, and the term quadriplegia denotes partial or complete weakness of all limbs. The same spinal abnormality can cause paraplegia or quadriplegia depending on the location of the injury. Cerebral abnormalities sometimes cause paraplegia. In such a case, all the limbs are weak. However, the leg weakness is so much greater than arm weakness, that paraplegia is the chief complain.

Weakness of both lower limbs without any involvement of the upper limbs, suggest an abnormality of either spinal cord or peripheral nerves. *Involvement of peripheral nerves* is characterized by a pattern of distal weakness and sensory loss, muscle atrophy and absent tendon reflexes. In contrast, *spinal paraplegia* causes spasticity, exaggerated tendon reflexes and a dermatomal level of sensory loss. Spinal cord paraplegia may be asymmetrical at first, and then the initial feature is monoplegia.

Paraplegia may result from a lesion in the spinal cord and may present as paraplegia in flexon or paraplegia in extension. The common causes in children are spinal cord compression and myelitis. It may also be caused by lesion in the anterior horn cells (e.g. poliomyelitis) or the peripheral nerves (e.g. Guillain-Barré Syndrome).

Table 13.9 : Causes of spinal paraplegia
Congenital malformations
Arachnoid cyst
Arteriovenous fistula
Atlantoaxial dislocation
Arnold-Chiari malformation
Meningomyelocele
Familial spastic paraplegia
Autosomal dominant, autosomal recessive and X-linked recessive
Infections
Guillain-Barré Syndrome
Poliomyelitis
Epidural abscess
Diskitis
Herpes zoster myelitis
Lupus myelopathy
Tuberculous osteomyelitis of spine
Metabolic disorders
Krabbe disease
Argininemia
Adrenoleucodystrophy
Transverse myelitis
Devic disease
Encéphalomyélites
Idiopathic
Traumatic
Concussion
Epidural hematoma
Fracture dislocation of spine
Tumors
Astrocytoma
Ependymoma
Ewing's sarcoma
Neuroblastoma

Clinical Manifestations

The common complaints of spinal paraplegia are clumsiness of gait, refusal to stand or walk, and loss of bladder or bowel control. Clumsiness of gait is the usual feature of slowly progressive disorders. Refusal to stand or walk is the symptom of an acute process.

During the stage of spinal shock which follows a rapidly developing severe lesion of the spinal cord, the normal reflex activity of the bladder and rectum is abolished resulting in retension of urine and feces. When reflex activity of the divided spinal cord is well established, in traumatic cases about 3 weeks after transaction, reflex evacuation of the bladder and rectum and reflex sweating occurs. Reflex emptying of the bladder can be facilitated by deep breathing and pressure over the hypogastrium. Reflex emptying of the rectum occurs in response to a volume of about 200 ml.

Scoliosis is a feature of many spinal cord disorders. It occurs with neural tube defects, spinal cord tumors and several degenerative disorders. It also occurs when the paraspinal muscles are weaker on one side of the spine than on the other side. The presence of scoliosis, in females before puberty, and in males of all age groups, should strongly suggest either a spinal cord disorder or a neuromuscular disease.

The first basis of differential diagnosis of paraplegia is on the basis of time taken for the paraplegia to develop. Paraplegia may be of acute, subacute or insidious onset depending on the time taken to develop.

Table 13.10 : Features and common causes of spinal paraplegia on the basis of onset

Features	*Acute onset*	*Sub acute onset*	*Insidious onset*
Onset	Sudden and progressive	Over 2 – 3 days	Over a period of month or more
Causes	Trauma	Acute myelitis	Spinal cord compression
	Hematomyelia Angioma	Tubercular spinal osteitis	Hereditary degenerative disorders
	Thrombosis of anterior spinal artery	Pyogenic extradural abscess	Hereditarty spastic paraplegia
	Secondary deposits in the spine		

Symptoms of a Focal Lesion at a Particular Level

Radicular Symptoms

A lesion of one of the *posterior spinal roots* cause pain referred to the corresponding dermatome, i.e., the area of the skin innervated by that root and also to the muscles which receive the sensory supply from it. Such root pains are likely to be made worse by coughing and sneezing, which raise the pressure within the spinal canal, and by movements of the neighbouring part of the spine. The dermatome is likely to be hyperalgesic and hyperaesthetic until the lesion interferes with the conduction in the root, when appreciation of light touch and pain are impaired over the dermatome.

A lesion of the *anterior spinal root* causes the symptoms of a lower motor neuron lesion in the muscles innervated by the corresponding spinal segment.

Sensory Impairment

A lesion of the *posterior columns* of the spinal cord leads to impairment of the appreciation of posture, passive movements of the joints, and vibration below the level of the lesion on the same side. A lesion involving the *spinothalamic tracts* causes impairment of appreciation of pain and temperature on the opposite side of the body.

Since the pathways conducting these forms of sensation take several segments to cross the spinal cord, the upper level of the area of sensory loss will be a corresponding number of dermatomes below segmental level of the lesion. This discrepancy will amount to two or three dermatomes below the segmental level of the lesion in the thoracic and lumbar regions and one in the cervical region.

Corticospinal Tract Lesion

Damage to the corticospinal tract will cause the symptoms of upper motor neuron lesion (weakness, spasticity, increased tendon reflexes, diminished abdominal reflex and an extensor plantar reflex) below the level of the lesion on the same side.

Anterior Horn Cell Lesion

Involvement of the anterior horn cells result in symptoms of lower motor neuron lesion, i.e., weakness, flaccidity, decreased or absent tendon reflexes.

Reflexes

A reflex whose arc passes through the segment involved will be impaired or abolished. Reflexes mediated by segments below the level of the lesion will show changes characteristic of corticospinal tract lesion.

Autonomic Involvement

Sweating will be abolished over the area of the skin which receives its sympathetic innervation from the segment of the spinal cord affected. Below the level there may be excessive sweating. A lesion of the cervical cord may result in excessive sweating over the whole body since the sympathetic outflow from the spinal cord is limited to the thoracic and first lumbar segments. Lesion below the first lumbar segment will not affect sweating.

A unilateral lesion involving one half of the spinal cord produces the *Brown-Sequard syndrome* which consists of ipsilateral weakness, spasticity and ataxia with contralateral loss of pain, temperature sensation.

Symptoms of Compression of Spinal Cord

The onset of symptoms is gradual when the cause is a spinal tumor, but is often rapid in case of secondary deposits of the spine. In tubercular disease of the spine onset is gradual but paraplegia may develop acutely.

The initial symptoms are sensory, the most common being pain radiating into the distribution of one or more spinal roots. Root pain is usually severe in vertebral collapse from all causes. It is also present in extramedullary spinal tumors. It is followed by a slowly progressive impairment of motor function. The functions of the corticospinal tract are impaired first.

When the thoracic cord is compressed, the clinical picture is that of a spastic paraplegia. In absence of sensory loss, the level of the lesion can be established by MRI. In case of cervical cord compression, the level of lesion can be determined by the sensory loss.

Laboratory Diagnosis

Examination of the CSF is of diagnostic value in spinal cord compression due to spinal tumors, infective causes like Guillain-Barré syndrome, myelitis, and trauma showing typical findings in each case.

In case of disease of the vertebral column, an X-ray examination of the spine may enable to discover the cause of compression.

Magnetic resonance imaging (MRI) is the procedure of choice for visualization of the spinal cord. **CT and radioisotope bone scanning** are useful for visualizing the vertebral column.

When anatomical localization between the spinal cord and peripheral nerves is difficult, *electromyogram* and *nerve conduction* studies are useful in making the distinction.

Acute Flaccid Paralysis (AFP)

Acute flaccid paralysis (AFP) is defined as paralysis of acute onset i.e. less than 4 weeks and that the affected limbs or limb is flaccid, i.e., floppy or limp. The deep tendon reflexes (DTR) are diminished or absent, sensation is not affected.

A *case of acute flaccid paralysis* is defined as any child below 15 years who has acute flaccid paralysis for which no obvious cause (e.g., severe trauma or electrolyte imbalance) is found or paralytic illness in any person of any age in whom polio is suspected.

Causes of AFP

1. Paralytic poliomyelitis.
2. Guillain-Barré syndrome.
3. Transverse myelitis in shock stage.
4. Traumatic neuritis.
5. Non-polio enteroviral infection:
   (a) Coxsakie A and B.
   (b) ECHO.
   (c) Enterovirus types 70 and 71.
   (d) Mumps.
6. Hypokalemia.
7. Peripheral neuropathies:
   (a) Drugs, e.g. INH, Vincristine.
   (b) Diabetes.
   (c) Toxins (lipids solvents, fish toxins).
   (d) Organophosphates pesticides.
   (e) Heavy metals (lead, mercury).
   (f) Post diphtheric paralysis.
   (g) Acute intermittent porphyria.
   (h) Acute motor axonal neuropathy (Chinese paralytic syndrome).

Pseudoparalysis

Pseudoparalysis is a condition where the presenting feature is inability to move a part of the body which is not due to paralysis. These conditions are not AFP. They may come in differential diagnosis of AFP. The causes of pseudoparalysis are as follows:

1. Unrecognized trauma from contusion, sprains, fractures.
2. Non-specific toxic synovitis.
3. Acute osteomyelitis.
4. Scurvy.
5. Acute pyogenic arthritis.
6. Acute rheumatic arthritis.
7. Congenital syphilitic osteomyelitis.

Common Differential Diagnosis

Paralytic Poliomyelitis

The median age group affected is 18 months (3 m–5 years). It is common during the hot and humid season.

(July to September). It is characterized by acute onset asymmetrical lower motor neuron paralysis. The muscle strength varies in different groups of muscles in different limbs. The maximum involvement occurs in first 4 days but may continue 4–7 days. Paralysis starts proximally at the trunk (at the shoulders or hip and progress downwards). Presence of fever just prior to paralysis– is a hallmark finding. There is muscle pain, absent or depressed DTR. There is no sensory loss.

Bulbar or bulbospinal forms will be associated with facial asymmetry, difficulty in swallowing, weakness or loss of voice, respiratory insufficiency and circulatory collapse.

Laboratory Diagnosis

Analysis of CSF: Pressure normal or increased, transparent or slightly turbid, protein 40-65 mg %, cells 20-300/cumm. Polymorpholeucocytosis initially, lymphocytosis later.

Guillain-Barré Syndrome (GBS)

It is an acute form of acquired peripheral neuropathy of autoimmune etiopathogenesis with demyelination as the prominent pathological process.

Frequently there is a preceding history of a respiratory tract infection, GI syndrome, surgery or immunization, 1-4 weeks (average 2 weeks) before the onset of symptoms. The identified agents in causation GBS include EB virus, cytomegalo virus, herpes virus, mycoplasma, campylobacter jejuni.

There is symmetrical weakness evolving rapidly over a period of days or weeks (< 4 weeks) then plateauing. The weakness starts in the distal part of lower limb and then ascends upwards. The weakness is more severe in the proximal muscles. Initially there is hyporeflexia then areflexia. There may be transient involvement of bladder and bowel. There is involvement of the cranial nerves, autonomic disturbances with sinus tachycardia, fluctuating BP, facial flushing etc. There is initial absence of fever. Complete recovery in majority of cases. Recovery starts at about 2-4 weeks after halt of progression.

Laboratory Diagnosis

CSF analysis after 1 week shows CSF protein upto 200 mg, WBC < 50 cells/cumm, PMN not > 2/cumm. There is albumino cytological dissociation. Nerve conduction velocity normal (after 3 weeks).

Sometimes it is clinically difficult to differentiate paralytic polio and GBS. Then it is recommended that CSF analysis be done at hospitalization and repeated a week later if it is equivocal. Nerve conduction velocity (NCV) after 3 weeks of onset of paralysis is the best way to differentiate between the two conditions. NCV is normal in GBS whereas it is abnormal in paralytic poliomyelitis.

Transverse Myelitis

Transverse myelitis is an immune mediated disease due to viral insult. The common age group affected is 4 years and above. Fever may be present before the onset of AFP but rarely during onset. The child complains of backache followed by symmetrical paralysis of the lower limbs with depressed or absent DTR. There is early onset of bladder and bowel dysfunction and profound anesthesia to all kind of sensation. Flaccidity usually changes to spasticity after several weeks and areflexia replaced by hyper reflexia.

Laboratory Diagnosis

CSF WBC normal, protein raised or normal. MRI shows swelling and hyperintensity of cord onT2 weighted images.

Traumatic Neuritis

There is history of injury to sciatic nerve by injection in gluteal region. The onset of weakness occurs 1 hr to 5 days after injection. It is associated with pain in the region of trauma or along the affected limb. Muscle tone is decreased or absent. Muscle power at hip and knee is normal. Child walks with foot drop. Knee jerk is present, Ankle jerk is absent. Atrophy of muscles may appear 40 to 60 days later (difference between calf circumferences does not exceed 0.5–1.5 cm). CSF analysis normal.

Non Polio Enterovirus

Non polio enterovirus infection is characterized by asymmetric lower motor neuron paralysis due to involvement of anterior horn cells. Most cases show a course of improvement with complete recovery. In some cases sequelae may mimic paralysis caused by wild polio.

Post Diphtheric Paralysis

Post diphtheric paralysis affects mainly unimmunized children. The clinical triad includes palatal palsy, loss of accommodation and polyneuritis. Palatal palsy presents in 2nd week with nasal twang, dysphagia and regurgitation of food. Ocular palsy manifest during 3rd week of illness. Involves muscles of accommodation, ciliary muscles and lateral rectus. General polyneuritis occurs after 3-6 weeks. There is bilateral symmetrical weakness of muscles of all extremities. Recovery is complete.

Heavy Metal Poisoning

Lead poisoning in childhood is associated with encephalopathy. Neuropathy occur in older children and adults. Wrist drop is present, associated with anorexia, hyperirritability, vomiting, constipation and abdominal pain. Lead line in gums.

Laboratory findings include basophilic stippling in the peripheral blood smear.

Arsenic and mercury poisoning are also associated with peripheral neuropathy.

Management

1. *Report* all cases of AFP to the DIO or Surveillance officer immediately.
2. *Collection of samples:* Two adequate samples (8 gms or the size of a thumb) of stool at the interval of 24–48 hours should be collected within 14 days of onset of paralysis. In cases seen late i.e. > 2 weeks stool specimen may be collected upto 60 days. Storage and transport of specimen should be at < 8°C.
3. *Monitoring of the child:* The parameters include pulse, BP, respiratory rate, and level of consciousness, extent of paralysis, bladder and bowel movement, autonomic instability.
4. *Care of bladder and bowel:* The bladder should be catheterized in case of urinary retention.

   Hot and cold compress or cholinergic drugs may be used in case polio is suspected. Constipation can be managed by giving mild laxatives or enema.

5. *Care of skin:* Skin should be kept clean. Frequent change of position of the child every 2–3 hours should be advised to prevent bedsores.
6. *Positioning of the affected limbs:* Child should lie on a firm bed to prevent sagging of the spine. The limbs should be placed in optimum position for relaxation of the paralyzed muscles. In case of lower limbs, hip should be kept in slight flexon, knee 5–10° flexon, and foot at 90°. Both legs should be supported from the lateral side with pillows to prevent external rotation of limbs. Rolled towels should be placed below the knee for positioning the hip and knee.

   The position of upper limbs is abduction of shoulder, moderate flexon at elbow with hand in functional position, i.e., extension of wrist, semiflexed fingers with thumb in opposition.
7. *Relief of pain and spasm:* Warm moist pack can be given by soft towel or flannel 3–4 times /day. Analgesics may be needed.
8. *Bed rest:* Complete bed rest to ensure that there is no stress on the affected muscles.
9. Massage and intramuscular injections are contraindicated during this period.
10. *Physiotherapy: Passive movement* of all joints of affected limbs should be given to prevent joint stiffness. Initially such movements should be within the limits of pain and should be done for 10 min 2 – 3 times a day.

    Active movements are started when the acute phase subsides and recovery of strength begins.
11. *Feeding*: Ensure proper nutrition and hydration. In bulbar and bulbospinal poliomyelitis nasogastric feeding may be required.
12. *Monitoring for respiratory paralysis in cases of polio and GBS*: Features to be monitored include brow sweating, anxiety, tachycardia, tachypnoea, inspiration in the middle of brief spoken sentences, low vital capacity (< 12–15 ml/kg), hypoxemia (Pa O_2 < 70 mm of Hg).

Indications for ICU Admission

1. Paralysis of intercostals muscles or diaphragm.
2. Involvement of vital centers in medulla.
3. Children with pharyngeal and laryngeal muscles paralysis.
4. Encephalitic type of poliomyelitis.

Specific Treatment

Specific treatment differs according to cause:

In cases with *paralytic poliomyelitis*, a careful assessment and recording of muscle power should to be done for use as a base line. Physiotherapy should continue to prevent deformities and contractures due to muscle imbalance or improper posture. Surgical intervention for various forms of deformities should be planned after 2 years of onset of paralysis. Guidance of pediatric physiotherapist, occupational therapist, social worker and vocational counselor is necessary in promoting a positive approach and adjustment.

For *transverse myelitis,* skin care is important while giving splints etc. Good skin care and posture should be maintained to prevent bed sores. Pulse IV methylprednisolone may be tried.

For *traumatic neuritis* physiotherapy is the mainstay. It may have to be continued for 3–9 months.

All cases of *Guillain-Barré syndrome* should be admitted to hospital for observation of progression of ascending paralysis because there may be involvement of respiratory muscles in the first 24 hours.

Patients with slow progression may be simply kept under observation for stabilization and spontaneous remission. In rapidly progressive cases who at presentation cannot walk independently or who have respiratory and / or bulbar involvement should be treated with IV IG (400 mg/kg/day IV infusion over 2 hours daily × 5 days or 2 gm/kg IV over 10–12 hours as a single dose). If the child improves but there is a relapse IV IG can be repeated. If there is no response, plasmapheresis can be tried. Combined administration of IV IG and interferon is effective in some patients. Supportive care viz. care of skin, bowel and bladder, respiratory support and antibiotics for secondary bacterial infection is important.

Recovery

Acute paralytic poliomyelitis: Maximal recovery occurs in the first 6 months with slow recovery upto 2 years. Degree of recovery ranges from minimal to complete.

Guillain-Barré syndrome: Complete recovery in majority of cases. Takes 3–6 months.

Transverse myelitis: With rapid onset, recovery begins several weeks to months later. Neurologic deficits remain. With slow onset taking several days for paralysis to develop, recovery begins in 1–3 days of symptom peak and recovery may be complete. May develop flaccid diplegia, atrophy after years.

Traumatic neuritis: Atrophy may appear 40–60 days later; but never reaches the level of polio. Children gradually recover with physiotherapy in 3–9 months.

Bell Palsy

Bell palsy is an acute unilateral facial nerve palsy that is not associated with other cranial neuropathies or brain stem dysfunction. It is a common disorder occurring at all ages from infancy through adolescence.

Etiology

The disease is believed to be a post infectious allergic or immune demyelinating facial neuritis than an active viral invasion of the nerve or its motor neurons of origin. It usually develops abruptly about two weeks after a systemic viral infection. The preceding infection is due to Epstein-Barr virus in about 20% cases. Lyme disease, herpes simplex virus, and mumps virus are identified in some other cases.

Clinical Manifestations

There is unilateral lower motor neuron paralysis of the face characterized by dropping of the angle of the mouth, inability to close the eyes, inability to frown the forehead and inability to blow the cheeks on the affected side.

Patients may develop an exposure keratitis on the side of the lesion as the eye remains open. Taste on the anterior two thirds of the tongue is lost on the involved side in about 50% cases.

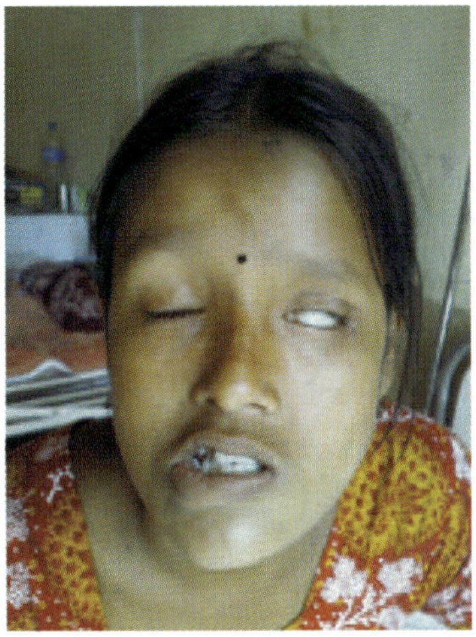

Fig. 13.12: Facial palsy (left side) lower motor neuron type

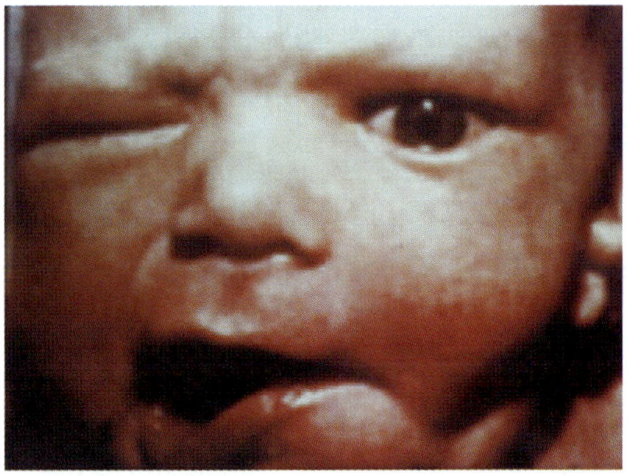

Fig. 13.13: Facial palsy (left side) in a newborn

Treatment

Protection of the eyes with an ocular lubricant, especially at night, is the only important supportive measure. Steroid therapy or surgical decompression of the facial canal is not of value and hence not recommended.

Prognosis

Prognosis is excellent. Spontaneous recovery occur in more than 85% cases without any residual facial weakness. Another 10% have mild facial weakness and only 5% are left with permanent severe facial weakness. If there is no sign of recovery within a few weeks, electrophysiologic examination of the facial nerve can help to determine the degree of neuropathy and regeneration. In chronic cases another cause of neuropathy should be considered. These include facial nerve tumours (neurofibroma, schwannoma), infiltration of facial nerve by leukemic cells, rhabdomyosarcoma of the middle ear, brainstem infarcts or tumours and traumatic injury.

Facial Palsy at Birth

Facial palsy in the newborn is usually caused by compression neuropathy from forceps application from which recovery is spontaneous in a few days or weeks in most cases. Facial palsy in the newborn needs differentiation from *congenital absence the depressor anguli oris muscle* which is characterized by facial asymmetry when an affected infant cries. It is a cosmetic defect and does not interfere with feeding. *Mobius syndrome* may present with bilateral or less commonly with unilateral facial palsy. It is a result of symmetric calcified infarcts in the tegmentum of the pons and medulla oblongata during the mid gestation or late fetal life. It may rarely be due to a developmental anomaly of the brainstem.

Muscular Dystrophies

Muscular dystrophies are a group of unrelated diseases, each transmitted by a different genetic trait and each differing in its clinical course and expression. A muscular dystrophy is characterized by the four obligatory criteria. They are: (1) It is a primary myopathy; (2) It has a genetic basis; (3) The course is progressive; (4) Degeneration and death of muscle fibres occur at some stage in the disease.

The muscular dystrophies include the following conditions: Duchenne and Becker muscular dystrophies, scapulohumeral muscular dystrophy, myotonic muscular dystrophy, limb girdle muscular dystrophy, facio-scapulohumeral muscular dystrophy and congenital muscular dystrophy. The most common condition, Duchenne and Baker muscular dystrophy is described in details.

DUCHENNE AND BECKER MUSCULAR DYSTROPHY

The most common hereditary muscular dystrophy is Duchenne muscular dystrophy. This disease is inherited as an X-linked recessive trait. The abnormal gene is on the X chromosome at the Xp21 locus. Becker muscular dystrophy is the same fundamental disease as the former, with a genetic defect at the same locus, but clinically with a milder and more protracted course.

Clinical Manifestations

On the basis of the inheritance, the boys manifest the disease and girls carry. The onset of the disease is rarely before early infancy although some may be already hypotonic. The gross motor development may be normal upto one year or mildly delayed. However, poor head control may be the first sign of weakness. Walking is achieved normally at one year of age but toddlers may assume a lordotic posture when standing to compensate the weakness of the glutei muscles. The Gower's sign is often evident by 3 years age and is fully expressed by the age of 5 – 6 years. The child has a waddling gait at the same time.

Gower's sign: Weakness in the hip girdle and proximal muscles of the lower limbs cause the child to use the hands to climb up the legs in order to assume an upright position, a maneuver called Gower's sign. The progression of muscle weakness continues into the second decade. The function of the distal muscles is relatively preserved well enough allowing the child to continue to use a pencil, computer key board and feeding utensils.

Respiratory muscle weakness is manifested by weak and ineffective cough, frequent pulmonary infections and decreasing respiratory reserve. Pharyngeal muscle weakness leads to episodes of aspiration, nasal regurgitation of liquids and nasal intonation. The function of the extra ocular muscles remains well preserved.

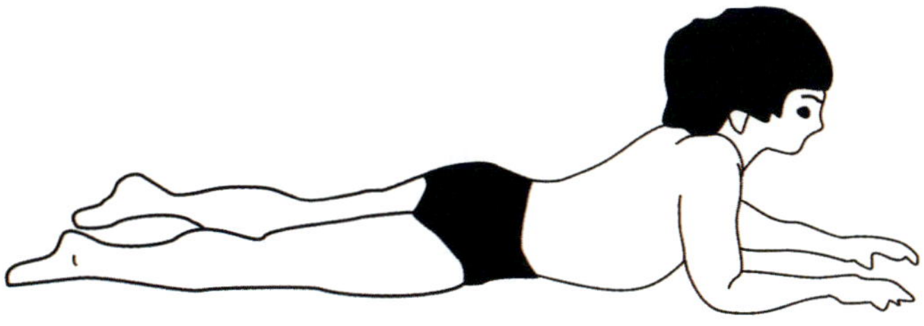

Sequence 1

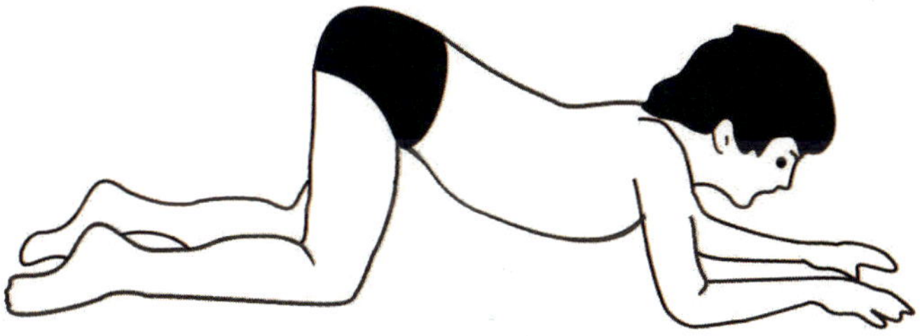

Sequence 2

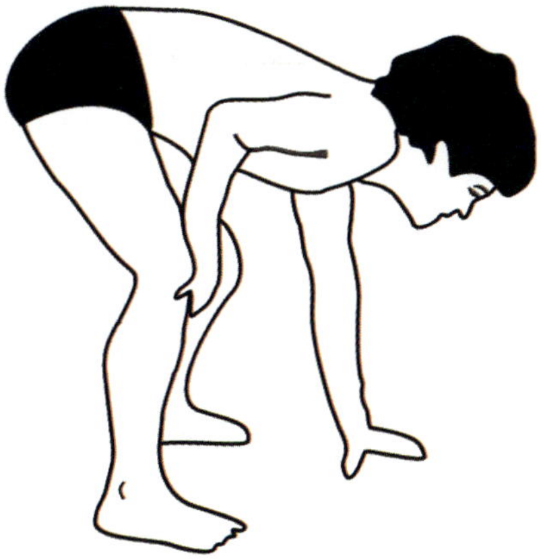

Sequence 3

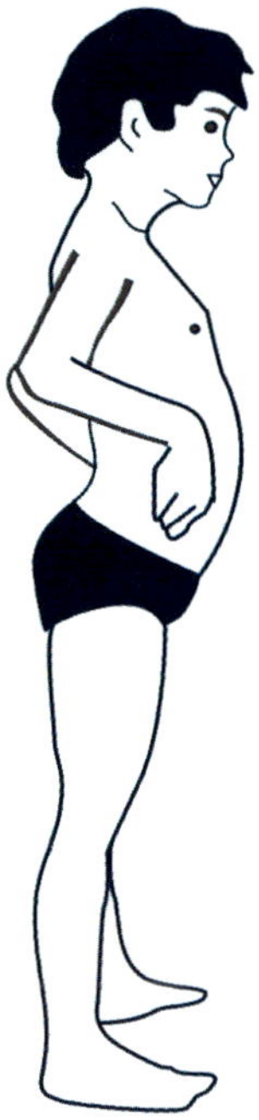

Sequence 4

Fig. 13.14: Showing the sequence of Gower's sign

Facial muscle weakness with a distinctive facies is a late event. Bowel and bladder incontinence is an uncommon and late event. Enlargement of calf muscles and wasting of the thigh muscles is a classic feature. The enlargement is caused by hypertrophy of some muscle fibres, infiltration of muscle by fat and proliferation of collagen. Muscular hypertrophy may also occur in the tongue and forearm. Cardiomyopathy is a constant feature of this disease. Some patients die early due to severe cardiomyopathy.

Scoliosis is common. The thoracic deformity compromises the pulmonary capacity and compresses the heart. Contractures most often involve the ankles, knees, hips and elbows.

In the lower limbs, the knee jerks are well preserved until about 6 years of age but are less brisk than the ankle jerk which remains normal till the terminal stage provided there are no severe contractures. In the upper extremities, the brachioradialis jerk is stronger than the biceps and triceps jerks.

Intellectual impairment occurs in all patients, although only 20–30% has an IQ less than 70. Majority has learning disabilities but still allow the child to function in a regular class room if remedial help is available. A few patients are severely mentally retarded. The incidence of epilepsy is slightly more in comparison to general pediatric population.

In the Becker muscular dystrophy, onset of weakness is much later and the patient remains ambulatory upto late adolescent or early adult life. Learning disabilities are less frequent. Other features are similar to Duchenne muscular dystrophy.

Laboratory Investigations

1. *Serum enzyme estimation:* The serum creatinine phosphokinase (CPK) level is consistently very high even in presymptomatic stages including at birth. The normal serum level is less than 160 IU/L. The usual serum level is 15,000 to 35,000 IU/L. In terminal stages, however the CPK value considerably lowers because there is less muscle to degenerate. The other lysosomal enzymes viz. serum aldolase and aspartate aminotransferase are also increased but are less specific.
2. X-ray PA view chest, ECG and Echocardiography should be done for cardiac assessment. It should be repeated periodically and once the diagnosis of cardiomyopathy is made, the child should be treated under supervision of a pediatric cardiologist.
3. Electromyography shows characteristic features of myopathy but is not specific. Motor and sensory nerve conduction velocities are normal. Both these investigations do not have any place in confirmation in diagnosis.
4. Polymerase chain reaction for the dystrophin gene mutation is the primary test, if the clinical features and the serum CPK level are consistent with the clinical diagnosis. If the blood PCR is diagnostic, muscle biopsy is deferred. If PCR is normal, dystrophin immunohistochemistry is performed on muscle biopsy sections.
5. Muscle biopsy is diagnostic and shows characteristic findings. The histological features include endomyseal connective tissue proliferation, scattered degenerating and regenerating myofibers, foci of mononuclear inflammatory cell infiltrates.

   Muscle biopsy is usually not necessary for diagnosis if there is a family history, with an affected brother whose diagnosis is confirmed. However, the first case in the family even if the presentation is typical needs confirmation with a biopsy study. The most common muscles sampled are the vastus lateralis (quadriceps femoris) and the gastrocnemius.
6. *Molecular genetic diagnosis:* It is possible by demonstration of deficient or defective dystrophin by

immunohistochemical staining of the sections of muscle biopsy tissue or by DNA analysis from peripheral blood. Ideally confirmation of the diagnosis by one of these methods should be done in every case.

Treatment

There is no specific treatment either for cure or for arrest of progression. Treatment of complications like cardiac failure and pulmonary infections can improve the child's quality of life. Cardiac failure can be treated with digoxin. Response is good in the early stages. Pulmonary infections should be promptly treated with proper antibiotics.

Physiotherapy delays but does not prevent contractures of joints. It contributes little to muscle strength. Exercise cannot increase muscle strength. Excessive exercise can actually accelerate the process of muscle fibre degeneration.

Preservation of a good nutritional status is important. Adequate supply of calcium is important to minimize osteoporosis in a child confined to a wheel chair. Obesity should be prevented by dietary restriction under supervision.

Pharmacotherapy includes use of glucocorticoids. Glucocorticoids decrease the rate of apoptosis or programmed cell death of myotubes during ontogenesis and can decelerate the myofibre necrosis in muscular dystrophy. Steroid therapy results in increase in strength initially but long term complications of prolonged steroid therapy may result in greater weakness than that which might have occurred in the natural course of the disease. Never the less, some patients treated early with steroids have appeared to have an improved long term prognosis as well as the short term improvement. Steroid treatment has helped to keep patients ambulatory for more years than expected without treatment. Prednisolone 0.75 mg/kg/day should be given for the first ten days of each month to avoid long term complications.

Another potential treatment which is still under investigation is intramuscular injection of antisense oligonucleotide drugs. These drugs induce exon skipping during mRNA splicing to restore the open reading frame in the Duchenne muscular dystrophy gene. Stem cell implantation or activation in muscle is theoretically plausible but has not proved practical.

Prognosis

The length of time the child remains ambulatory varies greatly. Some are confined to wheel chair by 7 years age. Most patients continue to walk with increasing difficulty until the age of 10 years. With orthotic bracing, physiotherapy and sometimes minor surgery (Achilles tendon lengthening), another 2 years ambulation can be added. In Duchenne muscular dystrophy, death occurs by about 18 years of age. The causes of death are respiratory failure in sleep, intractable heart failure, pneumonia or aspiration and bronchial obstruction. In Becker's type death occurs by mid or late twenties. Around 50% children may remain alive but with severe disabilities.

Suggested Reading

1. Mcintyre J, Robertson S, Norris E *et al*. Safety and efficacy of buccal midazolam versus rectal diazepam for emergency treatment of seizures in children: A randomized control trial. Lancet 2005; 366: 205-20.
2. Shorvon S. Status Epilepticus: Its clinical features and treatment in children and adults. Cambridge University Press, 1994.
3. Wolfe TR, Macfarlane TC. Intranasal midazolam therapy for pediatric status epilepticus. Am J Emerg Med 2006; 24: 343-346.
4. Kimberly D Statler, Colin B Van Orman. Status Epilepticus in Rogers' Textbook of Pediatric Intensive Care, 4th edition. Editor in chief David G Nichols, 2008 Lippincott Williams and Wilkins, Philadelphia.
5. Towne AR, Delorenzo RJ. Use of intramuscular midazolam for status epilepticus. J Emerg Med 1999; 17: 323-328.
6. Brain and Bannister's Clinical Neurology, 7th edition. Oxford Medical Publications, 1992.
7. Nelson Textbook of Pediatrics, 19th edition, 2011. W B Saunders Company.
8. The Development of the Infant and Young Child: Normal and Abnormal By Ronald S. Illingworth, 9th edition, 1987.
9. Nelson Textbook of Pediatrics, 10th edition, 1975. W B Saunders Company.
10. Nelson Textbook of Pediatrics, 17th edition, 2004. W B Saunders Company.
11. Essentials of Pediatric Neurology, 1st edition, 1997. Edited by B. Talukdar, New Age International (P) Limited.
12. Child Development and Developmental Diagnosis by A.K.Banga and Usha Banga, 1st edition, 1991. Jaypee Brothers Medical Publishers (P) Ltd.
13. Harrison's Principles of Internal Medicine, Volume II, 16th edition 2005. McGraw-Hill Medical Publishing Division.
14. Gerald M. Fenichel: Clinical Pediatric Neurology: A Signs and Symptoms Approach, 5th edition, Saunders.
15. Ira Bergman, Michael J. Painter. Disorders of consciousness. Nelson Essentials of Pediatrics, 4th edition, 2002, 776-783.
16. Singhi P and Singhi S. The Comatose Child in Medical Emergency in Children, 3rd edition, 2000. Sagar Publications, New Delhi.
17. Mathews L H and Frankel L R. Stabilization of the Critically Ill Child, Nelson Textbook of Pediatrics, 16th edition, 2000, 251-262.

14

Cardiology

OUTLINES

Evaluation of Congenital Heart Disease

The evaluation of congenital heart diseases involves a systemic approach, the three major steps of which are as follows:

1. Classification of the heart disease into acyanotic or cyanotic depending on the presence or absence of cyanosis which can be determined by physical examination and pulse oximetry.
2. Study of the character of heart sounds, presence of typical murmurs which will further help to narrow down the differential diagnosis.
3. Study of the chest radiograph by which the two groups can be further subdivided according to whether the chest radiograph shows evidence of increased, normal or decreased pulmonary vascular markings. This helps in further narrowing down the differential diagnosis.

An ECG can be used to determine whether right, left or biventricular hypertrophy exists. The final diagnosis is then confirmed by echocardiography or cardiac catheterization or by both.

Acyanotic Congenital Heart Diseases

Acyanotic congenital heart diseases can be classified into two groups on the basis of the physiologic load they produce on the heart: volume overload or pressure overload.

The common conditions that causes volume overload include the left to right shunts, atrioventricular valve regurgitation and cardiomyopathies.

The second group which causes pressure overload may be as a result of ventricular outflow obstruction (e.g. pulmonary and aortic stenosis) or less commonly obstruction to ventricular inflow (e.g. mitral or tricuspid stenosis and cor triatriatum) or narrowing of one of the great vessels (e.g. coarctation of aorta). Only the most common types viz. VSD, ASD, PDA and coarctation of aorta are only described in details.

Cyanotic Congenital Heart Diseases

Cyanotic congenital heart diseases can be subdivided on the basis whether the pulmonary blood flow is decreased (e.g. Tetralogy of Fallot, tricuspid atresia, total anomalous pulmonary venous return with obstruction) or increased (e.g. transposition of great arteries, single ventricle, persistent truncus arteriosus and total anomalous pulmonary venous return without obstruction). The most common type viz. Tetralogy of Fallot is described in details.

Characteristics

The common characteristics of *left to right shunts* are as follows:

1. Absence of cyanosis.
2. History of recurrent pneumonia.
3. Failure to thrive.
4. Presence of precordial bulge, shunt murmurs and diastolic flow murmurs.
5. Tendency for congestive heart failure.
6. Pulmonary plethora and cardiomegaly proportionate to the size of the shunt on a chest X-ray.

The common characteristics of *obstructive lesions* are as follows:

1. Absence of cyanosis or history of frequent chest infections.
2. Normal shape of precordium.
3. Heaving apex beat without cardiomegaly.
4. Presence of an ejection systolic murmur with a thrill. No diastolic murmurs unless associated with a valvular regurgitation.
5. A normal sized heart with normal or decreased pulmonary vasculature on a chest X-ray.
6. Right or left ventricular hypertrophy, depending on the size of lesion in the ECG.

The characteristics of a *cyanotic lesion* are as follows:

1. Presence of cyanosis and clubbing.
2. Polycythemia.

Ventricular Septal Defect

Ventricular septal defect is the most common cardiac anomaly and accounts for a worldwide incidence of 20-25% of all congenital heart disease. The All India Institute of Medical Sciences, New Delhi has recorded an incidence of 27% of all congenital heart diseases.

Anatomical Types

It is a communication between the left and right ventricles as a result of defect in the interventricular septum. 90% of the defects are located in the membranous part and the rest in the muscular part of the septum. The muscular type may be single or multiple. The membranous type may be associated with pulmonary stenosis or aortic insufficiency depending on the site of the defect in relation to the aortic or pulmonary valves.

Pathophysiology

The size of the left to right shunt depends on the size of the defect and the level of pulmonary vascular resistance in relation to systemic vascular resistance. When the communication is small (< 0.5 cm^2), the right ventricular pressure is normal. The higher pressure in the left ventricle drives the shunt from left to right. In large ventricular septal defects (> 1.0 cm^2), the right and left ventricular pressure is equalized. In these defects, the direction of the shunt and its magnitude are determined by the ratio of pulmonary to systemic vascular resistance.

The magnitude of intracardiac shunt is usually described by the pulmonary (Qp) to systemic blood flow (Qs) ratio. If Qp: Qs <1.75:1, the cardiac chambers are not appreciably enlarged and the pulmonary vascular bed is normal. If the Qp: Qs> 2:1, there is volume overload in the left ventricle, left atrium as well as right ventricle and pulmonary arterial hypertension. The main pulmonary artery, left atrium and the left ventricle are enlarged. When the Qp: Qs approaches1: 1, the shunt becomes bidirectional, the patient becomes cyanotic.

At birth, the pulmonary vascular resistance is high. The size of the shunt remains limited. With the decrease in the pulmonary pressure in the first few weeks, the size of the left to right shunt increases, and the symptoms and signs appear.

Hemodynamics

A ventricular septal defect results in shunting of oxygenated blood from the left to right ventricle. During systole, the left ventricle starts contracting before the right ventricle and blood from the left ventricle flows into the aorta and to the right ventricle through the defect. As the right ventricle is also contracting to empty into the pulmonary artery, the left to right shunt streams into the pulmonary artery almost directly. So a large volume of blood passes into the lungs. The increased volume of blood finally reaches the left atrium and then the left ventricle through the mitral valve.

The flow of blood from the left ventricle to the right ventricle start early, in the systole and a high pressure gradient is maintained between the two ventricles throughout the systole. This results in a *pansystolic murmur* which starts early masking the first heart sound and continues throughout systole in almost the same intensity. The pansystolic murmur ends beyond A_2 masking it completely. This is because at the end of systole, the left ventricular pressure becomes less than the aortic pressure and the aortic valve closes to produce the second sound. However, the left ventricular pressure is still higher than the right ventricular pressure and the shunt continues. The large volume of blood entering through the normal pulmonary artery produces an *ejection systolic murmur* and is recognized in the PA view chest X-ray as *pulmonary plethora*. Clinically, the ejection systolic murmur is recognized as a selective transmission of the pansystolic murmur to the upper left sternal border where its ejection character can be recognized as it does not mask the A_2. The large volume of blood passing through the normal mitral valve produces a *mid diastolic murmur* at the apex. During systole, the left ventricle has two outlets viz. to the aorta and the right ventricle; hence empties early. The aortic valve closes early. This results in early A_2. On the other hand, since the ejection into the pulmonary artery is increased, the P_2 is delayed. Therefore in patients with a large left to right shunt, the *second sound is accentuated as well as widely split but varies with respiration.*

Clinical Manifestations

The symptoms and signs of VSD vary according to the size of the defect, degree of pulmonary blood flow and pulmonary arterial pressure.

If the *VSD is very small*, the second sound is normally split and the pulmonary component is of normal intensity. A very small defect produces an early short systolic murmur. The very small VSD is the most common cause of a functional murmur, which disappear as the child grows up because of spontaneous closure.

With a *small VSD* (less than the size of the aortic orifice), the child is asymptomatic. Growth and development is normal. The cardiac lesion is detected during routine physical examination. The characteristic finding is a loud harsh, blowing holosystolic murmur best heard over the lower left sternal border, frequently accompanied by a thrill. The first and second sounds are masked by the murmur in the lower left sternal border. Second sound is normal, no cardiomegaly, no third heart sound, or flow murmur, normal ECG, and chest X-ray.

A *moderate sized defect* (approximately equal to the aortic orifice) is associated with features of a large VSD with or without pulmonary arterial hypertension.

With a *large VSD*, the child is symptomatic from early infancy with feeding difficulties, dyspnea, profuse perspiration, poor growth, recurrent pneumonia and cardiac failure in infancy. Cyanosis is absent but sometimes duskiness may be seen during crying or infections. Persistently present cyanosis and clubbing indicate reversal of shunt (Eisenmenger's syndrome).

Physical examination reveals a prominent and hyperdynamic left precordium, a left parasternal lift, laterally displaced apical impulse and a systolic thrill over the lower left parasternal region. A holosystolic murmur is present which is less harsh than that in a small VSD and more blowing in nature because of the absence of a significant pressure gradient across the defect. The murmur is usually not heard in the newborn period and later it may have an ejection systolic character. The pulmonic second sound is accentuated in presence of pulmonary hypertension. A low pitched, delayed diastolic murmur may be heard at the apex. It is caused by increased blood flow across the mitral valve and indicates a Qp: Qs ratio of 2:1 or greater.

X-ray studies: The size of the heart and the increase in pulmonary vascular markings relate to the magnitude of the left to right shunt.

With small VSD, the cardiac silhouette is normal and pulmonary vasculature is normal.

With moderate VSD, there is left ventricular and occasionally left atrial enlargement. An X-ray shows plethoric lungs.

In large VSD, there is gross cardiomegaly with prominence of ventricles, the left atrium and the pulmonary artery. The lungs are plethoric. There may be signs of pulmonary edema and pleural effusion. In presence of pulmonary obstructive vascular disease, the main pulmonary artery and hilar pulmonary arteries enlarge but the peripheral lung fields are ischemic.

The X-ray findings are prominent after 6 months of age with enlargement of the left ventricle. Initially there is the normal right ventricular dominance and in presence of the VSD, there is a slower decrease of the normal pulmonary vascular resistance.

Electrocardiography: The ECG findings also depend on the magnitude of the left to right shunt.

With small VSD, the ECG is normal. With moderate VSD, there is left ventricular hypertrophy. Left atrial hypertrophy may be occasionally seen. With large defects, the ECG shows biventricular hypertrophy. The axis is normal. In presence of pulmonary vascular obstructive disease, the ECG shows only right ventricular hypertrophy.

Echocardiography: A two dimensional and Doppler echo can identify the number, size and the exact location of the defect; estimate pulmonary arterial pressure; identify other associated defects and estimate the magnitude of the shunt.

Course and Complications

Small VSDs do not become bigger with age; rather they decrease in size. They close spontaneously, most frequently during the first two years of life. Small muscular VSDs are more likely to close than membranous ones. Most children with a small VSD remain asymptomatic, with no hemodynamic changes. The long term risk is infective endocarditis.

Infants with moderate to large VSD suffer repeated episodes of pneumonia and heart failure. Pulmonary vascular disease may develop as early as 6–12 months of age but the resulting right to left shunt usually does not develop until teenage. Infundibular stenosis may develop in some patients resulting in a decrease in the magnitude of the left to right shunt with an occasional production of a right to left shunt (acyanotic Fallot).

Management

In patients with large VSDs, the treatment is aimed at early control of heart failure and maintenance of normal growth. Heart failure is treated with digoxin and diuretics for 2–4 months. Frequent feedings with high calorie diet should be given. Anemia, if present should be corrected. If such treatment is successful and the child gains weight, the shunt may diminish in size with spontaneous improvement, especially during the first year of life. If initial medical management is not successful it should not be continued, surgery should be planned. In such cases pulmonary vascular disease can be prevented when surgery is performed within first year of life. Other indications for surgical closure are as follows:

1. Infants between 6 months and 1 year with large defects associated with pulmonary hypertension even if symptoms are controlled by medical management.
2. Patients older than 2 years with a Qp:Qs ratio greater than 2:1.
3. Patients with supra crystal VSD of any size because of the high risk of development of aortic valve regurgitation.

Severe pulmonary vascular disease, on the other hand is the contraindication of surgical intervention.

Atrial Septal Defect

Atrial septal defect is a communication between the left and right atrium. The reported Indian incidence is 13% of congenital heart disease with ostium secundum type, 10 times more than the ostium primum type. In western countries, isolated ostium secundum ASD account for approximately 7% of congenital heart defects.

Anatomical Types

There are three types of atrial septal defects. Ostium secundum defect, ostium primum defect and sinus venosus defect. Less commonly, the atrial septum may be nearly absent with the creation of a functional single atrium.

Ostium secundum defect is the most common type of ASD. This defect is located at the site of fossa ovalis. The ostium primum defect is situated inferior to the fossa ovalis. It is associated with a cleft in the anterior leaflet of the mitral valve with or without a cleft in the septal tricuspid valve. The sinus venosus defect is commonly located at the entry of the superior vena cava or rarely at the entry of inferior vena cava into the right atrium.

Hemodynamics

Atrial septal defect results in leak of oxygenated blood from left to right atrium in presence of minor difference of pressure between the two atria. The left to right shunt is therefore silent on auscultation.

In presence of the communication between the atria, the right atrium receives blood from the superior and inferior vena cava as well as the left atrium. To accommodate the extra volume of blood, the right atrium enlarges in size. The large volume of blood received by the right atrium passes through a normal sized tricuspid valve, producing a delayed diastolic murmur due to relative tricuspid stenosis. This murmur can be heard at the lower left sternal border. The right ventricle enlarges to accommodate this large volume of blood. When the large blood volume passes through the normal pulmonary valve, a pulmonary ejection systolic murmur is produced. It also results in a prolonged ejection phase of the right ventricle, late closure of the pulmonary valve and a delayed P_2. Normally the duration of right ventricular ejection varies with respiration. With an ASD, the right ventricular diastolic volume is constantly increased and the ejection time is prolonged throughout all phases of respiration. The second sound is, therefore, widely split and fixed. The P_2 is also accentuated and is well audible in the apex also. The left atrium may be enlarged, the left ventricle and aorta are normal in size.

The main pulmonary artery and its branches enlarge to accommodate the left to right shunt. The lung fields appear plethoric.

Clinical Manifestations

Ostium Secundum Defect

Children with ostium secundum defect are usually asymptomatic except for recurrent pneumonia. The lesion may be discovered during a routine physical examination. Even a large ASD rarely produces heart failure during childhood. The young children exhibit failure to thrive and older children have slender asthenic body build. The older children may also have mild effort intolerance which usually remains unnoticed until after surgical repair, when the child's growth and activity level increases.

The physical findings of ASD are characteristic but subtle and require a careful examination with special attention to the heart sounds.

There is a mild precordial bulge on the left side, a right ventricular systolic lift at the left sternal border. The first heart sound is loud. The second sound is widely split and fixed in both phases of respiration. A medium pitched ejection systolic murmur is heard best at the middle and upper left sternal border. A short rumbling mid diastolic murmur is audible at the lower left sternal border. Its presence indicates a Qp: Qs ratio of atleast 2:1.

X-ray Studies

Show varying degrees of cardiomegaly with enlargement of right atrium, right ventricle, and left atrium depending on the magnitude of the shunt. The pulmonary artery is large and there is pulmonary plethora.

Electrocardiography

The ECG shows right ventricular volume overload and right ventricular hypertrophy. The QRS axis may be normal or there may be right axis deviation and partial right bundle branch block.

Echocardiography

The location and size of the defect is easily appreciated by two dimensional echo. The shunt is confirmed by colour flow Doppler.

Ostium Primum Defect

The child with ostium primum defect exhibits failure to thrive from infancy. Frequent respiratory infections are usually severe. There may be episodes of heart failure.

On examination there is cardiomegaly with a displaced, heaving apex beat, a left parasternal heave due to right ventricular hypertrophy. With associated mitral incompetence, there is an apical pansystolic murmur associated with a thrill. There may be an apical mid diastolic murmur. The pulmonary second sound is widely split and fixed in both phases of respiration.

X-ray Studies

Show enlargement of right atrium, both ventricles. Enlargement of the pulmonary artery and pulmonary plethora.

Electrocardiography

The characteristic changes include left axis deviation, right ventricular hypertrophy and partial right bundle branch block. When mitral incompetence is marked, there may be evidence of left ventricular hypertrophy. Heart block may be present when there is persistent atrio-ventricular canal defect.

Echocardiography

Is confirmatory for diagnosis of the structural anomaly as well as confirmation of shunt.

Course and Complication

The overall rate of spontaneous closure of ostium secundum type of ASD is around 87%. An ASD of diameter > 8 mm rarely closes spontaneously. Ostium secundum defect are well tolerated during childhood. Symptoms usually do not appear until the third decade. Infective endocarditis is extremely rare in isolated defect. Rarely congestive cardiac failure can develop in infancy. Cerebrovascular accident, resulting from paradoxical embolism through an ASD is a rare complication.

Management

Medical management includes treatment of heart failure in infancy. No antibiotic prophylaxis for infective endocarditis is necessary for isolated ostium secundum defects.

Surgical or transcatheter closure is indicated in:

1. All symptomatic patients.
2. Asymptomatic patients with a Qp: Qs ratio of atleast 2:1.

The timing of elective closure is usually after 1st year and before entry to school. Surgery may be indicated during infancy if congestive heart failure does not respond to medical treatment.

Patent Ductus Arteriosus

During fetal life, ductus arteriosus connects the aorta and the pulmonary artery and most of the pulmonary arterial blood is shunted to the aorta. Functional closure of the ductus normally occurs soon after birth. It may remain patent even after the pulmonary vascular resistance falls when aortic blood is shunted to the pulmonary artery. Patent ductus arteriosus is associated with maternal Rubella infection during the first trimester of pregnancy. It is more common in females with a male: female ratio 1:2. It is a common problem in preterm babies.

Anatomy

Patent ductus arteriosus is a communication between the pulmonary artery and the aorta. The aortic end of the ductus is situated just distal to the origin of the left subclavian artery. The ductus enters the pulmonary artery at its bifurcation.

Hemodynamics

When the *pulmonary artery pressure is normal,* a pressure gradient is present throughout the cardiac cycle between the two great arteries. So the flow of blood through the patent ductus occurs both during the systole and diastole. The flow of blood results in a continuous murmur, which starts in systole, after the first sound and reaches a peak at the second sound. Thereafter, the murmur diminishes in intensity and audible during only a part of the diastole.

The continuous flow of blood results in systolic and diastolic overload of the pulmonary artery. This increased volume of blood passes through the lungs into the left atrium. The left atrium enlarges to accommodate the increased volume. The increased volume of blood enters the left ventricle in diastole through the normal mitral valve.

In presence of a large shunt, the passage of the large volume of blood through the normal mitral valve results in an accentuated 1st heart sound and a mitral delayed diastolic murmur. With a moderate shunt there is production of a third sound due to rapid early filling of the left ventricle. With a small shunt, the delayed diastolic murmur is absent.

The large volume of blood in the left ventricle has two effects. There is enlargement of the left ventricle and prolongation of the left ventricular systole. The prolongation results in delayed closure of the aortic valve and a late A_2. With a large left to right shunt, there may be a paradoxical split of the second sound. The large left ventricular volume ejected into the aorta results in dilatation of the arch of aorta, an aortic ejection click and an aortic ejection systolic murmur.

Children with PDA, tend to develop pulmonary arterial hypertension earlier than in those with VSD. With development of *pulmonary arterial hypertension*, the diastolic pressure difference between the aorta and the pulmonary artery is lost first. Therefore, with increasing pulmonary arterial hypertension, the diastolic component of the continuous murmur become shorter and may disappear altogether and the continuous murmur may be left with only an ejection systolic murmur.

PDA may be associated with hyperkinetic and obstructive types of pulmonary arterial hypertension. In both, the diastolic component of the murmur disappears and the P_2 is accentuated. The hyperkinetic type is associated with a large heart, and a mitral delayed diastolic murmur. The obstructive type is associated with a normal sized heart and absent mitral diastolic murmur. Severe pulmonary hypertension is associated with disappearance of the murmur, development of right to left shunt and differential cyanosis.

Clinical Manifestations

The children with a small PDA are asymptomatic. With large shunts there is physical retardation of growth, exertional dyspnea, and congestive cardiac failure.

The signs of PDA depend on the size and presence or absence of pulmonary arterial hypertension.

Large PDA without Pulmonary Arterial Hypertension

Signs of wide pulse pressure are present; most striking is bounding peripheral pulses. The precordium is hyperdynamic.The heart size is moderately or grossly enlarged. The apical impulse is left ventricular type. A systolic thrill may be palpable at the second left intercostal space. The first heart sound is accentuated. The second heart sound is paradoxically split. A third heart sound may be present. There is an ejection systolic murmur, best heard in the second left intercostal space, radiating to the clavicle or along the left sternal border. A low pitched mitral or tricuspid mid diastolic murmur may be audible at the apex.

Small to Moderate PDA

The heart size is normal. The apical impulse is prominent. A systolic or a continuous thrill may be palpable at the second left intercostal space. The second heart sound is normally split. There is a continuous murmur which is best heard in the second left intercostal space. It may radiate down the left sternal border or to the clavicle. It has a systolic and diastolic component. The harsh systolic murmur starts after the first heart sound and continues beyond the second heart sound masking it. It is followed by the diastolic component which is soft, smooth and decrescendo.

PDA with Pulmonary Arterial Hypertension

There is differential cyanosis (i.e. cyanosis in the lower half of the body). There is palpable suprasternal pulsation due to dilatation of the ascending and arch of aorta. A parasternal heave is present. The pulmonary second sound is accentuated. With moderate pulmonary arterial hypertension, the diastolic component of the continuous murmur decreases in duration and disappears with severe pulmonary arterial hypertension, so that there is only an ejection systolic murmur.

X-ray Studies

With a small PDA, the X-ray study may be normal. Larger shunts may show cardiomegaly of varying sizes with enlargement of left ventricle, left atrium, and ascending aorta. The pulmonary vascular markings are increased. With pulmonary arterial hypertension, the heart size is normal with marked prominence of the pulmonary artery segment and the hilar vessels.

Electrocardiography

The ECG is normal in case of a small PDA shunt. In moderate to large PDA, there may be left ventricular or biventricular hypertrophy.

Echocardiography

The PDA can be imaged and its size assessed by two dimensional echocardiography. Functional information can be obtained by Doppler studies.

Course and Complications

Spontaneous closure of a PDA does not usually occur in full term infants. This is because the PDA in term infants results from a structural abnormality of the ductal smooth muscles rather than a decreased responsiveness of the premature ductus to oxygen. With large shunts, there is recurrent pneumonia and/or congestive heart failure. Congestive heart failure occurs during infancy in case of large defects. It can occur at any age with a moderate sized defect. Pulmonary vascular obstructive disease may develop if a large PDA with pulmonary hypertension remains untreated. Infective endocarditis occur more with small PDA. Rarely, an aneurysm of PDA can develop and rupture.

Differential Diagnosis

A continuous murmur may also be present in the following conditions:

1. *Coronary arteriovenous fistula:* A continuous murmur is maximally heard along the right sternal border or upper left sternal border.
2. *Pulmonary arteriovenous fistula:* A continuous murmur is heard on the back. There is cyanosis and clubbing in absence of cardiomegaly.
3. *Venous hum:* It is heard as a continuous sound in the right and/or left infraclavicular and supraclavicular areas in the sitting position. It disappears in the supine position.
4. *Collaterals in coarctation of aorta or tetralogy of Fallot:* A continuous murmur is heard in the intercostal spaces, usually bilaterally.

5. *Persistent truncus arteriosus:* A continuous murmur is occasionally heard at the second right intercostal space or at the back in a cyanotic infant.
6. *Ruptured sinus of valsalva into right atrium:* The continuous murmur is present at the base.
7. *Total anomalous venous return into the right atrium:* A murmur similar to venous hum may be heard along the right sternal border in presence of mild cyanosis.
8. *Peripheral pulmonary artery stenosis:* A continuous murmur is audible all over the thorax.
9. *VSD with aortic regurgitation:* A combination of a pan systolic murmur and an early diastolic murmur is heard with a definite gap between the murmurs.
10. *Mitral regurgitation with aortic regurgitation:* A combination of a pansystolic and an early diastolic murmur can be heard but with a definite gap between the two murmurs.

Treatment

Irrespective of age, the PDA require surgical or catheter closure. This is done to prevent the complication which may arise if it is not closed.

Coarctation of Aorta

This vascular anomaly is characterized by constrictions of the aorta of varying degrees. It is a relatively common type of obstructive congenital anomaly. It is so amenable to surgical correction that palpation of the femoral artery should form a part of the physical examination of every patient from the newborn period and above. It is more common in males. 30% of cases with Turner's syndrome can have this anomaly.

Anatomy

The constrictions can occur at any point from the transverse arch to the iliac bifurcation but 98% occur just below the origin of the left subclavian artery at the origin of the ductus arteriosus. Coarctation of aorta may be associated with mitral valve abnormalities (supravalvular mitral ring or parachute mitral valve) and sub aortic stenosis. This group of left sided obstructive lesions is referred to as *Shone complex*.

Clinical Manifestations

Infants with coarctation may present with varying degrees of respiratory distress, oliguria or anuria, general circulatory shock and severe acidemia. Before ductal closure, there may be differential cyanosis because of right to left ductal shunt. Peripheral pulses are weak and there is a blood pressure differential, which becomes apparent after improvement of cardiac function with administration of ionotropes. The second heart sound is single and loud. A third heart sound gallop is usually present. An ejection systolic murmur is heard over the precordium which become louder after treatment.

Coarctation of aorta recognized after infancy is usually not associated with significant symptoms. Some children and adolescents complain of pain or weakness or both in the legs after exercise. Older children are suspected when they are found hypertensive on routine physical examination.

The classic sign of coarctation of the aorta is a disparity in the pulsation and blood pressure in the arms and legs. The femoral, popliteal, posterior tibial, and dorsalis pedis pulses are weak or absent in contrast to the bounding pulses of the arm and the carotid. The blood pressure in the lower limbs is lower than in the upper limbs and frequently it may be difficult to obtain. The differential in blood pressure is common in children above 1 year of age, majority of whom have a systolic hypertension in the upper extremities greater than 95th percentile for age. With involvement of the left subclavian artery in the coarctation, the pressure will be higher on the right limb than on the left. So blood pressure measurement should be done on all four limbs.

Other physical findings include palpable collaterals over the chest wall along the undersurface of the ribs over the back in the fifth to eight intercostal spaces and along the borders of the scapula, palpable aortic pulsations in the supra sternal notch, and an apical impulse of left ventricular type with varying degrees of left ventricular enlargement. The first heart sound is normal followed by an ejection click; the second heart sound is normally split with an accentuated aortic component. An ejection systolic murmur is present which is best heard in the left interscapular area but may be well heard in the apex.

X-ray Studies

Cardiac enlargement and pulmonary congestion are noted in infants with severe coarctation. During childhood, the heart size is normal until after 10 years of age when there is enlargement of the heart with a prominent ascending and arch of aorta. Notching of the inferior border of the ribs from pressure erosion by enlarged collaterals is seen in late childhood (Fig. 14.1). An E-shaped indentation on the barium filled esophagus (Fig. 14.2), or the "3 sign" suggests coarctation of aorta.

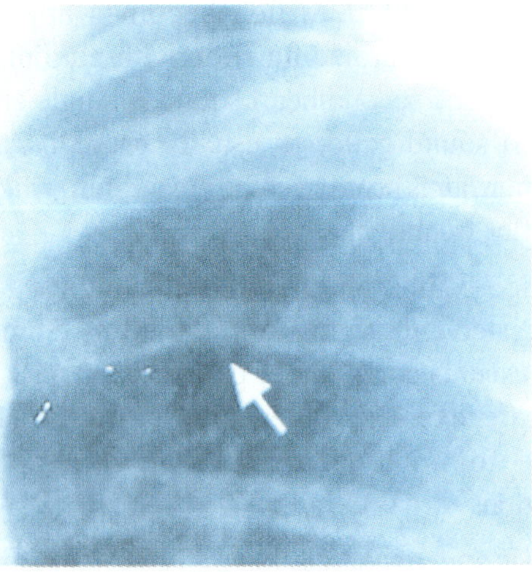

Fig. 14.1: Rib notching in coarctation of aorta

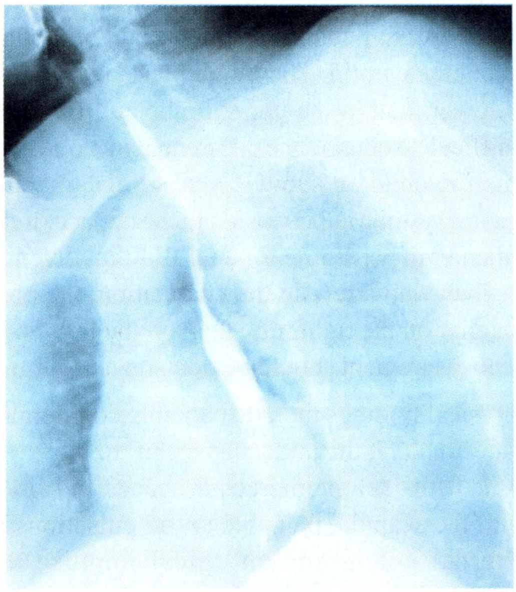

Fig. 14.2: Figure of E appearance in coarctation of aorta

Electrocardiography

Neonates and young infants show right or biventricular hypertrophy. It is normal in young children but reveals evidence of left ventricular hypertrophy in older children.

Echocardiography

Two dimensional echocardiography can visualize the segment of coarctation as well as the associated abnormalities of heart valves. Color Doppler is useful in demonstrating the specific site of the obstruction and disturbed flow distal to the coarctation.

Course and Complications

Left untreated, the majority of the older patients would succumb between the ages of 20–40 years. Some may live upto middle age without serious disability.

The common complications are related to systemic hypertension. These include hypertensive encephalopathy, intracranial hemorrhage (due to rupture of Berry's aneurysm of circle of Willis), heart failure and premature coronary artery disease. Infective endocarditis can occur on either the abnormal aortic valve or the coarctation. Aneurysm and rupture of the descending aorta can occur. In infants with severe coarctation, heart failure and hypoperfusion may be life threatening.

Treatment

In newborn with severe coarctation, closure of the ductus often results in hypoperfusion, acidosis and rapid deterioration. In such cases, prostaglandin E_1 infusion should be given to reopen ductus and reestablish adequate lower extremity blood flow. Once the diagnosis is confirmed and the infant is stabilized, surgical repair should be performed.

In the older child presenting with heart failure but good perfusion should be managed with decongestive therapy before surgery.

Between ages of 2–4 years elective surgical correction is indicated in coarctation of aorta with hypertension in the upper extremities or with a systolic pressure gradient of 20 mm or more between arms and legs. In older children surgery is indicated as soon as diagnosis is made.

Tetralogy of Fallot

Tetralogy of Fallot (TOF) is the most common cyanotic congenital heart disease seen in children beyond infancy.

Anatomy

The classical tetrad consists of a right ventricular outflow tract obstruction, a large ventricular septal defect with a right to left shunt, overriding of the aorta, and right ventricular hypertrophy.

The two main abnormalities are a VSD large enough to equalize the pressures in both ventricles and a right ventricular outflow obstruction. The right ventricular hypertrophy is secondary to right ventricular outflow obstruction and the VSD. The VSD in TOF is a perimembranous defect with an extension into the subpulmonary region. The right ventricular outflow tract obstruction is most frequently in the form of infundibular stenosis followed by a combination of infundibular stenosis and valvular stenosis. The valvular obstruction alone is rare. The main pulmonary artery is often small and various degrees of pulmonary artery branch stenosis may be present. There may be pulmonary atresia. A right sided aortic arch is present in 15–20% cases.

There are many variants of TOF depending on the type and degree of pulmonary stenosis, the size of VSD and the degree of overriding of aorta.

Hemodynamics

When the right ventricle contracts in the presence of marked pulmonary stenosis, blood is shunted across the VSD into the aorta. This results in persistent arterial desaturation and cyanosis. When pulmonary blood flow is severely restricted by obstruction to right ventricular outflow, it may be supplemented by the bronchial collateral circulation and by the PDA in the newborn. The peak systolic and diastolic pressures in both ventricles are similar and at the systemic level. There is a large pressure gradient across the obstructed right ventricular outflow tract. The pulmonary arterial pressure is normal or lower than normal.

The degree of right ventricular outflow obstruction determines the timing of onset of symptoms, the severity of cyanosis and the degree of right ventricular hypertrophy. When the obstruction to the right ventricular outflow is mild to moderate and a balanced shunt is present across the VSD, the patient may not have visible cyanosis. This condition is called acyanotic or pink tetralogy of Fallot.

Clinical Manifestations

Cyanosis, dyspnea on exertion, and paroxysmal hypercyanotic attacks (hypoxic or blue spells) are the usual presenting symptoms in children with TOF. Untreated cases with chronically less than 70% oxygen saturation have also delayed growth and development. Puberty is also delayed in such cases.

The onset and degree of cyanosis depends on the severity of right ventricular outflow obstruction. Central cyanosis may be present at birth in infants with severe degree of right ventricular obstruction. These babies are dependent on blood flow through the ductus arteriosus at birth. When the ductus closes within few hours after birth, severe central cyanosis and circulatory collapse can occur. Often cyanosis occurs later in latter part of infancy. Older children who have not undergone surgery have also marked clubbing of the fingers and toes. Infants with mild degrees of right ventricular outflow obstruction may initially present with heart failure as a result of the large VSD with left to right shunt. The child with acyanotic Fallot may be asymptomatic or may have signs of heart failure due to a large VSD.

Infants and toddlers may present with dyspnea on exertion. They can play actively for some time and then sit or lie down. Older children with significant cyanosis may be able to walk for a distance and then take rest assuming a squatting position and resume physical activity within a few minutes.

The *paroxysmal hypercyanotic attack* (also called cyanotic spell, hypoxic spell or "tet" spell) is associated with the reduction of an already compromised pulmonary blood flow which when prolonged results in systemic hypoxia and metabolic acidosis. Infants who have mild cyanosis at rest are often prone to develop anoxic spells because they have not acquired the homeostatic mechanism (polycythemia) to tolerate the rapid lowering of arterial oxygen saturation. In children with severe cyanosis, presence of polycythemia is protective.

Signs

Cyanosis and clubbing are present in varying degrees. The pulse is normal. A precordial bulge may be present in the left parasternal region due to right ventricular hypertrophy. The heart is not enlarged and the apical impulse may be difficult to locate. A systolic thrill may be felt along the left sternal border in the 3rd and 4th parasternal spaces in around 50% cases. The S_2 is single or the pulmonary component is soft. A grade 3–5 /6 systolic murmur is heard at the middle and upper left sternal border. The murmur is usually ejection systolic type (pulmonary stenosis) but may be holosystolic (VSD) towards the lower sternal border. The more severe the obstruction of the right ventricular outflow tract, the shorter and softer the systolic murmur. With pulmonary atresia, the ejection systolic murmur is absent and replaced by a continuous murmur of PDA. The murmur also becomes less prominent with a hypoxic spell.

In acyanotic Fallot, a long systolic murmur can be heard along the entire left sternal border as a result of infundibular stenosis and VSD. The auscultatory findings resemble those of a small VSD.

X-ray Studies

In cyanotic tetralogy of Fallot, the heart size is normal or smaller than normal, with the apex raised above the diaphragm (boot shaped heart). The main pulmonary artery segment is concave and the pulmonary vascular markings are diminished (oligemic lungs) (Fig. 14.3). The lung fields are "black" in TOF with pulmonary atresia. There may be presence of a right sided aortic arch and right atrial enlargement. In acyanotic Fallot, the X-ray findings are similar to those of a small to moderate VSD.

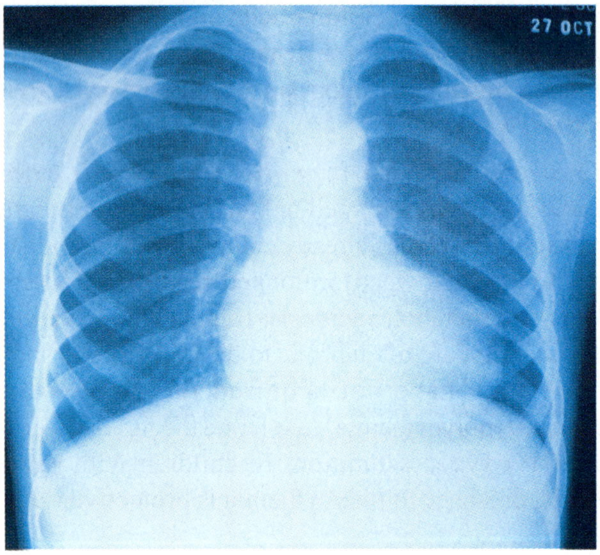

Fig. 14.3: Fallot's tetralogy

Electrocardiography

In cyanotic tetralogy of Fallot, the ECG shows marked right axis deviation (+ 120 to + 150 degrees) with right ventricular hypertrophy but strain pattern is unusual. There may be right atrial hypertrophy. In acyanotic tetralogy of Fallot, the QRS axis is normal and there is right ventricular hypertrophy rather than left ventricular hypertrophy or combined ventricular hypertrophy.

Echocardiography

Two dimensional echocardiography establishes the diagnosis. It provides information about the location and degree of the right ventricular outflow obstruction, extent of overriding of the septum, and the side of the aortic arch. It also helps to determine whether the PDA is supplying a portion of the pulmonary blood flow and presence of associated anomalies like ASD, anomalous position of the coronary arteries and persistence of left superior vena cava. Doppler studies estimate the pressure gradient across the obstruction.

Course and Prognosis

Infants with acyanotic TOF gradually becomes cyanotic. The children who are already cyanotic become more cyanotic. This is result of the worsening condition of the infundibular stenosis. Polycythemia develops secondary to cyanosis. Polycythemia can result in relative iron deficiency anemia.

Before correction, the children with TOF are susceptible to serious complications like cerebral thrombosis, brain abscess, bacterial endocarditis and heart failure. Thrombosis occurs most often in children younger than 2 years. Brain abscess is common above 2 years of age. Bacterial endocarditis may occur even after corrective or palliative surgery. Heart failure is not a usual feature in patients with cyanotic TOF. It may occur in a young infant with pink or acyanotic TOF. These children are at increased risk of hypoxic spells.

Treatment

Medical

Medical treatment consists of the following:

1. Administration of prostaglandin E_1, 0.05–0.20 microgram/kg/min I.V. It is a potent and specific relaxant of the smooth muscles of the ductus. It causes dilatation of the ductus arteriosus and provides adequate pulmonary blood flow until a surgery can be performed. Infants with severe TOF require medical treatment as well as surgical intervention in the neonatal period. The baby should be transferred to a centre with facilities for evaluation and treatment of congenital heart disease. It is important that a normal body temperature and oxygenation is maintained during transport. Intravenous administration of prostaglandin E_1 provides adequate pulmonary blood flow.
2. Recognition and treatment of hypercyanotic/hypoxic spell.
3. Oral propranolol therapy, 0.5 to 1.5 mg/kg every 6 hours, is used to prevent hypoxic spells while waiting for corrective surgery.
4. Maintenance of good dental hygiene and practice of antibiotic prophylaxis against infective endocarditis.
5. Detection and treatment of relative iron deficiency because cyanotic children with anemia are more susceptible to cerebrovascular complications.

Surgery

Severely cyanotic infants and children can be dramatically improved by means of a palliative surgery which consist of an anastomosis between systemic and pulmonary arteries which will augment the blood flow through the lungs. The most frequently employed anastomosis operation is the modified Blalock-Taussig shunt which consists of anastomosis of the subclavian artery and the homolateral branch of pulmonary artery or between the ascending aorta and the main pulmonary artery.

It is increasingly becoming the practice to carry out a complete correction of the defect as an initial procedure or following a previous shunt operation. In infants with less severe cyanosis, good growth and absence of hypoxic spells, primary repair is performed electively between 4 and 12 months age.

Hypoxic Spells

It is characterized by paroxysms of hyperapnea (rapid and deep respiration), irritability and prolonged crying, increasing cyanosis, and decreasing intensity of the heart murmur.

It is a problem particularly seen during infancy with a peak incidence between 2 and 4 months. The spells occur most frequently after awakening in the morning. The spells may last for a few minutes to few hours but is rarely fatal. Short episodes are followed by generalized weakness and sleep. Severe spells may progress to unconsciousness and occasionally to convulsions or hemiparesis.

Pathogenesis

The ratio of flows to the pulmonary and systemic circuits (Qp/Qs) from the right and left ventricle respectively is related to the ratio of resistance offered by the pulmonary resistance (PR) and the systemic vascular resistance (SVR). Either an increase in the PR or decrease in the SVR increases the degree of right to left shunt resulting in more severe arterial desaturation. Similarly, when the SVR increase and the PR decrease there is more blood flow though the pulmonary outflow obstruction.

In TOF, the VSD is so large that it equalizes the right and left ventricular pressures and the right and left ventricles may be treated as one chamber that ejects blood into the systemic and pulmonary circuits. Again, as pulmonary valve stenosis has a fixed resistance and the infundibular stenosis is relatively non-reactive, the PR remains fairly constant. Therefore, the degree of right to left shunt or the amount of pulmonary blood flow is controlled primarily by changes in the SVR. A decrease in SVR increases the right to left shunt and decreases the pulmonary blood flow resulting in increase in cyanosis and vice versa.

Therefore events that suddenly lower the SVR (viz. crying, defecation, or increased physical activity), may initiate a hypoxic spell. In addition, sudden tachycardia, hypovolemia can increase the right to left shunt through the VSD resulting in fall of systemic arterial oxygen saturation. The resulting hypoxia can initiate the hypoxic spell.

The Vicious Cycle

An increase in the right to left shunt results in fall in arterial PO_2, increase in PCO_2, and fall in pH which stimulates the respiratory centre and produces hyperapnea. Hyperapnea in turn increases the systemic venous return. In the presence a fixed pulmonary resistance or decreased SVR, the increased systemic venous return to the right ventricle passes through the VSD to the aorta. This leads to a further decrease in the arterial oxygen saturation and the vicious cycle continues.

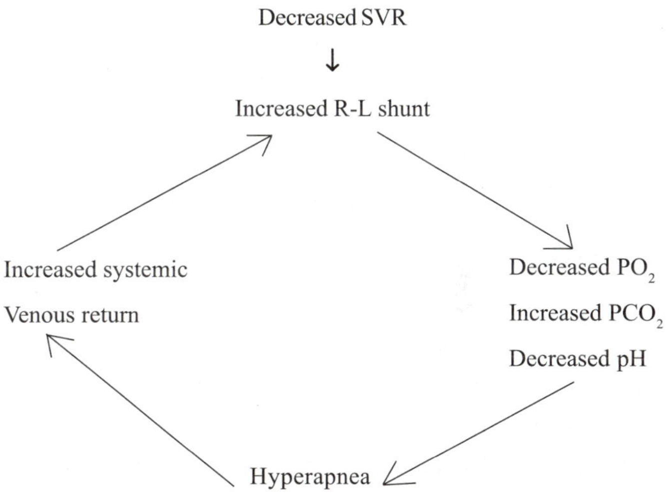

Fig. 14.4: The vicious cycle

Treatment

The aim of treatment is to break the vicious cycle of the spell. One or more of the following measures can be used to break the vicious cycle of the spell. The steps should be followed in a sequence as follows:

1. The infant should be held in a knee-chest position. This position traps the systemic venous blood in the legs and temporarily decreases the systemic venous return. The knee chest position can also increase the systemic vascular resistance by compressing the femoral arteries and reducing the arterial blood flow.

2. Morphine sulfate, 0.2 mg/kg administered subcutaneously or intramuscularly can suppress the respiratory centre and abolish hyperapnea and thus break the vicious cycle.
3. Acidosis should be corrected with sodium bicarbonate, 1 mEq/kg administered intravenously. The same dose can be repeated after 10 to 15 minutes. Sodium bicarbonate acts by reducing the stimulating effect of acidosis on the respiratory centre.
4. Oxygen can be administered but it has little effect on the arterial oxygen saturation.

   The infant usually responds to the above treatment with decreasing cyanosis and increase in the intensity of the murmur. If the condition does not improve fully, the following drugs can be tried.
5. Vasoconstrictors viz. phenylephrine, 0.02 mg/kg IV. It helps by raising the systemic arterial pressure.
6. Ketamine, 1–3 mg/kg IV over 1 minute. It increases the systemic vascular resistance and sedates the patient.
7. Propranolol 0.01 to 0.25 mg/kg slow IV. It reduces the heart rate and may reverse the spell. The mechanism of action is not clear. It may reduce the spasm of the right ventricular outflow tract and slow the heart rate. It may also increase the SVR.

ACQUIRED HEART DISEASE

The most common acquired heart disease in children is acute rheumatic fever and rheumatic heart disease. The other acquired heart diseases include cardiac arrhythmias, pericarditis and pericardial effusion, myocarditis and primary myocardial disease and systemic hypertension.

Acute Rheumatic Fever

Acute rheumatic fever is still a common cause of heart disease in developing countries. It is believed to be an immunologic lesion that occurs as a delayed sequelae of group A streptococcal pharyngitis. The serotypes of group A streptococcus, more frequently isolated from patients with acute rheumatic fever are M types 1, 3, 5, 6, 18 and 24. The attack rate of rheumatic fever after a streptococcal infection varies from 0.3% to 3%. The important predisposing factors include family history of acute rheumatic fever, poor socio-economic status, overcrowding, and inadequate treatment of streptococcal infection. The age group affected is 5–15 years and peak age is 8 years.

Pathology

The Aschoff bodies in the atrial myocardium are believed to be characteristic of rheumatic fever. These consist of inflammatory lesions associated with swelling and fragmentation of collagen fibers. The inflammatory lesions are also found in the joints, brain and skin. Valvular damage most commonly affects the mitral valves, less commonly the aortic and rarely the tricuspid and pulmonary.

Pathogenesis

Several theories have been proposed regarding the pathogenesis of rheumatic fever but only two are seriously considered: cytotoxicity theory and the immunologic theory.

The *cytotoxicity theory* focuses on enzyme streptolysin O which is shown to have a direct toxic effect on mammalian cells in tissue culture. This theory, however, fails to explain the latent period between the Group A streptococcal throat infection and the onset of acute rheumatic fever.

The *immunogenic theory* is supported by the clinical similarity of acute rheumatic fever to other illnesses produced by immunopathogenic processes and by the latent period between the Group A streptococcal infection and onset of rheumatic fever. Secondly the antigenicity of a large variety of Group A streptococcal products and constituents, as well as the immunologic cross-reactivity between the group A streptococcal components and mammalian tissues also lends support to this theory.

In addition, the involvement of group A streptococcal super antigen such as pyrogenic exotoxins has been proposed in the pathogenesis of acute rheumatic fever.

Clinical Manifestations

There is no single specific clinical manifestation or specific laboratory test that unequivocally establishes the diagnosis of rheumatic fever. A highly probable diagnosis of acute rheumatic fever is arrived at on the basis of modified Jones criteria. The recent recommendations of the American Heart Association are as follows:

Table 14.1: Modified Jones criteria for diagnosis of acute rheumatic fever (Updated 1992)

Major criteria	*Minor criteria*
Carditis	Fever
Migratory polyarthritis	Arthralgia
Erythema marginatum	Elevated acute phase reactants (ESR, CRP)
Chorea	
Subcutaneous nodules	Prolonged PR interval on an ECG
Plus	
Evidence of a preceding Group A streptococcal infection viz.	
• A positive throat culture or a rapid streptococcal antigen test.	
• An elevated or increasing streptococcal antibody titre.	

Interpretation

Diagnosis of initial attack of acute rheumatic fever.

Presence of two major or one major and two minor Jones criteria + Evidence of preceding streptococcal infection.

Diagnosis of Recurrent Rheumatic Fever

In presence of documented rheumatic heart disease or history of prior rheumatic fever, two minor Jones criteria + Evidence of preceding streptococcal infection suffices.

Points to be Noted in Application of the Jones Criteria

1. Two major criteria are always stronger than one major and two minor criteria for diagnosis of initial attack.
2. Arthralgia cannot be used as a minor criterion in presence of arthritis.
3. Prolonged PR interval cannot be used as minor criteria in presence of carditis.
4. The absence of evidence of an antecedent group A streptococcal infection is a warning that rheumatic fever is unlikely (except in cases of chorea).
5. The possibility of early suppression of full clinical manifestations with sub therapeutic doses of aspirin should be sought for during history taking.

Migratory Polyarthritis: It occurs in 75% cases of acute rheumatic fever. Polyarthritis involves larger joints, particularly knees, ankle, elbows and wrists. Rheumatic joints are hot, red, swollen and exquisitely tender. The joint involvement is migratory in character, i.e., a severely inflamed joint may become normal within 2–3 days without any treatment, as one or more joint become involved. Rheumatic arthritis dramatically responds even to a small dose of salicylates and it resolves without any residual deformity. A monoarticular involvement is unusual unless anti-inflammatory drug is started prematurely aborting the progression of migratory polyarthritis. Hence if a child is suspected to be suffering from acute rheumatic fever, salicylates should be withheld to observe the migratory progression. An absence of dramatic response to salicylates should suggest an alternative diagnosis.

Differential diagnosis: The other most important cause of polyarthritis is polyarticular type of juvenile idiopathic arthritis. The characteristic features are involvement of large and small joints including spine with an additive character rather than migratory. The joints are swollen without signs of inflammation. There is residual deformity. There is no dramatic response to salicylates.

The other causes of arthritis viz. Tubercular, pyogenic, post dysenteric are monoarticular.

Carditis: Carditis occurs in 40–80% of patients of acute rheumatic fever. It is a pancarditis involving the pericardium, myocardium and endocardium.The signs of carditis may include some or all of the following:

Signs of pericarditis include chest pain, pericardial friction rub and pericardial effusion.

Signs of myocarditis include tachycardia out of proportion of degree of fever, cardiomegaly, soft first heart sound, Carey Coomb's murmur and congestive heart failure.

In the past, myocarditis has been thought to be a determining factor for the morbidity and mortality in acute rheumatic fever. However, recent evidence shows that myocarditis per se plays a little role. Myocardial biopsy studies have failed to show significant myocardial damage. Echocardiography evaluation of left ventricle during acute rheumatic carditis has shown that the left ventricular contractility remains normal in presence of congestive failure indicating that the myocardial function is normal and not responsible for congestive failure. Thirdly, rapid control of congestive heart failure by surgical replacement of aortic and/ or mitral valves during acute rheumatic fever with decrease in size of the heart indicates that it is the acute hemodynamic overload secondary to mitral and /or aortic regurgitation which is responsible for the congestive heart failure and consequent mortality.

Signs of endocarditis include presence of murmurs as a result of valvulitis. The commonly affected valves are mitral and aortic. Isolated aortic valve involvement is rare. Tricuspid and pulmonary valve involvement is unusual. Isolated mitral insufficiency or a combination of mitral and aortic insufficiency is common during the acute phase. Presence of mitral stenosis or combination of mitral stenosis and regurgitation in acute stage may indicate a relapse because mitral stenosis is a lesion of the chronic stage.

Carditis may be mild (without cardiomegaly), moderate (with cardiomegaly without CCF), and severe (with CCF).

The surest signs of rheumatic carditis include presence of a pericardial friction rub and a murmur indicating involvement of both endocardium and pericardium, hence pancarditis.

Subcutaneous nodules are firm swellings of size varying from 0.2 to 2 cm. They are usually found symmetrically, singly or in clusters on the extensor surfaces of both large and small joints, over the scalp, or along the spine. They may last for weeks, and have a significant association with carditis.

Erythema marginatum is a transient manifestation. It is characterized by erythematous, serpiginous, macular, non- pruritic lesions with pale centres. It is seen primarily in the trunk and extremities and can be accentuated by warming the skin.

Chorea: It is called Sydenham chorea. It is a neuro-behavioral disorder which occurs in 10–15% cases of rheumatic fever. It occurs as an isolated disorder with a latent period more than that for arthritis or carditis. The onset is insidious and symptoms may remain unrecognized for several months.

The early clinical features include emotional lability, incoordination, poor school performance, uncontrollable movements and facial grimace which are exacerbated by stress and disappear with sleep.

The clinical signs to elicit chorea include:

1. *Milkmaid's grip:* Characterized by irregular contractions of the muscles of the hands while squeezing the examiners hands.
2. *Spooning and pronation of the hands:* When the patient's arms are extended.
3. Wormian movements of the tongue upon protrusion.
4. Presence of fine tremor while writing.

The child may present with florid chorea characterized by involuntary, purposeless movements of the limbs, body and face.

Diagnosis of isolated chorea is essentially clinical. A raised ASO titre is sometimes present. However, in patients with a long latent period, antibody level will be normal. Elevated titers of antineuronal antibodies, recognizing basal ganglia tissues, have been found in 90% of patients. Chorea is distressing in the acute phase but does not leave any permanent neurologic sequelae. It may be also associated with carditis when diagnosis of rheumatic chorea is evident.

Fever and arthralgia: Fever occurs early in the course of the illness. It is usually mild to moderate (102°F–104°F). Arthralgia refers to joint pain without the objective signs of arthritis.

An elevated acute phase reactants: An elevated acute phase reactants (ESR and C reactive protein) is an objective evidence of an inflammatory process.

A prolonged PR interval: A prolonged PR interval on the ECG is not specific of acute rheumatic fever.

Evidence of recent group a streptococcus infection: The supporting evidence of a recent group A streptococcal infection is an absolute requirement for the diagnosis of acute rheumatic fever. The clinical features of acute rheumatic fever typically appear 2–4 weeks after an acute episode of group A streptococcal pharyngitis.

However, around 1/3rd of patients may not have such a history at all. Moreover, clinical signs of pharyngitis are not present and only 10–20% cases have a positive throat culture when the child presents with acute rheumatic fever. Therefore, evidence of an antecedent group A streptococcal infection is based on elevated or increasing antistreptococcal antibody titres.

A rapid slide agglutination test (Streptozyme) has been introduced to detect antibodies against group A streptococcal antigens. This test is less standardized and less reproducible than the other tests and should not be used as a diagnostic test for an antecedent streptococcal infection.

If three antibody titres (ASO, anti-DNase B, and antihyaluronidase) are measured, 95–100% of patients with rheumatic fever have elevated titre whereas 80–85% patient have an elevation if only one antibody titre (i.e. usually ASO titre) is measured.

Except for patients of chorea, the clinical findings of acute rheumatic fever generally coincide with peak antistreptococcal titres. Even in cases of chorea, the antibody titres may be elevated but will be waning.

The diagnosis of acute rheumatic fever should not be made in children with elevated or increasing streptococcal antibody titres if they do not fulfill the Jones criteria. Such elevation may be coincidental, especially in young children, who may be suffering from group A streptococcal infection unrelated to acute rheumatic fever.

Management

Rest

All cases should be advised bed rest upto 2 weeks, during which the child should be examined daily for evolving signs of carditis. Carditis may develop in the first two weeks after onset. ESR is a useful guide to rheumatic activity and therefore to the duration of restriction of activities except in children with significant cardiac involvement. In carditis without failure, strict bed rest is required until the acute phase is over. In carditis with failure, strict bed rest should be advised until cardiac failure is controlled. Bed rest for 2 weeks to 3 months may be required for patients with carditis depending on the severity and evidence of progression or stabilization.

Anti Inflammatory Therapy

Cases with *rheumatic arthritis and carditis without cardiomegaly* should be treated with salicylates, 100 mg/kg/day in 4 to 6 divided doses (not to exceed 10 gms/day) for 2–3 weeks depending on response, clinical and laboratory (ESR, CRP). Then the dose should be reduced to 75 mg/kg /day and continued for 4–6 weeks. Clinical response is evidenced by absence of pain and swelling of joints and remission of fever. Laboratory evidence is a normal ESR and CRP.

Cases with *carditis with cardiomegaly alone or with congestive cardiac failure,* should be treated with prednisolone 2 mg/kg/day in divided doses for 2–3 weeks depending on response, clinical and laboratory, followed by tapering of the dose that reduces the dose by 5 mg/day every 2–3 days. While tapering steroids, should be treated with salicylates should be started in the dose of 75 mg/kg/day in 4 divided doses and continued for 6 weeks after stopping steroids.

Treatment of *congestive cardiac failure* consist of:

(a) Rest, oxygen, fluid restriction, sedation (morphine sulphate, 0.2 mg/kg, may be repeated 4–6 hourly in case of severe failure).

(b) Frusemide IV 1–2 mg/kg. This usually results in rapid diuresis and prompt improvement in clinical status, particularly if symptoms of pulmonary congestion are present.

(c) Digoxin in half the digitalizing dose when there is no response to above treatment.

(d) Valve replacement in case of intractable CCF.

Rebound: Occur after discontinuance of aspirin or more commonly after steroid therapy. Clinical rebound may manifest with arthralgia and fever or sometimes with frank arthritis and rarely as severe carditis. Sub-clinical rebounds may be detectable only by raised acute phase reactants.

The clinical manifestations of rebound usually resolve spontaneously or respond to salicylate therapy.

Treatment of Residual Streptococcal Throat Infection

The treatment of residual streptococcal infection may be done by one of the following:

1. Benzathene penicillin 1.2 million units (weight > 27 kg) and 0.6 million units (weight < 27 kg) deep IM stat after negative skin test done with benzyl penicillin. It may cause transient rise of ESR and interfere monitoring response on the basis of ESR.
2. Oral penicillin V, 250 mg 6 hourly × 10 days.
3. Erythromycin 40–50 mg/kg orally 8 hourly × 10 days if patient is allergic to penicillin.

Treatment of Chorea

The patient and parents should be reassured and told about the self limiting course of the disease. The child should be advised complete physical and mental rest. Anti inflammatory therapy is needed in presence of associated carditis. The child should be put on penicillin prophylaxis. For severe cases the following drugs may be used:

1. Phenobarbitone 15–30 mg 6–8 hourly.
2. *Haloperidol:* To start with 0.5 mg and increase upto 2.0 mg 8 hourly.

Continuous Anti Microbial Prophylaxis

The drugs used for continuous prophylaxis are benzathene penicillin G, oral phenoxymethyl penicillin, sulphadiazine and in children sensitive to penicillin and sulphadiazine, erythromycin.

Benzathene penicillin G is the drug of choice. It is given as 1.2 million units deep IM every 3 weeks after a negative skin test. The skin test should be done before every injection with benzyl penicillin. It may cause persistent pain at the site of injection for 1–2 days.

Phenoxymethyl penicillin V, 250 mg per oral 12 hourly may be used but is not much effective. It causes emergence of resistant strains of alpha hemolytic streptococci in the oral cavity where as benzathene penicillin and sulpha drugs does not. Presence of alpha hemolytic streptococci is a hazard for patients with RHD since they are at risk of infective endocarditis. Oral penicillin V is also not freely available. *Oral sulphadiazine* 500 mg (< 27 kg) and 1000 mg (> 27 kg) daily may be used. If child is allergic to penicillin and sulphadiazine, erythromycin 250 mg 12 hourly can be used.

Table 14.2: Chemoprophylaxis for recurrences of acute rheumatic fever

Drug	*Dose*	*Route*
Benzathene Penicillin	1.2 million units	Deep IM
Or, Penicillin V	250 mg 12 hourly	Oral
Or, Sulphadiazine	0.5 gm once daily (=/< 27 kg)	Oral
	1.0 gm once daily (> 27 kg)	Oral
For penicillin and sulphadiazine sensitivity		
Erythromycin	250 mg 12 hourly	Oral

The *duration of prophylaxis* differs according to the type of involvement. With only arthritis in the initial episode there is relatively a low risk of carditis with recurrences. In such cases penicillin prophylaxis can be discontinued when they reach 21 years of age or after at least 5 years have elapsed since the first attack of acute rheumatic fever. In patients with carditis without residual heart disease (valvular lesion) prophylaxis should be continued for 10 years or well into adulthood (25 years age) whichever is longer. In cases of carditis with residual heart disease prophylaxis should be continued for 10 years or atleast upto 40 years, preferably lifelong.

Advice on Discharge

There should be no restriction of physical activity except in patient with persistent cardiac enlargement who will usually tolerate moderate exercise but may not tolerate vigorous exercise or competitive sports. Patient with RHD is susceptible to infective endocarditis. They should be encouraged to maintain good oral and dental hygiene and should be protected against this condition during dental and other surgical procedures that may result in bacterimia. Maintenance of regular antimicrobial prophylaxis should be properly stressed.

Patient and Parental Guidance

When the diagnosis of acute rheumatic fever is confirmed, the physician should educate the patient and the parents about the disease and need to prevent subsequent streptococcal infection through continuous prophylaxis. The child needs follow-up at regular interval throughout life.

Acquired Valvular Heart Disease

Valvular heart disease may be congenital or acquired. The pathophysiology and clinical manifestations are similar. Almost all acquired valvular diseases are of rheumatic origin. The valvular lesions in rheumatic fever begin as small vegetations composed of fibrin and blood cells along the borders of one or more heart valves. As the inflammation subsides, the vegetations disappear leaving behind scar tissue. With repeated attacks of rheumatic fever, new vegetations form near the previous scars ultimately involving the mural endocardium and chordae tendinae.

Mitral valve involvement occurs in around 75% and aortic valve involvement in 25% of all cases of rheumatic heart disease. Isolated aortic stenosis of rheumatic origin without mitral valve involvement is extremely rare as also tricuspid valve involvement. Rheumatic pulmonary valve involvement never occurs.

MITRAL REGURGITATION

Mitral regurgitation is the most common valvular disease in children. The resultant chronic valvulitis following an attack of rheumatic fever is often mild or moderate in severity and the patient is asymptomatic. More than 50% of the patients who develop acute mitral insufficiency as a result of an attack of acute rheumatic fever cease to have the mitral murmur 1 year later. In children with severe chronic mitral regurgitation however, pulmonary arterial pressure is elevated and patient ultimately has congestive heart failure.

Hemodynamics

In mitral regurgitation, the left atrium receives a regurgitant stream of blood during ventricular systole in addition to the inflow from the pulmonary veins. With ventricular systole, the left atrial pressure rises but due to absence of obstruction at the mitral orifice there is no development of atrial diastolic hypertension. The left ventricle is overfilled in diastole by the augmented volume and an effective output into the aorta is maintained by rapid ejection. The increased stroke volume is expelled at relatively normal pressures and compensation is maintained by the left ventricle at the expense of only a slight increase in cardiac work.

Pulmonary congestion and pulmonary hypertension are not prominent features because pressures do not rise greatly above normal in the left heart except for a systolic peak in the left atrium. The hypervolumic state of the left heart is well tolerated and heart failure tends to develop late in the disease.

Mitral regurgitation which develops during an attack of acute rheumatic fever is of sudden onset. It is accompanied by myocarditis and a poorly functioning left ventricular myocardium. Hence left ventricular failure can occur with relatively moderate leaks as a result of increased left atrial pressure with resultant pulmonary congestion. Acute cardiac failure can lead to transient pulmonary hypertension from which the child recovers with recovery from acute rheumatic fever.

Clinical Manifestations

Symptoms

Children are usually asymptomatic during childhood. May complain of fatigue and palpitation in presence of arrhythmia. With severe mitral regurgitation or acute mitral regurgitation, the child may present with heart failure.

Signs

The signs depend on the severity of the valve involvement. With mild disease, the pulse is normal. The apical impulse is in the normal space corresponding to the age of the child. The precordium is quiet. Auscultation reveals a soft first heart sound, normal second heart sound and a pansystolic murmur in the mitral area which is radiated to the axilla.

With severe mitral regurgitation, there is tachycardia with a high pulse volume. The pulse pressure is wide. The precordium is hyperdynamic. The apical impulse is shifted downward and outward, has a forceful ill sustained character and may be associated with a systolic thrill. As the direction of the regurgitation stream is backward into the left atrium, and the left atrium is not palpable anteriorly, the murmur is usually not palpable as a thrill. The first heart sound is soft or normal; the second heart sound is normal but generally masked by the murmur. The second heart sound in the pulmonary area is widely split but the width of splitting is variable with phases of respiration; narrow during expiration and wider during inspiration. The wide splitting is due to the early aortic component of the second sound. The wide split disappears with failing left ventricle. A third sound is audible at the apex indicating increase early rapid filling of the left ventricle. Classically, there is a pansystolic murmur which radiates to the axilla and back (with involvement of the anterior valve leaflet) or to the lower left sternal border (with involvement of the posterior valve leaflet). There is also a delayed diastolic murmur starting with the third heart sound. This murmur is secondary to the large flow across the mitral valve during diastole.

X-ray Studies

The cardiac shadow is enlarged with a left ventricular configuration and the enlargement depends on the severity of valvular disease. The left atrium is also enlarged which is shown by an elevation of the left bronchus in the PA view and more clearly outlined in a barium swallow esophagus in the right anterior oblique view. In presence of left ventricular failure, there is presence of the prominence of the pulmonary veins in the hilar region and pulmonary congestion. With mild disease, the X-ray study is normal.

Electrocardiography

The ECG shows sinus tachycardia. The QRS axis may be normal or show left axis deviation. Signs of left ventricular hypertrophy are present in long standing cases and severe regurgitation. The ECG is normal in mild cases.

Echocardiography

Two dimensional echocardiography shows varying degrees of left atrial and left ventricular dilatation depending on the severity of mitral regurgitation. Doppler studies can assess the severity of regurgitation.

Course and Complications

Patients with mitral regurgitation are relatively stable for a long time. Mitral stenosis supervenes in some patients. Infective endocarditis is a rare complication. Cardiac failure is precipitated by progression of rheumatic process or infective endocarditis. The effects of chronic mitral regurgitation include congestive heart failure and ventricular arrhythmia which occur usually in adults.

Treatment

Medical

Prophylaxis against recurrence of acute rheumatic fever is all that is necessary in patients with mild mitral regurgitation. In cases with established valve lesion, prophylaxis against infective endocarditis for dental or other surgical procedures should be advised. Treatment of heart failure when necessary. After load reducing agents (captopril, hydralazine) may be used. They reduce the regurgitant volume and preserve left ventricular function.

Surgical

The indications of surgical treatment (i.e. valve replacement) include intractable heart failure due to rheumatic carditis, recurrent episodes of heart failure in spite of adequate medical therapy, dyspnea with moderate activity, and progressive cardiomegaly often with pulmonary hypertension.

MITRAL STENOSIS

Mitral stenosis of rheumatic origin is rare in children because it takes about 5–10 years from the initial attack to develop. In certain parts of the world like India where rheumatic fever is prevalent, severe mitral stenosis has been reported in children younger than 15 years. The mitral valve leaflets are thickened and there is fusion of the commissures. Calcification with immobility of the valve results over time.

Hemodynamics

The essential feature of mitral stenosis is obstruction to blood flow through the mitral valve orifice during diastole. Symptoms are not produced until the area of the valve orifice is reduced to approximately 2.5 cm^2. Signs however are present with lesser degree of stenosis. The patients become bedridden when the valve orifice area is less than 1 cm^2.

With *mild to moderate mitral stenosis,* the forward flow through the mitral valve remains normal. In significant mitral stenosis the blood flow to the left ventricle is diminished and the volume of blood and the pressure in the left atrium increases. High atrial pressure results in compensatory hypertrophy and increased contraction of the left atrium with resultant increased pressure gradient across the valve. This partially compensates for the obstruction. The left atrium is a thin walled chamber and the capacity for hypertrophy is limited. Later, pulmonary hypertension causes right ventricular hypertension and secondary right ventricular hypertrophy. The right ventricular hypertrophy is concentric without increase in the size.

Compensation occurs at the expense of muscular hypertrophy and increased work of the left atrium and right ventricle. Left atrial decompensation occur early because its walls are relatively thin. Atrial fibrillation is common. Left ventricular failure is followed by right heart failure.

With *significant mitral stenosis*, an adequate cardiac output can only be maintained with an elevation of left atrial pressure. As there are no valves at the openings of the pulmonary veins in the left atrium, the increased left atrial pressure is transmitted to the pulmonary veins. The increased pulmonary venous pressure results in pulmonary capillary engorgement, pulmonary congestion and increased pulmonary arterial pressure with constriction of pulmonary arterioles.

Clinical Features

The child with mitral stenosis may present with dyspnea on exertion, attacks of acute pulmonary edema, paroxysmal nocturnal dyspnea and orthopnoea.

Dyspnea on Exertion

Dyspnea on exertion may be of four grades. In grade I symptoms are provoked by more than average activity, e.g., running, walking up hills, playing outdoor games etc. In grade II symptoms occur on ordinary activity, e.g., walking at an average pace or upto two flights of stairs, dancing, carrying a shopping basket or any form of manual labour. In grade III symptoms develop with less than ordinary physical activity. Grade IV means total incapacity.

Acute Pulmonary Edema

Acute pulmonary edema occurs with an average grade of stenosis, relatively early in course before the protective mechanisms have time to develop.

The protective mechanisms or complications tending to prevent acute pulmonary edema in mitral stenosis are increase pulmonary vascular resistance, development of a capillary alveolar interstitial barrier, bronchopulmonary venous shunt and atrial fibrillation controlled by digitalis.

The precipitating factors are effort, emotion, respiratory infections, uncontrolled atrial fibrillation and anesthesia.

There is tachycardia, a rise in cardiac output, the left atrial pressure is raised with a normal pulmonary vascular resistance and altered capillary permeability (as a result of some neurogenic or chemical disturbance). There is increased capillary permeability and transudation of fluid into the interstitial space and alveoli. As the attack proceeds the arterial oxygen saturation falls. With severe anoxia there is a sharp rise in pulmonary vascular resistance which will lower the capillary pressure and terminate the attack.

Clinically, the attack starts insidiously and it can be divided into 4 stages. In stage I, there is dyspnea, orthopnoea and gentle repetitive cough. In stage II, suddenly dyspnea becomes severe accompanied by wheeze. The face becomes pale. There is tachycardia, blood pressure rises, and extremities turn cold and blue. In stage III, patient becomes greatly distressed and frightened. Widespread fine crepitations are present with expectoration of frothy white or pink sputum. In stage IV, there is increasingly lowering of oxygen saturation. Central cyanosis appears, blood pressure falls, and skin becomes grey, cold and wet, pulse imperceptible and respiration shallow.

Paroxysmal Dyspnea

Paroxysmal dyspnea is characterized by sudden attacks of dyspnea with wheeze. It may occur during the day but it is more common at night. The pathogenesis is similar to acute pulmonary edema with a difference. There is development of a physical barrier between the capillaries and alveoli. The capillary wall, interstitial tissue, and the alveolar basement membrane become thickened. When there is transudation of fluid it cannot enter the alveoli although it may pass into the interstitial space. These changes however, protect the patient from developing attacks of acute pulmonary edema.

Orthopnoea

Orthopnoea occurs in patients with grade III or IV dyspnea. The child is dyspneic in lying down position, gets relief in sitting posture. Sitting up especially with the legs down lowers the right atrial pressure and thus diminishes the output of the right ventricle. This in turn lowers the left atrial pressure and therefore the pulmonary venous and capillary pressures. In the horizontal position these effects are reversed which encourages transudation of fluid from the pulmonary capillaries into the interstitial tissue.

Signs

The signs of mitral stenosis consist of those directly related to the valve lesion and others to secondary hemodynamic disturbances.

1. The arterial pulse is small and blood pressure is often low. The jugular venous pulse show prominent 'a' waves when there is pulmonary hypertension with a regular rhythm. A general rise of venous pressure occurs when there is right heart failure.
2. With high pulmonary vascular resistance, there is peripheral cyanosis in the face and hands due to peripheral vasoconstriction secondary to low cardiac output. In advanced pulmonary hypertension the hands may be warm and the palms bright red as a result of impaired hepatic function.
3. There is often a bulging in the left precordium. A cardiac impulse may be seen in the left parasternal region (right ventricular hypertrophy). The apex is seen as a separate pulsation further to the left. The apex beat, on palpation, is localized in the region of the mid clavicular line or the anterior axillary line and felt as a sharp tap. It is commonly accompanied with a diastolic thrill. The tapping character is due to the loud first heart sound. A forceful and sustained pulsation (heave) in the left parasternal region and an epigastric pulsation may be felt due to right ventricular hypertrophy. The second sound is palpable over the pulmonary area. The presence of a parasternal heave and a palpable second sound is indicative of presence of pulmonary hypertension.
4. On auscultation, *the first sound is sharp and loud.* It can be heard all over the precordium but it is loudest at the mitral area. The late diastolic atrioventricular pressure gradient forces the mitral valve cusps to remain wide open to the end of diastole, so that when the left ventricular contraction starts the valve cusps suddenly close. This results in a loud first heart sound. The first heart sound may be soft when it is calcified. The second heart sound is loud in the pulmonary area. The pulmonary component is particularly loud in presence of pulmonary hypertension. An additional sound, *the opening snap,* occurs shortly after the second heart sound and is heard loudest just internal to the apex. It is present in cases with pure or dominant mitral stenosis. It is produced by the aortic cusp of the mitral valve when it is flung open into the cavity of the left ventricle as the atrioventricular pressure gradient is reversed at the end of the period of isometric relaxation. A *low pitched, rumbling mid diastolic murmur* follows the opening snap. This

murmur is best heard by the bell of the stethoscope placed lightly over the apex , with the patient reclining and slightly tilted to the left side. The mid diastolic murmur is short in mild cases, but in moderate and severe stenosis it continues throughout diastole. With normal rhythm, the mid diastolic murmur merges with a presystolic sharp, crescendo murmur which is readily heard after exercise. The murmurs may disappear in presence of severe pulmonary hypertension, atrial fibrillation and a very low cardiac output. The opening snap may be the only sign of mitral stenosis in such cases.

5. In combined mitral stenosis and regurgitation, the signs depend on relative dominance of regurgitation or stenosis. The signs of stenosis are modified in presence of regurgitation. The apex is less localized and it tends to be hyperdynamic as well as left ventricular in character. The first sound and the opening snap are softer. A pansystolic murmur is present, in addition to the mid diastolic murmur. With severe mitral regurgitation, the opening snap is replaced by presence of a third heart sound. Absence of an apical pansystolic murmur, on the other hand indicates that there is no significant regurgitation.
6. Clinical assessment of severity has been taken over by echocardiography which can provide a precise assessment of the severity. Clinically the following findings can help in assessment of severity.
   (a) Distance between the opening snap and the aortic component of the second sound. The closer the opening snap to the second sound, the more severe the stenosis.
   (b) Mild pulmonary arterial hypertension can be present in all degrees of mitral stenosis–mild, moderate and severe. Presence of severe pulmonary hypertension always indicates severe mitral stenosis.
   (c) The intensity or duration of the diastolic murmur does not correlate with the severity. Both mild and severe mitral stenosis can have soft murmurs.

X-ray Studies

There is enlargement of the left atrium, the left atrial appendage and the right ventricle. The left ventricle may be enlarged in presence of mitral regurgitation and severe carditis. A greatly enlarged right ventricle that is occupying the apex may erroneously interpret an apparent enlargement of the left ventricle. On a PA view chest X-ray, the enlarged left atrium may be seen as a hump below the right hilum giving a double contour of the right border of the heart and pushes the left bronchus upon the left side of the heart. In the lateral or oblique views the dilated left atrium displaces the barium filled esophagus backwards best seen in the right oblique view. The enlargement of the left atrial appendage is seen as a conspicuous bulge on the left border just below the pulmonary arc. It leads to straightening of the left border also described as mitralisation of the left border (Fig. 13.9). The enlargement of the right ventricle is more easily recognized clinically and by electrocardiography than by radiology. In advanced cases, the right atrium may also be enlarged. The aorta tends to be small and the pulmonary artery large. The dilatation of pulmonary artery is due to pulmonary hypertension and its degree is proportional to pulmonary vascular resistance.

The lungs show varying degrees of venous congestion. It is usually visible as a fan shaped mottling in the hilar region. The hilar shadows are large and the clear outline of vessels is usually blurred. The peripheral lung field loose normal translucency with redistribution of blood flow to the upper lobes and show a fine reticulation and occasionally large miliary shadows due to hemosiderosis. The lung parenchyma in the costophrenic angles shows horizontal threadlike lines in cases of long standing congestion (Kerley's lines). These are believed to represent edematous interlobular septa.

Electrocardiography

The P wave is bifid and widened to 0.12 second (called P mitrale) in lead II and left sided chest leads, in moderate and severe cases of mitral stenosis. The first peak represents right atrial activation and the second left atrial activation. The voltage is normal. The P wave is normal in mild cases. The P wave may be tall and peaked in mitral stenosis with pulmonary hypertension. The QRS complex is essentially normal in uncomplicated cases. It may show right axis deviation and right ventricular hypertrophy in presence of pulmonary hypertension.

Echocardiography

The echocardiography shows decreased EF slope, paradoxical posterior leaflet motion, left atrial enlargement and pulmonary arterial hypertension. 2D echo can identify the narrow mitral opening. Doppler echo provides transmitral gradient. An echocardiogram combined with Doppler study can give a precise assessment of severity of mitral stenosis.

Complications

The child with mitral stenosis may present with the following complications:

Hemoptysis

Hemoptysis may occur in various forms due to different causes. Sudden unexpected profuse hemorrhage, also known as pulmonary apoplexy is attributed to rupture of a small intrapulmonary bronchial vein or a dilated pleuro-hilar vein. Blood stained frothy sputum is associated with attacks of paroxysmal dyspnea and acute pulmonary edema which is also known as congestive hemoptysis. Frank blood hemoptysis may result due to pulmonary infarction.

Chest Pain

Chest pain is not a common feature in mitral stenosis. It may be psychogenic and reflects anxiety about the heart condition. It may be due to cardiac enlargement or a true ischemic pain as result of coronary insufficiency due to decreased cardiac output, pulmonary hypertension.

Dysphagia

Dysphagia may occur from pressure on the esophagus by an enlarged left atrium.

Left Recurrent Laryngeal Nerve Palsy

Left recurrent laryngeal nerve palsy *(Ortner's syndrome),* characterized by hoarseness of voice may occur due to paralysis of the left recurrent laryngeal nerve from pressure by the enlarged left atrium.

Peripheral Thromboembolism

Peripheral thromboembolism may occur in patients with mild mitral stenosis but occurs more commonly in patients with atrial fibrillation. The medium sized cerebral and limb vessels are frequently occluded. Aphasia with hemiplegia, a common sequel to middle cerebral artery embolism may be transient or permanent. Multiple emboli in the kidneys may cause systemic hypertension. Splenic and mesenteric infarction can occur. A massive clot can occlude the aorta causing severe pain in legs, buttocks and abdomen. Occasionally a massive clot may occlude the narrow mitral orifice and cause sudden death. Recurrent attacks of syncope may result from a ball valve thrombus causing intermittent occlusion of the mitral orifice.

Atrial Fibrillation

Atrial fibrillation occurs in majority of cases of mitral stenosis. Rare in children. *Bacterial endocarditis* is a very rare complication of mitral stenosis.

Management

Medical

Medical management include:

1. Good dental hygiene and antibiotic prophylaxis against infective endocarditis.
2. Prevention of recurrence of rheumatic fever by penicillin prophylaxis.
3. Treatment of acute pulmonary edema, heart failure.
4. Treatment of atrial fibrillation which consist of anticoagulation and cardioversion. Anticoagulation with warfarin should be started 3 weeks before cardio-version to prevent systemic embolisation of atrial thrombus. Anticoagulation is continued for 4 weeks after restoration of sinus rhythm. Digoxin is to be given to slow down ventricular rate and quinidine should be started 2 days before cardioversion. Quinidine may prevent recurrence.

Surgical

The indications of surgery include:

1. Symptomatic patients (dyspnea grade II or more, acute pulmonary edema, paroxysmal nocturnal dyspnea).
2. Recurrent atrial fibrillation, thromboembolic phenomenon and hemoptysis.

AORTIC REGURGITATION

Rheumatic valvulitis is the most common cause of aortic regurgitation. Isolated rheumatic aortic regurgitation is rare. Most cases have associated mitral valvular disease. The semi lunar valves are deformed and shortened and the valve ring is dilated so that the cusps fail to appose tightly. Bacterial endocarditis may be rarely a primary cause.

Hemodynamics

In aortic regurgitation, there is a backward leak of blood from the aorta into the left ventricle during diastole. This results in an increase in the left ventricular blood volume as well as increase in the size of the left ventricle. Because of the backward flow, the forward flow is impaired. There is compensatory peripheral vasodilatation as well as increased ejection from the left ventricle during early part of systole. There is a compensatory increase in systolic blood pressure and the diastolic pressure is low from the aortic backflow and peripheral vasodilatation. The resulting wide pulse pressure is manifested in the form of exaggerated arterial and arteriolar pulsations. The wider the pulse pressure more is the leak.

With mild regurgitation, pulse pressure is normal. In severe degree the diastolic pressure may be zero. Moderate degree regurgitation with good left ventricular myocardial function is tolerated well. With a failing left ventricular myocardium, the diastolic pressure goes up. This results in an increase in the left atrial pressure and pulmonary congestion.

Significant dilatation of the left ventricle will result in abnormal stress on the mitral valve–papillary muscle complex. This in turn will result in inadequate apposition of the mitral leaflets and mitral regurgitation.

Clinical Manifestations

Symptoms

A mild to moderate degree of aortic regurgitation does not produce symptoms. In severe degree, the initial symptom is dyspnea on exertion and palpitation. There may be excessive sweating and heat intolerance. Dyspnea on exertion can progress to pulmonary edema, paroxysmal dyspnea and orthopnoea if left ventricular failure is not treated. Angina may be precipitated by heavy exercise.

Signs

In mild cases an aortic early diastolic murmur may be the only sign of aortic regurgitation. In severe aortic regurgitation the combination of water hammer collapsing pulse, enlarged left ventricle and an early diastolic murmur are characteristic.

The pulse pressure is wide with a rise in the systolic pressure and a low diastolic pressure. With severe regurgitation, the diastolic pressure may be recorded zero. More is the leak wider is the pulse pressure.

The pulse rises steeply in systole and gives a characteristic tap to the palpating finger which is described as a water hammer. The rapid fall of pressure produces a collapsing quality. These signs are best appreciated by palpating the radial or brachial arteries with the flat of the fingers when the arm is elevated above the level of the heart. The other evidences of wide pulse pressure include prominent carotid pulsation (Corrigan's sign), visible pulsation in the peripheral arteries and arteriolar pulses in the nail beds, uvula, lips, ear lobes and retina. The other peripheral signs include:

1. *De Musset's sign* characterized by nodding of head with each systole due to sudden filling of carotid vessels in severe aortic regurgitation.
2. *Hill's sign,* an exaggeration of difference of systolic pressure between the brachial and femoral arteries. Normally the pressure difference is less than 20 mmHg, being more in the femorals. A systolic pressure difference more than 60 mmHg indicates severe aortic regurgitation. If the pressure difference is between 40 and 60 mmHg it suggests moderate and a pressure difference between 20 and 40 suggests mild aortic regurgitation.
3. *Pistol shot sound,* i.e., a sharp tapping sound can be heard over the femoral or brachial arteries on auscultation over these arteries in moderate and severe aortic regurgitation.
4. *Duroziez's sign* is characterized by presence of a combination of a systolic and diastolic murmurs over the brachial or femoral arteries. The systolic murmur can be heard on partial occlusion of the artery with pressure applied proximal to the chest piece and a diastolic murmur can be heard with pressure applied distal to the chest piece.

Examination of the Heart

The precordium is hyperdynamic. The heart is enlarged. The *apex* is shifted down and out. It is forceful and ill sustained. The size of the heart depends on the degree of the aortic leak. A *diastolic thrill* is occasionally present in the third left intercostal space. The first sound is decreased in intensity. The second sound is normal. There is an early diastolic murmur which begins immediately with the second heart sound and continues till late in diastole. It is heard loudest in the left 3rd and 4th intercostal space with radiation to the apex and beyond. It is a high pitched, decrescendo murmur. The murmur of aortic regurgitation is best heard in the 3rd and 4th left intercostal space because the aortic valves are situated below this area. With severe aortic regurgitation, there is also an ejection systolic murmur heard at the 2nd right intercostal space conducted to the neck and not infrequently associated with a systolic thrill. This murmur is a result of a large stroke volume passing across rough semi lunar valves. In some patients a short mid diastolic murmur may be heard at the mitral area–the *Austin Flint murmur*. It has been ascribed to the regurgitant flow from the aortic valve pushing back the aortic cusp of mitral valve in diastole, causing obstruction to the mitral orifice.

X-ray Studies

There is enlargement of the heart with left ventricular configuration with a dilated ascending aorta and a prominent aortic knob in severe cases. Pulmonary venous congestion develops if left ventricular failure supervenes.

Electrocardiography

The ECG is normal in mild cases. In moderate to severe cases there is left ventricular hypertrophy. Left atrial hypertrophy may be present in long standing cases.

Echocardiography

Can study the dimension of the heart chambers. Color Doppler examination can aid in estimating the severity of the regurgitation.

Course and Complications

Unlike mitral regurgitation, aortic regurgitation does not regress. Patients with combined lesion of aortic and mitral regurgitation during an attack of acute rheumatic fever may have only the aortic component after 1–2 years. Patients may remain asymptomatic for a long time, but once symptoms begin to develop, many patients deteriorate rapidly. Recurrence of rheumatic carditis may precipitate heart failure. Infective endocarditis is a rare complication.

Treatment

Medical

Medical treatment consist of:

1. Prophylaxis against recurrence of acute rheumatic fever and infective endocarditis.
2. Activity need not be restricted in mild cases, but moderate to severe degree aortic regurgitation requires avoiding hard physical effort especially competitive games.
3. Afterload reducers, viz., captopril, hydralazine when used on long-term basis has shown to reduce (or even reverse) the dilatation and hypertrophy of the left ventricle in children with aortic regurgitation without failure.

Surgical

The physical findings which have been used as indications for valve replacement are presence of:

1. Symptoms such as anginal pain or dyspnea on exertion.
2. Significant cardiomegaly (cardiothoracic ratio > 55% on chest X-ray), ejection fraction < 40%, or stress test induced symptoms even in asymptomatic patients.

AORTIC STENOSIS

Isolated aortic stenosis of rheumatic origin is extremely rare. It may occur in combination with aortic incompetence or mitral stenosis.

Hemodynamics

Changes in the circulation can occur when the orifice of the aortic valve is reduced to ¼ of the normal size. The ejection phase is prolonged and aortic valve closure is delayed. A systolic pressure gradient develops which may be any thing between a few mm upto 150 mm depending on the severity of stenosis. To maintain the stroke volume and cardiac output, great force is required. The left ventricle is initially hypertrophied and then dilated in the late stages. The low mean aortic pressure prevents the coronary blood flow from keeping pace with the increased demands of the left ventricle.

Clinical Manifestations

Symptoms

Mild to moderate aortic stenosis causes no symptoms. Severe stenosis causes characteristic symptoms which appear late in the course of the disease. Symptoms and signs result from decreased cardiac output, decreased coronary flow and heart failure.

Dyspnea on exertion is usually the first symptom and gradually progresses to orthopnoea, acute pulmonary edema and paroxysmal dyspnea as a result of left ventricular failure. There may be cardiac pain on effort which occurs as a result of coronary insufficiency due to low cardiac output. It is indistinguishable from angina pectoris. The reduced cardiac output may also result in attacks of dizziness; blackout or even syncope characteristically provoked by effort but may occur as a result of changes in posture, or peripheral vasodilatation without any provoking factor. Syncopal attacks may be severe and frequent.

Signs

1. The *pulse* is of small volume and slowly rising. The pulse tracing show a notch in the ascending limb (anacrotic pulse). The blood pressure is low or normal. The venous pulse is normal.
2. On palpation, the *apex beat* is normally placed or down and out indicating enlargement. It is heaving (i.e. forceful and sustained) in character and there may be a *systolic thrill* at the base of the heart which is well transmitted to the neck. On auscultation, the first and second sounds are normally heard in the mitral area. The aortic component of the second sound may be soft or absent in the aortic area. The physiological splitting of the second sound is seldom heard. This may be due to prolongation of left ventricular systole making the two sounds coincide, or to reversal of the normal order of valve closure making the earlier pulmonary component difficult to detect in the systolic murmur. There is an *ejection systolic murmur* of more than grade III in the aortic area conducted to the neck. The same murmur is transmitted to the apex where it may be as loud as in the aortic area, and occasionally may be loudest at the apex. The murmur is frequently preceded by an ejection click.
3. In acute rheumatic valvulitis, there is a soft or moderately loud ejection systolic murmur but no abnormal pulse or evidence of left ventricular hypertrophy.
4. A combined aortic stenosis and aortic regurgitation is frequent when the etiology is rheumatic. Regurgitation in the younger age group may change to dominant stenosis in later years. In such cases, the physical signs of both lesions may be present and the pulse frequently has a double impulse (pulsus bisferiens). The presence of pulsus bisferiens indicates dominance of aortic regurgitation. A decision regarding dominance is important to select cases for aortic valvotomy.
5. In combined aortic valve disease and mitral stenosis, the signs of dominant mitral valve stenosis damp all the signs of aortic valve disease which become more evident after mitral valvotomy.

X-ray Studies

In uncomplicated cases, the heart size is normal as there is pure concentric hypertrophy. The ascending aorta is usually prominent due to post stenotic dilatation which may be confined to the proximal part of the ascending aorta. If left ventricular failure has developed, then the heart enlarges due to dilatation and the radiological signs of left ventricular failure develop.

Electrocardiography

The ECG is helpful in assessing the degree of left ventricular hypertrophy and therefore the severity of aortic stenosis. The standard leads show the concordant pattern of left ventricular preponderance with tall R wave. Deep S-T depression and T wave inversion are a feature in the left sided chest leads. There may be left bundle branch block. The rhythm is usually normal but prolonged AV conduction and dissociation is not uncommon.

Course and Complications

The course of patients with aortic stenosis may be long and benign. A systolic murmur may have been heard in childhood and passed as innocent. An anacrotic pulse and left ventricular hypertrophy may not develop upto middle age. But once symptoms of cardiac failure develop, the course is usually downhill.

Bacterial endocarditis can occur at any time during the course, even in the early stages. Sudden death is not infrequent once symptoms have developed.

Treatment

Medical

1. Avoidance of hard physical effort, especially competitive games in mild to moderate cases.
2. Measures for prevention of recurrence of rheumatic fever and prevention of infective endocarditis.
3. Treatment of heart failure.

Surgical

Surgical treatment with valve replacement is indicated in severe aortic stenosis with ischemic pain, syncopal attacks and/or evidence of left ventricular failure.

TRICUSPID REGURGITATION

In majority of cases, tricuspid regurgitation is functional secondary to right ventricular dilatation with expansion of the tricuspid ring which may occur as a result of pulmonary hypertension or right ventricular failure due to any cause.

Clinical Manifestations

Symptoms

The child usually present with the symptoms of the underlying disease. The symptoms that are directly related to the leak are venous throbbing in the neck and abdomen. In advanced cases there may be symptoms of hepatic failure.

Signs

The physical signs include:

1. A systolic pulsation of the liver synchronous with the large *'v'* wave, best elicited by bimanual palpation of the liver.
2. A hyperdynamic, right ventricular thrust.
3. A pansystolic murmur with or without a thrill. The murmur may be heard anywhere from the left sternal edge to the apex. The intensity varies with respiration, being louder in inspiration. Sometimes there may be a short functional mid diastolic murmur as well.

X-ray Studies

Show dilatation of right atrium.

Electrocardiography

Electrocardiography may show right ventricular preponderance which is usually caused by the primary lesion.

Course and Prognosis

The course and prognosis depends on the primary lesion rather than the leak.

Treatment

1. Control of heart failure.
2. Treatment of the cause.

TRICUSPID STENOSIS

Majority of tricuspid valve stenosis is nearly always a result of rheumatic valvulitis but clinical tricuspid stenosis is infrequently recognized. It is nearly always accompanied by mitral stenosis and often by aortic valve disease. Acquired tricuspid stenosis is extremely rare. Congenital cases have been reported.

Clinical Manifestations

Symptoms

The first symptom may be discomfort in the neck due to the jugular venous pulsation. More often the venous pulse is seen in the mirror or noted by a relative. In severe cases there may be fatigue, obvious swelling of the abdomen due to enlargement of the liver and /or presence of ascites. Presence of tricuspid stenosis along with mitral stenosis relieves the patient of the distressing complications of mitral stenosis, viz., acute pulmonary edema, orthopnoea and paroxysmal dyspnea.

Signs

The signs of tricuspid stenosis include:

1. With normal rhythm, there is a giant *a* wave in the jugular venous pulse and a presystolic hepatic pulsation. In presence of atrial fibrillation, there is a prominent *v* wave with no *y* dip.
2. The precordium is quiet. The first heart sound in the tricuspid area is not convincingly loud. A tricuspid opening snap may be heard. The intensity of both these sounds is increased in inspiration. The pulmonary second sound is not accentuated. A presystolic or diastolic murmur which is sharply accentuated during inspiration can be heard at the left sternal edge in the 4th space. It is accompanied with a thrill.
3. In long standing cases, there may be recurrent ascites, hepatomegaly and signs of right heart failure.

X-ray Studies

Show enlargement of the right atrium without conspicuous dilatation of the pulmonary artery. The lung fields are relatively clear.

Electrocardiography

In cases with normal rhythm there is a combination of an unusually tall and wide P wave (Combined P pulmonale and P mitrale) and absence of right ventricular preponderance.

Treatment

Medical treatment includes treatment of edema and ascites. Pure or dominant stenosis should undergo surgery.

Cardiac Arrhythmias

Cardiac arrhythmias in children are not as common as in adults. The incidence of serious cardiac arrhythmias is around 5%. Increased vigilance of pediatricians and pediatric cardiologists and advances in recording technologies, viz., 24 hours ambulatory ECG monitoring have lead to increased recognition of arrhythmias in children. In addition, there is an increased incidence as more and more children undergo complex cardiac surgery for congenital heart disease.

The Conducting System

Cardiac arrhythmias are abnormalities of the conducting system of the heart. The conducting system comprise the sinoatrial (SA) node, internodal tracts connecting the SA node to the atrioventricular (AV) node, bundle of His and purkinjee fibres. These tissues have the ability to spontaneously generate impulses. The rate of impulse generation is fastest in the SA node and normally it dictates the rate and rhythm of the heart beat. The impulse generated in the SA node spreads throughout the atria and to the AV node, from where it passes via the bundle of His to supply both ventricles through the purkinjee fibres.

If the SA node ceases to function, the intrinsic rhythmicity of the AV node takes over at a slower rate (50–60/min in older children and 100/min in infants). If the AV node and bundle of His also cease to conduct impulse, the ventricles produce their own idioventricular rhythm (30–40/min). Cardiac arrhythmias can result from anomalous development or injury to any segment resulting in abnormal initiation or propagation of electrical activity.

Heart Rates in Normal Infants and Children

The cardiac arrhythmias are abnormalities of rate and rhythm. In children the normal heart rate is influenced by age, activity level and the clinical condition. Hence one should be aware of the normal heart rates.

Age	*Awake /min*	*Mean /min*	*Sleeping rate /min*
Newborn to 3 months	85 to 205	140	80–160
3 months to 2 years	100 to 190	130	75–160
2 years to 10 years	60 to 140	80	60–90
Above 10 years	60 to 100	75	50–90

Source: PALS provider manual.

The Electrocardiogram (ECG)

Most cardiac arrhythmias can be diagnosed by careful study of a standard 12 lead ECG with a long rhythm strip. The surface ECG is a graphic representation of the sequence of myocardial depolarization and repolarization. Each normal cardiac cycle consists of a P wave, a QRS complex and a T wave. The first deflection on surface ECG, the P wave represents the depolarization of both atria. The time required for depolarization to pass through the atria, the AV node, and the bundle of His is represented by the PR interval. The QRS complex represents depolarization of the ventricular myocardium. Ventricular repolarization is characterized as the ST segment and the T wave. On a normal ECG of good quality one can visualize the P waves, the QRS complexes and the T waves (Fig. 14.5).

The Normal ECG Tracings

The normal ECG tracings differ according to the age of the child. The ECG tracings of the newly borns and

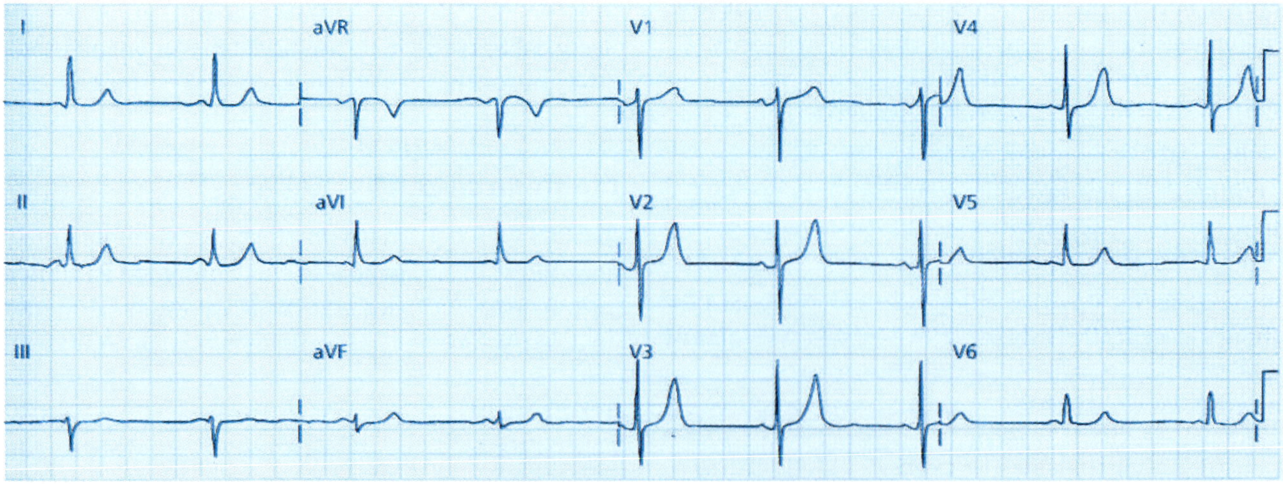

Fig. 14.5: Standard 12 lead normal ECG

neonates normally shows right axis deviation and right ventricular dominance (the right ventricular voltages are greater than the left, although they do not exceed normal limits). Between 1 month and 3 years of age, ECG tracings are intermediate, but usually show left ventricular dominance. Children three years and older should have ECG tracings that resemble that of an adult ECG.

The age related changes are mostly related to the changes in the ratio of left ventricle (LV) to right ventricle (RV) weight. At birth the right ventricle is thicker than the left ventricle. At birth, the LV/RV ratio is 1.5: 1. The ratio reaches to about 2:1 by 6 months of age and 2.5:1 by young adulthood.

Types of Cardiac Arrhythmias

The different types of cardiac arrhythmias common in children may be as follows:

1. **Sinus node dysfunction:** Sinus tachycardia, sinus bradycardia, sinus arrhythmia, extrasystoles, premature atrial complexes, and premature ventricular complexes.
2. **Tachyarrhythmias:** Supraventricular tachycardia (SVT), atrial flutter, atrial fibrillation, ventricular tachycardia and ventricular fibrillation.
3. **Bradyarrhythmias:** Sinoatrial block, sick sinus syndrome, atrioventricular block (first degree, second degree and complete heart blocks).

Sinus Tachycardia

Sinus tachycardia is defined as a sinus rhythm at a rate faster than that normal for age. The rate varies periodically with respiration, crying and struggling. It is commonly seen in conditions like fever, pain or anxiety, severe anemia, hypoxemia, hypovolemia, hyperthyroidism. To correct sinus tachycardia, the cause should be treated.

Sinus Bradycardia

Sinus bradycardia is defined as a slow sinus rhythm with a heart rate below 90/ minute in neonates and less than 60/minute thereafter. It may be seen in normal children and athletes and has no pathological significance. The other causes include excessive vagal stimulation (induced by suctioning or tracheal intubation), hypothermia, drugs (digoxin, calcium channel blockers or beta blocker overdose), congenital heart block, congenital heart surgery, myocarditis, increased intracranial pressure.

It should be differentiated from AV block. Children with sinus bradycardia are able to increase their heart rate with exercise to much higher than 100 beats / minute, whereas patients with AV block are usually unable to do so. Asymptomatic sinus bradycardia does not require any treatment. Symptomatic sinus bradycardia usually responds to intravenous atropine 0.6–1.2 mg.

Sinus Arrhythmia

Sinus arrhythmia is characterized by slowing of heart rate during expiration and acceleration during inspiration. It is the most common cause of irregular heartbeat in children. It is a consequence of normal parasympathetic nervous system activity. It is pronounced in the preterm infants, during recovery from febrile episodes and following drugs that enhance vagal tone.

The ECG shows varying RR intervals with normal QRS complexes preceded by a P wave and a constant PR interval.

Extrasystoles

Extrasystoles are produced by a discharge from an ectopic focus located anywhere in the atria, ventricles or junctional tissues. Isolated extrasystoles are of no clinical significance. It may occur due to digitalis toxicity and myocarditis.

Premature Atrial Complexes (PAC)

Premature atrial complexes are common during childhood. These may be present even in absence of heart disease. They are asymptomatic and do not require treatment. In infants frequent contractions may trigger supraventricular tachycardia or atrial fibrillation.

The ECG findings include a premature P wave having a different configuration from the normal P waves preceding a normal QRS complex. There is no compensatory pause.

Premature Ventricular Complexes (PVC)

Premature ventricular complexes may be seen in 15% of normal newborns and one third of normal adolescents in the absence of cardiac pathology. When PVCs are frequent, they may assume a definite rhythm, e.g., alternating with normal beats (bigamy) or occurring after two normal beats (trigamy).

PVCs in normal children can be caused by fever, anxiety, use of stimulants, caffeine, and electrolyte imbalance. In normal individuals they disappear during tachycardia or exercise. If they persist or become more frequent during exercise, the arrhythmia may have greater significance.

ECG characteristics include premature, widened, bizarre QRS complexes that are not preceded by a P wave. It is usually followed by a compensatory pause.

PVCs may degenerate into more severe arrhythmia when it is associated with an underlying heart disease. It is multifocal, increases with exercise, and associated with marked anxiety. Such patients need investigations and treatment. More than 50% of such cases are associated with evidence of organic heart disease. These patients require IV lidocaine drip followed by maintenance with antiarrhythmic drugs like propranolol.

Supraventricular Tachycardias (SVTs)

SVTs include a group of regular tachycardias that have a similar appearance on an ECG. Eighty percent of the affected children present in the first year of life. In approximately 70% cases, the heart is normal. An idiopathic type of SVT occurs in young infants. The remainder has associated congenital heart disease viz. Ebstein's anomaly, corrected TGA, and VSD, mitral valve prolapse, myocarditis or bacterial sepsis and following cardiac surgery.

SVTs involve components of the conduction system within or above the bundle of His and can be divided into three major categories: atrial tachycardia, nodal tachycardia and atrioventricular re-entrant tachycardia.

Atrioventricular re-entrant tachycardia is the most common mechanism of SVT and also the most common tachyarrhythmia in children. In SVT caused by reentry, two pathways are involved: one of these is the AV node and the other is an accessory pathway. The accessory pathway consists of an abnormal band of conducting tissue which connects the atria and ventricles (Bundle of Kent) or only a functional bypass tract. The band of conducting tissues resembles the Purkinjee tissue in its physiology, and in that it conducts very rapidly. Patients with accessory tract frequently have Wolff-Parkinson-White (WPW) syndrome.

Atrial tachycardia is a rare mechanism of SVT in which a rapid firing of a single focus in the atrium is responsible for the tachycardia. *Nodal tachycardia* may superficially resemble atrial tachycardia but the rate is relatively slower (120–200/minute).

Clinical Manifestations

Atrioventricular re-entrant SVT is characterized by an abrupt onset and cessation of tachycardia. It may be precipitated by an acute infection, exposure to sympathomimetic amines contained in decongestants. It usually occurs in the patient at rest. The attacks may last only for a few seconds or may persist for hours. The heart rate usually exceeds 180/minute but may be occasionally as rapid as 300/ minute. However, the clinical manifestation depends on the age of the child.

In the older child, the only complain may be awareness of the rapid heart rate. If the rate is exceptionally high and the attack is prolonged there may be precordial discomfort and heart failure may supervene.

Infants with SVT usually present with heart failure because the tachycardia goes unrecognized for a long time as they are unable to communicate. The heart rate during the paroxysm is 200–300/minute. If the attack continues for 6–24 hours or more with an extremely rapid heart rate, the child becomes acutely ill with restlessness, irritability, with an ashen colour. Tachypnea and hepatomegaly are the prominent signs of cardiac failure. There may be fever and leucocytosis.

If tachycardia occurs in the fetus, it can cause heart failure and hydrops fetalis.

The ECG shows a regular rate of 220–300/minute with narrow QRS complexes and absent or abnormal P waves. In about 5% cases, conduction within the ventricles is abnormal and the QRS complex is widened, mimicking ventricular tachycardia. SVT may be confused with sinus tachycardia. A heart rate above 220/minute and the paroxysms of abrupt onset and termination excludes sinus tachycardia.

The typical ECG tracings in WPW syndrome are usually seen when the patient is not having tachycardia. They include a short PR interval, and a slow upstroke of QRS (delta wave). This syndrome is most often present in a normal heart but it may be associated with congenital heart diseases like Ebstein's anomaly.

Treatment

Asymptomatic brief attacks do not require any treatment. To abolish the paroxysm, vagal stimulation is the mainstay of treatment. The safest and easiest method of vagal stimulation is to place of bag of ice cold water over the face. In the older children, this can be done by submersion of the face in iced saline. Older children may also be taught vagotonic maneuvers like valsalva maneuver, breath holding, carotid sinus massage and drinking ice water.

When these fail in a stable patient, adenosine is the drug of choice for pharmacological cardioversion. The starting

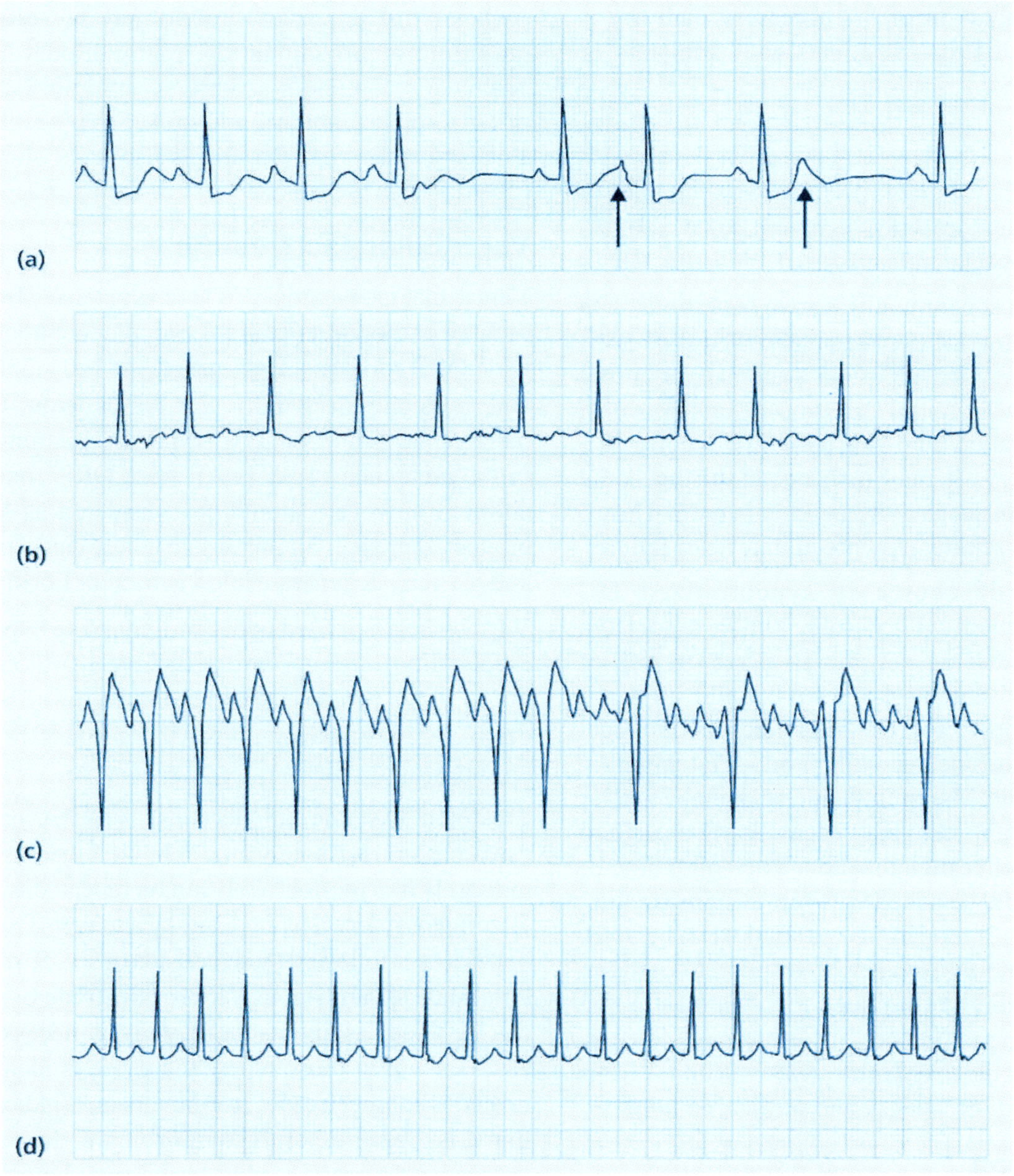

Fig. 14.6: ECG tracings in (a) Ectopic beats (b) Atrial fibrillation (c) Atrial flutter (d) AV junctional re-entrant tachycardia

dose is 100 microgram/kg, followed if necessary by increments of 50 micrograms/kg every 2 minutes as IV bolus till a maximum dose of 250 microgram / kg. Adenosine terminates SVT in 90–100% cases but reinitiation may occur in 25–30%. Verapamil (0.1–0.3 mg/kg rapidly over 15–30 seconds with a further half dose repeated after 10 minutes) may be used in children above one year of age. Below one year it is contraindicated because it can cause hypotension and cardiac arrest. Other drugs that have been used in initial treatment of SVT are phenylephrine or edrophonium. In cases with heart failure urgent cardioversion with synchronized DC cardioversion (0.5–2 W-sec/kg) is recommended as the initial management.

Once the patient has been converted to sinus rhythm, a long acting agent should be used for maintenance therapy to prevent recurrence. In patients without an antegrade accessory pathway, digoxin or propranolol is the drug of choice while children with WPW syndrome can be managed with propranolol. In resistant cases, the drugs that may be used include procainamide, quinidine, amiodarone etc. When there has been no recurrence after 6–12 months of therapy, the antiarrhythmic drug should be tapered and patient watched for recurrence.

Radiofrequency ablation of the accessory pathway is another treatment option in patients with refractory or poorly controlled SVT.

Atrial Flutter

Atrial flutter is characterized by a rapid heart rate of 250–400/minute or more with characteristic saw toothed flutter waves, best seen in leads II, III, aVF and V1.

Atrial flutter is most commonly seen in conditions with large, stretched atria due to congenital or acquired heart diseases. Examples include Ebstein's anomaly, tricuspid atresia, and rheumatic mitral valve disease and as a post operative complication following palliative or corrective intra atrial surgery. It may also occur during acute infectious illness. In neonates it can occur in normal heart. Uncontrolled atrial flutter may precipitate heart failure.

The treatment of choice is synchronized DC cardioversion. Patient with chronic flutter associated congenital heart disease may be at increased risk of thromboembolism and stroke. They should be given anticoagulant therapy before electric cardioversion. Vagal maneuvers or adenosine generally produce a temporary slowing of heart rate. The child should be digitalized after cardioversion. The rhythm may occasionally change to atrial fibrillation after digitalization. Then quinidine or procanamide should be added to revert to sinus rhythm. In refractory cases, amiodarone and sotalol can be used. In neonates with normal heart who respond to digoxin, the treatment should be continued for 6 months to one year if there is no recurrence. The other modalities of treatment used in older children with congenital heart disease include radiofrequency and surgical ablation.

Atrial Fibrillation

Atrial fibrillation is an uncommon condition in children and rare in neonates. It is characterized by a rapid heart rate 300 –700/minute and produces an irregularly irregular pulse. Most frequently it occurs in older children with rheumatic mitral valvular disease and is often the result of a chronically stretched atrial myocardium. It is also rarely seen as a complication of intra atrial surgery, in conditions producing atrial flutter and in patients with WPW syndrome. Conditions like thyrotoxicosis, pericarditis and pulmonary emboli should be suspected in a previously normal child or adolescent with atrial fibrillation.

Digitalization is the treatment of choice. However, digoxin should not be given in presence of WPW syndrome. In such a situation, sinus rhythm may be restored with quinidine or procainamide, with amiodarone or DC conversion. Patients with chronic atrial fibrillation are at risk of thromboembolism and stroke. They should undergo anticoagulation with warfarin as also cases where elective cardioversion is planned.

Ventricular Tachycardia

Ventricular tachycardia (VT) is characterized by presence of three or more premature ventricular contractions with wide QRS complexes, a heart rate of 120 – 200 / minute and complete atrioventricular dissociation. It may be paroxysmal or incessant. VT is rare in children compared to the incidence of SVT. All wide QRS complexes in children however, should be considered as VT unless proved otherwise. Acute cardiac failure can occur rapidly and VT may degenerate into ventricular fibrillation.

VT may be associated with conditions like hypokalemia, myocarditis, intramyocardial tumours, cardiomyopathy, mitral valve prolapse, anomalous origin of a coronary artery. It may follow corrective surgery for Fallot's tetralogy and VSD.

Treatment in stable patients consists of pharmacological cardioversion with lidocaine. The first loading dose is 1 mg/kg. If it is ineffective it can be repeated twice at 5 – 10 minutes interval using 2 mg/kg and then 3 mg/kg. The bolus dose is followed by an infusion of 30 –50 microgram/kg/minute. If unresponsive, procainamide or bretylium can be used. Maintenance therapy is necessary in all cases except in those where the cause is identified and treated. Prompt electrical cardioversion is indicated when there is hemodynamic compromise. In occasional unresponsive cases cardioversion may be achieved by repeating DC shock after loading with lidocaine. Pace maker insertion is the last resort for DC shock failures.

Ventricular Fibrillation

It is a tachyarrhythmia which is usually fatal unless an effective ventricular rate is rapidly re-established. The ECG shows a series of low amplitude, rapid irregular depolarization without identifiable QRS complexes.

Treatment consists of external cardiac massage with artificial ventilation and DC defibrillation. If defibrillation is not effective or fibrillations recur, amiodarone or lidocaine may be given IV and defibrillation repeated. After recovery the patient should be evaluated for the underlying cause and treated.

Sinoatrial Block

Sinoatrial block is characterized by a sudden pause in the heartbeat. It is a relatively rare condition in childhood; may occur as a manifestation of digoxin toxicity or following extensive atrial surgery. It is caused by a block in the conduction of impulses between the SA node and the surrounding atrium. It may or may not be symptomatic. With compromised cardiac function it may result in syncope.

Sick Sinus Syndrome

This condition results from abnormality in impulse generation from the SA node or impulse conduction through the atrium or both. It is characterized by cardiac standstill for a few cycles after which the heartbeat is initiated from an abnormal focus. The condition is most commonly seen after surgical correction of congenital heart disease viz. atrial switch operation for transposition of the great arteries.

The clinical manifestations depend on the heart rate. Most patients remain asymptomatic. Dizziness and syncope may occur during the periods of bradycardia. Sick sinus syndrome may be associated with SVT (Bradycardia-Tachycardia syndrome) which is characterized by symptoms of palpitation, exercise intolerance or dizziness.

Treatment consists of pacemaker therapy in patients who are symptomatic. With associated SVT, both drug therapy and pace maker therapy is necessary.

Atrioventricular Block

Atrioventricular block is caused by interference in the normal conduction of impulses from the atria to the ventricles through the AV node. It may be classified into three types.

First degree block: It is characterized by a prolonged PR interval. It is essentially an ECG diagnosis, is asymptomatic and does not require any treatment. It may be seen in patients suffering from acute rheumatic carditis, diphtheria, digoxin toxicity and Ebstein abnormality and L–TGA.

Second degree block: It may appear in otherwise normal children. The other causes are myocarditis, cardiomyopathy, congenital heart defect, and following cardiac surgery. There are two types:

Mobitz type I second degree AV block is characterized by progressive lengthening of successive PR intervals culminating in a drop beat. The cycle repeats. This is known as Wenckebach's phenomenon. It is usually the result of impaired conduction in the AV node itself. The underlying cause should be treated.

Mobitz type II second degree AV block is usually caused by disease of the bundle of His and purkinjee system and caries a risk of asystole. It is characterized by a constant PR interval with some P waves not conducted. Treatment of underlying cause may suffice but sometimes may require prophylactic pacemaker therapy.

Two to one (or higher) atrioventricular block is a condition where a QRS complex follows every second, third, or fourth P wave, resulting in 2:1, 3:1 or 4:1 AV block. The causes are similar to those of second degree heart block. Besides treatment of cause, pacemaker therapy may be occasionally necessary.

Third degree block (Complete heart block): Complete heart block may be congenital or acquired. The acquired type may be seen in myocardial diseases, cardiomyopathy, myocardial abscess secondary to infective endocarditis, complication of surgical correction of congenital heart defects like Fallot's tetralogy, VSD.

Congenital Complete Atrioventricular Block

The incidence of congenital heart block is 1 in 20,000–25,000 live births. It is often caused by autoimmune injury of the fetal conduction system by maternally derived IgG antibodies in a mother with overt or, more often, asymptomatic SLE. The complete heart block may not be present at birth but develops within the first 3–6 months. It is also seen associated with complex congenital heart disease and abnormal embryonic development of the conducting system. The infants with associated congenital heart disease and heart failure have a high mortality rate.

Diagnosis

Diagnosis of the condition in the fetus is possible by fetal echocardiography. Infants and toddlers may present with night terrors, tiredness with frequent naps and irritability. In the older children with an otherwise normal heart, the condition is commonly asymptomatic. Sometimes syncope and sudden death may occur. On examination the ventricular rate is usually 45–60/minute which may increase to 65–80/minute on exercise, pulse volume is high as a result of the compensatory large stroke volume and peripheral vasodilatation. The jugular venous pulse show cannon waves. The heart is enlarged, apex is forceful and there is an ejection systolic murmur along

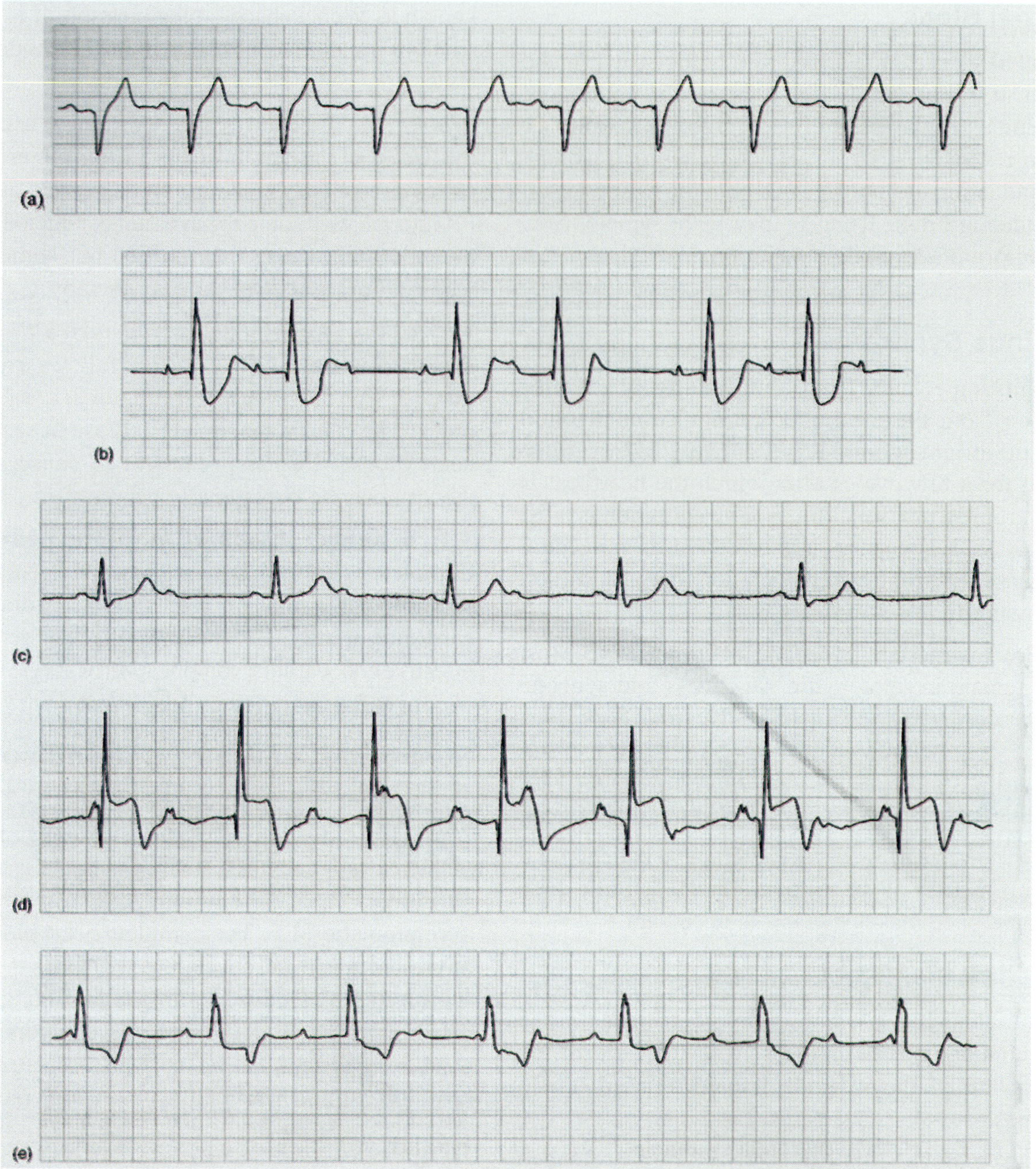

Fig. 14.7: Figure showing ECG changes in (a) First degree AV block, (b) Second degree AV block (Wenkebach type Mobitz type 1), (c) Second degree AV block at bundle branch level (Mobitz type 2), (d) Third degree AV block at the level of AV node (complete block), (e) Third degree AV block at bundle branch level (complete block)

the left sternal border and mid diastolic murmur at the apex.

The diagnosis is confirmed by ECG which shows that the P waves and QRS complexes have no constant relationship. The QRS duration may be prolonged or normal.

Treatment

Treatment is not required for children with asymptomatic congenital heart block. Neonates with heart rate 50 / minute or less, evidence of heart failure, wide complex rhythms and congenital heart disease needs cardiac pacing. Atropine, isoproterenol or epinephrine may be used to try to increase the heart rate temporarily until pacing can be arranged. Some patients may develop *Stokes Adam attacks* characterized by exercise intolerance, dizziness and syncope. Presence of such symptoms indicates implantation of a permanent pacemaker. Other indications of permanent pacemaker implantation include patients who develop progressive cardiac enlargement, prolonged pauses, and awake heart rates 40 /minute or less.

Prognosis

The prognosis of congenital complete heart block is usually favorable. Patients who have been observed upto 30–40 years have lived normal active life. Mortality is common in the first year; hence these patients need monitoring.

Congestive Heart Failure

Congestive heart failure (CHF) is a clinical syndrome characterized by inability of the heart to maintain an out put, at rest or during stress, necessary for the metabolic needs of the body (systolic failure), inability to receive blood into ventricular cavities at low pressure during diastole (diastolic failure) or a combination of both.

The basic defect is myocardial dysfunction which in children may be related to primary heart muscle disease, infiltrative disease of the myocardium and to altered loading conditions of pressure or volume overload.

Table 14.3 : Causes of acute and chronic heart failure

Acute heart failure	*Chronic heart failure*
1. Acute rheumatic carditis	1. Chronic valvular diseases
2. Myocarditis (viral, disphtheria, tetanus)	2. Dilated cardiomyopathy
3. Infective endocarditis	
4. Severe anemia	
5. Thyrotoxicosis	
6. Endocardial fibroelastosis	
7. Paroxysmal atrial tachycardia	
8. Fluid overload, severe hypoxia, acidosis, hypoglycemia and hypocalcemia (in newborn)	

Types of Heart Failure

Heart failure may be acute and chronic, low output or high output failure and systolic or diastolic failure. The common example of *acute heart failure* is acute rheumatic carditis. Other causes include myocarditis due to any cause (diphtheria, tetanus, viral), infective endocarditis, severe anemia, thyrotoxicosis, endocardial fibroelastosis, paroxysmal atrial tachycardia. In the newborn acute hear failure may be caused by fluid overload, severe hypoxia and acidosis, hypoglycemia, hypocalcemia.

Chronic heart failure is uncommon in children; commonly seen in chronic valvular disease, dilated cardiomyopathy.

Low output failure results from a low stroke volume (e.g. myocardial disease) and *high output failure* occurs as a result of high stroke volume (e.g. severe anemia, thyrotoxicosis). *Systolic heart failure* occurs when the heart is unable to pump out blood and *diastolic heart failure* results from decreased diastolic relaxation which leads to increased pressure in the pulmonary venous and arterial circulation.

Diastolic failure is uncommon in children. The causes include mitral and tricuspid stenosis, constrictive pericarditis, restrictive cardiomyopathy, acute mitral or aortic regurgitation, dilated cardiomyopathy, marked ventricular hypertrophy and myocardial ischemia. However, the last three causes lead to a mixed type of failure, i.e., systolic as well as diastolic. This diastolic dysfunction has specific management, e.g., valvuloplasty for valvular stenosis, pericardiectomy for constrictive pericarditis, surgery and symptomatic treatment for restrictive cardiomyopathy, valve repair of regurgitant valves in acute regurgitation. ACE inhibitors for marked cardiomegaly.

Etiology

The most common cause of heart failure in infants is congenital heart disease whereas in older children it is acute rheumatic fever and rheumatic heart disease. However, it should be remembered that if a child with congenital heart disease does not develop heart failure during the first year of life, it is not likely to happen in the next 10 years unless complicated by anemia, infection (Pneumonia) or infective endocarditis.

Congenital heart disease viz. ventricular septal defect (VSD), patent ductus arteriosus (PDA), and endocardial cushion defect (ECD), are the most common causes of heart failure in the first 6 months of life. The following facts have to be taken into consideration while analyzing the causes of CHF as a result of congenital heart disease:

1. Children with tetralogy of Fallot (TOF) do not develop CHF unless they undergo shunt procedures.
2. Atrial septal defect (ASD) rarely causes CHF in the pediatric age group.
3. Large left to right shunt lesions, viz., VSD and PDA; do not cause CHF before 6–8 weeks age because the pulmonary vascular resistance does not fall low enough

to cause a large left to right shunt until this age. The onset of CHF resulting from left to right shunt lesions may be earlier in premature infants (i.e., within the first month) because of earlier fall of vascular resistance in these infants.

Table 14.4 : The etiology of heart failure
Fetal
Severe anemia, supraventricular tachycardia, ventricular tachycardia, complete heart block.
Premature neonate
Fluid overload, PDA, VSD, corpulmonale (bronchopulmonary dysplasia), Hypertension.
Full term neonate
Asphyxial cardiomyopathy, arteriovenous malformation (vein of galen, hepatic), left sided obstructive lesions (coarctation of aorta, hypoplastic left heart syndrome), single ventricle, truncus arteriosus.
Infant-Toddler
VSD, anomalous left coronary artery, metabolic cardiomyopathy, hemolytic uremic syndrome, supraventricular tachycardia, viral myocarditis, Kawasaki disease.
Child-Adolescent
Acute rheumatic fever, glomerulonephritis, viral myocarditis, thyrotoxicosis, sickle cell anemia, endocarditis, corpulmonale (cystic fibrosis), hypertrophic and dilated cardiomyopathy, radiation and doxorubicin therapy, cardiomyopathy associated with muscular dystrophy and Friedreich's ataxia.

Table 14.5 : Causes of CHF resulting from CHD and age of onset

Age of onset	*Cause*
At birth	Hypoplastic left heart syndrome.
	Severe tricuspid or pulmonary regurgitation/atresia.
	Large systemic arteriovenous fistula.
First week	Transposition of great arteries.
	Patent ductus arteriosus in prematures.
	Total anomalous pulmonary venous return.
	Systemic arteriovenous fistula.
	Critical aortic stenosis/Pulmonary stenosis.
	Hypoplastic left heart syndrome.
1–4 weeks	Coarctation of aorta.
	Critical aortic stenosis.
	Large VSD, PDA in prematures.
	All other lesions previously listed.
4–6 weeks	Endocardial cushion defect.
6 weeks–4 months	Large VSD, PDA.
	Anomalous left coronary artery from pulmonary artery.

Pathophysiology

Heart failure is basically a compensatory mechanism. According to the Frank Sterling law, the force of myocardial contraction is equivalent to the end diastolic fibre length (EDFL) within the physiological limit. The EDFL depend on the end diastolic volume (EDV). The EDV, on the other hand depends on the end diastolic pressure. Therefore increase end diastolic pressure (EDP) will lead to increased EDV and thereby increase force of contraction.

A normal heart maintains cardiac output at normal end diastolic pressure, i.e., equal to 10 mmHg. In a failing heart, the basic defect lies in the contractile element of the heart. So it fails to maintain the cardiac output at the normal end diastolic pressure. Initially it tries to compensate by undergoing hypertrophy, but later on fails when the fibre length crosses the physiological limit. The failing heart then tries to maintain cardiac output at a higher EDP. When the EDP is 18–20 mmHg, it reflect back on pulmonary circulation and the patient complains of dyspnea and when it crosses 25 mm Hg pulmonary edema occurs.

The second compensatory mechanism is the neurohormonal mechanism. The neurohormonal responses include marked increase in the activity of the sympathoadrenal system, activation of renin angiotensin aldosterone system and secretion of ADH.

The effect of neurohormonal activation is seen by sinus tachycardia, retension of sodium and water, increase in peripheral vascular resistance and marked increase in myocardial energy and oxygen requirements. These changes are essential for survival during acute hemodynamic disturbances.

The atrial natriuretic hormone (ANH), secreted by the cardiac endocrine system produces natriuresis, vasodilatation, and inhibition of angiotensin II, aldosterone and ADH secretion thus reversing some of the above harmful effects. However, the increased levels of ANH are not adequate to counteract the changes effectively.

The first response to increased overload on the heart is hypertrophy of the ventricle concerned. The hypertrophy occurs before there is any increase in the venous pressure. This may be kept within physiological bounds by increased strength of contraction of heart muscles, and increased heart rate. Soon these mechanisms cease to be adequate resulting in increased venous filling pressure. The initial rise is physiological, but when the burden is excessive and the heart muscles become fatigued, the clinical signs of heart failure begin to appear.

The systemic venous pressure, in CHF, rises by several mechanisms, the primary one being due to decreased effectiveness of the heart muscles leading to a damming back of blood and a raised intra atrial pressure. Second factor is the reflex increase in sympathetic vasomotor tone, throughout the body, increasing the rate of flow through the veins to the right atrium. A third factor is the retension of fluid by the kidneys causing an augmentation of both interstitial fluid and blood volume.

Peculiarities in Children

In young children it is difficult to make a clear differentiation between left and right heart failure as in adults. The signs of right heart failure viz. liver enlargement can be readily identified than those of left viz. pulmonary congestion, some degree of which may be already present in children with intracardiac or vascular shunt. Hence, in children, it has been customary to rely more on the signs of right heart failure (particularly an enlarged, soft, tender liver) to make a diagnosis of failure even in patients whose primary cause is in the left heart.

In children, crepitations are uncommon. Instead, rhonchi are frequently heard. Cyanosis is common. Respiratory studies have shown a great increase in resistance to airflow. This is the result of rise in left ventricular, left atrial and pulmonary venous and capillary pressures. The lung becomes congested and less complacent. Transudates in the alveolar walls, alveoli and air passages may cause airflow obstruction and sufficient interference in oxygen transfer to reduce arterial oxygen and result in cyanosis.

Failure in infants and children is not accompanied by much fluid retention and hence edema. This may be due to the reason that edema is related, in some measure, to the length of time high capillary pressure has been maintained in the body. In children, the process of heart failure is generally acute and lead more promptly to death or improvement.

Unlike adults, infants and children are less dyspneic at night than in day time. This may be related to restlessness, irritability, crying and activity during the waking hours resulting in rise of blood pressure and therefore systemic resistance and thus an increase in load in the pulmonary circulation during the day. During night when the baby is asleep, the dyspnea is frequently less obvious.

In infants and children with congenital heart disease, as the heart muscle is originally healthy, the cardiac reserve is great. Hence digitalis produces excellent results.

Clinical Manifestations

The clinical features of congestive heart failure will depend on the degree of cardiac reserve. The presenting symptoms and signs differ according to the age of the child, viz., newborn, infants and the older child.

A critically ill infant or a child who has already exhausted the compensatory mechanisms will be symptomatic at rest. Others may be symptomatic either with mild activity or only with vigorous activity. It may be difficult for the parents to recognize the subtle changes which may occur in the newborn or infant over the course of days or weeks.

A thorough history is extremely important for both in making a diagnosis of CHF as well as in evaluating the possible cause.

Symptoms in Infants

Poor feeding of recent onset, tachypnoea that worsens during feeding, poor weight gain, irritability, and weak cry, noisy laboured respiration with intercostal and subcostal retraction as well as flaring of alae nasi, excessive perspiration are symptoms of CHF in the infants.

Signs of CHF in the Newborn

The signs of congestive heart failure in the newborn period are: Tachypnoea, tachycardia, enlarging soft tender liver, sudden unexplained weight gain. Jugular venous pressure cannot be evaluated because the newborn baby has a short neck. Cardiac signs of underlying disease are often present.

Signs Beyond Neonatal Period

The signs of CHF in infancy include tachycardia, gallop rhythm, tachypnea, wheeze, cardiomegaly, soft and tender hepatomegaly, generalized edema involving less often the legs and feet, more evident by sudden unexplained weight gain. Edema is difficult to elicit in infants because of an excess of subcutaneous fat in the limbs. In such situations one has to rely on signs like sudden unexplained weight gain in the infant as an indication of fluid retention. JVP cannot be assessed in infants because of a short neck. Cardiac signs of underlying disease are present.

Symptoms in Children Beyond Infancy

The symptoms of CHF include fatigue, effort intolerance, dyspnea, anorexia, abdominal pain and cough, decreased weight for height.

Signs of CHF in Children Beyond Infancy

The signs of CHF may be classified as follows, depending on the pathophysiologic mechanisms:

Compensatory responses to impaired cardiac function:

- Tachycardia, gallop rhythm, weak and thready pulse.
- Cardiomegaly: Absence of cardiomegaly almost rules out the diagnosis of CHF. It should however be noted that cardiomegaly may be already present in case of large left to right shunts.
- Signs of increased sympathetic activity viz. growth failure, perspiration, cold wet skin.

Signs of pulmonary congestion (left sided failure):

- Tachypnea.
- Dyspnea on exertion (poor feeding in infants).
- Orthopnea in older children.
- Wheeze and crackles in the lungs, cyanosis.

Signs of systemic congestion (right sided failure):

- Hepatomegaly: It is not always indicative of CCF. The liver may be palpable in presence of hyper inflated lungs (e.g., acute asthma, acute bronchiolitis etc.). Conversely, the absence of hepatomegaly does not exclude CCF because hepatomegaly may be absent in early failure (stage of pulmonary congestion).
- Puffy eyelids are common in infants.
- Distended neck veins and ankle edema.
- Splenomegaly, if present indicates presence of infection.

Laboratory Diagnosis

Cardiac failure is essentially a clinical diagnosis. Investigations may be necessary to find out the cause.

1. **X-ray studies:** Chest X-ray films are more reliable than physical examination in demonstrating cardiomegaly. All cases with CCF should have a CXR done.
2. **ECG:** ECG is not helpful in diagnosis of CCF but may help to determine chamber hypertrophy and thereby the etiology.
3. **Echocardiography:** Echocardiography may be done to determine the cause of CCF. It does not have a significant role in diagnosis of CCF.

Treatment

The treatment of congestive heart failure consists of:

(a) Control of heart failure state.
(b) Elimination of precipitating or contributing cause viz. infection, anemia, arrhythmias etc.
(c) Elimination of underlying cause.

Every patient with congestive cardiac failure should receive maximum medical treatment but continuing with long-term anticongestive measures is unwise if the heart defect can be repaired surgically. Medical treatment is primarily indicated to prepare the patient for surgery because it will provide a temporary relief and allow the patient time to wait for the surgery.

General Measures

1. **Bed rest:** Strict bed rest is often not necessary except in severe cases. However, the child should rest often and sleep adequately. An upright position should be maintained if the child feels comfortable. A cardiac chair or an infant chair may be used in case of an infant for the purpose.
2. **Oxygen inhalation:** Humidified oxygen (40–50%) should be administered to infants with respiratory distress.
3. **Sedation:** with morphine sulphate (0.1–0.2 mg/kg per dose subcutaneously every 4 hours as needed) or phenobarbital (2–3 mg/kg per dose orally or intramuscularly every 8 hourly as necessary) for the first 1–2 days may be indicated.
4. **Diet:** Infants having CHF usually fails to thrive. Increasing daily calories is an important aspect of their management. Severely ill infants may need nasogastric feeding. Breast milk feeding need supplementation of calories. Salt and fluid restriction is not indicated in infants. Use of potent diuretics has replaced these measures. Most older children can be managed with "no added salt diet (< 0.5 grams salt/day)" and avoidance of foods containing large amounts of sodium (chips, salted biscuits etc).
5. **Predisposing factors** viz. high fever, anemia and infection should be treated with antipyretics, antibiotics and packed cell transfusion (to raise hematocrit to 35% or more).
6. **Underlying causes:** viz. hypertension, arrhythmias, etc should be treated.
7. **Daily weight record** is essential in hospitalized patients.

Drug Therapy

Three major classes of drugs are used in treatment of CHF in children:

1. Diuretics.
2. Ionotropic agents.
3. After load reducing agents.

Diuretics

Patients with mild CCF may improve rapidly after a dose of fast acting diuretics.

(a) Frusemide is the drug of choice (1 mg/kg/dose IV, 2–3 mg/kg/day orally in 2–3 divided doses).

(b) Spironolactone (1–3 mg/kg/day orally in 2–3 divided doses) may be required in persistent CHF to prevent hypokalemia which is usually poorly tolerated. Diuretics are the first line drugs in treatment of CCF with rheumatic carditis.

Digitalis

Digoxin is the most commonly used preparation. It is worth mentioning that the pediatric dosage of digoxin is relatively larger than that used in adults. Pharmacokinetic studies indicate that infants and children require a larger dosage primarily because of a large volume of distribution and a more rapid clearance, including tubular secretion. Digitalization can be done by two methods viz. rapid and slow.

Rapid and Slow Digitalization

Rapid digitalization may be carried out intravenously (in critically ill child) or orally (in less critically ill child) and digitalization is completed within 24 hours.

Slow digitalization is usually done in immediate post operative period starting with the maintenance dose without a prior loading dose and digitalization is achieved in 7–10 days.

Table 14.6 : Oral digoxin dosage for CCF

Age	*Total digitalizing dose (microgram/kg)*	*Maintenance dose* (microgram/kg/day)*
Prematures	20	5
Term Newborn	30	8
<2 years	40–50	10–12
>2 years	30–40	8–10

* The maintenance dose is 25% of the total digitalizing dose to be given in two divided doses. The IV dose is 75% of the oral dose.

Step by Step Rapid Digitalization

1. A base line ECG (for rhythm and PR interval) and base line levels of electrolytes (K and Ca) should be obtained. Hypokalemia and hypocalcemia predispose to digoxin toxicity.
2. Two people should calculate the dosage independently and compare figures.
3. One half of the digitalizing dose should be given immediately, followed by one fourth then the final one fourth of the digitalizing dose at 6 to 8 hours intervals.
4. Maintenance dose should be started 12 hours after the final digitalizing dose. An ECG strip should be obtained before starting the maintenance dose.
5. Monitoring for digoxin toxicity should be done by ECG during the first 3–5 days after digitalization.

Precautions

1. Digoxin should be cautiously used in myocarditis, using half of the digitalizing dose because some patients with myocarditis are exquisitely sensitive to the drug. Rapid acting diuretics and ionotropes (in critically ill children) are safer and effective drugs in myocarditis.
2. In rheumatic carditis with CHF, steroids are the first line drugs. Anticongestive therapy with rapidly acting diuretics viz. frusemide usually suffices.
3. For long-term maintenance therapy digoxin should be given 5 days in a week to safeguard against the cumulative effect of digoxin.

Rapidly Acting Ionotropic Drugs

In critically ill infants with CHF, in those with renal dysfunction or in post operative cardiac patients with CHF, rapidly acting catecholamine with a short duration of action are preferable to digoxin.

(a) Dopamine (5–10 micrograms/kg/min IV) and dobutamine (2–8 microgram/kg/min IV) are the most commonly used preparations.

(b) Amrinone, a phosphodiesterase inhibitor, is useful in treating patients with low cardiac output, refractory to standard therapy. It has both positive ionotropic effects on the heart and significant peripheral vasodilator effects. It is generally used as an adjunct to dopamine or dobutamine therapy in an ICU setup. It is given at an initial loading dose of 0.75 mg/kg IV followed by an IV infusion of 5–10 microgram /kg/ min.

After Load Reducing Agents

This group of drugs reduces ventricular after load by decreasing peripheral vascular resistance, thereby improving myocardial performance. After load agents are usually used in conjunction with digoxin and diuretics. After load reducers are especially useful in children with CHF secondary to:

1. Dilated cardiomyopathy or doxorubicin induced cardiomyopathy.
2. Severe mitral regurgitation, aortic regurgitation; and
3. Large left to right shunts (VSD, PDA, AV canal defect).

The after load reducers are:

(a) Captopril (0.5–6 mg/kg/day in 2–3 divided doses) orally.

(b) Hydralazine (0.5–7.5 mg/kg/day in 3 divided doses) given orally.

(c) IV nitroprusside (0.5–8 microgram/kg/min) should be used in an intensive care setup in critically ill patient.

Beta Adrenergic Blockers

Beneficial effects of propranolol are reported in some infants with large left to right shunts and severe CHF who had failed to respond to conventional therapy. Propranolol (1–2 mg/kg) orally, decreases respiratory rate and heart rate and improves symptoms of CHF.

Surgical Management

Eliminating the underlying cause is the most desirable approach to treatment of CHF whenever possible. Surgical correction is the only way to treat CHF secondary to congenital heart disease. If medical treatment does not improve CHF within a few weeks to months, either a palliative or corrective surgery should be advised for the underlying cardiac defect viz. valvular surgery in valvular disease or a heart transplant in case of cardiomyopathy.

Infective Endocarditis

Infective endocarditis includes acute and sub-acute endocarditis which may be caused by bacteria as well as fungi.

Epidemiology

Infective endocarditis is often a complication of congenital or rheumatic heart disease but can also occur in a normal heart in children. It is rare in infancy but can occur in this age group following open heart surgery or associated with a central venous line. Surgical correction of congenital heart disease may reduce but does not eliminate the risk, with the exception of repair of ASD and PDA. Children who have undergone valve replacement or repair are particularly at high risk.

Etiology

Streptococcus viridens and staphylococcus aureus are the leading causative agents responsible for endocarditis in children. The organisms that cause endocarditis less frequently include group D enterococci, pseudomonas aeruginosa, serratia marcescens, coagulase negative staphylococcus and fungus.

Streptococcus viridens infection is more common after dental procedures. Staphylococcal infection is common in children with no underlying heart disease. Group D enterococci are seen more often after lower bowel and genitourinary manipulation. Pseudomonas aeruginosa or serratia is found more frequently in intravenous drug users and fungal endocarditis is seen after open heart surgery. Coagulase negative staphylococcus is the common organism in presence of an indwelling central venous catheter.

Pathogenesis

Almost all children who develop infective endocarditis have a history of an existing congenital or acquired heart disease. Drug addicts, however may develop endocarditis in a normal heart.

Two factors are important in the pathogenesis of infective endocarditis. Firstly, presence of structural anomalies of the heart or great arteries with a significant pressure gradient or turbulence which result in endothelial damage and platelet fibrin thrombus formation. Secondly, bacterimia which may be even transient. Vegetations usually form at the site of the endothelial or intimal erosion that result from the turbulent flow.

Ventricular septal defect, tetralogy of Fallot, aortic stenosis, patent ductus arteriosus, transposition of great arteries and Blalock-Taussig shunts, mitral valve prolapse, bicuspid aortic valves, rheumatic mitral and aortic regurgitation are the structural lesions associated with endocarditis.

Bacterimia can result from any localized infection, e.g., abscess, osteomyelitis, pyelonephritis. Bacterimia can also result from dental procedures, chewing or brushing teeth in children with carious teeth or gingivitis.

Pathology

The vegetations in infective endocarditis are irregular, large and friable. They more often cause perforation or erosion of underlying valve leaflet and sometimes erode the myocardium to produce para valvular abscesses. The vegetations are located near the lines of closure of the valve leaflets. In case of non valvular congenital defects, the vegetations tend to be located on the low pressure side of the defect, e.g. on the right ventricular margins of an interventricular septal defect.

The vegetations constitute masses of fibrin, blood cells, platelets and masses or colony formations of organisms.

Clinical Manifestations

The clinical manifestations of subacute and acute endocarditis are different. In the subacute form the onset is gradual. The symptoms are non-specific and consist of low grade fever with afternoon elevation which may be prolonged for several months, fatigue, myalgia, arthralgia, headache, chills, nausea and vomiting. In the acute type, onset is sudden with high intermittent fever, chills, weakness and lassitude.

There is presence of a murmur due to an underlying disease in the subacute form but sudden appearance and changing murmur during the course is common in acute form. The spleen is more often enlarged in the acute form.

Petechiae of the skin, mucous membrane, or conjunctivae are the most frequent skin lesions. The other skin lesions viz. Osler's nodes, Janeway's lesions, splinter hemorrhage are rarely found in children. Osler's nodes are tender; pea sized red nodes at the ends of the fingers or toes. Janeway's lesions are small, painless, hemorrhagic areas on the palms or soles. Splinter hemorrhages are linear hemorrhagic streaks beneath the nails. These lesions may represent vasculitis produced by circulating antigen antibody complexes.

Embolic phenomena to other organs include hematuria and renal failure, Roth's spot (oval retinal hemorrhage with pale centres near the optic disc), cerebral stroke, cerebral abscess, and cerebral hemorrhage. The neurological complications are most often associated with staphylococcal disease and are late manifestations. Meningismus, signs of raised intracranial tension, altered sensorium, and focal neurological signs are the manifestations of these complications. Pulmonary and systemic emboli are common in fungal infection.

Pericardial effusion may result from rupture of myocardial abscess in staphylococcal infection.

Carious teeth and gingival disease is frequently present. The child may present with signs of congestive heart failure.

Laboratory Diagnosis

1. A **complete blood count** shows anemia with hemoglobin levels lower than 12 gm/dl and polymorphonuclear leucocytosis. The ESR is increased. Hemoglobin levels and ESR may be normal in presence of polycythemia.
2. **Blood cultures** are positive in more than 90% cases in the absence of previous antimicrobial therapy. Pretreatment with antimicrobials reduces the yield to 50-60%. Blood specimens should be collected as early as possible. Three to five separate blood collections should be obtained over 24 – 48 hours, after careful preparation of the puncture site. The timing of specimen collection is not important as bacterimia is relatively constant.
3. **Urine examination** shows microscopic hematuria in 30% cases.
4. **Echocardiography:** Two dimensional or trans-esophageal echo can image vegetations of 3 mm in diameter. Negative echo does not rule out infective endocarditis. A false positive diagnosis is possible, especially with abnormal valves. Echo evidence of vegetation may persist for months or years after bacteriologic cure.

Management

Initial empirical therapy should be started, after collecting samples for blood culture, with antistaphylococcal semi-synthetic penicillin viz. Cloxacillin, an aminoglycoside viz. Gentamycin and Benzyl Penicillin. This combination will cover Staph aureus, gram negatives and Streptococcus Viridens. Vancomycin can be used in place of penicillin or semi-synthetic penicillin in penicillin allergic patients. The final selection of antibiotics will depend on the culture and sensitivity results. The drugs of choice according to the organism are as follows:

Table 14.7 : Drug dosage of commonly used drugs

Bacteria	*Drugs*	*Dose*	*Route*	*Duration of treatment*
S. viridens	Penicillin	2-3 lakh units/kg (max 20 million units/day)	IV 4 hrly	4–6 weeks
Penicillin allergy	Vancomycin	40–60 mg/kg/day (max 2 gms/day)	IV 8-12 hrly	4–6 weeks
Staph aureus	Cloxacillin +	100 mg/kg/day	IV 4–6 hrly	6–8 weeks
	Gentamicin	3–7.5 mg/kg	IV 8 hrly	2 weeks
MRSA (Methicillin resistant staph aureus)	Vancomycin	40–60 mg/kg/day (max 2 gm/day)	IV 8 – 12 hrly	4–6 weeks

Prevention

1. Maintenance of oral hygiene.
2. Antimicrobial prophylaxis before minor procedures.

An oral dose of antibiotic should be given 1 hour before and a parenteral dose 30 minutes before minor procedures.

In high risk patients one additional dose of antibiotic 6 hours after the procedure is completed.

Pericarditis and Pericardial Effusion

Pericarditis or inflammation of the pericardium which may be acute or chronic occurs as a primary disorder or as a part of a general disease. The acute form may be dry (fibrinous) or accompanied by effusion. Chronic pericarditis occurs as constrictive pericarditis or rarely as a chronic effusion. Chronic pericarditis is rare in children.

Pathophysiology

Pericardial inflammation may result in a local or generalized fibrinous pericarditis or an accumulation of fluid in the pericardial space. The fluid may be serous, serosanguinous, purulent or hemorrhagic. This depends on the etiology.

In fibrinous pericarditis, the surface of the pericardium is covered with exudates consisting of lymph, fibrin and inflammatory cells. The superficial layers of the myocardium may also show signs of inflammation in some cases. The exudates organize leaving varying degrees of slight pericardial thickening often with adhesions.

The pathogenesis of symptoms and signs of pericardial effusion depends on two factors–the speed of accumulation and the competence of the myocardium. In a healthy child, 10–15 ml of fluid is normally found in the pericardial space. A rapid accumulation of a large amount of pericardial fluid produces a serious circulatory embarrassment. A slow accumulation of a relatively small amount of fluid in presence of myocarditis may also result in cardiac tamponade. On the other hand, a slow accumulation of a large amount of fluid may be accommodated in the pericardial space by stretching of the pericardium, if the myocardium is intact. For every small increment of fluid, pericardial pressure rises slowly; but once a critical level is reached, pressure rises rapidly and culminates in severe cardiac compression.

With the development of cardiac tamponade, several compensatory mechanisms come into play. These include systemic and pulmonary venous constriction to improve diastolic filling, an increase in systemic vascular resistance to raise falling blood pressure and tachycardia to improve cardiac output. If left untreated in the compensatory phase, compromised cardiac output and shock occur.

Etiology

Infectious

(a) *Viral:* Coxsakie B, Echo, Epstein Barr, influenza, adeno.
(b) *Bacterial:* Streptococcus, pneumococcus, staphylococcus, meningococcus, mycoplasma, hemophilus influenzae.
(c) *Fungal:* Histoplasmosis, actinomycosis.
(d) *Parasitic:* Toxoplasmosis, echinococcus.

Connective Tissue Disorders

(a) Rheumatic fever.
(b) Juvenile rheumatoid arthritis.
(c) Systemic lupus erythematosus.
(d) Sarcoidosis.

Metabolic-Endocrine

(a) Uremia.
(b) Hypothyroidism.
(c) Chylopericardium.

Hematology-Oncology

(a) Bleeding diathesis.

(b) Primary or secondary metastasis.

(c) Radiotherapy induced.

Others

(a) Trauma.

(b) Post-cardiotomy (cardiac surgery).

(c) Idiopathic.

(d) Aortic dissection.

Viral pericarditis also known as acute benign pericarditis or idiopathic pericarditis is probably the most common cause. The common viruses implicated are coxsakie B and Echo. It is thought to be a hypersensitivity reaction to the viral disease. Most cases are mild and recover within several weeks with symptomatic treatment with non-steroidal anti-inflammatory drugs. In rare instances there may be cardiac tamponade. In some cases, the course may be chronic relapsing and need differential diagnosis with pericarditis due to collagen disease. Response to anti-inflammatory drugs in the latter patients is dramatic.

Purulent pericarditis is often associated with bacterial infections viz. pneumonia, epiglotitis, meningitis or osteomyelitis. The course is fulminant and if untreated, is terminated by acute cardiac tamponade and death.

Tuberculous pericarditis has an insidious onset and is an important cause of chronic constrictive pericarditis.

Pericarditis in *acute rheumatic fever* is a part of the pancarditis. It is associated with acute valvulitis. Cardiac tamponade is extremely rare.

Pericarditis is a common manifestation in *juvenile rheumatoid arthritis*. It may be the only manifestation and precede the onset of arthritis by months or years.

Uremic pericarditis occurs only in the presence of prolonged severe renal failure. It may lead to cardiac tamponade, usually respond to dialysis, may need pericardiectomy.

A *neoplastic pericardial effusion* is seen in association with Hodgkin's disease, lymphosarcoma and leukemia as a result of direct neoplastic invasion of the pericardium. Rarely infiltration may be the initial manifestation of a neoplastic disease. Cardiac tamponade may occur late in the course of the illness. Patients with neoplastic disease can also suffer from pericarditis as a result of radiation to the mediastinum.

Post-pericardiotomy pericardial effusion is a hypersensitivity reaction's to trauma to the pericardium and the epicardial surface of the heart. It is seen 1–2 weeks after open heart surgery. It should be suspected when a child becomes acutely ill within the first 4–6 weeks after cardiac surgery. The patient may initially have low grade fever, lethargy, loss of appetite or abdominal pain. Precordial or chest pain may or may not be present. Untreated cases may progress to cardiac tamponade. Most children respond to aspirin. More severe cases may require steroids. Treatment may have to be continued for 1–3 months. Recurrences may occur as long as 1 year postoperatively.

Clinical Features

Acute Fibrinous Pericarditis without Effusion

The child may be asymptomatic. The symptoms and signs may be submerged in those of the associated disease, e.g., rheumatic carditis. In some cases there may be distinctive features.

The first symptom is usually precordial pain. Pain varies in intensity and radiates to the left shoulder and back. It is sharp, stabbing in nature, may be aggravated by lying supine and relieved by sitting, especially leaning forward. There may be fever, abdominal pain, vomiting, cough and dyspnea.

The characteristic physical sign is a friction rub which occurs in systole and diastole, giving it a to and fro character. Friction rub is best heard towards the base of the heart.

Pericarditis with Effusion

The clinical picture varies with the amount of fluid and the rate at which it accumulates in the pericardial sac. With a small amount of fluid, the patient is asymptomatic. If it is large and accumulation is rapid the patient is anxious, restless and pale, complains of pain. Dyspnea and orthopnoea is present; the degree depends on the size of effusion.

The friction rub is present at the base of the heart in small effusion. With larger amount of fluid, the heart is quiet and hypodynamic, the extent of cardiac dullness increases and varies with the posture of the patient, the heart sounds are distant. With significant amount of fluid, there is interference with cardiac function (Cardiac tamponade).The signs of cardiac tamponade are tachycardia, increased pulsus paradoxus (> 20 mmHg), engorged neck veins, paradoxical inspiratory filling of the neck veins, hepatomegaly. Rapidly developing tamponade may cause peripheral circulatory failure and shock. Cardiac tamponade occurs more commonly in purulent pericarditis than in other forms of pericarditis.

X-ray Study

X-ray changes are seen when there is accumulation of fluid in the pericardial sac and are characterized by varying degrees of cardiomegaly.

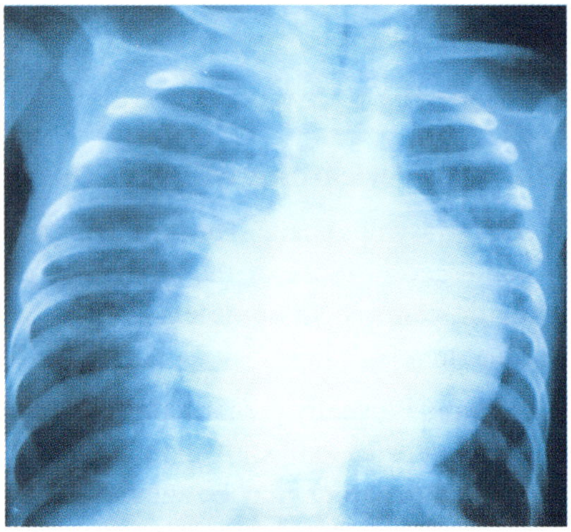

Fig. 14.8: Pericardial effusion

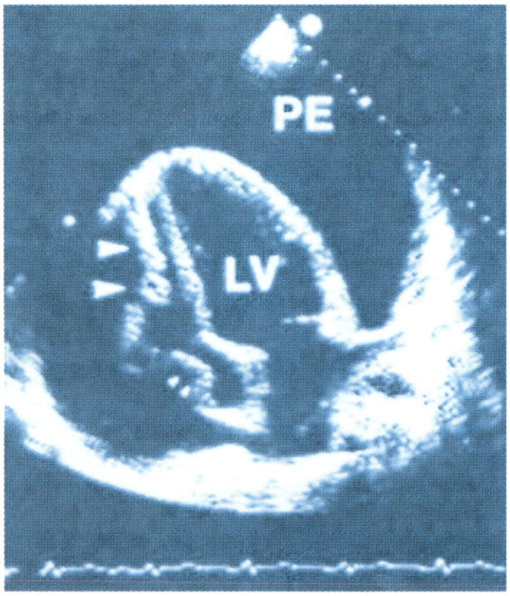

Fig. 14.9: Echo showing pericardial effusion (PE)

There is rounding of the heart shadow, becoming globular in some cases, with obliteration of the normal angulation along the left border, sharpening of the pericardiophrenic angles and a bulging into the retrocardiac space (best seen in the right oblique view). In cardiac tamponade, pulmonary vascular markings are increased, may be without increase in the cardiac shadow if it develops rapidly.

Electrocardiography

Due to widespread nature of the injury in acute pericarditis, ECG changes are present in all leads. The ST segment is elevated in all leads, showing more in some leads than in others. The T waves tend to become flattened and inverted. Inversion of T waves is sometimes seen in all standard leads and chest leads. The widespread nature of such a change is strong evidence of pericarditis. The QRS complex remains normal in form but the voltage is frequently diminished in all leads in pericardial effusion. The P waves are unaffected.

Echocardiography

It is the most sensitive technique for evaluation of the size and progression of pericardial effusion. A clear echo free space is recorded between the epicardium and pericardium. A posterior effusion is recorded behind the left ventricular epicardium and ends at the junction of the left ventricle and left atrium. Anterior effusion is recorded between the chest wall and the anterior right ventricular wall. The presence of both anterior and posterior effusion generally indicates a large collection of fluid. Flattening of the septal motion and collapse of right ventricular outflow during diastole are signs of pericardial tamponade.

Management

The management strategies will differ according to the cause of pericarditis. In suspected infective pathology, pericardiocentasis and pericardial fluid studies is mandatory. The pericardial fluid study should include physical; chemical (protein and glucose concentration) and cytological including total cell and differential count; gram and acid fast stains; viral, bacterial and fungal cultures as and when necessary.

Urgent surgical drainage of the pericardium is indicated when purulent effusion is suspected. This must be followed by IV antibiotic therapy for 4–6 weeks.

For cardiac tamponade also urgent decompression by surgical drainage or pericardiocentasis is indicated after emergency stabilization with IV infusion. Intravenous infusion will help to increase the central venous pressure and thereby improve cardiac filling.

There is no specific treatment for viral pericarditis. Treatment of the primary cause viz. uremia, collagen disease, gives relief of the pericarditis in these conditions.

Corticosteroid therapy is indicated in severe rheumatic pancarditis and post pericardiotomy syndrome.

Salicylates may be given for precordial pain. Digoxin is contraindicated in cardiac tamponade because it blocks tachycardia, the compensatory response to impaired venous return.

Constrictive Pericarditis

Constrictive pericarditis is a condition where essentially the pericardium is thickened, fibrotic and adherent which imposes a restrictive action on the heart so that diastolic filling is impeded, systolic ejection is diminished and there is development of venous congestion.

Etiology

Constrictive pericarditis may be associated with tubercular pericarditis, an earlier viral pericarditis, incomplete drainage of purulent pericarditis, hemopericardium, mediastinal radiation, and neoplastic infiltration or connective tissue disorders.

It is not an uncommon condition in children of our country. The common cause has been found to be tuberculous pericarditis. In most cases however, there is no history of previous pericarditis.

Pathogenesis

The heart is encased in a pericardium which is thickened from 2–10 mm with calcification. The heart muscle is essentially normal, but the superficial myocardium is frequently involved. The fibrous pericardium usually encases most of the heart and sometimes may extend to the great vessels. Occasionally it may also be localized.

The restrictive action of the pericardium on the heart results in decrease in diastolic filling, reduction in cardiac output, hypovolemia with retension of sodium and water. Hypovolemia also results in increased venous return which however cannot be accommodated by the constricted ventricles so that extreme congestion results.

Clinical Features

The onset of the disease is gradual. Symptoms are not prominent until the signs are well developed. The first complain may be dyspnea on exertion or swelling of the abdomen. Sometimes cough is a prominent symptom. Occasionally faintness on bending or coughing may be present.

The clinical signs include an elevated jugular venous pressure with equally prominent ‘a’ and ‘c’ waves and a ‘y’ descent. There is a paradoxical rise in venous pressure in inspiration (Kussmaul’s sign). The arterial pulse volume is low. There is increased pulsus paradoxus. The blood pressure is usually low. There may be peripheral cyanosis with cold extremities.

The precordium is quiet and the heart size is normal. The heart sounds are soft. There is presence of a diastolic pericardial knock. It is a short, high pitched sound related to the high pressure of ventricular filling. It is heard along the left sternal border.

Ascites is usually present. Its extent is in contrast to the much lesser degree of peripheral edema. Ascites is persistent and peritoneal tapping is followed by reaccumulation. The liver is moderately enlarged and pulsatile but may be small and cirrhotic in long standing cases. Pleural effusion of varying extent may be present. The disease runs a long chronic course with gradually increasing venous congestion, diminishing cardiac output and hepatic failure.

Laboratory Diagnosis

X-ray Studies

The heart size is normal. The angulations of the left border are smoothed out. The heart borders are ragged or shaggy. The superior vena caval shadow is prominent and merges with the right atrial margin. In many cases there is extensive calcification of the pericardium which is often best seen in oblique views. The lung vascularity is normal but small pleural effusions are common. Barium swallow esophagus may show left atrial enlargement in around 2/3rd of the cases.

Electrocardiography

The QRS complex is normal but may show a low voltage in around 75% cases. The ST segment is isoelectric but the T waves are flattened or inverted in several leads. Occasionally there may be right axis deviation and right ventricular hypertrophy pattern. Left atrial overload pattern may be present but uncommon.

Echocardiography

M–mode echo may reveal two parallel lines representing the thickened visceral and parietal pericardia or there may be multiple dense echoes. Two dimensional echo shows an immobile and dense appearance of the pericardium, abrupt displacement of the interventricular septum during early end-diastolic filling and dilatation of the hepatic veins and the inferior vena cava.

Cardiac catheterization reveals an elevated right and left atrial, ventricular end diastolic and pulmonary artery wedge pressures which are identical.

Treatment

Treatment consists of total resection of the pericardium. Symptomatic improvement occurs in 75% of cases. If tuberculous etiology is suspected a six weeks course of anti-tuberculous drug should be given pre-operatively followed by a full course post-operatively.

Myocarditis

Myocarditis refers to inflammation, necrosis, or myocytolysis of the myocardium. Severe myocarditis enough to be clinically recognized is rare, but mild and subclinical cases are not uncommon.

Causes

Viruses are probably the most common causes. Among viruses, adeno virus, coxsackie B virus, and echo viruses are the most common agents. *Other viruses* include polio, mumps, rubella, measles, CMV, HIV. *Immune mediated diseases* viz. rheumatic fever and Kawasaki disease, *bacterial infection* viz. diphtheria, tetanus, septicemia, infective endocarditis, *rickettsial diseases* viz. Rocky Mountain spotted fever and *parasitic and fungal diseases* like histoplasmosis, toxoplasmosis, coccidioidomycosis, hydatid cyst of pericardium can cause myocarditis.

Clinical Manifestations

The *newborn and infant* usually have an acute onset and present with symptoms like fever, respiratory distress, cyanosis, lethargy, vomiting, shock and signs like tachycardia disproportionate to fever, muffled heart sounds, gallop rhythm, signs of acidosis. Evidence of viral hepatitis, aseptic meningitis and rash may be present. In the most fulminant form, death may occur within 1–7 days.

An *older child* may present with acute onset, or commonly with a gradual onset congestive heart failure or a sudden onset of ventricular arrhythmia. In these patients, sometimes, the acute infectious phase has usually passed and the child presents as idiopathic dilated cardiomyopathy.

The *differential diagnoses* include carnitine deficiency, idiopathic dilated cardiomyopathy, pericarditis, endocardial fibroelastosis and anomalous origin of left coronary artery.

The *chest X-ray* shows an enormously enlarged heart and pulmonary edema. The *ECG* reveals sinus tachycardia, reduced QRS complex voltage, ST segment depression and T wave inversion in most leads. Arrhythmia in presence of fever and a large heart strongly suggest acute myocarditis. *ECHO* demonstrates poor ventricular function, pericardial effusion, and mitral regurgitation. Blood studies may show *elevated ESR and heart enzymes* (creatinine phosphokinase, LDH). *Serum viral titres* may be positive but a negative titre does not rule out diagnosis. Myocarditis can be confirmed by endomyocardial biopsy taken during cardiac catheterization.

Treatment

Supportive measures are the mainstay of treatment which includes treatment of congestive heart failure, treatment of arrhythmias. Digoxin should be started with half the normal dose and treatment of arrhythmias may require the use of IV amiodarone.

Steroids (Prednisolone 2 mg/kg/day tapered to 0.3 mg/kg daily over a period of 3 months) have been used in acute myocarditis with mixed results. Antiviral drug viz. pleconaril has been shown to be effective in neonates with acute myocarditis due to adeno virus. Cardiogenic shock may require inotropic drugs and ECMO. Refractory heart failure may require heart transplant.

Primary Myocardial Disease

Primary myocardial disease or cardiomyopathy is a disease of the heart muscle and is distinct from the specific heart muscle diseases of known cause. On the basis of anatomic and functional features, cardiomyopathy has been classified into three types viz. hypertrophic, dilated (or congestive) and restrictive. The three types of cardiomyopathies are functionally different from one another and hence demand different modalities of treatment.

Hypertrophic Cardiomyopathy

In hypertrophic cardiomyopathy (HCM), there is massive ventricular hypertrophy (characteristically left ventricle) with a smaller than normal ventricular cavity. Contractile function of ventricles is increased, but the filling is impaired by relaxation abnormalities. HCM is usually seen in adolescents and young adults occurring equally in both sexes. A transient form of HCM occurs in infant of diabetic mothers.

Clinical Manifestations

The symptoms include easy fatigability, dyspnea, palpitation, dizziness, and syncope or angina pain. Family history is present in 30–60% cases. Physical examination reveals a radial pulse with a sharp upstroke, a left ventricular lift, an apical thrill or a thrill along the left sternal border, a grade 1–3 / 6 ejection systolic, median pitch murmur at the apex or middle and lower left sternal border. A mitral holosystolic murmur is often present.

X-ray studies show a globular heart, mild left ventricular enlargement with normal pulmonary vascularity. The *ECG abnormalities* are LVH, abnormally deep Q waves (septal hypertrophy) with diminished or absent R waves in the precordial leads, negative T waves in left precordial leads (apical HCM). *Two dimensional ECHO* reveals concentric hypertrophy, localized central hypertrophy and asymmetrical septal hypertrophy. MRI is more helpful in diagnosis of apical HCM. It is a slowly progressive condition. Arrhythmia, cardiac dilatation and CHF may develop in later life. Sudden death may occur due to ventricular arrhythmia.

Treatment

Treatment may be medical or surgical.

Medical treatment includes restriction of moderate physical activity (outdoor games) and drugs viz. beta adrenergic blockers (propranolol), calcium channel blockers (nifedipine, Verapamil) in symptomatic patients. These agents reduce hyper contractile systolic function and improve diastolic filling. Digitalis is contraindicated as it increases the degree of obstruction.

Surgical treatment is indicated in patients who are not responding to medical treatment and who have severe obstruction with resting pressure gradient of greater than 50 mmHg. Morrow's myotomy—myectomy is the procedure of choice.

Dilated Cardiomyopathy

Dilated (or congestive) cardiomyopathy (DCM) is characterized by decreased systolic contraction of the ventricles associated with dilatation of all four cardiac chambers. Intracavity thrombus formation is common leading to pulmonary and systemic emboli. DCM may be idiopathic (in 60% cases) followed by familial and secondary. Many cases of unexplained cardiomyopathy may, infact, result from silent myocarditis. It is the most common form. Endocardial fibroelastosis and doxorubicin cardiomyopathy have clinical features similar to those of DCM.

Clinical Manifestations

There is a history of a viral infection prior to the onset of symptoms like fatigue, weakness and symptoms of left ventricular failure. Physical signs include tachycardia, pulmonary rales, weak peripheral pulses, engorged neck veins and hepatomegaly. There is cardiomegaly, a soft systolic murmur due to MR or TR with or without a gallop rhythm and a loud P2 if there is pulmonary hypertension.

X-ray studies show generalized cardiomegaly with predominant left ventricular enlargement and signs of pulmonary venous hypertension or pulmonary edema. The common *ECG abnormalities* are sinus tachycardia, LVH and ST elevation T inversion. There may be arrhythmias and AV conduction defects. *ECHO studies* reveal left ventricular enlargement with increased end diastolic and end systolic dimensions, reduced fractional shortening and ejection fraction. There may be pericardial effusion and intracavity thrombus. Progressive deterioration is the rule. About 30–40% of patients die within 4 years after onset of symptoms. Causes of death are CHF, ventricular arrhythmia and massive embolism.

Treatment

Treatment consists of treatment of CHF with bed rest, restriction of activity, digoxin and diuretics. Critically ill patients may require inotropic drugs and mechanical ventilation. Use of beta adrenergic blocking agents (propranolol) in chronic heart failure has shown to improve LV ejection fraction. Antiplatelet agents (aspirin) should be given to prevent thrombus formation. Arrhythmias may be treated with amiodarone. A cardiac pacemaker may be necessary with symptomatic bradycardia. Carnitine supplementation should be initiated in suspected carnitine deficiency. Many of the children with DCM may need cardiac transplant.

Endocardial Fibroelastosis

Primary endocardial fibroelastosis is a type of DCM occurring in infants. It is thought to be a consequence of viral myocarditis, interstitial myocarditis, carnitine deficiency and genetic factors. The child presents with symptoms and signs of CHF which develop in the first 10 months of life.

X-ray studies show marked generalized cardiomegaly with normal or congested pulmonary vascularity. The *typical ECG finding* is LVH with strain pattern. Arrhythmias and AV block may be present. ECHO reveals markedly dilated and poorly contracting left ventricle in absence of structural defects. The left ventricle is also dilated.

Treatment

Treatment consists of long continued therapy with digoxin, diuretics and afterload reducing agents. Digoxin should be continued for a minimum of 2–3 years and is then gradually discontinued if symptoms are absent, heart size is normal and ECG normal. An afterloading agent (hydralazine) has been reported to be beneficial. No surgical treatment is available.

With early and proper treatment, one-third of patients recover fully, one-third die of CHF and the rest survive with persistent symptoms.

Restrictive Cardiomyopathy

Restrictive cardiomyopathy is usually a result of infiltrative disease, denotes restriction of diastolic filling of the ventricles. The contractile functions of the ventricle may be normal, but there is marked dilation of both atria. It is a rare form of cardiomyopathy and constitutes only 5% of cardiomyopathy in children.

Clinical Manifestations

The presenting symptoms are exercise intolerance and dyspnea, or chest pain. Physical examination shows engorged jugular veins, gallop rhythm, and a systolic murmur of MR or TR. The *X-ray studies* show cardiomegaly, pulmonary venous congestion and occasional pleural effusion. The *ECG abnormalities* include atrial hypertrophy, atrial fibrillation, and supraventricular tachycardia. AV block may be present in familial type. The diagnostic *ECHO findings* are bilateral atrial enlargement with normal ventricles. LV systolic function is normal until late stage. Prognosis is generally poor.

Treatment

Treatment is supportive. Calcium channel blockers may be used to increase diastolic compliance. Anti-coagulants (warfarin) and antiplatelet agents (aspirin) may prevent thrombosis. Steroids and immunosuppressive drugs are suggested. A permanent pacemaker is indicated for complete heart block. Surgical option is cardiac transplant.

Systemic Hypertension

Systemic hypertension is commonly a disease of the adults. If left untreated it is a major risk factor for stroke, coronary artery disease and renal failure. In children, systemic hypertension is usually secondary to an underlying cause. Adolescents may acquire primary or essential hypertension (with no underlying cause) and the hypertension may track into adulthood. Therefore to increase early detection of hypertension, accurate blood pressure measurement should be a part of the routine annual examination of all children 3 years or older.

Definition

In children, hypertension is defined statistically because blood pressure levels vary with age and gender. The fourth report of the National High Blood pressure Education Programme (NHBPEP) working group on blood pressure in children and adolescents (2004) has recommended the following definitions:

1. Normal blood pressure is defined as average systolic and diastolic pressures below 90th percentile.
2. *Hypertension* is defined as systolic and / or diastolic pressure levels that are greater than the 95th percentile for age and gender on atleast three occasions. However, the adolescents with a blood pressure level 120 / 80 mm Hg or more are considered hypertensive even if they are less than the 95th percentile.
3. *Prehypertension* is defined as an average systolic and/or diastolic pressure between the 90th and 95th percentiles for age and gender.
4. When the blood pressure reading is above the 95th percentile, hypertension can be further classified into Stages 1 and 2 as follows:
   a. *Stage 1 hypertension* is present when the blood pressure readings are between the 95th and 99th percentiles.
   b. *Stage 2 hypertension* is present when the blood pressure readings are 5 mmHg or more above the 99th percentile values.
5. *White coat hypertension* is present when the blood pressure readings are greater than the 95th percentile in health care facilities but normal outside.

In children, blood pressure gradually increases with age. Therefore one should consult standard normograms for interpretation of blood pressure values. The fourth report on the diagnosis, evaluation and treatment of high blood pressure in children and adolescents published in Pediatrics 2004; 114: 555-76 has published blood pressure percentile charts by age and height percentile (See Appendix). These are claimed to be more useful than the former charts in relation to age only.

Etiology and Pathophysiology

Blood pressure is the product of cardiac output and peripheral vascular resistance. An increase in either cardiac output or peripheral resistance results in an increase in blood pressure. When the cause of this increase in pressure can be explained by an associated disease, the hypertension is referred to as secondary. When no underlying disease is present, the hypertension is referred to as primary or essential.

Primary or essential hypertension is commonly recognized in adolescents. It is often accompanied with a family history. The cause of essential hypertension is multifactorial. Many factors, including heredity, diet, stress, obesity, genetic alterations in calcium and sodium transport, vascular smooth muscle reactivity, the renin-angiotensin system and insulin sensitivity have been implicated in the causation of this disorder.

Secondary hypertension is common in infants and young children. It may be transient or sustained depending on the cause. The pathophysiology differs with involvement of different organs.

The common causes of chronic sustained hypertension, reported by the second task force on blood pressure control in children (1987) are as follows:

Newborns: Renal artery thrombosis, renal artery stenosis, congenital renal malformations, coarctation of aorta, bronchopulmonary dysplasia.

Below 6 years: Renal parenchymal disease, coarctation of aorta, renal artery stenosis.

6–10 years: Renal artery stenosis, renal parenchymal disease, essential hypertension.

Above 10 years: Primary hypertension, renal parenchymal disease.

Hypertension due to renal disorders accounts for the majority of causes of secondary hypertension. The mechanism of hypertension as a result of renal parenchymal disease and renal vascular disease is associated with sodium retension and increased renin secretion. The reduced glomerular filtration rate in renal parenchymal diseases (e.g. nephritis) result in salt and water retention, whereas mass lesion (tumour, cysts) may impair renal perfusion and stimulate renin production by the juxtaglomerular apparatus. Vascular lesions (e.g. renal artery stenosis) cause hypertension through stimulation of renin-angiotensin-aldosterone system.

Hypertension is a feature of endocrine disorders. Systolic hypertension and tachycardia are common in hyperthyroidism; diastolic pressure is usually not elevated. Hypercalcemia secondary to hyperparathyroidism results in mild hypertension because of an increase in vascular tone. Adrenocortical disorders may produce hypertension with increased mineral corticoid secretion. Pheochromocytoma of the adrenal medulla, a catecholamine secreting tumour presents with hypertension as a result of cardiac and peripheral vascular effects of epinephrine and norepinephrine.

Altered sympathetic tone can be responsible for acute or intermittent elevation of blood pressure in children with Guillain-Barré syndrome, poliomyelitis, burns and Stevens-Johnson syndrome.

Organic disease of the brain with rapidly expanding lesions, e.g., subarchnoid hemorrhage, hemorrhage into a brain tumour, may give rise to acute hypertension due to sudden increase in intracranial tension.

Table 14.8 : Causes of secondary hypertension

Table 14.8 : Causes of secondary hypertension
Transient hypertension
(a) *Renal:* APSGN, HUS, ATN, anaphylactoid purpura, pyelonephritis, trauma, after transfusion in patients with azotemia.
(b) *Drugs and poisons:* Corticosteroids, oral contraceptives, cyclosporin, Vitamin D intoxication, sympathomimetic agents, lead, mercury, cadmium, thallium.
(c) *Central and autonomic nervous system:* Increased ICT, Guillain-Barré syndrome, encephalitis, poliomyelitis.
(d) *Miscellaneous:* Hypercalcemia, white cell transfusion, extra-corporeal membrane oxygen (ECMO), chronic upper airway obstruction.
Sustained hypertension
(a) *Renal:* Chronic pyelonephritis, chronic glomerulonephritis, hydronephrosis, polycystic kidneys, vesicoureteral reflux, nephropathy, ureteral obstruction, renal trauma, tumours, rejection damage following transplant, connective tissue disorders.
(b) *Vascular:* Coarctation of aorta, renal artery obstruction, high umbilical artery catheterization, renal vein thrombosis.
(c) *Endocrine:* Cushing's syndrome, congenital adrenal hyperplasia, pheochromocytoma, primary hyperaldosteronism, hyperthyroidism, hyperparathyroidism, neural crest tumours.
(d) *Central nervous system:* Intracranial mass, hemorrhage, brain injury, quadriplegia.

Clinical Manifestations

Children with mild hypertension are asymptomatic. Children with severe hypertension can present with symptoms like headache, dizziness, nausea and vomiting, irritability, visual changes, epistaxis, anorexia, personality changes and seizures. Occasionally, congestive cardiac failure, renal dysfunction and stroke may be the presenting features.

Essential hypertension in children and adolescents is usually mild and is detected during routine examination or evaluation before athletic participation. The *diagnosis of essential hypertension* is suggested by the patient's age (usually above 10 years), mild blood pressure elevation, presence of mild to moderate degree of obesity, a positive family history and no signs of underlying disease.

Children with secondary hypertension can have blood pressure ranging from mild to severe degree. Unless the blood pressure has been sustained for some time or is rising rapidly, hypertension does not produce symptoms. Therefore, clinical manifestation of the underlying disease, e.g., failure to thrive in chronic renal disease are frequent presentations.

Hypertensive encephalopathy is suggested by the presence of vomiting, fever, ataxia, stupor and seizures. Young children and infants with unexplained heart failure should always have the blood pressure checked. Increasing irritability is often a complain in young children. Young children fail to recognize and communicate symptoms like headache, dizziness etc.

The *diagnosis of secondary hypertension* is suggested by the child's age (younger), mild to severe elevation of blood pressure, usually with growth failure except in disorders of the adrenal cortex which may present with obesity, and presence of features of the underlying disease.

The features suggesting an underlying disease may be as follows:

1. A family history of renal disease or early cardiovascular disease.
2. Failure to thrive.
3. History of intermittent febrile illness with documented UTI.
4. Presence of flank mass, abdominal bruit.
5. Difference in peripheral pulses and blood pressure in the extremities.
6. Medications viz. corticosteroids, oral contraceptives, nephrotoxic antibiotics, cold medications, heavy metals.
7. Habit of smoking.

Laboratory Investigations

Hypertension in children, in majority of cases is secondary to some cause, some of which may be amenable to complete cure. Therefore all children with hypertension should undergo investigations to rule out a secondary cause. The preliminary investigations should be directed towards detecting renal parenchymal disease, renovascular disease and coarctation of aorta and would comprise the following tests:

1. Urine analysis and urine culture.
2. A complete blood count.
3. Serum electrolytes, blood urea nitrogen, serum creatinine, serum uric acid.
4. Renal ultrasound.
5. An X-ray PA view chest.
6. An electrocardiogram and echocardiogram (in selected cases).

Urinalysis, urine culture, estimation of blood urea nitrogen, creatinine, uric acid should be done to exclude renal parenchymal disease. Presence of hypokalemia may indicate disorders viz. hyperaldosteronism, adrenogenital syndrome and renin producing tumours. An X-ray PA view chest can show notching of ribs indicating coarctation of aorta. An ECG and ECHO can rule out cardiac causes of hypertension. An ECG and an X-ray chest can also be done to record baseline data.

If the results of the preliminary tests are normal, and one suspect essential hypertension from history, the child should be advised for:

1. Serum lipid profile.
2. Fasting blood sugar.

More specialized tests may be required for detection of rare causes of secondary hypertension.

Renal Causes

1. Radionuclide scan.
2. Renal Doppler ultrasonography and renal angiography.
3. Renal vein plasma renin activity.
4. Abdominal aortogram.
5. Kidney biopsy, serum complement, serological tests.

Endocrine Causes

1. Urinary steroids viz. 17–ketosteroids and 17–hydroxycorticosteroids.
2. Urinary catecholamines viz. epinephrine and norepinephrine and their metabolites vanillylmandelic acid levels.
3. Serum and urinary aldosterone.
4. Plasma renin activity.

Renal Imaging

Renal ultrasonography provides a comparison of kidney size and a view of the anatomy of the collecting system as well as identification of a renal mass. A renal *radionuclide scan* is helpful in distinguishing variation in perfusion or scarring of the two kidneys. *Renal Doppler ultrasonography and angiography* can demonstrate lesions in the main arteries or in the segmental branches. Doppler ultrasonography may demonstrate abnormal arterial and venous flow. An *abdominal aortogram* helps in diagnosis of renovascular causes, coarctation of aorta, unilateral renal parenchymal disease, and pheochromocytoma. A careful selection of the tests is important depending on the nature of the abnormality.

Biochemical Tests for Endocrine Causes

Increased levels of urinary steroids viz. 17–ketosteroids and 17–hydroxycorticosteroids helps in diagnosis of Cushing's syndrome and adrenogenital syndrome. Increased urinary catecholamine levels and VMA indicate pheochromocytoma and neuroblastoma. Increased levels of aldosterone indicate hyperaldosteronism and renin producing tumours. Renal vein plasma renin activity is useful test for both renal parenchymal and renovascular diseases. A suppressed value suggests excess mineralocorticoid effect and an elevated value is associated with renal or renovascular involvement.

Course and Prognosis

The natural history of essential hypertension, detected in childhood or adolescence is still not clearly known. Many of these children continue to have hypertension as adults. The prognosis of secondary hypertension depends primarily on the underlying disease.

Prevention

Prevention of hypertension in the early years of life is an essential part of prevention of cardiovascular disease and stroke in adults. Other risk factors for cardiovascular illness include obesity, high dietary sodium intake, sedentary life style, elevated serum cholesterol levels, smoking and alcohol use. It is especially important to discourage cigarette smoking because of the pulmonary and cardiovascular consequences. The increase in arterial wall rigidity and blood viscosity that is associated with exposure to the components of tobacco may cause or exacerbate hypertension. Population based approaches for prevention of hypertension include reduction of sodium intake and an increase in physical activity.

Management

Principles

1. The goal of therapy for hypertension should be to reduce blood pressure to below 95th percentile. Two types of approaches to treatment are available viz. nonpharmacologic and pharmacologic. Both are useful in managing elevated blood pressure.
2. Secondary hypertension will require pharmacologic treatment until the cause is corrected.
3. Adolescents with essential hypertension are usually best managed initially with nonpharmacologic therapy.
4. For pharmacologic therapy, a pragmatic approach to selection of drugs is important. Only familiar drugs should be used. Monotherapy should be the aim. Drug regimen should be simple with use of long acting drugs. Trials of combination therapy may be necessary in patients with long standing poorly controlled, markedly elevated, labile hypertension. In such a situation co-administration of drugs with different sites and mechanism of action should be used.
5. To help compliance in children with sustained hypertension, there should be maintenance of drug calendars, parent's supervision, and patient-physician communication.

Nonpharmacologic Therapy

Nonpharmacologic therapy includes weight reduction, reduction in salt intake and a consistent programme of exercise and counseling.

Weight reduction may result in a reduction of upto 5–10 mm Hg of systolic and upto 5 mm Hg of diastolic pressure.

A *reduction of sodium intake* may similarly result in lowering of blood pressure upto 5 to 10 mm Hg. A restricted salt intake of 5-6 grams sodium chloride (85–100 mEq of sodium) per day is recommended.

A *consistent programme of exercises* viz. aerobics, yoga and relaxing exercises has been shown to reduce blood pressure.

Counseling of adolescents about the adverse effects of tobacco and alcohol on blood pressure may help them to comply with the advice to stop smoking, alcohol consumption.

In view of the beneficial effects of nonpharmacologic therapy and the undesirable effects of many anti-hypertensive drugs, a well supervised programme of non-pharmacologic therapy should be prescribed for young patients with essential hypertension.

Pharmacologic Therapy

When the patient is unable to cooperate with the non-pharmacologic approach or the reduction in blood pressure is not sufficient, antihypertensive agents should be prescribed. Young patients with essential hypertension who require drug therapy may be treated with a diuretic or a beta blocker (Propranolol). If the blood pressure is not lowered adequately, a calcium channel blocker (Nifedepine) may be added to the diuretic, and an ACE inhibitor (Enalapril) may replace the beta blocker. In adolescent with significant hypertension, ACE inhibitors and calcium channel blockers may be considered for initial therapy. In patients with long standing or poorly controlled hypertension, trials of combination of antihypertensive drugs may be required. The basic principle of combination antihypertensive therapy is the co-administration of drugs with different sites and mechanisms of action.

Table 14.9 : Common anti-hypertensive drugs

Drug	*Dosage*
1. Frusemide	1–3 mg /kg/day
2. Propranolol	1–2 mg /kg /day
3. Nefidepine	0.25–0.5 mg/kg/dose (max 10 mg) 4–6 hourly
4. Enalapril	Infant and children Per oral 0.1 mg–0.5 mg / kg/day in 1–2 doses IV 5–10 micrograms/ kg /dose 8 hourly Adolescents Per oral 2.5–5 mg/day titrated to a max 40 mg/1 day 12 hourly IV 0.0625–1.25 mg/kg (max 20 mg/day) 6 hourly.

About the Drugs Used for Control of Hypertension

Volume dependent hypertensive children usually show adequate response to diuretics. Those with high renin and high cardiac output usually respond to beta blockers. Chronic use of diuretics has been shown to cause elevation of serum lipids increasing the risk of ischemic heart disease in adults. Such a side effect is not confirmed in children. Beta blockers have also been associated with changes in serum lipids as well as mild reduction in exercise tolerance. Patients with reactive airway disease however cannot tolerate beta blockers.

Suggested Reading

1. Bedside Approach in the Diagnosis of Congenital Heart Diseases by R. Tandon, 1st edition, 1999. Churchill Livingstone Pvt Ltd., New Delhi.
2. Pediatric Cardiology for Practitioners by Myung K. Park with contribution by R. George Troxler, 4th (2002) and 5th edition (2007), Mosby Imprint of Elsevier, St. Louis, Missouri.
3. Paul Wood's Diseases of Heart and Circulation, 3rd edition. Reprinted 1968, 1969 Chapman and Hall Ltd, 1975, II New Fetter Lane, London EC4P 4EE. Printed in Great Britain by Whitstable Litho Ltd, Whitstable, Kent.
4. Nelson Textbook of Pediatrics edited by Berhman, Kliegman and Jenson, 17th edition, 2004 and 18th edition, 2006.
5. Practical Pediatric Problems by James Hutchison and Forrester Cockburn, 6th edition, 1986. P G Publishing Pvt Ltd, New Delhi.
6. PALS Provider Manual. American Heart Association.

15

Rheumatic Diseases

OUTLINES

Rheumatic diseases are a group of diseases which result from abnormally regulated immune responses that lead to inflammation of the target organs. They may present with a wide range of complaints because many different organs may be affected.

Early diagnosis is often difficult because diagnostic manifestations can take time to develop. Hence clinical evaluation may need to be repeated and occasionally an earlier diagnosis may need reconsideration.

There is a wide spectrum of rheumatic diseases in children. This chapter will discuss only some common types. They include juvenile idiopathic (rheumatoid) arthritis, Kawasaki disease, Henoch-Schönlein purpura, systemic lupus erythematosus (SLE) and Takayasu arteritis.

Juvenile Idiopathic Arthritis

Juvenile idiopathic arthritis (JIA), formerly known as Juvenile rheumatoid arthritis (JRA) is the most common rheumatic disease in children and the incidence is fast increasing in the developing countries as well. It is a major cause of disability in children. According to the classification criteria of American College of Rheumatology (ACR), juvenile rheumatoid arthritis is regarded as a category of diseases and not a single entity.

The *criteria for diagnosis* are as follows: Arthritis of one or more joints, onset before 16 years of age, arthritis persisting for 6 weeks, exclusion of other juvenile arthritis. *Arthritis* is described as swelling or effusion or presence of 2 or more of the following signs: Limitation of range of motion, tenderness or pain on motion, increased heat in one or more joints. It needs mention that although many other classifications have been proposed, only the ACR criteria have been statistically validated and meet the requirements of evidenced based medicine.

Three principal types have been proposed in the ACR classification viz. oligoarthritis or pauciarticular disease, polyarthritis rheumatoid factor +ve and polyarthritis rheumatoid factor – ve, and systemic arthritis.

Etiopathogenesis

The etiology is unknown. However, two necessary events have been postulated. These include an immunogenetic susceptibility and an external, presumably environmental trigger. Studies suggest an exaggerated immune reactivity in immunogenetically predisposed children, suspected to be in response to exposure to environmental antigens. It has been postulated that HLA typing would identify risk and protective factors. Polyarthritis is associated with HLA-DR4 and oligoarthritis with HLA-DR8. With a polygenic pathogenesis, JIA seldom results in multiple cases in a family. Studies of T-cell receptor expression confirm recruitment of T-cell specific for synovial non-self antigens that may be protective or associated with improved responsiveness to medical treatment. On the other hand, migration of T-cells whose surfaces bear molecules into the synovium can induce chronic activation of resident cellular components resulting in resistance to treatment. T-cell activation results in a cascade of events which leads to tissue damage in joints and other affected tissues. These include activation of B cells, complement consumption and immune complex formation and release of proinflammatory cytokines (viz., tumour necrosis factor (TNF)–alpha, interleukin 1 and 6). Inheritance of certain alleles may predispose to upregulation of the cytokine networks resulting in more severe articular and systemic disease.

JIA is characterized by synovitis of the peripheral joints which manifest as soft tissue swelling and effusion. Pathologically it is characterized by villous hypertrophy and hyperplasia with hyperemia and edema of the synovial tissues. There is vascular endothelial hyperplasia and infiltration of mononuclear and plasma cells. In advanced uncontrolled disease there is pannus formation. It is an inflammatory exudate over the synovial membrane which causes progressive erosion of the articular cartilage and the contiguous bone.

Clinical Manifestations

Early in the disease, symptoms may be subtle or acute. These often include morning stiffness, easy fatigability in the early afternoon after school followed by joint pain and swelling. The involved joints are warm but not erythematous, are painful on movements and resist full range of movement.

In the **oligoarthritis (pauciarticular disease)** type of onset, there is predominantly involvement of the joints of the lower extremities viz. the knees and ankles. At the onset often there is involvement of one joint. Inflammation of 4 or less joints is required as criteria for classification as pauciarticular disease. Isolated involvement of upper extremity large joint is not characteristic of this type of JIA. Extended oligoarthritis can occur with involvement of 5 or more joints after the first 6 months of the disease.

The **polyarthritis (polyarticular disease)** type is characterized by involvement of both large and small joints of both upper and lower extremities. Inflammation of 5 or more joints is required as criteria for classification of

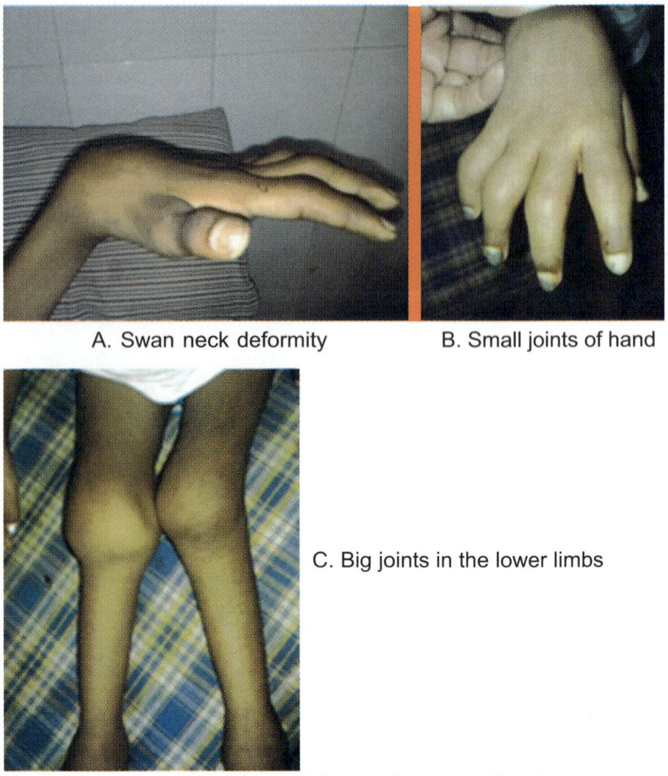

A. Swan neck deformity

B. Small joints of hand

C. Big joints in the lower limbs

Fig. 15.1: Involvement of joints in juvenile rheumatoid arthritis

this type. The involvement of the hip usually occurs later. Severe disease is associated with rheumatoid nodules on the extensor surfaces of the elbow and over the tendo achilles and micrognathia which reflects chronic temporomandibular joint disease. Cervical spine involvement occurs frequently with a risk of atlanto-axial subluxation and potential neurological deficit. Polyarthritis in children may be rheumatoid factor negative or associated with positive rheumatoid factor on 2 occasions at least 3 months apart.

The **systemic onset disease** is characterized by arthritis with or preceded by fever of 2 weeks or more duration, documented to be quotidian with temperature upto 39°C or more. Each febrile episode is accompanied by a characteristic faint, erythematous, macular rash which is nonpruritic. The rashes are salmon colored evanescent lesions, linear or circular, 2–5 mm in size distributed in groups commonly over the trunk and proximal extremities. A warm bath evokes reappearance of the rash. Characteristically, the rash is transient in nature with a group of lesions lasting for less than one hour.

The arthritis, fever are accompanied by one or more of the following features viz. rash, generalized lymphadenopathy, serositis (pericardial effusion) and hepatomegaly or splenomegaly.

Laboratory Diagnosis

Laboratory abnormalities characteristic of inflammation include raised ESR, C-reactive protein, leucocytosis, thrombocytosis and normocytic normochromic anemia.

Elevated ANA titres are present in atleast 40–85% of children with polyarticular or oligoarticular types. It is unusual in the systemic onset type. ANA positivity is associated with increased risk of development of chronic uveitis in children with oligoarthritis. The rheumatoid factor test may be positive in polyarticular disease. A positive rheumatoid factor test and presence of rheumatoid nodules are associated with an overall poor prognosis and eventual functional disability.

Early radiographic changes of arthritis include soft tissue swelling, regional osteoporosis, and periosteal new bone apposition about affected joints. Local bone growth may be decreased due to stimulation of regional epiphyseal closure. There may be limb length discrepancy due to acceleration of linear growth especially in the knee joint. In late stages there may be subchondral erosions and narrowing of cartilage space especially in small tubular bones, with varying degrees of bony destruction and fusion. Characteristic changes in the cervical spine are seen in the level of C 2-3 which may progress to atlanto-axial subluxation. An MRI is more helpful than a plain X-ray because it is more sensitive to early and minimal changes in bone and soft tissues.

Management

The objective of treatment is to establish a pattern of adaptation which is as normal as possible and achieve this with minimal side effects of the medications used. The goals of treatment are to achieve disease remission, prevent or halt joint damage, and foster normal growth and development. The treatment is individualized depending on the subtype and severity as well as response to treatment.

Oligoarthritis JIA: Most children suffering from this type respond to non-steroidal anti-inflammatory drugs (NSAIDs). Ibuprofen, 40-60 mg/kg/day (maximum 3.2 gm/day) or Naproxen 10-20 mg/kg/day (maximum 1gm/day) for 4-6 weeks are the drugs of choice. Those who have no or short lived improvement or those who have limitation of joint function or leg length discrepancy, benefit from intra articular corticosteroids. Triamcinolone hexacetonide is the steroid used. It provides a long lasting response. With inadequate response, intrarticular steroid may be repeated. However, it should not exceed 3 doses per year in a single joint. Response to treatment is indicated by clinical improvement of disease activity viz. joint swelling, but has no effect on laboratory indices. The children, who do not respond to NSAIDs and intra-articular corticosteroid injection, require treatment with disease modifying anti rheumatic drugs (DMARDs) as in polyarticular disease. Extended oligoarthritis should also be treated as polyarticular disease.

Polyarticular JIA: The child should be started on a NSAID and continued upto 4 - 6 weeks as in oligoarthritis. Oral steroids (Prednisolone 2 mg/kg/day) should be added as bridging medication initially awaiting response or during a flare up. If there is inadequate response after 6 weeks, oral methotrexate 10 mg/m^2/week should be started and steroid tapered. Failure to respond to methotrexate will need addition of a biologic DMARD.

Biologic medications inhibit pro-inflammatory cytokines such as tumour necrosis factor - alpha (TNF - alpha) and interleukin-1 (IL-1). In the event of inadequate response to methotrexate and in those with poor prognostic factors, biologic medication, TNF- alpha antagonist, Etanercept 0.8 mg/kg weekly (maximum dose 50 mg/week) given subcutaneously show significant clinical improvement after 3 months of therapy.

Systemic Onset JIA: NSAIDs alone rarely induce remission in children in systemic onset JIA. For treatment of fever ibuprofen 40-60 mg/kg/day (max 3.2 gm/day) or naproxen 10-20 mg/kg/day (max 1gm/day) should be given for 2 weeks. If response is inadequate prednisolone 1-2 mg/kg/day or I.V. methyl prednisolone 30 mg/kg/day (max 500 mg/day for 3 consecutive days, may be repeated after one week) should be considered. If the child responds, steroid should be tapered.

Methotrexate should be used as an adjunctive therapy. Failure to respond to methotrexate by 6 - 12 weeks needs addition of a biologic medication like Etanercept. Addition of IL-I receptor antagonist (Anakinra, 1- 2 mg/kg subcutaneously daily) during initiation of therapy often induces dramatic and rapid response.

Macrophage Activation Syndrome (MAS): Systemic JIA may be complicated with MAS. It is rare but occasionally fatal. It is characterized by acute development of profound anemia associated with leucopenia and thrombocytopenia, high spiking fever, lymphadenopathy, and hepatosplenomegaly. The patient may have purpura and mucosal bleeding, as well as elevated fibrin split product values and prolonged prothrombin time and partial thromboplastin time. A feature useful in distinguishing MAS from a flare of systemic disease is fall in ESR which results from hypofibrinogenemia and hepatic dysfunction. The diagnosis is confirmed by bone marrow examination demonstrating hemophagocytosis. Emergency treatment with high dose methyl prednisolone, cyclosporine or Anakinra has been generally effective. Severe cases need treatment similar to Hemophagocytic lymphohistiocytosis (HLS).

Use of Systemic Corticosteroids: Systemic corticosteroids are recommended only for management of severe systemic disease, for bridge therapy waiting for therapeutic response to a DMARD and for control of uveitis. Use of systemic corticosteroids, on long term basis, can be now well avoided with the advent of newer DMARDs because they impose the risk of severe toxic effects.

Periodic Ophthalmologic Examination: All cases of JIA should be screened for uveitis at regular intervals with periodic slit lamp ophthalmic examination. In oligoarticular disease, ophthalmological examination should be done initially, then 3 monthly for 2 years followed by 4-6 monthly for 5 years, and then annually. In polyarticular disease ophthalmological examination should be done initially, then 4-6 monthly for 5 years, and then annually. In systemic onset disease the initial examination should be followed by annual examinations.

Initial treatment of uveitis includes use of mydriatics and corticosteroids, topically, systemically or by periocular injection. Severe uveitis may warrant use of DMARDs and TNF-alpha antagonist (adalimumab and infliximab).

Rehabilitation

Rehabilitation of the child includes physiotherapy, advice for good nutrition and orthopedic intervention. The diet should ensure appropriate amount of calcium, vitamin D, protein and calorie. Physiotherapy and occupational therapy are invaluable adjuncts to the treatment programme of JIA.

Course and Prognosis

Some studies have shown that 30% of children suffering from JIA have significant active disease into adulthood. 50–60% has some form of disability or deformity in adulthood. 10% have major disabilities.

Marked systemic disease is difficult to control but is usually present during the first few years after onset and tends to regress over years. Thereafter, prognosis depends on the number of joints involved and the severity of arthritis.

The child with polyarticular disease often has a prolonged course with functional disability. The bad prognostic factors for functional disability include older age of onset, positive rheumatoid factor test, and presence of rheumatoid nodules and early development of bone erosions or disease of spine or hip.

Oligoarthritis is usually associated with chronic uveitis which may result in blindness. However, expert ophthalmological therapy has improved the outcome.

Kawasaki Disease

Kawasaki disease is an acute self limiting vasculitis of infancy and the young child. First described by Dr.Tomisaku Kawasaki in Japan in 1967, the disease is now known to occur in both endemic and community-wide epidemic forms in the Americas, Europe and Asia in children of all races. It is characterized by fever, bilateral non-exudative conjunctivitis, erythema of lips and oral mucosa, changes in the extremities, rash and cervical lymphadenopathy. Coronary artery aneurysm can develop in 15–25% of untreated children and may lead to ischemic heart disease or sudden death.

Pathogenesis

Kawasaki disease causes a severe vasculitis of all blood vessels but predominantly affecting the medium sized arteries, with predilection for the coronary arteries. The lesion in the arteries consists of edema of endothelial and smooth muscle cells with inflammatory infiltration of the vascular wall initially by polymorphonuclear cells followed by macrophages, lymphocytes (which are mostly CD 8 T-cells) and plasma cells which are mostly IgA cells. In the most severely affected arteries, inflammation involves all three layers of the vascular wall with destruction of internal elastic lamina. The vessel looses its structural integrity; they become weak resulting in dilatation or aneurysm formation. Thrombi may form in the lumen and obstruct blood flow. In the healing phase, there is progressive fibrosis with marked intimal proliferation resulting in stenotic lesion in the arteries.

An inflammatory infiltrate, including IgA plasma cells is also seen in non-vascular tissues like myocardium, upper respiratory tract, pancreas, kidney and biliary tract but without any sequelae.

There is a vigorous antibody response in the subacute form of illness which is suggested by elevated levels of all the serum immunoglobulins.

Clinical Manifestations

Kawasaki disease is generally divided into three clinical phases: acute febrile phase, subacute phase and convalescent phase. The *acute phase* usually lasts for 1–2 weeks. It is characterized by fever and other signs of acute illness. The *subacute phase* generally lasts until about 4th week. Fever and acute signs disappear except for irritability, conjunctival injection and anorexia. It is associated with desquamation of skin, thrombocytosis and development of coronary artery aneurysm and the highest risk of sudden death. The *convalescent phase* begins when all clinical signs of illness have disappeared and continue until the ESR return to normal, approximately 6–8 weeks after the onset of illness.

Diagnostic Criteria

Fever lasting for atleast 5 days.

Presence of atleast 4 of the following five signs:

1. Bilateral bulbar conjunctival injection, generally non-purulent.
2. Changes in the mucosa of the oropharynx, including injected pharynx, injected and/or dry fissured lips, and strawberry tongue.
3. Changes of the peripheral extremities, such as edema, and/or erythema of the hands or feet in the acute phase; or periungual desquamation in the subacute phase.
4. Rash, primarily truncal; polymorphous but non-vesicular.
5. Cervical adenopathy, > 1.5 cm, usually unilateral lymphadenopathy, not explained by other known disease process.

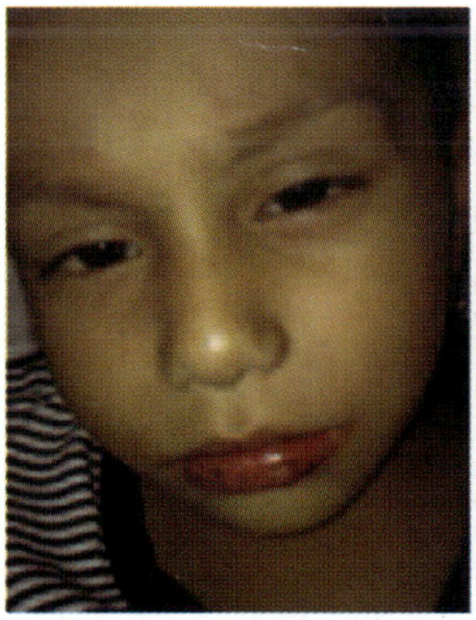

Fig. 15.2 : Cracked lips

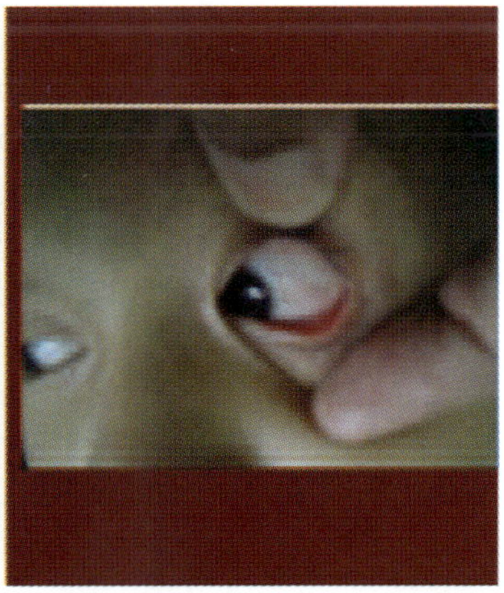

Fig. 15.3 : Non purulent conjunctivitis

Fever is generally high spiking (upto 104°F or higher), remittent, unresponsive to antibiotics. The duration of fever may be generally 1–2 weeks without treatment but may persist for 3–4 weeks. Prolonged fever has been shown to be a risk factor for the development of coronary artery disease.

The *rash* may be of various forms such as maculopapular, erythema multiformae or scarlatiniform. It is accentuated in the groin area. Perianal desquamation is common in the acute phase. Periungual desquamation of fingers and toes begins 1–3 weeks after the onset of illness and may progress to involve the entire hand and foot.

Besides the clinical criteria, the other associated symptoms which may be present during the first 10 days of illness include G.I. symptoms (vomiting, diarrhoea, or pain abdomen) in around 65% cases, respiratory features of interstitial pneumonia and effusion in 30% cases. Other clinical findings include significant irritability, especially in infants (which may due to aseptic meningitis), mild hepatitis, urethritis and meatitis with sterile pyuria, hydrops of gallbladder and arthritis.

Arthritis is more common in girls and may occur early in the illness with fever and other acute symptoms or may develop during the 2nd–3rd week. It generally affects hands, knees, ankles or hips.

Cardiac involvement which is the most important manifestation may be in form of myocarditis, pericarditis and coronary artery aneurysms. Coronary artery aneurysm develops during the 2nd–3rd weeks of illness and can be detected by 2D echocardiography. Valvular regurgitation and systemic artery aneurysm may develop but are uncommon. A giant coronary aneurysm (> / = 8 mm internal diameter) pose the greatest risk for rupture, thrombosis or stenosis and myocardial infarction.

Laboratory Diagnosis

There are no specific laboratory tests. However, certain laboratory findings are characteristics. Normocytic normochromic anemia is common. The leucocyte count is normal or elevated with increase of polymorphs and presence of immature forms. The platelet count is generally normal in the 1st week of illness but may increase upto 1,000,000/cumm by the 2nd–3rd week. The acute phase reactants viz. high ESR and C reactive protein is present in the acute phase and may persist for 4–6 weeks.

The antinuclear antibody and rheumatoid factor are negative. Sterile pyuria, mild elevation of liver transaminases and CSF pleocytosis may be present.

A 2D echo should be performed at diagnosis and again after 2–3 weeks of illness. If results are normal in both, a repeat study is performed 6–8 weeks after onset of illness, when the ESR is normal. There is no convincing evidence of long-term cardiovascular sequelae in children who do not develop coronary abnormalities within 2 months after the onset of illness. Therefore, if all the 3 studies are normal, additional follow-up studies are optional. For patients who develop coronary artery aneurysm, more frequent ECHO studies and angiography may be indicated. Such patients should be referred to a pediatric cardiologist.

Treatment

Patients in acute stage should be treated with intravenous immunoglobulin (IVIG) and high dose aspirin as soon as possible after diagnosis within 10 days of illness. Such a treatment will reduce the incidence of coronary artery disease to 2–4%. Treatment with aspirin alone, on the other hand will reduce the incidence to 20–25%. Treatment with IVIG and aspirin should be considered even if the diagnosis is made after 10 days if fever has persisted. However effect of such therapy on the risk of developing coronary artery aneurysm is unknown.

IVIG should be given in the dose of 2 gm / kg over 10–12 hours and aspirin 80–100 mg / kg / day divided into 4 doses and given 6 hourly. If there is partial or no response to the first dose, a second dose of IVIG 2 gm /kg should be considered. Use of corticosteroids in Kawasaki disease is controversial. It may be used if fever persists after 2 doses of IVIG.

The dose of aspirin should be reduced to 3–5 mg/kg/day once daily after the 14th day or the patient has been afebrile for 3–4 days. Aspirin in such doses should be continued for 6–8 weeks after the onset of illness.

Patients with small solitary aneurysm should continue aspirin (3–5 mg / kg / day) indefinitely. Patients with large or multiple small aneurysm may require the addition of dipyridamole, 4–6 mg / kg /day in 2–3 divided doses. Warfarin may be added in patients with high risk of thrombosis. The patients with aneurysm needs long-term follow-up with ECHO, stress tasting, and angiography. Coronary stenosis needs surgical intervention.

An attack of acute coronary thrombosis should be treated with prompt fibrinolytic therapy with urokinase or streptokinase under supervision of a pediatric cardiologist.

Prognosis

For patients who do not develop coronary artery disease, recovery is complete without any long-term effect. Recurrent illness occurs in 1–3% cases. The outcome of children with coronary abnormalities depends on the severity. Overall 50% of coronary artery aneurysm resolves echocardiographically by 1–2 years after illness. Giant aneurysms are most likely to lead to thrombosis or stenosis which necessitates surgical intervention including heart transplant.

Henoch-Schönlein Purpura

Henoch-Schönlein purpura also called anaphylactoid purpura is a vasculitis syndrome affecting the small non-muscular vessels of the body. It is characterized by purpuric rash, arthritis, abdominal pain and glomerulonephritis. The skin lesion is the most obvious sign; the visceral signs are less easily recognized but are far more serious.

Etiology

The cause is unknown. The syndrome can occur at any age but most cases occur between the age group of 2–8 years. Boys are affected twice as often as girls. Allergy or drug sensitivity is thought to play a role in some cases.

Pathology

In the skin, capillaries are most frequently affected. Small arterioles and venules may also be affected. There is infiltration of inflammatory cells viz. polymorphonuclear cells, round cells, eosinophils and RBCs surrounding the blood vessels.

Scattered debris, edema and swelling of the collagen fibrils are found adjacent to the affected vessels. Inflammation or hemorrhage may occur at other sites, like the synovium, gastrointestinal tract and the central nervous system.

In the kidney, the principal lesion is a proliferative change affecting endothelial and mesangial cells. These changes may be minor (focal and segmental glomerulitis), or there may be diffuse mesangial proliferation with extensive crescent formation, affecting all glomeruli. There are interstitial inflammatory changes; their severity is related to that of the glomerular lesions. Immunopathologic studies show deposition of IgA principally in the mesangium but occasionally in some of the capillary loops. There is also deposition of C_3, IgG and IgM in similar locations. Electron microscopy shows fine granular electron dense deposits within the mesangium and occasionally in relation to the glomerular basement membrane in sub-endothelial, intramembranous, or epimembranous locations.

Pathogenesis

The pathogenesis remains unknown. The disease appears to be mediated by formation of immune complexes containing polymeric IgA 1 within capillaries of the skin, intestines and glomerulus.

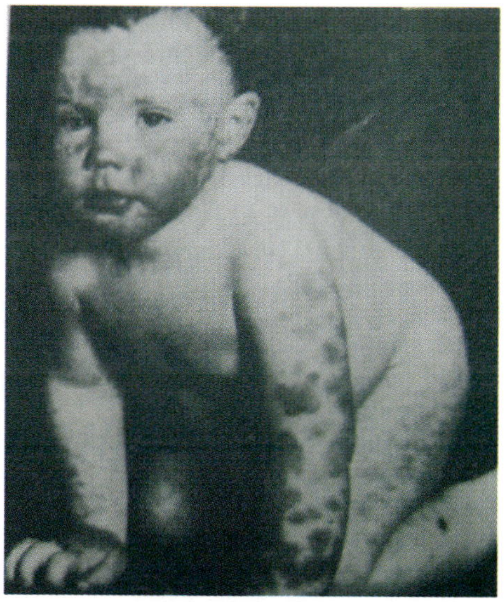

A. Face in infants

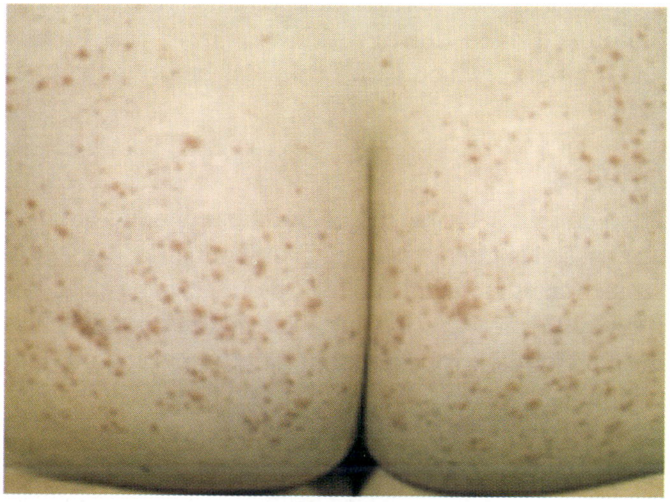

B. Buttocks

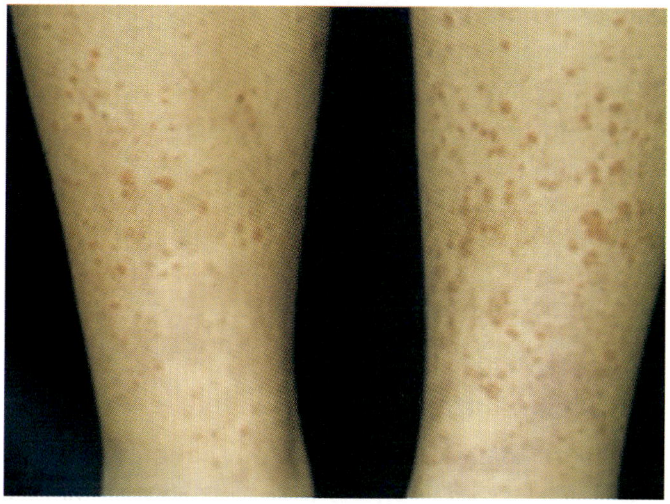

C. Legs

Fig. 15.4: Purpura in anaphylactoid purpura

Clinical Manifestations

The clinical manifestations include features of involvement of skin, joints, gastrointestinal and kidneys. The onset may be acute with simultaneous appearance of several manifestations or gradual with sequential appearance of different manifestations over a period of weeks.

The *skin lesions* usually appear on the lower extremities but may involve the buttocks, upper extremities, trunk and face as well. The skin manifestations are variable. The classic skin lesion begins as a small wheal or an erythematous maculopapule. Initially it blanches on pressure but later loses this ability and generally become petechial or purpuric. The purpuric areas become pink to purple, then rusty and eventually fades away. The skin lesions appear in crops; any one time a variety may be present. In addition to the characteristic lesions, the various patterns of erythema multiformae and erythema nodosum may occur. The skin lesions are rarely pruritic.

Angioedema involving scalp, eyelids, lips, dorsa of hands and feet, back and perineum is common especially in young children. Rarely an entire limb segment, such as the forearm, may be transiently swollen and tender.

Arthritis occurs in 75% of affected children. Large joints, particularly the knees and ankles are most commonly involved. The affected joints may be swollen, tender and painful on movement. There may be effusion which is serous with leucocytosis. Joint lesions usually resolve after a few days without residual deformity but may recur during the period of active disease.

Gastrointestinal symptoms occur in 75% of affected children. The most common complain is colicky abdominal pain, which may be severe and is often associated with vomiting. In around 50% patients there is gross or occult blood in stool and hematemesis. Failure to recognize the syndrome, may lead to a diagnosis of acute abdomen and unnecessary laparotomy.

Renal manifestations occur in 25–50% of children in the acute phase. The symptoms and signs appear 1–3 weeks after an acute upper respiratory infection. The child may present with gross hematuria, microscopic hematuria and proteinuria, with features of nephrotic syndrome, acute nephritis or renal insufficiency. Renal manifestations may occur upto 12 weeks after the onset of initial presentation. An uncommon presentation is associated with pain in the loin and renal colic as a result of ureteritis. Ureteritis is usually seen in children younger than 5 years of age and frequently leads to ureteral stenosis and hydronephrosis requiring surgical treatment.

Central nervous system manifestation is rare but serious. The child may present with seizures, paresis and coma.

Other manifestations include fever, malaise, hepatosplenomegaly, lymphadenopathy which may occur during the acute phase. Rarely intramuscular hemorrhage, cardiac involvement, eye involvement and testicular torsion have been reported.

Laboratory Diagnosis

Laboratory tests are not diagnostic.

1. The ESR is elevated. The white cell count is often increased. Eosinophilia may be present. Coagulation profile is normal.
2. With renal involvement, red cells, WBC, cast and protein are present in urine.
3. Stool may contain gross or occult blood.
4. Serum complement levels are normal or elevated. Serum IgA levels may be elevated.

Treatment

There is no specific treatment for HSP. Majority of patients require symptomatic treatment. Arthritis is managed with rest and NSAIDs. Systemic corticosteroids are indicated in patients with marked subcutaneous edema and severe rash, severe abdominal colic and orchitis. Prednisolone is administered in the dose of 1 - 2 mg/kg / day for 7 days, followed by gradual tapering in the subsequent 2 weeks. Therapy with oral corticosteroids is effective in reducing abdominal pain and joint pain. It does not prevent lupus nephritis.

Renal disease is mild in majority of cases and hence does not require specific therapy. There is complete recovery. Children with rapidly progressive glomerulonephritis and nephrotic range proteinuria require treatment with IV corticosteroids, cytotoxic drugs and in non responsive cases plasmapheresis.

Course

The course is variable. Often the disease is mild, lasting for a few days and manifested only by transient arthritis and few purpuric spots. In more severely affected children, the average duration of disease is 4–6 weeks. Subsequent exacerbations and remissions may occur. Sometimes the illness may smolder for 1 year or more.

Prognosis

Death may occur rarely during acute phase from gastrointestinal complications (viz. hemorrhage, intussusception and bowel infarction), acute renal failure or central nervous system involvement. The risk of chronic renal insufficiency after renal involvement is 2–5%. Presentation as nephrotic syndrome or acute nephritis carries the highest risk of chronic renal failure whereas a presentation with microscopic hematuria alone carries the best prognosis.

Systemic Lupus Erythematosus

Systemic lupus erythematosus (SLE) is a rheumatic disease of unknown cause. It is a condition which must be considered in the differential diagnosis of problems ranging from prolonged fever of unknown origin to arthralgia, anemia and nephritis. It should be suspected in patients with multiorgan symptoms with an abnormal complete blood count and urinalysis. The onset of disease is unusual before 8 years of age although it has been diagnosed even during infancy. There is a female predominance which varies from 4:1 before puberty to 8:1 afterward.

Etiology

It is a condition characterized by autoantibodies directed against self antigens resulting in inflammatory damage to target organs including kidneys, blood forming cells, and the central nervous system. The hallmark of SLE is autoantibody production, particularly antinuclear antibodies to DNA. Elevated levels of autoantibodies, particularly anti-double stranded DNA (anti-ds DNA) antibodies, are associated with circulating and tissue bound immune complexes that lead to complement fixation and recruitment of inflammatory cells resulting in tissue injury. Autoantibodies may precede the onset of disease by 9 years. This suggests a presymptomatic state of autoimmunity.

A genetic predisposition is suggested by the high frequency of SLE, other autoimmune disease, hypergammaglobulinemia and ANA in the family members. In addition, certain HLA types such as HLA-B8, HLA-DR2 and HLA-DR3 occur with increased frequency among patients with SLE. Congenital complement deficiency also acts as a predisposing factor.

Clinical Manifestations

The most common presentation in children includes prolonged fever, fatigue, anorexia, weight loss, arthralgia or arthritis, rash, hematologic abnormalities and renal disease. The symptoms may be intermittent or persistent.

The characteristic skin lesion is the malar or butterfly rash. It is frequently present and involves the cheeks and nasal bridge (Fig. 15.5). It varies from an erythematous blush to thickened epidermis to scaly patches. The rashes may be photosensitive and extend to all sun exposed part of the body. Other cutaneous lesions include erythematous macular eruptions (particularly on the fingers, palms and soles), purpura, livedo reticularis (lacelike bluish, purplish or erythematous discoloration of the skin indicating vascular instability) and Raynaud's phenomenon. Less commonly, there may be annular lesions, bullous or urticarial lesions and alopecia.

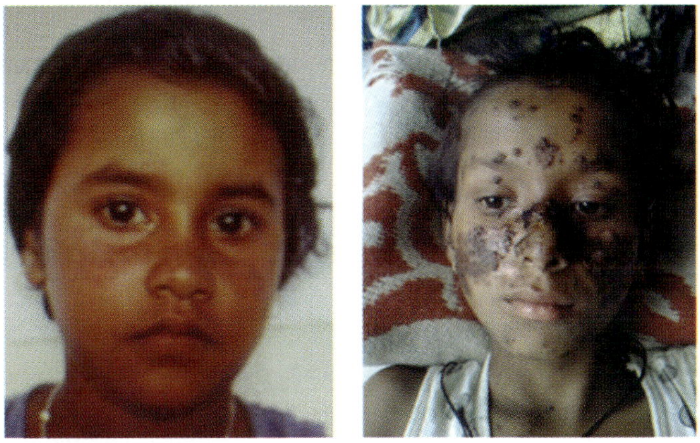

A. Erythematous blush B. Scaly patches

Fig. 15.5: Butterfly rash in SLE

The features pertaining to musculoskeletal system include arthralgia, arthritis (without residual affect), tendonitis and myositis.

There may be involvement of all the serous surfaces viz. pleural, pericardial and peritoneal. Often there is hepatosplenomegaly. Other GI symptoms include pain, diarrhoea, melena, inflammatory bowel disease and hepatitis.

Involvement of kidneys manifests with hypertension, nephrotic syndrome, or acute renal failure.

The features of cardiac involvement include verrucous endocarditis (Libman-Sacks disease), myocarditis, and thickening of heart valves. The child may present with heart failure, coronary artery vasculitis and thrombosis. The pulmonary manifestations include acute pulmonary hemorrhage, pulmonary infiltration often with superimposed infection and fibrosis. It needs mention that early signs of cardiopulmonary disease are clinically silent. It is detected by echocardiogram and deteriorating pulmonary function tests.

The common neurologic features are cognitive dysfunction, psychosis, arterial and venous thrombosis.

Differential Diagnosis

SLE may be considered in the differential diagnosis of problems characterized by prolonged fever, arthralgia, anemia and nephritis. The differential diagnosis includes acute post streptococcal glomerulonephritis, systemic onset JRA, acute rheumatic fever, infective endocarditis, leukemia, and immune thrombocytopenic purpura. However, SLE should be considered in patients with multiorgan symptoms especially if there are hematologic and urinary abnormalities.

Drug induced SLE is a SLE like disease that is precipitated by exposure to drugs like sulphonamides, antiarrhythmic agents and anticonvulscents. The typical symptoms of fever, rash and involvement of serous sacs spontaneously abate with discontinuation of the offending drug.

Laboratory Diagnosis

The degree of serologic disease activity is reflected by the increased levels of anti-double stranded DNA. It is more specific of SLE. Serum levels of total hemolytic component, C3 and C4 are decreased during active disease and provide a second measure of disease activity. Increased levels of ANA in children with active disease is an excellent screening tool, may not be specific of SLE because ANA can be raised without any disease or can be associated with rheumatic diseases and many other conditions. Hypergammaglobulinemia is common but non-specific.

Nephritis is present in most children suffering from SLE. The extent of renal involvement is usually disproportionate to the findings of urine analysis. Hence renal biopsy and staging can help determine the type of treatment in individual cases.

WHO Classification of Lupus Nephritis on the Basis of Biopsy

Class I : Normal.

I A : Negative by immunofluorescence (IF) and electron microscopy (EM).

I B : Normal by light microscopy (LM), deposits seen on IF and EM.

Class II : Mesangial hypercellularity (mesangial deposits on IF, EM).

II A : Mild hypercellularity.

II B : Moderate hypercellularity.

Class III : Focal proliferative glomerulonephritis, diffuse mesangial and focal subendothelial deposits on IF and EM.

Class IV : Diffuse proliferative glomerulonephritis, mesangial, subendothelial and subepithelial deposits on IF and EM.

Class V : Membranous nephropathy.

Class VI : Sclerosing glomerulonephritis.

Treatment

Systemic lupus erythematosus is a lifelong disease which requires monitoring indefinitely. The most important aspect of management is meticulous and frequent reevaluation of the clinical signs and laboratory data, especially for renal and serologic flares of the disease. Prompt detection and treatment of disease flares influence the disease outcome. The aim of treatment is to promote well-being in the patient. The nature of drug therapy depends on the severity of the disease. The WHO classification is useful in guiding treatment.

Class I disease do not require specific therapy. However, these patients should be under regular follow up for detection of exacerbation of the disease. They require management of the extra renal manifestations. *Hydroxychloroquine* is used to treat mild manifestations like skin lesions, fatigue, mild arthralgia and arthritis. Hydroxychloroquine (5 - 7 mg/kg/day) is recommended in all cases of SLE, if tolerated. In addition to treating mild manifestations like rash and mild arthritis, it prevents SLE flares, improves lipid profiles and may have a beneficial impact on mortality and renal outcome. In presence of skin lesions, sun exposure should be minimized by use of sunscreen. Arthralgia and arthritis require treatment with *non-steroidal anti-inflammatory agents*. It is important to keep in mind the potential toxic effects of the drugs.

Class II disease should be treated with prednisolone for induction of remission followed by maintenance therapy with low dose prednisolone + azathioprine. *Remission* is induced with prednisolone, 1 - 2 mg / kg/day for 4 - 6 weeks then gradually tapered. *Maintenance therapy* should consist of prednisolone, 0.2 - 0.3 mg/kg, + Azathioprine, 1 - 2 mg/kg/day for 2 - 3 years or more.

In Class III and IV disease, *remission* is induced with oral corticosteroid + cyclophosphamide. Prednisolone, 2 mg/kg/day for 4 weeks. Oral steroid is then gradually tapered to a maintenance dose of 0.2 - 0.3 mg/kg/day, for 4 - 5 years or more. If there is evidence of severe renal insufficiency, oral steroids may be preceded by 3 - 6 doses of IV methyl prednisolone (500 - 750 mg/m^2). Cyclophosphamide is administered preferably IV, 500 - 750 mg/m^2 every 3 - 4 weeks for 6 months or per oral 2 mg /kg/day for 3 - 4 months.

Maintenance therapy with small doses of Prednisolone (0.2 - 0.3/kg/day) + azathioprine (1 - 2 mg/kg/day) or mycophenolate mofetil (500 - 750 mg/m^2) should be continued for 2 - 3 years or more.

It needs mention that prednisolone should be tapered by 2.5 - 5 mg/week when prednisolone dose is 20 to 40 mg/day, 2.5 mg/week for a dose of 10 - 20 mg /day and 1 mg/every 2 - 4 weeks for doses 10 mg/day.

In Class V disease treatment has been tried with oral prednisolone + either cyclosporine / tacrolimus or mycophenolate mofetil. Class V disease is poorly responsive to treatment.

Class VI disease is advanced sclerosing nephritis with diffuse chronic damage suggesting progression to renal failure.

SLE resistant to standard medications has been treated with cyclosporine + rituximab + plasma exchange and IV immunoglobulin.

Prognosis

Childhood SLE was considered as a uniformly fatal disease. However, early diagnosis and treatment tailored to individual cases has improved the survival rate currently to > 90%. Untreated SLE may be followed by spontaneous remission, years of chronic disease or death of rapid onset.

Takayasu Arteritis

Takayasu arteritis is a common cause of renovascular hypertension in children. It is a chronic granulomatous disease of the aorta and its main branches. The involvement of the descending aorta and renal arteries is common.

Criteria for diagnosis: Presence of angiographic abnormalities of aorta or its main branches on CT or MRI with presence of atleast any one of the following:

1. Decrease peripheral artery pulse and / or claudication of extremities.
2. Bruit over the aorta and / or its main branches.
3. Blood pressure difference of more than 10 mm Hg.
4. Systemic hypertension.

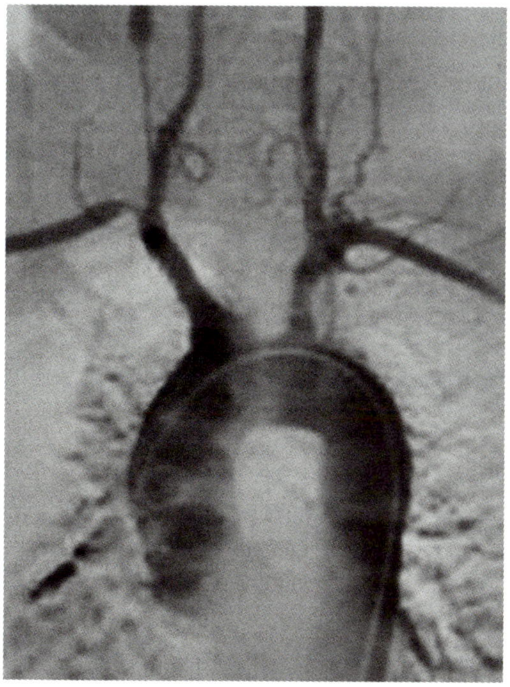

Fig. 15.6: CT angio showing complete occlusion of left common carotid artery

Clinical Manifestations

Some patients may have a past history or recent evidence of tuberculosis. An early phase of the disease is characterized by general features like fever, anorexia, weight loss, cough, pain in the joints and anemia. These features usually go unnoticed. Patients may complain of claudicating pain in the extremities. Subsequently the child may present with renovascular hypertension, hypertensive complications and congestive heart failure. The signs may be absence of pulses and presence of bruits.

The diagnosis is confirmed by angiography. It shows stenosis or occlusion of the involved vessels.

Treatment

Prednisolone (1 - 2 mg/kg/ day) during the acute phase followed by tapering and low dose maintenance for several months. A severe disease may occasionally require cytotoxic drugs. Hypertension should be treated using appropriate medications. Most cases are detected late because early signs are non-specific. If stenosis develops after the acute phase, reconstructive surgery or balloon angioplasty with or without stenting is often required.

Suggested Reading

1. Hashkes PJ, Laxer RM: Medical Treatment of Juvenile idiopathic arthritis. JAMA 2005; 294: 1671-1684.
2. Current Treatment of Juvenile Rheumatoid Arthritis. Pediatrics 2002; 109:109-1115.
3. Pediatric Kidney Diseases. Editor Chester M. Edelman Vol I and II 1st Edition 1978. Little Brown and Company.
4. Nelson Textbook of Pediatrics. Editors RM Kliegman, RE Behrman, HB Jenson and BF Stanton. 18th edition, 2007 Saunders, Philadelphia.
5. Nelson Textbook of Pediatrics. Editors RM Kliegman, RE Behrman, HB Jenson and BF Stanton. 19th edition, 2011 Saunders, Philadelphia.
6. Pediatric Nephrology. By R.N.Srivastava and Arvind Bagga. Fifth edition, 2011, Jaypee Brothers, Medical Publishers. New Delhi.

16

Endocrine and Metabolic Disorders

OUTLINES

Disorders of thyroid gland are among the most common endocrine problems in children. Goitre, hypothroidism, and less commonly hyperthyroidism are the three major forms of thyroid disorders in children.

The thyroid hormones influence growth, development and various biological and metabolic functions in the body. By virtue of their action on neuronal growth, differentiation and induction of nerve growth factor as well as neurotransmitter and enzyme systems, they play a crucial role in fetal and early post natal brain development. When diagnosis of congenital hypothyroidism is delayed beyond early infancy there is permanent impairment of intellectual and neurological function in later life. Beyond the age 3 years, when thyroid hormone dependent brain development is completed, the effects of thyroid deprivation are more evident on physical and skeletal maturation, with almost no impairment of intellectual functions. An early diagnosis of hypothyroidism is crucial.

Goitre

For epidemiological purposes WHO defines goitre as a thyroid gland where the size of the lateral lobes exceed the volume of the terminal phalanx of the subject examined.

Goitre may be congenital or acquired, endemic or sporadic. A child with goitre may have normal thyroid function, thyroid deficiency (hypothyroidism) or over production of thyroid hormones (hyperthyroidism).

Congenital Goitre

Congenital goitre is usually sporadic. It may result from defect in fetal thyroxine synthesis or administration of antithyroid drugs and iodides during pregnancy for the treatment of thyrotoxicosis.

Goitrogenic drugs and iodides cross the placenta and in high doses, may interfere in synthesis of thyroid hormone and cause hypothyroid in fetus. In women, with Graves disease treated with propylthiouracil, 100–200 mg/day such effects can occur. A women treated during pregnancy with amiodarone, an antiarrhythmic drug with 37% iodine content, can produce the same effect. All such newborn should undergo thyroid screen at birth because effected newborns should be administered thyroid hormone to treat clinical hypothyroidism, to hasten disappearance of goitre and prevent brain damage. However, thyroid hormone may be discontinued after a week when the antithyroid drug has been excreted by the newborn which usually takes around 7 days.

A large goitre may occasionally cause respiratory distress which interferes with breast feeding. The head may be maintained in extreme hyperextension which may even cause death.

An infant born to a mother suffering from Graves' disease is usually born with clinical signs of hyperthyroidism and goitre which is usually not large. The clinical signs include a restless, irritable, hyperactive, anxious and alert newborn that may be born preterm or small for date. There is exopthalmus, tachycardia, tachypnea and high temperature. If left untreated, weight loss occur in spite of increased appetite with hepatosplenomegaly and jaundice. There may be hypertension and cardiac decompensation. The infant may die if therapy is not instituted promptly. The serum TSH is low and serum T_4 is markedly elevated.

The condition is caused by transplacental passage of thyrotropin receptor stimulating antibody (TRS Ab). Very high levels of TRS Ab result in classical neonatal hyperthyroidism. The presence of thyrotropin binding antibody (TRB Ab) and intrauterine exposure to maternal antithyroid drugs may delay onset of symptoms of hyperthyroidism for several weeks.

Treatment consist of oral administration of propranolol (1–2 mg/kg/day in 3 divided doses) and propylthiouracil (5–10 mg/kg/day 8 hourly), and Lugols iodine (1 drop 8 hourly). In severe cases steroids and parenteral fluid therapy may be indicated. Heart failure should be treated with digoxin. After a euthyroid state is reached only propylthiouracil is continued. Most cases remit by 3–4 months of age; occasionally may persist upto childhood.

Iodine deficiency as a cause of congenital goitre is still prevalent in endemic areas of iodine deficiency in the developing countries. It is rare in developed countries.

Endemic Goitre

Etiology

Endemic goitre and cretinism results from dietary deficiency of iodine. Endemic goitre is rare in people living along the sea because sea water is rich in iodine and the iodine content of sea fish is also high. It is commonly seen in certain Alpine valleys, the Andes, Congo and the highlands of Papua New Guinea. In India it is highly prevalent along the foot hills of the Himalayas. With introduction of prophylaxis with iodized salt, endemic goitre has almost disappeared from many western countries. Iodine deficient goitre is common in girls than in boys.

Pathogenesis

The body overcomes a moderate degree of iodine deficiency with increased efficiency of synthesis of thyroid hormone. The iodine liberated in the tissues is returned rapidly to the gland which resynthesizes triiodothyronine at a high rate than normal. This increased activity is achieved by compensatory hypertrophy and hyperplasia of the thyroid gland. In areas where deficiency of iodine is severe, decompensation and hypothyroidism may result.

Clinical Manifestations

The clinical manifestation depends on the degree of iodine deficiency. In regions of mild deficiency, there is no noticeable enlargement of the thyroid except in periods of increase demand of the hormone, i.e., during periods of rapid growth, as in adolescence. In regions of moderate iodine deficiency, goitre appears in school children but disappears with maturity to reappear during pregnancy and lactation. In the hyper endemic areas nearly half the population has large goitres and endemic cretinism is common.

Laboratory Diagnosis

Serum T_4 levels are low but clinical hypothyroidism is rare. Serum T_3 levels are elevated. Serum TSH levels are only moderately elevated.

Endemic Cretinism

Endemic cretinism is the most serious consequence of iodine deficiency. Two types are described: the neurogenic type and the myxedematous type. The former is more frequently seen in South America and the south pacific region and the latter in Africa.

Pathogenesis

The neurological type occurs due to in utero iodine deficiency damaging the fetal brain during early embryogenesis before fetal thyroid has developed. The myxedematous type occurs due to in utero as well as post natal hypothyroidism. Iodine deficiency acting in conjunction with goitrogens may be responsible.

Clinical Manifestations

The *neurogenic syndrome* is characterized by mental retardation, deaf mutism, disturbances in gait, and upper motor lesion signs such as clonus of foot, exaggerated knee jerks and extensor plantar response. The affected child has goitre but euthyroid, have a normal pubertal development and adult stature. Physical signs of hypothyroidism, goitre, epiphyseal dysgenesis and biochemical alteration are absent. Such a situation can be prevented by iodine supplementation to the mother before conception.

In the *myxedematous syndrome*, the child has the typical hypothyroid facies and features of hypothyroidism such as coarse, dry skin and hair, hoarse voice, cold intolerance and constipation with severe growth retardation and mental deficiency. Radiological findings include epiphyseal dysgenesis and delay in bone age. There is no goitre instead thyroid atrophy. The myxedematous features are reversible by treatment with thyroid hormones but the mental retardation is not reversible.

A mixed type i.e. a combination of features of neurogenic and myxedematous type is seen commonly in the Himalayan endemic region. The neurologic type is also prevalent in this region.

Treatment

The endemic goitre and endemic cretinism require treatment with oral thyroxine as in cases with hypothyroidism. Clinical features of hypothyroidism will improve but neurological manifestations are unlikely to revert. A small goitre may disappear with treatment but a large goitre of long duration may not regress.

Iodine deficiency in endemic areas can be prevented with adequate daily intake of iodine. Iodized salt has been considered to be most appropriate vehicle for this, as it is consumed daily in small quantities by every one in reasonable amount.

Simple Goitre (Colloid Goitre)

Simple goitre is a condition of unknown cause, not associated with hypo or hyperthyroidism and not caused by inflammation or neoplasia. It is predominantly seen in girls with a peak incidence before and during pubertal years.

The goitre may be small or large. It is firm in consistency in 50% cases; occasionally asymmetric or nodular.

The serum TSH level is normal or low, scintiscans are normal and thyroid antibodies are absent.

The child may be treated with thyroxine which may help to avoid progression. The goitre may decrease in size in the natural course. Untreated cases should be under follow-up and re-evaluated periodically. This condition should be differentiated from lymphocytic thyroiditis.

Hypothyroidism

Hypothyroidism is a condition which results from deficient production of thyroid hormone or a defect in thyroid hormonal receptor activity. It may be congenital when manifestations are present at birth or acquired when manifestations appear after a period of normal thyroid function.

Congenital Hypothyroidism

Congenital hypothyroidism may be sporadic or familial, goitrous or non-goitrous. When the deficiency is severe, symptoms develop in the early weeks of life. In others where lesser degree of deficiency occurs, manifestations may be delayed for months.

The worldwide prevalence of hypothyroidism is 1 in 4000 infants. It is twice as common in girls.

Etiology

Thyroid dysgenesis in the form of aplasia, hypoplasia or an ectopic gland is the most common cause of congenital hypothyroidism accounting for 85% of cases. Aplasia is found in 30% of cases where radionuclide scans can find no remnants of thyroid tissue. Ectopic thyroid tissue may be lingual (at the base of the tongue), sublingual or subhyoid. The ectopic gland may function adequately in early infancy and childhood. Hence these infants may be missed on neonatal screening. But later on it fails to produce the adequate amount of thyroid hormones and manifestation of deficiency starts appearing.

Ninety-eight percent of thyroid dysgenesis occurs sporadically and 2% are familial with dominant or recessive inheritance. The male female ratio is 2:1. The exact cause of dysgenesis is unknown. Genetic predisposition and immunologic factors have been implicated. Immunologically mediated maternal/

transplacental factors cytotoxic to fetal thyroid are postulated but not proven. Inactivating mutations of TSH receptor gene or autosomal dominant PAX 8 gene is thought to be responsible in some cases. Dysgenesis is occasionally seen in infants with Down syndrome.

Dyshormonogenesis, i.e., defective synthesis of thyroxine may result from a variety of defects in biosynthesis of thyroid hormone. It is inherited as an autosomal recessive trait. Mutations in genes for thyroid peroxidase and thyroglobulin or rarely other genetic mutations may also be responsible.

The anatomically normal but functionally inadequate thyroid gland leads to excess TSH secretion causing hyperplasia and hypertrophy of the gland resulting in goitrous hypothyroidism. The goitre may be present at birth or may appear later.

The major forms of biosynthetic defects include defects in iodine trapping, iodide organification, coupling, deiodinase activity and abnormalities in thyroglobulin synthesis, storage or release, defects in peripheral tissue responsiveness to thyrotropin and thyroid hormones or thyroid hormone resistance. The clinical manifestations vary from euthyroid goitre to well marked goitrous hypothyroidism. An organification defect with associated deafness is described as Pendred syndrome.

Hypothalamic/Pituitary dysfunction is an uncommon cause of hypothyroidism. It is often associated with deficiency of other pituitary or hypothalamic hormones. It may result from anomalous pituitary hypothalamic development, or functional failure due to genetic mutations affecting the synthesis, release or action of TRH/TSH. Central isolated congenital hypothyroidism is rare and is caused by mutations of the TSH gene.

Clinical Manifestations

A high index of suspicion is essential as the classic symptoms and signs evolve gradually during the first few weeks of life. The clinical picture is fully developed by 3–6 months age. Further, when there is a partial deficiency of thyroid hormone, the symptoms may be milder and the onset of symptoms may be further delayed.

Most infants with congenital hypothyroidism are asymptomatic at birth as a result of transplacental passage of moderate amounts of maternal T_4. The low serum levels of T_4 and concomitantly elevated levels of TSH make it possible to screen and detect most hypothyroid neonates. In most developed countries, clinicians depend on neonatal screening for diagnosis of congenital hypothyroidism. This has made diagnosis possible in the newborn.

Early clinical diagnosis is difficult because in the newborn and early infancy the symptoms and signs are not sufficiently developed. The less characteristic manifestations that can help one to suspect a diagnosis of hypothyroidism are as follows:

Newborn

In the neonate, symptoms predominate over signs. Birth weight and length are normal but head size may be increased because of myxedema of brain. The posterior fontanels are wide open. There may be prolongation of physiological jaundice due to delayed maturation of glucoronide conjugation. This may be the earliest sign. Feeding difficulties such as sluggishness, lack of interest and choking spells are common during the first month of life. The tongue is large protruding out of the oral cavity resulting in apneic episodes, noisy respiration and nasal obstruction. The affected infants sleep much, cry little and are generally sluggish. The cry is hoarse. There may be constipation which does not respond to treatment.

The abdomen is large usually with a large umbilical hernia. The temperature is subnormal, often less than 35°C (95°F) and the skin particularly of the extremities may be cold and mottled. There is bradycardia. Heart murmurs, cardiomegaly and asymptomatic pericardial effusion are common. Edema of the genitals and extremities may be present. There is macrocytic anemia which does not respond to hematinic.

Beyond the Neonatal Period

The clinical signs become more obvious beyond neonatal period. Although thyroid hormones (particularly T_3) are

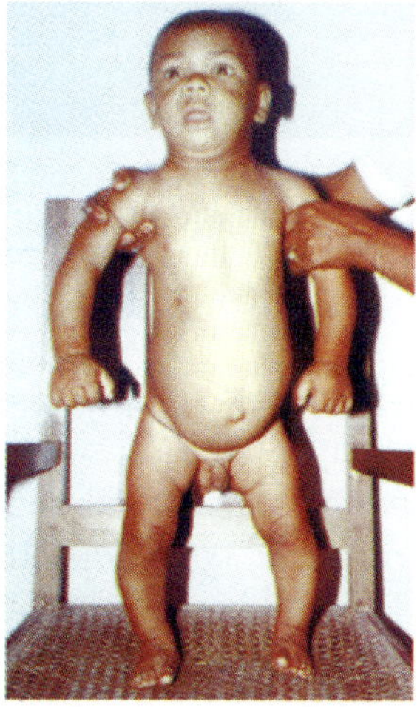

Fig. 16.1: Figure showing a cretin

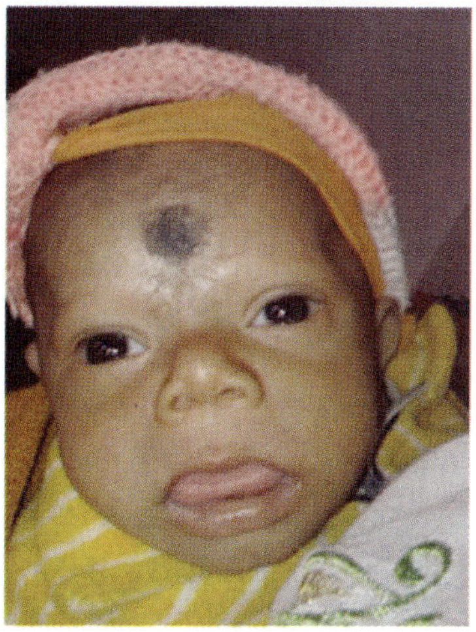

Fig. 16.2: Figure showing hypothyroid facies

excreted in breast milk, the amounts are inadequate to protect the breast fed infant.

The typical hypothyroid facies develop. It is characterized by wide apart eyes; depressed bridge of the broad nose, narrow palpebral fissure with swollen eye lids. The mouth is kept open, and the thick broad tongue protruding out.

The scalp is thickened, and the hair is coarse brittle and scanty. The hairline reaches far down the forehead. The forehead appears wrinkled especially when the child cries. The neck is short and thick and there may be deposits of fat above the clavicles and between the neck and the shoulders. The hands are broad and the fingers short. The skin is dry and scaly and there is little perspiration. Myxedema is manifested particularly in the skin of the eyelids, back of the hands and the external genitalia. Dentition is delayed. Carotenemia leads to a yellow skin with white scleras.

Hypothyroid infants appear lethargic. They are late in learning to sit and stand. The voice is hoarse and speech development is delayed. Sexual maturation may be delayed or may not take place at all.

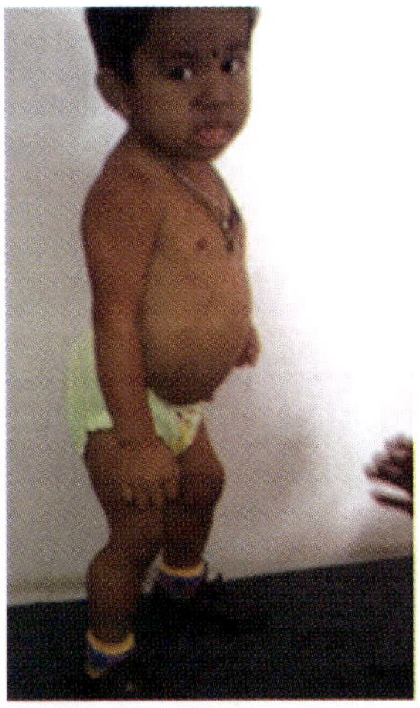

Fig. 16.3: Kocher debre semileinge syndrome

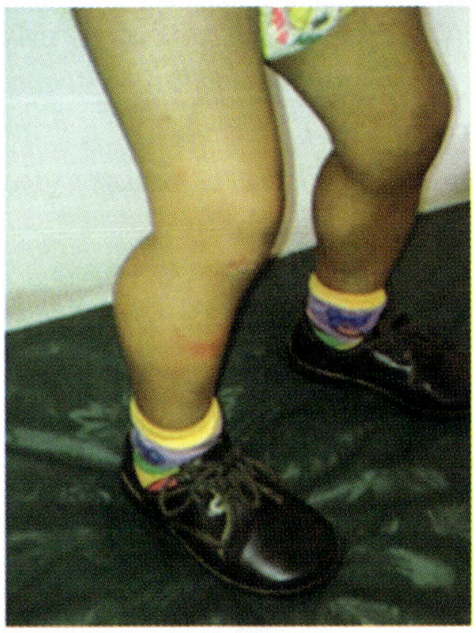

Fig. 16.4: Hypertrophied calf muscles

The muscles are hypotonic but in some cases there may be a generalized pseudohypertrophy of the muscles, particularly prominent in the calf muscles. This condition is known as *Kocher-Debre-Semilaigne syndrome*. It is more commonly seen in boys. The pathogenesis is not known but muscles become normal after treatment. It is seen in patients with severe deficiency and a longer duration of hypothyroid state.

Laboratory Diagnosis

Estimation of Thyroid Hormones

Estimation of thyroid hormones viz. T_4, T_3 and TSH is the mainstay for early diagnosis of congenital hypothyroidism. In developed countries, screening for hypothyroidism is done along with the metabolic screen. This measure has enabled diagnosis within 3–5 days after birth and starting of treatment within 2–3 weeks of age. This is important as this period of infancy coincides with the crucial phase of post natal brain development.

Both TSH and T4 levels are elevated on days 1 and 2 of life. The screening tests should be done between 3rd and 5th day of birth to decrease the false positive rates. If done before 24 hours of age it should be retested.

Majority of preterm, low birth weight infants may have T4 levels in hypothyroid levels. In addition, truly hypothyroid, low birth weight infants may demonstrate a delayed rise in TSH, 2–7 weeks after birth. Hence in all preterm babies with weight less than 1.5 kg, it is recommended to repeat tests at 2, 6, 10 weeks of life. If signs of congenital hypothyroidism appear in an infant, screening should be repeated if the original screening result is normal. The screening is performed by dried blood spot samples taken by heel prick.

One approach used for screening congenital hypothyroidism includes estimation serum T_4 followed by TSH if the former is low. This approach can identify infants with primary hypothyroidism, those with low levels of thyroxine binding globulin (TG), some cases with pituitary or hypothalamic hypothyroidism and infants with delayed increase in TSH levels. Another approach gaining acceptance is estimation of only serum TSH levels. This approach detects infants with primary hypothyroidism and may detect subclinical hypothyroid state but miss the other situations mentioned above.

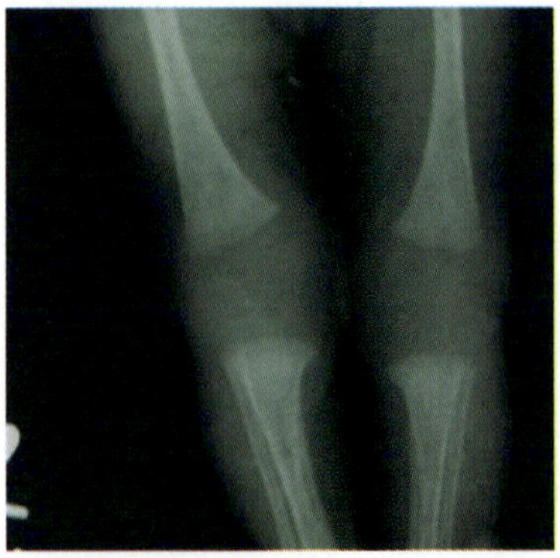

Fig. 16.5: Absence of distal femoral epiphysis

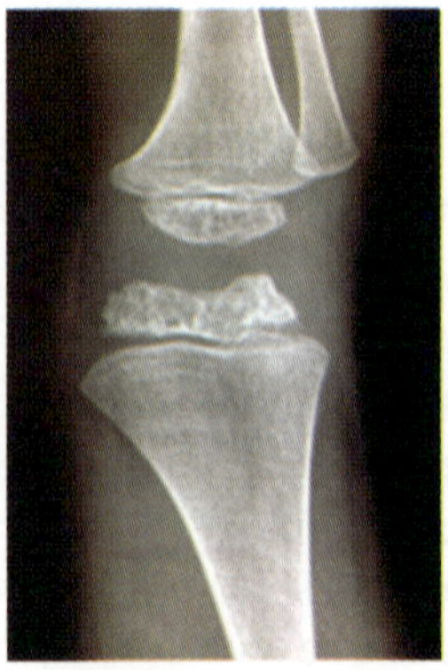

Fig. 16.6: Epiphyseal dysgenesis

Plain X-ray

The other investigations for hypothyroidism include plain X-ray to study the epiphysis, X-ray chest, thoracolumbar spine and skull, ECG, radionuclide study and USG.

There may be absence or delayed appearance or dysgenesis (epiphysis with multiple foci of ossification) of the epiphysis in about 60% cases of congenital hypothyroidism. For example the distal femoral epiphysis which is normally present at birth may be absent. Deformity of the 12th thoracic or 1st or 2nd lumbar vertebra is common. The X-ray of the skull shows large fontanels and wide sutures, intersutural (Wormian) bones. The sella turcica is often enlarged and round, rarely there may be erosions and thinning. The PA view chest may show cardiac enlargement or pericardial effusion.

The *ECG* may show low voltage P and T waves with diminished amplitude of QRS complex which suggest poor left ventricular function and pericardial effusion.

Scintigraphy with ^{123}I-sodium Iodide

Scintigraphy with ^{123}I-sodium iodide can help to pin point the underlying cause in infants with congenital hypothyroidism. USG examination of the thyroid is helpful for demonstration of thyroid tissue but it may fail to demonstrate some ectopic glands which may be shown by scintigraphy. Demonstration of ectopic thyroid is diagnostic of dysgenesis. A normally situated thyroid gland with normal uptake radionuclide indicates a defect in the thyroid hormone biosynthesis. Failure to demonstrate any thyroid tissue would suggest aplasia, TRB Ab and iodine trapping defect.

In children older than 2 years of age, the *serum cholesterol* level is usually elevated.

Treatment

Irrespective of the underlying cause of hypothyroidism, the treatment is same and should be initiated early. Treatment should not be delayed awaiting reports of scintigraphy or other investigation. The goal of therapy is to maintain the circulating serum T_4 level in the upper normal range for age (10–15 microgram/ dL in infancy) and normalize the elevated TSH level. Sodium L thyroxine given orally as a single dose is the preferred preparation because of its uniform potency, reliable absorption and good bioavailability. In the newborn, full replacement therapy can be initiated promptly. In long standing thyroid deficiency where diagnosis is delayed for months or occasionally for years, a quarter of the daily dosage is administered initially and stepped up gradually weekly or two weekly till the full replacement dose can be offered by 3–6 weeks or longer depending on the age of presentation.

Table 16.1 : Dose of L-thyroxine at different age

Age	*Dose*
Newborn	10–15 mcg/kg/day
6–12 months	6–8 mcg/kg/day or 50–75 mcg/day
Preschool	5–6 mcg/kg/day or 75–100 mcg/day
Older children	4–5 mcg/kg/day or 100–150 mcg/day
Adolescents	2–3 mcg/kg/day or 100–200 mcg/day

The daily dosage in older children and adolescents usually do not exceed 150–200 mcg/day. Alternatively, 100 mcg/ sq metre daily has been suggested. The required dose should be administered as a single dose in empty stomach to maximize absorption. The tablets should be kept in a cool place away from direct sunlight. The importance of regular therapy should be stressed irrespective of any other illness. Treatment should be continued lifelong.

Follow-up

The blood samples for T_3, T_4 and TSH estimation should be obtained 4 weeks after initiating therapy in the newborn and 5–6 weeks after reaching the final calculated dose in older infants and children. The test is repeated 2–3 monthly during infancy and 3–4 monthly during the second year and biannually or annually as the child grows. It should be checked after 6–8 weeks after any change in dose. The sample should be collected preferably 12–24 hours after the last dose of L-thyroxine. After initial stabilization, estimation of TSH and T_4 or additionally free T_4 will usually suffice. Serum T_4 should be maintained in the age related upper normal range with TSH in normal range.

Occasionally, in newborns or young infants where laboratory values are minimally abnormal and therapy has been started, treatment have to be continued under supervision for 2–3 years and then stopped for 5–6 weeks and child observed for appearance of symptoms and signs of hypothyroidism. Then only the decision for continuing life long therapy should be taken.

In addition to thyroid hormone studies, clinical evaluation and growth monitoring during therapy are equally important in follow-up.

Prognosis

Early diagnosis and adequate treatment from the first weeks of life result in normal linear growth and intelligence comparable with that of the unaffected sibling. However severely affected infants (very low serum T_4 levels and retarded skeletal maturation) have slightly reduced IQ, speech problems, short attention span, hypotonia or hypertonia. About 20% have a neurosensory hearing defect.

Without treatment, affected infants become profoundly mentally retarded dwarfs. Late diagnosis, failure to correct initial hypothyroid state rapidly, inadequate treatment and poor compliance in the first two years of life result in variable degree of brain damage.

When onset of hypothyroidism is after 2 years of age, normal development is much better even if diagnosis and initiation of therapy is delayed. On the other hand if early onset hypothyroidism is diagnosed after 2 years of age, replacement therapy improves only physical growth.

Acquired or Juvenile Hypothyroidism

Etiology

The most common cause of acquired hypothyroidism is chronic lymphocytic thyroiditis. Autoimmune thyroid disease may be a part of polyglandular syndromes. Children with Down, Turner and Klienfelter syndromes and celiac disease or diabetes are at higher risk of autoimmune thyroid disease.

Table 16.2 : Etiology of acquired hypothyroidism
Autoimmune thyroiditis: Hasimoto thyroiditis, polyglandular autoimmune syndrome
Congenital hypothyroidism of late onset
Endemic iodine deficiency: Goiterogens
Iatrogenic: Post thyroidectomy, drugs, ^{131}I therapy and cervical radiation
Systemic disease: Cystinosis, langerhans cell histiocytosis, iron overload
Hypothalamic/pituitary dysfunction
Miscellaneous: Chromosomal disorders (Down, Turner, Klinefelter syndromes, Large hemangioma)

Subtotal thyroidectomy or removal of ectopic thyroid tissue may result in hypothyroidism. Some patients with congenital thyroid dysgenesis or with incomplete genetic defects in thyroid hormone synthesis may not manifest until childhood and appear to have acquired hypothyroidism. These conditions however are now detected by the neonatal screening programme. Children with nephropathic cystinosis and Langerhans cell histiocytosis may result in hypothyroidism. Irradiation of the area of the thyroid, e.g. in Hodgkin's disease, for bone marrow transplant often results in thyroid damage. Protracted ingestion of medications containing iodide (e.g. amiodarone) can cause hypothyroidism often accompanied by goitre. A large hemangioma is associated with consumption of T_4 because of excess of local/type 3 deiodinase activity which converts T_4 to large amounts of biologically inactive reverse T_3 and T_3 to T_2. Although the condition corrects itself as the hemangioma shrinks over 1–2 years, replacement therapy with T_4 is advisable during infancy to prevent brain damage.

Clinical Manifestations

The onset of symptoms usually occurs in mid childhood. Growth failure is usually the first clinical manifestation but it often goes unrecognized. There is an insidious onset of symptoms like cold intolerance, constipation, lethargy, increased need for sleep. Scholastic performances do not suffer even in severe acquired hypothyroidism. The child may present with a classic myxedematous picture with pallor, dry skin, patchy alopecia and coarse and sparse hair and a dull look. Unexplained anemia may be a presenting feature. Tendon reflexes may show delayed relaxation. There is often strikingly delayed osseous maturation. Adolescents have delayed puberty whereas younger children may present with galactorrhea or pseudo precocious puberty (characterized by breast development in girls and enlargement of testis in boys).

In some children there is hyperplastic enlargement of the pituitary gland with suprasellar extension. This occurs after long standing hypothyroidism. These children may present with headache and visual problems. It may be mistaken for a pituitary tumour.

Laboratory Investigations and Treatment

Hormonal studies are same as for congenital hypothyroidism. Measurement of antithyroglobulin and antiperoxidase antibodies can clinch the diagnosis of autoimmune thyroiditis.

Treatment consists of administration of L thyroxine as described in congenital hypothyroidism. There may be deterioration of school work, poor sleep, restlessness, short attention span and behavioural problems during the first year of treatment. These manifestations are transient. Parents need a forewarning in this regard.

Hyperthyroidism

Hyperthyroidism is the result of excessive secretion of thyroid hormone. The most common cause in children is Graves' disease which is due to diffuse toxic goitre. Infants born to mothers with Graves' disease suffer from transient hyperthyroidism.

About 60% of the infiltrating lymphoid cells are T cells and about 30% has B cell markers. The T cells consists of helper (CD 4^+) and cytotoxic ($CD8^+$) cells. Presence or absence of goitre depends on the type of HLA haplotypes. Certain HLA haplotypes (HLA-DR4, HLA-DR5) are associated with an increased risk of goitre and thyroiditis whereas others (HLA-DR 3) are associated with the atrophic variety.

A number of other antibodies have also been demonstrated. Thyroid antiperoxidase antibodies (TPOAbs) are demonstrable in 90% children with lymphocytic thyroiditis. Antithyroid globulin antibodies (more common in adults) and thyrotropin receptor blocking antibodies (especially in cases with hypothyroidism) are also detected. It is now believed that Thyrotropin receptor blocking antibodies are related to the development of hypothyroidism and thyroid atrophy.

Clinical Manifestations

It is common in children above 6 years of age. Peak incidence is during adolescence. It may occur during the first 3 years of life also. There is usually a history of autoimmune thyroiditis in the parents or sibling.

The child most commonly presents with goitre and growth retardation. The goitre which may be small or large appears insidiously. In most patients, the thyroid is diffusely enlarged, firm in consistency and non-tender. In around 30% cases, the gland is lobular and may seem to be nodular. Most of the children are clinically euthyroid, some may have symptoms of pressure in the neck; some may have clinical signs of hypothyroidism and few may have hyperthyroidism. Another group of children may have signs of hyperthyroidism but with no laboratory evidence.

Autoimmune thyroiditis also tends to be associated with Down, Turner and Klinefelter syndrome. Anti-thyroid antibodies are also found in 20% of children with diabetes mellitus and congenital rubella syndrome.

Laboratory Diagnosis

Thyroid functions tests are usually normal. Thyroid ultrasound shows scattered hypoechogenecity in most patients. Majority of patients have serum antibody titres to TPO whereas antithyroid globulin test is positive in less than 50% cases. When both tests are done, approximately 95% of patients with thyroid autoimmunity can be detected. Thyroid scans reveal irregular and patchy distribution of radio isotope in 60% or more cases. The definitive diagnosis can be established by thyroid biopsy but is rarely indicated for clinical purpose alone.

Course

The goitre may become smaller or disappear spontaneously or it may remain unchanged with patient remaining euthyroid. Some patients acquire hypothyroidism gradually within months and years. Fifty percent of children with subclinical hypothyroidism revert to euthyroid while the other 50% develop overt hypothyroidism.

Treatment

The child needs treatment with L-thyroxine if there is evidence of hypothyroidism. As there are chances of spontaneous recovery, the child should be periodically evaluated to take decision on continued therapy. The goitre usually shows some decrease in size but may persist for years. Untreated patients should be checked periodically. If prominent nodules persist in spite of suppressive therapy, they should be examined histologically to exclude thyroid cancer.

Parathyroid

Primary disorders of the parathyroid glands are rare in children. There are four parathyroid glands which are situated in the neck. They develop from the third and fourth branchial pouches. The parathyroid hormone (PTH) is the major secretory product of the gland. PTH controls calcium and phosphate metabolism. When serum levels of calcium fall, secretion of PTH increases. PTH stimulates activity of 1 alpha hydroxylase in the kidney enhancing production of 1, 25 $(OH)_2$ D3.The increased levels of 1, 25 $(OH)_2$ D3 induces synthesis of calcium binding protein (calbindin-D) in the intestinal mucosa with resultant absorption of calcium. PTH also mobilizes calcium by directly enhancing bone resorption. The effects of PTH on bone and kidney are mediated through binding to specific receptors on the membranes of the target cells and through activation of a transduction pathway involving G protein coupled to the adenyl cyclase system.

Hypoparathyroidism

Hypoparathyroidism is a condition characterized by absent or low values of plasma PTH. It may be a result of decreased secretion or peripheral action of PTH.

Etiology

The causes of hypoparathyroidism are summarized below:

1. Transient deficiency of PTH
   (a) Early neonatal hypocalcemia (1st 12 - 72 hours of life).
   (b) Late neonatal hypocalcemia (2 - 10 days of life).
   (c) Transient idiopathic hypocalcemia (1 - 8 weeks).
2. Inadequate secretion
   (a) Aplasia or hypoplasia.
   (b) Autoimmune hypoparathyroidism.
   (c) Post surgical.
3. Suppression of PTH secretion from normal parathyroid gland
   (a) Maternal hyperparathyroidism.
   (b) Severe magnesium depletion.
4. PTH gene mutation (autosomal recessive)
5. Defective end organ response to PTH
6. Calcium sensing receptor defects (chromosome 3q12) (activating mutation-autosomal dominant)
7. Secretion of biologically inactive PTH (genetic defect in the proportion of the molecule that may impair processing of PTH)
8. Idiopathic
   (a) Sporadic.
   (b) Familial.

Clinical Manifestations

Mild deficiency may be detected only by laboratory investigations. Muscular pain and cramps may be the early manifestations. They may progress to numbness, stiffness and tingling of the hands and feet.

There may be only a positive Chvostek's or trousseau sign or laryngeal and carpopedal spasm. Seizures with or without loss of consciousness may occur at intervals of days, weeks or months. Seizure episodes may begin with abdominal pain followed by tonic rigidity and retraction of head and cyanosis. Hypoparathyroidism is frequently misdiagnosed as epilepsy. Headache, vomiting and papilledema may be associated with seizures suggesting a space occupying lesion.

In patients with long standing hypocalcemia, the eruption of teeth is delayed and eruption is irregular. The teeth may be unusually soft and enamel formation is irregular. The skin is dry and scaly. The nails of the fingers and toes may have horizontal lines. There may be candidal infection which most often involves the nails, oral mucosa, angles of the mouth and less often the skin. The candidal infection antedates the development of hypoparathyroidism.

With long standing untreated disease cataract and autoimmune keratoconjunctivitis may occur. Hypoparathyroidism may be associated with Addison disease, lymphocytic thyroiditis, pernicious anemia, alopecia areata or totalis, hepatitis and primary gonadal insufficiency. Permanent physical and mental deterioration occur if initiation of treatment is delayed for a long time.

Laboratory Findings

The serum calcium level is low (5 - 7 mg/dL), serum phosphorous is high (7 - 12 mg/dL), serum alkaline phosphatase is normal or low and the 1, 25 $(OH)_2$ D3 is usually low but may be high when hypocalcemia is severe. Serum calcium may be normal when there is associated Addison disease but hypocalcemia appears after effective treatment of Adrenal insufficiency. The level of serum magnesium should always be checked inpatients with hypocalcemia. It is usually low. Immunoassay reveals a low level of PTH.

X-ray of bones reveals an increased density limited to the metaphysis or an increased density of the lamina dura. ECG shows a prolongation of QT interval which disappears on correction of hypocalcemia. The EEG reveal widespread slow activity; which returns to normal after the serum calcium concentration has been within normal limit for a few weeks unless irreversible brain damage has occurred.

Treatment

Neonatal tetany should be treated with IV injection of 5 - 10 ml of 10% calcium gluconate at the rate of 0.5 - 1 ml/minute under monitoring of heart rate. In addition, 1, 25, dihydroxy cholecalciferol [1, 25 $(OH)_2$ D3] should be given. The initial dose is 0.25 microgram/day in two divided doses as the half life is short. The maintenance dose ranges from 0.01 - 0.10 microgram / day to a maximum of 1 - 2 microgram / day. After the calcium level comes to normal, therapy can be continued with Vitamin D2 in the dosage of 0.1 - 0.5 mg/day (1 mg of vitamin D2 has a biologic activity of 40,000 units) in infants and young children. Older children require 1.25 to 2.50 mg (50,000 to 1 lakh units) once daily.

An adequate intake of calcium should be ensured. Supplemental calcium can be given in the form of calcium gluconate to provide 800 mg of elemental calcium daily. Foods with high phosphorous content such as milk, eggs and cheese should be reduced in diet.

In the early stages of treatment, clinical evaluation and determination of serum calcium levels are indicated to determine the requirement of 1,25, dihydroxy cholecalciferol or Vitamin D2. If hypercalcemia occurs, treatment should be discontinued and resumed at a lower dose after the serum calcium level has returned to normal.

Transient Deficiency of PTH

Hypocalcemia during 12 - 72 hours of life is common especially in preterm, in infants with perinatal asphyxia and in infants of diabetic mothers. Between 2 - 10 days the type of feeding is also thought to be a determinant. In a group of infants with hypocalcemia at 1 - 8 weeks of age, a serum level of PTH is significantly lower than in normal infants. The exact cause is not known. Functional immaturity of the parathyroid gland has been thought to be one factor in the pathogenesis. It is thought that functional immaturity is a manifestation of a delay in development of enzymes that convert glandular PTH to secreted PTH.

Pseudohypoparathyroidism (Albright Hereditary Osteodystrophy)

This is a condition where the parathyroid glands are normal or hyperplastic. Serum levels of immunoreactive PTH are elevated even when the patient has hypocalcemia and may be elevated when the patient is normocalcemic. Neither endogenous nor administered PTH raises the serum calcium level or lowers the serum phosphorous level. The genetic defect is in the hormone receptor adenylate cyclase system.

Clinical Features

Usually manifestations appear around the age of 8 years. They have mental retardation and specific somatic features of Albright hereditary osteodystrophy viz. short stature, round facies, short neck, obesity, subcutaneous calcification and shortening of metacarpal and metatarsal bones. There may be other skeletal abnormalities like exostosis, short and wide phalanges, and general demineralization. Basal ganglia calcification and cataract may be present. They have symptomatic hypocalcemia with tetany as the presenting features.

Laboratory Features

Serum calcium levels are low with elevated phosphorous and alkaline phosphatase levels. PTH levels are elevated in presence of normocalcemia or hypocalcemia. The confirmatory test is demonstration of deficient urinary cAMP and phosphorous excretion following administration of IV synthetic PTH. Definitive diagnosis is established by demonstration of the mutated G protein.

Treatment

It is essentially the same as in idiopathic hypoparathyroidism

Hyperparathyroidism

Hyperparathyroidism is a condition of excessive production of parathyroid hormone. It may be primary or secondary. Primary type results from a primary defect of the parathyroid glands such as an adenoma or hyperplasia. An increased production of PTH which is compensatory and aimed at correcting hypocalcemia due to different causes is termed as secondary hyperparathyroidism.

Etiology

Hyperparathyroidism is rare in children. It is usually due to a single benign adenoma. It usually manifests after 10 years of age.

Severe hyperparathyroidism in newborn has been reported in few cases. Severe neonatal hyperparathyroidism may be homozygous or heterozygous for the mutation in the calcium sensing receptor gene. Most individuals with one copy of this mutation exhibit autosomal dominant familial hypocalciuric hypercalcemia.

Hyperparathyroidism can occur as a part of the constellation known as multiple endocrine neoplasia (MEN) syndrome or of the hyperparathyroidism / jaw tumour syndrome. MEN type I is an autosomal dominant disorder characterized by hyperplasia or neoplasia of the endocrine pancreas, the anterior pituitary, and the parathyroid glands. It is rare below the age of 18 years and common above 50 years age. MEN type II may be associated with hyperparathyroidism.

Hyperparathyroidism/jaw tumour syndrome is an autosomal dominant disorder. The condition affects adults primarily but it has been diagnosed in children as early as 10 years.

Transient neonatal hyperparathyroidism has occurred in infants born to mothers with hypoparathyroidism (idiopathic or surgical) or with pseudohypoparathyroidism. The cause of this condition is chronic intra uterine exposure to hypocalcemia with resultant hyperplasia of the fetal parathyroid glands.

Clinical Manifestation

In neonatal hyperparathyroidism, symptoms develop shortly after birth and consist of irritability, lethargy, constipation, refusal to feed and failure to thrive. Radiographs reveal subperiosteal bone resorption, osteoporosis and pathologic fractures. Symptoms may be mild, resolving spontaneously or may have a rapidly fatal course if diagnosis and treatment are delayed.

Clinical presentations in infants include failure to thrive, poor feeding and hypotonia.

The symptoms in the older age group are those of hypercalcemia which include muscular weakness, anorexia, nausea, vomiting, constipation, polydypsia, polyuria, loss of weight and fever. When hypercalcemia is prolonged there is nephrocalcinosis with progressive renal dysfunction. Renal calculi may form and produce renal colic and hematuria. Osseous changes may produce pain in the back or extremities, disturbance of gait, genu valgum, fractures and tumours. Abdominal pain is occasionally a prominent presentation. It may be associated with acute pancreatitis. Parathyroid crisis may occur characterized by progressive oliguria, azotemia, stupor and coma with a serum calcium level greater than 15 mg/dL. Long standing hypercalcemia may result in sequalae like mental retardation, seizures and blindness.

Laboratory Findings

The serum calcium level is elevated. With adenomas it may be as high as 12 mg/dL. In parathyroid hyperplasia it may be 15 - 20 mg/dL; may go upto 30 mg/dL. Even when serum calcium level is border line or only slightly elevated the ionized calcium level is often increased. The serum phosphorous level is reduced to about 3 mg/dL or less. Serum magnesium is low.

The urine specific gravity is low and fixed. Serum levels of non-protein nitrogen and uric acid may be elevated. In patients with adenoma and skeletal involvement serum alkaline phosphatase level is increased but may be normal in cases with hyperplasia but with associated skeletal involvement it will be high. Serum levels of PTH are elevated.

Resorption of subperiosteal bone, best seen along the phalanges of the hands, is the most consistent and characteristic radiographic finding. There may be gross trabeculation or granular appearance, resulting from rarefaction, in the skull. The lamina dura may be absent. In advanced disease there may be generalized rarefaction, cysts, tumours, fractures and deformities. In about 10% cases there may be radiological signs of rickets. X-ray of abdomen may show renal calculi and nephrocalcinosis.

Treatment

Adenomas should be removed. Severe neonatal hypercalcemia requires total parathyroidectomy.

Prognosis

Prognosis is good if early diagnosis and surgical treatment is possible. Extensive osseous lesions cause deformities which are permanent.

Cushing's Syndrome

Cushing's syndrome is a condition resulting from abnormally high levels of cortisol or other glucocorticoids as a result of adrenocortical hyperfunction. It can be iatrogenic or the result of endogenous cortisol secretion.

Etiology

The most common cause of Cushing's syndrome in children is prolonged exogenous administration of glucocorticoid hormones in high doses for treating another condition. The common cause of endogenous disease is Cushing's disease, in which there is excessive ACTH secretion due to a pituitary adenoma. The other rare causes in children which result in ectopic ACTH production include adrenocortical tumour: benign or malignant, neuro-blastoma, Wilms' tumour, islet cell carcinoma of pancreas. These are extremely rare in children.

Clinical Manifestations

The clinical presentation differs according to the cause and age of onset. The condition appears to be severe and clinical findings very obvious in infants. The face is rounded with prominent cheeks and flushed appearance (moon facies). There is generalized obesity which is more common in young children. In children with adrenal tumours, signs of abnormal masculinization are frequent. These include hirsutism on the face and the trunk, pubic hair, acne, deepening of voice. The length may fall below 3rd percentile or be accelerated when significant virilization is present. Hypertension is common and may lead to heart failure. Increased susceptibility to infection may lead to fatal sepsis.

In older children, a gradual onset obesity and deceleration or cessation of growth may be the early manifestation. The obesity is more severe in the trunk and face compared to the limbs.

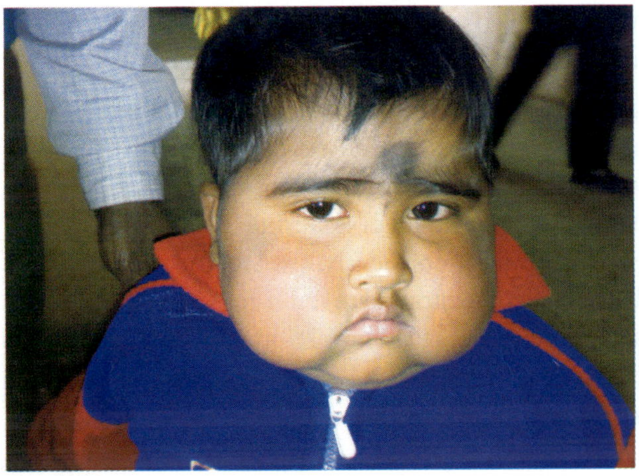

Fig. 16.10: Cushing's syndrome (moon facies)

The other features include weakness, headache and emotional lability. Onset of puberty is delayed or there may be amenorrhea in post pubertal girls. Purple colored striae are common over the abdomen and thighs. Hypertension and hyperglycemia are usually present and hyperglycemia may progress to diabetes. Osteoporosis is common. The cardinal signs to suspect Cushing's syndrome in children include obesity, growth retardation, hypertension, psychosis, hirsutism and unexplained osteoporosis.

Laboratory Diagonsis

The laboratory investigations may be divided into those for diagnosis of Cushing's syndrome and those for diagnosis of the cause.

For Diagnosis of Cushing's Syndrome

1. *8 am and midnight cortisol level estimation:* Except in infants and young children in whom the diurnal rhythm is not always established, the cortisol levels in blood are normally elevated at 8 am and decrease to less than 50% by midnight. In patients with Cushing's syndrome this diurnal variation is lost and the cortisol levels at 8 am and mid night are comparable. If night blood sample collection is difficult, salivary levels can be measured. A high night time salivary cortisol may be a good screening test for screening obese children.
2. *Urinary excretion of free cortisol:* This is best done in a 24-hour collection of urine and is expressed as a ratio of micrograms of cortisol per gram of creatinine. The urinary excretion of free cortisol is increased.
3. *A single dose dexamethasone suppression test:* In normal individuals, when a single dose of dexamethasone in a dose of 25–30 microgram/ kg (maximum of 2 mg) is given at 11 pm it results in a plasma cortisol of less than 5 microgram/dL at 8 am. It does not occur in patients with Cushing's syndrome.
4. The insulin levels are elevated and the glucose tolerance test is often abnormal.

For Diagnosis of Cause

After the diagnosis of Cushing's syndrome is established, the next step is to determine whether it is caused by a pituitary adenoma, an ectopic ACTH secreting tumour or a cortisol secreting tumour.

1. ACTH levels are usually suppressed in patients with cortisol secreting tumours. They are very high in ectopic ACTH secreting tumours and may be normal in ACTH secreting pituitary adenomas.
2. After an intravenous bolus dose of corticotrophin releasing hormone (CRH), patients with ACTH dependent Cushing's syndrome have an exaggerated ACTH and cortisol response but with adrenal tumours show no increase.
3. Two step dexamethasone suppression tests consist of administration of dexamethasone 30 and 120 microgram / kg / day in 4 divided doses, on consecutive days. In children with pituitary Cushing's syndrome, the larger dose suppresses serum levels of cortisol. There is no such effect with ACTH independent Cushing's syndrome.
4. *Neuroimaging:* Adrenal tumours in children are large and can be easily detected by USG. A CT scan can

detect virtually all adrenal tumours larger than 1.5 cm in diameter. An MRI can detect ACTH secreting pituitary adenomas. Contrast studies with gadolinium increases the detection.

5. Bilateral inferior petrosal sinus blood sampling to measure concentration of ACTH before and after CRH administration, is the test which may be performed to localize the tumour when a pituitary adenoma is not visualized by neuroimaging.

Management

Management of Cushing's syndrome includes treatment of cause and supportive care for hypercortisolism.

For adrenal lesions, in children, resection is the recommended treatment with preoperative stress dose and post operative maintenance dose of hydrocortisone. The stress dose consists of hydrocortisone 100 mg/metre^2 /day in 4 divided doses. The dose should be tapered to 25 mg / metre^2/day over the first 2–3 days after surgery. A maintenance dose of hydrocortisone (8–10 mg/metre^2/ day) should be continued for atleast 6 months. Adrenal carcinoma is highly malignant and does not respond to post surgery chemotherapy.

Pituitary adenomas are treated with trans-sphenoidal resection. It is a highly successful procedure. Children with recurrence after surgery may be treated with repeat surgery, bilateral adrenelectomy or cranial irradiation.

In cases with Cushing's syndrome, where no cause has been established after detailed evaluation, the treatment options include bilateral adrenelectomy and medical management. Medical treatment with cyproheptadine, ketokonazole, aminoglutethimide etc has been tried but results in children are not encouraging.

Primary Aldosteronism

Primary aldosteronism is a condition which results from excessive secretion of aldosterone independent of renin-angiotensin system. It is characterized by hypertension, hypokalemia, and suppression of renin angiotensin system.

It is a rare condition in children. Aldosterone secreting adenomas are common in females and have been reported as early as 3.5 years of age. Multinodular adrenocortical hyperplasia, which are bilateral, are seen in older children and are common in males. Glucocorticoid suppressible hyperaldosteronism which occurs in a small percentage of congenital adrenal hyperplasia is a very rare condition.

Clinical Manifestations

Many children are asymptomatic, incidentally diagnosed with moderate hypertension. Others may present with severe hypertension (upto 240/150 mm Hg) with complains of headache, dizziness and visual disturbances. Patients with chronic hypokalemia may present with polyuria, polydipsia, nocturia and enuresis. With severe hypokalemia there may be muscle weakness, tetany, and intermittent paralysis, fatigue and growth failure.

Laboratory Diagnosis

The urine is normal or alkaline and there is kaliuresis. There is increase in the 24 hours excretion of aldosterone. Urinary levels of 18-oxocortisol and 18-hydroxycortisol may be increased but to the extent as in cases of glucocorticoid suppressible hyperaldosteronism.

Blood pH is increased. There is hypokalemia, hypomagnesaemia and decreased serum chloride. Serum levels of calcium is normal even in presence of tetany. Plasma aldosterone level is normal or elevated. Plasma levels of renin is persistently low and the ratio of plasma aldosterone concentration to renin activity is high. Plasma levels of 18-oxocortisol and 18-hydroxycortisol may be increased.

Treatment

The treatment of aldosterone producing adenoma is surgical removal. Cases of bilateral adrenal hyperplasia may be treated with spironolactone which often results in normalization of blood pressure and serum potassium levels. Unilateral adrenelectomy may be indicated if the patient cannot be controlled medically or the side effects of spironolactone are unacceptable.

Hypopituitarism

Hypopituitarism can occur as a result of deficiency of growth hormone with or without deficiency of other pituitary hormones.

Etiologic Classification of Hypopituitarism

Isolated Growth Hormone Deficiency

1. Genetic forms of growth hormone deficiency and growth hormone resistance.
2. Acquired growth hormone deficiency; idiopathic and post radiation.

Multiple Pituitary Hormone Deficiency

1. Genetic.
2. Acquired:
   (a) *Tumours:* Craniopharyngioma, optic gliomas, pituitary adenoma.
   (b) *Trauma:* Motor vehicle injuries.
   (c) *Inflammatory:* Histiocytosis, hypophisitis, tuberculosis.
3. Pituitary hypoplasia of uncertain etiology:
   (a) Isolated.
   (b) In association with developmental anomalies viz. anencephaly, holoporencephaly, cleft lip and palate etc.

Clinical Manifestations

Classic growth hormone deficiency should be suspected in cases with length/height more than 3 SD below the mean for age and sex. Acquired growth hormone deficiency can occur at any age. When it is of short duration, the height may be normal. A strong clinical suspicion is therefore necessary for diagnosis.

The children with *multiple pituitary hormone deficiencies* and those with genetic defects of growth hormone has a birth length that average 1 SD below the mean. With severe defects in growth hormone production or action, they are more than 4 SD below the mean by 1 year of age. With less deficiency, the child may have regular but slow growth in height, with increments always less than the normal percentiles. Periods of lack of growth may alternate with short spurts of growth. Without treatment, adult height is 4–12 SD below the mean.

Infants with *congenital defects of the pituitary or hypothalamus* usually present with neonatal emergencies such as apnea, cyanosis and severe hypoglycemia with or without seizure. There may be persistent neonatal jaundice with elevation of both unconjugated and conjugated bilirubin. Presence of microphallus in boys is an important diagnostic clue.

The child presents with proportionate short stature with small hands and feet. The head is round; the face is short and broad. The frontal bone is prominent. The nose is small and saddle shaped but the nasolabial folds are well developed. The eyes are protuberant. The mandible and chin are underdeveloped. The eruptions of teeth are delayed and are over crowded. The neck is short. The voice is high pitched and remains high pitched after puberty. The genitals are usually under developed for the child's age. Sexual maturation is delayed or absent. Symptomatic hypoglycemia, usually after fasting occurs in 10–15% of children with panhypopituitarism and those with isolated growth hormone deficiency. Intelligence is usually normal.

In *acquired hypopituitarism*, the child is normal initially. The manifestations appear gradually and progress. A tumour of the brain is identified as the most common cause of acquired hypopituitarism and craniopharyngioma is the most common tumour in children. The clinical features of craniopharyngioma include visual defects, optic atrophy, papilledema and cranial nerve palsy and growth failure. Slowing of growth may antedate neurological features. In some cases neurological manifestations may precede the endocrine manifestation or signs of pituitary insufficiency may appear after surgery. If the lesion is an expanding tumour, the presenting features include headache, vomiting, visual disturbances, pathologic sleep patterns, decreased school performance, seizures, and polyuria and growth failure.

When there is complete destruction of the pituitary, the signs of pituitary insufficiency are present. The atrophy of the adrenal cortex, thyroid and gonads results in loss of weight, sensitivity to cold, and absence of sweating. Sexual maturation fails to take place or regresses if already present. There may be atrophy of the gonads and genital tract with amenorrhea and loss of pubic and axillary hair. There may be diabetes insipidus.

Differential Diagnosis

The conditions for differential diagnosis include familial short stature, constitutional growth delay, primary hypothyroidism, emotional deprivation and systemic diseases like inflammatory bowel disease, celiac disease, occult renal disease and anemia. A few children may be detected who are otherwise normal but are short (> 3 SD below the mean for age) and growth velocity is 5 cm or less / year. The provocative tests are normal.

Laboratory Investigations

Growth Hormone Provocative Tests

The diagnosis of growth hormone deficiency is based on eliciting a growth hormone peak in response to physiological conditions like exercise and sleep or provocation by pharmacologic stimulation. The pharmacologic agents used are insulin, clonidine, L-dopa, arginine, glucagon or GNRH. A diagnosis is based on demonstration of absent or low levels of growth hormone in response to stimulation. Peak levels of growth hormone less than 10 microgram/L in each of the two provocative tests are compatible with growth hormone deficiency.

Pituitary Function Tests

The hormones to be estimated for establishing other pituitary functions include levels of TSH, T_4, ACTH, cortisol, dihydroepiandrosterone sulphate, gonadotrophin, and gonadal steroids. This will help to find out the level of lesion causing the pituitary dysfunction.

Radioimaging

A plain X-ray of the skull is helpful when there is a destructive or space occupying lesion. The changes include evidence of ICP, enlargement of sella, with ballooning and erosion, calcifications within or above the sella. Radioimaging can also help in detection of bone age which tends to be approximately 75% of chronological age. X-ray long bones reveal slender bones and osteopenia.

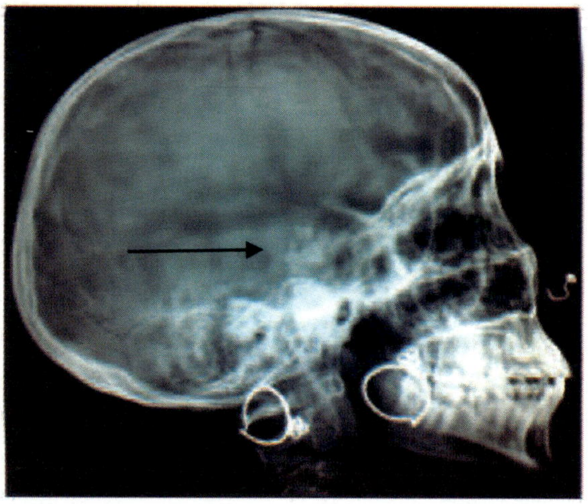

Fig. 16.11 : Suprasellar calcification

An MRI is helpful not only in providing detail about a SOL but also in defining the size of the anterior and posterior pituitary lobes and the stalk. It can also differentiate a full from an empty sella. It is also helpful in confirmation of suspected hypopituitarism in a newborn with hypoglycemia and micropenis. MRI is superior to CT scan in the evaluation.

Treatment

In children with classic growth hormone deficiency, treatment should be started as soon as possible to accrue the maximum effect on mature height. The recommended dose of human growth hormone is 0.18–0.3 mg/kg /week. It is administered subcutaneously in 6–7 divided doses. Therapy should be continuous until near final height is achieved. Criteria for stopping treatment include a growth rate less than 2.5 cm per year and a bone age greater than 14 years in girls and greater than 16 years in boys. Maximal response to growth hormone occurs in the first year of treatment. The response tends to decrease with successive years.

There should be simultaneous replacement of the other hormonal deficiency when detected. However, in case of partial deficiency therapy can be deferred until growth has been completed. In patients with gonadotrophin deficiency, gonadal steroids should be started when bone age reaches the age at which puberty usually takes place. For infants with micropenis, one or two 3 monthly course of monthly intramuscular injection of 25 mg testosterone enanthate or cypionate may bring the penis to normal size without any effect on osseous maturation.

Precocious and Delayed Puberty

Precocious puberty means early pubertal development. It represents the effect of elevated sex steroids viz. estrogen in girls and testosterone in boys. Delayed puberty is a commonly encountered problem in pediatrics. It can be a manifestation of a wide variety of systemic, nutritional and endocrine disorders.

Normal Pubertal Development

The age of onset of puberty varies and is more closely related to osseous maturation than with chronological age. In girls, the breast bud is usually the first sign of puberty (10–11 years age) followed by the appearance of pubic hair, 6–12 months later. The menarche occurs usually 2–2.5 years later but the interval may be as long as 6 years.

In boys, the growth of testes (> 3 cm in volume or 2.5 cm in the longest diameter) and thinning of the scrotum is the first sign followed by pigmentation of the scrotum and growth of penis and then appearance of pubic hair. Axillary hair appears in mid puberty. The voice deepens and there is acceleration of growth.

PRECOCIOUS PUBERTY

Puberty is generally considered to be precocious when physical changes of sexual maturation appear before the age of 8 years in girls and 9 years in boys.

Classification

Precocious puberty may be classified as gonadotrophin dependent, also called true or central precocious puberty and gonadotrophin independent, also called precocious pseudopuberty or peripheral precocious puberty.

True precocious puberty is always isosexual and results from activation of hypothalamic-pituitary-gonadal (HPG) axis. The gonadotrophin mediated increase in size and activity of the gonads leads to increasing sex hormone secretion and progressive sexual maturation. Precocious pseudopuberty is heterosexual or isosexual. In precocious pseudopuberty, there is appearance of some of the secondary sexual characteristics, but there is no activation of the normal hypothalamic-pituitary-gonadal axis.

Table 16.3: Causes of precocious puberty
True precocious puberty
Idiopathic
Organic brain lesions: Hypothalamic hamartoma, brain tumours, hydrocephalous, severe head trauma, myelomeningocele, prolonged and untreated hypothyroidism.
Precocious pseudopuberty
Females
Isosexual (feminizing) conditions: McCune Albright syndrome, ovarian cysts, ovarian tumours, feminizing adrenocortical tumour, exogenous estrogen.
Heterosexual (masculinizing) conditions: Congenital adrenal hyperplasia, adrenal tumours, ovarian tumours, glucorticoid receptor defect, exogenous androgen.
Males
Isosexual (masculinizing) conditions: Congenital adrenal hyperplasia, adrenocortical tumour, Leydig cell tumour, familial male precocious puberty, hCG secreting tumours, teratoma, glucocorticoid receptor defect, exogenous androgen.
Heterosexual (feminizing) conditions: Feminizing adrenocortical tumours, exogenous estrogen.

True Precocious Puberty

Clinical Manifestations

It is usually a sporadic condition, seen in about 10 times more in girls. Some cases may be familial. In more than 90% of sexual precocity in girls, no cause can be detected. However in boys, a structural central nervous system abnormality can be detected in 25–75% cases.

Sexual development may begin at any age and generally follows the sequence observed in normal puberty.

In girls, however, the early menstrual cycles may be more irregular than they are in normal puberty. The initial cycles are usually anovulatory, but pregnancy has been reported as early as 5 years. In boys erections are common and nocturnal emissions may occur. Testicular biopsy shows stimulation of all elements of the testes and spermatogenesis has been observed as early as 5 – 6 years.

In affected girls and boys, the height, weight and osseous maturation is advanced. The increased rate of bone maturation results in early closure of epiphysis affecting the ultimate height. Without treatment, approximately 30% and even larger percentage of boys achieve a height less than 5th percentile as adults.

Mental development is usually compatible with the chronological age. Emotional behaviour and mood swings are common, but serious psychological problems are rare.

The clinical course is variable. Three patterns have been observed: *rapidly progressive* (common in girls with onset below 6 years of age and most boys) affecting ultimate height, *slowly progressive* (commonly seen in girls above 6 years of age) with preserved height potential and a spontaneously *regressive or unsustained* type seen in a small percentage of girls.

Laboratory Diagnosis

Serum estradiol levels in girls are low or undetectable in the early phase of precocity. In the boys, serum testosterone levels are detectable or clearly elevated particularly in early morning samples. Normally serum Luteinizing hormone (LH) is undectable in prepubertal children. They become detectable in 50–70% of children with precocity. Serial measurement of LH in blood samples obtained during sleep reveals pulsatile secretion of LH and is more reliable than a single level.

Gonadotrophin releasing hormone stimulation test (GnRH stimulation test) or a leuprolide (GnRH antagonist) stimulation test is a helpful diagnostic tool particularly in boys. There is a brisk LH response (LH peak > 5–10 IU/ L) with predominance of LH over FSH after intravenous administration of GnRH. In girls, however, the nocturnal LH secretion and LH response to GnRH may be quite low at breast stage II–early stage III (LH peak < 5 IU/L) and the LH: FSH ratio may remain low until mid puberty. In such girls central precocious puberty can be proved by detecting pubertal levels of estradiol (> 50 pg/ml) 20–24 hours after stimulation with leuprolide.

Osseous maturation is variably advanced, often more than 2–3 SD. Pelvic ultrasonography in girls shows progressive enlargement of the ovaries, followed by enlargement of the uterus to pubertal size.

A CT or MRI scan usually demonstrates physiologic enlargement of the pituitary gland, as seen in normal puberty and other organic causes.

Treatment

Use of GnRH agonists is the treatment of choice in central precocious puberty. They desensitize the gonadotrophic cells of the pituitary to the stimulatory effect of the endogenous GnRH and thereby effectively halt the progression of central sexual precocity. Triptorelin and leuprolide are depot preparations of GnRH analogues which are administered intramuscularly every month. Discontinuation of therapy leads to resumption of puberty.

Such treatment is required for rapidly progressive precocious puberty. Girls with slowly progressive puberty however, do not seem to benefit from such therapy in terms of height prognosis. GnRH therapy is very costly. The other drugs which are used when GnRH therapy is not feasible include medroxyprogesterone acetate, cyproterone acetate and aromatase inhibitors.

Precocious Pseudopuberty

Clinical Manifestations

Precocious pseudopuberty occurs in association with some other conditions which may be different for the boys and girls. The most common cause in girls is idiopathic followed by estrogen producing granulosa cell tumors. Congenital adrenal hyperplasia is the common cause in boys.

Precocious pseudopuberty is characterized by increased estrogen or testosterone production in the setting of low basal gonadotrophin levels and lack of pubertal response to GnRH stimulation. There is appearance of only secondary sexual characteristics like thelarche, pubarche, vaginal bleeding, and growth acceleration etc together with the features of the parent disease.

Treatment

Underlying cause of precocious pseudopuberty should be treated. In addition, medroxyprogesterone acetate (100 mg/m^2 every 2–3 weeks IM or orally 10 mg twice a day) may be given. Cyproterone acetate (75–100 mg/m^2 in 2–3 divided doses) is also useful for stopping cyclical bleeding and regressing secondary sexual characters.

Incomplete or Partial Precocious Puberty

The common forms of incomplete precocious puberty are premature thelarche and premature pubarche. Premature menarche is a rare entity in this subgroup.

Premature Thelarche

Premature thelarche denotes isolated premature breast development. There are two peaks of breast enlargement. It could occur in the first 2–4 years and then at 6 years. Occasionally, persistence or progression of breast tissue may also be noted from birth.

In the first 2–4 years the enlargement is thought to be due to oversensitivity of infant's breast tissues to ovarian estrogens. This usually regresses but may persist without progression.

In the second group, enlargement may be asymmetric to begin with and is often unilateral. The cause is thought to be a temporary increase in ovarian estrogen production. Rarely an ovarian cyst or follicle may be detected but this does not persist. The condition is usually benign. However, it needs follow-up to rule out combined peripheral and central precocious puberty as it may be the initial manifestation of gonadotrophin mediated precocious puberty.

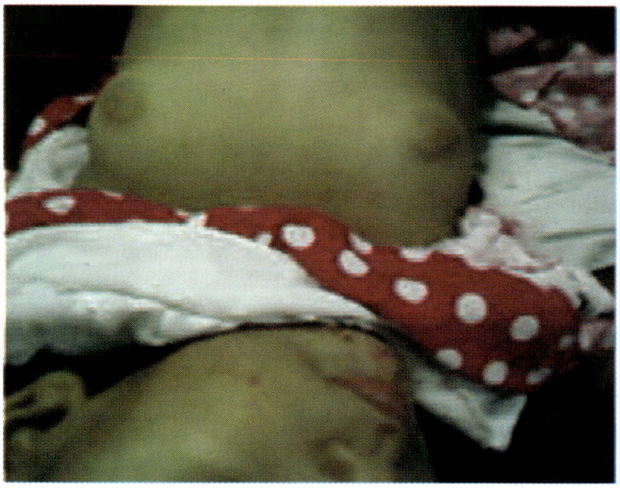

Fig. 16.12: Premature thelarche

Premature Pubarche

Premature pubarche denotes early development of sexual hair. It is thought to be due to premature adrenarche, i.e., early onset of adrenal androgen production. It is more common in girls and rare before 6 years age. Isolated pubarche is usually nonprogressive. Early pubic hair may be accompanied by acne, oily skin, adult body sweaty odour and occasionally axillary hair. Subsequent growth and pubertal development occur at normal age and proceed normally.

Premature Menarche

It is a rare entity in which girls present with isolated vaginal bleeding in absence of other secondary sexual characters. They have only 1–3 episodes of bleeding. Puberty occurs in the usual time and menstrual cycle is normal. More common causes of vaginal bleeding such as vulvovaginitis, foreign body, or sexual abuse should be excluded. It is thought to be the result of increased sensitivity of endometrium to circulating estrogen levels too low to produce breast development.

DELAYED PUBERTY

Puberty is said to be delayed if pubertal changes do not start by the age of 13 years in girls and by 14 years in boys.

Delayed puberty is less common in girls. It is more likely to be associated with an underlying disorder. Puberty in girls is said to be delayed when Tanner stage II for breast development is not achieved by the age of 13 years. A girl with delayed pubertal progression, i.e., no menarche within 5 years of thelarche needs evaluation for delayed puberty. Constitutional delay of puberty is rare in girls. Incomplete variations of delayed puberty like isolated amenorrhea, or amenorrhea without pubarche can occur in girls.

The prevalence of delayed puberty is higher in boys. The likelihood of identifying an associated disorder is much lower compared to girls. Testicular volume is the most reliable marker of pubertal onset. A volume more than 4 ml suggest onset of puberty. Constitutional delay of puberty and growth is the most common cause of delayed puberty in boys.

Delayed puberty in both boys and girls can be classified into hypogonadotropic hypogonadism or disorders of HPG axis (disorders associated with low gonadotrophin levels) and hyper gonadotrophic hypogonadism or ovarian disorders (girls) and testicular disorders (boys). Gonadotrophin levels are therefore very helpful in differentiating these disorders.

Table 16.4 : Causes of delayed puberty

Hypogonadotropic hypogonadism

Transient

1. Constitutional delay in growth and pubertal development.
2. Chronic systemic diseases: Renal failure, liver disease, renal tubular acidosis, cystic fibrosis.
3. Nutritional disorders: PEM, anorexia nervosa, bulimia nervosa.
4. Endocrine disorders: Hypothyroidism, hyperprolactinemia, type 1 diabetes mellitus.

Contd.

Contd.

Permanent

Isolated hypogonadotropic hypogonadism

1. Genetic disorders, e.g., Kallmann syndrome.
2. Dysmorphic syndromes, e.g., Prader Willi syndrome.

Multiple pituitary hormone deficiency

1. *Congenital malformations:* Holoporencephaly, midline defects.
2. *Genetic disorders:* LH gene deletions.
3. *Brain tumours:* Craniopharyngioma, gliomas, germinoma.
4. *CNS insults:* Surgery, infection, radiation and trauma.
5. *Infiltrative diseases:* Histiocytosis, sarcoidosis, Hemochromatosis, autoimmune.

Hypergonadotropic hypogonadism

Boys

1. *Chromosomal abnormality:* Klinefelter syndrome, gonadal dysgenesis.
2. *Steroidogenic defects*: Congenital adrenal hyperplasia.
3. *Testicular insults:* Radiotherapy, chemotherapy, trauma, torsion, infection.
4. *Malformations:* Vanishing testis syndrome (anorchia), cryptorchidism.
5. *Inefficient testosterone action:* 5, alpha reductase deficiency, androgen sensitivity syndrome.

Girls

1. *Gonadal dysgenesis*: Turner syndrome, trisomy 13, 18, 21.
2. *Steroidogenic defects*: 17, alpha hydroxylase, aromatase deficiencies.
3. *Ovarian insults*: Surgery, radiation, alkalyting agents, infections.
4. *Ovarian failure:* Autoimmune polyendocrinopathy.
5. *Gonadotrophin resistance*: LH and FSH receptor mutations.

Isolated amenorrhea due to

1. *Structural malformation*: Vaginal septum, imperforate hymen, mullerian agenesis.
2. *Inefficient androgen action*: Complete androgen insensitivity syndrome.

Evaluation

The first step in evaluation in both girls and boys is confirmation of delay by careful evaluation of the components of puberty by SMR. The second step should aim at exclusion of an underlying systemic disorder. This can be achieved by the help of a thorough history and physical examination including a neurological examination with special emphasis on focal neurological signs, signs of increased intracranial pressure, fundoscopy. The girls, in addition should undergo a thorough local examination of the introitus, hymen and clitoris to identify any structural anomalies. Growth velocity, and symptoms and signs of specific syndromes should be looked for.

Investigations

Initial investigations should aim at excluding systemic disease such as complete hemogram, renal function test, liver function test, malabsorption studies and blood gases. This should be followed by a skeletal survey to determine bone age. The girls must also have a pelvic USG done to assess uterine size, shape and endometrial thickness. The hormonal studies should be deferred till the age of 14 years in boys. In girls with bone age less than 11 years, gonadotrophin levels should be interpreted with caution as the HPG feedback is immature.

A basal gonadotrophin level helps to differentiate between hypo and hyper gonadotrophic hypogonadism. In case the levels are inconclusive, the GnRH stimulation test should be performed. The further investigation is different for boys and girls.

Girls

Low gonadotrophin levels: Check prolactin levels.

Prolactin levels:

Normal: MRI head and pituitary function.

Elevated: Advise MRI (to exclude tumor of the hypothalamic pituitary region), thyroid function test (to exclude hypothyroidism), drugs.

Elevated gonadotrophin levels: Check karyotype for Turner syndrome.

Abnormal: Turner syndrome.

Normal: Advise for USG pelvis, antiovarian antibodies (for autoimmune Oophoritis), and estimation of steroid metabolites (to exclude steroidogenic defects).

Boys

Low gonadotrophin levels: Constitutional delay of puberty and growth (CDPH)/Hypogonadotropic hypogonadism (HH).

Advise GnRH agonist test, morning testosterone levels and DHEAS (dehydroepiandrosterone sulphate).

CDPH: Positive response to GnRH agonist, morning testosterone levels > 20 ng/dL, low DHEAS.

HH: High DHEAS.

High gonadotrophin levels: Advise testosterone levels.

Low testosterone levels: Advise karyotyping.

Abnormal (47, XXY): Klinefelter syndrome.

Normal: Testicular insult, cryptorchidism, anorchia (hCG stimulation test), gonadal dysgenesis (testicular biopsy), disorders of steroidogenesis (estimation of steroid metabolites).

High testosterone levels: Advise testosterone: DHT ratio.

High: Androgen insensitivity syndrome (AIS).

Low: 5, alpha reductase deficiency.

Management

The aims of treatment include management of underlying disorder and attainment of appropriate pubertal development and reproductive potential.

Treatment of Underlying Disorders

Treatment of the underlying systemic disorders viz. malnutrition, eating disorders etc. is often associated with progression of puberty. Correction of hyperprolactinemia, hormone replacement in endocrine disorders like hypothyroidism, hypopituitarism, steroid supplementation in steroidogenic defects and congenital adrenal hyperplasia is expected to result in pubertal development. Boys with anorchia should be offered prosthetic testis for psychological support.

Induction of Puberty

Induction of puberty should be deferred till the bone age is greater than 12 years in girls and 13 years in boys to avoid premature closure of epiphysis and compromised final height.

Girls

Treatment should be started with low dose estrogen (5 microgram ethinyl estradiol or 0.3 mg conjugated estrogen daily) doubling the dose every six months to achieve the maximum adult dose by 2 years. Estrogen patch can be used with the advantage of continued exposure and good compliance. The child should be followed up for growth and pubertal development. When the endometrial thickness becomes > 5 mm or there is withdrawal bleeding, cyclical estrogen progesterone should be started. Estrogen should be continued from day 1 to 21. Medroxyprogesterone should be added from day 11–21.

Boys

The most commonly used drug is testosterone injections (testosterone enanthate, propionate or cypionate). It should be started at a low dose (100 mg / month) and gradually increased to adult doses (100 mg/week). Long acting testosterone implants are now more commonly used because they do not need frequent injections. In boys with hypogonadotropic hypogonadism, therapy with hCG (2000 IU biweekly) should be combined with testosterone for 6 months for proper growth of testis and growth of pubic hairs.

Boys with CDPG should receive short course testosterone (testosterone enanthate 100 mg IM 3 – 6 monthly) together with an aromatase inhibitor, oxandrolone, 0.25 mg/kg (maximum dose 10 mg) to minimize effect of testosterone on skeletal growth and ultimate height. Aromatase inhibitor therapy has been shown to decrease the progression of bone age advancement and increase height potential in boys with CDPG treated with testosterone.

Management of Fertility

Therapy should be planned only when fertility is considered. In vivo fertilization and embryo transfer is a viable fertility option in both girls and boys.

Girls with hypogonadotropic hypogonadism, after treatment with combination of human chorionic gonadotrophin (hCG) and human menopausal gonadotrophin (hMG) become potentially fertile.

Treatment with combination of hCG and hMG has been shown to be effective in increasing the sperm count and potential for fertility in boys with hypogonadotropic hypogonadism.

This treatment is very costly and not always affordable. Hence in vivo fertilization is a better option in both sexes.

Diabetes Mellitus

Diabetes mellitus is a chronic, metabolic syndrome characterized by chronic hyperglycemia as a cardinal biochemical feature, resulting from an absolute or relative deficiency of insulin.

Two major forms of diabetes are Type 1 diabetes mellitus which is caused by deficiency of insulin secretion due to pancreatic beta cell damage and Type 2 diabetes mellitus which is a consequence of insulin resistance occurring at the level of skeletal muscles, liver and adipose tissue.

Classification of Diabetes Mellitus

Type 1 diabetes mellitus: Type 1 A and Type 1 B.

Type 2 diabetes mellitus.

Other specific types

Pancreatic diseases: Fibrocystic pancreatic disease, cystic fibrosis, thalassemia major.

Endocrine diseases: Cushing's syndrome, thyrotoxicosis, growth hormone excess.

Drugs: Steroids, diphenylhydantoin, pentamidine, thiazides, diazoxide.

Infection: Congenital rubella, entero virus, rotavirus.

Genetic defects of insulin secretion and action.

Auto antibodies against insulin receptors and insulin.

Associated with genetic syndromes: Turner, Klinefelter, Lawrence Moon-Biedl, Prader-Willi syndromes.

TYPE 1 DIABETES MELLITUS

Type 1 diabetes mellitus is the most common form seen in childhood and adolescence; although increase in the incidence of Type 2 diabetes mellitus is reported in the obese adolescents. It is characterized by low or absent levels of endogenously produced insulin and dependence on exogenous insulin. The child may present at any age. However, the onset occurs predominantly in childhood with peak at 7–15 years.

Classification

Type 1 diabetes is subclassified as Type 1A and Type 1B. The former constitutes nearly 90% of Type 1 diabetes mellitus. It is due to an autoimmune destruction of the pancreatic beta cells by T lymphocytes and macrophages infiltrating the islets. The latter which constitute the rest 10% cases, such antibodies are absent and the cause of beta cell destruction is not known. Hence it is also called idiopathic type. Such cases may form a larger proportion of Type 1 diabetes mellitus in the Indians and Japanese.

Etiopathogenesis

Type 1 diabetes mellitus also called insulin dependent diabetes mellitus (IDDM) is a chronic autoimmune disease resulting from a T cell mediated destruction of beta cells of the pancreas. Genetic predisposition and environmental factors have been identified in the etiopathogenesis.

The pathogenesis can be divided into certain arbitrary phases: interaction between predisposing genes and environment, initiation of autoimmunity and a pre diabetic phase of progressive beta cell destruction and finally the clinical appearance of diabetes.

Genetic Predisposition

Genetic predisposition is evidenced by 50% rate of concordance of the disease in monozygotic twins and an increased prevalence in the first degree relatives. Type 1 diabetes mellitus is found in approximately 5% of siblings and 3% of parents of the patient. The inheritance is complex and multiple genes are likely to be involved. The strongest association has been found with the HLA region (IDDM 1 locus). About 50% of the genetic susceptibility is due to this region. Another 10% is found to be associated with the promoter region of the insulin gene (IDDM 2 locus). Two other loci which have been recently identified include the cytotoxic T-lymphocyte antigen 4 (CTLA 4, IDDM 12 locus) and gene encoding lymphoid tyrosine phosphatase (PTPN22).

Environment

Environment has been found to play an important role in the pathogenesis of Type 1 diabetes mellitus. This is evidenced by recent increase in the incidence as well as the seasonal variation in its occurrence. The different environmental factors have been identified but their exact modes of action have not been identified.

The environmental factors implicated for are as follows:

1. Viruses: Rubella, enteroviruses, rotavirus.
2. Early weaning to cow's milk.
3. Early weaning to cereals.
4. Deficiency of Vitamin D.
5. Stress.

Among the viruses implicated, congenital rubella has definite evidence of involvement in the pathogenesis. Among the dietary factors, shorter duration of breast feeding and early weaning to cow's milk and early introduction of cereals may act as a predisposing factor. Vitamin D deficiency has also been identified as a risk factor. Stress is more likely to act as a precipitating factor by increasing insulin resistance through its effect on glucose counter regulatory hormones.

Initiation of Autoimmunity

The process by which autoimmunity against beta cells is triggered is not clear. A specific T cell response against one or more beta cell antigen may be initiated against a foreign antigen like a virus infecting another tissue. Cytotoxic T cells can directly attack the pancreatic tissue already infected, aided by helper T cell. These helper T cells are activated by antigens presented to them by infected macrophages. Alternatively, infection of the beta cells by a virus could lead to expression of the viral protein on the beta cell surface triggering attack on the cytotoxic T cells. With the initiation of the autoimmune attack, various cytokines are liberated which amplify the immune response. These include interleukin 1 and 6, gamma interferon, and tumour necrosis factor (TNF). These amplify the immune response. Cytokines act by direct beta cell destruction, diminishing insulin secretion from the beta cells and activating cytotoxic T cells. They also enhance the expression of HLA class 1 molecules on the beta cells thus increasing their vulnerability. Damage to beta cells may be mediated also through production of radicals like superoxide and high concentration of nitric oxide.

Prediabetic Phase

In this phase, the child would be asymptomatic, but there will be evidence of autoimmunity in the form of T-cell responses and antibodies against various islet antibodies. The antibodies do not cause beta cell destruction but they are important markers for the autoimmune process. These antibodies can be detected many years prior to clinical onset of diabetes.

The earliest functional abnormality is a diminished first phase insulin response to intravenous glucose. This progresses to impaired glucose tolerance and later to elevated fasting plasma glucose. The prediabetic phase may last for months to many years.

Clinical Appearance of Diabetes

Diabetes usually becomes overt in the presence of a precipitating event such as a viral infection. After treatment of hyperglycemia with insulin and disappearance of the acute stress, insulin sensitivity normalizes. The patient may again enter into a phase where endogenous insulin secretion is adequate to control hyperglycemia (honeymoon phase). This phase may last for weeks to months, before insulin secretion further diminishes, requiring permanent insulin therapy.

Clinical Manifestation

The clinical presentations depend on the degree of insulinopenia and hyperglycemia. The typical presentations include polyuria, polydipsia, nocturia, enuresis, increased appetite, loss of weight and weakness. Initially polyuria and nocturia is intermittent. With increasing insulinopenia and chronic hyperglycemia, it becomes more persistent and polydipsia becomes more apparent. Female patients may present with monilial vaginitis due to chronic glycosuria. If the condition is not recognized at this stage, the child develops features of ketoacidosis viz. abdominal discomfort, nausea, vomiting. There is dehydration, Kussmaul respiration (deep heavy rapid breathing) fruity odour of the breath, diminished neurocognitive function and coma. As in any hyperosmotic state, the degree of dehydration may be clinically underestimated because intravascular volume is conserved at the expense of intracellular volume.

About 20–40% of children with new onset diabetes progress to ketoacidosis before diagnosis.

This entire progression happens much more quickly in younger children probably due to a more aggressive destruction of beta cells. In adolescents, the course is usually prolonged. In any case, progression of symptoms may be accelerated by stress situations like intercurrent illness or trauma.

Laboratory Criteria for Diagnosis

Laboratory diagnosis is usually simple because glucose levels in blood and urine are typically very high. The normal venous plasma glucose is < 100 mg/dL and normal value of 2 hours post glucose is < 140 mg/dL in children. In presence of clinical symptoms, the following laboratory parameters clinch the diagnosis:

Any random venous plasma glucose = / > 200 mg/dL with classical symptoms of polyuria, polydipsia and weight loss, or

Fasting (after 8 hours fast) plasma glucose = / > 126 mg/dL, or

Two-hour plasma glucose level during glucose tolerance test = / > 200 mg/dL (after glucose loading of 1.75 gm/kg).

Other Investigations

A baseline glycohemoglobin (HbA_{1c}) estimation allows assessment of the duration of hyperglycemia. It also provides an initial value to compare the effectiveness of subsequent therapy. The child should be screened for other autoimmune diseases like thyroiditis, celiac disease.

Routine screening of healthy and at risk children with determination of post prandial blood glucose or screening oral glucose tolerance test have not yielded good detection rates. Hence screening procedures are not recommended in children. However, if a child has transient hyperglycemia with glucosuria while under substantial physical stress, this child should be monitored for development of symptoms of persistent hyperglycemia and tested if such symptoms appear.

Treatment

The goals of therapy in non-ketotic new onset diabetes, for excellent diabetes control include (1) maintenance of balance between blood glucose control and avoiding hypoglycemia, (2) elimination of polyuria and nocturia, (3) prevention of ketoacidosis, (4) normal growth and development.

Therapy encompasses initiation and adjustment of insulin therapy, teaching of the child and caretakers and reestablishment of the routine of life. The treatment can be initiated on OPD basis in a diabetic clinic with complete staff under supervision of a pediatric endocrinologist. Otherwise, the child should be admitted to hospital for initial therapy.

Insulin Therapy

The initial dose insulin/ kg body weight /day, required to control hyperglycemia depends on several factors. The dose requirement is higher in pubertal children and in those who have to restore greater deficits of body glycogen, protein and fat. On the other hand those children with new onset diabetes in the honeymoon phase will require fewer doses because they have some residual beta cell function which reduces the need for exogenous insulin. The optimal dose of insulin for individual cases can be determined empirically, with frequent blood glucose monitoring and insulin adjustment.

Insulin therapy should be started as soon as the diagnosis is made. In the initial 4–6 weeks, insulin requirements tend to be higher but once stabilized , most children need 0.5–1.0 units of insulin /kg/day.

Types of Insulin Therapy

Two modes of insulin therapy are practised: The conventional and intensive therapy.

The *conventional insulin therapy* involves giving a mixture of short acting and intermediate acting insulin two times daily in the ratio of 1:2 of regular to intermediate acting insulin. Approximately two thirds of the total daily dose is given 20–40 minutes before breakfast and the rest one third before dinner. Subsequently the dose is adjusted according to the blood glucose patterns seen in the individual. This regimen is easy and cost effective and works in a large proportion of children especially in the mid childhood where the eating and activity patterns are predictable. In toddlers, in whom the timing and amount of food and activity are unpredictable, and in adolescents, who may desire flexibility, conventional therapy is not suitable.

Table 16.5 : Goals of therapy in diabetes

	Conventional therapy	*Intensive therapy*
Fasting blood glucose	120–160 mg/dL	80–120 mg/dL
2 hrs post-meal	Post meal not monitored	< 180 mg/dL
Bedtime	> 100 mg/dL	> 100 mg/dL
Hb_{1c}	7%–8%	6%–7%

The *intensive insulin therapy* has the advantage of strict blood glucose control which is the most important strategy for prevention of long-term complications of diabetes. The intensive insulin therapy usually uses the basal bolus principle giving four or more injections of insulin per day or by using an insulin pump. This regimen necessitates 4–6 blood glucose tests with meal planning and daily exercise regimen with constant access to a multi-disciplinary diabetic team. Used properly, these regimen offer greater flexibility, tighter control, lesser hypoglycemia but it needs motivation of family and is costly. Intensive therapy is suitable for toddlers and adolescents.

The basal needs for insulin are met with a once or twice daily dose of a long acting insulin analogue, glargine / detemir insulin. Blood glucose is checked before each meal and depending on the sugar level and the size of the meal; the dose of rapid or short acting insulin is decided.

Inhaled and oral insulin is being evaluated in adults with Type 1 and Type 2 diabetes. The preliminary data is promising. It will need further evaluation and monitoring before regular use.

Diet

The recommended diet for a child with diabetes is a healthy, balanced, normal diet in which large amounts of simple sugars are avoided. The total calories should be enough to maintain ideal body weight and promote growth.

The *calorie* requirement can be roughly calculated by the formula of 1000 calories at 1 year age plus 100 calories per year of age after that. Since many children present with weight loss at presentation, their calorie needs may be quite high initially. Subsequently care should be taken to avoid obesity. Ten to 20% of the total calories should be provided by protein. Fats should contribute 25–30% of the calories, of which less than one third should be saturated fats. Carbohydrates should constitute 55% of total calorie; 70% of which should be complex carbohydrate. Fibre content should be > 20 gms/day. *Protein* intake should be 2.0 gm/kg/day for infants to 0.9 gm/kg for teenagers. Sucrose and sugars should be restricted but not be forbidden. Non-nutritive sweeteners can be used safely.

Food should be divided into three main meals viz. breakfast, lunch and dinner and two to three between meal snacks.

The total daily calories should be distributed as follows: Breakfast: 20%, Mid morning snacks: 10%, Lunch: 20%, Evening snacks: 10%, Dinner: 30%. Bed time: 10%. The snacks are not important with rapid acting and peakless insulin regimens. An adequate fibre intake (whole grains, fruits, salads, sprouts) regulates glucose absorption from the gut, promotes satiety and thus reduces hyperglycemia, obesity and dyslipidemia.

The families should be provided with food exchange lists which contain food items with equivalent calorie content. This will help the child to have variety in meals. Food with low glycemic index should be preferred over foods with high glycemic index. The glycemic index is a measure of the rate of rise of blood sugar after a particular type of food is eaten, in comparison to glucose which is taken as 100. Examples of healthy low glycemic index foods are dal, lentils with the skin (red kidney beans or rajma), chapatti (made from mix of wheat flour and gram flour), oat porridge, noodles, green vegetables and fruits such as apple, guava, peach and orange. The intelligent and highly motivated parents and the older child who are on intensive regimen may be also explained the concept of carbohydrate counting for insulin adjustment.

The child should not be made to feel different in public. This improves the likelihood of a well adjusted and responsible adolescent and young adult. They should be allowed occasional treats especially birthdays and festivals.

Exercise

All kinds of physical exercise should be encouraged. Aerobic exercise (such as all outdoor games or an exercise bicycle) should be preferred to exercise like weightlifting. The child should exercise 30 – 45 minutes in the form of brisk walking, jogging, cycling, swimming, badminton, football, dancing, hockey or tennis. There should be provision for extra calories before vigorous exercise to prevent hypoglycemia. Exercise however should be avoided during periods of hypoglycemia or ketosis.

Monitoring

1. *Home monitoring of blood glucose (HMBG)* helps to detect instances as well as pattern of high blood

sugar, safeguard against hypoglycemia and achieve normal blood glucose in those on intensive therapy. HMBG should be done pre meal (i.e. fasting, pre-lunch and pre-dinner) and at bed time and at 2–3 am two times a month. The insulin dose can be adjusted according to the blood glucose levels. Blood glucose testing is painful and costly. Urine glucose testing is cheaper but is a poor alternative because its correlation with blood sugar is poor and it cannot detect hypoglycemia.

2. *Glycosylated hemoglobin (HbA_{1c})* must be tested every 3–4 months in order to check for the overall glycemic control over the preceding period. The normal value is 4%–6%.
3. *Height, weight, pubertal development* should be reviewed 2–4 times a year. In addition, blood pressure, injection sites, thyroid gland, feet for corns and abrasions, peripheral pulses and sensations should be examined. It should be remembered that hypertension, obesity, short stature, delayed puberty could have the onset after 10–15 years of onset of diabetes.
4. *Screening for complications:* A baseline fundus examination should be performed soon after diagnosis and subsequently annually after 3–5 years of diagnosis. Microalbuminuria should be tested at diagnosis and annually after 5 years of diabetic state. Serum lipids should be estimated after glucose control. If found to be normal, the test should be repeated every 5 years. Thyroid function test should be tested at the onset of diabetic state and subsequently periodically if growth velocity is slow or if there is repeated hypoglycemia. Testing for celiac disease is relevant in case of poor weight and height gain, anemia, or frequent abdominal symptoms like pain, diarrhoea and vomiting.
5. *Monitoring during sick days:* More frequent monitoring is necessary when the child is sick for prevention of ketoacidosis. Insulin dose should not be omitted but may be adjusted according to the blood glucose levels. Blood glucose and urinary ketones should be checked 4 hourly. The child should be hospitalized if there is excessive vomiting, anorexia; decreasing or dark colored urine; there is breathlessness or drowsiness and ketones are rising in spite of extra insulin.

Diabetes Education

Education is the most important aspect in the management of diabetes. The parents, the older child and adolescent should be aware of the disease in simple language and the importance of good control for prevention of complications. They should be informed about the different types of insulin and the technique of using and talked in details about the diet. They should be made aware of causes and management of hypoglycemia and discussed the importance of exercise and advised accordingly. Sick day rules should be discussed and indications of hospitalization should be told. The child should be directed to carry the diabetes identity card and some candy to use in case of hypoglycemia attacks.

The parents as well as the adolescents should be discussed about the special issues to be taken care of during this period. The hormonal changes during adolescence lead to increase requirement of insulin and this requirement lasts for 2–3 years. Adolescence is a turbulent phase of life. Adolescents seek independence but is incapable of accepting full responsibility. Presence of a chronic illness like diabetes may be difficult to cope. An understanding attitude, emotional support and formal sex education must be provided to them. Further, the responsibility should be relinquished by the parents gradually and overall parental involvement should be continued. In view of the erratic food and activity pattern during this period, the need for flexible and individualized insulin, exercise and meal programme in adolescents should be emphasized.

Diabetes Ketoacidosis

Diabetes ketoacidosis (DKA) is a state of acute metabolic decompensation characterized by the triad of hyperglycemia, ketonuria, and metabolic acidosis occurring in patients of IDDM. The biochemical criteria include a blood glucose level > 300 mg / dl, ketonuria > 1: 2 dilutions or absolute value > 3 meq / L and a blood pH <7.3 or HCO_3 < 15 meq/L. Euglycemic ketoacidosis may occur in patients who have had prolonged vomiting, poor oral intake or partial treatment with insulin before presentation.

Most episodes of DKA occur in patients with known IDDM. In these patients DKA is precipitated by infections viz. pneumonia, UTI, acute gastroenteritis; omission/error in recommended insulin dosage. Other causes include trauma, psychological stress, pancreatitis, steroid therapy. In 25-30% of cases, DKA may be the first manifestation of IDDM especially in the age group of less than 2 years and more than 10 years.

Pathophysiology

Diabetes ketoacidosis is characterized by hyperglycemia and ketonuria which results from absolute or relative deficiency associated with elevated levels of some or all of the stress hormones. Hyperglycemia results in increased serum osmolarity and causes osmotic diuresis with loss of fluid and electrolytes and activation of renin-angiotensin-aldosterone mechanism with accelerated potassium loss. If hyperglycemia and dehydration are severe and prolonged for several hours, there is cerebral edema.

Increased catabolic process result in cellular loss of sodium, potassium and phosphate. Loss of phosphate depletes the red cells of 2, 3-diphosphoglycerol (2, 3-DPG), shifting the oxygen dissociation curve to the left. Ketonemia causes loss of sodium and potassium along with ketone bodies in urine. There is ileus with vomiting which further aggravates dehydration and electrolyte imbalance. Ketone bodies being organic acids are buffered by bicarbonate. This leads to depletion of bicarbonate and resultant acidosis. Severe acidosis has a negative inotropic effect and causes peripheral vasodilatation thereby accentuating shock. Shock and tissue hypoxia lead to secondary lactic acidosis.

Clinical Manifestation

DKA is more common in a female child. In addition to the general features of IDDM, there will be features of ketoacidosis.

General Features of IDDM

These include history of progressive polyuria, polydipsia, polyphagia and weight loss, onset of enuresis in a previously toilet trained child and recurrent pyogenic infection and monilial vaginitis especially in adolescent girls.

Features of Ketoacidosis

Symptoms include increasing polyuria and polydipsia, pain abdomen and vomiting, lethargy, irritability followed by drowsiness, seizures and coma. *Signs* include dehydration, tachycardia, low volume pulse, hypotension, hypothermia, acidotic breathing, fruity odor of breath, abdominal distention, and rigidity, and features of metabolic encephalopathy.

DKA must be considered in the differential diagnosis of a child presenting with dehydration and polyuria, acute abdominal signs, respiratory distress or coma.

Investigation

For Rapid Confirmation of Diagnosis

1. Blood glucose (dextrosticks, also blood sample for confirmation).
2. Blood ketones.
3. Urine ketones.

Evaluation of the Extent of Metabolic Derangement

1. Serum sodium, potassium, bicarbonate, chloride, lactate.
2. Serum creatinine and urea.
3. Blood pH, ECG (for rapid documentation of potassium imbalance).

Classification of Diabetes Ketoacidosis

Parameters	*Normal*	*Mild*	*Moderate*	*Severe*
Clinical	No change	Oriented alert but fatigued	Kussmaul respiration oriented, but sleepy, arousable	Kussmaul / depressed resp, sleepy to depressed sensorium to coma
Laboratory				
CO_2 (mEq/L, venous)	20 – 28	16 – 20	10 – 15	< 10
p H (venous)	7.35 – 7.45	7.25 – 7.35	7.15 – 7.25	< 7.15

* Severe hypernatremia (corrected serum sodium > 150 mEq/L) should also be classified as severe DKA.

Source: Nelson Text Book of Pediatrics, 18th edition, 2007.

To Rule Out Infection and Other Causes

1. TC (WBC), DLC, HB% (TC > 25,000/cu mm is suggestive of infection).
2. Blood culture, urine culture and sensitivity, CSF analysis after fundoscopy.
3. X-ray chest.

Follow-up Investigation

1. Blood glucose hourly at bedside.
2. Serum electrolytes 2–4 hourly till stabilized.
3. Serum pH, bicarbonate, urea, hematocrit, osmolarity, anion gap 2–6 hourly.
4. ECG for evidence of hyperkalemia/ hypokalemia and arrhythmias.
5. 24 hours fluid intake and urine output.

Management

Therapy in diabetic ketoacidosis must aim at correction of insulinopenia and rehydration simultaneously. Insulin should be given at the beginning of therapy to accelerate movement of glucose into cells, decrease hepatic glucose production, and halt the movement of fatty acids from the periphery to the liver. Rehydration also lowers glucose levels by improving renal perfusion and enhancing renal excretion.

The combination of these therapies usually causes a rapid initial decline in serum glucose levels. Once glucose goes below 180 mg /dL, the osmotic diuresis stops. It should be noted that repair of hyperglycemia occurs well before correction of acidosis. Therefore, insulin should be continued to control release of fatty acids after normal glucose levels are reached. In order to prevent hypoglycemia, glucose should be added to the infusion as 5% solution when the serum glucose level is decreased to about 250 mg/dL. The glucose infusion rate can also be lowered once hyperglycemia has resolved.

Initial Resuscitation

The child should be preferably treated in a pediatric intensive unit especially when age is below 5 years, child in shock or with altered sensorium.

The first priority is maintenance of airway, breathing and circulation.

If a child presents with coma, with depressed airway reflexes or paralytic ileus, emergency measures like endotracheal intubation, gastric decompression and urinary catherization should be a priority. In all other cases, the first action should be to replenish fluid on the basis of degree of dehydration and start insulin therapy and potassium replacement 30–60 minutes after fluid therapy is started.

Fluid and Electrolyte Therapy

Calculation of fluid deficits using clinical signs is difficult in children with DKA because intravascular volume is better maintained in hypertonic state. Assessed by any sign of dehydration, a child with DKA will be more dehydrated than the child with normotonic fluid deficit.

Milwaukee protocol is being in use for last 20 years and is acclaimed to be a very efficient protocol for treatment of DKA. It is designed to restore most electrolytes deficits, to reverse the acidosis and to rehydrate the ill child. When treated with this protocol, children with milder DKA recover in 10 to 20 hours (hence need less total IV fluid before switching to oral intake) whereas children with more severe DKA require 30 to 36 hours. It needs mention that a child with severe hypernatremia should be classified as severe DKA and hence treated with longer duration of fluid therapy.

According to this protocol, a standard fluid deficit of 85 ml/kg (to correct 8.5% dehydration) is assumed. To this amount the maintenance fluid is added and the total amount of fluid for 24 hours is calculated.

The appropriate maintenance fluid therapy required can be calculated as 1500 ml/sq metre or as

< 10 kg: 100 ml/kg;

10-20 kg: 1000 ml+ 50 ml/kg for each kg in excess of 10 kg;

> 20 kg: 1500 ml + 20 ml/kg for each kg in excess of 20 kg.

Fluid therapy can be done through a peripheral venous access. A central line placement and CVP measurement should be performed when absolutely indicated as there is risk of thrombosis in DKA.

First Hour

For all children an initial bolus of 20 ml/kg of normal saline/ ringers lactate should be infused in 1 hour. This ensures a quick volume expansion. It may be repeated if quick clinical improvement is not seen. Mannitol should be kept at bedside; to be pushed 1 gm /kg IV for cerebral edema.

Second Hour Onwards

Therapy, second hour onwards includes remainder fluid therapy, correction of potassium imbalance and acidosis and monitoring. The intravenous fluid rate second hour onwards until resolution of DKA is calculated as follows:

$$\text{IV rate} = \frac{85 \text{ ml/kg} + \text{maintenance} - \text{bolus}}{23 \text{ hours}}$$

The fluid to be used second hour onwards is 0.45% saline. This helps to repair the free water deficits to allow intracellular rehydration and to allow a more appropriate replacement of ongoing hypotonic urine losses.

Once the blood glucose goes below 180 mg/dl, the osmotic diuresis stops and rehydration accelerates without further increase in the infusion rate. 5% dextrose should be added when blood glucose comes down to < 250 mg/dL and 10% dextrose if the blood glucose goes below 150 mg dL.

Any child can be easily transitioned to oral intake and subcutaneous insulin when DKA has essentially resolved which is indicated by total CO_2 > 15 meq/L, pH > 7.3, sodium stable between 135 and145 mEq/L and no emesis. At this point, IV insulin therapy should be stopped and child given the first dose of subcutaneous insulin with a meal.

Hypokalemia with serum K < 3.5 mEq/L should be treated with 40–60 mEq potassium/L of fluid. If serum K level is between 3.5–5.0 mEq/L, the dose of potassium is 30–40 mEq/L. If the initial serum K level is less than 3 mEq/L, IV potassium should be increased to 80 mEq/L. Oral potassium can be given in the dose of 0.5–1 mEq/kg/day.

Acidosis should be suspected if there is symptomatic hyperkalemia or if pH < 6.9 with circulatory instability 1 hour after fluid therapy. The dose of 7.5% sodium bicarbonate is 1–2 mEq / kg diluted with equal amount of distilled water or normal saline and infused very slowly over 1–2 hours.

Monitoring

Patients should be closely monitored. For all but the mildest cases, clinical monitoring should include:

1. Neurological examination for signs of increasing intracranial pressure which include change of consciousness, depressed respiration, worsening headache, bradycardia, apnea, pupillary changes, abnormalities of tone, seizure, papilledema.
2. Laboratory parameters to be monitored include estimation of serum electrolytes, glucose and pH. Blood testing should be done every 1–2 hours for children with severe DKA and every 3–4 hours for those with mild to moderate DKA.

Insulin Therapy

Only regular or rapid acting insulin analogues are used in management of DKA. Continuous low grade infusion is the preferred method. It is simple, effective, physiological, and easily titrable with less chance of hypoglycemia and hypokalemia. It is usually started in the second hour. 50 units of regular insulin are added to 500 ml normal saline and running off 50–60 ml in order to saturate insulin binding sites in the infusion tubing. This solution yields a concentration of 0.1 unit/ml. This is infused through an infusion pump to provide 0.1 unit/kg/hour. Blood sugar should be monitored 2 hourly. If blood sugar does not fall by 50–100 mg/dl in 2 hours, the rate of infusion is doubled. The insulin infusion should be continued till acidosis is corrected (blood pH > 6.9, bicarbonate > 15 mmol/L). Thereafter insulin infusion should be discontinued. A subcutaneous dose of regular insulin 0.25 units / kg should be given half an hour before discontinuation of insulin infusion. Following this, a regimen of regular and intermediate acting insulin in two or more daily doses can be started as described for Type 1 diabetes.

Oral Feeds

Oral fluids can be started as soon as the patient is conscious, vomiting has stopped, there is no abdominal distension, there is normal bowel sounds and the child is willing to eat. Normally fluid can be started by 4–12 hours. Initially, clear fluids are offered, then soft solids and finally normal diet. Oral potassium supplement should be continued till patient regains original body weight.

Complications

The most serious complication in DKA is cerebral edema. It is common in children below 5 years age. It usually develops 4–16 hours after starting treatment. It must be suspected if sudden neurological deterioration occurs after initial favourable response to treatment. The signs of cerebral edema include headache, seizure, altered consciousness and delirium. Bradycardia, tachypnea may be the early signs. Papilledema, unequal pupils are signs of herniation of brainstem.

At the detection of the earliest sign, the IV fluid rate should be reduced and head end elevated to 30°. Mannitol

(0.25–1.0 gm./kg over 20 minutes) or 3% hypertonic saline (5–10 ml/kg over 30 minutes) should be started and intubation and ventilation planned for hyperventilation. Symptomatic cerebral edema carries a high mortality.

Post Acidotic Phase

Diabetic ketoacidosis is usually corrected within 36–48 hours of appropriate treatment. The post acidotic phase usually lasts 5–10 days. During this period one should try to recognize and treat precipitating factors, e.g., infection, achieve near normal metabolic control by adjusting insulin dosage, institute appropriate nutritional pattern and educate parents regarding management and complications.

INBORN ERRORS OF METABOLISM

The term "inborn errors of metabolism" was first used by Garrod in 1908 when he described four diseases viz. albinism, alkaptonuria, cystinuria and pentosuria. He also noted the frequency of consanguineous marriage in the pedigrees of his patients and correctly inferred the genetic origin of these orders. He further suggested that these diseases arose through the medium of defective enzyme activities. With the introduction of new biochemical techniques there has been a remarkable increase in the knowledge of inborn errors of metabolism.

An Approach to Inborn Errors of Metabolism

Inborn errors of metabolism are a group of hereditary biochemical disorders caused by gene mutation that encode specific proteins. These mutations can result in the alteration of primary protein structure or the amount of protein synthesized. The functional ability of the protein, whether it is an enzyme, receptor, transport vehicle, membrane or structural element, may be relatively or seriously compromised.

At present, it is technologically possible to screen for a large number of metabolic conditions during the first few days of life, before any clinical manifestation of the disease become apparent.

Diagnosis of inborn errors of metabolism is facilitated by considering the disorders presenting in the neonatal period and later period of life separately.

Neonatal Period

A history of consanguinity and/or death in the neonatal period should always raise the suspicion, especially when the neonate is sick, because most of the inborn errors are inherited as autosomal recessive traits. Again some of these disorders are more prevalent in certain specific population groups. Therefore knowledge of the ethnic background may help in diagnosis.

Clinical findings are usually nonspecific and similar to those seen in infants with sepsis. An inborn error should be considered in the differential diagnosis of a severely ill neonate. These infants should undergo special investigation.

Infants with metabolic disorders are usually normal at birth. Symptoms and signs like lethargy, poor feeding, vomiting and seizures may however develop as early as few hours after birth. A history of clinical deterioration in a previously normal neonate should suggest an inborn error. Physical examination reveals nonspecific findings. Most signs are related to the central nervous system. Hepatomegaly is a feature in many inborn errors. Occasionally an unusual odour of urine may help to clinch a diagnosis. Some of the diseases and odours are shown in a tabular form:

Table 16.6 : Some amino acid disorders and associated abnormal odour

Inborn error of metabolism	*Urine odour*
Maple syrup urine disease	Maple syrup
Phenyl ketonuria	Mousy or musty
Tyrosinemia	Boiled cabbage, rancid butter
Hypermethionemia	Boiled cabbage
Glutaric acidemia	Sweaty feet

Beyond Neonatal Period

They are milder variants and hence causes no symptoms in the first few days of life. They escape detection in the neonatal period. Early clinical manifestations in children beyond neonatal period are commonly nonspecific and are attributed to unidentified perinatal insults. Onset of symptoms is gradual. An inborn error of metabolism should be considered in any child with one or more of the following features:

1. Unexplained mental retardation, developmental delay or regression, motor deficits or seizures.

2. Intermittent episodes of unexplained vomiting, acidosis, mental deterioration or coma.
3. Unusual odour especially during an acute illness.
4. Hepatomegaly.
5. Renal stones.
6. Muscle weakness or cardiomyopathy.

Diagnosis

Diagnosis usually necessitates a battery of specific laboratory tests. The following investigations help in differentiating major causes of inborn errors. They are measurements of serum concentrations of glucose, ammonia, bicarbonate and the pH.

Observations

1. Elevation of blood ammonia levels is usually caused by defects in urea cycle enzymes.
2. Elevation of blood ammonia with severe acidosis indicates organic acidemias.
3. When blood ammonia, pH, and bicarbonate are normal one should suspect other aminoacidopathies.
4. Hypoglycemia with normal blood ammonia, pH and bicarbonate indicate galactosemia.

A specific diagnosis is facilitated by the following tests:

1. Direct biochemical assays of metabolites or their metabolic byproducts. Or of an enzyme function.
2. DNA analysis of the gene.
3. Neuroradiology, biopsy or post mortem examination.

Most of the inborn errors of metabolism presenting in the neonatal period are lethal if specific treatment is not started immediately. Neonatal metabolic screening with tandem mass spectroscopy can identify many disorders in the asymptomatic stage.

Clinical approach to a newborn with suspected metabolic disorder

(Adapted from Nelson Text Book of Pediatrics, 17th edition)

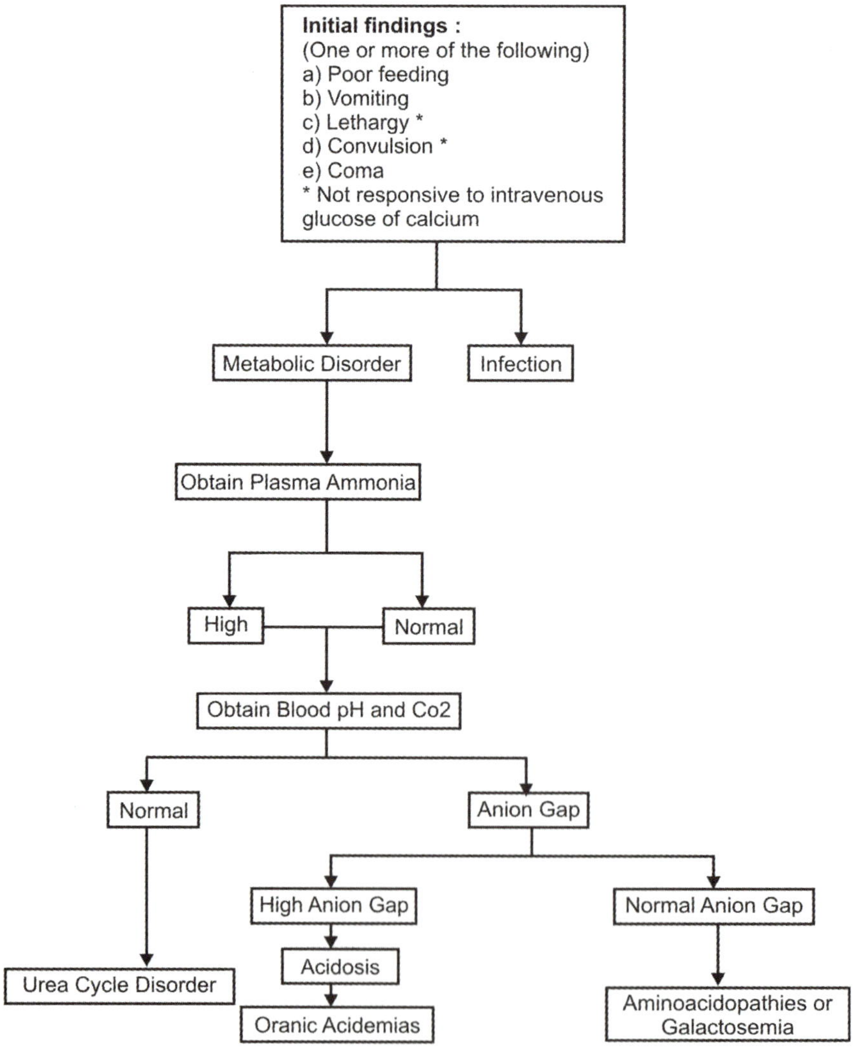

Flowchart

Two common and preventable inborn errors of metabolism have been described viz. Galactosemia and Phenylketonuria.

Galactosemia

Galactosemia denotes elevated levels of galactose levels in blood. It is found in three distinct inborn errors of galactose metabolism defective in one of the following enzymes viz. galactose-1-uridyl transferase, galactokinase and uridine diphosphate galactose 4 epimerase. It is an autosomal recessive disorder.

Galactose-1-Phosphate Uridyl Transferase Deficiency

The term galactosemia generally designates the galactose -1- uridyl transferase deficiency disease. In this type two forms of deficiency exist: infants with complete deficiency of the enzyme (Classic galactosemia) and the other with partial transferase deficiency. The incidence is 1/60,000.

Pathogenesis

The newborn infant receives high amount of lactose (upto 40% in breast milk) which consists of equal amounts of glucose and galactose. Without the enzyme galactose -1-uridyl transferase, the infant is unable to metabolize galactose -1- phosphate to glucose -1-phosphate. Accumulation of galactose-1-phosphate results in injury to kidneys, liver and brain. This injury may begin in fetal life by the transplacental galactose derived from the diet of a heterozygous mother or by endogenous production of galactose in the fetus.

Clinical Features

Classical galactosemia is a serious disease with the onset of symptoms typically by the second half of the first week of life after milk feeding has been started. The diagnosis should be considered in the newborn or infant if any one of the following features is present: vomiting, diarrhoea, lethargy, irritability, jaundice, poor weight gain or failure to gain birth weight, nuclear cataracts, hepatomegaly and splenomegaly, hypoglycemia, seizures. When the diagnosis is not made at birth, damage to liver (cirrhosis) and brain (mental retardation) becomes increasingly severe and irreversible. These patients are at increased risk of E. coli sepsis. Death from liver and renal failure and sepsis may follow within days after birth. All the abnormal features may regress rapidly on a galactose free diet save mental retardation.

Partial transferase deficiency is generally asymptomatic. It is more frequent than the classic type. It is usually diagnosed in newborn screening. When symptomatic, onset of disease is later. The features are same as in the classic type.

Laboratory Diagnosis

The preliminary diagnosis can be made by demonstration of nonglucose reducing substance in urine while the patient is receiving breast milk or lactose containing milk formula. The Benedicts test is positive but the Clinistix urine test results are negative because it is specific for glucose as it is based on the action of glucose oxidase. The reducing substance can be specifically identified by chromatography or by specific enzymatic test for galactose. Semi quantitative assay of blood for galactose-1-phosphate uridyl transferase is helpful in diagnosis. This test is also used for newborn screening.

Treatment

Treatment consists of substituting a lactose free formula for breast feeding and later a galactose free diet.

Prognosis

Prognosis is excellent when diagnosis is made before starting breast feeding and the infant is supplemented on a lactose free milk formula. Elimination of galactose from diet reverses growth failure as well as renal and liver dysfunction and regression of cataract. However, on long term follow up patient manifests ovarian failure with primary or secondary amenorrhea, decreased bone mineral density, developmental delay and learning disabilities which increase with increasing age. With classic galactosemia, around 80 to over 90% of female patients are reported to suffer from hypergonadotrophic hypogonadism and the majority of women are infertile. Most patient manifest speech disorders and impaired motor function and balance with or without ataxia.

Galactokinase Deficiency

This is also an autosomal recessive disorder which results from deficiency of the enzyme galactokinase which normally catalyzes the phosphorylation of galactose to galactose -1-phosphate. The principal metabolites accumulated are galactose which results in an elevated blood level of galactose and galactitol which accumulates in the lens leading to development of cataract. Two genes have been reported to encode galactokinase viz. GK1 on chromosome 17q24 and GK2 on chromosome 15.

The sole *manifestation* is cataract. Pseudomotor cerebri is a rare complication. The child is otherwise asymptomatic. Heterozygotes may be at risk of presenile cataract. There is an increased concentration of blood galactose level provided the patient has been fed on breast milk or a lactose containing formula.

The *diagnosis* is made by demonstration of absence of galactokinase activity in erythrocytes or fibroblasts. The galactose-1-phosphate uridyl transferase activity is normal.

Treatment is dietary restriction of galactose.

Uridine Diphosphate Galactose-4-Epimerase Deficiency

The gene of UDP galactose - 4- epimerase is located on chromosome 1 at 1p36. This enzyme deficiency results in abnormal accumulation of metabolites similar to those in transferase deficiency. In addition, there is also an increase in cellular UDP-galactose.

There are two types of epimerase deficiency. The first one is a benign form which is discovered incidentally through neonatal screening programs. The enzyme deficiency is limited to leucocytes and erythrocytes. The affected ones are asymptomatic. No treatment is required. However, it is advisable to follow up with examination of urine for reducing substances and exclude aminoaciduria within a few weeks of diagnosis while the infant is on a lactose containing diet.

In the second form, the enzyme deficiency is generalized. It is a severe disease and clinical manifestations are similar to classic galactosemia with additional symptoms of hypotonia and nerve deafness.

Diagnosis is confirmed by assay of epimerase in erythrocytes. Carrier detection is possible by measurement of epimerase activity in the erythrocytes. Prenatal diagnosis of the severe form is possible by enzyme assay of cultured amniotic fluid cells.

Treatment is restriction of dietary galactose.

Phenylketonuria

Phenylketonuria is an inborn error of the amino acid metabolism. It is transmitted as an autosomal recessive trait, so that in a family in which the disease has appeared the chances of future children being affected will be 1 in 4. The gene for enzyme phenylalanine hydroxylase is located on chromosome 12q24.1. Many disease causing mutations have been identified. The majority of patients are compound heterozygotes for two different mutant alleles.

Pathogenesis

Phenylalanine is an essential amino acid. In normal individuals phenylalanine is converted in the liver to tyrosine by the activity of phenylalanine hydroxylase. Deficiency of this enzyme or its cofactor tetrahydrobiopterin causes accumulation of phenylalanine in the body fluids and brain within 2 - 3 weeks after birth. The severity of hyperphenylalaninemia depends on the degree of enzyme deficiency. It may vary from plasma concentration of >20 mg/dL to mildly elevated levels of 2 - 6 mg/dL. In affected infants with plasma concentration of > 20 mg/dL, the excess phenylalanine is metabolized to phenyl ketones (phenyl pyruvate and phenyl acetate) giving the condition the name phenyl ketonuria (PKU). Phenylalaninemia is the term applied to lower levels of phenylalanine (< 20 mg/dL). The brain is the main organ affected. The CNS damage in affected patients is caused by elevated concentrations of phenylalanine in brain tissue. The high blood levels of phenylalanine saturate the transport system across the blood brain barrier causing inhibition of uptake of other amino acids like tyrosine and tryptophan. The exact mechanism of brain damage is however, not known.

Classical Phenylketonuria (PKU)

Classical PKU is characterized by a plasma phenylalanine level of >20 mg/dL. Severe hyperalaninemia, if untreated, results in development of signs and symptoms.

Clinical Manifestations

The affected infant is normal at birth. The infants are however, lighter in their complexion compared to their siblings. They are frequently blue eyed, fair haired. Some may have a mild eczematoid or seborrhoeic rash which disappears as the child grows older. These children have an unpleasant odour described as mousy or musty. This is the odour of phenylacetic acid. Severe vomiting may be sometimes an early symptom.

The infant may present with seizures, spasticity, tremors. In untreated children, the common presentations include microcephaly, prominent maxillae with widely spaced teeth, enamel hypoplasia. Profound mental retardation develops gradually if the infant remains untreated. 50 to 70% will have an IQ below 35 whereas 88 - 90% below 65%. Only 2 - 5% of untreated cases may have normal IQ. Older untreated children become hyperactive with autism. They may also present with purposeless hand movements, rhythmic rocking, and athetosis. It needs mention that clinical manifestations of classical PKU are rarely seen in countries where neonatal screening programmes for detection of PKU exist.

Milder Forms of Hyperphenylalaninemia/Non-PKU Hyperphenylalaninemia

These are a group of infants detected in screening programmes with plasma phenylalanine levels of <20 mg/dL above the normal i.e. 2 mg/dL.These infants do not excrete phenylketones. Although with low levels of plasma phenylalanine, these children require dietary therapy on the basis of their untreated phenylalanine level.

Diagnosis

The diagnostic criteria for PKU include the following: (i) On a normal diet, phenylalanine level in excess of 20 mg/dL/24 hours on two occasions; (ii) Blood tyrosine level more than 5 mg/dL; and (iii) Presence of abnormal urinary metabolites of phenylalanine.

Identification and measurement of phenyl ketones in urine by ferric chloride test (Guthrie's test) may offer a simple test for diagnosis of PKU in infants with developmental and neurologic abnormalities. It is a bed side test. Addition of 10% ferric chloride solution to fresh urine of patient results in an emerald green color, which fades in 20 minutes. In countries where the screening programme exists, a child is detected to have hyperphenylalaninemia on screening. The diagnosis is confirmed by quantitative measurement of plasma phenylalanine concentration by fluorometric assay. Then additional studies for biopterin metabolism should be performed to rule out biopterin deficiency as the cause of hyperphenylalaninemia.

Neonatal Screening for Hyperphenylalaninemia

The test is done on a few drops of blood collected on a filter paper. It is recommended that the blood for screening should be collected in the first 24 - 48 hours of life after feeding protein in order to reduce the possibility of false negative results especially in the milder forms of the conditions. Guthrie test is useful in newborn. The method of choice however, is tandem mass spectrometry which identifies all types of hyperphenylalaninemia with a low false positive rate. Diagnosis must be confirmed by measurement of plasma phenylalanine concentration. Blood phenylalanine may rise in affected infants to diagnostic levels as early as four hours after birth even in the absence of protein feeding.

Molecular probes are now available for prenatal diagnosis.

Treatment

Long term care of these patients is best achieved by a team of experienced professionals viz. physician, nutritionist, neurologist, geneticist and psychologist in a regional treatment centre. The goal of therapy is to reduce phenylalanine levels in plasma and brain.

All infants with a plasma phenylalanine levels of >6 mg/dL should be treated with a phenylalanine restricted diet. The diet should be started as soon as diagnosis is established. The current recommendation from 2001 National Institutes of Health Consensus Development panel is that the phenylalanine restricted diet should be continued for life because it has been shown that discontinuation of such diet even in adulthood cause deterioration of IQ and cognitive performance. Further, it is also recommended that the plasma phenylalanine levels are to be maintained between 2 and 6 mg/dL in neonates through 12 years of age and between 2 and 15 mg/dL in older individuals.

Formulas low in phenylalanine for infants and special food items low in phenylalanine for children and adults are available commercially for dietary treatment. It should be noted that as phenylalanine is not synthesized endogenously the diet should not be phenylalanine free because it may result in phenylalanine deficiency. The signs of deficiency include failure to thrive, lethargy, anorexia, anemia, rashes diarrhoea and sometimes even death.

Oral administration of tetrahydrobiopterin (BH4), the cofactor of enzyme phenylalanine hydroxylase (PAH) has been tried. It may result in reduction of plasma phenylalanine in some patients with PAH deficiency. Sapropterin, a synthetic form of BH4 is being used in the dose of 10 mg/kg/day. It acts as a cofactor in patients with residual PAH activity. It reduces phenylalanine levels in upto 50% patients.

Suggested Reading

1. Textbook of Endocrinology edited by Robert H. Williams, 4th edition 1974, W B Saunders Company, Philadelphia, USA.
2. Pediatric Endocrine Disorders edited by Meena P Desai, PSN Menon, Vijaylakshmi Bhatia, Second edition 2008, Orient Longman, Hyderabad.
3. American Diabetes Association, 2007. Clinical practice recommendation. ADA website www.diabetes.org.
4. Wolfsdorf JN Glaser MA Sperling. Diabetes ketoacidosis in infants, children and adolescents. A consensus statement from American Diabetes Association, Diab Care 29: 1150-59.
5. Nelson Textbook of Pediatrics, 18th edition, 2004 edited by Behrman, Kliegman and Jenson.

17

Oncology

OUTLINES

An Approach to Diagnosis of Childhood Cancer

Malignant disorders are relatively infrequent in children accounting for 1–3% of all cancers. Though precise data is not available, a conservative estimate would suggest that 35–40 thousand children develop cancer each year in India.

Statistics from the western countries reports a 5-year survival rate of 70% in children with cancer below the age of 15 years. It also indicates that the number of cancer cases rise as the countries develop. The types of cancer in children are totally different from those in adults. The response to therapy is also different.

Acute leukemia is the most common cancer in children. Pre-B ALL in the low risk group has a complete remission rate of 90% and an event free probability of 79%. Even in high risk ALL; the cure rate is now 50–70%. In India, lost to follow-up of children under treatment is a common problem which has contributed to the poor results of treatment. This is mainly because of two reasons, high rate of poverty and lack of awareness regarding the status of childhood cancers.

The role of primary care health personnel, in the management of children with cancer, revolves around early detection and prompt referral and follow-up care. It needs mention that 85% of pediatric cancers are associated with symptoms viz. irregular fever, pallor, pain, lymphadenopathy, purpura, mass, which may be associated with so many other common diseases. Hence early diagnosis is possible with vigilance and high index of suspicion. Early referral to a cancer center is always better for optimal care. Precise anatomical or clinical staging or sub group classification is an essential foundation for planning treatment. Delays in diagnosis and work up prior to starting therapy can push a low risk patient into a high risk one. Once treatment is initiated it should continue uninterrupted for the schedule time. Primary care health personnel can play a significant role at this point.

Common Pediatric Tumours

Pediatric malignancy are essentially classified as hematological (leukemia and lymphomas) or solid tumours (neuroblastoma, Wilms' tumour etc.).

Hematological

(a) *Leukemias:* ALL, ANLL, CML.

(b) *Lymphomas:* NHL (lymphoblastic, undifferentiated) Hodgkin's Disease (HD).

Solid Tumours

(a) *CNS tumours:* Medulloblastoma (cerebral and cerebellar), ependymoma, astrocytoma, craniopharyngioma.

(b) *Abdominal tumours:* Neuroblastoma (NBL), Wilm's tumour, hepatoblastoma, lymphoma, mesoblastic nephroma.

(c) *Gonadal tumours:* Yolk sac tumour, teratoma, rhabdomyosarcoma.

(d) *Thoracic tumours:* Neuroblastoma, teratoma, lymphoma, leukemias.

(e) *Others:* Ewing's sarcoma, retinoblastoma.

When to Suspect?

A systematic approach, which should include a detailed history, a meticulous physical examination, appropriate investigations coupled with awareness, is the key to a timely diagnosis.

Most of the symptoms and signs of childhood cancers are either a consequence of involvement of the bone marrow or due to a mass and its effect on the surrounding normal tissues. The cardinal signs of cancer in children are anemia, bone tenderness, lymphadenopathy, abdominal mass, and headache, visual and neurological abnormalities. It is evident that these symptoms and signs are non-specific and could easily be interpreted to denote infectious illnesses which are widely prevalent in our country. The existence of these symptoms, however, must alert the attending physician to include malignant disorders in the differential diagnosis.

Fever: Fever, in malignant disorders, may be because of the disease itself, a concomitant infection, or as a consequence of hemorrhage or necrosis in a solid tumour. Prolonged fever more than 2 weeks duration, which does not respond to an antibiotic, high fever associated with neutropenia, could be a lead to the existence of a neoplasia.

Lymphadenopathy: A lymph node is considered enlarged if it is more than 10 mm in its greatest diameter. However, inguinal nodes are not considered abnormal unless they are > 15 mm, whilst epitrochlear nodes of 5 mm or more are pathological. Adenopathy in the epitrochlear and supraclavicular or post auricular area is definitely abnormal. A diagnostic work up would be warranted in the following situations:

1. Progressive increase in size of the glands.
2. Persistence of nodes for more than 4–6 weeks.
3. Mediastinal lymphadenopathy.
4. Nodes that fail to respond to antibiotics or anti-tubercular drugs.
5. Nodes associated with an abnormal chest film, hepatosplenomegaly, anemia, unexplained fever or thrombocytopenia.
6. Localized lymphadenopathy which is firm, rubbery or matted.

Pallor: Pallor due to nutritional deficiency is common in our children. In a child with pallor, the following features may indicate a lymphoreticular malignancy:

1. Rapidly progressive anemia in absence of blood loss.
2. Repeated fall in hematocrit over days in spite of packed red cells transfusions.
3. Associated with features viz. bleeding, lymphadenopathy, abdominal or mediastinal mass, bone pains or arthritis.

Bone pain and arthritis: 10–15% of cases of acute lymphoblastic leukemia have arthritis as a prominent feature. Such cases are often mistaken for acute rheumatic fever or juvenile rheumatoid arthritis. The pain may be intermittent which increase in severity with time. The presence of anemia or leucopenia with arthritis or bone pain should prompt a bone marrow examination. This is particularly essential if steroid therapy is contemplated. Bone pains are a frequent manifestation also in neuroblastoma.

Headache: With complains of repeated headache one should rule out increased intracranial tension. The best method of screening for tumour in a patient with headache is a careful neurological examination. Tests like CT scan, MRI no doubt rule out intracranial tumours but it is not possible to recommend such tests routinely to all children with headache. Radiological examination is necessary in the following situations:

1. Recurrent early morning headache that awaken the child.

2. Recurrent incapacitating headache.
3. Headache associated with vomiting, visual or visual field defect, papilledema, neurological deficits, or diabetes insipidus.

Bleeding: Bleeding manifestation is an uncommon initial sign in children suffering from cancer. Significant bleeding as a presenting sign should be evaluated with a bone marrow examination. Bleeding per vagina may be the only symptom of vaginal rhabdomyosarcoma or endodermal sinus tumour. Periorbital ecchymosis, unilateral or bilateral indicates metastasis of neuroblastoma.

Abdominal mass: Any mass in the abdomen of a child should be considered malignant until proved otherwise. A palpable, firm, abdominal mass is the most common sign that would suggest a diagnosis of a malignant solid tumour.

Eye changes: The following two eye signs should lead one two suspect a malignant condition:

1. A yellow white (cat's eye) reflex seen through the pupil, particularly when associated with a family history of an eye tumor.
2. Proptosis, unilateral or bilateral, without signs of inflammation.

Mediastinal masses: May be:

1. Asymptomatic discovered on routine chest X-ray.
2. Associated with symptoms secondary to compression of adjacent structures viz. respiratory tract (cough, dyspnea, stridor), esophagus (dysphagia), and superior vena cava (engorged neck and chest wall veins, facial puffiness).
3. Often associated with hemorrhagic pleural effusion and /or pericardial involvement.

The most common malignancies in children which involves the mediastinum are NHL, ALL, HD and NBL. The location of the mass in one of the anatomic regions of the mediastinum can be a clue to the nature of the mass. For example a mass in the anterior mediastinum indicates NHL, ALL and HD. Posterior mediastinal masses usually indicates neurologic tumours e.g. neuroblastoma, NHL.

Chronic ear discharge: Chronic suppurative otitis media is a common cause of ear discharge in children. However, ear discharge associated with skin rash, seborrhea, skull defects, hepatosplenomegaly or lymphadenopathy should raise the possibility of a malignant condition like Langerhans' cell histiocytosis (LCH).

The Investigational Approach

Should be aimed at:

1. Establishment of clinical diagnosis.
2. Determination of extent of disease.

Establishment of Diagnosis

(a) Hematological malignancies

1. Examination of peripheral blood smears.
2. Estimation of hemoglobin.
3. A complete blood count viz. TLC, DLC, Platelet, reticulocyte counts.
4. Bone marrow examination: Indications are:
   i. Significant depression of one or more cell lines or abnormalities of blood counts in absence of infectious causes.
   ii. Association of abnormal blood counts with unexplained lymphadenopathy or hepatosplenomegaly.
   iii. Presence of atypical cells or blast cells in peripheral blood smears.

Points to be Noted

1. Anemia, leucopenia, and thrombocytopenia can occur alone or in combination.
2. Leucocytosis with counts in excess of 100x 10^9 /L can also occur.
3. Besides leukemia, the other tumours which can involve the bone marrow are NHL, NBL and LCH.
4. Pancytopenias have been described frequently with Salmonella typhi infection, visceral Leishmaniasis and megaloblastic anemia. Hence infections have to be ruled when evaluating a case with pancytopenia.

(b) Solid tumours

1. *FNAC* has proved to be effective in identifying the nature of the tumour and the histological type in majority of cases. It can be used safely for deeply situated mass lesions or mediastinal nodes with aspirations being guided by USG or CT scan. FNAC has established itself as a valuable, reliable and cost effective diagnostic procedure for solid tumours. An excisional or incisional biopsy should be advised in the following situations:
   i. When the mass is localized to an organ with no evidence of metastasis and total removal of the mass is the plan of treatment.

ii. When there is a strong clinical suspicion of neoplastic disease and FNAC from an enlarged lymph node shows features of reactive hyperplasia. In such a situation, the most firm and the largest node is to be removed for examination.

iii. When FNAC fails to identify the precise tumour type and further studies like immunochemistry or immunophenotyping are indicated.

2. *Biochemical markers* are useful in differentiating between some types of solid tumors, as well as to confirm remissions and recurrence of the disease process. The useful markers are serum alpha feto protein (elevated in germ cell tumours and some cases of hepatoblastoma), beta human chorionic gonadotrophin (elevated in germ cell tumours) and urinary catecholamines (elevated in neuroblastoma).

Determination of Extent of Disease

It is important to document the extent of disease before initiating therapy. Involved sites must be also re-evaluated after an adequate period of therapy to ensure that a complete remission has been attained before continuing with further treatment. The following investigations should be done with this aim:

1. Examination of a cytocentrifuged specimen of CSF in cases with acute lymphoblastic leukemia and NHL to exclude CNS leukemia.
2. Testicular FNAC in cases with painless testicular enlargement.
3. A skeletal survey can be done in cases with significant bone pain. However, the number of bone involvement does not alter prognosis or a change in plan of treatment.
4. An X-ray chest, skull, and long bones, USG, CT, MIBG bone scans, bone marrow aspirates and trephine bone biopsy are the investigations to be used for staging of solid tumours.

The Dos and Donots

The incidence of malignancy in children is low. However, it is imperative that a diagnosis established at the earliest so that therapy can be instituted at earlier stages of the disease when the child's general condition has not deteriorated significantly. The dos and donots to be remembered in diagnosis of pediatric cancer are:

- Steroids should not be administered in suspected cases of JRA without doing a bone marrow examination.
- It is preferable to do a bone marrow examination before starting steroids in ITP.
- One should not start ATT in a patient with lymphadenopathy without a definite diagnosis.
- If lymphadenopathy is significant and FNAC is reported as reactive hyperplasia, a lymph node biopsy should be planned.
- A blood transfusion should be given prior to diagnosis only if Hb % is < 5 gm % or if there are impending or overt features of congestive heart failure.

Leukemias

The leukemias may be described as a group of malignant diseases in which genetic abnormalities in a hemopoetic cell give rise to a clonal proliferation of cells. The leukemic cells have a growth advantage over the normal cellular elements owing to an increased rate of proliferation, a decreased rate of spontaneous apoptosis or both. The result is a disruption of normal marrow function and, ultimately marrow failure.

The leukemias account for about 41% of all malignancies that occur in children younger than 15 years of age.

Classification

The leukemias are classified on the basis of two main criteria, the clinical course of the disease and the type and degree of differentiation of the predominant leukemic cell populations, into acute and chronic and lymphoid and myeloid respectively.

Acute Leukemia

It is the most common malignancy encountered in pediatric practice. It generally pursues an aggressive clinical course which, unless modified by treatment, rapidly results in death in the great majority of patients.

A group of French, American and British hematologists has described a classification system which has achieved a high degree of acceptance. It is called the *FAB classification* and is based on blood and bone marrow morphological features defined by Romanovsky and cytochemical stains. In this system leukemia is described as acute when there are more than 30% blast cells in bone marrow. According to cell type it is classified into acute lymphoblastic which accounts for 70–80% and acute myeloid or acute non-lymphoblastic leukemia which accounts for 20–30% of acute leukemias. It further divides acute lymphoblastic leukemia into three subgroups and acute myeloid leukemia into seven subgroups.

Table 17.1 : Acute leukemias: FAB classification

Acute lymphoblastic leukemia (ALL)	
L 1	Homogenous small lymphoblasts with scanty cytoplasm, regular round nuclei, inconspicuous nucleoli.
L 2	Heterogenous lymphoblasts with variable amounts of cytoplasm, irregular or cleft nuclei, large nucleoli.
L 3	Large homogenous lymphoblasts with basophilic cytoplasm, round nuclei, prominent nucleoli, cytoplasmic vacuolation.
Acute myeloid leukemia (AML) or Acute non-lymphoblastic leukemia (ANLL)	
M 1	Myeloblastic leukemia without maturation
M 2	Myeloblastic leukemia with maturation
M 3	Hypergranular promyelocytic leukemia
M 4	Myelomonocytic leukemia
M 5	Monocytic leukemia
M 6	Erythroleukemia
M 7	Megakaryocytic leukemia

Chronic Leukemias

Chronic leukemias are also divided into chronic lymphocytic and chronic myelocytic types. Chronic myelocytic leukemia accounts for 1–2% of the cases in children. Chronic lymphocytic leukemia is non-existent in children.

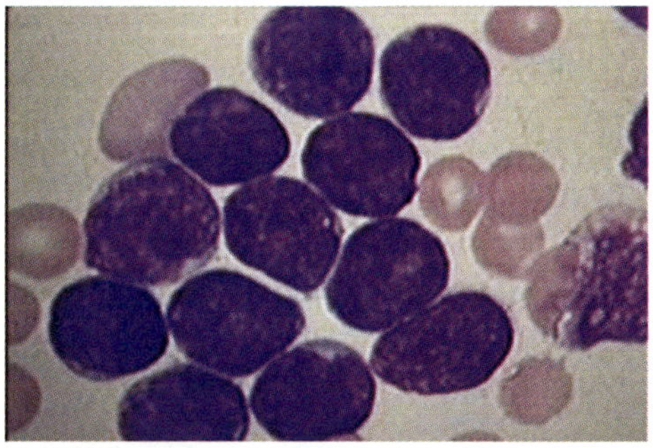

Fig. 17.1: PBS showing ALL, L_1

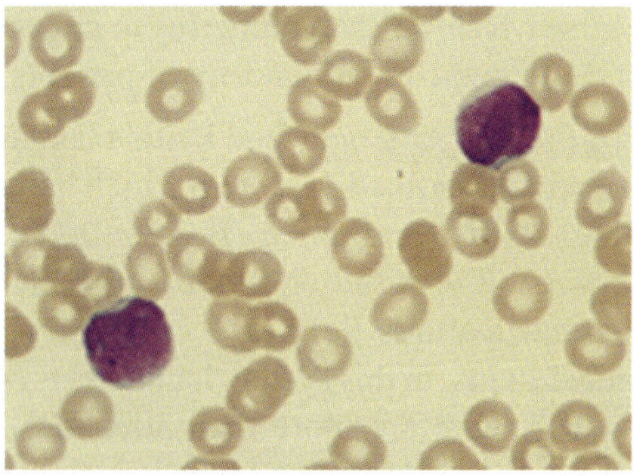

Fig. 17.2: PBS showing ALL, L_2

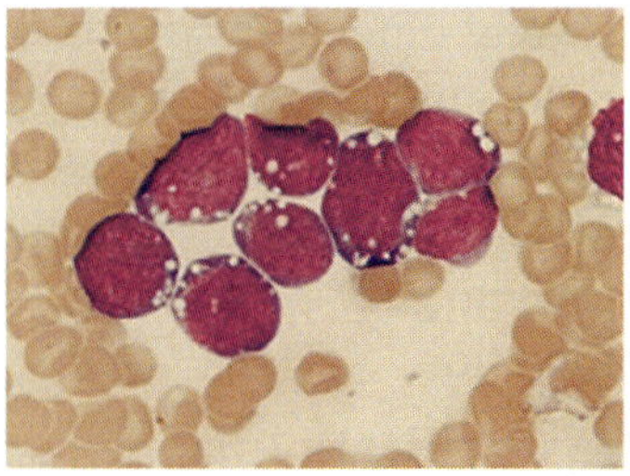

Fig. 17.3: PBS showing All, L_3

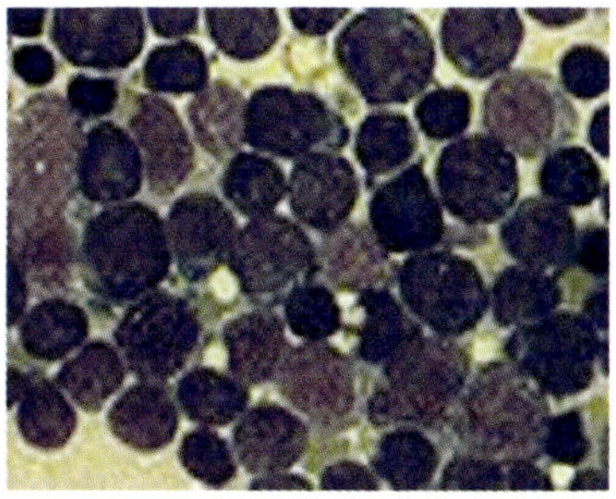

Fig. 17.4: Bone marrow showing ALL

ACUTE LYMPHOBLASTIC LEUKEMIA

Acute leukemia in children, especially in young children, is usually lymphoblastic type. It is the first disseminated cancer shown to be curable.

Epidemiology

In many parts of the world, an increasing number of cases have been reported in the last four decades. This is partly thought to be due to a more accurate diagnosis. The peak incidence is between 2–6 years of age. The disease occurs more commonly in males and this disparity becomes more obvious with increasing age.

Etiology

Several genetic and environmental factors are believed to be associated with childhood leukemia although in virtually all cases, the etiology remains unknown. A genetic predisposition is indicated by the association of the disease in children with certain chromosomal disorders (viz. Down syndrome, Bloom syndrome), ataxia telangiectasia and Fanconi syndrome. The risk is around 20 times higher in these children than normal controls. Further, among identical twins, the risk to the second twin if one develops leukemia is greater than in the general population irrespective of the zygosity.

Among the environmental factors, exposure to medical radiation both in utero and in childhood has been incriminated. Recent studies have implicated association between B cell ALL and Epstein-Barr viral infection and human T cell lymphoma leukemia virus (HTLV) in causation of leukemia.

Clinical Manifestations

The onset of symptoms may be abrupt or insidious. However, an abrupt onset is more common in children. The most common presenting features are fever, pallor and bleeding manifestations such as petechiae, bruise and hemorrhage. Fever is associated with malaise, rigors, generalized aches and the temperature as high as 39–41°C is not uncommon. In about 50% of cases there is a history of an upper respiratory infection in the preceding 1–2 months.

Less commonly the onset may be insidious and symptoms may be localized to bones or joints. As the disease progresses, signs and symptoms of bone marrow failure become more obvious with occurrence of pallor, fatigue, purpura/petechiae or epistaxis as well as fever which may be caused by infection.

There may be mild to moderate enlargement of liver and spleen and lymph glands. Because of the frequency of oral and pharyngeal sepsis, the cervical nodes are more often enlarged than other areas and are often tender. The lymph nodes may not be palpable or slightly enlarged when the child first presents.

The features of bones and joints involvement include tenderness over the sternum, most marked over the lower end. In few cases there may be associated swelling, redness and tenderness usually close to joints, simulating osteomyelitis. Joint manifestation include migratory joint pain, persistent joint pain in one or more joints associated with local signs of inflammation such as heat, redness and swelling.

The child may present with cardiovascular symptoms like precordial pain due to pericarditis which may occur due to leukemic infiltration, hemorrhage or infection, bacterial or viral.

Meningeal involvement is often seen during hematological remission where there has been no effective cranial prophylaxis. Meningeal leukemia is manifested by signs of raised intracranial pressure, with headache, irritability, vomiting, meningismus and cranial nerve palsy and papilledema. These can occur singly or together. The possibility of meningeal leukemia should be considered in a child who develops unexplained headache or vomiting, either in remission or relapse. Infrequently the child may present with focal neurological signs or paraplegia due to spinal cord compression.

Respiratory distress may occur as a result of severe anemia. It may also occur due to airway obstruction as a result of a large mediastinal mass which is common in adolescent males with T cell ALL.

Laboratory Diagnosis

Examination of *peripheral blood* for hemoglobin and peripheral blood smear for cell morphology study, total leucocytic count, differential leukocyte count, reticulocyte count and platelet count usually suffices for a diagnosis of ALL. The diagnosis should be confirmed by a *bone marrow aspiration* study.

The type of leukemia can be determined by the morphological features of the leukemic cells in the peripheral blood and marrow as seen in the Romanovsky stained film. *Cytochemical stains and estimation of serum lysozyme* give supplementary information. Study of *cell markers* has become particularly useful in acute lymphoblastic leukemia to determine the immunophenotypes on the basis of the cell surface and intracellular markers. These subtypes do not necessarily conform to the morphologically defined subgroups in the FAB classification and the various cell surface marker patterns have clinical and prognostic implications.

Blood Picture

The typical blood picture is of anemia and thrombocytopenia, with a moderate or marked increase in white cells, the majority of which are blast cells. The red cells are moderately anisocytic and poikilocytic with mild polychromasia. A moderate increase in reticulocytes upto 5% can occur, and a small number of nucleated red cells may be seen in the blood film. Thrombocytopenia with platelet counts well below 50×10^9/l is common. In about 25% patients, the TLC is reduced at the onset and ranges from 1 to 4×10^9/l. In advanced cases it may exceed 100×10^9/l. In occasional patient with low white cell counts, blasts cells may be present in very small numbers. In these cases, a film made from the buffy coat of centrifuged blood may enable blast cells to be detected more easily. In rare cases, no immature cells may be detected even after a careful inspection of the blood film. In very rare instances, the white cell count remains low but blast cells cannot be found in any stage of the disease.

Bone Marrow

Because of hypercellularity or associated fibrosis in the bone marrow, a blood tap is not uncommon, and occasionally a dry tap occurs. Blast cells are usually the outstanding feature and cells in mitosis are common.

Erythropoetic cells are reduced and sometimes completely absent. There may be dyserythropoesis characterized by presence of erythroblasts, larger than normal with megaloblastic features. Megakaryocytes are reduced or absent. On the basis of the FAB classification, presence of blast cells 30% or more is essential for a diagnosis of acute leukemia.

These criteria apply to most cases of acute leukemia but occasionally the marrow may be even normocellular or hypocellular.

Examination of bone marrow chromosomes reveals abnormalities in upto 75% cases. The nature of karyotype has a relationship to prognosis. For example presence of Philadelphia chromosomes or translocations between chromosomes 4 and 11, or chromosomes 8 and 14 have been suggested to be an independent prognostic factor for poor prognosis in ALL.

Examination of Romanovsky stained blood film helps in the study of the morphological features of the blast cells and enable one to classify ALL by the FAB classification.

Cytochemical stains help to categorize ALL as an adjunct to Romanovsky staining. The most useful cytochemical stains and their reaction patterns are:

1. Myeloperoxidase and Sudan black is negative in lymphoid cells.
2. Periodic acid Schiff (PAS) is positive in immature lymphoid cells.
3. Acid phosphatase test shows a focal positive reaction in T-cell ALL blast cells.

Cell surface markers used for classification of ALL are:

1. Immunoglobulin bound to the cell surface membrane (SIg), a B lymphoid cell marker.
2. A T lymphoid cell surface marker equating with T11 surface antigen with sheep erythrocyte rosette formation.
3. Surface and internal antigens, detected by the use of specific antibodies, which include the common acute lymphoblastic leukemia (c ALL) antigen, T and B lymphoid cell surface antigens, and cytoplasmic u chains (whose presence in the absence of SIg serves as an index of pre-B cell status).

Estimation of deoxynucleotidyl transferase (TdT) by immunofluorescence after reaction with monoclonal anti TdT is also useful in the diagnosis of ALL. The levels are high in contrast to most cases of acute myeloblastic leukemia.

Table 17.2 : Immunophenotypes of acute lymphoblastic leukemia

Type	*Characteristic features*
Common ALL	c ALL antigen Pan B antigen
T ALL	E rosette formation Pan T antigen
Pre T ALL	No E rosette formation Pan T antigen
B ALL	SIg
Pre-B ALL	Cytoplasmic u chains only
Null ALL	No definite marker

Differential Diagnosis

Differential diagnosis will include disorders with:

1. Similar clinical findings which include:
   (a) Causes of ulceration of the throat (infectious mononucleosis, agranulocytosis, acute follicular tonsillitis, diphtheria, and Vincent's angina). Among these, the major problem is infectious mononucleosis which also presents with fever, ulceration of the throat, lymphadenopathy and splenomegaly associated with presence of atypical cells in the blood. However, all these conditions can be differentiated by specific hematological and microbiological tests.
   (b) Other causes of joint and bone pain viz. acute rheumatic arthritis and osteomyelitis. Although acute rheumatic arthritis may present with similar clinical findings, polymorphonuclear leucocytosis is usual in this condition whereas neutropenia is the rule in leukemia. Osteomyelitis may be suspected when there is marked reddening, swelling or tenderness of one joint.
   (c) Other causes of fever which include subacute bacterial endocarditis, typhoid, septicemia, lymphoma and brucellosis. A proper history, clinical examination and examination of blood will help differentiate.
   (d) Cases of ALL may present with acute abdominal pain, respiratory difficulty due to mediastinal obstruction, or nervous system involvement. They need differentiation from the other causes of such conditions.
2. Similar blood picture may be present in conditions like myelodysplastic syndromes, leukemoid reaction and other causes of pancytopenia. *Myelodysplastic*

syndromes are uncommon in children. They are characterized by significant anemia, neutropenia, and thrombocytopenia, accompanied by blast cells in the peripheral blood. They can be distinguished from the bone marrow examination where the blasts cells are less than 30%. A *leukemoid blood picture*, seen in infectious mononucleosis, is most commonly confused with ALL. The causes of *pancytopenia* should be differentiated from subleukemic acute leukemia where few or no blast cells are observed in peripheral blood. The bone marrow examination is diagnostic in these conditions.

Treatment

The aims of treatment are eradication of the leukemic process and control of complications viz. anemia, infection and hemorrhage.

Eradication of leukemic process involves the use of antileukemic drugs, usually in combination with supplementary measures like cranial prophylaxis to destroy the disease in sanctuary sites viz. central nervous system.

Most children are treated on clinical trials conducted by national and international working groups. The drug regimen depends on whether the child falls in the average risk or high risk group. A patient between 1–10 years of age, and with a initial leukocyte count of less than 50,000 / cu mm is widely used to define average risk. A patient considered to be at high risk is child below 1 year and above 10 years or who have an initial leukocyte count more than 50,000 / cu mm. Clinical trials have also demonstrated that good response to therapy is also an indication of average risk and better prognosis. Further, ALL (L1) and c ALL have average risk. ALL (L2 & L3), T cell ALL and patients with chromosomal abnormalities fall in high risk category. Drug trials have shown that outcome of patients at higher risk can be improved by administration of more intensive therapy and that children with chromosomal abnormalities have a higher risk of relapse in spite of intensive therapy.

The treatment is mainly divided into three phases viz. Induction of remission followed by CNS prophylaxis and a maintenance phase. Many regimens also have a consolidation phase after induction of remission which is an attempt to prevent relapse of the disease. This aspect of management is currently the subject of research in the field of treatment of ALL. The consolidation phase consists of further systemic chemotherapy in an attempt to eradicate or continually suppress any residual leukemic cells. This is especially of merit in ALL associated with poor prognostic factors viz. L3 morphologic features, T cell surface antigen and presence of the Philadelphia chromosome.

Conservative approaches to management of ALL have been generally superseded by aggressive combination chemotherapy combined with supportive measures like antibiotic therapy and platelet transfusion to combat infection and bleeding respectively. However, present evidence indicates that very intensive chemotherapy is of lesser importance in children with good prognostic factors.

Induction of Remission

The induction phase is generally for 4 weeks. It consists of administration of 4 weekly doses of vincristine, daily oral prednisolone for 28 days to tail of in another 2 weeks, and twice weekly doses of L-aspariginase (total 10 doses). A patient with high risk factors should receive 4 weekly doses of daunorubicin in addition. With this approach, 98% of patients are in remission after 4 to 5 weeks of treatment.

Complete remission means return to good health with loss of abnormal physical signs attributable to acute leukemia, return of neutrophil count and platelet count to near normal and in the bone marrow blast cells are less than 5%. *Partial remission* means return to reasonable good health, significant improvement in abnormal physical signs attributable to leukemia, a return of atleast two of the three peripheral blood elements to normal value and a significant reduction in the degree of blast cells in the bone marrow.

Monitoring of Effects of Chemotherapy

The effect of chemotherapy is monitored by the following:

1. Counts of leukemic cells, neutrophils and platelets in blood.
2. Disappearance of leukemic cells from blood and bone marrow.

The majority of remissions occurs after one or two courses of treatment, and is followed by a progressive rise in counts of neutrophils and platelets and hemoglobin level to normal values. There is also disappearance of leukemic cells from the peripheral blood and bone marrow. Persistence of leukemic cells is regarded as an indication for continuation of active treatment.

Consolidation Phase

The consolidation phase usually includes drugs not included in the initial induction therapy such as cytosine arabinocide, cyclophosphamide, 6 mercaptopurine etc.

CNS Prophylaxis

The second phase of therapy focuses on CNS therapy. It should be started within one month of attaining remission with cranial irradiation and multiple twice weekly intrathecal injections of methotrexate during the course of cranial irradiation. Presently it has been shown that approximately the same results are achieved by administration of methotrexate alone. This regimen consists of repeated intrathecal injections of methotrexate given in conjunction with intensive chemotherapy. However, those patients who have lymphoblasts in the CSF and an elevated CSF leukocyte count at the time of diagnosis should also receive irradiation to brain and spinal cord together with intrathecal methotrexate.

Maintenance Phase

The third phase or maintenance phase consists of daily dose of oral 6 mercaptopurine and weekly doses of oral methotrexate together with intermittent doses of vincristine and prednisolone. The maintenance phase lasts for 2–3 years. It should commence after the blood picture has returned to normal after induction of complete remission. During maintenance phase the drug dosage is modified to avoid depression of the leukocyte below 3000/mm^3.

The dose of methotrexate should be titrated if TC < 3500 / cumm, ANC < 1000/ cumm as follows: (a) TC 3500–3000/cumm: less by 25% (b) TC 3000–2500/ cumm: less by 50% (c) TC 2500–2000/ cumm: less by 75% and (d) 2000–1500/ cumm: stop till TC 2000/ cumm.

Table 17.3 : Common drugs and dosage

Drug	*Dosage*
Vincristine	1.5 mg / m^2 body surface/ day IV
Prednisolone	40 mg/m^2 body surface / day orally
Daunorubicin	25 mg / m^2 body surface / day IV
Adriamycin	25 mg/ m^2 body surface / day IV
L-Asparaginase	6000 units / m^2 body surface / day IM
6 mercaptopurine	60 mg / m^2 body surface / day orally
Methotrexate PO	15 mg / m^2 body surface / week orally
Methotrexate IT	10 mg (below 2 years), 12.5 mg (2–8 years), 15 mg (9 years and above)
Cytosine arabinoside	100 mg/ m^2 body surface IV infusion
Cyclophosphamide	500 mg/m^2 body surface IV infusion

Prophylactic Therapy

Lysis of malignant cells is sometimes sufficiently rapid to result in increased production of uric acid leading to a rapid onset of impaired renal function. Certain prophylactic measures should be instituted before and during remission induction therapy especially in cases where the leukemic blood count is high and where there is marked splenomegaly or lymphadenopathy.

These include administration of *allopurinol* in order to depress urate formation as a result of rapid lysis of neoplastic cells, *increased fluid intake* to facilitate removal of purine degradation products in the urine and *alkalization of urine* to prevent urate deposition in the renal tubules.

Supportive Care

Supportive care is essential for successful administration of aggressive chemotherapy. Patients with a large tumour burden (e.g. T cell ALL) are prone to tumour lysis syndrome. Many chemotherapeutic agents (e.g. daunorubicin, doxorubicin and cytosine arabinoside) often produce severe myelosuppression which may require red cell and platelet transfusion. The hemoglobin level should be kept above 7 gm/dl, absolute neutrophil count above 1800/ mm^3 and platelet count above 20,000 /mm^3 during induction remission phase. Platelet transfusion should be given when the platelet count is less than 20,000/mm^3.

Antimicrobial nasal spray and mouth rinse and oral administration of nystatin and/or ketokonazole are generally employed as a means of reducing the load of pathogen in the GI tract and reduce local oropharyngeal infection. Isolation of patient or reverse barrier nursing has not shown to be particularly effective in preventing infection as many infections are derived from flora in the patient's GI tract.

Aggressive empirical antimicrobial therapy should be initiated in patients with fever and neutropenia after sending samples for confirmation of sepsis. If a child with febrile neutropenia does not respond to the sensitive antibiotic administered in adequate doses, samples for fungal culture should be sent and antifungal drugs should be started.

All patients should also receive prophylaxis for pneumocystis carinii pneumonia with cotrimoxazole during chemotherapy and for several months after completing treatment.

Treatment of Relapse

A relapse carries the most serious implication when it occurs during or shortly after completion of therapy.

A *bone marrow relapse* should be treated with intensive chemotherapy regimen including drugs not used previously in the patient followed by allogenic stem cell transplant. It can result in long-term survival in some patients. The relapse rate is much less than in those patients treated with chemotherapy alone. With only chemotherapy, remission may be obtained but the duration of remission tends to be shorter than following the first remission and progressively increasing difficulty is experienced in achieving subsequent remissions. CNS prophylaxis should be given if not given earlier. The maintenance therapy should include additional chemotherapeutic agents.

A *CNS relapse* is characterized by signs and symptoms of raised intracranial pressure and isolated cranial nerve palsies. The diagnosis is confirmed by demonstration of presence of leukemic cells in the CSF. The treatment includes intrathecal methotrexate and cranial irradiation. Intrathecal methotrexate should be given twice weekly for two weeks and then weekly till the CSF is free of leukemic cells. As these patients are at high risk of a bone marrow relapse systemic chemotherapy should also be used.

Testicular relapse occurs in 1–2% of boys with ALL. It occurs usually after completion of therapy. It presents with unilateral or bilateral, painless swelling of the testis. The diagnosis is confirmed by biopsy of the affected testis. Treatment includes local irradiation and systemic chemotherapy. Treatment is usually successful and survival rate is good.

Course and Prognosis

The improvement in the treatment of childhood ALL is one of the major successes of modern pediatric oncology. With current treatment, 60–70% of newly diagnosed children can anticipate prolonged (> 5 years) disease free survival and most of these are likely to be cured. In those with good risk factors, the survival rates may approach 90%. It should be noted that response to treatment is the only genuine prognostic factor. Untreatable ALL is always fatal.

Acute Myeloblastic Leukemia

Acute myeloblastic leukemia (AML) also called acute non-lymphoblastic leukemia (ANLL) account for about 20–30% of all childhood leukemia. Morphologically AML is classified into 7 types (see Table 16.1). AML occur uniformly in children between 1–10 years age group. Several predisposing factors have been identified. These include chromosomal and genetic disorders like Down syndrome, Bloom syndrome and Fanconi's anemia. AML can develop as second malignancy after treatment of other malignant conditions with alkalyting agents. It can also evolve in patients with preleukemic states or myeloproliferative disorders.

Clinical Manifestations

The patients with AML can present with any or all of the findings associated with marrow failure as in ALL. Besides, the patient with AML can present with certain specific features like gingival hypertrophy, subcutaneous nodules, chloromas and features of disseminated intravascular coagulation.

Gingival hypertrophy is characteristic of myelomonocytic (M4) and monocytic (M5) types. It can occur less commonly in the other forms as well. It represents tissue infiltration by leukemia. Chloromas (Fig. 17.5) are periocular tumours named as such because of the greenish hue derived from myeloperoxidase within the blasts. Chloromas can occur in other sites like skin and spinal cord. Rarely they may be the first sign of AML. Involvement of CNS at diagnosis may be present in 5–15% cases. Hepatosplenomegaly may be present in 50% of cases.

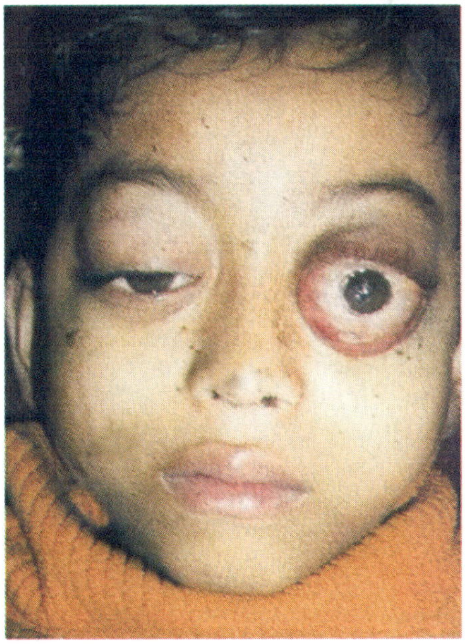

Fig. 17.5: Acute myeloblastic leukemia (Chloroma left eye)

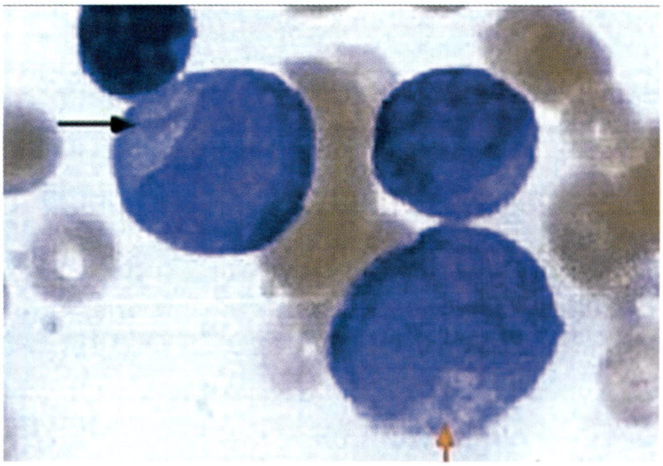

Fig. 17.6: Figure showing AML M_1

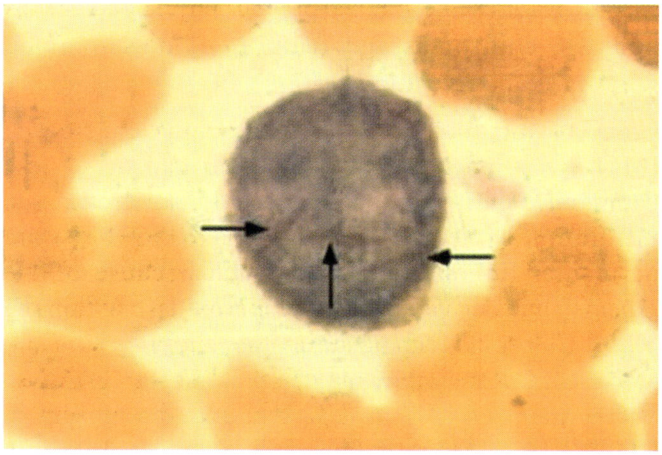

Fig. 17.7: Figure showing auer bodies

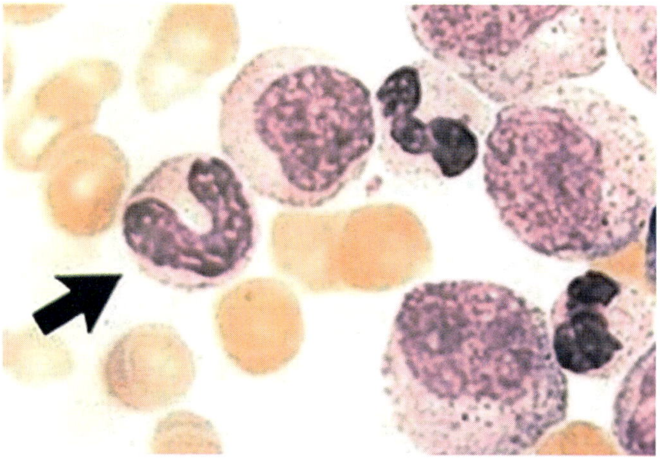

Fig. 17.8: Figure showing chronic myelocytic anemia

Laboratory Diagnosis

Usually there is leucopenia, anemia and thrombocytopenia with presence of blasts cells. Occasionally, there may be very high white cell count with intravascular clumping and the patient may present with somnolence or stroke.

Bone marrow examination is confirmatory. The FAB classification designates a proportion of blast cells of 30 % or more as an essential criterion for diagnosis of AML. In erythroleukemia (M6), the erythroid series make up a large proportion of bone marrow cells. Cytochemical stains reveal AML 1 to be peroxidase positive whereas promyelocytic (M3) type peroxidase negative but non-specific esterase positive. The myeloblasts in AML 1 are characterized by cells with prominent nucleoli and cytoplasmic granules. There is presence of Auer bodies which consist of azurophilic granule material.

The commonly occurring chromosomal translocations include 15; 17 in M3 and 1; 22 in M7 subtypes.

The poor prognostic factors include WBC count > 100,000 /mm^3, extramedullary manifestation at diagnosis and monosomy 7 and requirement of more than one course for complete remission.

Treatment

The treatment of AML is also done in phases as in cases of ALL. The supportive care needs are basically same as for ALL. However, the very intensive therapy required in AML produces prolonged bone marrow suppression with a very high incidence of serious infection.

Treatment Protocol for AML

Induction

1. Cytosar 100 mg/sq m/day × 7 days.
2. Daunorubicin 45 mg/sq m /day × 3 days.

Consolidation

1. Cytosar 3 gm / sq m/ dose 12 hourly day 1,3,5.

Induction Failure

1. Cytosar 3 gm/sq m /dose × 1,3,5.
2. Mitoxantrone 12 mg/sq m/day 2,4,6.

Induction of Remission

The induction regimen most commonly used is a combination of cytosine arabinoside (100 mg/m^2 /day) given as a continuous infusion, for 7 days and daunorubicin (45 mg / m^2 /day) for three days. Examination of bone marrow should be done 3 weeks after the commencement of the treatment. It provides a useful guide to assessment of response.

About 60% of cases attain meaningful remissions following treatment with this regimen. About two thirds of these respond after one course. In the remaining one third, remission is usually attained after a second course of treatment in which cytosine arabinoside is administered for 5 days and daunorubicin for 2 doses. Persistence of leukemic cells after the second course is usually taken as an indication of refractory disease, and alternative forms of treatment are considered in such cases. Use of transretinoic acid has resulted in better response in AML 3. Allogenic bone marrow transfusion in first remission has given long-term disease free survival.

CNS prophylaxis should be given as in ALL with intrathecal methotrexate and cranial irradiation.

Maintenance Therapy

A variety of regimens have been tried with an aim to reduce the incidence of relapse. These include one or more further courses of the successful induction regimen soon after the onset of remission, intermittent courses of moderately intense chemotherapy with different agents in a cyclical manner. However, none has been successful as a means for reduction of the rate of recurrence.

CHRONIC MYELOCYTIC LEUKEMIA

Chronic myelocytic leukemia (CML) also known as chronic myeloid leukemia accounts for 2–3% of all leukemias in children. Two types have been described: adult type and the juvenile type.

Adult Type CML

The adult type is the common type seen in children. The hallmark of the disease is the presence of Philadelphia chromosome (Ph), which involves a translocation of chromosome 22 and 9. The disease has been associated with exposure to ionizing radiation.

Clinical Manifestations

The disease is characterized clinically by an initial chronic phase which terminates 3 – 4 years after the onset and moves into the accelerated or blast crisis phase.

The initial chronic phase has an insidious onset with non-specific symptoms like fever, fatigue, weight loss and anorexia. There is massive enlargement of the spleen resulting in pain in the upper left quadrant of abdomen. The other presenting features include arthritis, priapism, retinopathy, and skin infiltration. The patient is in a stable condition in the chronic phase.

The blast crisis phase is commonly associated with symptoms of malaise, fatigue, anorexia, night sweats, bone pain, and splenic discomfort. The important physical signs are weight loss, pallor, pyrexia, sternal tenderness, appearance of lymphadenopathy. Death usually occurs from hemorrhage or infection or combination of both.

The average life span of a patient in chronic phase is about 3 years with a range of 1–10 years whereas in acute blast crisis phase, it is extremely short.

Laboratory Diagnosis

The blood picture reveals anemia, thrombocytosis and leucocytosis as high as > 100000 / mm^3. The bone marrow is hyperplastic with erythroid to myeloid ratio of 1:10 to 1:50. There is predominance of granulocyte cells in all stages of maturation.

The acute blast crisis can be of lymphoblastic origin or myeloid origin. In this phase the child has severe anemia, thrombocytopenia, a rapidly rising white cell count and increase of blast cells in the blood as well as bone marrow. The blast cells may constitute 80% or more of the bone marrow cells. In majority of cases, the blast cells are myeloid in type, but in 20–30% the blasts have lymphoblastic features.

Treatment

In the chronic phase, the blood counts are usually controlled by busulphan or hydroxyurea. About 80–90% of the children will ultimately become drug resistant or have a blast crisis with increasing anemia, thrombocytopenia and continuing increase of blast cells in the blood and bone marrow resulting in death.

The lymphoid blast crisis can be controlled with vincristine and prednisolone but the myeloid blast crisis does not respond to the standard treatment of AML.

Interferon has shown good result in prolonging remission. Bone marrow transfusion in chronic phase has better results than done during blast crisis phase.

Juvenile CML

Juvenile chronic myelocytic leukemia (JCML) is rare, constituting less than 2% of childhood leukemia. It occurs in children below 2 years age. The patients with this disease do not have the Philadelphia chromosome (Ph) that is characteristic of CML. The children with neurofibromatosis have a predilection for this type of CML.

The patients with JCML present with rashes, lymphadenopathy and splenomegaly. The peripheral blood often shows a high white cell count but less than 100000/mm^3, thrombocytopenia and presence of erythroblasts. The bone marrow shows a myelodysplastic type of picture.

The response to chemotherapy is poor. Stem cell transplant is promising but less than for the adult type.

DIAGNOSTIC APPROACH TO LYMPHADENOPATHY

The initial approach to a patient with a lymphoid tumour is to consider the possibility that lymphadenopathy might be due to some infective, inflammatory or chemical cause. The common causes of lymph node enlargement are shown in Table 17.4.

Table 17.4 : Causes of lymph node enlargement

Bacterial
Acute bacterial infection
Tuberculosis
Viral
Infectious mononucleosis
Cytomegalovirus
Acquired immunodeficiency syndrome
Other infections
Toxoplasmosis
Cat-Scratch fever
Chemical
Hydantoin pseudolymphoma
Others
Sarcoidosis
Autoimmune diseases like juvenile rheumatoid arthritis
SLE
Neoplastic
Non-Hodgkin's lymphoma
Hodgkin's disease
Secondary neoplastic lymphadenopathy

The most common conditions for lymph node enlargement are acute bacterial infection and tuberculosis. Three conditions viz. infectious mononucleosis, toxoplasmosis and cytomegalovirus present a very similar picture with pyrexia, lymph node enlargement, usually generalized, and characteristic atypical lymphocytes in the peripheral blood like in malignant lymphoma.

In case of lymphadenopathy associated with HIV infection, a clinical suspicion should be aroused if the child belongs to the high risk group like a hemophiliac, thallassemic, an intravenous drug user or any one who has received a blood transfusion within the past few years. The protean manifestations include weight loss, respiratory infection, diarrhoea, and thrombocytopenia which are common to lymphoma. Appropriate blood tests can exclude. On occasions, however, a lymph node biopsy may be required to exclude lymphoma.

In cat scratch disease there is history that the patient has a cat as a pet although a history a scratching may not be collected. The common site of lymph node enlargement is the epitrochlear group, to a lesser extent the adjacent axilla, and sometimes in the posterior triangle or inguinal region. The nodes are hot, tender and indurated.

Tuberculosis should be considered when the lymph node enlargement is in the tonsillar or jugulodiagastric group. The glands are characteristically firm and matted. Diagnosis can be confirmed by a FNAC and/or excision biopsy.

Enlargement of nodes may occur in the vicinity of the involved joints in juvenile rheumatoid arthritis and systemic lupus erythematosus. The other typical features of the respective disease will help in differential diagnosis (e.g. butterfly rash in SLE).

The clinical features which may be helpful in diagnosis of sarcoidosis are presence of iritis or iridocyclitis, parotid enlargement, erythema nodosum. An X-ray chest shows hilar lymph node enlargement. There is also hyperglobulinemia, hypercalcemia or an increased excretion of urinary calcium.

In hydantoin pseudolymphoma, the clinical and histologic pictures closely resemble non-Hodgkin's lymphoma. However, there is a history of exposure to the drug. It is usually seen in patients who have been receiving mesantoin or hydantoin for many months. The patient may have fever and skin rash in addition to marked lymphadenopathy with occasional enlargement of the spleen.

Thus in every case of suspected malignant lymphoma, the establishment of tissue diagnosis is mandatory to exclude non-malignant causes of lymph node enlargement, and to determine the subgroup of lymphoma to which the patient's disease belongs.

Lymphomas

Lymphomas are result of neoplastic proliferation of cells of lymphoid series. The two major categories of malignant lymphomas include non-Hodgkin's lymphoma and Hodgkin's disease. They constitute 10% of all childhood malignancy.

Non-Hodgkin's Lymphoma

Non-Hodgkin's lymphoma (NHL) is a group of biologically related diseases that include precursor B-NHL (5%), mature B-cell NHL (60%) and T cell-NHL (25%). These are indistinguishable at the cellular level from their leukemic counterparts. Irrespective of clinical symptoms, the disease is classified as leukemia by the presence of more than 30% of lymphoblasts in the bone marrow. The annual incidence of NHL is approximately 0.8 per 100,000 children below 15 years of age. Boys predominate over girls by 3:1. There is no clear age related incidence peak.

In general, T-cell NHL has a mediastinal location of lymphomas and mature B-NHL have an abdominal location. Although lymph node enlargement is the usual clinical presentation, extra nodal involvement is not uncommon, especially in the bone marrow, CNS, skin, liver and spleen. The malignant cell division rate is extremely rapid. Patients may develop life threatening tracheal compression, intestinal obstruction or spinal cord infiltration in a few days.

Pathogenesis

Most cases of NHL in children are high grade, diffuse neoplasms. Although elaborate classifications have been developed, they have little application in pediatric disease. Three histologic subtypes have been recognized: lymphoblastic, usually of T-cell origin, small non-cleaved cell lymphoma (SNCCL), with Burkitt or non-Burkitt subtypes and of B-cell origin; and a large cell lymphoma (LCL), with diffuse and anaplastic subtypes and of T- and B-, or indeterminate cell origin.

Both environmental and genetic factors have been implicated. EB virus infection is thought to have a major role in pathogenesis of Burkitt' type of SNCCL, but how EB virus contributes to the pathogenesis is not clearly known. Congenital and acquired immunodeficiency is identified as predisposing factors for development of NHL. Epidemiological studies have also implicated pesticide exposure as a possible risk factor. Different chromosomal translocations are specific for some histologic subtypes. For example in SNCCL (Burkitt type) there may be one of the three translocations viz. t (8; 22), t (8; 14) or t (2;8).

Clinical Manifestations

Non-Hodgkin's disease can occur at any age. Males are affected approximately twice as commonly as females. The rapidity of onset and spread varies widely according to the histological types.

The lymphoblastic type of NHL often presents as an intrathoracic tumour, usually a mediastinal mass. The symptoms and signs include dyspnea, chest pain, dysphagia, pleural effusion and superior vena caval syndrome. There may be associated cervical or axillary lymphadenopathy in around 80% cases. Primary involvement of bone, bone marrow, testis or skin is not uncommon. The central nervous system may also be involved.

The SNCCL type of NHL usually presents as an abdominal tumour. The presenting features are abdominal pain or distension, intestinal obstruction, change in bowel habit, intestinal bleeding or rarely intestinal perforation. There may be also involvement of the central nervous system, bone marrow and peripheral nodes. The jaw involvement is seen in Burkitt's type.

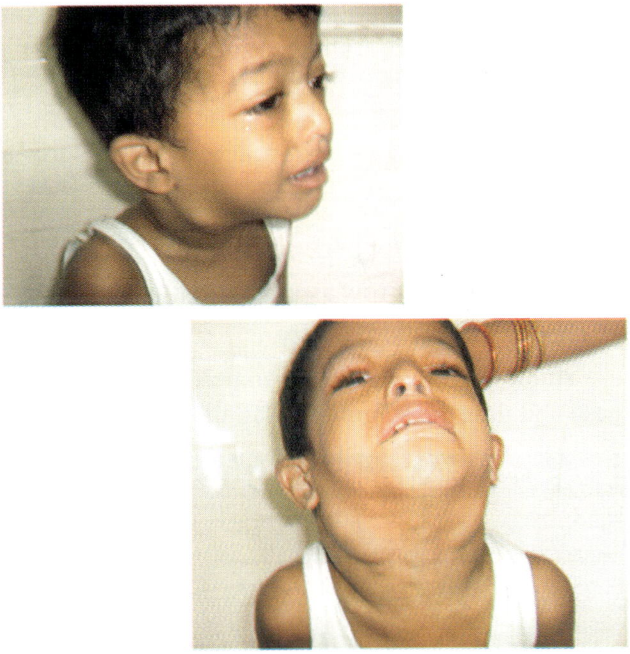

Fig.17.9: Cervical lymphadenopathy in non-Hodgkin's lymphoma

The large cell lymphoma type can occur in many sites including abdomen, mediastinum, skin, bone and soft tissues. Central nervous system involvement is rare.

Laboratory Diagnosis

A tissue diagnosis by means of lymph node biopsy is the

confirmatory test. It should be planned after exclusion of the non-malignant causes of lymphadenopathy on the basis of history, clinical examination and relevant laboratory findings or when doubt remains regarding the cause. It should be performed on a palpable superficial lymph node.

In case of solitary mediastinal involvement, scalene node biopsy sometimes establishes the diagnosis. If a superficial lymph node is not palpable sometimes it may be necessary to wait until a superficial node is sufficiently large. Occasionally, a diagnostic laparotomy may be necessary.

Staging of the Disease

The staging of the disease or assessment of extent of the disease is the next question after establishment of the histological diagnosis. The staging helps to plan the appropriate treatment. For example localized disease can be treated with radiotherapy whereas presence of disease in organs like lungs or bone marrow needs planned chemotherapy. The pretreatment studies for staging NHL include the following:

1. Complete blood count.
2. Serum electrolytes, uric acid, lactate dehydrogenase, creatinine, calcium, phosphorous.
3. Liver function tests.
4. Chest radiograph and CT.
5. Abdominal and pelvic USG and/or CT.
6. Gallium scan and/or bone scan.
7. Bilateral bone marrow aspirate and biopsy.
8. Cerebrospinal fluid cytology.

These studies will help to determine the extent of the disease and thus the staging to plan the treatment.

Table 17.5 : Staging of non-Hodgkin's lymphoma

Stage I
A single tumour (extra nodal) or single anatomic area (nodal), with the exclusion of mediastinum or abdomen.
Stage II
A single tumour (extra nodal) with regional node involvement.
Two or more nodal areas on the same side of the diaphragm.
Two single (extra nodal) tumours with or without regional node involvement on the same side of the diaphragm.
A primary gastrointestinal tract tumour, usually in the ileocecal area, with or without involvement of associated mesenteric nodes only.

Contd.

Contd.

Stage III
Two single tumours (extra nodal) on opposite sides of the diaphragm.
Two or more nodal areas above or below the diaphragm.
Any primary intrathoracic tumour (mediastinal, pleural, or thymic).
Any extensive primary intra-abdominal disease.
Stage IV
Any of the above, with initial involvement of the central nervous system and/or bone marrow at the time of diagnosis.
Source:
From St. Jude staging system of childhood non-Hodgkin's source lymphoma from Semin Oncol 1980; 7:332-99.

This system of staging defines the tumour extent. Stage I applies to localized disease, stage II regional disease, stage III to extensive disease, and stage IV to disseminated disease.

Treatment

NHL is considered a disseminated disease from the time of diagnosis even in patients with apparently localized disease. The NHL is exquisitely chemosensitive. Hence chemotherapy is the mainstay of treatment.

Patients with stage I and II disease, irrespective of the histologic type, are effectively treated with six cycles of COMP (cyclophosphamide, vincristine, methotrexate and prednisolone) regimen or three cycles of COPA (cyclophosphamide, vincristine, prednisolone, and adriamycin) except in case of T cell lymphoblastic NHL which should be treated with the regimen employed for treatment of high risk ALL.

Patients with stage III and IV disease are best treated with therapy based on the histologic subtype. SNCCL respond well with short duration intensive multiagent chemotherapy protocols. One such regimen is CAOP (cyclophosphamide, adriamycin, vincristine, and prednisolone) which is repeated every 3 weeks together with intrathecal therapy (similar to acute lymphoblastic leukemia). A relapse, if it occurs, is rapidly progressive and relatively resistant to additional therapy. Lymphoblastic lymphomas require longer duration therapies similar to acute lymphoblastic leukemia. Early relapse requires allogenic bone marrow transplant. The large cell lymphoma of T cell origin is treated with chemotherapy regimen similar to those used for lymphoblastic lymphoma. B cell derived large cell lymphoma can be treated with the same regimen used for SNCLL with a 6-year event free survival as high as 95%.

Hodgkin's Disease

Hodgkin's disease is currently one of the most curable malignancies in children and adolescents. It is more common in developing countries than in developed countries. Hodgkin's disease in children shows a male predominance and a lower age at diagnosis. The incidence before 5 years of age is reported in as many as 20–30% in developing countries in comparison to only 5% in industrialized countries. Lymphomas are the third most common childhood cancers in the developing world with about 50% are Hodgkin's disease whereas in western countries it is the sixth most frequent childhood malignancy.

Etiology

The etiology is not established. The role of Epstein-Barr virus is supported by serologic studies and the frequent presence of EBV genome in the biopsy material. An apparent increased risk in twins and first degree relatives can be accounted for by a genetic predisposition or exposure to the same etiologic agent. Pre-existing immunodeficiency, either congenital or acquired, increases the risk of developing Hodgkin's disease.

Pathology

The histopathological features of Hodgkin's disease include a partial or total effacement of nodal architecture and replacement by inflammatory cells like histiocytes, lymphocytes, eosinophils and plasma cells along with the Reed-Sternberg cell which is considered the hallmark of Hodgkin's disease. It is a large cell with multiple or multilobulated nuclei. The infiltrate of inflammatory cells surround the Reed-Sternberg cell and varies with the histologic type.

The WHO classification is a modification of the Rye morphologic classification (Lukes *et al.*, 1966) with addition of immunological markers. It includes two biologically and clinically distinct entities: nodular lymphocytic predominance Hodgkin's lymphoma and classical Hodgkin's lymphoma.

In the nodular lymphocytic predominance type the lymphocytic-histiocytic cells are characterized by a complete or nearly complete B cell phenotype, leukocyte common antigen positive, while CD15 and CD30 are negative.

On the other hand, the tumour cells of the classical type are characterized by a CD 3 positive, frequently CD 15 positive and CD45 negative phenotype while T cell and B cell associated antigens are usually negative. The classical type includes four subtypes viz. lymphocyte predominant, nodular sclerosing, mixed cellularity and lymphocyte depleted. The most common subtype found in children from developing countries is mixed cellularity.

Pathogenesis

Hodgkin's disease appears to arise in lymphoid tissue and spreads to adjacent lymph node areas in a relatively orderly manner. There is also involvement of the liver, spleen, bone, bone marrow or brain as a result of hematogenous spread when it is usually associated with systemic symptoms. There is also elevation of various cytokine levels in patient sera viz. interleukin 1 and 2 and tissue necrosis factor (TNF). They may be responsible for systemic symptoms of fever and night sweats (IL 1 and 2) and weight loss (TNF) as well as influences the proliferation of Reed-Sternberg cells and induces immunosuppression.

Clinical Manifestations

The most common presentation of Hodgkin's disease in children is enlarged, painless cervical or supra clavicular lymph nodes, usually unilateral, firm and rubbery in consistency. Inguinal or axillary lymphadenopathy is uncommon. Mediastinal adenopathy is seen in over 50% of the patients and may be responsible for superior mediastinal syndrome. Splenic involvement is found in 30 – 40%. Spread of disease below the diaphragm is a sign of advanced disease. The constitutional symptoms include fever above 38°C (100° F) for atleast three consecutive days, night sweats and weight loss greater than 10% in last six months and rarely pruritus. The presence of atleast one constitutional symptom correlates with poor prognosis.

Staging

Modified Ann Arbor staging system:

Stage I	Involvement of a single lymph node region or of a single extra lymphatic organ or site.
Stage II	Involvement of two or more lymph node regions, on the same side of the diaphragm or localized involvement of an extra lymphatic organ or site and one or more lymph node regions on the same side of the diaphragm.
Stage III	Involvement of lymph node regions on both sides of the diaphragm, which may be accompanied by involvement of the spleen or by localized involvement of an extra lymphatic organ.

Contd.

Contd.

Stage IV	Diffuse or disseminated involvement of one or more extra lymphatic organs or tissues with or without associated lymph node involvement.
Stages are further categorized as:	
A	No symptoms.
B	Unexplained fever, night sweats or weight loss or weight loss of more than 10% of body weight in the previous 6 months.
Bulky disease	Based on mediastinal mass larger than one third thoracic diameter; lymph node masses equal to or bigger than 10 cm diameter and / or four or more nodal regions involved.

From Lister TA, Crowther D, Sutcliffe SB *et al.*: Report of a committee convened to discuss the evaluation and staging of patients with Hodgkin's disease: Cotswold's meeting. J Clin Oncol 1989; 7: 1630-36.

Laboratory Studies for Staging

1. Complete blood count.
2. ESR, serum ferritin, serum copper.
3. Liver function tests.
4. Chest X-ray with measurement of mediastinal ratio.
5. Chest CT with contrast medium enhancement.
6. Neck CT if cervical nodes are palpable.
7. Abdominal CT or MRI.
8. Gallium scan.
9. Bone marrow biopsy with advanced disease or "B" symptoms.
10. Bones scan with elevated serum alkaline phosphatase level or bone pain.

Treatment

The optimal treatment strategy in children remains controversial, especially in cases of advanced disease. Combination chemotherapy (in which two different chemotherapy are alternated) and combined modality therapy (CMT) in which combined chemoradiotherapy is used has been tried with success.

Combined chemotherapy regimens include protocols containing alkalyting agents e.g. COPP (cyclophosphamide, vincristine, procarbazine, prednisolone); COMP (cyclophosphamide, vincristine, methotrexate, prednisolone); CVPP (cyclophosphamide, vinblastine, procarbazine, prednisolone) and protocols containing anthracyclin and epipodophyllotoxin e.g. ABVD (adriamycin, bleomycin, vinblastine, dacarbazine); VAMP (vinblastine, doxorubicin, methotrexate, prednisolone).

Children with bulky mediastinal disease are best treated with CMT rather than chemotherapy or radiotherapy alone.

Treatment of early stage disease (I and IIA) shows excellent results with either CMT or chemotherapy alone with disease free or event free survival more than 90%. Stage II B and III A need more intensive chemotherapy. Treatment of advanced disease requires more aggressive chemotherapy by increasing the dose intensity of treatment. Regimens using COPP alternating with ABVD provide disease control in about 75 % of stage II B–IV patients without radiotherapy. However, the stage IV patients do poorly even when combined with radiotherapy.

Treatment of Relapses

Most relapses occur within first three years, although a relapse as late as 10 years has been diagnosed. Cases with relapses can be treated with high dose chemotherapy regimens containing different drugs like ifosfamide, epirubicin, etoposide, cisplatin and melphalan with a high risk of treatment related morbidity. Stem cell transplant is an alternative.

Brain Tumors

Tumors of the brain and spinal cord are the most frequent solid tumors occurring in children under 15 years of age, and the second most prevalent group of malignancy in this age group after leukemia and lymphoma. In contrast to other childhood malignancies, the improvement in the overall prognosis of children affected by a primary CNS neoplasm has been modest. The five-year survival is slightly above 70% for astrocytoma and 50% for P NET and ependymoma. Malignant gliomas and notably glioblastoma multiformae remain incurable disease. Differences in survival by treatment centres have been reported with a survival advantage for those children treated in tertiary care centres.

CNS neoplasms cannot be considered a single entity as they encompass quite a heterogenous group of tumors. The International Classification of Childhood Cancer (ICCC), which groups all childhood malignancies, describes CNS neoplasms in six sub categories:

1. Ependymoma including the choroid plexus tumors.
2. Astrocytoma.
3. Primitive neuroectodermal tumours (P NET).
4. Other gliomas.

5. Other specified neoplasms including cranio-pharyngioma, pituitary adenoma, pineal parenchymal tumours, meningiomas.
6. Unspecified neoplasms.

Astrocytoma is by far the most frequent histological subtype. It represents a family of neoplasms ranging from indolent tumors such as pilocytic astrocytoma to the most malignant glioblastoma multiformae. However, in children, the non-malignant types are more common. *P NET* are the second most common frequent subtype. The term P NET encompasses a group of neoplasms of which medulloblastoma is the most frequent subtype.

According to the WHO classification of tumors of CNS and meninges, 5 categories viz. juvenile pilocytic astrocytoma, medulloblastoma/primitive neuroectodermal tumor (P NET), diffuse astrocytomas, ependymoma and craniopharyngioma constitute 80% of all pediatric brain tumors.

The incidence of CNS tumours is higher in infants and young children upto 7 years age in comparison to older children and adolescence. There are age related differences in primary location of tumor. Within the first year of life, supratentorial tumors predominate and include most commonly choroid plexus tumors and teratomas. From 1–10 years of age, infratentorial tumors predominate, owing to the high incidence of juvenile pilocytic astrocytoma and medulloblastoma. After 10 years of age, once again supratentorial tumors predominate, with diffuse astrocytomas most common. Tumors of the optic pathway and hypothalamus region, the brainstem and pineal midbrain region occur with greater incidence in children and adolescence.

Table 17.6 : Age related differences in primary location of common tumors

Age	*Location*	*Tumors*
Within first year	Supratentorial	Choroid plexus tumors, astrocytoma, teratomas
1–10 years age	Infratentorial	Juvenile pilocytic astrocytoma medulloblastoma
Above 10 years	Supratentorial	Diffuse astrocytoma

Etiology

Little is known about the etiology of brain tumors. Existence of some predisposing familial syndromes is well-known. However, CNS neoplasm associated with cancer predisposing syndromes represents a minority of brain tumors. It may provide newer insights into a possible genetic association. Recent studies have documented families where multiple first degree relatives have primary bone tumors. There is also increasing recent evidence of chromosomal abnormalities that are specific to certain childhood brain tumors. Among other plausible factors implicated relate to environmental factors, occupational exposure, viruses and post natal irradiation.

Clinical Manifestations

Central nervous system tumors generally have subtle presenting features initially. It is only in the late stages, a full blown picture becomes obvious.

The clinical presentation of patients depends on the location of the tumor, type of tumor and the age of the child. The presentations are related to raised intracranial pressure as a result of obstruction of CSF flow and /or focal brain dysfunction characterized by focal neurological signs and seizures. In children, the frequent tumor location in or adjacent to the cerebral midline structures makes raised intracranial pressure a common initial event.

Signs and symptoms of increased intracranial pressure are age dependent, being usually non-specific in very young age group.

Infants with open cranial sutures may present with signs of raised intracranial pressure viz. irritability, vomiting and lethargy. For slow growing tumors, infants may show disproportionately accelerated rates of head circumference increase. Downward, divergent deviation of the eyes may occur with severely raised intracranial pressure in infants. In older children, increased ICP may herald insidiously with subtle personality changes and / or poor school performance. Morning headache, vomiting without nausea, diplopia and papilledema are late signs of increased ICP.

The *midline or infratentorial tumors* present with the classical triad of headache, nausea and /or vomiting, and papilledema. The presence of neck pain and stiffness, especially when associated with head and neck extension, visual failure, altered consciousness, episodes of decerebrated posturing and altered cardiorespiratory functions are symptoms of severe intracranial pressure which requires immediate intervention.

Seizures are relatively uncommon presenting features of childhood brain tumors. Focal neurological signs depend on the location of the tumor.

The *infratentorial tumor* may also present with disorders of equilibrium, gait and coordination, blurred vision, diplopia and nystagmus.

The presentation of *primary brainstem tumors* includes gaze palsy, cranial nerve palsy and upper motor neurone motor deficits.

Supratentorial tumors are associated with focal disorders viz. motor disorders, sensory changes, speech disorders, seizures and reflex abnormalities.

Optic pathway tumors present with decreased visual acuity, Marcus Gunn pupil, nystagmus and / or visual field defects.

Suprasellar and third ventricle region tumors may present with diabetes insipidus, hypothyroidism, growth hormone deficiency as well as panhypopituitarism.

The *diencephalic syndrome* is characterized by failure to thrive, emaciation, increased appetite, and sometimes behavioural problems which occur almost exclusively in infants (below one year of age) with a midline supratentorial tumor involving the hypothalamus.

Parinaud syndrome is the classical presentation of pineal region tumors. It is characterized by paresis of upward gaze, pupillary dilatation, reactive to accommodation but not to light, nystagmus to convergence or retraction and eyelid retraction.

Spinal cord tumors or spinal cord dissemination of brain tumors may present with long nerve tract motor or sensory deficits, bowel and bladder deficits and back or radicular pain.

Meningeal metastatic disease from brain tumors or leukemia may present with signs and symptoms similar to those in case of infratentorial tumors.

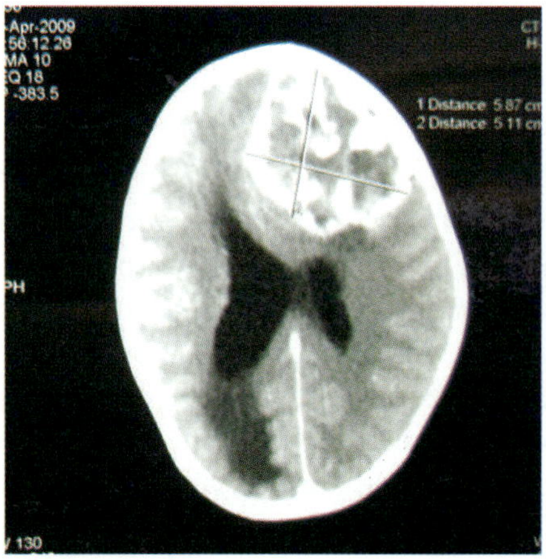

Fig. 17.10: CT scan showing astrocytoma

Laboratory Diagnosis

The final and definitive confirmation of CNS tumor relies on neuroimaging. Computed axial tomography (CAT) still remains an essential tool for investigation in case of brain tumors primarily because of easier accessibility and particularly in special circumstances, e.g., study of calcifications and lesions in the base of the skull.

However, for almost all CNS tumors, *MRI* is the method of choice for defining tumor extension within the brain and spinal cord. A preoperative MRI helps in treatment decision making and planning as well as assessing the outcome of therapeutic intervention. *MR spectroscopy*, an advancement of MRI, helps for investigating the presence of selected metabolites within the tumour. This methodology has refined the contribution of MRI in the management of brain tumors. Single-photon-emission tomography and positron- emission tomography are often used for differential diagnosis of residual disease from recurrent tumor.

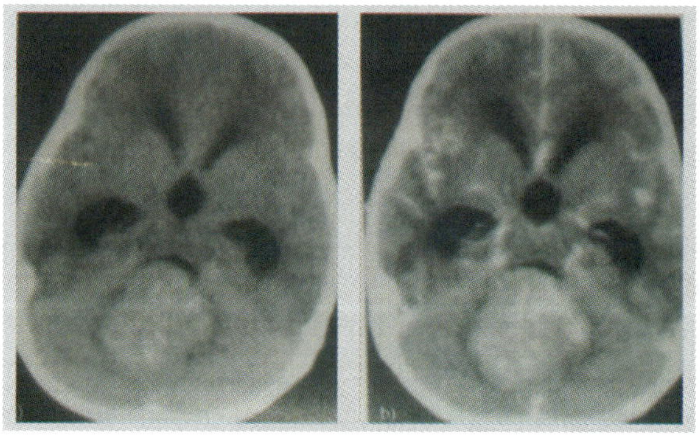

Fig. 17.11: Axial CT scan of the brain showing a large posterior fossa mass enhancing after contrast, associated with triventricular hydrocephalous

Treatment

The treatment of childhood CNS neoplasms represents an organizational challenge. An articulated multi-disciplinary dedicated team of experts (viz. neurosurgeons, neuroradiologists, neuropathologists, radiotherapists, neurooncologists and specialist nurses, neuropediatrician, ophthalmologist, clinical psychologist endocrinologist and occupational therapists) is the basis of an effective pediatric neurooncology programme.

Surgery, radiotherapy and chemotherapy are the conventional therapeutic tools for treatment of childhood CNS neoplasms. However, the treatment approaches vary according to the different histological types.

It should be noted that in children many of the intracranial tumors are either benign or slow growing that can be compatible with a long life expectancy. Some of the tumours remain stable for years. Others grow, slowly but definitively and some others can go through spontaneous regression. Therefore the treatment philosophy adopted for treating children with malignant CNS neoplasm is clearly different from that adopted for managing a slow growing neoplasm.

Surgery is the cornerstone for pilocytic astrocytoma which is the prototype of a slow growing neoplasm. But when the primary tumor involves the optic pathway and complete resection is not possible, then use of chemotherapy and radiotherapy is recommended. Again, regardless of the age of the patient, chemotherapy is the treatment of choice in children with a progressive or symptomatic pilocytic astrocytoma in a child with neurofibromatosis type 1.

Clinical trials for treatment of malignant CNS neoplasm can be tracked down only for medulloblastoma which is a highly malignant neoplasm with a special propensity for leptomeningial dissemination. Maximum reasonable surgery, craniospinal radiotherapy and cisplatin based maintenance chemotherapy is the uniformly accepted standard treatment of medulloblastoma. In young children however, complete resection of the tumor followed by post operative systemic and intrathecal chemotherapy have shown promising results. Glioblastoma multiformae have a very poor prognosis. Complete resection may be possible but these tumors are very poorly radio and chemosensitive. Ependymoma are treated with surgery followed by radiotherapy but role of chemotherapy is still controversial.

Solid Tumors

Solid tumors (excluding brain tumors and lymphoma) account for approximately 45% of all malignant disease in children. The solid tumours may present: (i) as a localized mass presenting in soft tissues, bone or a palpable organ (e.g. Wilms' tumour presenting as a mass in the kidney); or (ii) with the consequences of pressure from a mass or local structure or adjacent tissue (e.g. airway obstruction secondary to a mediastinal mass); or (iii) with the consequences of disseminated disease (e.g. symptoms attributable to bone marrow infiltration or to systemic ill-health).

The types of solid tumours seen in children are very different from those in adults in whom carcinomas of breast, lung, gut and skin predominate. Such diagnoses are rare in children. Many of the solid tumors seen in children are distinctive embryonal tumors which arise almost exclusively in early childhood. Further, the frequency of different tumors varies with age. For example, the peak incidence of neuroblastoma and Wilms'tumor is in early childhood whereas bone tumors occur more frequently in adolescence.

Table 17.7 : Common solid tumors in children

Types
Neuroblastoma
Wilms' tumor
Rhabdomyosarcoma
Other soft tissue sarcoma
Bone tumors
Extracranial germ cell tumors
Retinoblastoma
Liver tumors
Carcinoma and melanoma

Etiology

In most cases, the precise etiology is unclear, but it is likely to represent an interaction between environmental factors (e.g. radiation, viruses) and host genetic susceptibility (e.g. gene mutation). Most cancers occur as a result of mutations in cellular genes (oncogenes and tumor suppressor genes) which may be either inherited or sporadic. One example of inherited cancer is bilateral retinoblastoma which is associated with a deletion of chromosome 13.

Laboratory Diagnosis

Solid tumors are identified and localized on ultrasound, X-rays, CT and MR scans. Nuclear medicine imaging (e.g. radiolabelled technetium bone scan) may be useful to identified metastatic disease.

Tumor marker studies are helpful in neuroblastoma in which there is increased urinary catecholamines excretion and for germ cell and liver cell tumor, in which there is increased alpha fetoprotein production.

The diagnosis, however, should be confirmed histologically by biopsy or by bone marrow sampling. The differentiation between some solid tumors may be sometimes difficult with standard microscopy, and further differentiation usually requires immunohistochemistry and sometimes electron microscopy.

NEUROBLASTOMA

Neuroblastoma arises from neural crest tissues in the adrenal medulla and elsewhere in the sympathetic nervous system. It is most common before the age of 5 years with a median age at presentation around 2 years. The disease presents a spectrum of aggression from benign ganglioneuroma, through ganglioneuroblastoma, to malignant neuroblastoma. It may also show a pattern of spontaneous regression in very young infants.

Most children present with an abdominal mass, typically of adrenal origin, but the primary can lie anywhere along the sympathetic chain from the neck to the pelvis. At presentation, the tumor mass is often large and may cross the midline and envelope major blood vessels. Paravertebral tumors may extend through an adjacent intervertebral foramen and cause spinal cord compression. In children over 2 years of age, clinical symptoms are mainly from metastatic disease, particularly bone pain and bone marrow suppression.

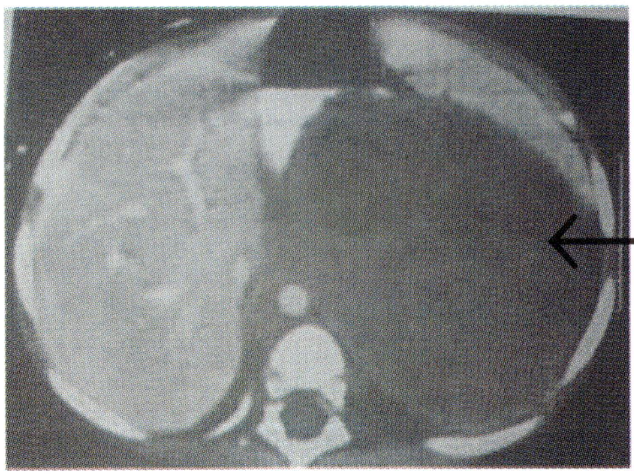

Fig. 17.12: Typical cross-sectional CT scan image of abdominal neuroblastoma

The diagnosis can often be made from characteristic clinical and radiological features and raised urinary catecholamines. Confirmation is by biopsy. Evidence of metastatic disease can be detected by bone marrow examination, bone scan and radioisotope labeled MIBG (meta iodo benzyl guanidine) scan.

The majority of the children over one year presents with advanced disease and have a poor prognosis. Their treatment consists of initial chemotherapy followed by surgery to resect residual primary disease. The risk of relapse is high even with aggressive chemotherapy and the prospect of cure is very poor in children with metastatic disease. Attempt to reduce relapse include use of 13-cis-retinoic acid at the end of conventional chemotherapy.

The few children who present with localized primary disease can often be cured with surgery alone. A subgroup of infants aged less than 1 year present with localized primary tumor but with evidence of skin, liver and/or bone marrow disease. The prognosis of these patients is very good. Spontaneous regression can occur and cure is often possible with minimal therapy.

WILMS' TUMOR (NEPHROBLASTOMA)

Wilms' tumor/nephroblastoma, is a complex, mixed embryonal neoplasm of the kidney. It comprises approximately 6% of pediatric cancers and is the second most common malignant abdominal tumour in childhood. It usually occurs in children between 2–5 years of age. Although a rare diagnosis after 10 years, it has been reported in neonates and adolescents.

A small number of children have associated congenital abnormalities like aniridia, genital anomalies, hemi hypertrophy and Beckwith Wiedemann syndrome (characterized by Omphalocele, macrosomia and hypoglycemia). It is now clear that there are several genes responsible for both the genetic and sporadic forms of Wilms' tumor although less than 1% of patients have a family history.

Most children present with a large abdominal mass, often detected incidentally in an otherwise well child. Occasionally, children have symptoms of poor appetite and poor weight gain. Hemorrhage into the mass can cause abdominal pain and pallor. Macroscopic hematuria is uncommon but an important mode of presentation. Hypertension is common at diagnosis and may persist, requiring treatment, until nephrectomy.

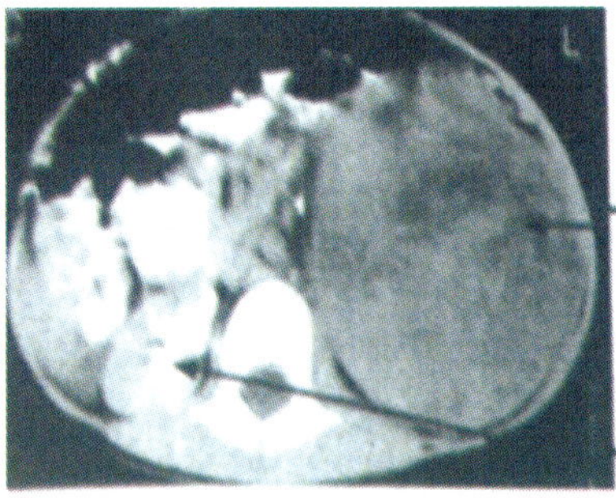

Fig.17.13: Cross-sectional CT scan image of left Wilms' tumor

Overall prognosis in Wilms' tumor is good and more than 80% of the patients can be cured. Pre-nephrectomy chemotherapy is the favoured approach at present because it gives an opportunity to tailor subsequent treatment to initial chemotherapy response and may reduce the risk of tumor rupture during primary nephrectomy. Radiotherapy is required only in a minority of patients including those with lung metastasis and with extensive intra-abdominal disease. The cure rate even for those with metastatic disease at presentation is around 60% but the salvage of children with relapse is still a great challenge.

RHABDOMYOSARCOMA

Soft tissue sarcoma accounts for 7–8% of all cancer in children. The most common subtype is rhabdomyosarcoma. Other soft tissue sarcomas, often described as non-rhabdo soft tissue sarcomas, are a heterogenous group of tumors that are generally more common in adults.

Rhabdomyosarcoma (RMS) is the most common soft tissue sarcoma in children. It originates from the primitive mesenchymal tissue. There are two major subtypes: embryonal (approximately 80%) and alveolar (approximately 20%).

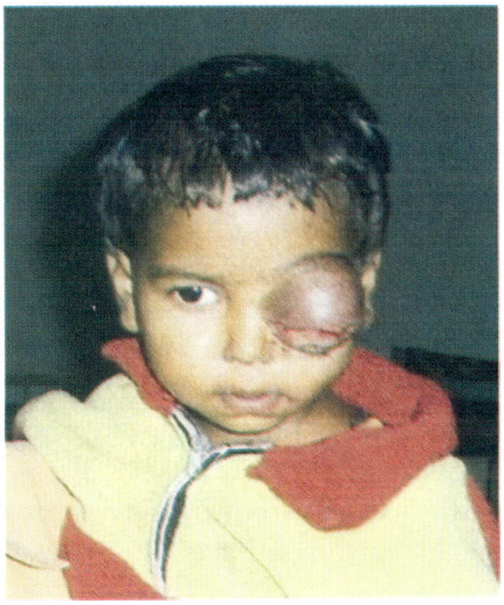

Fig. 17.14: Rhabdomyosarcoma

RMS occurs at a wide variety of primary sites resulting in a range of different presentations. Head and neck are the most common sites with presenting features like proptosis, nasal obstruction and blood stained nasal discharge. Genitourinary tumors are the next common and cause dysuria and urinary obstruction or blood stained vaginal discharge. Metastatic disease in the lungs, liver, bone marrow or bone may be present in about 15% cases at diagnosis and is associated with a particularly poor prognosis.

Confirmation of diagnosis is by biopsy and histology. The distinction of the two major subtypes is usually possible by standard light microscopy but the presence of a characteristic translocation between chromosome 2 (or less commonly chromosome 1) and 13 offers confirmation of the alveolar type.

As the tumor margins are often deceptively ill defined, attempts at primary surgical excision are often unsuccessful. Surgery is therefore discouraged unless this can be achieved without mutilation or irreversible organ damage. RMS is a chemosensitive tumor. A minority of patients with completely resected local disease require only a short course of chemotherapy. The majority patients require aggressive combination chemotherapy and some form of local treatment, often including radiotherapy.

LANGERHANS CELL HISTIOCYTOSIS

Langerhans cell histiocytosis (LCH), previously known as histiocytosis X, is a rare condition characterized by an abnormal proliferation of histiocytes. It is no longer believed to be a truly malignant condition. LCH can present as a localized disease or a systemic disease. The pathogenesis of LCH is uncertain but an atypical immunological response to presumed infection is postulated. It includes the clinical entities of eosinophilic granuloma, Hand-Schuller-Christian disease and Letterer-Siwe disease.

Eosinophilic Granuloma

Eosinophilic granuloma, a localized disease of bone is common and may present at any age with pain, swelling or rarely a fracture.

Diabetes insipidus is a well-known association with LCH and probably occurs more frequently in patients where disease affects the base of the skull. It may be the only presenting symptom in an otherwise asymptomatic child.

Plain X-ray reveals a characteristic lytic lesion with a well defined border (Fig. 17.15). A full skeletal survey should be done to exclude multiple lesions. Multiple bone lesions can occur at any site and frequently involve the skull.

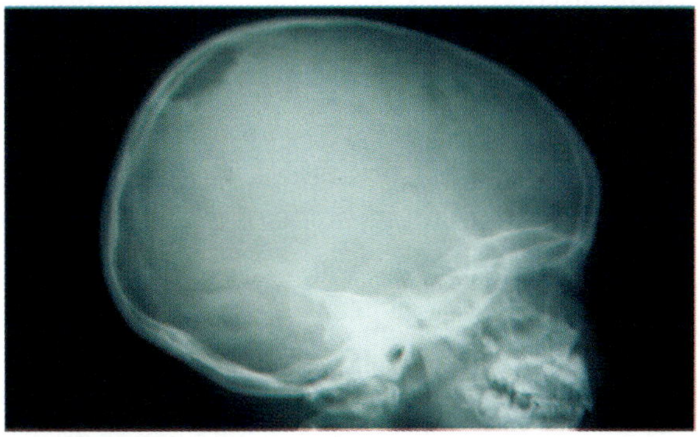

Fig. 17.15: Characteristic lytic lesion in the skull in eosinophilic granuloma

For a definitive diagnosis, biopsy on standard microscopy should be supplemented by the demonstration of CD1a epitopes on the cell surface by immunohistochemistry and/or demonstration of cytoplasmic Birkbeck granules by electron microscopy.

Curettage of the lesion, intra cavity steroid injection and radiotherapy are all successful forms of treatment although biopsy itself may be sufficient to initiate healing in many cases. Asymptomatic lesions may not require any treatment. For diabetes insipidus long-term treatment with desmopressin is usually required.

Hand-Schüller Christian Disease

Hand-Schüller Christian disease is a systemic form of the disease with visceral involvement. The rare form is characterized by the triad–exophthalmos, diabetes insipidus and large defects in the membranous bones of the skull as visualized in X-ray. Commonly the child may present with anemia, hepatosplenomegaly, spinal and limb pains (due to multiple bone deposits), swollen and necrotic gums with loose teeth, and honey comb lungs. Various rashes may develop such as maculopapules, reddish yellow lumps or yellow crusts over the scalp. Otorrhoea due to mastoid involvement is common. The defects in the skull may become palpable soft swelling. Hydrocephalus and papilledema can develop.

Treatment consists of radiotherapy which may relieve pain and chemotherapy may induce long remission. Diabetes insipidus can be controlled with desmopressin. It may have a less favorable prognosis.

Letterer-Siwe Disease

Letterer-Siwe disease, a systemic form of the disease is seen in the infants. Typically it is characterized by a seborrhoeic rash, most commonly affecting the skull. The soft tissue involvement is variable affecting the gums, ears, lungs, liver, spleen, lymph nodes and bone marrow. This form of LCH is usually progressive and requires combination chemotherapy although spontaneous regression may occur. The outlook is variable but most patients are cured although some may experience long-term sequelae.

Treatment

The course of single system disease (e.g. bone, lymph node and skin) is generally benign with a high chance of spontaneous remission. Treatment in single system disease should be directed at arresting the progression of lesion (e.g. bone lesion). Curettage or low dose local radiation therapy (5 - 6 Gy) may be sufficient. For multisystem disease, treatment consists of systemic chemotherapy with vinblastine or etoposide which has been found to be very effective. The experimental therapies suggested for unresponsive disease include therapy with cyclosporine / antithymocyte globulin and modalities like stem cell transplant.

OSTEOSARCOMA

Malignant bone tumors more commonly affect adolescents than children. Osteosarcoma is the most common primary malignant bone tumor followed by Ewing's sarcoma. In children younger than 10 years of age, Ewing's sarcoma is more common than osteosarcoma. Both tumor types occur most frequently in the second decade of life.

The cause of osteosarcoma is not known. Certain genetic or acquired conditions seem to predispose to its development. For example, patients with hereditary retinoblastoma have a significantly increased risk of developing osteosarcoma. It can also be induced by exposure to radiation such as after radiotherapy treatment for Ewing's sarcoma, craniospinal radiation for brain tumors or high dose irradiation for other malignancies. Certain benign conditions like Paget's disease, multiple hereditary exostoses and fibrous dysplasia are associated with malignant transformation to osteosarcoma.

Pathologically, there are three subtypes: osteoblastic, chondroblastic and telangiectatic, although no significant difference in outcome is associated. The pathological diagnosis is made by demonstration of a highly malignant, pleomorphic, spindle cell neoplasm associated with the formation of malignant osteoid and bone.

Pain and swelling are the most common presenting symptoms. Initial complaints may be attributed to sports injury or sprain as these tumors occur most commonly in active adolescents. The diagnosis should be suspected in a patient with deep bone pain, often causing nighttime awakening, not responding to conservative therapy within a reasonable amount of time. Additional clinical findings may include limitation of movements, joint effusion, tenderness and warmth.

The complete blood counts are usually normal. Serum alkaline phosphatase and lactic dehydrogenase levels may be elevated.

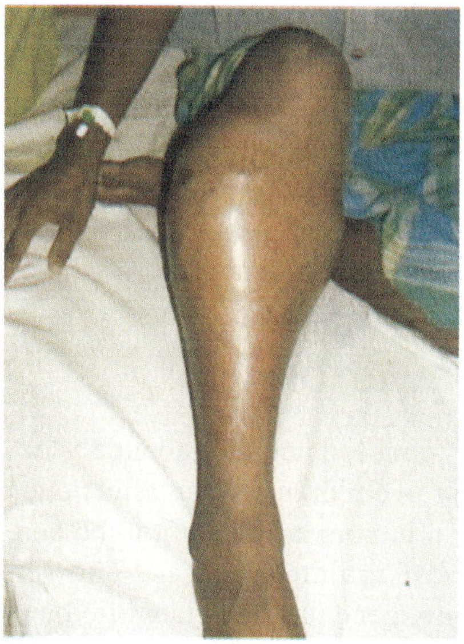

Fig. 17.16: Osteosarcoma

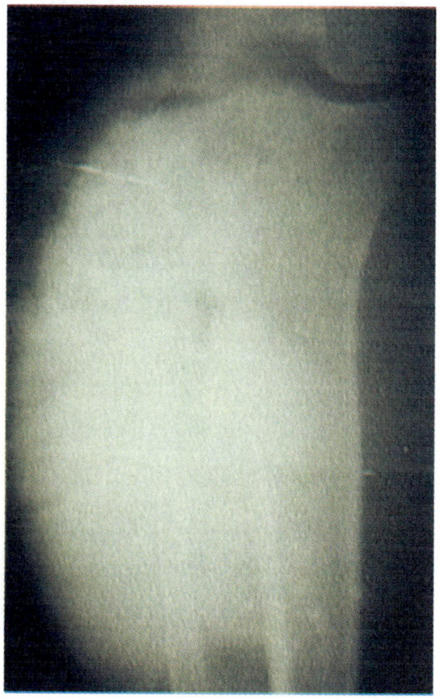

Fig. 17.17: X-ray findings (Sunburst appearance)

The classic radiographic appearance of osteosarcoma is called the *sun burst* appearance with mixed lytic and blastic appearance and new bone formation. The differential diagnosis of the lytic bone lesion includes histiocytosis, Ewing's sarcoma, lymphoma and bone cyst.

An incisional biopsy is needed to confirm the diagnosis. Before the biopsy, an MRI of the primary lesion and the entire bone should be performed to evaluate the tumor for its proximity to nerves and blood vessels and soft tissue and joint extension. The metastatic work-up consists of a CT of the chest and radionuclide bone scan which should be performed before biopsy.

The current approach to treatment is preoperative chemotherapy in an attempt to facilitate limb salvage surgery. It is important to resume chemotherapy as soon as possible after surgery. Lung metastasis present at diagnosis should be resected at some time during the course of treatment. The chemotherapeutic agents used include doxorubicin, cisplatin, methotrexate and ifosfamide. After limb salvage surgery, intensive rehabilitation and physical therapy is necessary to ensure maximal functional outcome.

EWING'S SARCOMA

Ewing's sarcoma family includes Ewing's sarcoma and peripheral primitive neuroectodermal tumor (PPNET). It refers to a group of small round cell undifferentiated tumors of childhood. It is thought to be of neural crest origin. The classical bony Ewing's sarcoma and PPNET both are characterized by the presence of the same molecular genetic abnormality. Ewing's sarcoma, an undifferentiated sarcoma of bone may also rise from soft tissue. The anatomic sites of involvement include extremities, pelvis, and spine and chest wall.

The clinical presentations of Ewing's sarcoma are similar to osteosarcoma and include pain, swelling, limitation of movements, and tenderness over the involved bone or soft tissue. It is often associated with systemic manifestations like fever and weight loss and the patient may undergo treatment for a presumptive diagnosis of osteomyelitis. The patient may present with respiratory distress in case of huge chest wall primary tumours. Paraspinal or vertebral tumors may present with symptoms of spinal compression. Sometimes there may be a delay in diagnosis when pain and swelling is attributed to a sports injury.

The characteristic radiographic finding is a primary lytic lesion with periosteal reaction (onion skinning appearance). An MRI/CT will show a soft tissue mass. The MRI of the tumor and entire length of the bone should be done in order to examine the extent of the soft tissue and bony mass and the proximity of the tumor to neurovascular structures. CT guided biopsy of the lesion confirms the diagnosis. Enough tissue should be obtained for special stains, cytogenetics, and molecular studies. Thorough evaluation of metastatic disease should be done which includes CT of the chest, radionuclide bone scan and bone marrow aspirate and biopsy from atleast two sites.

Ewing's sarcoma is radiosensitive. Local control can be achieved with surgery or radiotherapy. Radiation therapy is however, associated with a risk of radiation induced second malignancy especially osteosarcoma as well as bone growth failure in skeletally immature patients. Radiotherapy has a place when surgical resection is not possible or incomplete, for example in the pelvis or spine. Surgery followed by multidrug chemotherapy regimen is preferred by many centres as the mode of treatment. The standard drug combination is vincristine, doxorubicin, and cyclophosphamide. Addition of ifosfamide and etoposide improves the outcome of non-metastatic disease. The patients with bone marrow / bone disease have a poor survival.

LIVER TUMORS

Liver tumors are rare. Primary liver tumors in the newborn and in the first few months of life are more likely to be benign, e.g., a hemangioma. The primary malignant tumors are mostly hepatoblastoma and hepatocellular carcinoma (HCC). The latter are seen in countries with high incidence of hepatitis B infection. It can also occur in children with other forms of preexisting liver disease.

The hepatic tumors generally present with an abdominal mass. As the disease progresses, anorexia, weight loss, vomiting and abdominal pain may ensue. Metastatic spread of hepatoblastoma most commonly involves the regional lymph nodes and lungs. Hepatocellular carcinoma can present as an acute abdominal crisis with rupture of the tumor and hemoperitoneum.

Serum alpha feto protein (AFP) level is an important tumor marker for diagnosis and monitoring of hepatic tumors. The AFP level is elevated in almost all hepatoblastomas and 60% cases of hepatocellular carcinomas. Anemia is common. LFT is normal in hepatoblastoma. Liver enzymes may be elevated but serum bilirubin is normal in HCC. Hepatitis B and C serology are normal in hepatoblastoma, may be positive in HCC in endemic areas.

A plain X-ray and ultrasonography of abdomen can characterize the hepatic mass. Ultrasonography can differentiate malignant hepatic masses from benign vascular lesions. A CT/MRI can accurately define the extent of intrahepatic tumor involvement and the potential for surgical resection. Evaluation of metastatic disease should include a CT of the chest and bone scan.

Treatment includes surgery and adjuvant chemotherapy. As much as 85% of liver can be resected. Hepatic regeneration is noted within 3–4 months of surgery. Cisplatin in combination with vincristine and 5-fluorouracil or doxorubicin is effective treatment for hepatoblastoma. Same drugs have shown some activity against HCC but improved long-term outcome has been difficult to achieve.

RETINOBLASTOMA

Retinoblastoma accounts for about 5% of severe visual impairment in children. It may affect one or both eyes. All bilateral tumors are thought to be hereditary as are upto 20% of unilateral cases. The retinoblastoma susceptibility gene has been identified on chromosome 13. The pattern of inheritance is dominant but with incomplete penetrance. Most cases present within first three years of life.

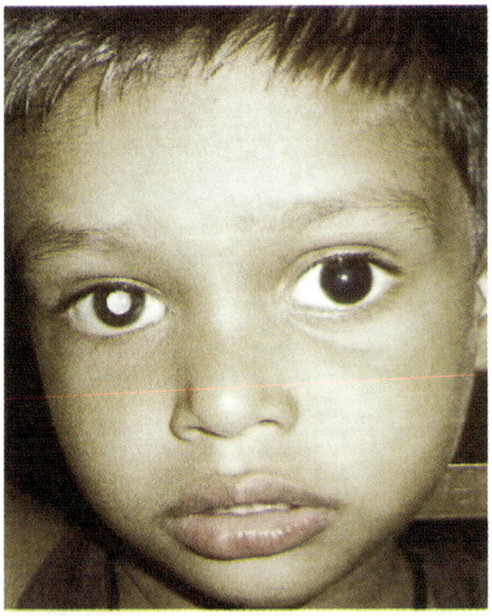

Fig. 17.18: Retinoblastoma

Retinoblastoma classically presents with leukoria, a white reflex which is often first noticed when a red reflex is not present at routine newborn or well child examination or in a flash photograph of the child. Strabismus is commonly the initial presenting complain. Orbital inflammation, hyphema, and pupil irregularity are signs of advance disease. About 10% cases are detected by routine ophthalmologic screening in the context of a positive family history.

Diagnosis is established by characteristic findings on ophthalmoscopic examination of both eyes under general anesthesia. It also facilitates photographing and mapping of the tumors.

Orbital sonography and CT or MRI are used to evaluate the extent of intraocular disease and extraocular spread. CSF analysis, bone marrow examination and bone scan may be necessary as and when indicated.

The primary goal of treatment is cure and secondary goal is preservation of vision. In most unilateral disease the tumor is large and enucleation is undertaken if there is no potential for useful vision. In bilateral disease, the traditional approach involves enucleation of the more severely affected eye and irradiation of the remaining eye in hope of salvaging some useful vision. Small tumors can be treated with laser photocoagulation or cryotherapy. With the availability of effective chemotherapy, attempt has been made to salvage both eyes with some degree of functional vision. Large tumors often respond to multiagent chemotherapy, including vincristine, etoposide and carboplatin.

Suggested Reading

1. De Gruchy's Clinical Hematology in Medical Practice. Editors Frank Firkin, Colin Chesterman and Bryan Rush, 5th edition, 1989, Reprinted 2006.
2. IAP speciality series on Pediatric Hematology and Oncology. Editors M R Lokeshwar, Nitin K. Shah, Bharat Agarwal, Anupam Sachdeva. Printed and published by Indian Academy of Pediatrics, Kailash Darsan, Kennedy Bridge, Bombay, 2006.
3. PHO review volume 1–10, Indian Academy of Pediatrics subspeciality chapter on Pediatric Hematology-Oncology 1988–1997.
4. Practical Pediatric Hematology, Reference manual, National training project, 1st edition. Editor Anupam Sachdeva, Pediatric Hematology Oncology chapter, 2006. Child Oncology. Annales Nestle, vol 63, number 3, 2005, Nestec Ltd, Avenue Nestle 55, CH-1800 Vevey, Switzerland.
5. Nelson Textbook of Pediatrics, Editors Behrman, Kliegman and Jenson, 17th edition, 2004. Saunders, Philadelphia, Pennsylvania 19106.

18

Common Chromosomal Disorders

OUTLINES

Chromosomal Abnormalities

The chromosomes are made up of DNA and other protein complexes and contain most of the genetic information that is passed from one generation to the next. Cytogenetics arranges chromosomes by size in pairs– the largest being chromosome 1 and the smallest, chromosome 22 and then the sex chromosomes.

A *gene* is that portion of a chromosome which codes for a character. The position of a gene on a chromosome is called its locus. Corresponding loci on the two members of a pair chromosome carry genes for the same character. The character coded by the two chromosomes may have different forms. For example, one of them may code for a black iris and the other a blue iris. Such alternative forms of a gene are known as *alleles*. If the alleles code for the same traits, these are said to be present in homozygous state. If they code for different traits, they are in heterozygous state. A gene is called a *dominant gene* if an allele clinically manifests itself even in the heterozygous state. A *recessive gene* is one which does not express itself clinically when the other allele from the other parent is normal. The genetic make up of a person is called the genotype and the clinically manifest character is called phenotype. *Genetic polymorphism* is a term used when a gene express itself in several slightly modified forms without adverse effect on the health of the individual.

Karyotyping means visual display of chromosomes and is obtained after the chromosomes are arrested during cell division in prophase and are photographed and arranged according to size. The normal karyotype is 46 XX for females and 46 XY in males. A description of the karyotype consists of three parts: the number of chromosomes, the sex chromosome constitution and any abnormalities found.

Chromosomal abnormalities are an important cause of mental retardation and congenital abnormalities. Chromosomal anomalies include abnormalities of number and structure. The most common abnormalities of chromosome number are trisomies. These occur when there are three representatives of a particular chromosome instead of two. Trisomies are usually the result of meiotic non-disjunction, i.e., failure of a chromosome pair to separate. Trisomy may be present in all cells or may occur in mosaic form. Most individuals with trisomies exhibit a consistent and specific phenotype depending on the chromosome involved. The most frequent trisomy in humans is trisomy 21 or Down syndrome. Trisomies of chromosome 13 and chromosome 18 are also relatively common and are associated with mental retardation and a characteristic set of congenital anomalies. The common sex chromosome anomaly is Turner's syndrome. The other anomalies include Klinefelter syndrome, 47 XXY male, Fragile X syndrome. Only the most common types of chromosomal anomalies viz. Down syndrome and Turner's syndrome is described.

Down Syndrome

The incidence of Down syndrome in general population is 1 in 600–800 live births. The incidence is greater than twice this frequency when all conceptions are considered since more than half of the trisomy 21 fetuses are spontaneously aborted during early pregnancy.

About 95% of cases of Down syndrome have three freestanding copies of chromosome 21. Approximately 1% of individuals are mosaic with some normal cells and approximately 4% have a translocation involving chromosome 21. However, translocation account for 9% of the children with Down syndrome born to mothers younger than 30 years of age.

There is an increase risk of trisomy 21 in women older than 35 years. It is an indication for prenatal diagnosis. Fifty percent of the translocations arise in the individual itself and the other half are inherited from a translocation carrier parent. Parents who are carriers of translocation produce three types of viable offsprings: normal phenotype and karyotype, a phenotypically normal translocation carrier, and the translocation trisomy 21. The phenotype in translocation Down syndrome is not distinguishable from regular trisomy 21 Down syndrome. Hence chromosome study must be performed in all children with Down syndrome. If a translocation is identified, chromosome studies should be performed in parents to identify translocation carriers. These carriers have a high recurrence risk for a chromosomally abnormal child and also family members at risk.

Clinical Manifestations

The clinical features are same irrespective of the mode of inheritance, i.e., whether it is a trisomy, translocation or mosaic.

The features of Down syndrome are so characteristic that the diagnosis is always possible at birth. The skull appears small, brachycephalic with a flat occiput. The hair is usually straight and sparse. The face is flat. The palpebral fissure has an upward slant with epicanthic folds which are confined to the inner angles in contrast to those seen in the mongoloid race which includes most of the upper eye lid. The bridge of the nose is flat and there is hypertelorism. The iris is speckled (Brushfield spots). The lips are thin. The tongue is normal in shape and pointed and frequently protrudes out from the unduly small oral cavity. As years go by the tongue become deeply fissured transversely (scrotal tongue). The palate is high arched.

Features of Down Syndrome

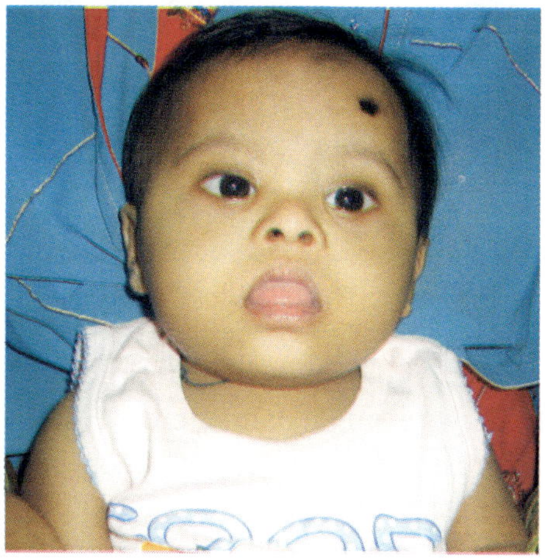

Fig. 18.1: The facies

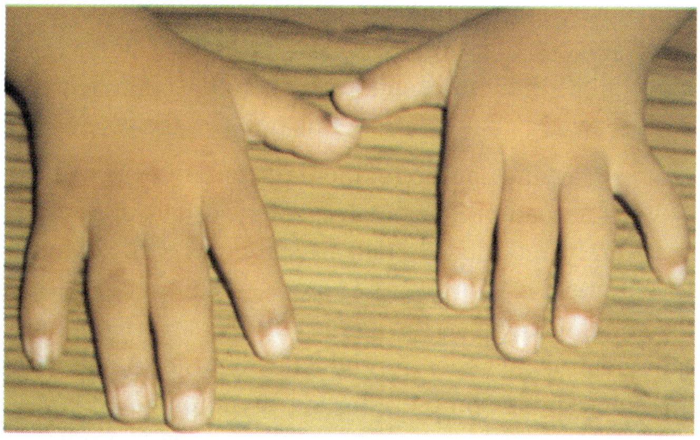

Fig. 18.2: Clinodactyly of little finger

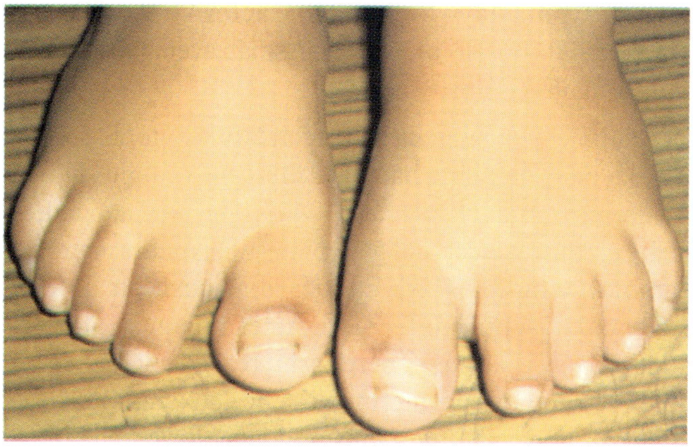

Fig. 18.3: The sandle gap

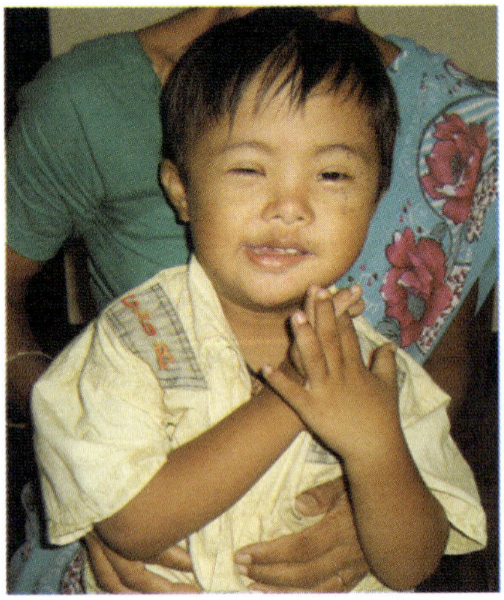

Fig. 18.4: The cheerful Down child

The hands are short with broad fingers. The palm frequently shows a single palmer crease (simian crease) and a single crease on finger 5. The little finger is incurved due to hypoplasia of the middle phalanx (clinodactyly). There are also characteristic abnormalities of the dermatoglyphic patterns. Most fingers have ulnar loops with radial loops on fingers 4 and 5. The axial triradius is distal and the atd angle is large. There is a wider gap between the great toe and the second toe (sandle gap) in the feet with a skin crease at this point in the sole.

There is varying degrees of mental retardation as well as growth retardation. The mental status is usually moderate to severely retarded though in some cases the rate of development may be normal upto 3–4 years age and then decelerate. However, the child is usually an affectionate individual, always cheerful and fond of music. A common characteristic is marked muscular hypotonia and laxity of ligaments. However, muscle tone tends to improve with age and development slows. Radiography reveals pelvic dysplasia which is characteristic of Down syndrome. It consists of broad ilia, small acetabular angles and elongated ischia.

Development of genitalia and secondary sexual characters is delayed. The pubic hairs are thin and straight. Down syndrome is usually associated with congenital anomalies of the cardiovascular and gastrointestinal malformations; common examples are endocardial cushion defect, ventricular septal defect, PDA, esophageal atresia, duodenal atresia etc. There is increased incidence of juvenile type of chronic myelocytic leukemia in these children. Older children have evidence of biochemical hypothyroidism. The incidence increases with increasing age probably due to thyroid autoantibodies. Hence it has been recommended that thyroid function test should be undertaken in these children on the first contact and then every year.

Risk of Recurrence

When parents are normal and child has trisomy 21, the risk of recurrence in subsequent siblings is 1%. If the mother is a carrier of a translocated chromosome, the risk is 10%. If the father is a carrier, the risk of recurrence is 5%. Sporadic cases have little chance of recurrence. Even in young mothers, Down syndrome is more often due to trisomy rather than translocation.

Prenatal Diagnosis

Prenatal diagnosis is indicated in women older than 35 years of age and if there is a sibling history of Down syndrome. The screening tests for the purpose include estimation of maternal serum alpha fetoprotein and prenatal ultrasonography. A low maternal serum alpha fetoprotein is an indicator of Down syndrome. Prenatal ultrasonography may detect a thickened nuchal fold, absence nasal bone, a short femur, cardiac and gastrointestinal anomalies. The confirmatory test is examination of fetal chromosomes by amniocentesis or chorionic villus sampling.

Treatment

There is no definite treatment. Physiotherapy, early stimulation programme, speech therapy plays an important role in improving performance. Regular ENT, ophthalmic and cardiac evaluation should be done in all cases for early detection of problems relating to them. However, it should be noted that muscle tone spontaneously improves whereas the rate of development decreases with age. Social performance is usually achieved as that expected for mental age. The children with Down syndrome generally behave as good babies and happy children, like mimicry, are friendly, have a good sense of rhythm and like music.

The special issues in management include presence of congenital heart disease, proneness to develop acute leukemia, lymphocytic thyroiditis and presence of atlanto-axial instability.

The incidence of *congenital heart disease* is high (around 40%). The common defects are AV canal defect, VSD and PDA. They have a greater propensity to early development of pulmonary vascular disease. A routine ECHO and early intervention is important.

Acute leukemia is 14 times more frequent than in normal population. The incidence of ALL and AML is same as in normal population as well as the expected outcome. They are sensitive to methotrexate and other antimetabolites. More toxicity is seen with standard doses. After induction, they require less intensive therapy for better results.

Long-term outcome is better with > 80% survival rate.

Lymphocytic thyroiditis is caused by lymphocytic infiltration or by thyroid growth stimulating immunoglobulin. Thyroid screening is indicated for all children with Down syndrome. Administration of L thyroxin may be required to improve mental outcome.

Atlantoaxial instability is caused by odontoid hypoplasia and joint laxity. Extension of the neck routinely used to maintain and intubate the airway for administration of anesthesia may cause cervical dislocation and spinal cord trauma. A lateral neck X-ray in extension and flexion should be ordered before anesthesia.

Genetic counseling and prenatal diagnosis are good ways to prevent Down syndrome.

Turner's Syndrome

Turner's syndrome is a sex chromosomal anomaly consisting of sexual infantilism, webbed neck and cubitus vulgus with complete or partial absence of the second X chromosome with or without mosaicism. Turner's syndrome occurs in about 1 in 1500–2500 live born females. The frequency of the 45 X karyotype at conception is about 3% but 99% of these are spontaneously aborted. The mosaic Turner's syndrome survives.

Fifty percent of cases with Turner's syndrome have a 45X chromosomal complement. About 15% are mosaics for 45X and a normal cell line. The single X is of maternal origin in 50–70% patients. The mechanism of chromosome loss is not known. The risk of syndrome does not increase with maternal age. In Turner syndrome the normal process of disappearance of oocytes in the ovary is accelerated. Nearly all oocytes disappear from the ovary by two years. The ovaries are described as streaks and consist only of connective tissue with few germ cells.

Clinical Manifestations

The characteristic features of Turner's syndrome at birth include edema of the dorsa of the hands and feet and loose skin folds at the nape of the neck. The infant is born low birth weight and the length is decreased.

The clinical manifestations in childhood include webbing of the neck, a low posterior hair line, small mandible, prominent ears, epicanthal folds, high arched palate, and broad chest with widely spaced nipples, cubitus valgus, and hyper convex finger nails. The diagnosis in childhood is often first suspected at puberty when sexual maturation fails to occur.

In some girls the only finding may be short stature with minimal other manifestations. The growth deceleration begins in infancy and young childhood and gets progressively more pronounced in later childhood and adolescence. There is developmental delay but intelligence is normal in most cases. Patients with a 45 X karyotype whose X chromosome is of paternal origin are significantly better adjusted and have superior verbal and higher order executive function skills. An increased carrying angle at the elbow is a characteristic finding but may not be always clinically significant. Scoliosis is seen in adolescent girls.

Sexual maturation fails to occur at the expected age, but 10–20% of girls have spontaneous breast development and a small percentage may have menstrual periods.

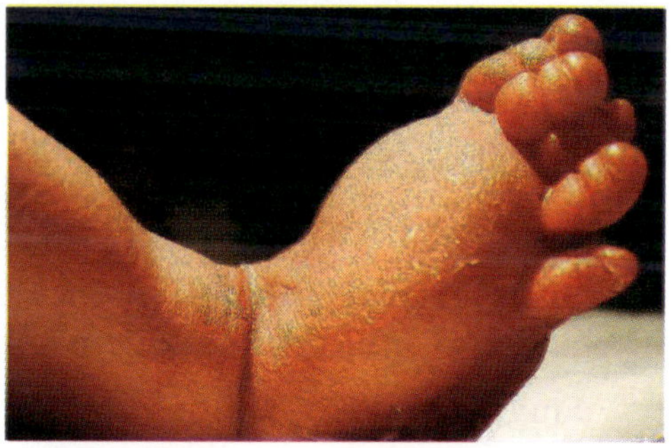

Fig. 18.5: Edema of feet (newborn)

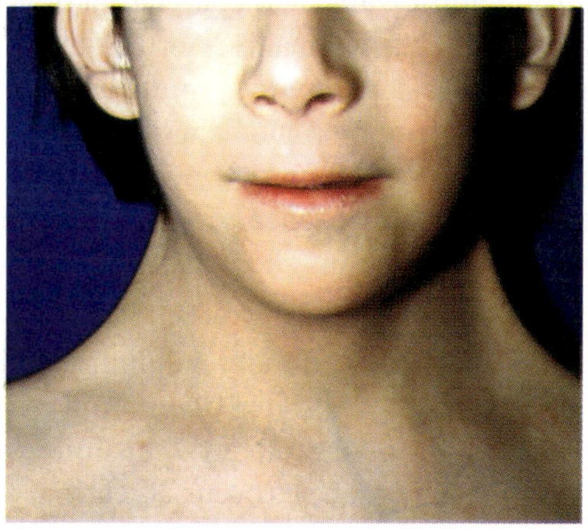

Fig. 18.6: Webbed neck in Turner's syndrome

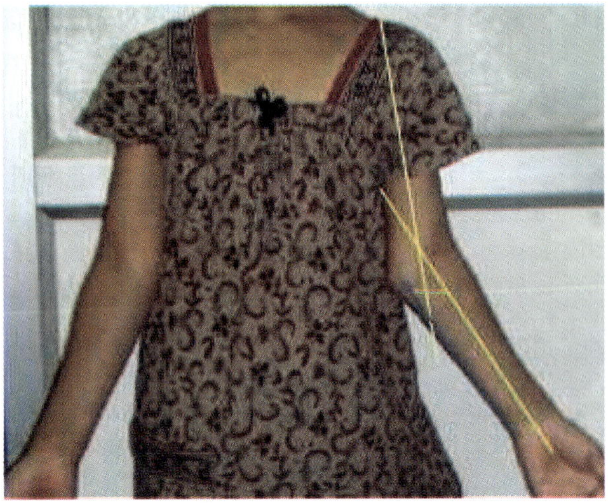

Fig. 18.7: An increased carrying angle

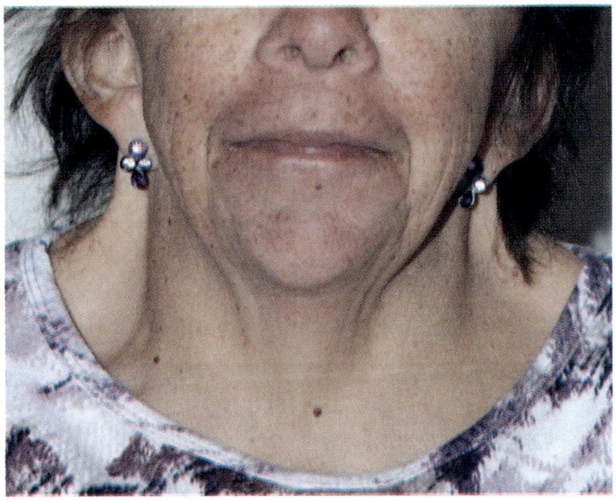

Fig. 18.8: Web neck

Pregnancies have been reported in spontaneously menstruating patients with Turner's syndrome.

Associated congenital abnormalities are common. Cardiovascular and renal abnormalities are commonly seen. Bicuspid aortic valve and coarctation of aorta are common cardiovascular anomalies. Aortic stenosis, mitral valve prolapse, and anomalous pulmonary venous drainage are the less common anomalies found. Congenital anomalies of renal system include pelvic kidney, horse shoe kidney, complete absence of one kidney, uretero pelvic junction obstruction. There may be dysgenesis of anterior chamber and keratoconus in the eyes.

Primary hypertension is common. Autoimmune thyroid disease with or without goiter occur in 10–30% of patients. Abnormal glucose tolerance, insulin resistance and rarely frank type 2 diabetes occur. Recurrent bilateral otitis media is common as also sensorineural hearing defects.

In patients with mosaicism, the abnormalities are less prominent and fewer. Short stature may be the only manifestation of Turner's syndrome other than signs of ovarian failure.

Laboratory Diagnosis

Chromosomal analysis is the mainstay for confirmation of diagnosis of Turner's syndrome. It should be considered in all cases of girls with short stature. Patients with a marker chromosome in some or all cells should be tested for DNA sequences.

Ultrasonography of kidneys and ovaries and echocardiography of the heart should be done in all confirmed cases to exclude associated anomalies.

Radiography: Radiological anomalies detected are shortening of the 4th metatarsal and metacarpal bones, epiphyseal dysgenesis in the joints of knees and elbows, scoliosis and Madelung deformity. In older children, there is inadequate osseous mineralization.

Hormone studies: Plasma levels of *follicle stimulating hormone* (FSH) are markedly elevated during infancy, at 2–3 years age. A progressive decrease in levels occurs until a nadir is reached at 6–8 years of age. By 10–11 years the level again rise to adult castrate levels.

Thyroid antiperoxidase antibodies should be checked periodically. If positive, thyroid profile should be obtained. *Growth hormone* secretion defects are seen in adolescent period.

Treatment

Treatment in Turner's syndrome includes hormone therapy and psychosocial support. Treatment with recombinant growth hormone increases height velocity and ultimate stature in most girls. Replacement therapy with estrogen can be started in these girls at 12–13 years of age. In girls, in whom growth hormone treatment is not started until late childhood or adolescence, estrogen therapy may need to be delayed until 14–15 years. This will help in greater gains in height.

Psychosocial support for these girls and their family is an integral part of treatment.

Genetic Counseling

Most of the genetic disorders are not easily treatable, but are preventable by proper understanding and counseling. Hence the importance of genetic counseling as an integral part of management of genetic disorders has to be realized by all clinicians.

The American Society of Human Genetics in 1975 has defined genetic counseling as the communicative process which deals with human problems associated with the occurrence and/or recurrence of a genetic disorder in a family.

Objective

The main objective of Genetic counseling is to assist the individual and the family understand the scientific information about the disease, its course, possible management, risk of recurrence and facility of prenatal diagnosis, if available. Helping the patient and family to cope with the problem of genetic disorder is equally important.

Indications

The indications of genetic counseling include the following:

1. Advanced parental age, i.e., mother >35 years, father >50 years.
2. Previous child with or family history of congenital abnormality, dysmorphism, mental retardation, isolated birth defects, metabolic disorder, chromosome abnormality, single gene disorder.
3. Consanguinity.
4. Teratogenic exposure (occupational or abuse).
5. Repeated pregnancy loss or infertility.
6. Abnormal pregnancy screening, e.g., increased maternal serum alpha feto protein, multiple positive triple screen, abnormalities in fetal USG, abnormal fetal karyotype.
7. Adult onset genetic disorder like cancer , Huntington's disease.
8. Heterozygote screening based on ethnic risk for Sickle cell anemia ,Thalassemia, Gaucher's disease, Tay-Sachs disease.
9. Follow-up of abnormal genetic testing.
10. When a child has got two major malformations, one major and two minor or three or more minor malformations.

Genetic Disorders

It is essential to have knowledge about genetic disorders and types of inheritance for proper counseling and to explain the risk of recurrence.

Chromosomal Disorders

These disorders are generally sporadic and occur in 0.5% of all live newborns. The risk of their recurrence is low except in situation where either parent is a balanced translocation carrier. Chromosomal disorders include non-disjunction (e.g., Trisomies -21, 18, 13) Mosaicism, translocation and deletion.

Single Gene Disorder

In this disorder, a mutant gene exhibit one of the four following Mendelian inheritance patterns:

Autosomal dominant: The autosomal dominant disorders have the following characteristics:

The disorder is transmitted from affected heterozygous parents in a vertical pattern (parent to child), appearing in multiple generations.

An affected individual has a 50% (1 in 2) chance of passing on the deleterious gene for each pregnancy.

Unaffected individuals (family members who do not manifest the trait) do not pass the disorder to their children.

Males and females are equally affected.

The finding of male to male transmission essentially confirms autosomal dominant inheritance. Many patients with such a disorder do not have a history of affected family member. Possible reasons for this may be new mutations, incomplete penetrance, variable expression and somatic mutation.

Autosomal recessive: The autosomal recessive disorders have the following characteristics:

Transmission occurs from two affected heterozygous carrier parents to a child. There is also horizontal transmission in multiple affected family member of a kindred in the same generation.

There is 25% chance of being homozygous, 50% chance of being heterozygous carrier, 25% chance being normal.

Male and female equally affected.

There is increased frequency in presence of consanguinity.

Sometimes there may be pseudodominant inheritance if homozygous affected individual has a partner who is a heterozygous carrier.

X-linked recessive: The X-linked disorders have the following characteristics:

Transmission usually occurs to the sons through carrier mothers. Female carriers are generally unaffected.

Affected male will have only carrier daughters there is no chance of effected son (no male to male transmission).

There is 50% chance for the son to be affected and equal chance to be normal and 50% chance for the daughter to be carrier and equal chance for the daughter to be normal.

Females may occasionally exhibit signs of an X-linked trait similar to male. It occurs owing to non-random activation; homozygosity for an X-linked trait or presence of sex chromosome abnormality (45X or 46XY female).

X-linked dominant inheritance: Both male and female are effected, more severe in male. Female carriers typically manifest abnormal findings.

Affected male will have only affected daughters and unaffected sons and half of the off springs of effected women will be effected.

Examples of Common Single Gene Disorders

Autosomal Dominant	*Autosomal Recessive*	*X-linked Recessive*	*X-linked Dominant*
Achondroplasia	Albinism	Hemophilia A, B	Vitamin D resistant hypophos-phatemic Rickets
Hereditary spherocytosis	Galactosemia, phenyl ketonuria, Gaucher disease	Duchenne muscular dystrophy	Incontinentia pigmenti (lethal in males)
Huntington chorea	Wilson's disease	G-6-PD deficiency	
Marfan syndrome	Ataxia telangiectasia	Hunter's syndrome	
Tuberous sclerosis	Cystic fibrosis		

Polygenic and Multifactorial Inheritance

Transmission, as a result of additive and interactive effect of one or more genes plus environmental factors is called polygenic and multifactorial inheritance. Examples are congenital heart diseases, cleft lip, cleft palate, congenital hypertrophic pyloric stenosis, Hirschsprung disease, diabetes and hypertension. Characteristics of polygenic and multifactorial inheritance are as follows:

Risk of recurrence is higher if malformation is more severe. For example recurrence risk of Hirschsprung disease is increased with increased length of the aganglionic segment.

When these diseases have marked sex predilection, the risk of recurrence is high, e.g., congenital hypertrophic pyloric stenosis (M: F=5:1).

There is similar rate of recurrence (3–5%) among all 1st degree relative (parents, siblings, offsprings of the affected child).

Risk of recurrence is related to incidence of the disease. It is increased when multiple family members are affected. The risk in identical twin is 21–63%.

Non-Traditional Inheritance

Non-traditional inheritance is observed in the following conditions:

Mitochondrial disorders: This exhibit maternal inheritance; a woman with a mitochondrial genetic disorder will have only affected offsprings of either sex, while an affected father will have no affected offsprings.

Triplets repeat expansion disorder, examples of which are Huntington's disorder, Fragile X syndrome.

Genomic imprinting, examples are Prader-Willi syndrome, Angelman syndrome.

Pseudogenetic inheritance and familial clustering is possible due to environmental factors and teratogens, e.g., multiple siblings with asthma due to cigarette smoking.

Laboratory Diagnosis

The tests include hematological and imaging investigations, chromosomal analysis, enzyme assay, metabolite measurement, DNA analysis. Investigation of parents and family members should also be done particularly in autosomal dominant disorders.

Chromosome Analysis

Indications of chromosome analysis:

1. Child with multiple congenital anomalies and/or dysmorphic features.
2. Two major malformations and/or 3 minor malformations.
3. Pregnant women with advanced maternal age >35 years.
4. Problem in early growth and development including ambiguous genitalia and mental retardation.
5. Fertility problem or recurrent miscarriage (>3), still birth, neonatal death.
6. A first degree relative with known or suspected structural chromosomal abnormality.

DNA analysis is currently available for thalassemia, hemoglobinopathies, hemophilia etc.

Syndrome Diagnosis

It can be done with the help of books like Smiths Recognizable Patterns of Human Malformations (JONES, 2005), Radiology of Syndrome, Metabolic Disorder and Skeletal Dysplasia by Taybi and Lachman or by online computerized database.

Steps in Genetic Counseling

First step in genetic counseling is accurate diagnosis. Diagnosis is done on the basis of history taking and physical examination followed by diagnostic tests for confirmation of clinical diagnosis.

A systematic family history can ascertain the mode of genetic transmission and the risks to family members. It can identify common environmental and behavioral factors that influence the occurrence of disease. Family history can help to prepare a family pedigree. A pedigree provides a graphic depiction of a family's structure and medical history. Antenatal and birth history can give informations regarding exposure to teratogens and radiation.

Physical examination of both affected and apparently unaffected individuals in the family should be done. A complete physical examination from head to toe and relevant anthropometric measurements such as weight, height, head circumference, body proportions, and photographs of dysmorphic child should be taken.

Discuss the Prognosis and Risk of Recurrence

Genetic counselor should interpret the anticipated risk of recurrence of the inherited disorder in the future siblings in a meaningful manner, so that the family can arrive at a rational decision.

Discuss the Options Available to Couple

The options may include the following: no further action, restrict family size, adoption, artificial insemination by donor, ovum donation or preimplantation diagnosis, prenatal diagnosis by USG, CVS (chorionic villous sampling), amniocentesis, cord blood sampling.

For handicap, options are *MTP*, *neonatal treatment* as corrective surgery (should discuss with paediatric surgeon) and *euthenics*, a system of treatment for genetic disorders by modification of the environment to allow the genetically abnormal individual to develop normally and to live a relatively normal life, e.g., diet control in PKU, use of human growth hormone for growth disorder. The other options are gene therapy, enzyme replacement therapy and organ transplantation.

Counseling

Skillful communication is of paramount importance in genetic counseling. It should be carried out in strict privacy.

The counselor should provide the information in simple, non-technical and local language and unbiased manner and in writing. It should cover all aspect of disease, i.e., etiology, diagnosis, treatment, course and prognosis but the depth of explanation should commensurate with educational background of the couple. The risk of recurrence should be explained, if necessary with the help of diagrams.

It is essential that genetic counseling is non-directive, non-judgmental, non-coercive. Non-directiveness is an art of presenting facts without influencing decision. The couple's decision should be respected and supported.

Finally the couple should be informed about support group and follow-up session should be arranged to reinforce information provided in earlier session, to answer new queries, to provide updates and for psychological support to the family.

Prevention of Genetic Disorders

Prenatal Diagnosis

Prenatal diagnosis of genetic disease continues to improve. The genetic or developmental basis for many disorders is emerging, along with increased test accuracy. Two types of tests are available: screening tests and diagnostic procedures. A relevant family history, a positive screening test or a questionable ultrasound examination may lead to consideration for a diagnostic procedure.

Screening Tests

These are done during pregnancy. They can individualize a woman's risk of carrying a fetus with neural tube defect (NTD) or a chromosomal anomaly viz. Down's syndrome, Edward syndrome.

Maternal serum alpha fetoprotein (MSAFP): Measurement between 15 and 22 weeks of gestation screens for NTDs. MSAFP elevated above 2.5 multiples of the median for gestation age occurs in 70 - 85% of fetuses with open spina bifida and 95% of fetuses with anencephaly. Low level of MSAFP is also associated with chromosomal abnormalities.

Triple/Quad panel: A triple screen includes estimation of serum levels of human chorionic gonadotrophin (hCG), unconjugated estriol (UE3) and inhibin; alteration of levels of which are associated with chromosomal abnormalities. In a quad screen, MSAFP is added. In a pregnancy with a fetus with trisomy 21, there are increased levels of hCG and decreased levels of UE3. A serum panel in combination with maternal age can estimate the risk trisomy 21 for an individual woman. In a woman less than 35 years of age, 5% will have a positive serum screen, but 98% of which will not have a fetus with trisomy. Approximately only 70% of fetus with trisomy 21 will have a positive maternal triple screen compared to 80% with a positive quad screen.

Nuchal lucency screening: First trimester ultrasonographic assessment of the fluid collected at the nape of the neck is a sensitive marker of trisomy. An enlarged nuchal lucency can detect 70 - 80% of trisomy and also other structural abnormalities like cardiac defects.

Diagnostic Procedures

Diagnostic tests are considered in women with a positive family history of genetic diseases, a positive screening test or at risk USG.

Chorionic villous sampling (CVS): It should be performed at or after 10 weeks. A sample of placental tissue is obtained through a catheter placed either transcervically or transabdominally under ultrasonographic guidance. CVS provides the earliest possible detection of a genetically abnormal fetus through analysis of trophoblast cells. The transabdominal CVS can be used as late as the third trimester when amniotic fluid is not available or fetal blood sampling cannot be performed. Karyotyping can be done in direct preparations of rapidly dividing cytotrophoblasts or cultured trophoblast cells. Results are available in the former method in 2 days while it takes 8-12 days in the latter method.

Amniocentesis: Amniocentesis is performed as a follow up study after CVS to analyze fetal cells because CVS acquired cells reflect placental constitution and in around 2% cases, it may identify both karyotypically normal and abnormal cells. Around 20 ml of amniotic fluid is removed from around the fetus through a USG guided needle. The removed amount is replaced by the fetus within 24 hours.

The possible complications of CVS and amniocentesis are similar. If done before 10 weeks of gestation a pregnancy loss rate of 1 - 2 % and if done in the second trimester (16 - 20 weeks) the pregnancy loss is 0.5 - 1% can occur. So it is usually performed in the second trimester.

Amniotic fluid can be analyzed for alphafeto protein (AFP), acetylcholine esterase (AChE), bilirubin, and pulmonary surfactant.

Increased levels of AFP along with presence of AChE identify NTDs with more than 98% sensitivity when the fluid sample is not contaminated with fetal blood. The AFP levels are also elevated when the fetus has abdominal wall defects, congenital nephrosis, or intestinal atresia. In cases with isoimmune hemolysis, increased levels of bilirubin in the amniotic fluid indicate RBC destruction. Amniotic fluid bilirubin proportional to the degree of hemolysis is dependent upon the gestational age and can be used to predict fetal well-being (Liley curve). Pulmonary surfactant can be measured once or sequentially to determine the lung maturity (see HMD in Chapter 7).

Fetal cells in amniotic fluid are analyzed for chromosomal and genetic make up. These tests include karyotyping and DNA analysis (direct and indirect DNA studies and DNA sequencing).

Karyotyping abnormalities relating to Chromosomes 13, 18, 21, X and Y can be rapidly detected by using fluorescent in situ hybridization (FISH) with sensitivity in the range of 90%.

DNA analysis helps in diagnosis of Tay-Sachs disease, alpha and beta thalassemia, cystic fibrosis and phenylketonuria.

DNA sequencing for many genetic disorders has revealed that a multitude of different mutations within a gene can result in the same clinical disease. For example cystic fibrosis can result from more than1000 different mutations.

Preimplatation biopsy: In early gestation (eight cell stage of human embryo) one or two cells can be removed without known harm to the embryo. This procedure is helpful in the following situations:

In women who are at risk of X linked recessive disorders, determination of XX containing embryos, FISH can enable transfer of only female embryos through assisted reproduction.

In an elderly woman or when one member of a couple carries a balanced translocation, only those embryos that screen negative for chromosomal abnormality in question is transferred.

Free fetal DNA analysis in maternal circulation: It is a non-invasive method; hence it would eliminate the potential procedure related loss of normal pregnancy. Analysis of free fetal DNA which is present in large quantities in the maternal circulation is likely to be a beneficial procedure than study of fetal cells in maternal circulation because of its limited number.

It needs mention that when a significant malformation or a genetic disease is diagnosed prenatally, the information gives the obstetrician and the pediatrician time to educate the parents, discuss the options, and establish an initial neonatal treatment plan before delivery of the infant.

Carrier Screening

Carrier screening assist in detection of carrier state of a genetic disease and thereby counselling for mate selection or procreation thereby limiting the spread of the genetic disorder. The carrier state of a large number of autosomal recessive and X linked recessive disorders has been detected by carrier screening. Few examples are high serum levels enzyme creatinine phospho-kinase in female carriers, relatively low levels of enzyme G6PD in erythrocytes in female carriers and high levels of HbA2 levels in carriers of Beta thalassemia trait.

Metabolic Screening

In the western countries, newborn infants are routinely screened for some inborn errors of metabolism. It is important for early detection of the metabolic disorders in the newborn period and thereby early intervention to prevent or minimize the handicaps arising out of it. Few examples of preventable metabolic disorders are galactosemia, phenylketonuria, Tyrosinosis and congenital hypothyroidism.

Prevention of Neural Tube Defects (NTD)

It is now proved beyond doubt that use of folic acid prior to conception prevents NTD. It is recommended that all expectant mothers should consume about 0.4 mg of folic acid daily to prevent first occurrence of NTD. To prevent recurrence the dose of folic acid is 4 mg/day. It should be started one month prior to and continued for 3 months after conception. Food fortification with folic acid has also been considered.

Suggested Reading

1. Nelson Textbook of Pediatrics, 18th Edition, Vol. 1, 2008, 485-525, 786-89.
2. Practical Pediatric Problems edited by James H. Hutchinson and Forrester Cockburn 6th edition, 1986. Published by P G Publishing Pte Ltd. New Delhi, Singapore, Hong Kong.
3. Forfar and Arniel's Textbook of Pediatrics, 6th Ed, 438-439.
4. Phadke SR Genetic Counseling, Indian J. Pediatrics 2004; 71: 151-156.

19

Common Pediatric Surgical Problems

OUTLINES

Cleft Lip and Palate

Clefts of lip, alveolus and hard and soft palate are the most common congenital abnormalities of the orofacial structures. They frequently occur as isolated deformities but may be associated with other congenital anomalies, particularly congenital heart disease.

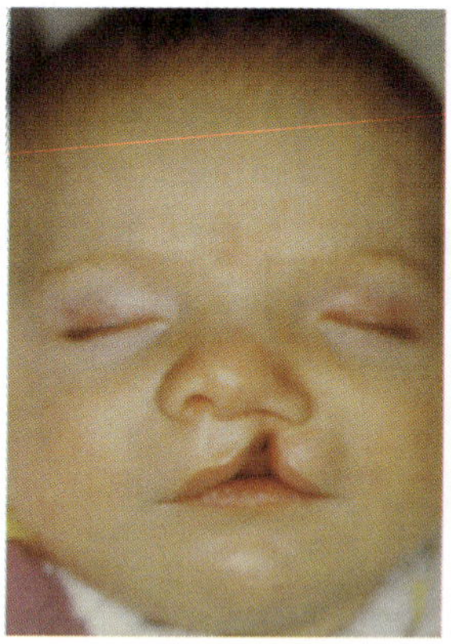

Fig. 19.1: Cleft lip

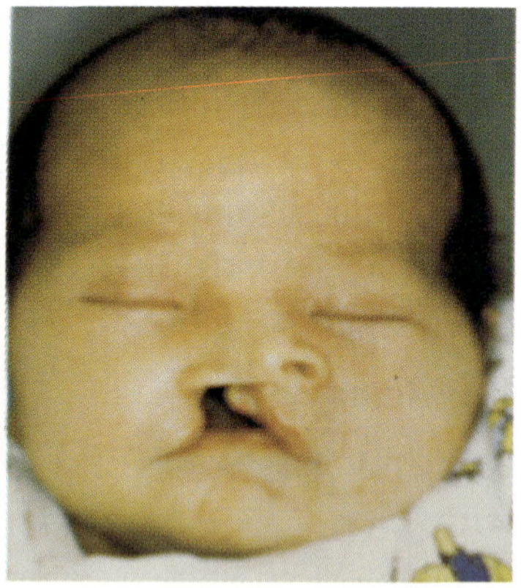

Fig. 19.2: Unilateral cleft lip and palate

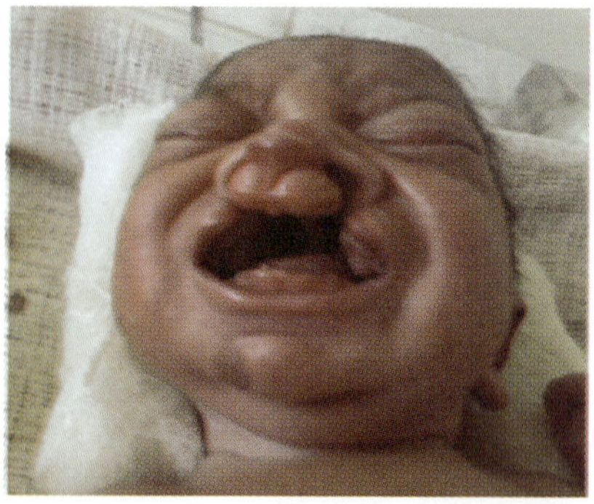

Fig. 19.3: Bilateral cleft lip and palate

Several distinct subgroups exist with difference in incidence. They are cleft lip alone (15%), cleft lip and palate (45%) and isolated cleft palate (40%). Cleft lip and palate predominates in males, whereas cleft palate alone appears more common in females. Cleft lip may be unilateral or bilateral. When unilateral, the deformity affects the left side in 60% cases.

Etiology

Both cleft lip palate and isolated cleft palate have a genetic predisposition and environmental component. A family history of cleft lip and palate in the first degree relative increases the risk to 1 in 25 live births. However, genetic predisposition is more significant in cleft lip palate. Environmental factors exert a greater influence in isolated cleft palate. The environmental factors implicated are maternal epilepsy and drugs, e.g., steroids, diazepam and phenytoin. The beneficial affect of antenatal folic acid supplementation to prevent clefts still remain equivocal. Pierre Robin syndrome which comprises isolated cleft palate, retrognathia and glossoptosis, is the most common associated sequence with cleft palate. It is associated with respiratory difficulty and feeding difficulty in the neonatal period.

Management

An antenatal diagnosis of cleft lip, unilateral or bilateral is possible by USG after 18 weeks of gestation. Isolated cleft palate cannot be diagnosed antenatally. When diagnosis is confirmed antenatally, the mother needs counseling.

Problems Immediately After Birth

Problems may occur with feeding the baby. The baby with Pierre Robin syndrome may have respiratory difficulty. Many mothers can successfully breast feed if the cleft is incomplete and confined to the lip. In others expressed breast milk can be fed with a spoon or dropper. Feeding plates, constructed from a dental impression of the upper jaw is rarely necessary.

The baby with Pierre Robin syndrome should be nursed in the prone position to prevent intermittent airway obstruction. More severe and persistent airway obstruction can be managed by retained nasopharyngeal intubation to maintain the airway. Surgical adhesion of the tongue to the lower lip is an alternative measure but less commonly practised.

Timing of Repair

Cleft lip repair is commonly performed between 3–6 months of age and cleft palate repair is frequently performed between 6 and 18 months.

Choanal Atresia

Choanal atresia consists of a bony or membranous septum between the nose and the pharynx. It may be unilateral or bilateral. In most cases the atresia is a combination of membranous and bony septum. Nearly 50% of affected infants have other congenital anomalies, which is more common in bilateral defects.

Clinical Manifestations

With unilateral atresia, the infant may be asymptomatic until the first upper respiratory infection when the diagnosis may be suggested by persistent nasal obstruction on one side. Bilateral choanal atresia is usually diagnosed in the neonatal period. The neonate has a variable ability for mouth breathing. Those who have difficulty in mouth breathing, make vigorous attempts to breathe and often develops cyanosis which is relieved on crying. This occurs cyclically. Those who are able to breathe through their mouths experience difficulty in sucking, swallowing and become cyanotic when they attempt to feed.

The diagnosis is confirmed by inability to pass a firm catheter through each nostril 3–4 cm into the nasopharynx. The anatomy is best evaluated by using high resolution CT.

Treatment

The initial step is to establish an oral airway and the neonate fed with a orogastric tube. If the infant do not have any other serious medical problem, transnasal repair is done in the neonatal period. A stent is however kept for weeks after repair to prevent closure or stenosis. An infant with associated life threatening problems needs a tracheostomy.

The surgical repair of unilateral atresia may be deferred for several years. In both unilateral and bilateral atresia restenosis is common. Reoperation or dilatation is commonly required. Mitomycin C has been used to help prevent the development of granulation tissue and stenosis.

Congenital Esophageal Atresia

Congenital esophageal atresia is usually associated with a tracheo esophageal fistula (TEF). There are five different types (Fig. 19.4). The most common type is the one in which the lower segment of esophagus communicates with the trachea, the upper segment being blind (87%).

It is important to diagnose this condition within 48 hours of birth because subsequent surgical correction is the only hope of survival.

Clinical Manifestations

An esophageal atresia should be suspected in all cases with hydramnios which is present in 50% of cases with atresia. Neonates with atresia presents with excessive secretions at birth and need repeated suctioning during resuscitation. There is excessive and continuous frothing from the mouth. In such neonates a nasogastric tube should be introduced before feeding is started.

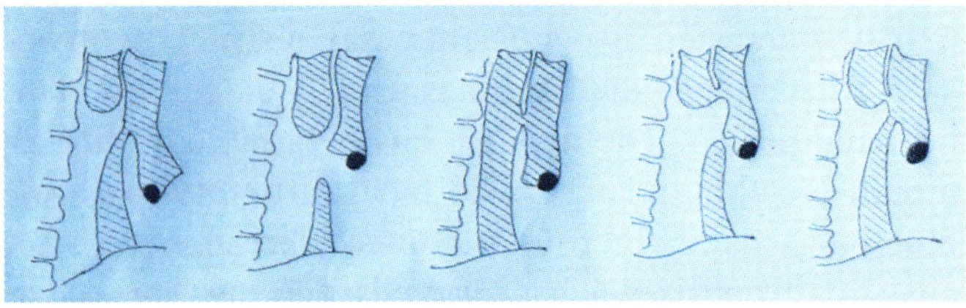

A (87 %) B (8 %) C (4 %) D (< 1 %) E (< 1 %)

Fig. 19.4: Different types of esophageal atresia

Type A: Blind upper segment with TEF, **Type B:** Blind upper and lower segments with no TEF, **Type C:** H type, **Type D:** Lower segment blind with TEF, **Type E:** TEF with both upper and lower segment.

The diagnosis is virtually certain if the tube cannot be introduced beyond 8–10 cm. Feeding leads to attacks of coughing and cyanosis and aspiration pneumonia.

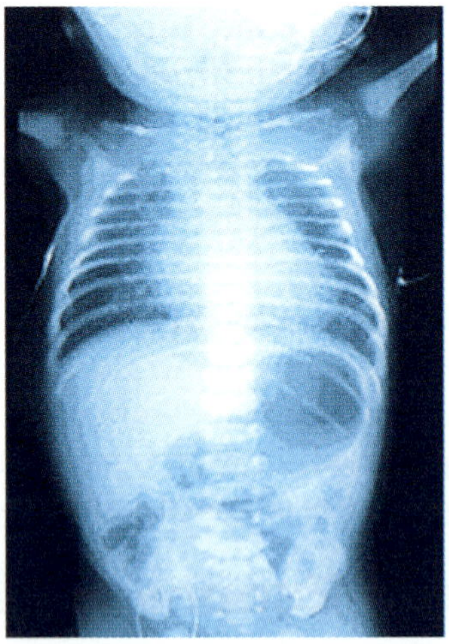

Fig. 19.5: X-ray chest and abdomen showing feeding tube unable to move beyond and upper esophageal pouch with air in stomach (esophageal atresia with TEF)

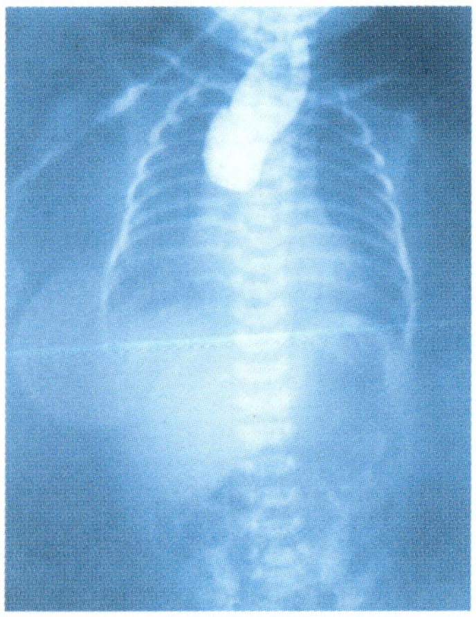

Fig. 19.6: Contrast medium filled pouch and gas in the stomach

Radiological confirmation can be done on a lateral chest X-ray which shows a lucent proximal pouch that may displace the trachea anteriorly. Presence of bowel gas indicates a fistula connecting the distal segment to the trachea. In doubtful cases, air (preferable) or a small amount of contrast medium can be injected through the nasogastric tube.

Treatment

Corrective surgery is normally performed shortly after the diagnosis is made. Preoperative management consists of nil orally, IV fluid, continuous oral suction to avoid aspiration.

Prognosis

Following recovery from the immediate post-operative period, the long-term prognosis is excellent. The post-operative complications include pneumonia and leakage from the anastomosis.

Congenital Hypertrophic Pyloric Stenosis

Congenital hypertrophic pyloric stenosis is a condition in which there is failure of the pylorus to relax leading to muscular hypertrophy. The incidence is approximately 3 cases per 1000 births. It is common in males, the ratio being male: female is equal to 4 : 1. There seems to be a familial association. In such families, the mother is found to be affected in 50% of cases. Ten percent of male siblings and 2% of female siblings are affected.

The classical pathological feature is that the musculature of the pylorus and adjacent antrum is grossly

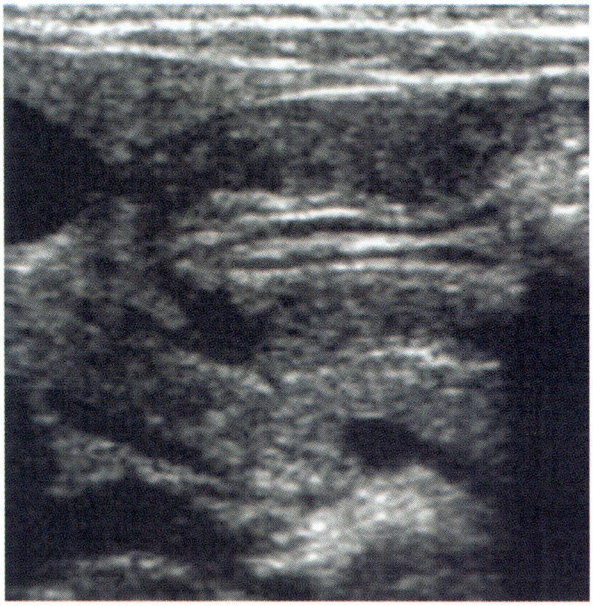

Fig. 19.7: USG longitudinal section of pylorus showing thickened circular muscles, elongated pyloric canal and narrow pyloric canal

hypertrophied, the hypertrophy being maximum in the pylorus. The mucosa is compressed such that only a probe can be inserted.

Clinical Manifestations

The most commonly affected is the first born male child. The condition most commonly presents at 4 weeks after birth. It may however present as early as 3rd week and rarely as late as 7th. Vomiting is the presenting symptom which becomes forcible and projectile after 2–3 days of onset. The vomitus contains milk without bile. Immediately after vomiting the child is hungry. There is significant weight loss and the infant rapidly becomes emaciated and dehydrated.

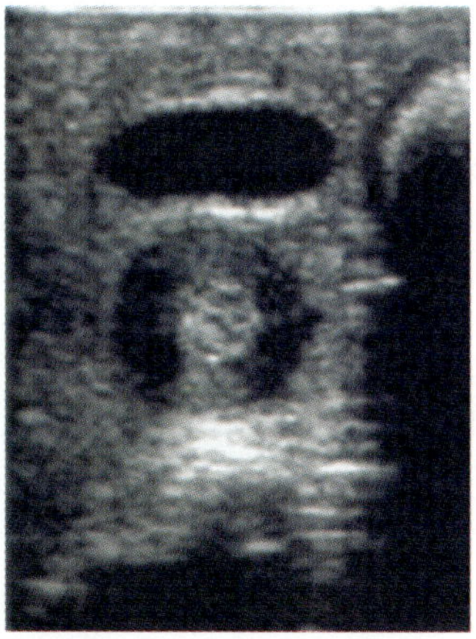

Fig. 19.8: USG transverse section of pylorus showing target sign

Diagnosis can be made with a test feed. Feeding produces characteristic peristalsis that can be seen to pass across the upper abdomen from left to right. At the same time, the abdomen is palpated to detect a lump.

Ultrasonography is the investigation of choice as it can detect the classical features of the pyloric canal.

The common condition which needs to be differentiated includes gastroesophageal reflux, feeding problems, raised intracranial pressure and urinary tract infection. Duodenal atresia and intestinal obstruction is normally not confused because of the absence of bile in the vomitus.

Treatment

The first step is correction of the metabolic abnormalities. The child should be rehydrated with dextrose-saline- and potassium. There is no role of conservative treatment because with surgery recovery is virtually 100%. The surgical procedure of choice is Ramstedt's operation.

The nasogastric tube can be removed after the operation. Feeding can be commenced on the morning after the operation.

Congenital Umbilical Hernia

A congenital umbilical hernia is presumed to be due to intrauterine epithelisation of a small exomphalos. A fully developed umbilical hernia is rarely present at birth. It gradually develops during early part of infancy. The hernia is partially the result of failure of the round ligament (obliterated umbilical vein) to cross the umbilical ring and partially from the absence of Richet fascia.

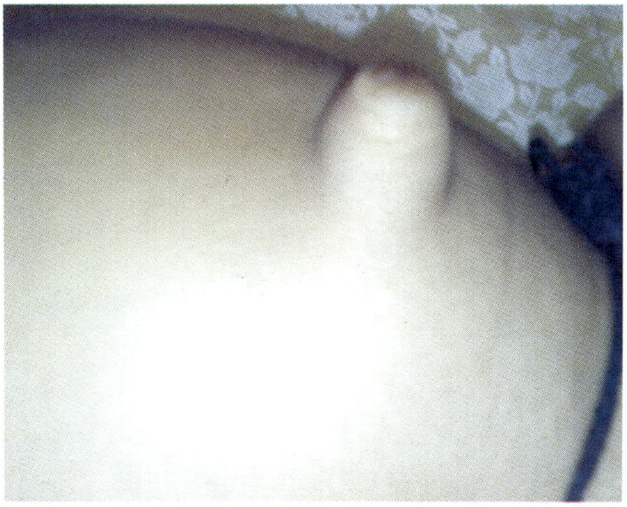

Fig. 19.9: Umbilical hernia

The hernia is often symptomless but increases in size on crying and assumes a classical conical shape. Obstruction and strangulation is extremely uncommon below the age of 3 years.

Treatment

Most umbilical hernias that appear before the age of 6 months disappear spontaneously by one year of age. Even large hernias (5–6 cm in all dimensions) have been known to disappear by 5–6 years age. Strangulation is extremely rare. Strapping is ineffective. Surgery is indicated when the hernia persist upto the age of 4–5 years, causes symptoms, strangulation or becomes progressively larger after the age of 1–2 years.

Exomphalos (Omphalocele)

Exomphalos or omphalocele is a condition in which the abdominal contents protrude out through the umbilicus. It results due to failure of all or part of the midgut to return to the coelom during early fetal life. It may be divided into those with a fascial defect less than or greater than 4 cm. In the smaller defect there may be a small loop of intestine. In the large defects, the liver, spleen, stomach, pancreas, colon or bladder may be seen through the covering membrane. The covering membrane is thin but consists of two layers–outer layer of amniotic membrane and an inner layer of peritoneum. The umbilical cord joins the hernia sac at some point. Occasionally the sac may rupture. Exomphalos may be associated with congenital anomalies of the other systems. A large exomphalos may be associated with respiratory distress.

Exomphalos needs immediate surgical repair before infection has taken place and before the tissues have been damaged by drying. Saline soaked sterile dressings should be applied immediately to prevent drying. In preterm infants with a large intact sac or infants when an early major operation is not possible, the intact sac is painted with a desiccating antiseptic solution (1% mercurochrome). This helps in epithelialisation over the sac followed by growth of granulation tissue from the periphery. The subsequent ventral hernia is repaired later. A synthetic material may be used to cover the viscera if the sac has ruptured or if excessive mobilization of skin would be necessary to cover the mass and its intact sac.

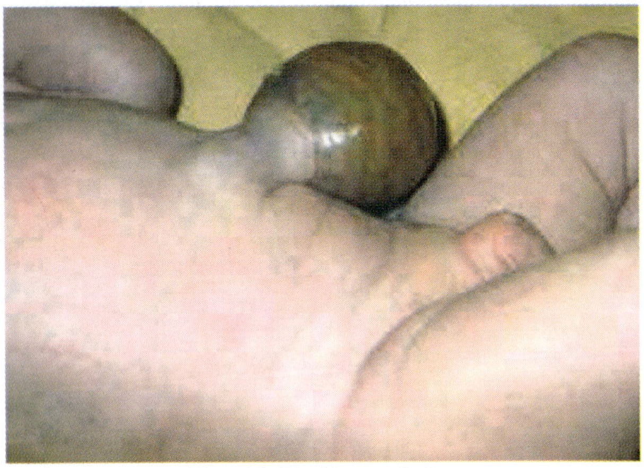

Fig. 19.10: Exomphalos

Gastroschisis

Gastroschisis is a condition where the abdominal contents herniated out through the abdominal wall lateral to the umbilical cord. The abdominal wall defect is usually less than 5 cm and herniated viscera usually consist of colon and small intestine not covered with peritoneal sac. The protruded intestinal loops may have associated atresia or stenosis. There are no associated congenital malformations as in case of exomphalos.

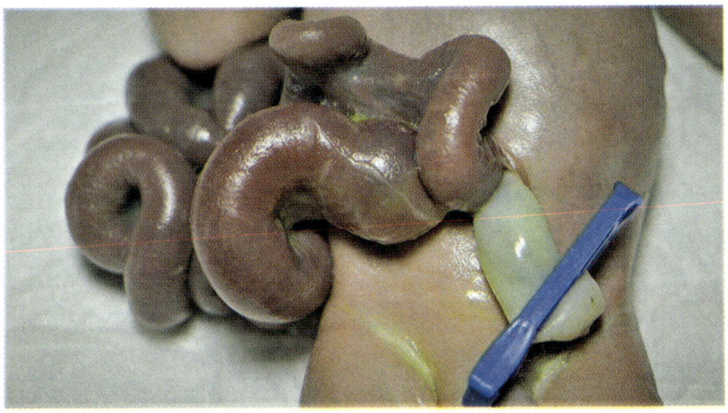

Fig. 19.11: Gastroschisis

The exposed intestines should be covered with warm saline soaked gauze, an IV drip and nasogastric aspiration started soon after birth. Because of the absence of the sac, the primary closure should be attempted as an emergency procedure. These patients require pre and post operative intensive medical care and parenteral nutrition.

Congenital Diaphragmatic Hernia

It is a neonatal emergency. There is herniation of abdominal contents through the diaphragm. Most often the hernia occurs through the posterolateral part of the diaphragm usually on the left side. Less frequently the hernia may occur through the anterolateral or retrosternal diaphragm. It is a condition amenable to surgical repair. Hence an early recognition is important.

The acute emergency that arises in great majority of infants is due to the lungs being prevented from expanding by the intestines, spleen and other abdominal organs. Further, the entry of air into the intestine after birth causes the heart to be displaced and the opposite lung to be embarrassed.

Clinical Manifestations

There is rapidly increasing dyspnea and cyanosis which may be further aggravated by bag and mask ventilation during resuscitation. On examination, the heart may be found on the right side, simulating dextrocardia. Percussion note may be dull or tympanitic depending on the intestinal contents fluid or gas. On auscultation, diminished breath sounds, or bowel sounds may be heard. The abdomen

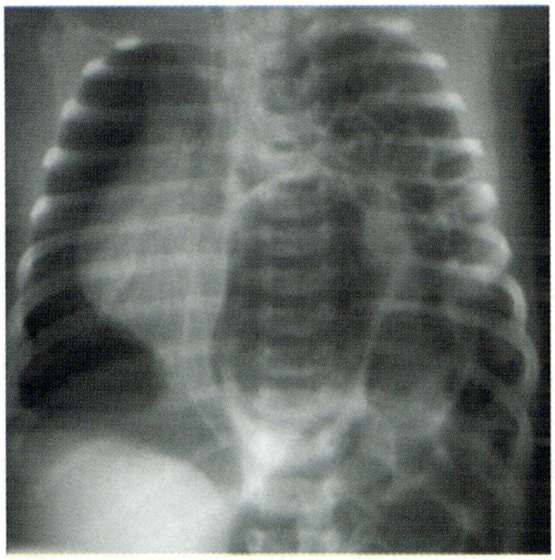

Fig. 19.12: X-ray showing features of diaphragmatic hernia

may be scaphoid. When the hernia occur retrosternally, there is no neonatal emergency. The symptoms have a later onset with respiratory problems. The plain X-ray findings include shifting of the heart and mediastinum to the opposite side, absence of the diaphragm and presence of a non-homogenous opacity on the same side of the hemithorax.

The diagnosis can be confirmed by a plain X-ray. However, a barium meal X-ray may be required in case of a retrosternal type because the X-ray finding is puzzling in such cases.

Management

No bag and mask ventilation should be done for a baby with suspected diaphragmatic hernia. If neonate is asphyxiated, intubation and bag and tube ventilation should be used.

A large diameter NG tube should be inserted and left open ended to prevent upper intestinal gaseous distension

Surgery should be performed promptly after stabilization. It consists of repair of the defect.

Inguinal Hernia

Inguinal hernias in children are almost always indirect and due to a patent processus vaginalis. They are frequently seen in male infants especially when born preterm. Around 15% of inguinal hernias are bilateral.

Clinical Manifestations

The common presentation is appearance of an intermittent swelling in the groin or scrotum on crying or straining. Some inguinal hernias present as a firm, tender lump in the groin or scrotum due to obstruction at the external ring. The infant may be vomiting and irritable.

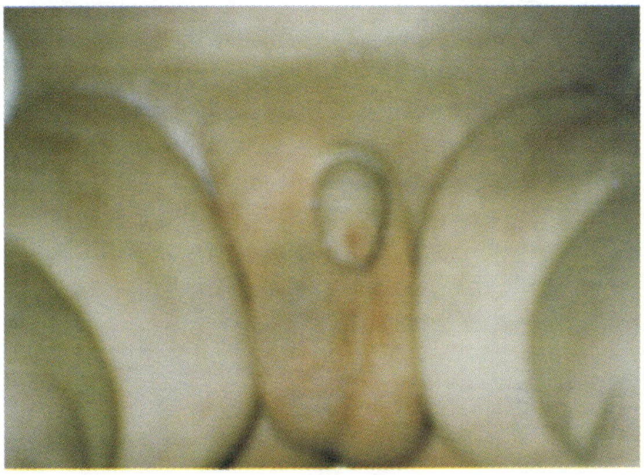

Fig. 19.13: Inguinal hernia (right side)

Treatment

In infants, inguinal hernias should be repaired promptly to prevent strangulation. Incarcerated hernias can be reduced by gentle pressure. Surgery is delayed for 24–48 hours to allow resolution of edema. If reduction is impossible emergency surgery is indicated to prevent strangulation of bowel (or ovary) and damage to the testis.

Hydrocele

Hydrocele is collection of fluid around the testis. It results from tracking down of peritoneal fluid through a patent processus vaginalis. Hydroceles may be unilateral or bilateral, asymptomatic, nontender scrotal swelling. They may be tense or lax but typically transilluminate.

The majority of hydrocele spontaneously resolves. Surgery is recommended if the hydrocele persists beyond 2 years of age.

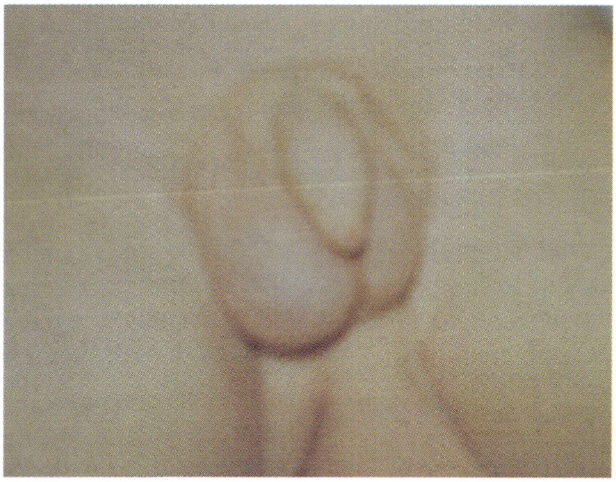

Fig. 19.14: Figure showing hydrocele (right side)

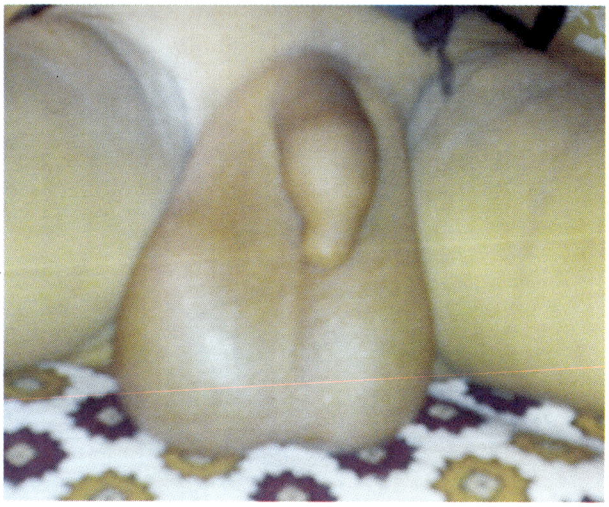

Fig. 19.15: Figure showing bilateral hydrocele

Undescended Testis

The testis may be retractile, ectopic or undescended. The retractile testis is typically present in the scrotum in early infancy and can be manipulated into the bottom without tension but tends to be pulled up by the cremasteric muscle. With time the testis resides permanently in the scrotum. However, rarely, the testis subsequently ascends into the inguinal canal. An ectopic testis lies outside its normal line of descend; most often in the perineum or femoral triangle. An undescended testis may be palpable in the groin or at the neck of the scrotum or it may be impalpable if absent or located in the abdomen or the inguinal canal.

Undescended testis occurs when the testis has been arrested along its normal pathway of descent. At birth about 3% of term male infants have unilateral or bilateral undescended testes but by 3 months of age this figure goes down to 1% and it changes little thereafter. The incidence is higher in preterm infants because the testis descends through the inguinal canal during the last trimester of pregnancy.

Investigation

Laparoscopy is the optimum investigation for the impalpable testis. USG is helpful but has limited role in detecting inguinal testis in obese boys. In case of bilateral impalpable testes, the presence of testicular tissue can be confirmed by human chorionic gonadotrophin stimulation test. There is rise of serum testosterone in response to intramuscular human chorionic gonadotrophin.

Treatment

The current recommendation is that the testis should be brought down before one year of age in order to improve fertility and reduce chance of testicular malignancy. To optimize spermatogenesis, the testis needs to be in the scrotum below the body temperature at a young age. The undescended testes are histologically abnormal and are at increased risk of malignancy. The greatest risk is with bilateral intra-abdominal testes.

Phimosis and Paraphimosis

Phimosis refers to inability to retract the prepuce. Normally at birth, the foreskin is adherent to the surface of the glans penis. These adhesions separate spontaneously with time allowing the foreskin to become retractile. At one year age, approximately 50% of boys have a non-retractile foreskin, by 4 years it declines to 10% and by 16 years to 1%. Physiological ballooning of a non-retractile foreskin can occur during micturition. There may be accumulation epithelial debris under the infantile prepuce. It is not pathologic and do not require surgical treatment. Phimosis may be also pathologic in older boys resulting from inflammation and scarring at the tip of the foreskin. A cicatricial scar may also result from forceful retraction of the prepuce on one or more occasions preventing subsequent retraction of the foreskin.

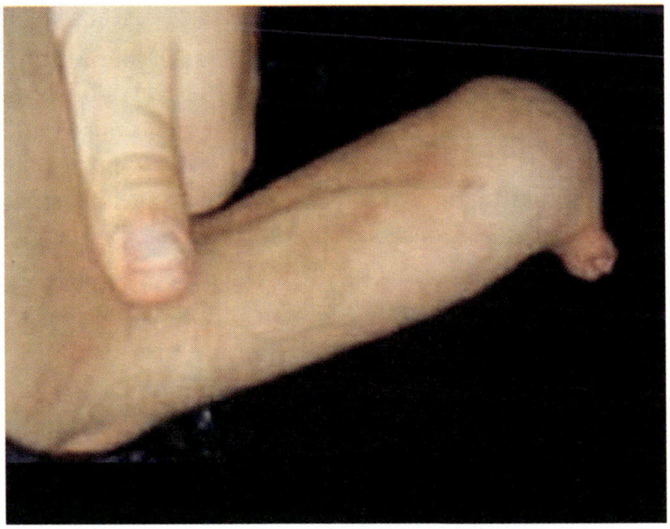

Fig. 19.16: Figure showing phimosis

In boys with persistent physiologic or pathologic phimosis, application of a corticosteroid cream to the foreskin three times daily for one month loosens the phimotic ring in around 70% cases. If there is ballooning during micturition or phimosis exist beyond 10 years age, circumcision is indicated. The other indications of circumcision are recurrent balanoposthitis and recurrent urinary tract infection.

Paraphimosis is a condition when the foreskin is retracted behind the coronal sulcus and the prepuce cannot be pulled back over the glans. There is edema due to venous stasis in the retracted foreskin which results in pain and inability to reduce the foreskin.

Treatment includes lubrication of the foreskin and glans and compressing the glans to retract the prepuce beyond the coronal sulcus. In rare cases emergency circumcision may be indicated.

Hypospadias

Hypospadias is a condition characterized by a ventral urethral meatus, a hooded foreskin and a variable degree of chordae (a ventral curvature of the penis most apparent on erection). In most cases, the urethra open just proximal to the glans penis, but in severe cases it may be on the penile shaft or in the perineum. Severe forms may be associated with additional genitourinary abnormalities and intersex disorders.

Glandular hypospadius may be a cosmetic concern but proximal varieties impair function. Surgical correction should be undertaken before 2 years of age.

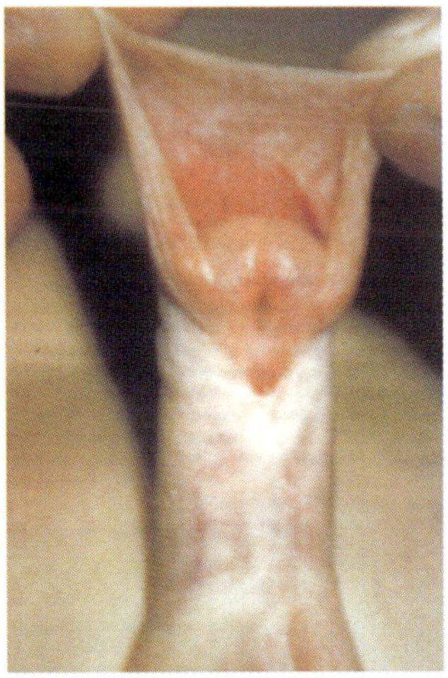

Fig. 19.17: Figure showing hypospadias

Imperforate Anus

Imperforate anus is divided into two main groups–high and low depending on whether the termination of the bowel is above or below the pelvic floor. The low abnormalities include a covered anus, ectopic anus, anal stenosis and membranous anal stenosis. The high abnormalities include anorectal agenesis, rectal atresia and cloaca.

The low abnormalities are easy to diagnose and relatively simple to treat and outlook is good. The high varieties have a fistula into the urinary tract or vagina together with a defect in the pelvic floor and are difficult to treat and post-operative function tends to be poor.

All newborns at birth should be examined for the presence of the anus. This will help early detection of imperforate anus. Later, with high abnormalities the infant may present with passage of meconium/stool through the urethra or vagina (in females).

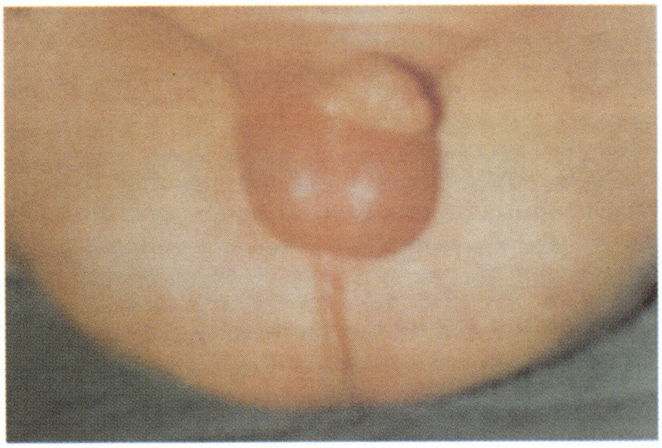

Fig. 19.18: Figure showing imperforate anus

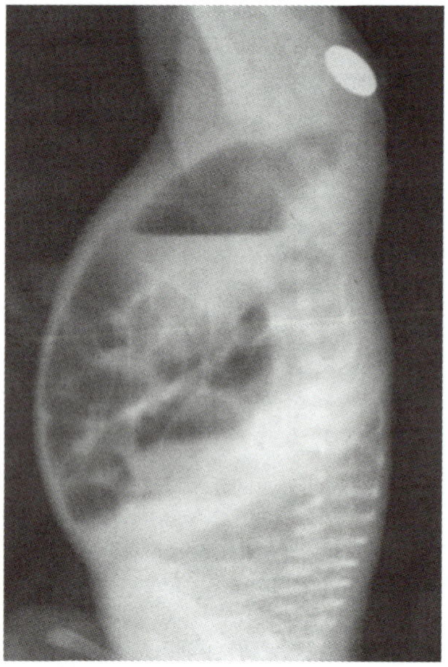

Fig 19.19: Invertogram showing a high type of imperforate anus

Radiological examination can be done 24 hours after birth when sufficient air may have collected in the large intestine. A lateral prone radiograph with a metal indicator strapped to the site of the anus can determine the distance between the blind end of the rectum and the indicator. If the distance is more than 2.5 cm, the abnormality is of the high type.

Treatment

Low abnormalities can be treated soon after birth. High or complex abnormalities need a preliminary colostomy followed by detailed investigations; a reconstructive surgery at a few months of age.

Hirschsprung Disease

Hirschsprung disease is a condition caused by absence of ganglia in the myenteric plexus of the intestinal wall usually of the distal hind gut. This is believed to result from a failure of migration of neuroblasts into the gut from the vagal nerve trunks at the end of the first trimester of fetal life.

The loss of ganglion cells extends for a variable distance above the anorectal junction. The most common part to be involved is the rectum and lower sigmoid. Involvement may also be in the form of short segments in the lower rectum. Involvement of the whole intestine has also been reported. It should be noted that the severity of symptoms is not always consistent with the length of the intestinal segment involved and may be related to the number of acetylcholinesterase positive nerve fibres.

The absence of the ganglion cells gives rise to a contracted non-peristaltic segment with a dilated hypertrophied segment of normal colon above it.

Clinical Manifestations

The clinical manifestations vary from acute intestinal obstruction in the neonates to chronic constipation in later life.

In the neonates, delayed passage of meconium beyond first 24 hours of life together with abdominal distension following feeds and bilious vomiting are features to suspect Hirschsprung disease. It is often complicated with enterocolitis, which may result in perforation and septicemia and a high mortality.

In the first few weeks of life, the complain may be chronic constipation. The classic picture of gross abdominal distension, chronic constipation and failure to thrive is becoming rare due to increasing awareness of the condition. A per rectal examination reveals an empty rectum and passage of stool and gas giving temporary relief.

Beyond infancy, there may be a series of incomplete large bowel obstruction characterized by acute episodes of abdominal distension. There is no absolute constipation. Severe diarrhoea may occur due to development of ulcerating colitis with accompanying abdominal distension.

Severe constipation without soiling in an otherwise healthy child can be caused by a shorter spastic segment. Fecal soiling is not usually a feature of this condition.

Laboratory Diagnosis

A *plain X-ray* in erect and supine position can give the following informations: distended large and small intestine loops with fluid levels consistent with low intestinal obstruction, intramural gas and free peritoneal gas indicating enterocolitis and perforation respectively.

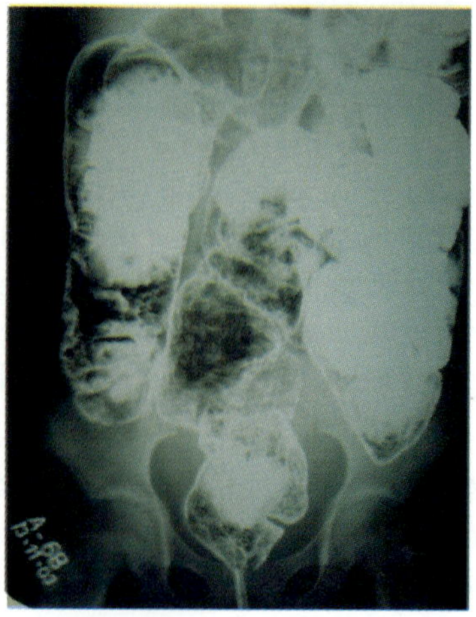

Fig. 19.20: Barium enema with dilated colon and conical end

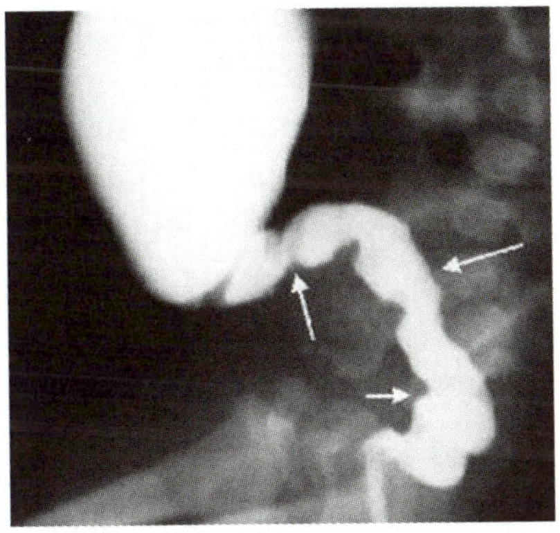

Fig. 19.21: Barium enema showing the spastic segment

An *enema* using a water soluble contrast medium will confirm the diagnosis and indicate the length and site of the involved intestine. The important positive findings include coning down of the transitional zone, dilated colon irregularity of the mucosa and narrow spastic distal segment.

Rectal biopsy is confirmatory with histological demonstration of aganglionosis and hypertrophic nerve fibres in the nerve plexus.

Anorectal manometry is a useful screening test in a child with constipation who is otherwise fit.

Treatment

The treatment is surgical repair. The operative options are to perform a definitive procedure as soon as the diagnosis is established or perform a temporary colostomy and wait until the infant is 6–12 months old to perform the definitive repair.

Acute Intussusception

Acute intussusception is a condition in which one portion of the gut becomes invaginated within an immediately adjacent segment. The invagination is invariably proximal into distal bowel.

Etiology

The condition is common in children with a peak incidence at 3–9 months. Most of the cases occur without a cause (idiopathic). An associated illness such as gastroenteritis or urinary tract infection is found in 30% cases. It is believed that hyperplasia of the Peyer's patches in terminal ileum, secondary to weaning may be the initiating event. The peak incidence is in spring and summer. It may be related to infection by pathogens like adenovirus or rotavirus.

In the older children intussusception is associated with a lead point like Meckel's diverticulum, polyp, intestinal duplication, Henoch-Schönlein purpura or the appendix.

Anatomically intussusception may be defined as ileo ileal, ileocecal and ileocolic depending on the site and extent of invagination. The ileocolic is the most common variety.

Clinical Manifestations

The clinical presentation of intussusception is classical. An otherwise healthy, well male child of 3–9 months age, develops sudden onset of screaming associated with drawing up of the legs. The attacks last for a few minutes recur every 15 minutes and become progressively severe. During attacks, the child has facial pallor while between episodes the child is listless and drawn. Vomiting may or may not occur at the outset but becomes conspicuous with time. Initially, there is passage of normal stool followed by stools containing blood and mucus described as red currant jelly stools.

Examination should be done between episodes of pain without disturbing the child. The abdomen is not distended. A lump may be felt that hardens on palpation in about 50–60% cases. There may be an associated feeling of emptiness in the right iliac fossa (sign of Dance). On rectal examination, blood stained mucus may be found in the finger. Occasionally, in extensive ileocolic or colocolic intussusception, the apex may be palpable or even may protrude from the anus.

If the condition is left untreated, pain will become continuous. There will be profound vomiting and abdominal distension. Ultimately death occurs from small intestinal obstruction or peritonitis secondary to gangrene.

Laboratory Diagnosis

A plain X-ray of abdomen usually reveals evidence of small or large bowel obstruction with absent cecal gas shadow and crescent sign in ileoileal or ileocolic cases. A barium enema shows 'claw sign' in ileocolic or colocolic types. Equivocal cases of ileoileal type may be further evaluated by USG which should show the presence of a small intestinal mass.

Treatment

Treatment consist of hydrostatic reduction and operative management when the former fails or is contraindicated. However, immediately on diagnosis the child should be put nil per oral, nasogastric suction and intravenous fluid.

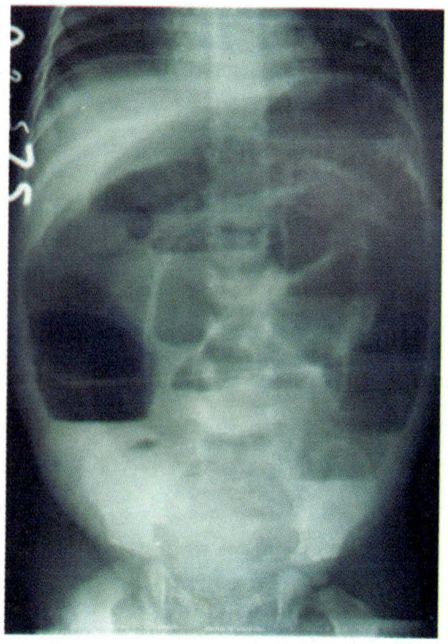

Fig. 19.22: Multiple air fluid levels as in intestinal obstruction

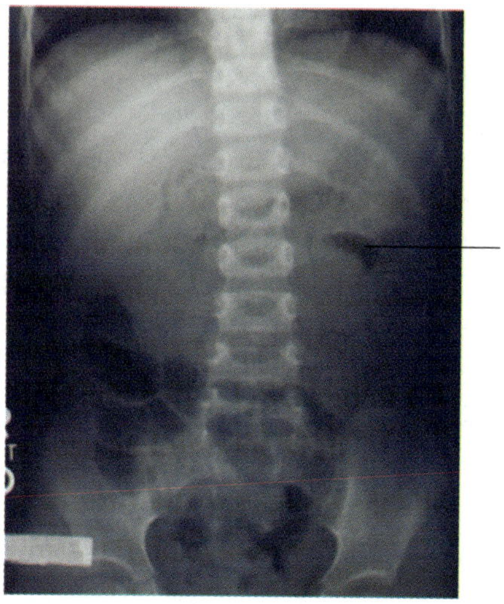

Fig. 19.23: 'Crescent sign' in intussusception

Acute Appendicitis

Inflammation of the vermiform appendix results in the clinical syndrome of acute appendicitis. Acute appendicitis is relatively rare in infants, and becomes increasingly common in childhood and early adult life. It is the most common cause of an acute abdomen in young adults. Incidence is equal in both sexes before puberty. Later the incidence increases in males.

Etiology

The exact etiology is not known. Decreased dietary fibre and increased consumption of refined carbohydrates are considered as important. Appendicitis is associated with bacterial proliferation within the appendix but no single organism is found to be responsible. A mixed growth of aerobic and anaerobic organism is usually found. The initiating event causing bacterial proliferation is not established. Obstruction of the lumen by fecolith or stricture has been observed in majority of cases. Intestinal parasites, particularly oxyuris vermicularis (pin worm) can proliferate in the appendix and occlude the lumen.

Clinical Manifestations

Symptoms start with poorly localized colicky abdominal pain. The pain is frequently first noticed in the periumbilical region. It is associated with anorexia, nausea and usually one or two episodes of vomiting which follow the onset of pain. About one third of children with appendicitis have a similar history in the first degree relative.

With the progression of inflammation pain becomes intense and localized to the iliac fossa. Coughing and sudden movement exacerbates the pain. An inflamed appendix in the pelvis may cause suprapubic discomfort and tenesmus. Tenderness can be elicited only on rectal examination. If the inflamed appendix is in contact with the bladder the child may complain of increased frequency of micturation. After about six hours of onset of pain, there is mild fever with corresponding increase in pulse rate. A temperature greater than 38.5°C suggests other causes, e.g., mesenteric adenitis. In around 20% cases there is no fever.

Acute obstructive appendicitis is characterized by an abrupt onset, generalized abdominal pain, vomiting resembling acute intestinal obstruction. These cases require urgent surgery to prevent perforation.

The cardinal signs include low grade pyrexia, localized abdominal tenderness, muscle guarding and rebound tenderness. Superficial palpation will detect the maximum point of tenderness muscle guarding in the right iliac fossa (McBurney's point). Rebound tenderness can be elicited at this point by asking the child to cough or by gentle percussion. Deep palpation of the left iliac fossa may cause pain in the right iliac fossa (Roving's sign). If the inflamed appendix lies on the psoas muscle, the patient will lie with the right hip flexed for relief of pain (Psoas sign). If the inflamed appendix is in contact with the obturator internus, flexon and internal rotation of the hip will cause pain in the hypogastrium (Obturator test).There may be cutaneous hyperesthesia over the iliac fossa.

In case, the appendix is retrocecal in position, deep tenderness is present in the loin and psoas test is positive.

Rarely the inflamed appendix may lie behind the terminal ileum. The diagnosis is difficult because the pain may not shift, there is diarrhoea and retching. Tenderness, if any is illdefined, though it may be present immediately to the right of the umbilicus.

Diagnosis of appendicitis in children below 3 years is usually delayed because a proper history cannot be obtained. Therefore the incidence of perforation and post-operative morbidity is high. Diffuse peritonitis can develop due to the underdeveloped greater omentum which is unable to localize the inflammation.

The diagnosis of acute appendicitis is essentially clinical. The most widely used scoring system is the Alvarado score. A score of 7 or more is strongly predictive of acute appendicitis.

Table 19.1 : The Alvarado score

Symptoms	*Score*
Migratory RIF* pain	1
Anorexia	1
Nausea and vomiting	1
Signs	
Tenderness (RIF)	2
Rebound tenderness	1
Elevated temperature	1
Laboratory	
Leucocytosis	2
Shift to left (segmented neutrophils)	1
Total	10

* RIF: right iliac fossa.

Laboratory Diagnosis

In a patient with an unequivocal score (5–6) an abdominal USG or a contrast enhanced CT examination can help in confirmation. Abdominal USG is more helpful in children. Both will show a distended, edematous appendix, presence of lumen obstruction (e.g. by a fecolith), intramural gas (in CT scan).

Treatment

The treatment of appendicitis is appendicectomy. There should not be unnecessary delay in surgery especially in the younger age group to prevent perforation and peritonitis. However, a short period of preoperative preparation helps in the high risk group. The child should be started on IV fluids to maintain a normal urine output and intravenous antibiotics covering gram positive and gram negative organisms as well as anerobics. Pyrexia should be treated with paracetamol.

However, when obstructive appendicitis is diagnosed, operation should not be deferred longer than it takes to optimize the patient's condition.

Congenital Talipes Equinovarus (CTEV)

Congenital talipes equinovarus or club foot is a condition that has been recognized for thousand years and was described by Hippocrates. It is more commonly seen in boys. Most cases are idiopathic. Some may be the result of multifactorial inheritance. The risk of club foot increases by 20 times if a first degree relative has the condition. It may be associated with syndromes or neuromuscular conditions like arthrogryposis. These cases are difficult cases to treat. The apparently idiopathic cases which recur may be associated with spinal problems which need evaluation.

The condition can be diagnosed antenatally by USG. It is usually obvious at birth. However, the mobility of the foot should be assessed. In a true CTEV, the hind foot is in fixed equines and varus. If the foot is lifted by the toes it will be noted that the heel is not in line with the leg. The fore foot is adducted and may be supinated. There may be a cavus deformity of the foot with a palpable tight band in the sole.

The infant should also be examined for associated abnormalities particularly of the hip and spine.

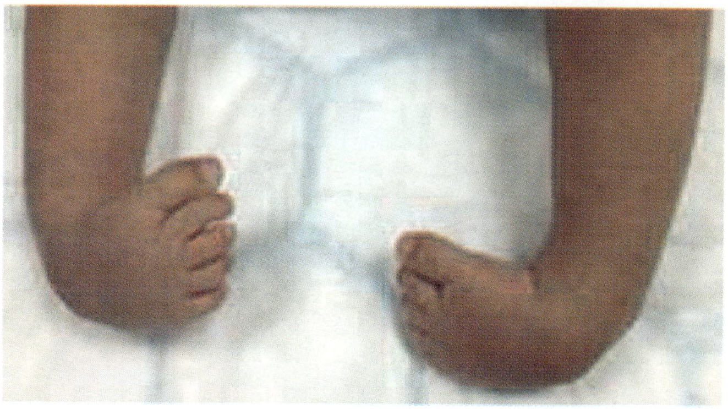

Fig. 19.24: Talipes equinovarus

Treatment

Mild cases may respond to conservative treatment, whereas severe cases are likely to need surgery. However, the foot cannot be made normal, except in mild cases. In severe cases, the foot is likely to be smaller and stiffer than the other side with a thin calf muscle. The criteria of successful treatment include a foot, particularly the heel goes flat on the ground, the ability to wear normal shoes and preservation of as much mobility as possible. The parents should be given a careful explanation of the condition.

Conservative treatment include stretching, strapping, serial splintage, and special boots. Gentle stretching should be started as soon as possible after birth. It should be supplemented by the other modes of treatment. Surgical treatment is indicated when the conservative treatment is ineffective. Conservative treatment should be continued and surgery planned at about 7 months.

Rectal Prolapse

Rectal prolapse may be partial or complete. In partial rectal prolapse the mucous membrane and the submucosa of the rectum protrude outside the anus for approximately 1–4 cm. A partial rectal prolapse is thought to represent the head of a rectal intussusception and is the early manifestation of a complete rectal prolapse.

The condition occurs mostly in children between 1–3 years age. In infants the predisposing factors include (i) the direct downward course of the rectum due to the as yet underdeveloped sacral curve and (ii) reduced resting anal tone which offers diminished support to the mucosal lining of the anal canal. In children partial prolapse usually occurs after an attack of diarrhoea, severe whooping cough or from severe protein energy malnutrition which results in diminution of fat in the ischio-rectal fossa. It may be associated with fibrocystic disease, neurological causes and maldevelopment of pelvis.

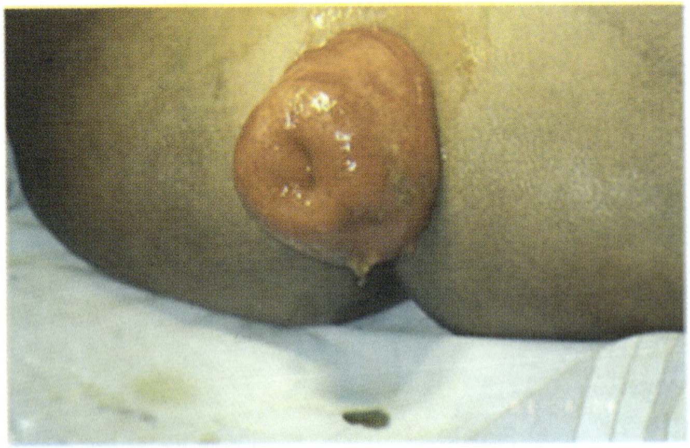

Fig. 19.25: Complete rectal prolapse

In complete rectal prolapse the protrusion consist of all layers of the rectal wall which is more than 4 cm in length. When more than 5 cm in length it contains a pouch of peritoneum anteriorly placed containing small intestine. It is usually associated with a weak pelvic floor.

The prolapse is thought to commence as a rectal intussusception which gradually descends to protrude outside the anus. Complete rectal prolapse is uncommon in children.

Treatment

For partial rectal prolapse, digital reposition by parents helps in correction of the condition. The parent is taught to replace the protrusion. The distal two thirds of the index finger is wrapped with tissue paper. The finger is inserted into the protrusion and the mass is eased into place. The finger is then gently withdrawn leaving the tissue paper to disintegrate. Correction of malnutrition should be done by dietary advice.

If digital reposition fails after a trial for 6 weeks, submucous injection of a sclerosing agent (hypertonic saline) may be carried out under general anesthesia. Surgery may be necessary occasionally.

Treatment of complete rectal prolapse is surgery.

Labial Adhesions

In this condition, there is a central line of adhesion in the labia minora from an area immediately inferior to the clitoris to the fourchette. Labial adhesions are commonly seen in children younger than 6 years of age and it is usually asymptomatic. The child may suffer from recurrent urinary tract infection. This results from pooling of urine in the vagina and recurrent vulvovaginitis.

Topical estrogen cream application once a day for 7 days is the treatment of choice. It is effective in 90% cases. It should be followed by cleansing and application of an ointment containing zinc oxide for 1–2 months after the adhesions separate to prevent recurrence. Mechanical separation of adhesion is advised only if the adhesions appear to separate easily and if it does not cause significant trauma. There is no place of surgical treatment.

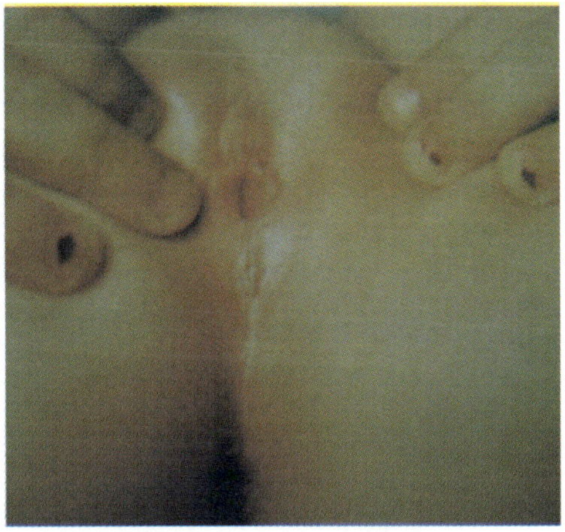

Fig. 19.26: Labial adhesions

Anal Fissure

Anal fissure is a small laceration of the mucocutaneous junction of the anus. It is mainly seen in infancy. It is an acquired lesion secondary to the forceful passing of a hard stool. Fissures are usually the consequence of constipation. Once a fissure is formed, the patient retains stool voluntarily to avoid the painful bowel movement. It exacerbates constipation and in turn the fissure and creates a vicious cycle.

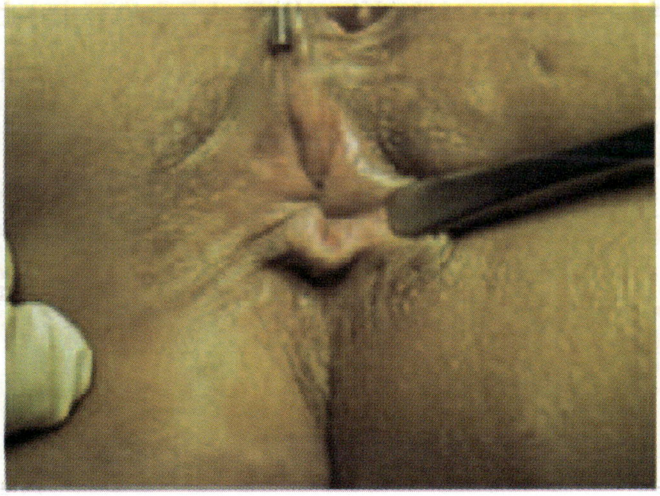

Fig. 19.27: Showing external anal fissure

Clinical Manifestations

There is usually a history of constipation. The child may present with pain during defecation and bright red blood on the surface of the stool. On local examination, a minor laceration can be seen. For the local examination, the infant's hips are held in flexion, the buttocks are separated to expand the folds of the perianal skin when the fissure becomes evident. Sometimes peripheral to the laceration there is a tag. This is a skin appendage that actually represents epithelialized granulomatous tissue secondary to the chronic inflammation.

Treatment

The parents should be explained the cause. The constipation should be treated by stool softeners to prevent stretching the anus. The dose should be adjusted to keep the stool soft and not cause diarrhoea. Simultaneously the cause of constipation should be investigated and treated.

Congenital Dislocation of Hip

Congenital dislocation of hip (CDH) has an incidence which varies from 10 - 20 / 1000 live birth. Bilateral involvement is seen in around 30 - 40% of cases.

Etiology

The exact etiology is unknown. It is seen more commonly in the first born, post term and large for date and female infants delivered following breech presentation. A family history of increased frequency of hip abnormalities may indicate a genetic predisposition. A prolonged gestation is associated with increase in maternal hormones which may account for the laxity of the hip joint.

Clinical Manifestations

Routine examination of hips in all neonates by Ortolani-Barlow maneuver helps in early diagnosis. Asymmetry of gluteal and shortening of leg on the affected side is a clue to diagnosis. The femoral pulse may not be readily felt on the affected side. An X-ray should be advised to be taken with both hips extended and legs held in 450 abduction and full internal rotation. The conventional skiagrams of hip may not show any abnormalities. An ultrasound examination of the hip joint provides diagnostic information after one month age. It needs mention that there is high incidence of false positive report during neonatal period.

Examination of hips: A routine examination of the hip is necessary to exclude congenital dislocation of hip in every baby. It should be left to the end of examination of newborn because it is uncomfortable for the baby. Babies at greater risk of hip dislocation include females, presence of family history, born by breech extraction, primipara with extended breech delivery. The steps of examination of the hip are as follows:

The infant is made to lie on the back with the legs towards the examiner. The baby should be undressed from waist downward. It is preferable to examine one hip at a time.

The examiner steadies the pelvis of the baby by putting his thumb over the symphysis pubis and fingers under the sacrum.

On the side of the hip to be examined, the thigh is flexed keeping the knees bend. It is grasped by the examiner's hand by placing the middle finger on the outer side over the greater trochanter and the thumb on the inner side of the thigh opposite the lesser trochanter.

Test for dislocation: Pressure is applied over the greater trochanter with the middle finger in an attempt to relocate the displaced femoral head back into the acetabulum. If the head is felt to move with or without a palpable or audible clunk it confirms dislocation.

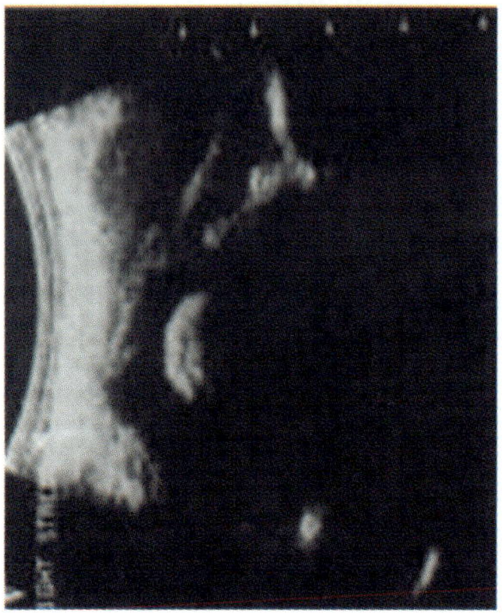

Fig. 19.28: USG showing 'black hole sign' in congenital dislocation of right hip

Test for subluxation: With the thumb placed in the inner side of the thigh, backward and outward pressure is applied to the head of the femur in an attempt to dislocate it. If the femoral head is felt to move backwards over the rim of the acetabulum for a distance of 0.5 cm, with or without a palpable or audible clunk the hip is said to be dislocatable.

Treatment

Early management is essential of optimal functional recovery. Treatment may be medical or surgical.

The legs are maintained in a position of abduction and external rotation by the use of Von Rosen splint. To treat classic cases of CDH, the Pavlik harness has been effectively used to keep the hips flexed and abducted. The recovery takes about 3 - 4 months time.

Open surgical reduction of the dislocation is indicated in cases of CDH where the femoral head does not relocate into acetabulum on flexion and abduction and Ortolani's sign is absent and in unilateral cases where there is shortening of the limb on the affected side.

Suggested Reading

1. Bailey and Love's Short Practice of Surgery, 24th edition, 2004. Edited by R.C.G. Russel, Norman S. Williams and Christopher J.K. Bulstrode, Arnold.
2. Practical Pediatric Problems, 6th edition, 1986. James H. Hutchison and Forrester Cockburn. P.G. Publishing Pte Ltd. Singapore, Hongkong, N. Delhi.
3. Nelson Textbook of Pediatrics, 17th edition, 2004, edited by Behrman, Kliegman and Jenson, Saunders.

20

Poisoning in Children

OUTLINES

A poison has been defined as a substance which when introduced into or absorbed by the living organism causes injury or death. Childhood poisoning includes accidental ingestion in the toddlers and preschoolers, falling prey to curiosity and intentional overdoses and homicidal poisoning in adolescents.

Epidemiology and Approach to Management

Epidemiology

The reported incidence of childhood poisoning in India varies from 0.3–7.6%. Eighty-five percent poisoning occurs in children below 5 years of age with a peak incidence in the second year of life. Male children predominate. It is accounted for by their greater degree of activity. Almost all these exposures are unintentional and reflect the propensity for children in this age group to put virtually anything in their mouth. Majority of the toxic exposures in children occur at home and most involve only a single substance. Ingestion is the most common route of exposure. The other routes of exposure are dermal, ophthalmic and inhalation. Poisoning exposures in children 6–12 years age are very uncommon. Toxic exposures in adolescents are primarily intentional (suicide or abuse) or occupational. The incidence also tends to be higher among children from lower socio-economic strata owing to poor storage facility in such households and among children from large families due to parental negligence.

Most of the poisoning exposures in children can be managed without direct medical intervention because either the product involved is not inherently very toxic or the quantity of material involved is not sufficient to produce significant toxic effects. The common non-drug products include cosmetics, cleaning substances, plants, foreign bodies and hydrocarbons. Fortunately, 75% of poisoning episodes involve ingestion of substances which are non-toxic or less toxic unless otherwise ingested in large quantities. In these cases, only reassurance is required.

The list of non-toxic/low toxic substances include cosmetics (hair oil, cream emulsion, eyebrow pencil, lipstick and mascara), shampoo, tooth paste, shaving cream, toilet soaps, lead pencils, match sticks, cigarettes, candles, chalk, clay, water colors, adhesives, ball point pen ink, dry indoor paint, slaked lime, latex emulsion, some drugs (antacids, antibiotics, oral contraceptives, mercury of thermometer), house lizards discovered in food and non-nitrite containing fertilizers.

Poison prevention education should be an integral part of visits in the well baby clinic, even before the child is mobile.

Approach to Management

The approach will include both legal and medical management. The legal duties of a medical practitioner in case of suspected poisoning includes the following:

Legal Duties

1. A government medical officer is required to report to police all cases of suspected poisoning, whether accidental, suicidal, or homicidal attended in the hospital. If such a patient dies, the doctor should not issue a death certificate but inform the police.
2. If a private practitioner is convinced that the patient is suffering from homicidal poisoning, he is bound to inform the police or magistrate. If he/she is sure that the patient is suffering from suicidal or accidental poisoning, he is not bound to inform the police. But if the practitioner is summoned by the investigating police officer, he is bound to give all informations regarding the case or he is liable to be prosecuted under law.
3. Hence it is pertinent that all medical officers should keep detailed records about the particulars of the patient, number of visits, the symptoms and signs observed at presentation and treatment given.

Medical Management

Medical management should start with obtaining a detailed history and physical examination. Simultaneously, supportive therapy should be started to maintain homeostasis.

The informations to be obtained include description of the toxin, amount ingested, and time of exposure, progression of symptoms and presence of any underlying disease. History is often unreliable so one has to depend on physical signs to unreveal the identity of the poison.

Table 20.1 : Physical signs relating to common poisons
Eyes
Miosis: Opium, barbiturates, anticholine esterase inhibitors.
Mydriasis: Dhatura, carbon monoxide, sympathomimetics.
Partial/Total blindness: Methyl alcohol.
Blurring of vision: Dhatura, alcohol, ergot.
Face and scalp
Alopecia: Arsenic, lead, ergot.
Facial twitching: Lead, mercury, phenothiazines.
Skin and mucus membrane
Pallor: Sympathomimetics, insulin, aniline derivatives, pilocarpine.
Cyanosis: Carbon monoxide, morphine, sulphonamides, drugs causing methemoglobinemia.
Sweating: Physostigmine, pilocarpine.
Dry, hot skin: Dhatura, botulinum.
Gastrointestinal
Nausea, vomiting, diarrhoea, dehydration: Phenol, corrosives, heavy metals, mushrooms, salicylates, morphine.
Nervous system
Headache: Carbon monoxide, phenol, atropine, scorpion bites.
Convulsion: Carbon monoxide, dhatura, mushroom, salicylates.
Delirium: Dhatura, DDT, lead, physostigmine.
Respiratory system
Pulmonary edema: Carbon monoxide, narcotics, salicylates.
Cardiovascular system
Bradycardia, AV block: Organophosphorous, digitalis, tricyclic depressants.
Ventricular tachyarrhythmia: Antipsychotics, lithium, heavy metals.

Points to be Noted

If a child presents with unexplained unconsciousness, respiratory or circulatory collapse acute poisoning should be considered. However, other causes of altered sensorium such as head trauma, metabolic abnormalities and intracranial infection should be excluded.

The pertinent examination related to acute poisoning include measurement of blood pressure, pulse rate and volume, temperature, pupil size, presence or absence of sweating and peristaltic movements.

Toxic Syndromes

Several syndromes have been described with specific symptoms and signs which help diagnosis of the acute poisoning. They are as follows:

Anticholinergic Syndrome

The anticholinergic syndrome is caused by belladonna alkaloids, dhatura, antihistaminics, tricyclic antidepressants and some mushrooms.

The symptoms include thirst, flushed face, mydriasis, blurring of vision, hyperthermia, urinary retention, delirium, hallucinations, tachycardia and respiratory insufficiency.

Cholinergic Syndrome

It is caused by organophosphate and carbamate insecticides, some mushrooms, and severe black widow spider bites.

The symptoms include nausea, vomiting, diarrhoea, muscle fasciculations, miosis, weakness or paralysis, bronchospasm, tachycardia or bradycardia, convulsions and coma.

Extrapyramidal Syndrome

The most common cause is overdose of metoclopramide. Other drugs are phenothiazines and haloperidol.

The symptoms include tremor, rigidity, torticollis, dysphonia, oculogyric crisis and dysphonia.

Hypermetabolic Syndrome

Common causes are ingestion of overdose of salicylates, ingestion of phenol and chlorophenoxy herbicides.

The symptoms are characterized by fever, tachypnea, tachycardia, restlessness, convulsions and metabolic acidosis.

Narcotic Syndrome

The causes include all narcotics, heroin.

It is characterized by CNS depression, hypothermia, hypotension, hypoventilation and miosis.

Sympathomimetic Syndrome

The causes include drugs like amphetamines, cocaine, phenylpropanolamine, methylphenidate, theophylline and caffeine.

The symptom complex consists of excitation, psychosis, seizures, hypertension, tachypnea, hyperthermia and mydriasis.

Withdrawal Syndrome

This results from withdrawal of alcohol, barbiturates, benzodiazepines and narcotics.

It is characterized by abdominal cramps, diarrhoea, lacrimation, sweating, yawning, tachycardia, restlessness and hallucinations.

Principles of General Management

The patient may be treated at home or immediately shifted to a hospital. When domestic treatment is planned, followup assessment should be made at half hour, one and four hours. In case of any change in the patient's condition, the decision to transfer should be taken. The transportation should be preferably in an ambulance well equipped for emergency care. The poison container should be transported with the patient. If the patient vomits, the vomitus should be brought along with the patient.

The principles of general management include initial medical care, prevention of absorption of poison, and enhancing elimination by different methods.

Initial Medical Care

The initial attention should be focused on life support i.e. maintenance of airway, breathing and circulation.

A clear airway is maintained by proper positioning, suctioning and use of airway to prevent fallback of tongue if necessary. Breathing is maintained by oxygen inhalation when the child is having spontaneous respiration, intubation and intermittent positive pressure ventilation when respiration is inadequate. The ABG should be monitored and mechanical ventilation started when indicated. Continuous IV doxapram infusion may be required for severe respiratory depression. Circulation is maintained by institution of the proper amount of IV fluids.

Treatment of shock, dysrhythmias, acid-base disturbances, hypothermia and seizures should be done in the usual lines. Treatment of poisoning is mainly symptomatic and supportive because antidotes exist only for few poisons.

Table 20.2 : Antidotes for some common poisons

Antidote	*Use*	*Dose*	*Route*
Atropine	Organophosphate	0.05 mg/kg repeated every 5–10 minutes as needed	IV
N-acetylcysteine	Acetaminophen	140 mg/kg loading followed by 70 mg/ kg 6 hourly for 17 doses	PO
Flumazenil	Benzodiazepine	0.2 mg over 30 secs. If response inade-quate, repeat every 1 minute to maxi-mum 1 mg	IV
Physostigmine	Anticholinergics	0.02 mg/kg; slow push, may repeat every 5–10 min to max 2 mg	IV/IM
Methylene blue	Methemoglobi-nemia	0.1–0.2 ml/kg of 1% solution. Slow infusion, may be repeated every 30–60 minutes	IV
Diphenhydramine	Extrapyramidal symptoms	5 mg/kg/day 8 hourly maximum 300 mg/day	IV/PO
Desferrioxamine	Iron	Infusion 15 mg/kg /hr, max 6 gm/24 hr	IV
		90 mg/kg/ dose 8 hourly, max 6g / 24 hrs	IM
Pyridoxine	Isoniazid	dose = dose of isoniazid	IV
	Mushrooms	25 mg/kg body weight	

Prevention of Absorption of Poison

Development of major toxicity may be prevented by prompt action to remove the source of poison and minimize the contact with the absorptive surface.

Dermal and ocular decontamination can be done by flushing the effected area with tepid water for a minimum of 10 minutes; some chemicals like alkaline corrosives may require more time. For dermal exposures, mild soap and water can be used. For inhaled poisons, decontamination is generally done by moving the patient to fresh air or if necessary by administration of oxygen.

Several procedures like emesis, gastric lavage, use of activated charcoal, cathartics and whole bowel irrigation are used to prevent absorption of a poison from the gastro-intestinal tract.

Emesis with syrup ipecac as a method to prevent absorption of ingested poison has declined in the past two decades. It has a delayed onset of action and can remove only about one third of the stomach contents.

Gastric lavage is the procedure most commonly used but it is not so efficacious in children. The procedure consists of aspiration of stomach contents followed by flushing with aliquots of normal saline. It should be used only in older children and in select situations.

The use of *activated charcoal*, on the other has increased because of its efficacy. Activated charcoal is specially prepared to have a large adsorptive surface area. The usual dose is 10 – 30 grams for a child and 30 -100 grams in adolescents. If it is given through a nasogastric tube, the placement of the tube in the stomach should be confirmed because instillation of charcoal directly into the lungs is disastrous. Activated charcoal is commercially available mixed with water or a solution of sorbitol, a cathartic. With life threatening symptoms, repeated doses may be necessary.

Cathartics are commonly used in conjunction with activated charcoal to hasten clearance of charcoal-toxin complex. However, no evidence has shown that it is of value. The commonly used cathartics are sorbitol (max dose 1 gm / kg), magnesium citrate (max dose 250 mg/kg). Cathartics should be used with caution in young children as it may cause dehydration and electrolyte imbalance.

Whole bowel irrigation is a technique useful for removing slowly absorbed toxin. This method can be combined with use of activated charcoal. In young children, there is a risk of dehydration and electrolyte imbalance. It is done by instillation of large volumes of polyethylene glycol electrolyte solution into the stomach to cleanse the entire gastrointestinal tract.

Methods for Enhancing Elimination

Elimination of toxins can be enhanced by several methods like diuresis, dialysis and hemoperfusion.

Diuresis along with increasing the pH of urine with IV sodium bicarbonate increases elimination of salicylates and phenobarbitone.

Dialysis, both hemodialysis and peritoneal dialysis has been used with success to treat selected poisonings. Although hemodialysis is more efficient, peritoneal dialysis is easier to perform in children and is usually sufficient. Dialysis is useful when large quantities of salicylates and theophylline are ingested. Others include methanol, ethylene glycol poisonings. Hemoperfusion may be used in adolescents to treat large ingestions of salicylates and theophylline. It is rarely used in children because of the associated risk.

Laboratory Investigations

Only in some poisonings blood levels are integral part of the treatment plan. They are salicylates, acetaminophen, iron, methanol and ethylene glycol. For others it may help in diagnosis only.

Kerosene Poisoning

It is the most common accidental poisoning in children. The reported incidence varies from 30–60%. Preschool children (commonly 1–3 years age group) are the most common victims. The reason for being common is the easy availability of kerosene in most households. Kerosene poisoning can occur following ingestion, inhalation, dermal exposure and ocular exposure. However, kerosene poisoning most commonly occurs due to ingestion.

Pathogenesis

Kerosene is not well absorbed from the gastrointestinal tract. Systemic toxicity generally results from absorption via lungs following aspiration. There is early chemical pneumonia, which may progress to atelectasis, pneumothorax and pleural effusion. The resulting interference in gaseous exchange in the lungs leads to hypoxia which leads to involvement of the CNS and other systems. The fatal dose is 30 ml and fatal period is 24 hours.

Clinical Manifestations

After ingestion, usually there is burning in the throat, sensation of choking, colicky abdominal pain, cough, nausea, vomiting and diarrhoea. In severe cases there may be gastrointestinal hemorrhage, acute renal failure, cardiac arrhythmia, and fever with tachypnea and respiratory difficulty, drowsiness and coma. Contact with skin can cause irritation, burn or necrosis.

An X-ray of the chest shows evidence of pneumonia, within two hours in severe cases and within 6–8 hours in 90% cases. There may be pneumatoceles and later pneumothorax.

Treatment

Many children asymptomatic after ingestion of kerosene may develop symptoms of toxicity even after 24 hours. Therefore the child should be kept under observation for atleast 24 hours.

Treatment is mainly supportive. Evacuation of stomach by gastric lavage or emesis do not benefit the child, rather they may increase the chances of aspiration and therefore not indicated routinely. Gastric lavage with a cuffed tube may be indicated in comatose patients. Oxygen inhalation through hood or mask should be administered in cases with respiratory symptoms like tachypnea and cyanosis. Prophylactic antibiotics are not necessary. It is indicated in presence of evidence of bacterial pneumonia.

Dhatura Poisoning

Dhatura is a plant which grows in wild all over India. All the parts of the plant are poisonous but seeds and fruits are most toxic. The children can ingest dhatura fruits mistaking them as common edible fruits but it is usually used to stupefy people mostly for robbery, kidnapping or even rape. The lethal dose of dhatura alkaloids is 4 mg and death usually occurs within 24 hours.

Pathogenesis

The active principle is called dhaturine and contains the three alkaloids viz. hyoscine, levohyoscyamine, and traces of atropine. After ingestion of the fruit or seeds, the alkaloids are absorbed from the intestine. They antagonize the actions of acetyl choline. The chief site of action is the cholinergic muscarinic receptors of the post ganglionic parasympathetic nerves at the cortical and subcortical levels in the brain. However, the cholinergic nicotinic receptors at neuromuscular junctions remain unaffected in dhatura poisoning.

Clinical Features

Symptoms usually appear within half an hour after ingestion. The features due to peripheral anti-muscarinic effects include excessive thirst, blurring of vision and difficulty in swallowing. There is tachycardia, flushing of skin and symmetrical pupillary dilatation. The skin and mucous membrane is dry. Ingestion of large quantities may lead to fever or even hyperpyrexia, urinary retension, and diminished bowel sounds. The terminal events are hypertension and arrhythmias.

The features of central antimuscarinic effect include agitation, confusion, and disorientation, and visual incoordination, auditory and visual hallucination. There may be muttering delirium which is characterized by continuous muttering of indistinct words. The child appears to grasp at imaginary objects picks at his clothing and tries to pull imaginary threads from the nail beds. This is followed by drowsiness within an hour. Seizures and coma and respiratory paralysis are terminal events.

Treatment

Children with only peripheral features usually completely recover spontaneously within 24–48 hours. They do not require active treatment but should be admitted to hospital and kept under observation for 48 hours. Cases with severe poisoning should be admitted to hospital. They require gastrointestinal decontamination by gastric lavage, specific antidote and supportive care.

Gastric lavage is done with normal saline. It is effective when patient comes within 48 hours of ingestion. After lavage, activated charcoal (1–2 g/kg) is left in the stomach.

The specific antidote of dhatura poisoning is physostigmine. It is indicated in patients with hallucination, seizures or supraventricular tachycardia. The dose is 0.5 mg IV slowly over a period of 3–5 minutes and may be repeated every 10 minutes to a maximum of 2 mg. Side effects may be controlled with atropine 0.5 mg subcutaneously for each mg of physostigmine administered. Physostigmine crosses the blood brain barrier; hence reverses both peripheral as well as central antimuscarinic effects of dhatura.

Supportive care includes maintenance of airway, breathing and circulation in the comatose patient. An IV line should be secured. Hyperpyrexia should be treated with cold sponging, convulsion with diazepam and hypotension with IV fluid bolus and vasoactive drugs. Hypertension is usually transient; hence do not require anti-hypertensives.

Organophosphate Poisoning

Organophosphates are used as insecticides. They are inhibitors of cholinesterase enzymes. Most organophosphate poisonings occur as a result of accidental exposure to insecticides in and around the home or paddy fields. Organophosphates are rapidly absorbed through skin, conjunctiva and inhalation. In children it is usually an accidental ingestion or contamination of skin.

Pathogenesis

Acetyl choline is responsible for neurotransmission by receptor sites in parasympathetic and sympathetic ganglia and nerve endings to sweat glands; neuromuscular junction and certain sites of CNS. Normally, acetyl choline after release is hydrolyzed to inactive choline and acetic acid by acetyl choline esterase. Organophosphates bind to cholinesterase enzymes, preventing the degradation of acetyl choline resulting in accumulation at nerve synapses stimulating neurotransmission. The enzymes affected are acetyl choline esterase (found in red cell), pseudocholine esterase (found in plasma) and neurotoxic esterase (found in nervous system). If left untreated, organophosphates form a permanent bond to these enzymes. This process occurs within 2–3 days after exposure but takes weeks to months to regenerate inactivated enzymes.

Clinical Features

The clinical symptoms and signs are a result of continuous stimulation of muscarinic and nicotinic receptor sites. In most cases these appear within 24 hours of exposure. However, with highly soluble newer organophosphate compounds, clinical features may develop after several days.

The *muscarinic clinical features* include emesis and urinary and fecal incontinence, diaphoresis, drooling, bronchospasm, miosis, hypotension and bradycardia. *Nicotinic features* include muscle weakness, fasciculations, tremors, hypoventilation, hypertension, tachycardia and dysrhythmias. Central nervous system effects include malaise, confusion, delirium, seizures and coma. The commonly used acronym for the most common symptoms is SLUDGE which stands for *salivation, lacrimation, urination, defecation, gastrointestinal cramps and emesis.* The classic findings of massive cholinergic overdrive is represented by the acronym DUMBBELLS which stands for *diarrhoea, urination, miosis, bradycardia, broncho secretions, emesis, lacrimation and salivation.*

RBC cholinesterase and pseudocholine esterase can be measured. It can document exposure to the poison but do not correlate well with the symptoms.

Table 20.3 : WHO hazard classification for clinical presentation of organophosphate poisoning

Mild	*Moderate*	*Severe*
Anorexia, headache, dizziness, weakness, anxiety, tremor of tongue and eyelids, miosis, impairment	Nausea, salivation, lacrimation abdominal cramps, vomiting sweating, slow pulse, tremor of muscles	Diarrhoea, pin point and non-reacting pupils, respiratory difficulty, pulmonary edema, loss of sphincter control convulsion, coma and heart block

Treatment

Mild cases may need only observation. Severely intoxicated patients require aggressive treatment in the form of maintenance of airway, breathing and circulation, decontamination, antidote and supportive care.

Airway can be easily compromised by muscular weakness. Some patients may require oxygenation, intubation and mechanical ventilation in presence of signs of respiratory failure. Circulation should be maintained with intravenous fluid and vasoactive drugs.

Decontamination can be done by gastric lavage with potassium permanganate (1: 5000) solution and use of cathartics. The persons who are incharge of nursing the child should wear gloves. All the clothings of the child should be removed and the contaminated clothes should be laundered. Skin and hair should be washed thoroughly with soap and water including finger nails and skin folds. Contaminated leather shoes should be discarded.

Antidotes include atropine and pralidoxime (20- PAM, Protopam). Atropine blocks muscarinic receptor and acetyl choline in CNS but has no effect on neuromuscular junction. Atropine may be administered in a dose of 0.05 mg/kg IV initially and repeated at 5–15 minutes interval (maximum dose 10–12 mg in 24 hours). The clinical sign of atropine effect is drying of all secretions. The pupils however, may not dilate. So this sign should not be taken as an end point. Atropine sulphate nebulization, 2 mg 6 hourly have been tried and found effective. Atropine should be avoided in cyanosed patients as it may cause ventricular fibrillation. In such cases mechanical ventilation must precede atropinization.

Pralidoxime primarily counteracts nicotinic effects. It should be preferably started within 12 hours following exposure but it continues to be effective even if given thereafter. The dose of PAM is 25–50 mg / kg IV as a 5% solution in isotonic saline over 5–10 minutes followed by continuous infusion @ 7.5 mg /kg/ hour started after 4 hours.

Supportive care includes treatment of convulsion, shock, hemodialysis in seriously ill patients and close monitoring. Diazepam is preferred over other anticonvulscents. Phenobarbitone should be avoided. Phenothiazines should not be used as it can potentiate the effect of the organophosphorous compounds.

Close monitoring is necessary as relapse of symptoms may occur even after full apparent recovery.

Acetaminophen Poisoning

Acetaminophen (Paracetamol) is the most widely used analgesic and antipyretic in children. Poisoning is mostly accidental. It is common in children below 6 years of age. The recommended dose of paracetamol is 10–15 mg/kg body weight at 4 hours interval. The fatal dose is 20–25 gm.

The acute toxic dose of acetaminophen is generally considered to be more than 200 mg/kg in children younger than 12 years of age. A single ingestion of more than 7.5 grams is considered a minimum toxic dose in adolescents. Repeated administration of acetaminophen at doses exceeding the recommended doses may lead to hepatic damage or failure in some children.

Parents should be warned not to exceed the recommended doses prescribed and beware of its presence in combination products. However, it needs mention that even if hepatoxicity develops, the mortality rate is less than 0.5% and patients who recover have no sequelae.

Pathogenesis

With therapeutic doses, acetaminophen is rapidly absorbed. It produces a peak plasma level in half to one hour. With normal liver function, the plasma half life is 1–3 hours. Acetaminophen is primarily metabolized in the liver to sulphate or glucoronide conjugates, which are metabolically inert. Around 4% of a therapeutic dose of acetaminophen is metabolized by hepatic cytochrome p-450 enzymes to a highly reactive intermediate metabolite to N-acetyl-p-benzoquinoneimine (NAPQI) which is immediately conjugated with glutathione to form a harmless mercapturic acid conjugate. A small amount of acetaminophen is excreted unchanged in urine.

With overdoses, when hepatic stores of glutathione are depleted to less than 70% of the normal, there is excess amount of NAPQI which combine with hepatic macromolecules and cause cellular damage.

Clinical Manifestations

Patients who are acutely overdosed pass through four stages of toxicity as follows:

Stage I: Symptoms appear half to 24 hours after ingestion. They include non-specific symptoms like anorexia, nausea, vomiting, malaise, pallor and diaphoresis. Laboratory investigations are normal.

Stage II: Symptoms develop after 24–48 hours. There is resolution of the above symptoms with appearance of right upper quadrant abdominal pain and tenderness, oliguria with elevated serum bilirubin, hepatic enzymes and prothrombin time.

StageIII: Symptoms develop after 72–96 hours of ingestion. Anorexia, nausea, vomiting may reappear with increased laboratory findings of abnormal liver function. Acute liver failure and death can occur in less than 1% cases.

StageIV: Symptoms appear 4 days to 2 weeks after ingestion. There is resolution of hepatic dysfunction with normal liver function tests. The serum SGPT may remain elevated for few days.

As the early signs of toxicity are non-specific, when toxic ingestion is suspected, a plasma acetaminophen level should be measured. It should be done 4 hours or later to determine the severity of an overdose and determine whether antidotal treatment is indicated.

Treatment

Treatment includes decontamination, antidote and supportive measures. If the child reports within 4 hours of ingestion, gastric lavage should be done with normal saline. Activated charcoal should be left in the stomach.

The specific antidote of acetaminophen is N-acetylcysteine and it is the drug of choice. It can be given orally or intravenously, but it is more effective orally. The oral loading dose is 140 mg/ kg followed by 70 mg/ kg 4 hourly for 17 doses. If the patient vomits within one hour of administration of a dose, it should be repeated. To mask the unpleasant odour of the drug and reduce nausea and vomiting following administration, N-acetyl cysteine should be diluted to a concentration of 5% solution and fruit juices or carbonated beverages may be added. Laboratory investigations should be repeated during the course of treatment. If liver failure sets in, N acetyl cysteine is contraindicated. It should be treated in the usual line. Renal function should also be monitored and if renal failure occurs it should be treated.

Oleander Poisoning

Oleander is a shrub with worldwide distribution. All parts of the plant are poisonous but fruits and seeds cause most toxic effects. The fatal dose is one leaf or one seed and fatal period is 6 days. Oleander poisoning is accidental in children but may be suicidal in adolescents.

The common oleander has atleast 5 cardiac glycosides which have some structural similarity to digitoxin. The resulting toxic syndromes resemble digitalis poisoning. After absorption from the GIT, glycosides are concentrated mainly in the heart.

Clinical Manifestations

Child with oleander poisoning predominantly have gastrointestinal and cardiac symptoms. Nausea, vomiting, diarrhoea, and mucosal erythema develop within one hour of ingestion. There may be perioral paresthesia, dizziness, progressive muscle weakness and excessive salivation in the early phase. Cardiac symptoms include hypotension, sinus bradycardia, supraventricular tachycardia, conduction defects like A-V block and complete heart block, ventricular tachycardia and ventricular fibrillation. The common metabolic effects may be hypokalemia, hyperkalemia and hypomagnesaemia.

Treatment

A child, who has ingested less than half of a leaf or flower, should be given an emetic and kept under observation at home. Symptomatic patient or a patient who has ingested more than one leaf or seed should be hospitalized. Emesis and gastric lavage should be done as early as possible followed by administration of charcoal.

The child should be kept under cardiac monitoring for early detection of cardiac features of poisoning. Hypotension responds to crystalloid and vasopressor agents. Sinus bradycardia should be treated with atropine (0.02–0.05 mg /kg/dose). The arrhythmias usually resolve by 24 hours but may persist for 3–6 days. They are refractory to drugs. Majority requires temporary pacing.

Anti-digoxin FAB fragment have been recommended for treatment of cardiac features. It rapidly reverses the cardiac symptoms. It is safe. The dose is 400 – 800 mg in 200 ml saline and is administered by intravenous infusion over 20 minutes. The patient should be monitored for signs of anaphylaxis.

Naphthalene Poisoning

Naphthalene is used as deodorant in lavatories, as pesticide in moth balls and in the dye industries. Poisoning with naphthalene in children is usually accidental. It may occur either from ingestion of moth balls or inhalation from bed clothes. Toxicity following exposure to blankets stored with naphthalene has also been reported in infants.

The toxic metabolite of naphthalene is alpha naphthol. It causes hemolysis with subsequent hepatic necrosis and renal tubule blockage. However, hemolysis occurs in those children with hereditary deficiency of glucose 6 phosphate dehydrogenase deficiency in the red cells. The fatal dose is about 2 grams and fatal period may be from few hours to 2-3 days. Absorption in children is more rapid hence fatality is more.

Clinical Manifestations

The effects of naphthalene poisoning include hemolytic anemia, acute nephritis, optic neuritis and jaundice. Hemolytic anemia is the most common among these.

In the newborn, the usual presentation is that of acute hemolytic anemia with anemia and jaundice progressing to kernicterus.

In the older child, the clinical manifestations are different after ingestion and after inhalation. After ingestion, symptoms start with nausea, vomiting and abdominal pain due to gastric irritation. Other manifestations include hemoglobinuria (dark brown or black urine), pain in the loin and suprapubic region, burning micturition, strangury, convulsion, coma and death.

Inhalation results in headache, malaise, nausea, vomiting, conjunctivitis, mental confusion and visual disturbances.

Three important laboratory findings include anisocytosis and fragmented red cells in the peripheral blood smear, presence of hemoglobin and albumin in urine and methemoglobinemia.

Treatment

Treatment consists of emesis if patient comes within 2 hours of ingestion and gastric lavage with warm water or normal saline and administration of activated charcoal.

Milk and fatty food should be avoided for 2–3 hours because naphthalene is fat soluble. The urine should be maintained alkaline with administration of IV fluids and sodi bi carb so as to prevent precipitation of acid hematin crystals in the renal tubules. The patient should be monitored for hemolysis for atleast one week after exposure. Hydrocortisone may be used to limit hemolysis. However, severe hemolysis may require red cell transfusion. Methemoglobinemia should be treated with methylene blue. Liver and kidney failure if present should be treated in the usual lines.

Iron Poisoning

Iron is one of the most common causes of childhood poisoning death. The potential severity of exposure is based on the amount of elemental iron ingested. The elemental iron present in different formulation is given in the composition. It is different for different salts e.g. ferrous sulphate contains 20%, ferrous gluconate 12%, and ferrous fumerate 33% elemental iron. Greater than 60 mg/kg of elemental iron is generally considered a toxic dose.

Pathophysiology

Iron is a corrosive to the gastrointestinal mucosa. It also accumulates in the mitochondria and tissues to produce systemic toxicity. Iron causes venodilation and increased capillary permeability which results in hypotension. Reduced peripheral perfusion and mitochondrial damage result in accumulation of lactic and citric acid causing metabolic acidosis. Serious poisoning also causes hepatic necrosis which results in abnormal liver function and coagulopathy. Drowsiness and coma may develop as a result of hemodynamic instability or possibly a direct toxic effect of iron in the CNS.

Clinical Manifestations

The hallmark of iron poisoning viz. nausea, vomiting, diarrhoea and abdominal pain develops usually within 30 minutes to 6 hours after ingestion of the toxic dose. In more serious poisoning, the child may have hematemesis and bloody diarrhoea. The gastrointestinal symptoms and signs subside over 6 - 12 hours. The child should however be kept under observation to monitor systemic toxic signs viz. hypotension or drowsiness. Systemic signs are more common in patients with severe gastrointestinal signs. Gastric scarring and pyloric stenosis can develop 2 - 4 weeks after a large ingestion or when iron tablets remain in prolonged contact with the gastrointestinal mucosa. Pyloric stenosis may be symptomatic requiring surgery.

Laboratory Investigations

Serum iron levels should be estimated about 4 hours after ingestion. Levels above 500 microgram/dL indicate that significant toxicity is likely. Serum glucose level, liver function tests, coagulation tests and blood gas levels should be monitored in these patients.

An abdominal X-ray may confirm ingestion as iron is radio opaque. A repeat X-ray may help assessment of efficiency of gastric decontamination. A negative result however does not rule out iron ingestion because only undissolved tablets are radio opaque. Moreover tablets containing multivitamin and iron are not visualized because of the low iron content and rapid dissolution.

Treatment

Specific Therapy

The specific iron chelator is deferoxamine. It acts as an antidote for moderate to severe intoxication. It is indicated when serum iron level is greater than 500 microgram / dL, regardless of symptoms or presence of moderate to severe symptoms regardless of serum iron levels. It should be administered by continuous intravenous infusion in the dose of 15 mg/kg/hour (max 6 gm/day).

Supportive Therapy

Ipecac induced vomiting may be used to remove the tablets from the stomach. Gastric lavage is not recommended in young children as it cannot remove the large sized tablets. Whole bowel irrigation may be of benefit. If tablets adhere to the gastric mucosa then removal by endoscopy or gastrotomy or aggressive bowel irrigation can be attempted.

Oral bicarbonate (2%), dilute phospho-soda (1:4) and magnesium hydroxide when administered orally react with iron to form poorly absorbed iron salts but this technique is of questionable clinical benefit.

Snake Bite

Snake bite remains a public health problem worldwide except probably in the polar region, New Zealand and some islands. There are more than 3,000 known species of snakes. Only 200 snakes are poisonous to human. Ninety percent of the poisonous snakes belong to one of the three families: the Hydrophidae or poisonous sea snakes, elapidae which includes cobra, king cobra and krait and the viperidae or true vipers viz. pit viper, Russell's viper.

The snake venom is modified saliva containing a mixture of about 26 enzymes viz. phospholipases, phosphatases, proteases, esterases (acetylcholine esterase) and toxins (neurotoxin, cardiotoxin, myotoxin and hemorrhagens). This property of snake venom is responsible for the spectrum of clinical manifestations like neuromuscular blockade, systemic cardiovascular toxicity, local tissue injury, hemolysis and bleeding tendency.

Majority of snake bites are reported in young male children. This is because of their increased outdoor activity, curiosity and carelessness. As the children have a smaller body mass for venom distribution, they have a more serious systemic reaction to envenomation and account for high mortality.

Pathogenesis

The composition of snake venom is species specific. Venom from elapidae and the Hydrophidae is primarily neurotoxic and has a curare like effect by blocking neurotransmission at the neuromuscular junction. Death results from respiratory depression. Death from pit viper bites result from hemorrhagic shock, renal failure and adult respiratory distress syndrome.

Differences Between Poisonous and Non-Poisonous Snakes

Features	*Poisonous*	*Non-poisonous*
Head	Large and triangular with small scales	Small and oval with small scales
Pupils	Vertically elliptical	Round
Belly scales	Large and covering entire breath	Small not covering entire breath
Pit*	Present between eye and nostril	Not present
Fangs	Present 2 numbers, large, long recurvated	Absent
Tail	Compressed	Not compressed
Bite	Distinct fang marks and small teeth marks	Series of tiny punctures and scratches

* A heat responsive organ to localize prey.

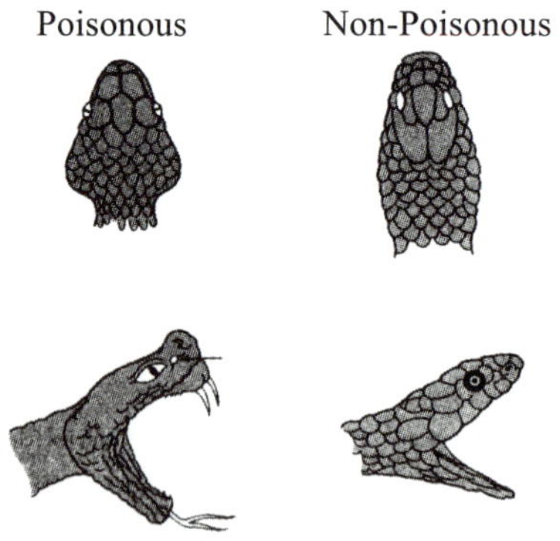

Fig. 20.1: Identification of poisonous and non-poisonous snakes (From Nelson Textbook of Pediatrics, 17th edition)

Clinical Manifestations

The clinical manifestations of snake bite may be divided into local and systemic features, which may vary in degree depending on the species of snake. The most common and earliest symptom following snake bite however is fright features which may include excitability, transient, pallor, sweating, vomiting, sometimes diarrhoea, shock and even death.

The local symptoms at the site of bite include pain, swelling, ecchymosis, bullae, serosanguinous discharge, bleeding and gangrene of subcutaneous tissue and regional lymphadenitis.

The general systemic manifestations include fever, headache, muscle cramps and diaphoresis. The systemic features relating to the different systems are as follows:

- Nausea, vomiting, colicky abdominal pain and rarely jaundice.
- Bleeding and severe anemia.
- Tingling numbness around the mouth, scalp and fingers, muscle fasciculation, ptosis, and paralysis of skeletal muscles.
- Acute tubular necrosis, glomerulonephritis, acute cortical necrosis.
- Cardiac arrhythmias, shock and asystole, pulmonary edema and respiratory failure.

In pit viper bites, which usually occur in the extremities, there is pain and swelling at the site of bite within minutes followed by edema and ecchymosis and in severe bites there is bulla formation and tissue necrosis. Systemic symptoms include nausea, vomiting, diaphoresis, weakness, tingling around the face and fasciculations. Rarely, the patient may present with shock or arrhythmias and bleeding diathesis.

In bites of elapidae, there is less pain locally because the venom has no cytotoxin. The symptoms may rapidly progress from drowsiness to cranial nerve palsies, and death from respiratory paralysis.

Diagnosis and Laboratory Test

The diagnosis of the type of snake (poisonous or non-poisonous) from bite marks is fallacious. Hence not of much use. A positive 20-minute whole blood clotting test can be used to confirm the biting species as viperine because elapidae species do not cause anti-hemostatic symptoms.

The 20-minute whole blood coagulation test is adopted as a standard test for coagulopathy. A few ml of fresh venous blood is taken in a clean, new, dry test tube and is left undisturbed for 20 minutes and then gently tilted. If the blood is still liquid it is an evidence of coagulopathy.

First Aid Treatment

The first aid recommended is based on the mnemonic "Do it R.I.G.H.T." which consist of the following:

R = Reassurance to the patient. Seventy percent of all snake bites are from non-poisonous snakes. Only 50% poisonous snakes actually envenomate the patient.

I = Immobilization of the part in the same way as in case of a fractured limb. Young children can be carried. No application of tight ligatures, tourniquet. They do not work and can be dangerous. Clean the wound with sterile saline water and cover with a sterile dressing.

GH = Get to hospital immediately. Traditional remedies have no proven benefit in treating snake bite.

T = Tell the doctor of any systemic symptoms like ptosis that manifest on way to hospital.

Criteria for Administration of Anti Snake Venom (ASV)

Anti-venom is most effective if administered within 4 hours of the bite. It is of little value if delayed beyond 12 hours. ASV should be administered only when there is evidence of systemic envenomation. Anti-venom is contraindicated if there is a history of atopy and child is sensitive to equine anti-serum. The indications are as follows:

1. Positive 20-minute whole blood clotting time and presence of spontaneous bleeding.
2. Presence of ptosis.
3. Severe local symptoms such as swelling rapidly crossing a joint or involving half the bitten limb. When a tourniquet has been used, if the swelling continues after it has been removed for more than 1 hour.

Dosage Guidelines for Anti-Venom

Degree	*Clinical features*	*No. of vials*
Mild	Progressive swelling with or without lymphadenitis with local ecchymosis/ purpura.	5
Moderate	Mild systemic signs like nausea, vomiting and bradycardia or coagulation defect or hematological changes.	5–15
Severe	Rapidly progressive swelling with extensive local effect, systemic features, DIC, encephalopathy, shock, paralysis.	15–20

Reconstitution and Administration

Each anti-venom vial is diluted with 10 ml of distilled water or isotonic saline and then given at the rate of 4 mg/ minute. Reconstituted anti-venom can also be diluted with 3 volumes of normal saline and infused slowly at first and with increased rate if tolerated over 1 hour. Thereafter, depending on the response vials may be added till all systemic symptoms disappear or the progression of swelling ceases.

ASV test doses have been abandoned because they have been shown to have no predictive value and may presensitize the patient.

Reactions of Anti Snake Venom

Reactions usually occur within 10–180 minutes. The reactions comprise of anaphylaxis, hypotension, and bronchospasm and angioneurotic edema. The reactions are managed by administration of epinephrine (1: 1000), 0.01mg/kg IM. In addition, to provide longer protection against anaphylactoid reactions, hydrocortisone (2 mg/kg) IV and a H1 antihistamine (0.2 mg/kg) IV should be administered.

Adrenaline by IM route reaches necessary blood plasma levels in 8 minutes. If after 10–15 minutes, the patient's condition does not improve or is worsening, a second dose of adrenaline should be administered. A third dose may be required but usually 2 doses are sufficient.

The anti-venom infusion should be stopped till the reaction subsides then restarted slowly for 10–15 minutes. The patient should be closely monitored and then the normal drip rate resumed. In cases with severe envenomation, anti-venom can be readministered even in presence of reaction under cover of adrenaline and hydrocortisone.

Repeat Doses of ASV

In antihemostatic bites, after the initial dose of ASV, the 20 minutes whole blood clotting test should be repeated every 6 hours. The result will determine if additional doses are required. In case of neurotoxic bites, after the first dose, a neostigmine test is given and the patient closely monitored. If the patient has not improved after 1–2 hours or has worsened then a second dose and final dose should be given. After this if the patient does not improve they will require mechanical ventilation.

Supportive Therapy

Supportive treatment should be available when need arises. Treatment of shock, acute renal failure, pulmonary edema and respiratory failure should be provided in the usual lines.

Bee and Wasp Sting

Bees and wasps have a sting attached to the end of the abdomen through which venom is injected. The venom is stored in a venom gland. The venom of both contains proteins and vasoactive substances. It is not very potent and usually causes only local reaction. A small percentage of population is sensitized and is at risk of immediate hypersensitivity reaction. Reaction is severe in young children and those who have been stung before.

Clinical Manifestations

Most cases present with local reactions like intense pain, itching, formation of wheal and erythema. Edema may occur in areas with loose connective tissue like eyelids, genitalia. Local reactions usually subside by few hours but may remain upto a day or two. Stings on the head, face, neck, pharynx and tongue can lead to severe edema and death due to respiratory obstruction. Bells palsy has been reported as a result of sting in the facial nerve.

A previously sensitized child may present with urticaria, abdominal cramps, nausea and vomiting, angioedema, bronchospasm, hypotension, convulsion, coma leading to death. This type of severe reaction is more common in children with a history of atopy and a child with a previous sting.

Treatment

A local reaction can be treated with cold compress, analgesic and topical application of antihistamine. Cold compress helps to retard absorption of venom as well as release of histamine from damaged cells.

Acute systemic reaction should be treated with IV crystalloids, oxygen and epinephrine (1:1000), 0.1 mg/kg I.M. Hydrocortisone (2 mg/kg I.V.) is useful in cases with laryngeal edema and bronchospasm. Hypotension and shock should be treated with crystalloids and vasopressor. Respiratory failure needs mechanical ventilation.

Spider Bites

Spider envenomation can lead to death in young children. Black widow spider, a species which is often found in the tropical region is particularly dangerous. However, majority of spider bites are painful but not dangerous.

Clinical Features

There is burning at the site of bite after envenomation. After about an hour, there is generalized muscular spasm,

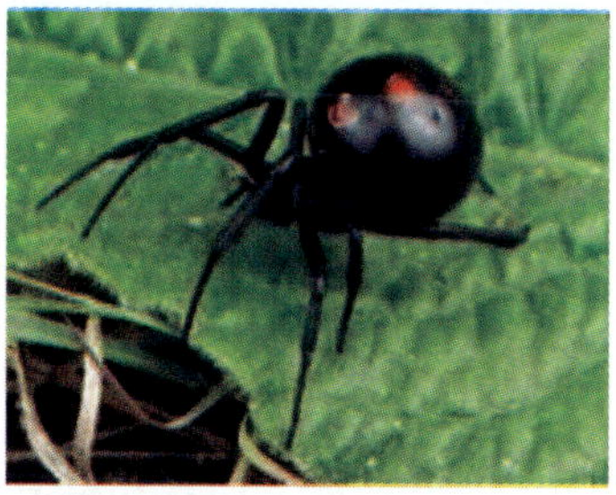

Fig. 20.2: Figure showing black widow spider

nausea, vomiting, pain, tenderness and rigidity of the abdomen. It may mimick an attack of acute appendicitis. Fever, sweating and shock can occur later.

Treatment

The site of bite should be washed thoroughly with hot water. Muscular spasm can be treated with 10% calcium gluconate or diazepam. Anti-venom is indicated in cases with severe systemic reaction. The dose is 2.5 ml diluted in 50 ml of saline and given IV over 15 minutes. It may be repeated if symptoms recur. Shock should be treated with crystalloids and vasopressors.

Lizard Bites

Venomous lizards are not found in India. Therefore lizard bites in India requires only reassurance. No treatment is necessary.

The venom of a venomous variety of lizard is neurotoxic in nature. Envenomation can occur by contamination of a wound. The clinical presentations include local features like excruciating pain, massive edema and erythema as a result of tissue injury. Systemic features are nausea, vomiting and hematemesis, blurring of vision, dyspnea, dysphonia, hyperesthesia and profound weakness. Systemic manifestation usually last for 3–4 days. Hyperesthesia may persist for several weeks.

Treatment comprises application of a tourniquet, incision and suction and cooling of the site of bite. Local anesthetics may be infiltrated locally to relieve pain. No anti-venom is available.

Food Poisoning

Food poisoning is a term used to describe a number of illnesses in which gastrointestinal symptoms arise within 24 hours or so of eating food contaminated with bacteria, bacterial toxins or irritant chemicals.

Food poisoning may be bacterial and nonbacterial (chemicals and mushroom).

Bacterial Food Poisoning

The causative agents for bacterial food poisoning include staphylococcus aureus, bacillus cereus, clostridium perfringens, vibrio cholerae, enterotoxigenic E. coli, salmonella, shiegella, vibrio para hemolyticus.

Clinical Manifestation

The clinical manifestations differ according to the organisms. It is shown in a tabular form:

Organisms	*Onset of symptoms*	*Symptoms*	*Common food sources*
Staphylococcus aureus	1–6 hrs	Nausea, vomiting, diarrhoea	Poultry, ham, potato or egg Salad, cream pastries, mayonnaise
Bacillus cereus	1–6 hrs	Nausea, vomiting, diarrhoea	Fried rice
	8–16 hrs	Abdominal cramps, diarrhoea	Meat, vegetables, dried beans, cereals
Clostridium perfringens	8–16 hrs	Abdominal cramps, diarrhoea	Beef, poultry, legumes
Vibrio cholerae	> 16 hrs	watery diarrhoea	Fish
Salmonella	> 16 hrs	Inflammatory diarrhoea	Eggs, poultry, beef, dairy products
Shiegella	> 16 hrs	Blood and mucus	Potato, egg salad, raw vegetables

Diagnosis

The occurrence of severe vomiting in a group of people who have partaken of the same meal a few hours before the onset of symptoms is strongly suggestive of the diagnosis of food poisoning. The time of onset of diarrhoea after a meal and the type of meal taken can provide clues to the bacterial cause. Confirmation may be done by examination of the vomitus/stool or the food if available.

Treatment

The mainstay of treatment is adequate rehydration with oral rehydration solution and IV fluids as indicated.

If vomiting is severe or persistent, a parenteral injection of an antiemetic may be indicated. Antibiotics are rarely indicated. There is no evidence that they shorten the course of illness. They may prolong the carrier state in salmonella food poisoning.

Chemical Food Poisoning

Chemical food poisoning is usually accidental. It may follow the use of inadequately cleaned containers or action of acids on inferior enamel ware. Lead, tin, zinc and antimony poisoning can occur in these ways.

Clinical Manifestation

The main feature suggestive of chemical food poisoning is the short interval between ingestion and the appearance of symptoms. The patient usually complains of an abnormal taste, often metallic, within minutes, accompanied by nausea and abdominal pain followed by vomiting and diarrhoea within half an hour.

Neurological symptoms have followed ingestion of food contaminated with pesticides. DDT causes paraesthesiae and limb twitching. Endrin and similar agricultural sprays cause convulsion. Consumption of ortho-tricresyl phosphate, mistaken for edible oil, cause flaccid paralysis after 2–3 weeks of ingestion. Sodium fluoride ingested, when used in error for baking powder, can cause diarrhoea and vomiting rapidly followed by paresis.

Treatment

Treatment is symptomatic and supportive.

Mushroom Poisoning

Mushrooms are common food items. There are poisonous and non-poisonous types. Poisoning is usually accidental when one cannot identify the poisonous species. There are many species of mushrooms. Most poisoning however is due to amanita (phylloides, muscaria and bresa) and galerina venenata.

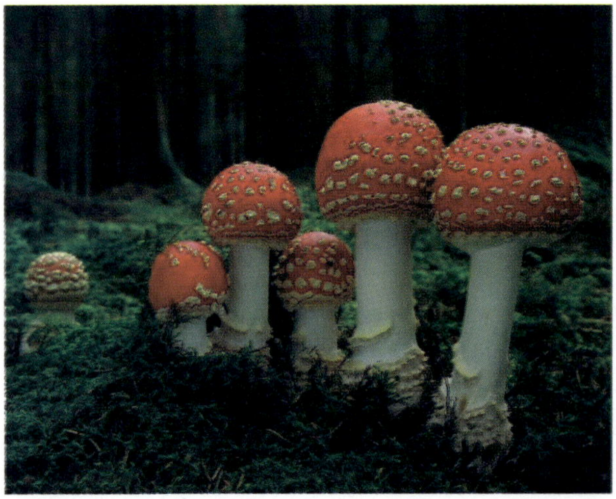

Fig. 20.3: Figure showing amanita muscaria mushroom

Clinical Manifestations

The clinical manifestations produced by amanita/galerina appear after a latent period of 6–12 hours. There is nausea, vomiting and severe abdominal pain followed by profuse watery diarrhoea which may persist for 12–24 hours. After 24 to 48 hours, jaundice (with elevated transaminases), renal failure and coma occur. Death may occur in 4–7 days after ingestion.

Treatment

In the initial phase, fluid therapy on the basis of degree of dehydration is the mainstay of treatment. In the late phase treatment for renal failure and hepatic failure is also necessary.

The specific treatment for amanita poisoning aims to remove the toxin rapidly and to block binding at its target sites. Initially activated charcoal and lactulose should be given orally along with fluid therapy. Intravenous penicillin G (250 mg/kg/day) combined with silibinin (20–50 mg/kg/day) should be administered as a continuous intravenous infusion. This helps to inhibit binding of toxins and to interrupt enterohepatic recirculation of amanitotoxin.

Hemodialysis and hemoperfusion are also recommended for intoxicated children. Cases with severe hepatic failure may require orthotopic liver transplant.

Drowning

Drowning is a preventable cause of death in children. It is a form of asphyxial death, within 24 hours of the incident, resulting from suffocation caused by submersion in water. Complete submersion is not necessary because submersion of the nose and mouth alone for a sufficient period can cause death from drowning. After drowning, consciousness is usually lost within three minutes of submersion. However, struggle for life with rising and sinking of the body goes on for a variable period until constant submersion occurs. This is followed by convulsive movements, coma or suspended animation and death.

Drowning may be of several types. *Wet drowning* is death as a result of inhalation of water where death occurs within minutes of submersion secondary to cardiac arrest and ventricular fibrillation. *Dry drowning* is a type when water does not enter the lungs but death occurs due to immediate sustained laryngospasm due to inrush of water into the nasopharynx or larynx. It is commonly seen in children. *Near drowning* refers to a submersion victim who is resuscitated and survives for atleast 24 hours regardless of the eventual outcome.

Pathophysiology

The sequence of events after submersion comprises an initial period of panic, violent struggle, automatic swimming movements followed by breath holding or laryngospasm. The respiratory disturbance depends more on the amount of water aspirated than on the water composition. The pulmonary alveolar lining is semi-permeable. When water enters the alveoli of the lungs, there is exchange of water through the alveolar lining. The extent and direction of this exchange depends on the difference of the osmotic pressure of the blood and the type of water, i.e., fresh water or sea water.

Fresh water (0.6% sodium chloride) is hypotonic in comparison to blood. In case of fresh water drowning, water is rapidly absorbed across the alveoli into the circulation leading to hypervolemia, hemodilution, hypoelectrolytemia and hemolysis. *Sea water* (over 3% sodium chloride) is hypertonic in comparison to blood. In case of sea water drowning, water is drawn into the lung from the circulation resulting in pulmonary edema, hypovolemia, hyper-electrolytemia and hemoconcentration.

Prolonged submersion results in global hypoxic injury. There is endothelial damage resulting in excessive capillary permeability and loss of protein rich fluid into the third space. Most victims are therefore hypovolemic.

There is seriously compromised oxygen uptake and carbon dioxide elimination resulting in hypoxia and hypercarbia and subsequently combined respiratory and metabolic acidosis caused by hypercapnia and anaerobic metabolism.

If the victim is rescued before aspiration of fluid occurs, the lung damage and pathophysiologic changes are minimum and the hypoxia and acidosis tend to resolve rapidly. On the other hand, aspiration of fluid into airway results in persistently abnormal gas exchange. There is significant ventilation perfusion mismatch and diffusion defect leading to intrapulmonary shunting. The surfactant system is also affected. Fresh water aspiration causes the surfactant to denature and become non-functional. Sea water aspiration either dilutes or washes the surfactant out of the alveoli entirely. This results in alveolar instability, atelectasis and decreased lung compliance.

There is decrease stroke volume and decreased arterial oxygen content. Cardiogenic shock can occur as a result of hypoxic damage of the myocardium and impairment of myocardial function by metabolic acidosis. Hypoxemia may result in ventricular tachycardia and fibrillation and asystole.

Hypoxic ischemic insult can lead to acute tubular necrosis in the kidney, liver dysfunction and DIC, sloughing and perforation of GIT.

Injury to the central nervous system results from increased intracranial pressure, cytotoxic cerebral edema, excessive accumulation of cytosolic calcium and oxygen derived free radical damage. There is depletion of ATP which is the cause of primary insult at the biochemical level.

An oxygen conserving adaptation occurs in response to submersion in the form of the diving reflex. Cerebral flow is maintained while blood flow to the GIT, skin, muscles etc is markedly reduced.

The resultant severe hypothermia following submersion has an important effect i.e. decrease in energy utilization. Cerebral metabolism is depressed and oxygen consumption is reduced. The oxyhemoglobin dissociation curve is shifted to the left. Hypothermia decreases WBC function and decrease production of insulin resulting in increased risk of infection and hyperglycemia respectively.

Management

Management at the Site

The first step in management of a rescued victim of drowning is institution of cardiopulmonary resuscitation immediately at the site of rescue. If the victim is not breathing and pulse less on evaluation mouth to mouth breathing and closed chest compression should be started after removing any debris in the oropharynx. No attempt should be made to drain the water from the lungs before pulmonary resuscitation as this fluid will get absorbed. The mouth and nostrils should be cleaned and air passage kept clear by suction. The body should be wrapped in warm blankets.

The goal is to improve tissue oxygen delivery as soon as possible in order to minimize hypoxic ischemic damage. CPR should continue during transport of the victim to the hospital.

If the victim is far away from the shore or the side of a pool, pulmonary resuscitation should be started on the spot where the victim is retrieved instead of rushing the victim to the shore and then starting CPR. It should be noted that success or failure of cardiopulmonary resuscitation (CPR) at the site of the accident often determines the outcome.

Mouth to Mouth Breathing and Closed Chest Cardiac Compression

To give *mouth to mouth breathing*, the patient is made to lie on the back with the head hyper extended. The operator takes a deep breath and then breathes directly mouth to mouth. The patient is allowed to exhale passively. This should be repeated 15 – 20 times per minute and continued for an hour or till natural respiration is restored.

For *closed chest cardiac compression*, the patient is made to lie on the back. The operator places his hands one on the top of the other on the lower third of the sternum. Forcible rhythmic compressions are made at the rate 60 to 80 per minute. The force of compression must be sufficient to produce pulsation in the carotid and femoral arteries.

The respiratory and heart rates for CPR in newborn shall be different (30 /minute and 90 /minute respectively, ratio 1: 3).

Management in the Hospital

Priority should be given to maintenance of airway, breathing and circulation. Other forms of associated trauma viz. injury to head, cervical spine and other areas should be considered. A neurological examination should be done after respiratory and circulatory stability has been achieved.

Oxygen saturation should be monitored. Continuous ECG monitoring is necessary to detect arrhythmias. The modified Glasgow coma scale should be noted as a base line. Central venous pressure (CVP) should be monitored for assessment and management of intravascular volume. An orogastric tube should be inserted and the stomach is aspirated and emptied of swallowed water.

If the patient has adequate respiratory effort, supplemental oxygen is all that is indicated. Endotracheal intubation and mechanical ventilation is indicated in the following situations:

1. Cardiorespiratory arrest.
2. Depressed consciousness with loss of airway protective reflexes.
3. Severe respiratory distress or severe hypoxia in spite of supplemental oxygen.
4. Severe hypothermia (Core temperature < 30° C).
5. A deteriorating neurological status.
6. PaO_2 less than 60 mmHg while on 50% oxygen, oxygen saturation less than 90% or worsening hypercapnia.

Most often a high PEEP is required. High frequency ventilation may be required if respiratory failure is unresponsive to conventional ventilation. Extracorporeal life support may be required in treatment of severe lung injury.

In presence of *hypothermia*, which is common, efforts at rewarming should be instituted at the earliest. All wet clothes are removed. Active external rewarming using electric warming devices, hot water bags, warm beddings and radiant warmers (for neonates) should be started in patients with a core temperature more than 30°C. If the core temperature is less than 30°C active internal rewarming is necessary by using warmed intravenous fluids, warmed humidified oxygen, gastric or rectal lavage and peritoneal lavage with warm fluids.

Hypovolemia is managed by bolus doses of crystalloids (Sodium chloride 20 ml/kg) and inotropic drugs. Hypothermia slows renal and hepatic excretion of drugs and hence cardiotonic drugs should be used with caution.

Mild to moderate *acidosis* is corrected with oxygenation and tissue perfusion. In more severe cases sodium bicarbonate administration may be required. Cerebral edema and increased ICP should be managed with usual measures to reduce ICP.

Arrhythmias are common with fresh water drowning. Arrhythmias require defibrillation. Hypothermic heart is resistant to the effects of defibrillation. Hence the patient should be rewarmed before defibrillation or the attempt repeated.

Fulminant sepsis and pneumonia due to S. pneumoniae can occur. Empiric antibiotics should be administered to patients with severe cardiopulmonary deterioration especially after a period of stability. Routine prophylactic antibiotic is not necessary.

Prognosis

Most victims, who resume spontaneous respiration at the site, become responsive, have a sinus rhythm and have been submerged for less than 5 minutes in water warmer than 5°C, survive without neurological sequalae. Victims submerged in warm water and present with cardiac arrest may return to normal circulation within 10 minutes with aggressive pre-hospital care. Poor prognostic factors of death or severe neurological sequalae include: (i) Unresponsive on arrival at the hospital; (ii) Elevated blood glucose level; (iii) Fixed pupils; (iv) Cardiac arrest requiring more than 25 minutes of advanced life support; (v) Initial GCS score less than 5; and (vi) Presence of seizure and flaccidity.

Suggested Reading

1. Textbook of medical jurisprudence and toxicology by C.K. Parikh, 5th edition, 1995.
2. The pediatric management of snake bites: The national protocol. Indian Pediatrics 2007: 44, pp 173–175.
3. Poisoning in children by Utpal Kant Singh, FC Layland, Sanjay Suman and Rajniti Prasad. 2nd edition, 2001, Jaypee Brothers Medical Publishers (P) Ltd.
4. Nelson Textbook of Pediatrics, 17th edition, 2004. Edited by Behrman, Kliegman and Jenson. Saunders, Philadelphia.
5. IAP Journal of Practical Pediatrics, Vol 3, 1995.
6. Price's Textbook of the practice of Medicine. Edited by Sir Ronald Bodley Scott, 11th edition, 1973, ELBS and Oxford University Press.
7. Harrison's Principles of Internal Medicine edited by Anthony S. Fauci, Eugine Braunwald, Kurt J. Isselbacher *et al.* 14th edition, 1998. McGraw-Hill, Health Professions Division.

Appendices

Blood Pressure Levels for BOYS by Age and Height Percentile

Age (Year)	BP Percentile ↓	Systolic BP (mmHg) ← Percentile of Height →							Diastolic BP (mmHg) ← Percentile of Height →						
		5th	10th	25th	50th	75th	90th	95th	5th	10th	25th	50th	75th	90th	95th
1	50th	80	81	83	85	87	88	89	34	35	36	37	38	39	39
	90th	94	95	97	99	100	102	103	49	50	51	52	53	53	54
	95th	98	99	101	103	104	106	106	54	54	55	56	57	58	58
	99th	105	106	108	110	112	113	114	61	62	63	64	65	66	66
2	50th	84	85	87	88	90	92	92	39	40	41	42	43	44	44
	90th	97	99	100	102	104	105	106	54	55	56	57	58	58	59
	95th	101	102	104	106	108	109	110	59	59	60	61	62	63	63
	99th	109	110	111	113	115	117	117	66	67	68	69	70	71	71
3	50th	86	87	89	91	93	94	95	44	44	45	46	47	48	48
	90th	100	101	103	105	107	108	109	59	59	60	61	62	63	63
	95th	104	105	107	109	110	112	113	63	63	64	65	66	67	67
	99th	111	112	114	116	118	119	120	71	71	72	73	74	75	75
4	50th	88	89	91	93	95	96	97	47	48	49	50	51	51	52
	90th	102	103	105	107	109	110	111	62	63	64	65	66	66	67
	95th	106	107	109	111	112	114	115	66	67	68	69	70	71	71
	99th	113	114	116	118	120	121	122	74	75	76	77	78	78	79
5	50th	90	91	93	95	96	98	98	50	51	52	53	54	55	55
	90th	104	105	106	108	110	111	112	65	66	67	68	69	69	70
	95th	108	109	110	112	114	115	116	69	70	71	72	73	74	74
	99th	115	116	118	120	121	123	123	77	78	79	80	81	81	82
6	50th	91	92	94	96	98	99	100	53	53	54	55	56	57	57
	90th	105	106	108	110	111	113	113	68	68	69	70	71	72	72
	95th	109	110	112	114	115	117	117	72	72	73	74	75	76	76
	99th	116	117	119	121	123	124	125	80	80	81	82	83	84	84
7	50th	92	94	95	97	99	100	101	55	55	56	57	58	59	59
	90th	106	107	109	111	113	114	115	70	70	71	72	73	74	74
	95th	110	111	113	115	117	118	119	74	74	75	76	77	78	78
	99th	117	118	120	122	124	125	126	82	82	83	84	85	86	86
8	50th	94	95	97	99	100	102	102	56	57	58	59	60	60	61
	90th	107	109	110	112	114	115	116	71	72	72	73	74	75	76
	95th	111	112	114	116	118	119	120	75	76	77	78	79	79	80
	99th	119	120	122	123	125	127	127	83	84	85	86	87	87	88
9	50th	95	96	98	100	102	103	104	57	58	59	60	61	61	62
	90th	109	110	112	114	115	117	118	72	73	74	75	76	76	77
	95th	113	114	116	118	119	121	121	76	77	78	79	80	81	81
	99th	120	121	123	125	127	128	129	84	85	86	87	88	88	89
10	50th	97	98	100	102	103	105	106	58	59	60	61	61	62	63
	90th	111	112	114	115	117	119	119	73	73	74	75	76	77	78
	95th	115	116	117	119	121	122	123	77	78	79	80	81	81	82
	99th	122	123	125	127	128	130	130	85	86	86	88	88	89	90

Contd.

Blood Pressure Levels for BOYS by Age and Height Percentile (*Contd.*)

Age (Year)	BP Percentile ↓	Systolic BP (mmHg) ← Percentile of Height →							Diastolic BP (mmHg) ← Percentile of Height →						
		5th	10th	25th	50th	75th	90th	95th	5th	10th	25th	50th	75th	90th	95th
11	50th	99	100	102	104	105	107	107	59	59	60	61	62	63	63
	90th	113	114	115	117	119	120	121	74	74	75	76	77	78	78
	95th	117	118	119	121	123	124	125	78	78	79	80	81	82	82
	99th	124	125	127	129	130	132	132	86	86	87	88	89	90	90
12	50th	101	102	104	106	108	109	110	59	60	61	62	63	63	64
	90th	115	116	118	120	121	123	123	74	75	75	76	77	78	79
	95th	119	120	122	123	125	127	127	78	79	80	81	82	82	83
	99th	126	127	129	131	133	134	135	86	87	88	89	90	90	91
13	50th	104	105	106	108	110	111	112	60	60	61	62	63	64	64
	90th	117	118	120	122	124	125	126	75	75	76	77	78	79	79
	95th	121	122	124	126	128	129	130	79	79	80	81	82	83	83
	99th	128	130	131	133	135	136	137	87	87	88	89	90	91	91
14	50th	106	107	109	111	113	114	115	60	61	62	63	64	65	65
	90th	120	121	123	125	126	128	128	75	76	77	78	79	79	80
	95th	124	125	127	128	130	132	132	80	80	81	82	83	84	84
	99th	131	132	134	136	138	139	140	87	88	89	90	91	92	92
15	50th	109	110	112	113	115	117	117	67	62	63	64	65	66	66
	90th	122	124	125	127	129	130	131	76	77	78	79	80	80	81
	95th	126	127	129	131	133	134	135	81	81	82	83	84	85	85
	99th	134	135	136	138	140	142	142	88	89	90	91	92	93	93
16	50th	111	112	114	116	118	119	120	63	63	64	65	66	67	67
	90th	125	126	128	130	131	133	134	78	78	79	80	81	82	82
	95th	129	130	132	134	135	137	137	82	83	83	84	85	86	87
	99th	136	137	139	141	143	144	145	90	90	91	92	93	94	94
17	50th	114	115	116	118	120	121	122	65	66	66	67	68	69	70
	90th	127	128	130	132	134	135	136	80	80	81	82	83	84	84
	95th	131	132	134	136	138	139	140	84	85	86	87	87	88	89
	99th	139	140	141	143	145	146	147	92	93	93	94	95	96	97

BP, blood pressure

* The 90th percentile is1.28 SD, 95th percentile is 1.645 SD, and the 99th percentile is 2.326 SD over the mean.

For research purposes, the standard deviations in Appendix Table B-1 allow one to compute BP Z-scores and percentiles for boys with height percentiles given in Table 3 (i.e., the 5th,10th, 25th, 50th,75th, 90th and 95th percentiles). These height percentiles must be converted to height Z-scores given by (5% = -1.645; 10% = -1.28; 25% = -0.68; 50%= 0; 75% = 0.68; 90% = 1.28; 95% = 1.645) and then computed according to the methodology in steps 2-4 described in Appendix B. For children with height percentiles other than these, follow steps 1-4 as described in Appendix B.

From the Fourth Report on the Diagnosis, Evaluation and Treatment of High Blood Pressure in Children and Adolescents. Pediatrics 2004;114:555-76.

Blood Pressure Levels for GIRLS by Age and Height Percentile

Age (Year)	BP Percentile ↓	Systolic BP (mmHg) ← Percentile of Height →							Diastolic BP (mmHg) ← Percentile of Height →						
		5th	10th	25th	50th	75th	90th	95th	5th	10th	25th	50th	75th	90th	95th
1	50th	83	84	85	86	88	89	90	38	39	39	40	41	41	42
	90th	97	97	98	100	101	102	103	52	53	53	54	55	55	56
	95th	100	101	102	104	105	106	107	56	57	57	58	59	59	60
	99th	108	108	109	111	112	113	114	64	64	65	65	66	67	67
2	50th	85	85	87	88	89	91	91	43	44	44	45	46	46	47
	90th	98	99	100	101	103	104	105	57	58	58	59	60	61	61
	95th	102	103	104	105	107	108	109	61	62	62	63	64	65	65
	99th	109	110	111	112	114	115	116	69	69	70	70	71	72	72
3	50th	86	87	88	89	91	92	93	47	48	48	49	50	50	51
	90th	100	100	102	103	104	106	106	61	62	62	63	64	64	65
	95th	104	104	105	107	108	109	110	65	66	66	67	68	68	69
	99th	111	111	113	114	115	116	117	73	73	74	74	75	76	76
4	50th	88	88	90	91	92	94	94	50	50	51	52	52	53	54
	90th	101	102	103	104	106	107	108	64	64	65	66	67	67	68
	95th	105	106	107	108	110	111	112	68	68	69	70	71	71	72
	99th	112	113	114	115	117	118	119	76	76	76	77	78	79	79
5	50th	89	90	91	93	94	95	96	52	53	53	54	55	55	56
	90th	103	103	105	106	107	109	109	66	67	67	68	69	69	70
	95th	107	107	108	110	111	112	113	70	71	71	72	73	73	74
	99th	114	114	116	117	118	120	120	78	78	79	79	80	81	81
6	50th	91	92	93	94	96	97	98	54	54	55	56	56	57	58
	90th	104	105	106	108	109	110	111	68	68	69	70	70	71	72
	95th	108	109	110	111	113	114	115	72	72	73	74	74	75	76
	99th	115	116	117	119	120	121	122	80	80	80	81	82	83	83
7	50th	93	93	95	96	97	99	99	55	56	56	57	58	58	59
	90th	106	107	108	109	111	112	113	69	70	70	71	72	72	73
	95th	110	111	112	113	115	116	116	73	74	74	75	76	76	77
	99th	117	118	119	120	122	123	124	81	81	82	82	83	84	84
8	50th	95	95	96	98	99	100	101	57	57	57	58	59	60	60
	90th	108	109	110	111	113	114	114	71	71	71	72	73	74	74
	95th	112	112	114	115	116	118	118	75	75	75	76	77	78	78
	99th	119	120	121	122	123	125	125	82	82	83	83	84	85	86
9	50th	96	97	98	100	101	102	103	58	58	58	59	60	61	61
	90th	110	110	112	113	114	116	116	72	72	72	73	74	75	75
	95th	114	114	115	117	118	119	120	76	76	76	77	78	79	79
	99th	121	121	123	124	125	127	127	83	83	84	84	85	86	87
10	50th	98	99	100	102	103	104	105	59	59	59	60	61	62	62
	90th	112	112	114	115	116	118	118	73	73	73	74	75	76	76
	95th	116	116	117	119	120	121	122	77	77	77	78	79	80	80
	99th	123	123	125	126	127	129	129	84	84	85	86	86	87	88

Contd.

Blood Pressure Levels for BOYS by Age and Height Percentile (*Contd.*)															
Age (Year)	BP Percentile ↓	Systolic BP (mmHg)							Diastolic BP (mmHg)						
		← Percentile of Height →							← Percentile of Height →						
		5th	10th	25th	50th	75th	90th	95th	5th	10th	25th	50th	75th	90th	95th
11	50th	100	101	102	103	105	106	107	60	60	60	61	62	63	63
	90th	114	114	116	117	118	119	120	74	74	74	75	76	77	77
	95th	118	118	119	121	122	123	124	78	78	78	79	80	81	81
	99th	125	125	126	128	129	130	131	85	85	86	87	87	88	89
12	50th	102	103	104	105	107	108	109	61	61	61	62	63	64	64
	90th	116	116	117	119	120	121	122	75	75	75	76	77	78	78
	95th	119	120	121	123	124	125	126	79	79	79	80	81	82	82
	99th	127	127	128	130	131	132	133	86	86	87	88	88	89	90
13	50th	104	105	106	107	109	110	110	62	62	62	63	64	65	65
	90th	117	118	119	121	122	123	124	76	76	76	77	78	79	79
	95th	121	122	123	124	126	127	128	80	80	80	81	82	83	83
	99th	128	129	130	132	133	134	135	87	87	88	89	89	90	91
14	50th	106	106	107	109	110	111	112	63	63	63	64	65	66	66
	90th	119	120	121	122	124	125	125	77	77	77	78	79	80	80
	95th	123	123	125	126	127	129	120	81	81	81	82	83	84	84
	99th	130	131	132	133	135	136	136	88	88	89	90	90	91	92
15	50th	107	108	109	110	111	113	113	64	64	64	65	66	67	67
	90th	120	121	122	123	125	126	127	78	78	78	79	80	81	81
	95th	124	125	126	127	129	130	131	82	82	82	83	84	85	85
	99th	131	132	133	134	136	137	138	89	89	90	91	91	92	93
16	50th	108	108	110	111	112	114	114	64	64	65	66	66	67	68
	90th	121	122	123	124	126	127	128	78	78	79	80	81	81	82
	95th	125	126	127	128	130	131	132	82	82	83	84	85	85	86
	99th	132	133	134	135	137	138	139	90	90	90	91	92	93	93
17	50th	108	109	110	111	113	114	115	64	65	65	66	67	67	68
	90th	122	122	123	125	126	127	128	78	79	79	80	81	81	82
	95th	125	126	127	129	130	131	132	82	83	83	84	85	85	86
	99th	133	133	134	136	137	138	139	90	90	91	91	92	93	93

BP, blood pressure

* The 90th percentile is 1.28 SD, 95th percentile is 1.645 SD, and the 99th percentile is 2.326 SD over the mean.

For research purposes, the standard deviations in Appendix Table B-1 allow one to compute BP Z-scores and percentiles for girls with height percentiles given in Table 4 (i.e., the 5th,10th, 25th, 50th,75th, 90th and 95th percentiles). These height percentiles must be converted to height Z-scores given by (5% = -1.645; 10% = -1.28; 25% = -0.68; 50%= 0; 75% = 0.68; 90% = 1.28; 95% = 1.645) and then computed according to the methodology in steps 2-4 described in Appendix B. For children with height percentiles other than these, follow steps 1-4 as described in Appendix B.

From the Fourth Report on the Diagnosis, Evaluation and Treatment of High Blood Pressure in Children and Adolescents. Pediatrics 2004;114:555-76.

Weight-for-age BOYS Birth 5 to 10 years (Percentiles)						
Year-Month	Months	3rd	15th	Median	85th	97th
0.0	0	2.5	2.9	3.3	3.9	4.3
0.1	1	3.4	3.9	4.5	5.1	5.7
0.2	2	4.4	4.9	5.6	6.3	7.0
0.3	3	5.1	5.6	6.4	7.2	7.9
0.4	4	5.6	6.2	7.0	7.9	8.6
0.5	5	6.1	6.7	7.5	8.4	9.2
0.6	6	6.4	7.1	7.9	8.9	9.7
0.7	7	6.7	7.4	8.3	9.3	10.2
0.8	8	7.0	7.7	8.6	9.6	10.5
0.9	9	7.2	7.9	8.9	10.0	10.9
0.10	10	7.5	8.2	9.2	10.3	11.2
0.11	11	7.7	8.4	9.4	10.5	11.5
1.0	12	7.8	8.6	9.6	10.8	11.8
1.1	13	8.0	8.8	9.9	11.1	12.1
1.3	15	8.4	9.2	10.3	11.6	12.7
1.4	16	8.5	9.4	10.5	11.8	12.9
1.5	17	8.7	9.6	10.7	12.0	13.2
1.6	18	8.9	9.7	10.9	12.3	13.5
1.7	19	9.0	9.9	11.1	12.5	13.7
1.8	20	9.2	10.1	11.3	12.7	14.0
1.9	21	9.3	10.3	11.5	13.0	14.3
1.10	22	9.5	10.5	11.8	13.2	14.5
1.11	23	9.7	10.6	12.0	13.4	14.8
2.0	24	9.8	10.8	12.2	13.7	15.1
2.1	25	10.0	11.0	12.4	13.9	15.3
2.2	26	10.1	11.1	12.5	14.1	15.6
2.3	27	10.2	11.3	12.7	14.4	15.9
2.4	28	10.4	11.5	12.9	14.6	16.1
2.5	29	10.5	11.6	13.1	14.8	16.4

WHO Child Growth Standards

Source: de Onis M, Garza C, Onyango AW, Martorell R. WHO child growth standards. *Acta Paediatrica* (Suppl) 200 450: 1-110 and www.who.int/childgrowth/standards/en/

Weight-for-age BOYS 5 to 10 years (Percentiles)						
Year-Month	**Months**	**3rd**	**15th**	**Median**	**85th**	**97th**
5.1	61	14.6	16.2	18.5	21.2	23.8
5.2	62	14.7	16.4	18.7	21.4	24.0
5.3	63	14.8	16.5	18.9	21.6	24.3
5.4	64	15.0	16.7	19.0	21.9	24.5
5.5	65	15.1	16.8	19.2	22.1	24.8
5.6	66	15.3	17.0	19.4	22.3	25.1
5.7	67	15.4	17.1	19.6	22.5	25.3
5.8	68	15.5	17.3	19.8	22.7	25.6
5.9	69	15.7	17.4	19.9	23.0	25.8
5.10	70	15.8	17.6	20.1	23.2	26.1
5.11	71	16.0	17.7	20.3	23.4	26.4
6.0	72	16.1	17.9	20.5	23.6	26.7
6.1	73	16.3	18.1	20.7	23.9	26.9
6.2	74	16.4	18.2	20.9	24.1	27.2
6.3	75	16.5	18.4	21.1	24.3	27.5
6.4	76	16.7	18.6	21.3	24.6	27.8
6.5	77	16.8	18.7	21.5	24.8	28.1
6.6	78	17.0	18.9	21.7	25.0	28.3
6.7	79	17.2	19.1	21.9	25.3	28.6
6.8	80	17.3	19.2	22.1	25.5	28.9
6.9	81	17.5	19.4	22.3	25.8	29.2
6.10	82	17.6	19.6	22.5	26.0	29.5
6.11	83	17.8	19.8	22.7	26.3	29.8
7.0	84	17.9	19.9	22.9	26.5	30.1
7.1	85	18.1	20.1	23.1	26.8	30.4
7.2	86	18.2	20.3	23.3	27.0	30.7
7.3	87	18.4	20.5	23.5	27.3	31.1
7.4	88	18.5	20.6	23.7	27.5	31.4
7.5	89	18.7	20.8	23.9	27.8	31.7
7.6	90	18.8	21.0	24.1	28.1	32.0

WHO Child Growth Standards

Weight-for-age BOYS 5 to 10 years (Percentiles)						
Year-Month	Months	3rd	15th	Median	85th	97th
7.7	91	19.0	21.2	24.3	28.3	32.3
7.8	92	19.1	21.3	24.6	28.6	32.7
7.9	93	19.3	21.5	24.8	28.9	33.0
7.10	94	19.5	21.7	25.0	29.1	33.3
7.11	95	19.6	21.9	25.2	29.4	33.7
8.0	96	19.8	22.0	25.4	29.7	34.0
8.1	97	19.9	22.2	25.6	30.0	34.4
8.2	98	20.1	22.4	25.9	30.2	34.7
8.3	99	20.2	22.6	26.1	30.5	35.1
8.4	100	20.4	22.7	26.3	30.8	35.5
8.5	101	20.5	22.9	26.5	31.1	35.8
8.6	102	20.7	23.1	26.7	31.4	36.2
8.7	103	20.8	23.3	27.0	31.7	36.6
8.8	104	21.0	23.5	27.2	32.0	37.0
8.9	105	21.1	23.6	27.4	32.3	37.4
8.10	106	21.3	23.8	27.6	32.6	37.8
8.11	107	21.4	24.0	27.9	32.9	38.2
9.0	108	21.6	24.2	28.1	33.2	38.6
9.1	109	21.8	24.4	28.3	33.5	39.0
9.2	110	21.9	24.6	28.6	33.8	39.4
9.3	111	22.1	24.7	28.8	34.2	39.8
9.4	112	22.2	24.9	29.1	34.5	40.3
9.5	113	22.4	25.1	29.3	34.8	40.7
9.6	114	22.6	25.3	29.6	35.2	41.1
9.7	115	22.7	25.5	29.8	35.5	41.6
9.8	116	22.9	25.7	30.1	35.8	42.0
9.9	117	23.1	25.9	30.4	36.2	42.5
9.10	118	23.2	26.1	30.6	36.6	43.0
9.11	119	23.4	26.3	30.9	36.9	43.5
10.0	120	23.6	26.6	31.2	37.3	43.9

WHO Child Growth Standards

Weight-for-age GIRLS Birth to 5 years (Percentiles)						
Year-Month	**Months**	**3rd**	**15th**	**Median**	**85th**	**97th**
0.0	0	2.4	2.8	3.2	3.7	4.2
0.1	1	3.2	3.6	4.2	4.8	5.4
0.2	2	4.0	4.5	5.1	5.9	6.5
0.3	3	4.6	5.1	5.8	6.7	7.4
0.4	4	5.1	5.6	6.4	7.3	8.1
0.5	5	5.5	6.1	6.9	7.8	8.7
0.6	6	5.8	6.4	7.3	8.3	9.2
0.7	7	6.1	6.7	7.6	8.7	9.6
0.8	8	6.3	7.0	7.9	9.0	10.0
0.9	9	6.6	7.3	8.2	9.3	10.4
0.10	10	6.8	7.5	8.5	9.6	10.7
0.11	11	7.0	7.7	8.7	9.9	11.0
1.0	12	7.1	7.9	8.9	10.2	11.3
1.1	13	7.3	8.1	9.2	10.4	11.6
1.2	14	7.5	8.3	9.4	10.7	11.9
1.3	15	7.7	8.5	9.6	10.9	12.2
1.4	16	7.8	8.7	9.8	11.2	12.5
1.5	17	8.0	8.8	10.0	11.4	12.7
1.6	18	8.2	9.0	10.2	11.6	13.0
1.7	19	8.3	9.2	10.4	11.9	13.3
1.8	20	8.5	9.4	10.6	12.1	13.5
1.9	21	8.7	9.6	10.9	12.4	13.8
1.10	22	8.8	9.8	11.1	12.6	14.1
1.11	23	9.0	9.9	11.3	12.8	14.3
2.0	24	9.2	10.1	11.5	13.1	14.6
2.1	25	9.3	10.3	11.7	13.3	14.9
2.2	26	9.5	10.5	11.9	13.6	15.2
2.3	27	9.6	10.7	12.1	13.8	15.4
2.4	28	9.8	10.8	12.3	14.0	15.7
2.5	29	10.0	11.0	12.5	14.3	16.0

WHO Child Growth Standards

Weight-for-age GIRLS Birth to 5 years (Percentiles)						
Year-Month	Months	3rd	15th	Median	85th	97th
2.6	30	10.1	11.2	12.7	14.5	16.2
2.7	31	10.3	11.3	12.9	14.7	16.5
2.8	32	10.4	11.5	13.1	15.0	16.8
2.9	33	10.5	11.7	13.3	15.2	17.0
2.10	34	10.7	11.8	13.5	15.4	17.3
2.11	35	10.8	12.0	13.7	15.7	17.6
3.0	36	11.0	12.1	13.9	15.9	17.8
3.1	37	11.1	12.3	14.0	16.1	18.1
3.2	38	11.2	12.5	14.2	16.3	18.4
3.3	39	11.4	12.6	14.4	16.6	18.6
3.4	40	11.5	12.8	14.6	16.8	18.9
3.5	41	11.6	12.9	14.8	17.0	19.2
3.6	42	11.8	13.1	15.0	17.3	19.5
3.7	43	11.9	13.2	15.2	17.5	19.7
3.8	44	12.0	13.4	15.3	17.7	20.0
3.9	45	12.1	13.5	15.5	17.9	20.3
3.10	46	12.3	13.7	15.7	18.2	20.6
3.11	47	12.4	13.8	15.9	18.4	20.8
4.0	48	12.5	14.0	16.1	18.6	21.1
4.1	49	12.6	14.1	16.3	18.9	21.4
4.2	50	12.8	14.3	16.4	19.1	21.7
4.3	51	12.9	14.4	16.6	19.3	22.0
4.4	52	13.0	14.5	16.8	19.5	22.2
4.5	53	13.1	14.7	17.0	19.8	22.5
4.6	54	13.2	14.8	17.2	20.0	22.8
4.7	55	13.4	15.0	17.3	20.2	23.1
4.8	56	13.5	15.1	17.5	20.4	23.3
4.9	57	13.6	15.3	17.7	20.7	23.6
4.10	58	13.7	15.4	17.9	20.9	23.9
4.11	59	13.8	15.5	18.0	21.1	24.2
5.0	60	14.0	15.7	18.2	21.3	24.4

WHO Child Growth Standards

Weight-for-age GIRLS 5 to 10 years (Percentiles)						
Year-Month	**Months**	**3rd**	**15th**	**Median**	**85th**	**97th**
5.1	61	14.2	15.8	18.3	21.3	24.3
5.2	62	14.3	16.0	18.4	21.5	24.6
5.3	63	14.4	16.1	18.6	21.7	24.9
5.4	64	14.5	16.3	18.8	21.9	25.1
5.5	65	14.7	16.4	19.0	22.2	25.4
5.6	66	14.8	16.5	19.1	22.4	25.7
5.7	67	14.9	16.7	19.3	22.6	25.9
5.8	68	15.0	16.8	19.5	22.8	26.2
5.9	69	15.2	17.0	19.6	23.0	26.5
5.10	70	15.3	17.1	19.8	23.2	26.7
5.11	71	15.4	17.2	20.0	23.5	27.0
6.0	72	15.5	17.4	20.2	23.7	27.3
6.1	73	15.6	17.5	20.3	23.9	27.5
6.2	74	15.8	17.7	20.5	24.1	27.8
6.3	75	15.9	17.8	20.7	24.3	28.1
6.4	76	16.0	17.9	20.9	24.6	28.4
6.5	77	16.1	18.1	21.0	24.8	28.7
6.6	78	16.3	18.2	21.2	25.0	28.9
6.7	79	16.4	18.4	21.4	25.3	29.2
6.8	80	16.5	18.5	21.6	25.5	29.5
6.9	81	16.6	18.7	21.8	25.7	29.8
6.10	82	16.8	18.8	22.0	26.0	30.1
6.11	83	16.9	19.0	22.2	26.2	30.4
7.0	84	17.0	19.2	22.4	26.5	30.8
7.1	85	17.2	19.3	22.6	26.7	31.1
7.2	86	17.3	19.5	22.8	27.0	31.4
7.3	87	17.5	19.7	23.0	27.3	31.7
7.4	88	17.6	19.8	23.2	27.5	32.1
7.5	89	17.8	20.0	23.4	27.8	32.4
7.6	90	17.9	20.2	23.6	28.1	32.8

WHO Child Growth Standards

Weight-for-age GIRLS 5 to 10 years (Percentiles)						
Year-Month	Months	3rd	15th	Median	85th	97th
7.7	91	18.1	20.4	23.9	28.4	33.1
7.8	92	18.2	20.6	24.1	28.7	33.5
7.9	93	18.4	20.7	24.3	28.9	33.8
7.10	94	18.6	20.9	24.5	29.2	34.2
7.11	95	18.7	21.1	24.8	29.5	34.6
8.0	96	18.9	21.3	25.0	29.8	34.9
8.1	97	19.1	21.5	25.3	30.2	35.3
8.2	98	19.2	21.7	25.5	30.5	35.7
8.3	99	19.4	21.9	25.8	30.8	36.1
8.4	100	19.6	22.1	26.0	31.1	36.5
8.5	101	19.8	22.3	26.3	31.4	36.9
8.6	102	20.0	22.6	26.6	31.8	37.4
8.7	103	20.1	22.8	26.8	32.1	37.8
8.8	104	20.3	23.0	27.1	32.5	38.2
8.9	105	20.5	23.2	27.4	32.8	38.6
8.10	106	20.7	23.4	27.6	33.2	39.1
8.11	107	20.9	23.7	27.9	33.5	39.5
9.0	108	21.1	23.9	28.2	33.9	40.0
9.1	109	21.3	24.1	28.5	34.2	40.4
9.2	110	21.5	24.4	28.8	34.6	40.9
9.3	111	21.7	24.6	29.1	35.0	41.3
9.4	112	21.9	24.8	29.4	35.3	41.8
9.5	113	22.1	25.1	29.7	35.7	42.3
9.6	114	22.3	25.3	30.0	36.1	42.7
9.7	115	22.6	25.6	30.3	36.5	43.2
9.8	116	22.8	25.8	30.6	36.9	43.7
9.9	117	23.0	26.1	30.9	37.3	44.2
9.10	118	23.2	26.3	31.2	37.7	44.7
9.11	119	23.4	26.6	31.5	38.1	45.2
10.0	120	23.7	26.9	31.9	38.5	45.7

WHO Child Growth Standards

Length-for-age BOYS Birth to 2 years (Percentiles)						
Year-Month	**Months**	**3rd**	**15th**	**Median**	**85th**	**97th**
0.0	0	46.3	47.9	49.9	51.8	53.4
0.1	1	51.1	52.7	54.7	56.7	58.4
0.2	2	54.7	56.4	58.4	60.5	62.2
0.3	3	57.6	59.3	61.4	63.5	65.3
0.4	4	60.0	61.7	63.9	66.0	67.8
0.5	5	61.9	63.7	65.9	68.1	69.9
0.6	6	63.6	65.4	67.6	69.8	71.6
0.7	7	65.1	66.9	69.2	71.4	73.2
0.8	8	66.5	68.3	70.6	72.9	74.7
0.9	9	67.7	69.6	72.0	74.3	76.2
0.10	10	69.0	70.9	73.3	75.6	77.6
0.11	11	70.2	72.1	74.5	77.0	78.9
1.0	12	71.3	73.3	75.7	78.2	80.2
1.1	13	72.4	74.4	76.9	79.4	81.5
1.2	14	73.4	75.5	78.0	80.6	82.7
1.3	15	74.4	76.5	79.1	81.8	83.9
1.4	16	75.4	77.5	80.2	82.9	85.1
1.5	17	76.3	78.5	81.2	84.0	86.2
1.6	18	77.2	79.5	82.3	85.1	87.3
1.7	19	78.1	80.4	83.2	86.1	88.4
1.8	20	78.9	81.3	84.2	87.1	89.5
1.9	21	79.7	82.2	85.1	88.1	90.5
1.10	22	80.5	83.0	86.0	89.1	91.6
1.11	23	81.3	83.8	86.9	90.0	92.6
2.0	24	82.1	84.6	87.8	91.0	93.6

WHO Child Growth Standards

Height-for-age BOYS 2 to 5 years (Percentiles)						
Year-Month	Months	3rd	15th	Median	85th	97th
2.0	24	81.4	83.9	87.1	90.3	92.9
2.1	25	82.1	84.7	88.0	91.2	93.8
2.2	26	82.8	85.5	88.8	92.1	94.8
2.3	27	83.5	86.3	89.6	93.0	95.7
2.4	28	84.2	87.0	90.4	93.8	96.6
2.5	29	84.9	87.7	91.2	94.7	97.5
2.6	30	85.5	88.4	91.9	95.5	98.3
2.7	31	86.2	89.1	92.7	96.2	99.2
2.8	32	86.8	89.7	93.4	97.0	100.0
2.9	33	87.4	90.4	94.1	97.8	100.8
2.10	34	88.0	91.0	94.8	98.5	101.5
2.11	35	88.5	91.6	95.4	99.2	102.3
3.0	36	89.1	92.2	96.1	99.9	103.1
3.1	37	89.7	92.8	96.7	100.6	103.8
3.2	38	90.2	93.4	97.4	101.3	104.5
3.3	39	90.8	94.0	98.0	102.0	105.2
3.4	40	91.3	94.6	98.6	102.7	105.9
3.5	41	91.9	95.2	99.2	103.3	106.6
3.6	42	92.4	95.7	99.9	104.0	107.3
3.7	43	92.9	96.3	100.4	104.6	108.0
3.8	44	93.4	96.8	101.0	105.2	108.6
3.9	45	93.9	97.4	101.6	105.8	109.3
3.10	46	94.4	97.9	102.2	106.5	109.9
3.11	47	94.9	98.5	102.8	107.1	110.6
4.0	48	95.4	99.0	103.3	107.7	111.2
4.1	49	95.9	99.5	103.9	108.3	111.8
4.2	50	96.4	100.0	104.4	108.9	112.5
4.3	51	96.9	100.5	105.0	109.5	113.1
4.4	52	97.4	101.1	105.6	110.1	113.7
4.5	53	97.9	101.6	106.1	110.7	114.3
4.6	54	98.4	102.1	106.7	111.2	115.0
4.7	55	98.8	102.6	107.2	111.8	115.6
4.8	56	99.3	103.1	107.8	112.4	116.2
4.9	57	99.8	103.6	108.3	113.0	116.8
4.10	58	100.3	104.1	108.9	113.6	117.4
4.11	59	100.8	104.7	109.4	114.2	118.1
5.0	60	101.2	105.2	110.0	114.8	118.7

WHO Child Growth Standards

Height-for-age BOYS 5 to 19 years (Percentiles)						
Year-Month	Months	3rd	15th	Median	85th	97th
5.1	61	101.6	105.5	110.3	115.0	118.9
5.2	62	102.1	106.0	110.8	115.6	119.5
5.3	63	102.6	106.5	111.3	116.2	120.1
5.4	64	103.1	107.0	111.9	116.7	120.7
5.5	65	103.5	107.5	112.4	117.3	121.3
5.6	66	104.0	108.0	112.9	117.8	121.8
5.7	67	104.4	108.5	113.4	118.4	122.4
5.8	68	104.9	109.0	113.9	118.9	123.0
5.9	69	105.4	109.4	114.5	119.5	123.5
5.10	70	105.8	109.9	115.0	120.0	124.1
5.11	71	106.2	110.4	115.5	120.5	124.7
6.0	72	106.7	110.8	116.0	121.1	125.2
6.1	73	107.1	111.3	116.4	121.6	125.8
6.2	74	107.6	111.8	116.9	122.1	126.3
6.3	75	108.0	112.2	117.4	122.6	126.9
6.4	76	108.4	112.7	117.9	123.1	127.4
6.5	77	108.8	113.1	118.4	123.6	127.9
6.6	78	109.3	113.6	118.9	124.2	128.5
6.7	79	109.7	114.0	119.4	124.7	129.0
6.8	80	110.1	114.5	119.8	125.2	129.5
6.9	81	110.5	114.9	120.3	125.7	130.1
6.10	82	111.0	115.4	120.8	126.2	130.6
6.11	83	111.4	115.8	121.3	126.7	131.1
7.0	84	111.8	116.3	121.7	127.2	131.7
7.1	85	112.2	116.7	122.2	127.7	132.2
7.2	86	112.6	117.1	122.7	128.2	132.7
7.3	87	113.0	117.6	123.1	128.7	133.3
7.4	88	113.4	118.0	123.6	129.2	133.8
7.5	89	113.8	118.4	124.1	129.7	134.3
7.6	90	114.3	118.9	124.5	130.2	134.8
7.7	91	114.7	119.3	125.0	130.7	135.3
7.8	92	115.1	119.7	125.5	131.2	135.9
7.9	93	115.5	120.2	125.9	131.7	136.4
7.10	94	115.9	120.6	126.4	132.2	136.9
7.11	95	116.2	121.0	126.8	132.6	137.4

WHO Child Growth Standards

Height-for-age BOYS 5 to 19 years (Percentiles)						
Year-Month	Months	3rd	15th	Median	85th	97th
8.0	96	116.6	121.4	127.3	133.1	137.9
8.1	97	117.0	121.8	127.7	133.6	138.4
8.2	98	117.4	122.2	128.2	134.1	138.9
8.3	99	117.8	122.7	128.6	134.6	139.4
8.4	100	118.2	123.1	129.0	135.0	139.9
8.5	101	118.6	123.5	129.5	135.5	140.4
8.6	102	119.0	123.9	129.9	136.0	140.9
8.7	103	119.3	124.3	130.4	136.4	141.4
8.8	104	119.7	124.7	130.8	136.9	141.9
8.9	105	120.1	125.1	131.3	137.4	142.4
8.10	106	120.5	125.5	131.7	137.9	142.9
8.11	107	120.9	125.9	132.1	138.3	143.4
9.0	108	121.3	126.3	132.6	138.8	143.9
9.1	109	121.6	126.7	133.0	139.3	144.4
9.2	110	122.0	127.1	133.4	139.7	144.9
9.3	111	122.4	127.6	133.9	140.2	145.4
9.4	112	122.8	128.0	134.3	140.7	145.8
9.5	113	123.2	128.4	134.7	141.1	146.3
9.6	114	123.5	128.8	135.2	141.6	146.8
9.7	115	123.9	129.2	135.6	142.1	147.3
9.8	116	124.3	129.6	136.1	142.5	147.8
9.9	117	124.7	130.0	136.5	143.0	148.3
9.10	118	125.0	130.4	136.9	143.5	148.8
9.11	119	125.4	130.8	137.3	143.9	149.3
10.0	120	125.8	131.2	137.8	144.4	149.8
10.1	121	126.2	131.6	138.2	144.8	150.3
10.2	122	126.5	132.0	138.6	145.3	150.7
10.3	123	126.9	132.4	139.1	145.8	151.2
10.4	124	127.3	132.8	139.5	146.2	151.7
10.5	125	127.7	133.2	140.0	146.7	152.2
10.6	126	128.1	133.6	140.4	147.2	152.7
10.7	127	128.5	134.0	140.8	147.7	153.2
10.8	128	128.9	134.4	141.3	148.1	153.7
10.9	129	129.2	134.9	141.7	148.6	154.2
10.10	130	129.6	135.3	142.2	149.1	154.7
10.11	131	130.0	135.7	142.7	149.6	155.3

WHO Child Growth Standards

Height-for-age BOYS 5 to 19 years (Percentiles)

Year-Month	Months	3rd	15th	Median	85th	97th
11.0	132	130.5	136.1	143.1	150.1	155.8
11.1	133	130.9	136.6	143.6	150.6	156.3
11.2	134	131.3	137.0	144.1	151.1	156.8
11.3	135	131.7	137.5	144.5	151.6	157.4
11.4	136	132.1	137.9	145.0	152.1	157.9
11.5	137	132.6	138.4	145.5	152.6	158.4
11.6	138	133.0	138.8	146.0	153.1	159.0
11.7	139	133.4	139.3	146.5	153.7	159.5
11.8	140	133.9	139.8	147.0	154.2	160.1
11.9	141	134.3	140.3	147.5	154.8	160.7
11.10	142	134.8	140.7	148.0	155.3	161.2
11.11	143	135.3	141.2	148.5	155.9	161.8
12.0	144	135.8	141.7	149.1	156.4	162.4
12.1	145	136.2	142.2	149.6	157.0	163.0
12.2	146	136.7	142.8	150.2	157.6	163.6
12.3	147	137.2	143.3	150.7	158.2	164.2
12.4	148	137.7	143.8	151.3	158.8	164.8
12.5	149	138.3	144.4	151.9	159.4	165.5
12.6	150	138.8	144.9	152.4	160.0	166.1
12.7	151	139.3	145.5	153.0	160.6	166.7
12.8	152	139.9	146.0	153.6	161.2	167.4
12.9	153	140.4	146.6	154.2	161.8	168.0
12.10	154	141.0	147.2	154.8	162.5	168.7
12.11	155	141.5	147.8	155.4	163.1	169.4
13.0	156	142.1	148.3	156.0	163.7	170.0
13.1	157	142.6	148.9	156.7	164.4	170.7
13.2	158	143.2	149.5	157.3	165.0	171.3
13.3	159	143.8	150.1	157.9	165.7	172.0
13.4	160	144.3	150.7	158.5	166.3	172.6
13.5	161	144.9	151.3	159.1	166.9	173.3
13.6	162	145.4	151.8	159.7	167.5	173.9
13.7	163	146.0	152.4	160.3	168.2	174.6
13.8	164	146.6	153.0	160.9	168.8	175.2
13.9	165	147.1	153.6	161.5	169.4	175.8
13.10	166	147.6	154.1	162.1	170.0	176.5
13.11	167	148.2	154.7	162.6	170.6	177.1

WHO Child Growth Standards

Height-for-age BOYS 5 to 19 years (Percentiles)

Year-Month	Months	3rd	15th	Median	85th	97th
14.0	168	148.7	155.2	163.2	171.2	177.6
14.1	169	149.2	155.7	163.7	171.7	178.2
14.2	170	149.7	156.3	164.3	172.3	178.8
14.3	171	150.3	156.8	164.8	172.8	179.3
14.4	172	150.7	157.3	165.3	173.3	179.9
14.5	173	151.2	157.8	165.8	173.9	180.4
14.6	174	151.7	158.3	166.3	174.4	180.9
14.7	175	152.2	158.7	166.8	174.8	181.4
14.8	176	152.6	159.2	167.2	175.3	181.9
14.9	177	153.0	159.6	167.7	175.8	182.3
14.10	178	153.5	160.0	168.1	176.2	182.8
14.11	179	153.9	160.5	168.5	176.6	183.2
15.0	180	154.3	160.9	169.0	177.0	183.6
15.1	181	154.7	161.3	169.4	177.4	184.0
15.2	182	155.1	161.6	169.7	177.8	184.4
15.3	183	155.4	162.0	170.1	178.2	184.8
15.4	184	155.8	162.4	170.5	178.6	185.1
15.5	185	156.1	162.7	170.8	178.9	185.5
15.6	186	156.5	163.1	171.1	179.2	185.8
15.7	187	156.8	163.4	171.5	179.6	186.1
15.8	188	157.1	163.7	171.8	179.9	186.4
15.9	189	157.4	164.0	172.1	180.1	186.7
15.10	190	157.7	164.3	172.4	180.4	187.0
15.11	191	158.0	164.6	172.6	180.7	187.3
16.0	192	158.3	164.8	172.9	181.0	187.5
16.1	193	158.5	165.1	173.1	181.2	187.7
16.2	194	158.8	165.3	173.4	181.4	188.0
16.3	195	159.0	165.6	173.6	181.6	188.2
16.4	196	159.3	165.8	173.8	181.8	188.4
16.5	197	159.5	166.0	174.0	182.0	188.6
16.6	198	159.7	166.2	174.2	182.2	188.7
16.7	199	159.9	166.4	174.4	182.4	188.9
16.8	200	160.1	166.6	174.6	182.6	189.0
16.9	201	160.3	166.8	174.7	182.7	189.2
16.10	202	160.5	166.9	174.9	182.8	189.3
16.11	203	160.6	167.1	175.0	183.0	189.4

WHO Child Growth Standards

Height-for-age BOYS 5 to 19 years (Percentiles)

Year-Month	Months	3rd	15th	Median	85th	97th
17.0	204	160.8	167.2	175.2	183.1	189.5
17.1	205	160.9	167.4	175.3	183.2	189.6
17.2	206	161.1	167.5	175.4	183.3	189.7
17.3	207	161.2	167.6	175.5	183.4	189.8
17.4	208	161.3	167.7	175.6	183.5	189.9
17.5	209	161.4	167.8	175.7	183.5	189.9
17.6	210	161.5	167.9	175.8	183.6	190.0
17.7	211	161.7	168.0	175.8	183.7	190.0
17.8	212	161.7	168.1	175.9	183.7	190.1
17.9	213	161.8	168.2	176.0	183.8	190.1
17.10	214	161.9	168.3	176.0	183.8	190.1
17.11	215	162.0	168.3	176.1	183.9	190.2
18.0	216	162.1	168.4	176.1	183.9	190.2
18.1	217	162.2	168.5	176.2	183.9	190.2
18.2	218	162.2	168.5	176.2	183.9	190.2
18.3	219	162.3	168.6	176.3	184.0	190.2
18.4	220	162.4	168.6	176.3	184.0	190.3
18.5	221	162.4	168.7	176.4	184.0	190.3
18.6	222	162.5	168.7	176.4	184.0	190.3
18.7	223	162.6	168.8	176.4	184.1	190.3
18.8	224	162.6	168.8	176.4	184.1	190.3
18.9	225	162.7	168.9	176.5	184.1	190.3
18.10	226	162.7	168.9	176.5	184.1	190.3
18.11	227	162.8	168.9	176.5	184.1	190.3
19.0	228	162.8	169.0	176.5	184.1	190.3

WHO Child Growth Standards

Length-for-age GIRLS Birth to 2 years (Percentiles)						
Year-Month	Months	3rd	15th	Median	85th	97th
0.0	0	45.6	47.2	49.1	51.1	52.7
0.1	1	50.0	51.7	53.7	55.7	57.4
0.2	2	53.2	55.0	57.1	59.2	60.9
0.3	3	55.8	57.6	59.8	62.0	63.8
0.4	4	58.0	59.8	62.1	64.3	66.2
0.5	5	59.9	61.7	64.0	66.3	68.2
0.6	6	61.5	63.4	65.7	68.1	70.0
0.7	7	62.9	64.9	67.3	69.7	71.6
0.8	8	64.3	66.3	68.7	71.2	73.2
0.9	9	65.6	67.6	70.1	72.6	74.7
0.10	10	66.8	68.9	71.5	74.0	76.1
0.11	11	68.0	70.2	72.8	75.4	77.5
1.0	12	69.2	71.3	74.0	76.7	78.9
1.1	13	70.3	72.5	75.2	77.9	80.2
1.2	14	71.3	73.6	76.4	79.2	81.4
1.3	15	72.4	74.7	77.5	80.3	82.7
1.4	16	73.3	75.7	78.6	81.5	83.9
1.5	17	74.3	76.7	79.7	82.6	85.0
1.6	18	75.2	77.7	80.7	83.7	86.2
1.7	19	76.2	78.7	81.7	84.8	87.3
1.8	20	77.0	79.6	82.7	85.8	88.4
1.9	21	77.9	80.5	83.7	86.8	89.4
1.10	22	78.7	81.4	84.6	87.8	90.5
1.11	23	79.6	82.2	85.5	88.8	91.5
2.0	24	80.3	83.1	86.4	89.8	92.5

WHO Child Growth Standards

Height-for-age GIRLS 2 to 5 years (Percentiles)						
Year-Month	**Months**	**3rd**	**15th**	**Median**	**85th**	**97th**
2.0	24	79.6	82.4	85.7	89.1	91.8
2.1	25	80.4	83.2	86.6	90.0	92.8
2.2	26	81.2	84.0	87.4	90.9	93.7
2.3	27	81.9	84.8	88.3	91.8	94.6
2.4	28	82.6	85.5	89.1	92.7	95.6
2.5	29	83.4	86.3	89.9	93.5	96.4
2.6	30	84.0	87.0	90.7	94.3	97.3
2.7	31	84.7	87.7	91.4	95.2	98.2
2.8	32	85.4	88.4	92.2	95.9	99.0
2.9	33	86.0	89.1	92.9	96.7	99.8
2.10	34	86.7	89.8	93.6	97.5	100.6
2.11	35	87.3	90.5	94.4	98.3	101.4
3.0	36	87.9	91.1	95.1	99.0	102.2
3.1	37	88.5	91.7	95.7	99.7	103.0
3.2	38	89.1	92.4	96.4	100.5	103.7
3.3	39	89.7	93.0	97.1	101.2	104.5
3.4	40	90.3	93.6	97.7	101.9	105.2
3.5	41	90.8	94.2	98.4	102.6	106.0
3.6	42	91.4	94.8	99.0	103.3	106.7
3.7	43	92.0	95.4	99.7	103.9	107.4
3.8	44	92.5	96.0	100.3	104.6	108.1
3.9	45	93.0	96.6	100.9	105.3	108.8
3.10	46	93.6	97.2	101.5	105.9	109.5
3.11	47	94.1	97.7	102.1	106.6	110.2
4.0	48	94.6	98.3	102.7	107.2	110.8
4.1	49	95.1	98.8	103.3	107.8	111.5
4.2	50	95.7	99.4	103.9	108.4	112.1
4.3	51	96.2	99.9	104.5	109.1	112.8
4.4	52	96.7	100.4	105.0	109.7	113.4
4.5	53	97.2	101.0	105.6	110.3	114.1
4.6	54	97.6	101.5	106.2	110.9	114.7
4.7	55	98.1	102.0	106.7	111.5	115.3
4.8	56	98.6	102.5	107.3	112.1	116.0
4.9	57	99.1	103.0	107.8	112.6	116.6
4.10	58	99.6	103.5	108.4	113.2	117.2
4.11	59	100.0	104.0	108.9	113.8	117.8
5.0	60	100.5	104.5	109.4	114.4	118.4

WHO Child Growth Standards

Height-for-age GIRLS 5 to 19 years (Percentiles)						
Year-Month	Months	3rd	15th	Median	85th	97th
5.1	61	100.6	104.7	109.6	114.5	118.6
5.2	62	101.1	105.1	110.1	115.1	119.2
5.3	63	101.5	105.6	110.6	115.7	119.7
5.4	64	102.0	106.1	111.2	116.2	120.3
5.5	65	102.4	106.6	111.7	116.8	120.9
5.6	66	102.9	107.1	112.2	117.3	121.5
5.7	67	103.3	107.5	112.7	117.8	122.0
5.8	68	103.8	108.0	113.2	118.4	122.6
5.9	69	104.2	108.5	113.7	118.9	123.1
5.10	70	104.6	108.9	114.2	119.4	123.7
5.11	71	105.1	109.4	114.6	119.9	124.2
6.0	72	105.5	109.8	115.1	120.4	124.8
6.1	73	105.9	110.3	115.6	120.9	125.3
6.2	74	106.3	110.7	116.1	121.4	125.8
6.3	75	106.8	111.2	116.6	122.0	126.4
6.4	76	107.2	111.6	117.0	122.5	126.9
6.5	77	107.6	112.0	117.5	123.0	127.4
6.6	78	108.0	112.5	118.0	123.5	127.9
6.7	79	108.4	112.9	118.4	124.0	128.5
6.8	80	108.9	113.4	118.9	124.5	129.0
6.9	81	109.3	113.8	119.4	125.0	129.5
6.10	82	109.7	114.3	119.9	125.5	130.0
6.11	83	110.1	114.7	120.3	126.0	130.6
7.0	84	110.5	115.1	120.8	126.5	131.1
7.1	85	110.9	115.6	121.3	127.0	131.6
7.2	86	111.4	116.0	121.8	127.5	132.1
7.3	87	111.8	116.5	122.2	128.0	132.7
7.4	88	112.2	116.9	122.7	128.5	133.2
7.5	89	112.6	117.4	123.2	129.0	133.7
7.6	90	113.1	117.8	123.7	129.5	134.3
7.7	91	113.5	118.3	124.1	130.0	134.8
7.8	92	113.9	118.7	124.6	130.5	135.3
7.9	93	114.4	119.2	125.1	131.0	135.9
7.10	94	114.8	119.6	125.6	131.5	136.4
7.11	95	115.2	120.1	126.1	132.1	136.9

WHO Child Growth Standards

Height-for-age GIRLS 5 to 19 years (Percentiles)

Year-Month	Months	3rd	15th	Median	85th	97th
8.0	96	115.7	120.5	126.6	132.6	137.5
8.1	97	116.1	121.0	127.0	133.1	138.0
8.2	98	116.5	121.5	127.5	133.6	138.5
8.3	99	117.0	121.9	128.0	134.1	139.1
8.4	100	117.4	122.4	128.5	134.6	139.6
8.5	101	117.9	122.9	129.0	135.2	140.2
8.6	102	118.3	123.3	129.5	135.7	140.7
8.7	103	118.7	123.8	130.0	136.2	141.2
8.8	104	119.2	124.3	130.5	136.7	141.8
8.9	105	119.6	124.7	131.0	137.2	142.3
8.10	106	120.1	125.2	131.5	137.8	142.9
8.11	107	120.5	125.7	132.0	138.3	143.4
9.0	108	121.0	126.2	132.5	138.8	144.0
9.1	109	121.5	126.6	133.0	139.4	144.5
9.2	110	121.9	127.1	133.5	139.9	145.1
9.3	111	122.4	127.6	134.0	140.4	145.6
9.4	112	122.8	128.1	134.5	141.0	146.2
9.5	113	123.3	128.6	135.0	141.5	146.8
9.6	114	123.8	129.1	135.5	142.0	147.3
9.7	115	124.2	129.5	136.1	142.6	147.9
9.8	116	124.7	130.0	136.6	143.1	148.4
9.9	117	125.2	130.5	137.1	143.6	149.0
9.10	118	125.7	131.0	137.6	144.2	149.5
9.11	119	126.1	131.5	138.1	144.7	150.1
10.0	120	126.6	132.0	138.6	145.3	150.7
10.1	121	127.1	132.5	139.2	145.8	151.2
10.2	122	127.6	133.0	139.7	146.4	151.8
10.3	123	128.1	133.5	140.2	146.9	152.4
10.4	124	128.5	134.0	140.7	147.5	152.9
10.5	125	129.0	134.5	141.3	148.0	153.5
10.6	126	129.5	135.0	141.8	148.6	154.1
10.7	127	130.0	135.5	142.3	149.1	154.6
10.8	128	130.5	136.0	142.9	149.7	155.2
10.9	129	131.0	136.6	143.4	150.2	155.8
10.10	130	131.5	137.1	143.9	150.8	156.3
10.11	131	132.0	137.6	144.5	151.3	156.9
11.0	132	132.5	138.1	145.0	151.9	157.5

WHO Child Growth Standards

Height-for-age GIRLS 5 to 19 years (Percentiles)						
Year-Month	Months	3rd	15th	Median	85th	97th
11.1	133	133.0	138.6	145.5	152.4	158.1
11.2	134	133.5	139.1	146.1	153.0	158.6
11.3	135	134.0	139.7	146.6	153.5	159.2
11.4	136	134.5	140.2	147.1	154.1	159.8
11.5	137	135.0	140.7	147.7	154.6	160.3
11.6	138	135.5	141.2	148.2	155.2	160.9
11.7	139	136.0	141.7	148.7	155.7	161.4
11.8	140	136.5	142.2	149.2	156.3	162.0
11.9	141	136.9	142.7	149.7	156.8	162.5
11.10	142	137.4	143.2	150.2	157.3	163.1
11.11	143	137.9	143.7	150.7	157.8	163.6
12.0	144	138.4	144.1	151.2	158.3	164.1
12.1	145	138.8	144.6	151.7	158.8	164.6
12.2	146	139.3	145.1	152.2	159.3	165.1
12.3	147	139.7	145.5	152.7	159.8	165.6
12.4	148	140.2	146.0	153.1	160.3	166.1
12.5	149	140.6	146.4	153.6	160.7	166.5
12.6	150	141.0	146.8	154.0	161.2	167.0
12.7	151	141.4	147.3	154.4	161.6	167.4
12.8	152	141.8	147.7	154.8	162.0	167.9
12.9	153	142.2	148.1	155.2	162.4	168.3
12.10	154	142.6	148.4	155.6	162.8	168.7
12.11	155	143.0	148.8	156.0	163.2	169.1
13.0	156	143.3	149.2	156.4	163.6	169.4
13.1	157	143.7	149.5	156.7	163.9	169.8
13.2	158	144.0	149.9	157.1	164.3	170.1
13.3	159	144.3	150.2	157.4	164.6	170.5
13.4	160	144.6	150.5	157.7	164.9	170.8
13.5	161	144.9	150.8	158.0	165.2	171.1
13.6	162	145.2	151.1	158.3	165.5	171.4
13.7	163	145.5	151.4	158.6	165.8	171.7
13.8	164	145.8	151.6	158.8	166.0	171.9
13.9	165	146.0	151.9	159.1	166.3	172.2
13.10	166	146.3	152.1	159.3	166.5	172.4
13.11	167	146.5	152.4	159.6	166.8	172.6
14.0	168	146.7	152.6	159.8	167.0	172.8

WHO Child Growth Standards

Height-for-age GIRLS 5 to 19 years (Percentiles)						
Year-Month	**Months**	**3rd**	**15th**	**Median**	**85th**	**97th**
14.1	169	146.9	152.8	160.0	167.2	173.0
14.2	170	147.2	153.0	160.2	167.4	173.2
14.3	171	147.3	153.2	160.4	167.6	173.4
14.4	172	147.5	153.4	160.6	167.7	173.6
14.5	173	147.7	153.6	160.7	167.9	173.8
14.6	174	147.9	153.7	160.9	168.1	173.9
14.7	175	148.0	153.9	161.0	168.2	174.0
14.8	176	148.2	154.0	161.2	168.3	174.2
14.9	177	148.3	154.2	161.3	168.5	174.3
14.10	178	148.5	154.3	161.4	168.6	174.4
14.11	179	148.6	154.4	161.6	168.7	174.5
15.0	180	148.7	154.5	161.7	168.8	174.6
15.1	181	148.8	154.6	161.8	168.9	174.7
15.2	182	149.0	154.8	161.9	169.0	174.8
15.3	183	149.1	154.8	162.0	169.1	174.9
15.4	184	149.2	154.9	162.0	169.1	174.9
15.5	185	149.2	155.0	162.1	169.2	175.0
15.6	186	149.3	155.1	162.2	169.3	175.0
15.7	187	149.4	155.2	162.3	169.3	175.1
15.8	188	149.5	155.2	162.3	169.4	175.1
15.9	189	149.6	155.3	162.4	169.4	175.2
15.10	190	149.6	155.4	162.4	169.5	175.2
15.11	191	149.7	155.4	162.5	169.5	175.3
16.0	192	149.8	155.5	162.5	169.6	175.3
16.1	193	149.8	155.5	162.6	169.6	175.3
16.2	194	149.9	155.6	162.6	169.6	175.3
16.3	195	149.9	155.6	162.6	169.6	175.3
16.4	196	150.0	155.7	162.7	169.7	175.4
16.5	197	150.0	155.7	162.7	169.7	175.4
16.6	198	150.0	155.7	162.7	169.7	175.4
16.7	199	150.1	155.8	162.7	169.7	175.4
16.8	200	150.1	155.8	162.8	169.7	175.4
16.9	201	150.2	155.8	162.8	169.8	175.4
16.10	202	150.2	155.9	162.8	169.8	175.4
16.11	203	150.2	155.9	162.8	169.8	175.4
17.0	204	150.3	155.9	162.9	169.8	175.4

WHO Child Growth Standards

Height-for-age GIRLS 5 to 19 years (Percentiles)						
Year-Month	**Months**	**3rd**	**15th**	**Median**	**85th**	**97th**
17.1	205	150.3	155.9	162.9	169.8	175.4
17.2	206	150.3	156.0	162.9	169.8	175.5
17.3	207	150.4	156.0	162.9	169.8	175.5
17.4	208	150.4	156.0	162.9	169.8	175.5
17.5	209	150.4	156.1	162.9	169.8	175.5
17.6	210	150.5	156.1	163.0	169.9	175.5
17.7	211	150.5	156.1	163.0	169.9	175.5
17.8	212	150.5	156.1	163.0	169.9	175.5
17.9	213	150.5	156.1	163.0	169.9	175.5
17.10	214	150.6	156.2	163.0	169.9	175.5
17.11	215	150.6	156.2	163.0	169.9	175.5
18.0	216	150.6	156.2	163.1	169.9	175.5
18.1	217	150.7	156.2	163.1	169.9	175.5
18.2	218	150.7	156.2	163.1	169.9	175.5
18.3	219	150.7	156.3	163.1	169.9	175.5
18.4	220	150.7	156.3	163.1	169.9	175.5
18.5	221	150.7	156.3	163.1	169.9	175.5
18.6	222	150.8	156.3	163.1	169.9	175.5
18.7	223	150.8	156.3	163.1	169.9	175.5
18.8	224	150.8	156.3	163.1	169.9	175.5
18.9	225	150.8	156.4	163.1	169.9	175.5
18.10	226	150.8	156.4	163.2	169.9	175.5
18.11	227	150.8	156.4	163.2	169.9	175.5
19.0	228	150.9	156.4	163.2	169.9	175.5

WHO Child Growth Standards

Head circumference-for-age BOYS Birth to 5 years (Percentiles)

Year-Month	Months	3rd	15th	Median	85th	97th
0.0	0	32.1	33.1	34.5	35.8	36.9
0.1	1	35.1	36.1	37.3	38.5	39.5
0.2	2	36.9	37.9	39.1	40.3	41.3
0.3	3	38.3	39.3	40.5	41.7	42.7
0.4	4	39.4	40.4	41.6	42.9	43.9
0.5	5	40.3	41.3	42.6	43.8	44.8
0.6	6	41.0	42.1	43.3	44.6	45.6
0.7	7	41.7	42.7	44.0	45.3	46.3
0.8	8	42.2	43.2	44.5	45.8	46.9
0.9	9	42.6	43.7	45.0	46.3	47.4
0.10	10	43.0	44.1	45.4	46.7	47.8
0.11	11	43.4	44.4	45.8	47.1	48.2
1.0	12	43.6	44.7	46.1	47.4	48.5
1.1	13	43.9	45.0	46.3	47.7	48.8
1.2	14	44.1	45.2	46.6	47.9	49.0
1.3	15	44.3	45.5	46.8	48.2	49.3
1.4	16	44.5	45.6	47.0	48.4	49.5
1.5	17	44.7	45.8	47.2	48.6	49.7
1.6	18	44.9	46.0	47.4	48.7	49.9
1.7	19	45.0	46.2	47.5	48.9	50.0
1.8	20	45.2	46.3	47.7	49.1	50.2
1.9	21	45.3	46.4	47.8	49.2	50.4
1.10	22	45.4	46.6	48.0	49.4	50.5
1.11	23	45.6	46.7	48.1	49.5	50.7
2.0	24	45.7	46.8	48.3	49.7	50.8
2.1	25	45.8	47.0	48.4	49.8	50.9
2.2	26	45.9	47.1	48.5	49.9	51.1
2.3	27	46.0	47.2	48.6	50.0	51.2
2.4	28	46.1	47.3	48.7	50.2	51.3
2.5	29	46.2	47.4	48.8	50.3	51.4

WHO Child Growth Standards

Head circumference-for-age BOYS Birth to 5 years (Percentiles)						
Year-Month	**Months**	**3rd**	**15th**	**Median**	**85th**	**97th**
2.6	30	46.3	47.5	48.9	50.4	51.6
2.7	31	46.4	47.6	49.0	50.5	51.7
2.8	32	46.5	47.7	49.1	50.6	51.8
2.9	33	46.6	47.8	49.2	50.7	51.9
2.10	34	46.6	47.8	49.3	50.8	52.0
2.11	35	46.7	47.9	49.4	50.8	52.0
3.0	36	46.8	48.0	49.5	50.9	52.1
3.1	37	46.9	48.1	49.5	51.0	52.2
3.2	38	46.9	48.1	49.6	51.1	52.3
3.3	39	47.0	48.2	49.7	51.2	52.4
3.4	40	47.0	48.3	49.7	51.2	52.4
3.5	41	47.1	48.3	49.8	51.3	52.5
3.6	42	47.2	48.4	49.9	51.4	52.6
3.7	43	47.2	48.4	49.9	51.4	52.7
3.8	44	47.3	48.5	50.0	51.5	52.7
3.9	45	47.3	48.5	50.1	51.6	52.8
3.10	46	47.4	48.6	50.1	51.6	52.8
3.11	47	47.4	48.6	50.2	51.7	52.9
4.0	48	47.5	48.7	50.2	51.7	53.0
4.1	49	47.5	48.7	50.3	51.8	53.0
4.2	50	47.5	48.8	50.3	51.8	53.1
4.3	51	47.6	48.8	50.4	51.9	53.1
4.4	52	47.6	48.9	50.4	51.9	53.2
4.5	53	47.7	48.9	50.4	52.0	53.2
4.6	54	47.7	49.0	50.5	52.0	53.3
4.7	55	47.7	49.0	50.5	52.1	53.3
4.8	56	47.8	49.0	50.6	52.1	53.4
4.9	57	47.8	49.1	50.6	52.2	53.4
4.10	58	47.9	49.1	50.7	52.2	53.5
4.11	59	47.9	49.2	50.7	52.2	53.5
5.0	60	47.9	49.2	50.7	52.3	53.5

WHO Child Growth Standards

Head circumference-for-age GIRLS Birth to 5 years (Percentiles)						
Year-Month	Months	3rd	15th	Median	85th	97th
0.0	0	31.7	32.7	33.9	35.1	36.1
0.1	1	34.3	35.3	36.5	37.8	38.8
0.2	2	36.0	37.0	38.3	39.5	40.5
0.3	3	37.2	38.2	39.5	40.8	41.9
0.4	4	38.2	39.3	40.6	41.9	43.0
0.5	5	39.0	40.1	41.5	42.8	43.9
0.6	6	39.7	40.8	42.2	43.5	44.6
0.7	7	40.4	41.5	42.8	44.2	45.3
0.8	8	40.9	42.0	43.4	44.7	45.9
0.9	9	41.3	42.4	43.8	45.2	46.3
0.10	10	41.7	42.8	44.2	45.6	46.8
0.11	11	42.0	43.2	44.6	46.0	47.1
1.0	12	42.3	43.5	44.9	46.3	47.5
1.1	13	42.6	43.8	45.2	46.6	47.7
1.2	14	42.9	44.0	45.4	46.8	48.0
1.3	15	43.1	44.2	45.7	47.1	48.2
1.4	16	43.3	44.4	45.9	47.3	48.5
1.5	17	43.5	44.6	46.1	47.5	48.7
1.6	18	43.6	44.8	46.2	47.7	48.8
1.7	19	43.8	45.0	46.4	47.8	49.0
1.8	20	44.0	45.1	46.6	48.0	49.2
1.9	21	44.1	45.3	46.7	48.2	49.4
1.10	22	44.3	45.4	46.9	48.3	49.5
1.11	23	44.4	45.6	47.0	48.5	49.7
2.0	24	44.6	45.7	47.2	48.6	49.8
2.1	25	44.7	45.9	47.3	48.8	49.9
2.2	26	44.8	46.0	47.5	48.9	50.1
2.3	27	44.9	46.1	47.6	49.0	50.2
2.4	28	45.1	46.3	47.7	49.2	50.3
2.5	29	45.2	46.4	47.8	49.3	50.5

WHO Child Growth Standards

Head circumference-for-age GIRLS Birth to 5 years (Percentiles)						
Year-Month	Months	3rd	15th	Median	85th	97th
2.6	30	45.3	46.5	47.9	49.4	50.6
2.7	31	45.4	46.6	48.0	49.5	50.7
2.8	32	45.5	46.7	48.1	49.6	50.8
2.9	33	45.6	46.8	48.2	49.7	50.9
2.10	34	45.7	46.9	48.3	49.8	51.0
2.11	35	45.8	47.0	48.4	49.9	51.1
3.0	36	45.9	47.0	48.5	50.0	51.2
3.1	37	45.9	47.1	48.6	50.1	51.3
3.2	38	46.0	47.2	48.7	50.1	51.3
3.3	39	46.1	47.3	48.7	50.2	51.4
3.4	40	46.2	47.4	48.8	50.3	51.5
3.5	41	46.2	47.4	48.9	50.4	51.6
3.6	42	46.3	47.5	49.0	50.4	51.6
3.7	43	46.4	47.6	49.0	50.5	51.7
3.8	44	46.4	47.6	49.1	50.6	51.8
3.9	45	46.5	47.7	49.2	50.6	51.8
3.10	46	46.5	47.7	49.2	50.7	51.9
3.11	47	46.6	47.8	49.3	50.7	51.9
4.0	48	46.7	47.9	49.3	50.8	52.0
4.1	49	46.7	47.9	49.4	50.9	52.1
4.2	50	46.8	48.0	49.4	50.9	52.1
4.3	51	46.8	48.0	49.5	51.0	52.2
4.4	52	46.9	48.1	49.5	51.0	52.2
4.5	53	46.9	48.1	49.6	51.1	52.3
4.6	54	47.0	48.2	49.6	51.1	52.3
4.7	55	47.0	48.2	49.7	51.2	52.4
4.8	56	47.1	48.3	49.7	51.2	52.4
4.9	57	47.1	48.3	49.8	51.3	52.5
4.10	58	47.2	48.4	49.8	51.3	52.5
4.11	59	47.2	48.4	49.9	51.4	52.6
5.0	60	47.2	48.4	49.9	51.4	52.6

WHO Child Growth Standards

Weight-for-length BOYS Birth to 2 years (Percentiles)					
cm	3rd	15th	Median	85th	97th
45.0	2.1	2.2	2.4	2.7	2.9
45.5	2.1	2.3	2.5	2.8	3.0
46.0	2.2	2.4	2.6	2.9	3.1
46.5	2.3	2.5	2.7	3.0	3.2
47.0	2.4	2.5	2.8	3.1	3.3
47.5	2.4	2.6	2.9	3.2	3.5
48.0	2.5	2.7	2.9	3.2	3.5
48.5	2.6	2.8	3.0	3..3	3.6
49.0	2.7	2.9	3.1	3.4	3.7
49.5	2.7	2.9	3.2	3.5	3.8
50.0	2.8	3.0	3.3	3.7	4.0
50.5	2.9	3.1	3.4	3.8	4.1
51.0	3.0	3.2	3.5	3.9	4.2
51.5	3.1	3.3	3.6	4.0	4.3
52.0	3.2	3.4	3.8	4.1	4.5
52.5	3.3	3.6	3.9	4.3	4.6
53.0	3.4	3.7	4.0	4.4	4.7
53.5	3.5	3.8	4.1	4.5	4.9
54.0	3.6	3.9	4.3	4.7	5.0
54.5	3.8	4.0	4.4	4.8	5.2
55.0	3.9	4.2	4.5	5.0	5.4
55.5	4.0	4.3	4.7	5.1	5.5
56.0	4.1	4.4	4.8	5.3	5.7
56.5	4.3	4.6	5.0	5.4	5.9
57.0	4.4	4.7	5.1	5.6	6.0
57.5	4.5	4.8	5.3	5.8	6.2
58.0	4.6	5.0	5.4	5.9	6.4
58.5	4.8	5.1	5.6	6.1	6.5
59.0	4.9	5.2	5.7	6.2	6.7
59.5	5.0	5.4	5.9	6.4	6.9
60.0	5.1	5.5	6.0	6.5	7.0
60.5	5.3	5.6	6.1	6.7	7.2
61.0	5.4	5.8	6.3	6.8	7.4

WHO Child Growth Standards

Weight-for-length BOYS Birth to 2 years (Percentiles)					
cm	3rd	15th	Median	85th	97th
61.5	5.5	5.9	6.4	7.0	7.5
62.0	5.6	6.0	6.5	7.1	7.7
62.5	5.7	6.1	6.7	7.3	7.8
63.0	5.8	6.2	6.8	7.4	8.0
63.5	5.9	6.3	6.9	7.5	8.1
64.0	6.0	6.5	7.0	7.7	8.2
64.5	6.1	6.6	7.1	7.8	8.4
65.0	6.4	6.8	7.4	8.1	8.7
65.5	6.5	6.9	7.6	8.2	8.9
66.0	6.6	7.1	7.7	8.4	9.0
66.5	6.7	7.2	7.8	8.5	9.1
67.0	6.8	7.3	7.9	8.6	9.3
67.5	6.9	7.4	8.0	8.7	9.4
68.0	7.0	7.5	8.1	8.9	9.5
68.5	7.1	7.6	8.2	9.0	9.7
69.0	7.2	7.7	8.4	9.1	9.8
69.5	7.3	7.8	8.5	9.2	9.9
70.0	7.4	7.9	8.6	9.4	10.1
70.5	7.5	8.0	8.7	9.5	10.2
71.0	7.6	8.1	8.8	9.6	10.3
71.5	7.7	8.2	8.9	9.7	10.5
72.0	7.8	8.3	9.0	9.8	10.6
72.5	7.8	8.4	9.1	10.0	10.7
73.0	7.9	8.5	9.2	10.1	10.8
73.5	8.0	8.6	9.3	10.2	11.0
74.0	8.1	8.7	9.4	10.3	11.1
74.5	8.2	8.8	9.5	10.4	11.2
75.0	8.3	8.9	9.6	10.5	11.3
75.5	8.4	9.0	9.7	10.6	11.4
76.0	8.5	9.0	9.8	10.7	11.6
76.5	8.5	9.1	9.9	10.8	11.7
77.0	8.6	9.2	10.0	10.9	11.8
77.5	8.7	9.3	10.1	11.0	11.9
78.0	8.8	9.4	10.2	11.1	12.0
78.5	8.8	9.5	10.3	11.2	12.1

WHO Child Growth Standards

Weight-for-height BOYS 2 to 5 years (Percentiles)					
cm	3rd	15th	Median	85th	97th
79.0	8.9	9.5	10.4	11.3	12.2
79.5	9.0	9.6	10.5	11.4	12.3
80.0	9.1	9.7	10.6	11.5	12.4
80.5	9.2	9.8	10.7	11.6	12.5
81.0	9.3	9.9	10.8	11.8	12.6
81.5	9.3	10.0	10.9	11.9	12.8
82.0	9.4	10.1	11.0	12.0	12.9
82.5	9.5	10.2	11.1	12.1	13.0
83.0	9.6	10.3	11.2	12.2	13.1
83.5	9.7	10.4	11.3	12.3	13.3
84.0	9.8	10.5	11.4	12.5	13.4
84.5	9.9	10.6	11.5	12.6	13.5
85.0	10.1	10.7	11.7	12.7	13.7
85.5	10.2	10.9	11.8	12.8	13.8
86.0	10.3	11.0	11.9	13.0	13.9
86.5	10.4	11.1	12.0	13.1	14.1
87.0	10.5	11.2	12.2	13.2	14.2
87.5	10.6	11.3	12.3	13.4	14.4
88.0	10.7	11.4	12.4	13.5	14.5
88.5	10.8	11.5	12.5	13.6	14.6
89.0	10.9	11.7	12.6	13.8	14.8
89.5	11.0	11.8	12.8	13.9	14.9
90.0	11.1	11.9	12.9	14.0	15.1
90.5	11.2	12.0	13.0	14.1	15.2
91.0	11.3	12.1	13.1	14.3	15.3
91.5	11.4	12.2	13.2	14.4	15.5
92.0	11.5	12.3	13.4	14.5	15.6
92.5	11.6	12.4	13.5	14.7	15.7
93.0	11.7	12.5	13.6	14.8	15.9
93.5	11.8	12.6	13.7	14.9	16.0
94.0	11.9	12.7	13.8	15.0	16.1
94.5	12.0	12.8	13.9	15.2	16.3
95.0	12.1	12.9	14.1	15.3	16.4
95.5	12.2	13.1	14.2	15.4	16.6

WHO Child Growth Standards

Weight-for-height BOYS 2 to 5 years (Percentiles)					
cm	3rd	15th	Median	85th	97th
96.0	12.3	13.2	14.3	15.6	16.7
96.5	12.4	13.3	14.4	15.7	16.9
97.0	12.5	13.4	14.6	15.9	17.0
97.5	12.7	13.5	14.7	16.0	17.2
98.0	12.8	13.6	14.8	16.1	17.3
98.5	12.9	13.8	14.9	16.3	17.5
99.0	13.0	13.9	15.1	16.4	17.7
99.5	13.1	14.0	15.2	16.6	17.8
100.0	13.2	14.1	15.4	16.7	18.0
100.5	13.3	14.2	15.5	16.9	18.2
101.0	13.4	14.4	15.6	17.1	18.4
101.5	13.6	14.5	15.8	17.2	18.5
102.0	13.7	14.6	15.9	17.4	18.7
102.5	13.8	14.8	16.1	17.6	18.9
103.0	13.9	14.9	16.2	17.7	19.1
103.5	14.0	15.0	16.4	17.9	19.3
104.0	14.2	15.2	16.5	18.1	19.5
104.5	14.3	15.3	16.7	18.2	19.7
105.0	14.4	15.4	16.8	18.4	19.9
105.5	14.5	15.6	17.0	18.6	20.1
106.0	14.7	15.7	17.2	18.8	20.3
106.5	14.8	15.9	17.3	19.0	20.5
107.0	14.9	16.0	17.5	19.1	20.7
107.5	15.1	16.2	17.7	19.3	20.9
108.0	15.2	16.3	17.8	19.5	21.1
108.5	15.3	16.5	18.0	19.7	21.3
109.0	15.5	16.6	18.2	19.9	21.5
109.5	15.6	16.8	18.3	20.1	21.7
110.0	15.8	16.9	18.5	20.3	22.0
110.5	15.9	17.1	18.7	20.5	22.2
111.0	16.1	17.2	18.9	20.7	22.4
111.5	16.2	17.4	19.1	20.9	22.6
112.0	16.3	17.6	19.2	21.1	22.9

WHO Child Growth Standards

Weight-for-height BOYS 2 to 5 years (Percentiles)					
cm	3rd	15th	Median	85th	97th
112.5	16.5	17.7	19.4	21.4	23.1
113.0	16.6	17.9	19.6	21.6	23.4
113.5	16.8	18.1	19.8	21.8	23.6
114.0	17.0	18.2	20.0	22.0	23.8
114.5	17.1	18.4	20.2	22.2	24.1
115.0	17.3	18.6	20.4	22.4	24.3
115.5	17.4	18.7	20.6	22.7	24.6
116.0	17.6	18.9	20.8	22.9	24.8
116.5	17.7	19.1	21.0	23.1	25.1
117.0	17.9	19.3	21.2	23.3	25.3
117.5	18.0	19.4	21.4	23.6	25.6
118.0	18.2	19.6	21.6	23.8	25.8
118.5	18.4	19.8	21.8	24.0	26.1
119.0	18.5	20.0	22.0	24.2	26.3
119.5	18.7	20.1	22.2	24.5	26.6
120.0	18.8	20.3	22.4	24.7	26.8

WHO Child Growth Standards

Weight-for-length GIRLS Birth to 2 years (Percentiles)					
cm	3rd	15th	Median	85th	97th
45.0	2.1	2.2	2.5	2.7	2.9
45.5	2.2	2.3	2.5	2.8	3.0
46.0	2.2	2.4	2.6	2.9	3.1
46.5	2.3	2.5	2.7	3.0	3.2
47.0	2.4	2.6	2.8	3.1	3.3
47.5	2.4	2.6	2.9	3.2	3.4
48.0	2.5	2.7	3.0	3.3	3.5
48.5	2.6	2.8	3.1	3.4	3.7
49.0	2.7	2.9	3.2	3.5	3.8
49.5	2.8	3.0	3.3	3.6	3.9
50.0	2.8	3.1	3.4	3.7	4.0
50.5	2.9	3.2	3.5	3.8	4.1
51.0	3.0	3.2	3.6	3.9	4.3
51.5	3.1	3.4	3.7	4.0	4.4
52.0	3.2	3.5	3.8	4.2	4.5
52.5	3.3	3.6	3.9	4.3	4.7
53.0	3.4	3.7	4.0	4.4	4.8
53.5	3.5	3.8	4.2	4.6	5.0
54.0	3.6	3.9	4.3	4.7	5.1
54.5	3.7	4.0	4.4	4.9	5.3
55.0	3.9	4.1	4.5	5.0	5.4
55.5	4.0	4.3	4.7	5.2	5.6
56.0	4.1	4.4	4.8	5.3	5.8
56.5	4.2	4.5	5.0	5.5	5.9
57.0	4.3	4.6	5.1	5.6	6.1
57.5	4.4	4.8	5.2	5.7	6.2
58.0	4.5	4.9	5.4	5.9	6.4
58.5	4.6	5.0	5.5	6.0	6.5
59.0	4.8	5.1	5.6	6.2	6.7
59.5	4.9	5.2	5.7	6.3	6.9
60.0	5.0	5.4	5.9	6.5	7.0
60.5	5.1	5.5	6.0	6.6	7.2
61.0	5.2	5.6	6.1	6.7	7.3

WHO Child Growth Standards

Weight-for-length GIRLS Birth to 2 years (Percentiles)					
cm	**3rd**	**15th**	**Median**	**85th**	**97th**
61.5	5.3	5.7	6.3	6.9	7.5
62.0	5.4	5.8	6.4	7.0	7.6
62.5	5.5	5.9	6.5	7.2	7.8
63.0	5.6	6.0	6.6	7.3	7.9
63.5	5.7	6.1	6.7	7.4	8.0
64.0	5.8	6.2	6.9	7.5	8.2
64.5	5.9	6.3	7.0	7.7	8.3
65.0	6.1	6.6	7.2	8.0	8.6
65.5	6.2	6.7	7.4	8.1	8.8
66.0	6.3	6.8	7.5	8.2	8.9
66.5	6.4	6.9	7.6	8.3	9.0
67.0	6.5	7.0	7.7	8.5	9.2
67.5	6.6	7.1	7.8	8.6	9.3
68.0	6.7	7.2	7.9	8.7	9.4
68.5	6.8	7.3	8.0	8.8	9.5
69.0	6.9	7.4	8.1	8.9	9.7
69.5	7.0	7.5	8.2	9.0	9.8
70.0	7.0	7.6	8.3	9.1	9.9
70.5	7.1	7.7	8.4	9.3	10.0
71.0	7.2	7.8	8.5	9.4	10.1
71.5	7.3	7.9	8.6	9.5	10.3
72.0	7.4	7.9	8.7	9.6	10.4
72.5	7.5	8.0	8.8	9.7	10.5
73.0	7.6	8.1	8.9	9.8	10.6
73.5	7.6	8.2	9.0	9.9	10.7
74.0	7.7	8.3	9.1	10.0	10.8
74.5	7.8	8.4	9.2	10.1	10.9
75.0	7.9	8.5	9.3	10.2	11.1
75.5	8.0	8.6	9.4	10.3	11.2
76.0	8.0	8.6	9.5	10.4	11.3
76.5	8.1	8.7	9.6	10.5	11.4
77.0	8.2	8.8	9.6	10.6	11.5
77.5	8.3	8.9	9.7	10.7	11.6

WHO Child Growth Standards

Weight-for-height GIRLS 2 to 5 years (Percentiles)					
cm	3rd	15th	Median	85th	97th
78.0	8.4	9.0	9.8	10.8	11.7
78.5	8.4	9.1	9.9	10.9	11.8
79.0	8.5	9.2	10.0	11.0	11.9
79.5	8.6	9.2	10.1	11.1	12.1
80.0	8.7	9.3	10.2	11.2	12.2
80.5	8.8	9.4	10.3	11.4	12.3
81.0	8.9	9.5	10.4	11.5	12.4
81.5	9.0	9.6	10.6	11.6	12.6
82.0	9.1	9.7	10.7	11.7	12.7
82.5	9.2	9.9	10.8	11.9	12.8
83.0	9.3	10.0	10.9	12.0	13.0
83.5	9.4	10.1	11.0	12.1	13.1
84.0	9.5	10.2	11.1	12.2	13.3
84.5	9.6	10.3	11.3	12.4	13.4
85.0	9.7	10.4	11.4	12.5	13.5
85.5	9.8	10.5	11.5	12.7	13.7
86.0	9.9	10.6	11.6	12.8	13.8
86.5	10.0	10.8	11.8	12.9	14.0
87.0	10.1	10.9	11.9	13.1	14.1
87.5	10.2	11.0	12.0	13.2	14.3
88.0	10.3	11.1	12.1	13.3	14.4
88.5	10.4	11.2	12.3	13.5	14.6
89.0	10.5	11.3	12.4	13.6	14.7
89.5	10.6	11.4	12.5	13.8	14.9
90.0	10.8	11.5	12.6	13.9	15.0
90.5	10.9	11.7	12.8	14.0	15.2
91.0	11.0	11.8	12.9	14.2	15.3
91.5	11.1	11.9	13.0	14.3	15.5
92.0	11.2	12.0	13.1	14.4	15.6
92.5	11.3	12.1	13.3	14.6	15.8
93.0	11.4	12.2	13.4	14.7	15.9
93.5	11.5	12.3	13.5	14.9	16.1

WHO Child Growth Standards

Weight-for-height GIRLS 2 to 5 years (Percentiles)					
cm	**3rd**	**15th**	**Median**	**85th**	**97th**
94.0	11.6	12.4	13.6	15.0	16.2
94.5	11.7	12.6	13.8	15.1	16.4
95.0	11.8	12.7	13.9	15.3	16.5
95.5	11.9	12.8	14.0	15.4	16.7
96.0	12.0	12.9	14.1	15.6	16.9
96.5	12.1	13.0	14.3	15.7	17.0
97.0	12.2	13.1	14.4	15.8	17.2
97.5	12.3	13.3	14.5	16.0	17.3
98.0	12.4	13.4	14.7	16.1	17.5
98.5	12.6	13.5	14.8	16.3	17.7
99.0	12.7	13.6	14.9	16.4	17.8
99.5	12.8	13.8	15.1	16.6	18.0
100.0	12.9	13.9	15.2	16.8	18.2
100.5	13.0	14.0	15.4	16.9	18.3
101.0	13.1	14.1	15.5	17.1	18.5
101.5	13.3	14.3	15.7	17.2	18.7
102.0	13.4	14.4	15.8	17.4	18.9
102.5	13.5	14.5	16.0	17.6	19.1
103.0	13.6	14.7	16.1	17.8	19.3
103.5	13.8	14.8	16.3	17.9	19.5
104.0	13.9	15.0	16.4	18.1	19.7
104.5	14.0	15.1	16.6	18.3	19.9
105.0	14.2	15.3	16.8	18.5	20.1
105.5	14.3	15.4	16.9	18.7	20.3
106.0	14.5	15.6	17.1	18.9	20.5
106.5	14.6	15.7	17.3	19.1	20.7
107.0	14.7	15.9	17.5	19.3	21.0
107.5	14.9	16.1	17.7	19.5	21.2
108.0	15.0	16.2	17.8	19.7	21.4
108.5	15.2	16.4	18.0	19.9	21.6
109.0	15.4	16.6	18.2	20.1	21.9
109.5	15.5	16.7	18.4	20.3	22.1
110.0	15.7	16.9	18.6	20.6	22.4
110.5	15.8	17.1	18.8	20.8	22.6

WHO Child Growth Standards

Weight-for-height GIRLS 2 to 5 years (Percentiles)					
cm	3rd	15th	Median	85th	97th
111.0	16.0	17.3	19.0	21.0	22.8
111.5	16.2	17.4	19.2	21.2	23.1
112.0	16.3	17.6	19.4	21.5	23.4
112.5	16.5	17.8	19.6	21.7	23.6
113.0	16.7	18.0	19.8	21.9	23.9
113.5	16.8	18.2	20.0	22.2	24.1
114.0	17.0	18.4	20.2	22.4	24.4
114.5	17.2	18.5	20.5	22.6	24.7
115.0	17.3	18.7	20.7	22.9	24.9
115.5	17.5	18.9	20.9	23.1	25.2
116.0	17.7	19.1	21.1	23.4	25.5
116.5	17.9	19.3	21.3	23.6	25.7
117.0	18.0	19.5	21.5	23.8	26.0
117.5	18.2	19.7	21.7	24.1	26.3
118.0	18.4	19.9	22.0	24.3	26.5
118.5	18.6	20.1	22.2	24.6	26.8
119.0	18.7	20.3	22.4	24.8	27.1
119.5	18.9	20.5	22.6	25.1	27.4
120.0	19.1	20.6	22.8	25.3	27.6

WHO Child Growth Standards

BMI-for-age BOYS 5 to 19 years (Percentiles)						
Year-Month	**Months**	**3rd**	**15th**	**Median**	**85th**	**97th**
5.1	61	13.1	14.0	15.3	16.7	18.1
5.2	62	13.1	14.0	15.3	16.7	18.1
5.3	63	13.1	14.0	15.3	16.7	18.1
5.4	64	13.1	14.0	15.3	16.7	18.1
5.5	65	13.1	14.0	15.3	16.7	18.1
5.6	66	13.1	14.0	15.3	16.7	18.1
5.7	67	13.1	14.0	15.3	16.7	18.2
5.8	68	13.1	14.0	15.3	16.8	18.2
5.9	69	13.1	14.0	15.3	16.8	18.2
5.10	70	13.1	14.0	15.3	16.8	18.2
5.11	71	13.2	14.0	15.3	16.8	18.3
6.0	72	13.2	14.0	15.3	16.8	18.3
6.1	73	13.2	14.0	15.3	16.8	18.3
6.2	74	13.2	14.1	15.3	16.9	18.4
6.3	75	13.2	14.1	15.3	16.9	18.4
6.4	76	13.2	14.1	15.4	16.9	18.4
6.5	77	13.2	14.1	15.4	16.9	18.5
6.6	78	13.2	14.1	15.4	16.9	18.5
6.7	79	13.2	14.1	15.4	17.0	18.5
6.8	80	13.2	14.1	15.4	17.0	18.6
6.9	81	13.2	14.1	15.4	17.0	18.6
6.10	82	13.2	14.1	15.4	17.1	18.7
6.11	83	13.3	14.2	15.5	17.1	18.7
7.0	84	13.3	14.2	15.5	17.1	18.8
7.1	85	13.3	14.2	15.5	17.1	18.8
7.2	86	13.3	14.2	15.5	17.2	18.8
7.3	87	13.3	14.2	15.5	17.2	18.9
7.4	88	13.3	14.2	15.6	17.2	18.9
7.5	89	13.3	14.2	15.6	17.3	19.0
7.6	90	13.3	14.3	15.6	17.3	19.0
7.7	91	13.4	14.3	15.6	17.3	19.1
7.8	92	13.4	14.3	15.6	17.4	19.2
7.9	93	13.4	14.3	15.7	17.4	19.2

WHO Child Growth Standards

BMI-for-age BOYS 5 to 19 years (Percentiles)

Year-Month	Months	3rd	15th	Median	85th	97th
7.10	94	13.4	14.3	15.7	17.4	19.3
7.11	95	13.4	14.3	15.7	17.5	19.3
8.0	96	13.4	14.4	15.7	17.5	19.4
8.1	97	13.4	14.4	15.8	17.5	19.4
8.2	98	13.5	14.4	15.8	17.6	19.5
8.3	99	13.5	14.4	15.8	17.6	19.5
8.4	100	13.5	14.4	15.8	17.7	19.6
8.5	101	13.5	14.4	15.9	17.7	19.7
8.6	102	13.5	14.5	15.9	17.7	19.7
8.7	103	13.5	14.5	15.9	17.8	19.8
8.8	104	13.5	14.5	15.9	17.8	19.9
8.9	105	13.6	14.5	16.0	17.9	19.9
8.10	106	13.6	14.5	16.0	17.9	20.0
8.11	107	13.6	14.6	16.0	17.9	20.0
9.0	108	13.6	14.6	16.0	18.0	20.1
9.1	109	13.6	14.6	16.1	18.0	20.2
9.2	110	13.7	14.6	16.1	18.1	20.2
9.3	111	13.7	14.6	16.1	18.1	20.3
9.4	112	13.7	14.7	16.2	18.2	20.4
9.5	113	13.7	14.7	16.2	18.2	20.5
9.6	114	13.7	14.7	16.2	18.3	20.5
9.7	115	13.8	14.7	16.3	18.3	20.6
9.8	116	13.8	14.8	16.3	18.4	20.7
9.9	117	13.8	14.8	16.3	18.4	20.8
9.10	118	13.8	14.8	16.4	18.5	20.8
9.11	119	13.8	14.8	16.4	18.5	20.9
10.0	120	13.9	14.9	16.4	18.6	21.0
10.1	121	13.9	14.9	16.5	18.6	21.1
10.2	122	13.9	14.9	16.5	18.7	21.1
10.3	123	13.9	15.0	16.6	18.7	21.2
10.4	124	14.0	15.0	16.6	18.8	21.3
10.5	125	14.0	15.0	16.6	18.8	21.4
10.6	126	14.0	15.1	16.7	18.9	21.5
10.7	127	14.0	15.1	16.7	19.0	21.6
10.8	128	14.1	15.1	16.8	19.0	21.6
10.9	129	14.1	15.2	16.8	19.1	21.7

WHO Child Growth Standards

BMI-for-age BOYS 5 to 19 years (Percentiles)						
Year-Month	**Months**	**3rd**	**15th**	**Median**	**85th**	**97th**
10.10	130	14.1	15.2	16.9	19.1	21.8
10.11	131	14.2	15.2	16.9	19.2	21.9
11.0	132	14.2	15.3	16.9	19.3	22.0
11.1	133	14.2	15.3	17.0	19.3	22.1
11.2	134	14.3	15.3	17.0	19.4	22.2
11.3	135	14.3	15.4	17.1	19.4	22.2
11.4	136	14.3	15.4	17.1	19.5	22.3
11.5	137	14.4	15.4	17.2	19.6	22.4
11.6	138	14.4	15.5	17.2	19.6	22.5
11.7	139	14.4	15.5	17.3	19.7	22.6
11.8	140	14.5	15.6	17.3	19.8	22.7
11.9	141	14.5	15.6	17.4	19.8	22.8
11.10	142	14.5	15.6	17.4	19.9	22.9
11.11	143	14.6	15.7	17.5	20.0	23.0
12.0	144	14.6	15.7	17.5	20.1	23.1
12.1	145	14.6	15.8	17.6	20.1	23.1
12.2	146	14.7	15.8	17.6	20.2	23.2
12.3	147	14.7	15.9	17.7	20.3	23.3
12.4	148	14.8	15.9	17.8	20.3	23.4
12.5	149	14.8	16.0	17.8	20.4	23.5
12.6	150	14.8	16.0	17.9	20.5	23.6
12.7	151	14.9	16.1	17.9	20.6	23.7
12.8	152	14.9	16.1	18.0	20.6	23.8
12.9	153	15.0	16.2	18.0	20.7	23.9
12.10	154	15.0	16.2	18.1	20.8	24.0
12.11	155	15.0	16.3	18.2	20.9	24.1
13.0	156	15.1	16.3	18.2	20.9	24.2
13.1	157	15.1	16.4	18.3	21.0	24.3
13.2	158	15.2	16.4	18.4	21.1	24.4
13.3	159	15.2	16.5	18.4	21.2	24.5
13.4	160	15.3	16.5	18.5	21.3	24.6
13.5	161	15.3	16.6	18.6	21.3	24.7
13.6	162	15.4	16.6	18.6	21.4	24.8
13.7	163	15.4	16.7	18.7	21.5	24.9
13.8	164	15.5	16.7	18.7	21.6	24.9
13.9	165	15.5	16.8	18.8	21.7	25.0

WHO Child Growth Standards

BMI-for-age BOYS 5 to 19 years (Percentiles)						
Year-Month	Months	3rd	15th	Median	85th	97th
13.10	166	15.5	16.8	18.9	21.7	25.1
13.11	167	15.6	16.9	18.9	21.8	25.2
14.0	168	15.6	16.9	19.0	21.9	25.3
14.1	169	15.7	17.0	19.1	22.0	25.4
14.2	170	15.7	17.0	19.1	22.0	25.5
14.3	171	15.8	17.1	19.2	22.1	25.6
14.4	172	15.8	17.2	19.3	22.2	25.7
14.5	173	15.9	17.2	19.3	22.3	25.8
14.6	174	15.9	17.3	19.4	22.4	25.8
14.7	175	16.0	17.3	19.5	22.4	25.9
14.8	176	16.0	17.4	19.5	22.5	26.0
14.9	177	16.1	17.4	19.6	22.6	26.1
14.10	178	16.1	17.5	19.6	22.7	26.2
14.11	179	16.1	17.5	19.7	22.7	26.3
15.0	180	16.2	17.6	19.8	22.8	26.4
15.1	181	16.2	17.6	19.8	22.9	26.4
15.2	182	16.3	17.7	19.9	23.0	26.5
15.3	183	16.3	17.7	20.0	23.0	26.6
15.4	184	16.4	17.8	20.0	23.1	26.7
15.5	185	16.4	17.8	20.1	23.2	26.7
15.6	186	16.4	17.9	20.1	23.2	26.8
15.7	187	16.5	17.9	20.2	23.3	26.9
15.8	188	16.5	18.0	20.3	23.4	27.0
15.9	189	16.6	18.0	20.3	23.5	27.0
15.10	190	16.6	18.1	20.4	23.5	27.1
15.11	191	16.7	18.1	20.4	23.6	27.2
16.0	192	16.7	18.2	20.5	23.7	27.3
16.1	193	16.7	18.2	20.6	23.7	27.3
16.2	194	16.8	18.3	20.6	23.8	27.4
16.3	195	16.8	18.3	20.7	23.9	27.5
16.4	196	16.8	18.4	20.7	23.9	27.5
16.5	197	16.9	18.4	20.8	24.0	27.6
16.6	198	16.9	18.5	20.8	24.0	27.7
16.7	199	17.0	18.5	20.9	24.1	27.7
16.8	200	17.0	18.5	20.9	24.2	27.8
16.9	201	17.0	18.6	21.0	24.2	27.8

WHO Child Growth Standards

BMI-for-age BOYS 5 to 19 years (Percentiles)						
Year-Month	**Months**	**3rd**	**15th**	**Median**	**85th**	**97th**
16.10	202	17.1	18.6	21.0	24.3	27.9
16.11	203	17.1	18.7	21.1	24.3	28.0
17.0	204	17.1	18.7	21.1	24.4	28.0
17.1	205	17.2	18.7	21.2	24.5	28.1
17.2	206	17.2	18.8	21.2	24.5	28.1
17.3	207	17.2	18.8	21.3	24.6	28.2
17.4	208	17.3	18.9	21.3	24.6	28.2
17.5	209	17.3	18.9	21.4	24.7	28.3
17.6	210	17.3	18.9	21.4	24.7	28.4
17.7	211	17.4	19.0	21.5	24.8	28.4
17.8	212	17.4	19.0	21.5	24.8	28.5
17.9	213	17.4	19.1	21.6	24.9	28.5
17.10	214	17.4	19.1	21.6	24.9	28.6
17.11	215	17.5	19.1	21.7	25.0	28.6
18.0	216	17.5	19.2	21.7	25.0	28.6
18.1	217	17.5	19.2	21.8	25.1	28.7
18.2	218	17.5	19.2	21.8	25.1	28.7
18.3	219	17.6	19.3	21.8	25.2	28.8
18.4	220	17.6	19.3	21.9	25.2	28.8
18.5	221	17.6	19.3	21.9	25.3	28.9
18.6	222	17.6	19.4	22.0	25.3	28.9
18.7	223	17.7	19.4	22.0	25.4	29.0
18.8	224	17.7	19.4	22.0	25.4	29.0
18.9	225	17.7	19.5	22.1	25.5	29.0
18.10	226	17.7	19.5	22.1	25.5	29.1
18.11	227	17.8	19.5	22.2	25.5	29.1
19.0	228	17.8	19.5	22.2	25.6	29.1

WHO Child Growth Standards

BMI-for-age GIRLS 5 to 19 years (Percentiles)

Year-Month	Months	3rd	15th	Median	85th	97th
5.1	61	12.9	13.8	15.2	16.9	18.6
5.2	62	12.9	13.8	15.2	16.9	18.6
5.3	63	12.9	13.8	15.2	17.0	18.7
5.4	64	12.9	13.8	15.2	17.0	18.7
5.5	65	12.9	13.8	15.2	17.0	18.7
5.6	66	12.8	13.8	15.2	17.0	18.7
5.7	67	12.8	13.8	15.2	17.0	18.8
5.8	68	12.8	13.8	15.3	17.0	18.8
5.9	69	12.8	13.8	15.3	17.0	18.8
5.10	70	12.8	13.8	15.3	17.0	18.9
5.11	71	12.8	13.8	15.3	17.1	18.9
6.0	72	12.8	13.8	15.3	17.1	18.9
6.1	73	12.8	13.8	15.3	17.1	19.0
6.2	74	12.8	13.8	15.3	17.1	19.0
6.3	75	12.8	13.8	15.3	17.1	19.0
6.4	76	12.8	13.8	15.3	17.2	19.1
6.5	77	12.8	13.8	15.3	17.2	19.1
6.6	78	12.8	13.8	15.3	17.2	19.2
6.7	79	12.8	13.8	15.3	17.2	19.2
6.8	80	12.8	13.8	15.3	17.3	19.3
6.9	81	12.8	13.9	15.4	17.3	19.3
6.10	82	12.9	13.9	15.4	17.3	19.3
6.11	83	12.9	13.9	15.4	17.3	19.4
7.0	84	12.9	13.9	15.4	17.4	19.4
7.1	85	12.9	13.9	15.4	17.4	19.5
7.2	86	12.9	13.9	15.4	17.4	19.6
7.3	87	12.9	13.9	15.5	17.5	19.6
7.4	88	12.9	13.9	15.5	17.5	19.7
7.5	89	12.9	13.9	15.5	17.5	19.7
7.6	90	12.9	14.0	15.5	17.6	19.8
7.7	91	12.9	14.0	15.5	17.6	19.8
7.8	92	13.0	14.0	15.6	17.6	19.9
7.9	93	13.0	14.0	15.6	17.7	20.0

WHO Child Growth Standards

BMI-for-age GIRLS 5 to 19 years (Percentiles)						
Year-Month	**Months**	**3rd**	**15th**	**Median**	**85th**	**97th**
7.10	94	13.0	14.0	15.6	17.7	20.0
7.11	95	13.0	14.0	15.7	17.8	20.1
8.0	96	13.0	14.1	15.7	17.8	20.2
8.1	97	13.0	14.1	15.7	17.9	20.2
8.2	98	13.1	14.1	15.7	17.9	20.3
8.3	99	13.1	14.1	15.8	18.0	20.4
8.4	100	13.1	14.2	15.8	18.0	20.4
8.5	101	13.1	14.2	15.8	18.1	20.5
8.6	102	13.1	14.2	15.9	18.1	20.6
8.7	103	13.2	14.2	15.9	18.2	20.7
8.8	104	13.2	14.3	15.9	18.2	20.7
8.9	105	13.2	14.3	16.0	18.3	20.8
8.10	106	13.2	14.3	16.0	18.3	20.9
8.11	107	13.3	14.4	16.1	18.4	21.0
9.0	108	13.3	14.4	16.1	18.4	21.1
9.1	109	13.3	14.4	16.1	18.5	21.1
9.2	110	13.3	14.4	16.2	18.5	21.2
9.3	111	13.4	14.5	16.2	18.6	21.3
9.4	112	13.4	14.5	16.3	18.7	21.4
9.5	113	13.4	14.5	16.3	18.7	21.5
9.6	114	13.4	14.6	16.3	18.8	21.6
9.7	115	13.5	14.6	16.4	18.8	21.6
9.8	116	13.5	14.6	16.4	18.9	21.7
9.9	117	13.5	14.7	16.5	18.9	21.8
9.10	118	13.6	14.7	16.5	19.0	21.9
9.11	119	13.6	14.7	16.6	19.1	22.0
10.0	120	13.6	14.8	16.6	19.1	22.1
10.1	121	13.6	14.8	16.7	19.2	22.2
10.2	122	13.7	14.9	16.7	19.3	22.2
10.3	123	13.7	14.9	16.8	19.3	22.3
10.4	124	13.7	14.9	16.8	19.4	22.4
10.5	125	13.8	15.0	16.9	19.5	22.5
10.6	126	13.8	15.0	16.9	19.5	22.6
10.7	127	13.9	15.1	17.0	19.6	22.7
10.8	128	13.9	15.1	17.0	19.7	22.8
10.9	129	13.9	15.1	17.1	19.8	22.9

WHO Child Growth Standards

BMI-for-age GIRLS 5 to 19 years (Percentiles)						
Year-Month	Months	3rd	15th	Median	85th	97th
10.10	130	14.0	15.2	17.1	19.8	23.0
10.11	131	14.0	15.2	17.2	19.9	23.1
11.0	132	14.0	15.3	17.2	20.0	23.2
11.1	133	14.1	15.3	17.3	20.0	23.3
11.2	134	14.1	15.4	17.4	20.1	23.4
11.3	135	14.2	15.4	17.4	20.2	23.5
11.4	136	14.2	15.5	17.5	20.3	23.6
11.5	137	14.2	15.5	17.5	20.4	23.7
11.6	138	14.3	15.6	17.6	20.4	23.8
11.7	139	14.3	15.6	17.7	20.5	23.9
11.8	140	14.4	15.7	17.7	20.6	24.0
11.9	141	14.4	15.7	17.8	20.7	24.1
11.10	142	14.5	15.8	17.9	20.8	24.2
11.11	143	14.5	15.8	17.9	20.8	24.3
12.0	144	14.6	15.9	18.0	20.9	24.4
12.1	145	14.6	15.9	18.1	21.0	24.5
12.2	146	14.7	16.0	18.1	21.1	24.6
12.3	147	14.7	16.1	18.2	21.2	24.7
12.4	148	14.7	16.1	18.3	21.3	24.8
12.5	149	14.8	16.2	18.3	21.3	24.9
12.6	150	14.8	16.2	18.4	21.4	25.0
12.7	151	14.9	16.3	18.5	21.5	25.1
12.8	152	14.9	16.3	18.5	21.6	25.2
12.9	153	15.0	16.4	18.6	21.7	25.3
12.10	154	15.0	16.4	18.7	21.8	25.4
12.11	155	15.1	16.5	18.7	21.8	25.5
13.0	156	15.1	16.5	18.8	21.9	25.6
13.1	157	15.2	16.6	18.9	22.0	25.7
13.2	158	15.2	16.7	18.9	22.1	25.8
13.3	159	15.3	16.7	19.0	22.2	25.9
13.4	160	15.3	16.8	19.1	22.3	26.0
13.5	161	15.3	16.8	19.1	22.3	26.1
13.6	162	15.4	16.9	19.2	22.4	26.1
13.7	163	15.4	16.9	19.3	22.5	26.2
13.8	164	15.5	17.0	19.3	22.6	26.3
13.9	165	15.5	17.0	19.4	22.6	26.4

WHO Child Growth Standards

BMI-for-age GIRLS 5 to 19 years (Percentiles)						
Year-Month	**Months**	**3rd**	**15th**	**Median**	**85th**	**97th**
13.10	166	15.6	17.1	19.4	22.7	26.5
13.11	167	15.6	17.1	19.5	22.8	26.6
14.0	168	15.6	17.2	19.6	22.9	26.7
14.1	169	15.7	17.2	19.6	22.9	26.8
14.2	170	15.7	17.3	19.7	23.0	26.8
14.3	171	15.8	17.3	19.7	23.1	26.9
14.4	172	15.8	17.4	19.8	23.2	27.0
14.5	173	15.8	17.4	19.9	23.2	27.1
14.6	174	15.9	17.4	19.9	23.3	27.1
14.7	175	15.9	17.5	20.0	23.4	27.2
14.8	176	15.9	17.5	20.0	23.4	27.3
14.9	177	16.0	17.6	20.1	23.5	27.4
14.10	178	16.0	17.6	20.1	23.5	27.4
14.11	179	16.0	17.6	20.2	23.6	27.5
15.0	180	16.1	17.7	20.2	23.7	27.6
15.1	181	16.1	17.7	20.3	23.7	27.6
15.2	182	16.1	17.8	20.3	23.8	27.7
15.3	183	16.2	17.8	20.4	23.8	27.7
15.4	184	16.2	17.8	20.4	23.9	27.8
15.5	185	16.2	17.9	20.4	23.9	27.9
15.6	186	16.2	17.9	20.5	24.0	27.9
15.7	187	16.3	17.9	20.5	24.0	28.0
15.8	188	16.3	18.0	20.6	24.1	28.0
15.9	189	16.3	18.0	20.6	24.1	28.1
15.10	190	16.3	18.0	20.6	24.2	28.1
15.11	191	16.4	18.0	20.7	24.2	28.2
16.0	192	16.4	18.1	20.7	24.2	28.2
16.1	193	16.4	18.1	20.7	24.3	28.2
16.2	194	16.4	18.1	20.8	24.3	28.3
16.3	195	16.4	18.1	20.8	24.4	28.3
16.4	196	16.5	18.2	20.8	24.4	28.4
16.5	197	16.5	18.2	20.9	24.4	28.4
16.6	198	16.5	18.2	20.9	24.5	28.4
16.7	199	16.5	18.2	20.9	24.5	28.5
16.8	200	16.5	18.3	20.9	24.5	28.5
16.9	201	16.5	18.3	21.0	24.6	28.5

WHO Child Growth Standards

BMI-for-age GIRLS 5 to 19 years (Percentiles)						
Year-Month	Months	3rd	15th	Median	85th	97th
16.10	202	16.6	18.3	21.0	24.6	28.6
16.11	203	16.6	18.3	21.0	24.6	28.6
17.0	204	16.6	18.3	21.0	24.7	28.6
17.1	205	16.6	18.3	21.1	24.7	28.6
17.2	206	16.6	18.4	21.1	24.7	28.7
17.3	207	16.6	18.4	21.1	24.7	28.7
17.4	208	16.6	18.4	21.1	24.8	28.7
17.5	209	16.6	18.4	21.1	24.8	28.7
17.6	210	16.6	18.4	21.2	24.8	28.8
17.7	211	16.6	18.4	21.2	24.8	28.8
17.8	212	16.7	18.4	21.2	24.8	28.8
17.9	213	16.7	18.5	21.2	24.9	28.8
17.10	214	16.7	18.5	21.2	24.9	28.8
17.11	215	16.7	18.5	21.2	24.9	28.9
18.0	216	16.7	18.5	21.3	24.9	28.9
18.1	217	16.7	18.5	21.3	24.9	28.9
18.2	218	16.7	18.5	21.3	25.0	28.9
18.3	219	16.7	18.5	21.3	25.0	28.9
18.4	220	16.7	18.5	21.3	25.0	28.9
18.5	221	16.7	18.5	21.3	25.0	28.9
18.6	222	16.7	18.5	21.3	25.0	29.0
18.7	223	16.7	18.6	21.4	25.0	29.0
18.8	224	16.7	18.6	21.4	25.1	29.0
18.9	225	16.7	18.6	21.4	25.1	29.0
18.10	226	16.7	18.6	21.4	25.1	29.0
18.11	227	16.7	18.6	21.4	25.1	29.0
19.0	228	16.7	18.6	21.4	25.1	29.0

WHO Child Growth Standards

Intra Uterine Growth Weight Chart
Both Sexes (AIIMS, New Delhi)

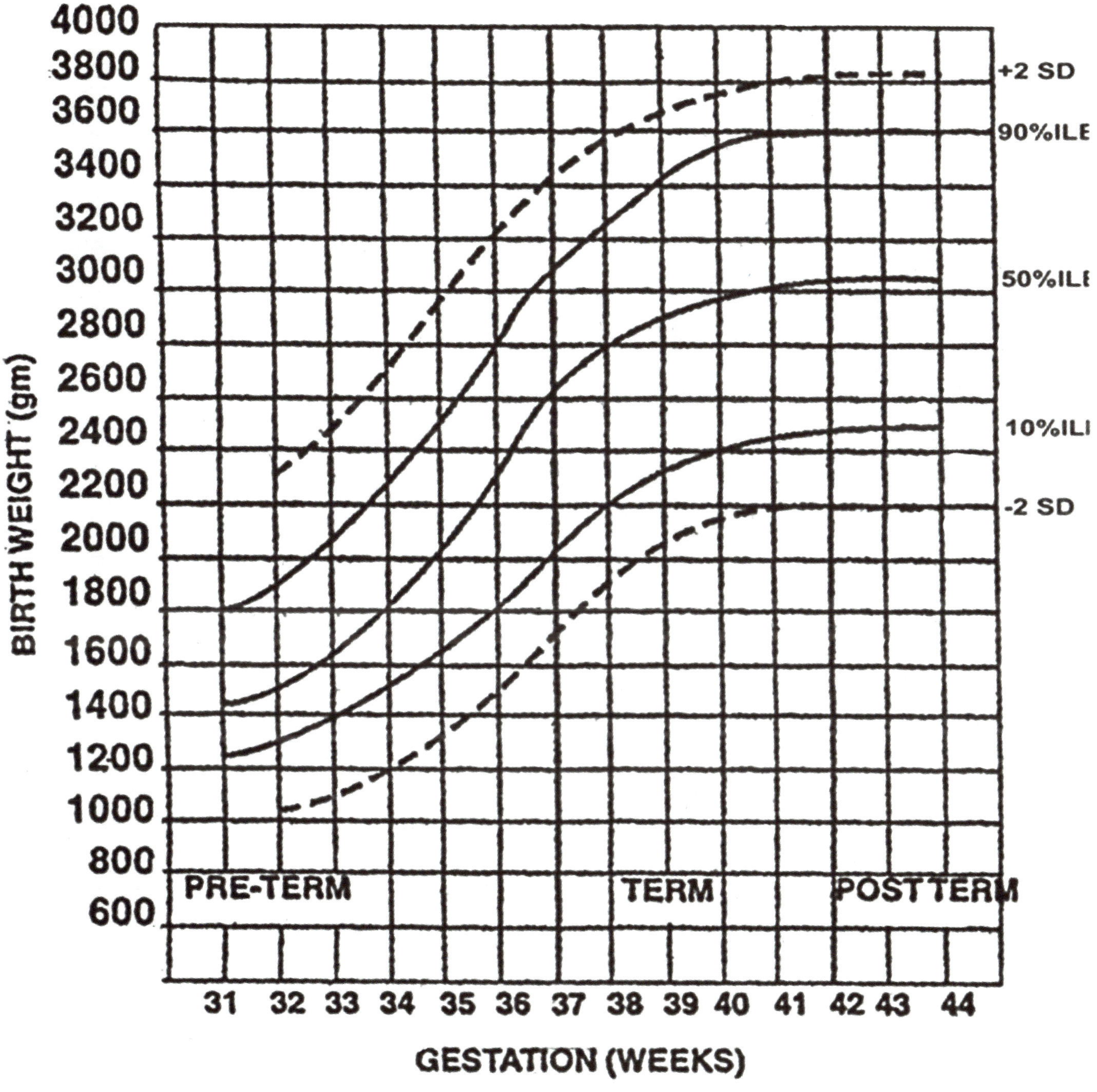

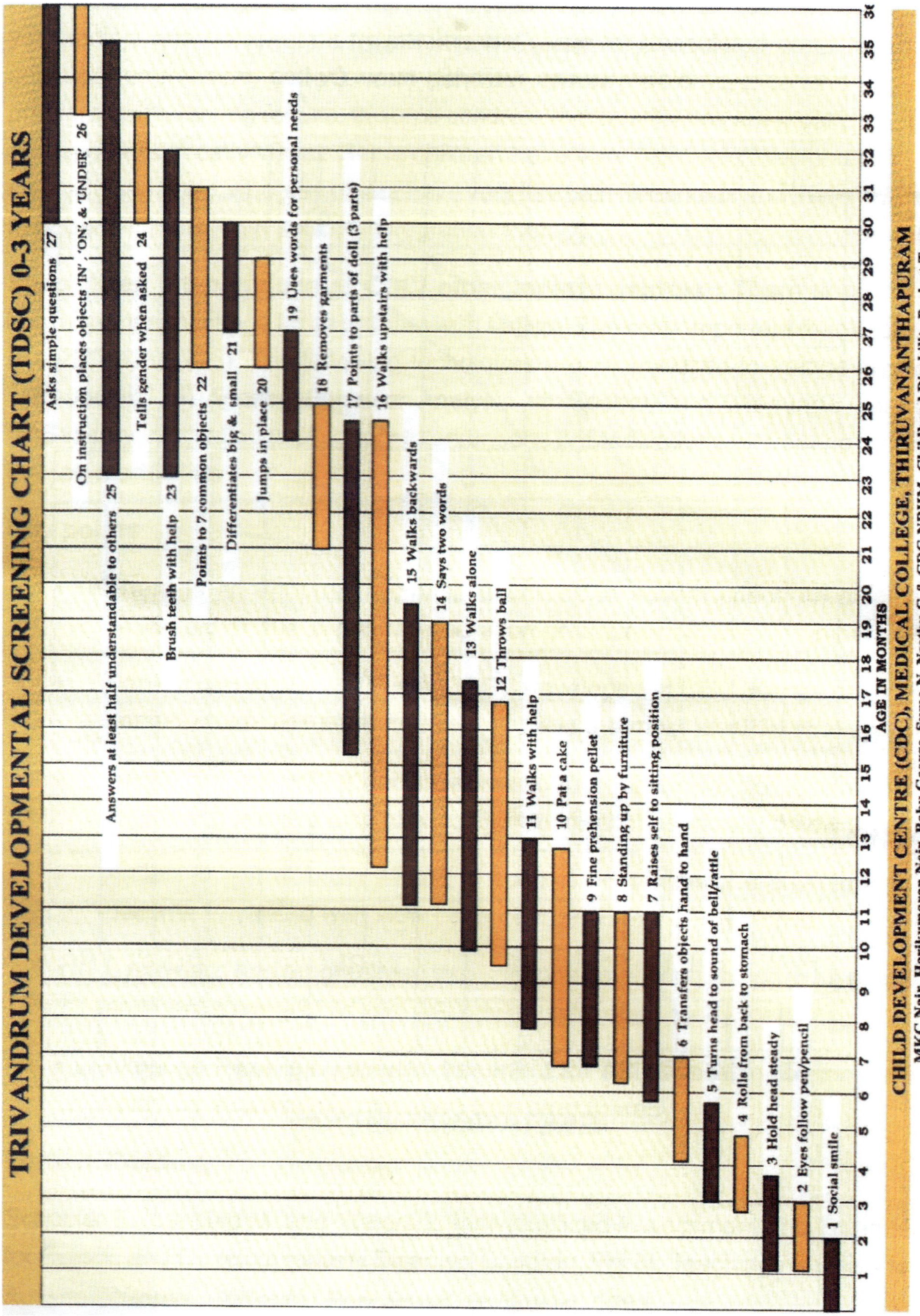

Indian Pediatrics - August 1991, Vol. 28, Number 8

BMI-for-age BOYS

Birth to 5 years (percentiles)

World Health Organization

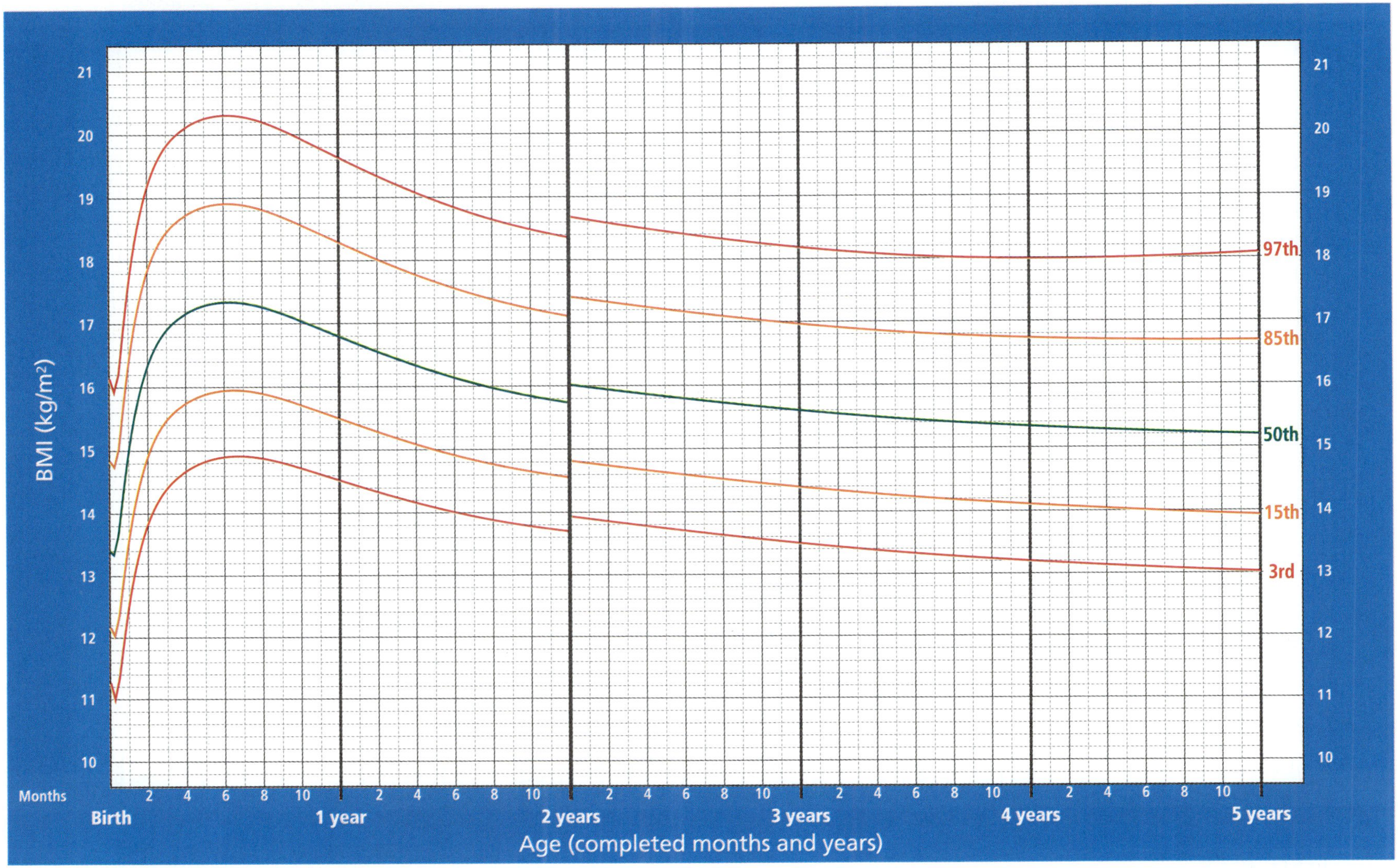

WHO Child Growth Standards

BMI-for-age GIRLS

5 to 19 years (percentiles)

World Health Organization

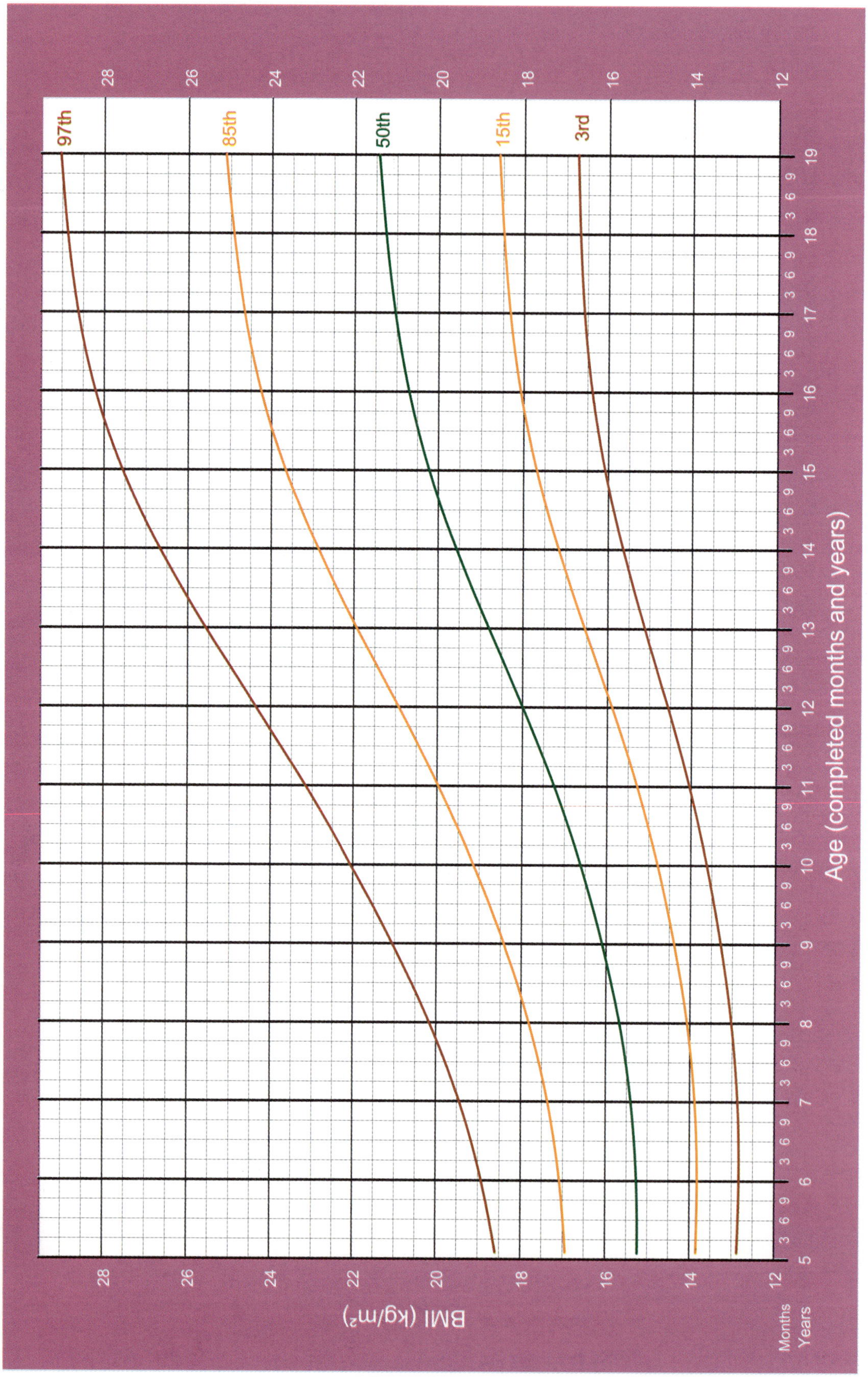

2007 WHO Reference

BMI-for-age GIRLS

Birth to 5 years (percentiles)

World Health Organization

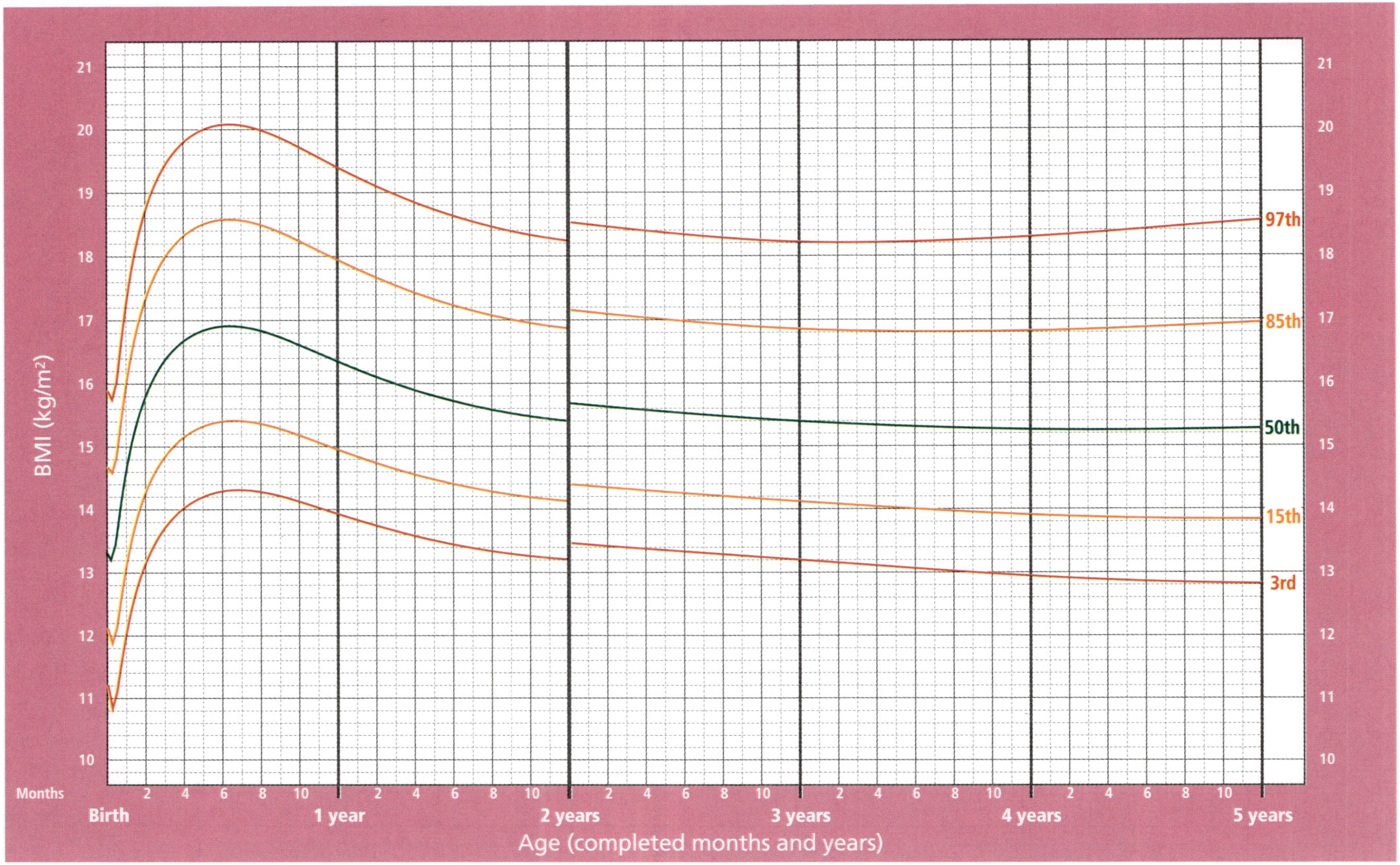

WHO Child Growth Standards

Head circumference-for-age GIRLS

Birth to 5 years (percentiles)

World Health Organization

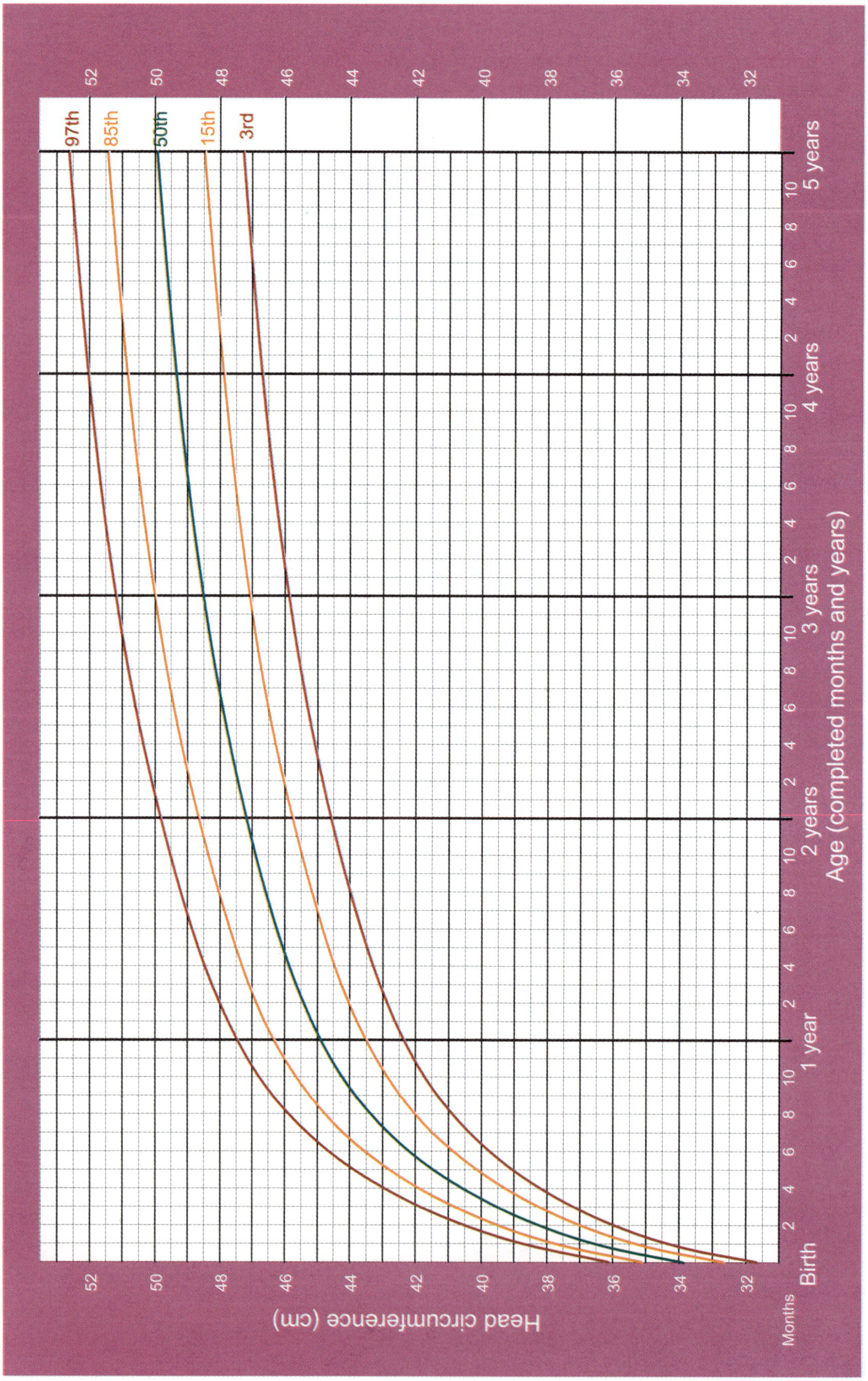

WHO Child Growth Standards

Head circumference-for-age GIRLS

World Health Organization

Birth to 2 years (percentiles)

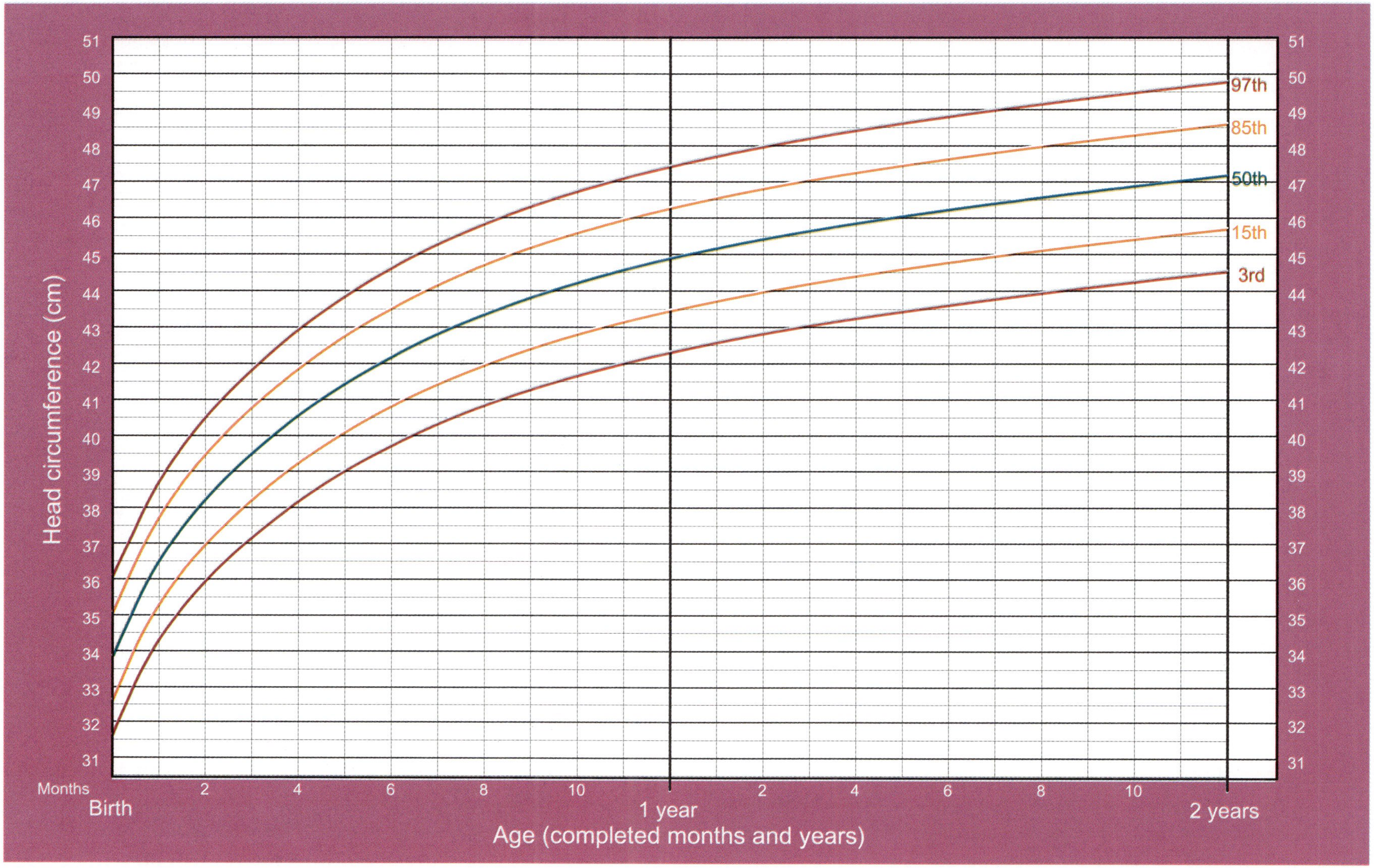

WHO Child Growth Standards

Head circumference-for-age GIRLS

World Health Organization

Birth to 13 weeks (percentiles)

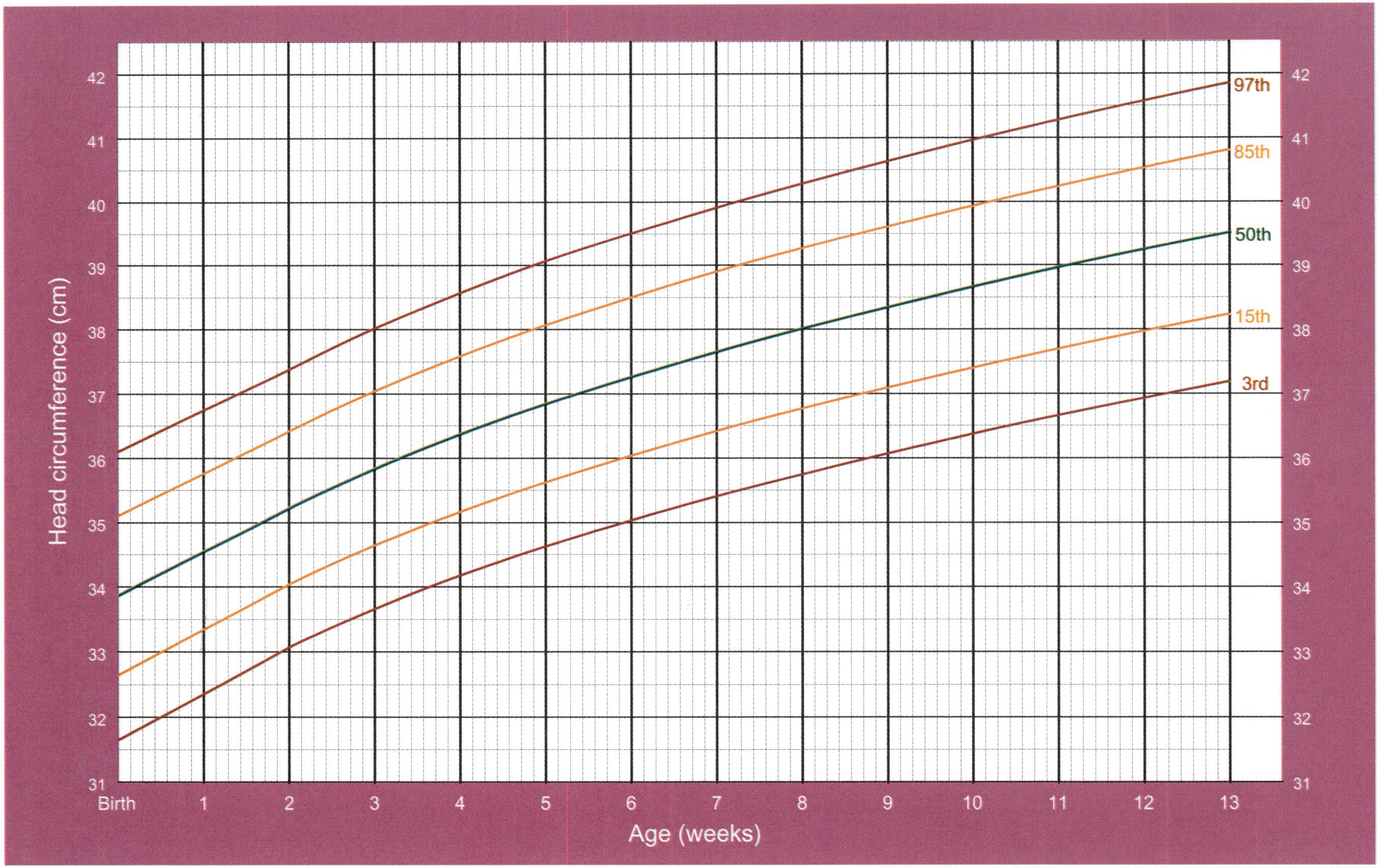

WHO Child Growth Standards

Length-for-age BOYS

6 months to 2 years (percentiles)

World Health Organization

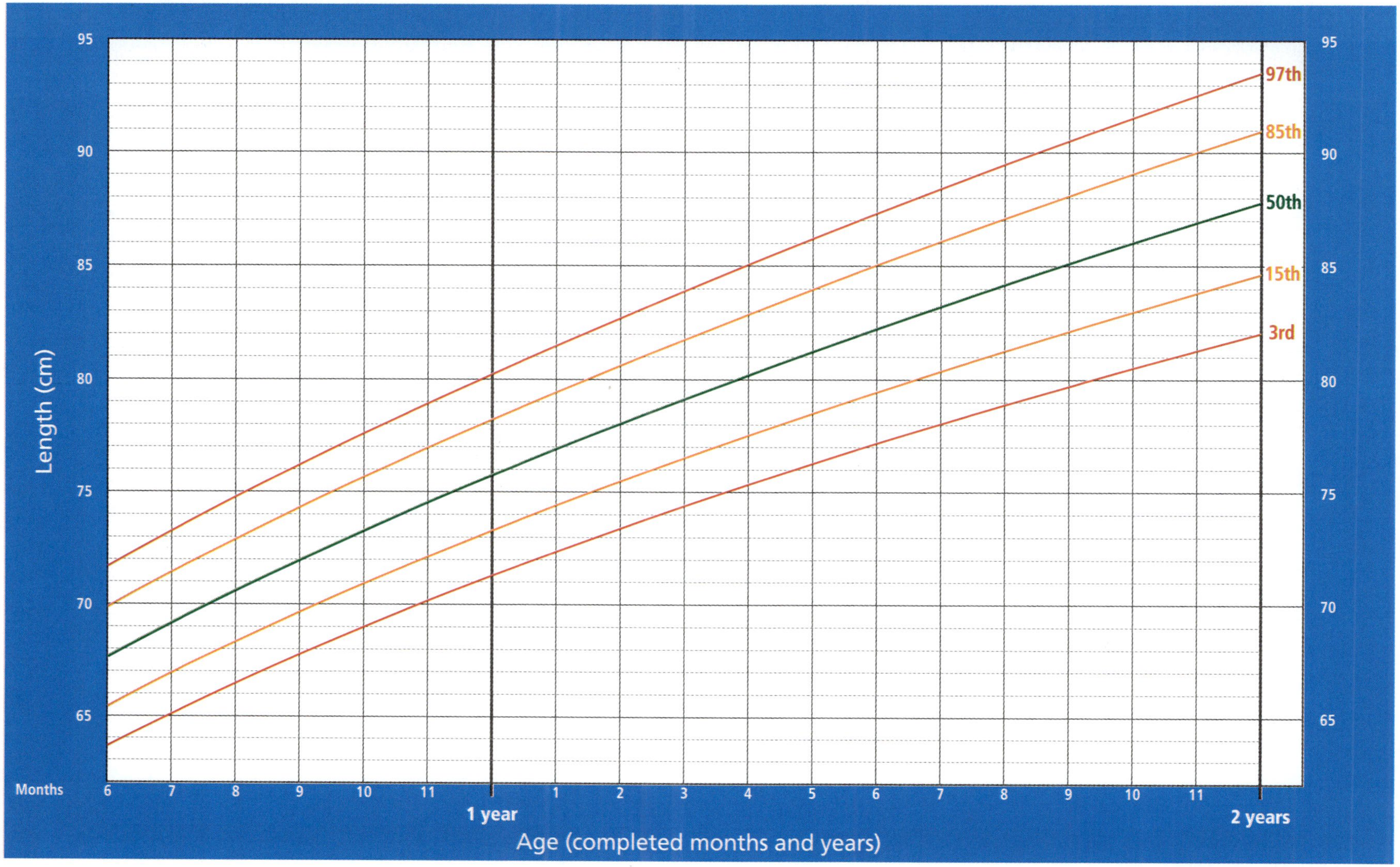

WHO Child Growth Standards

Length-for-age BOYS

World Health Organization

Birth to 6 months (percentiles)

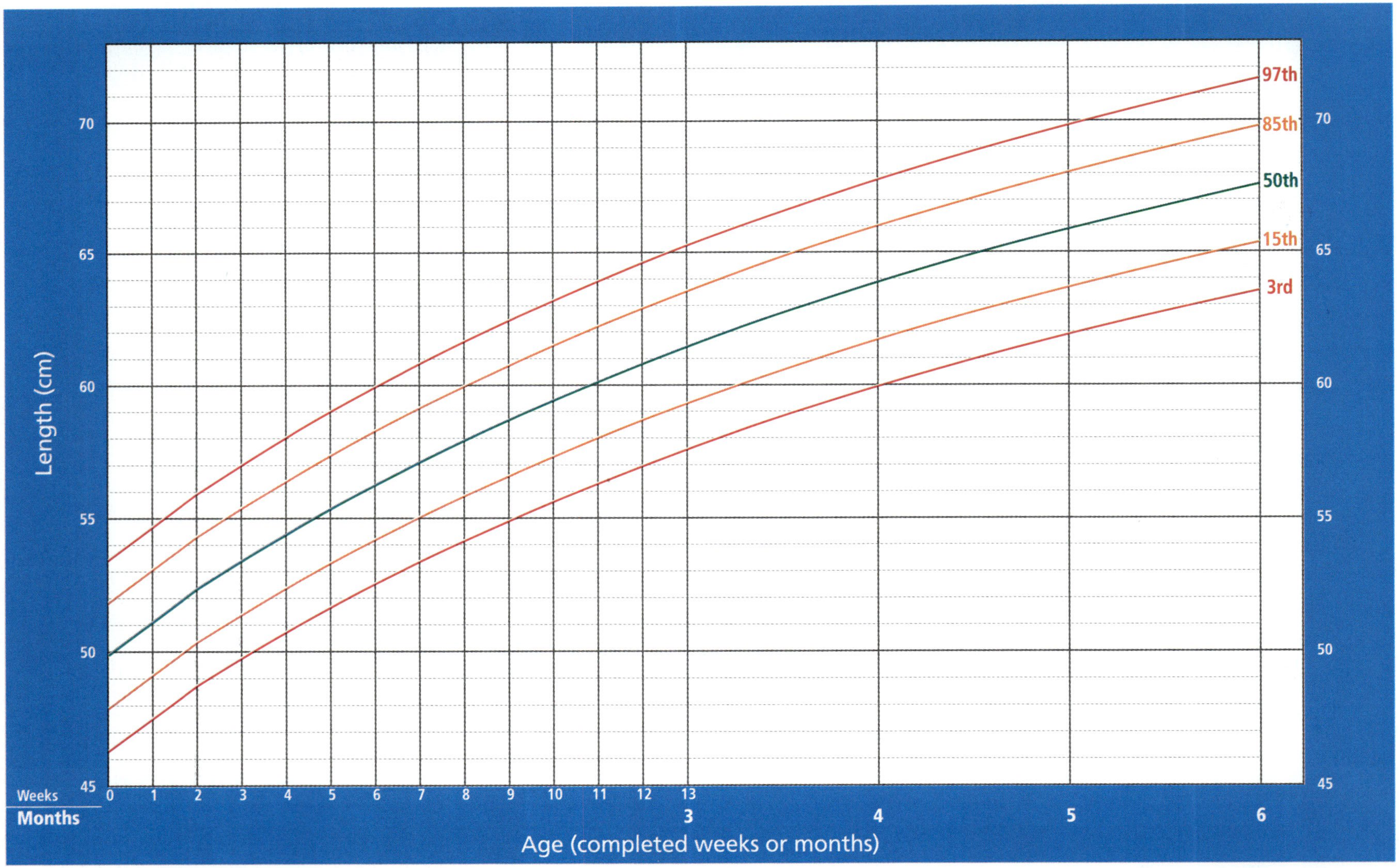

WHO Child Growth Standards

Length-for-age GIRLS

Birth to 6 months (percentiles)

World Health Organization

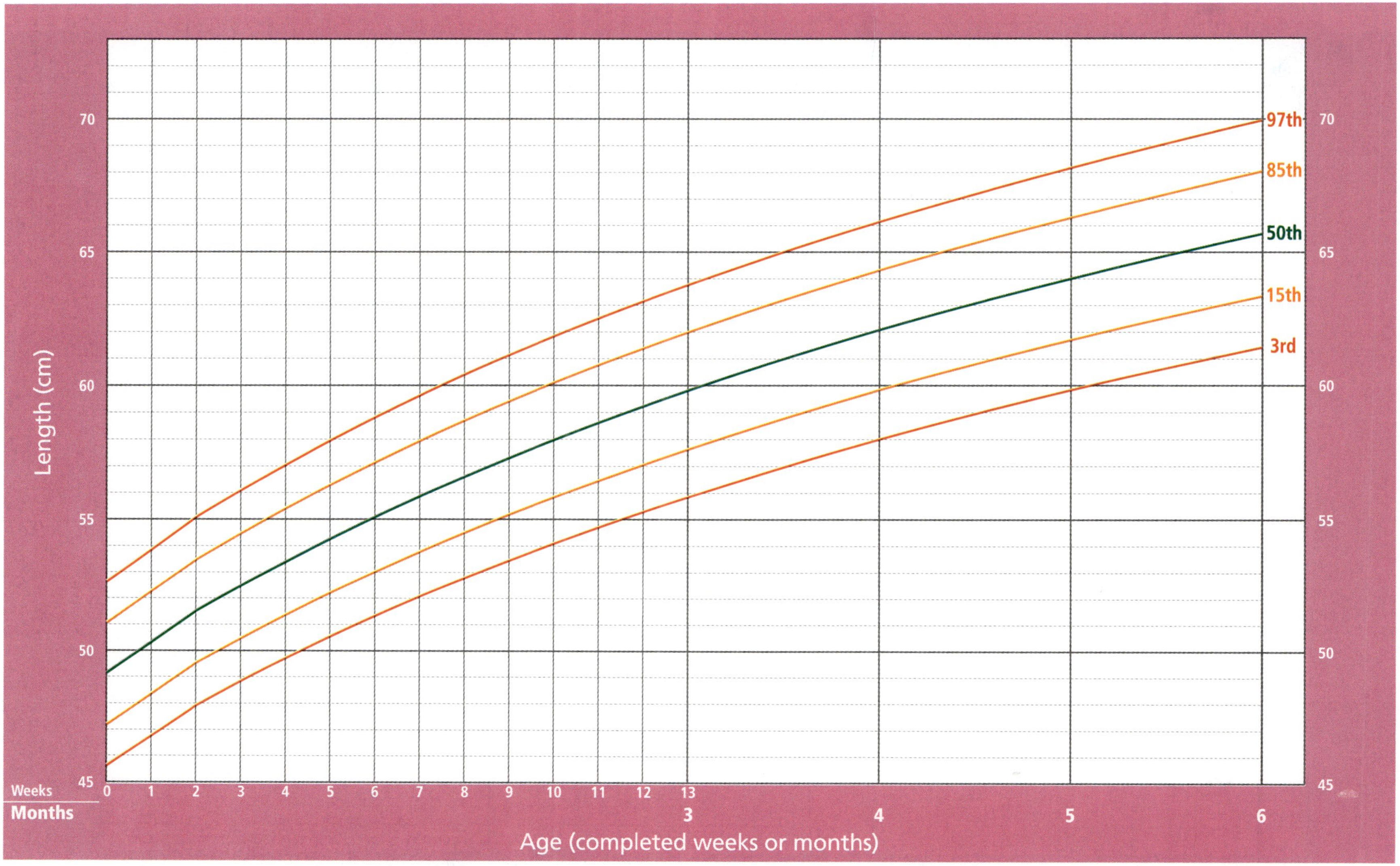

WHO Child Growth Standards

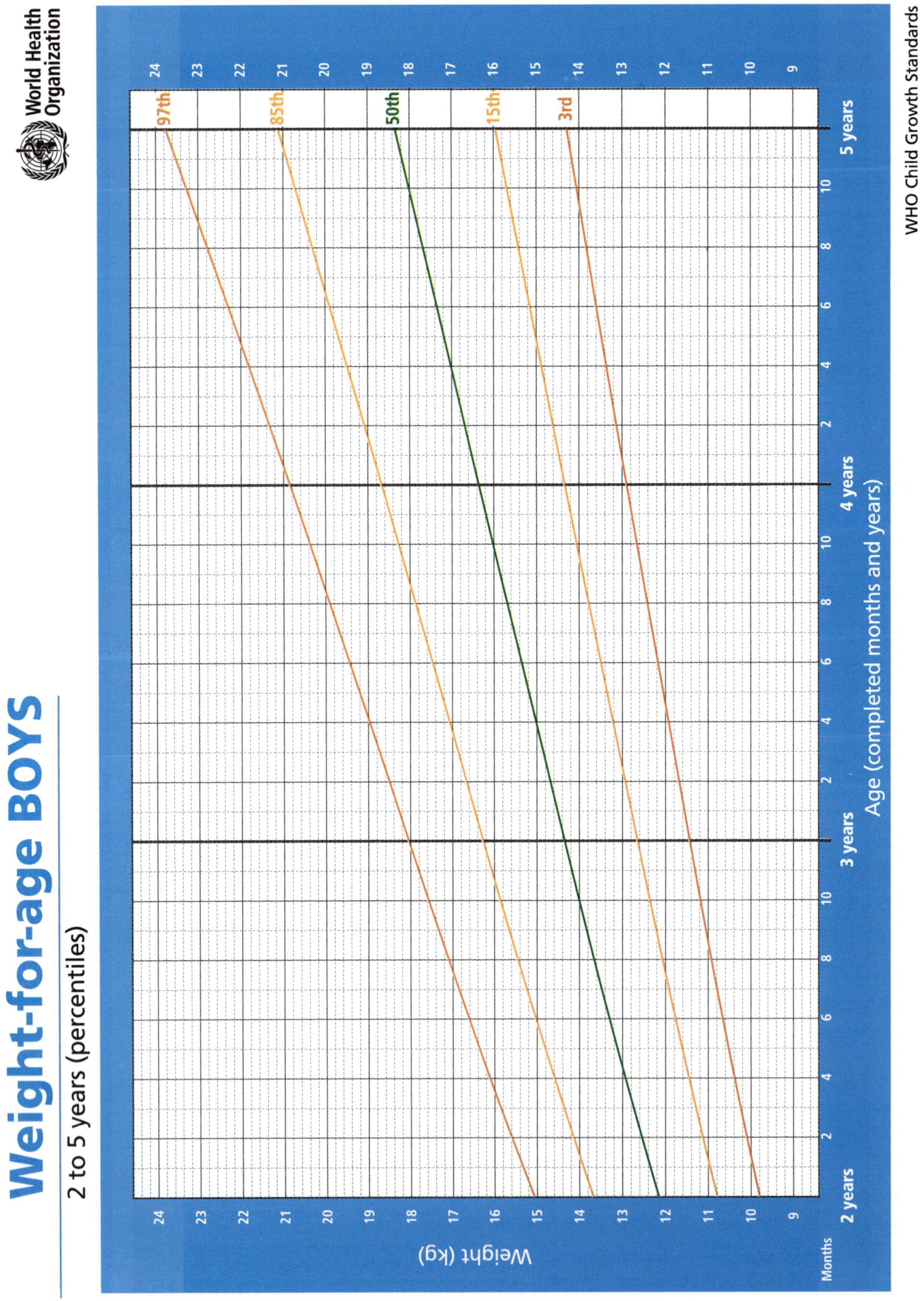

Weight-for-age BOYS
2 to 5 years (percentiles)
World Health Organization
97th
85th
50th
15th
3rd
Weight (kg)
24
23
22
21
20
19
18
17
16
15
14
13
12
11
10
9
Months
2 years
2
4
6
8
10
3 years
4 years
5 years
Age (completed months and years)
WHO Child Growth Standards

Weight-for-age BOYS

6 months to 2 years (percentiles)

World Health Organization

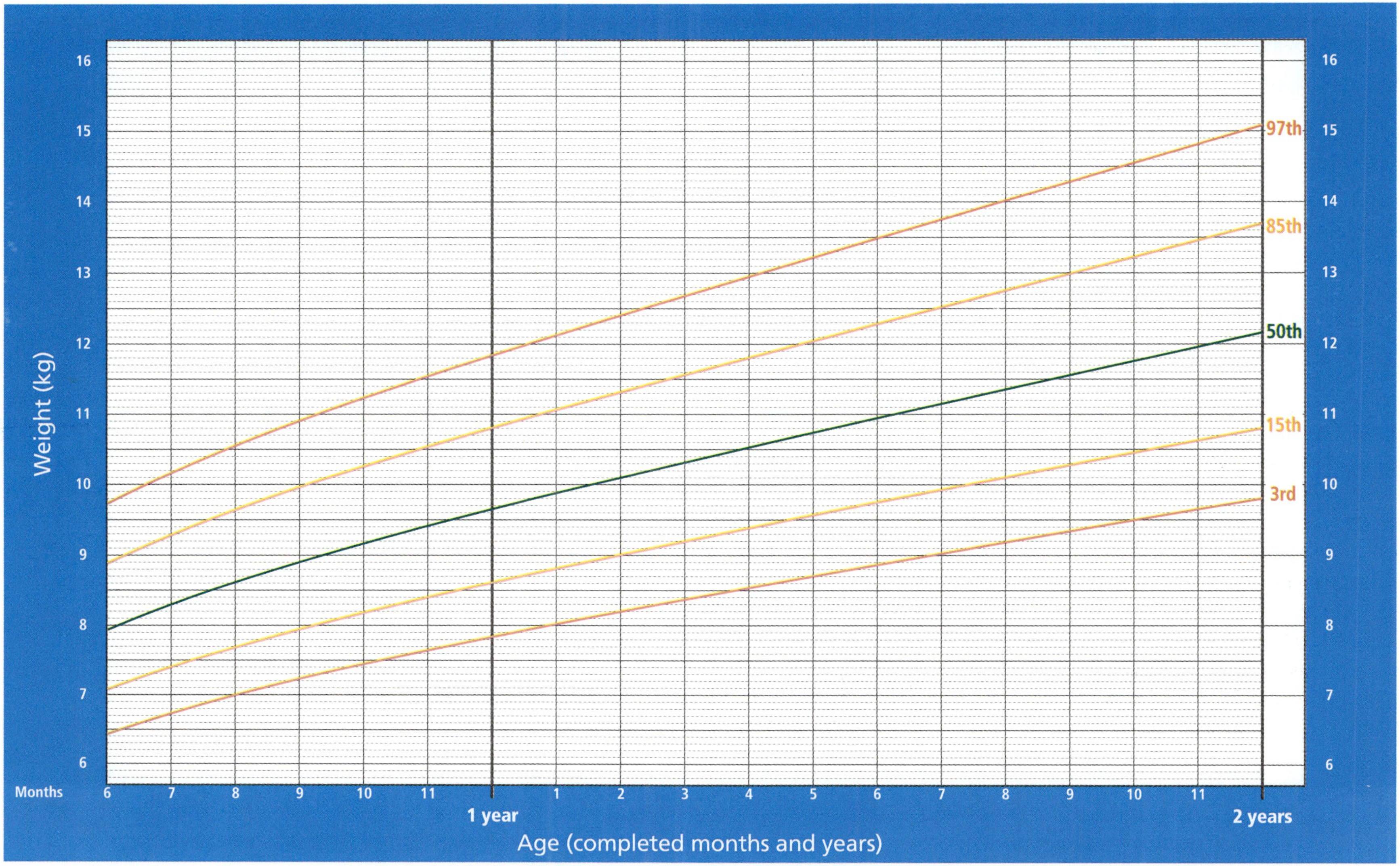

WHO Child Growth Standards

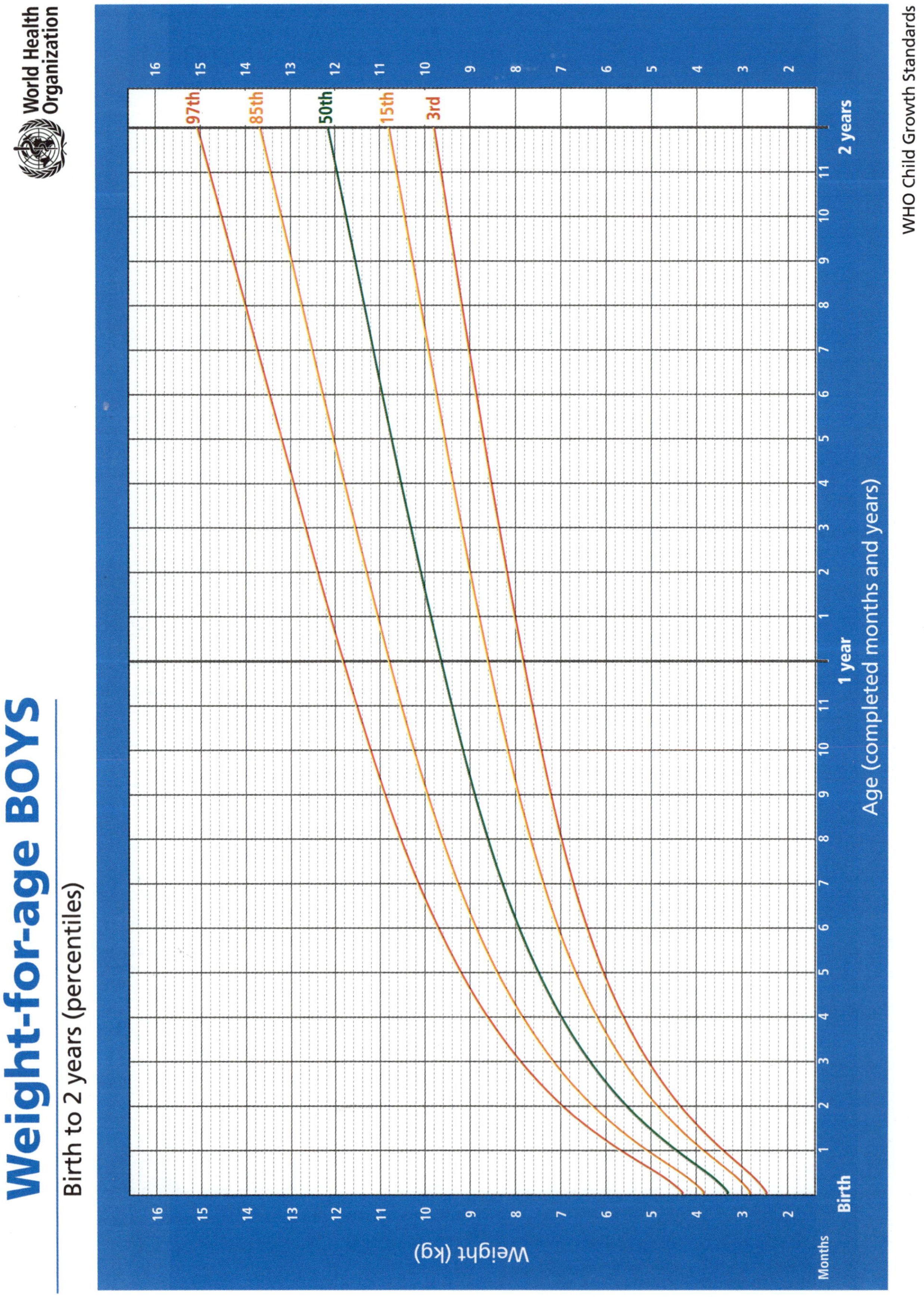
Weight-for-age BOYS
Birth to 2 years (percentiles)
World Health Organization
97th
85th
50th
15th
3rd
Weight (kg)
Months
Birth
1 year
2 years
Age (completed months and years)
WHO Child Growth Standards

Weight-for-height BOYS

2 to 5 years (percentiles)

World Health Organization

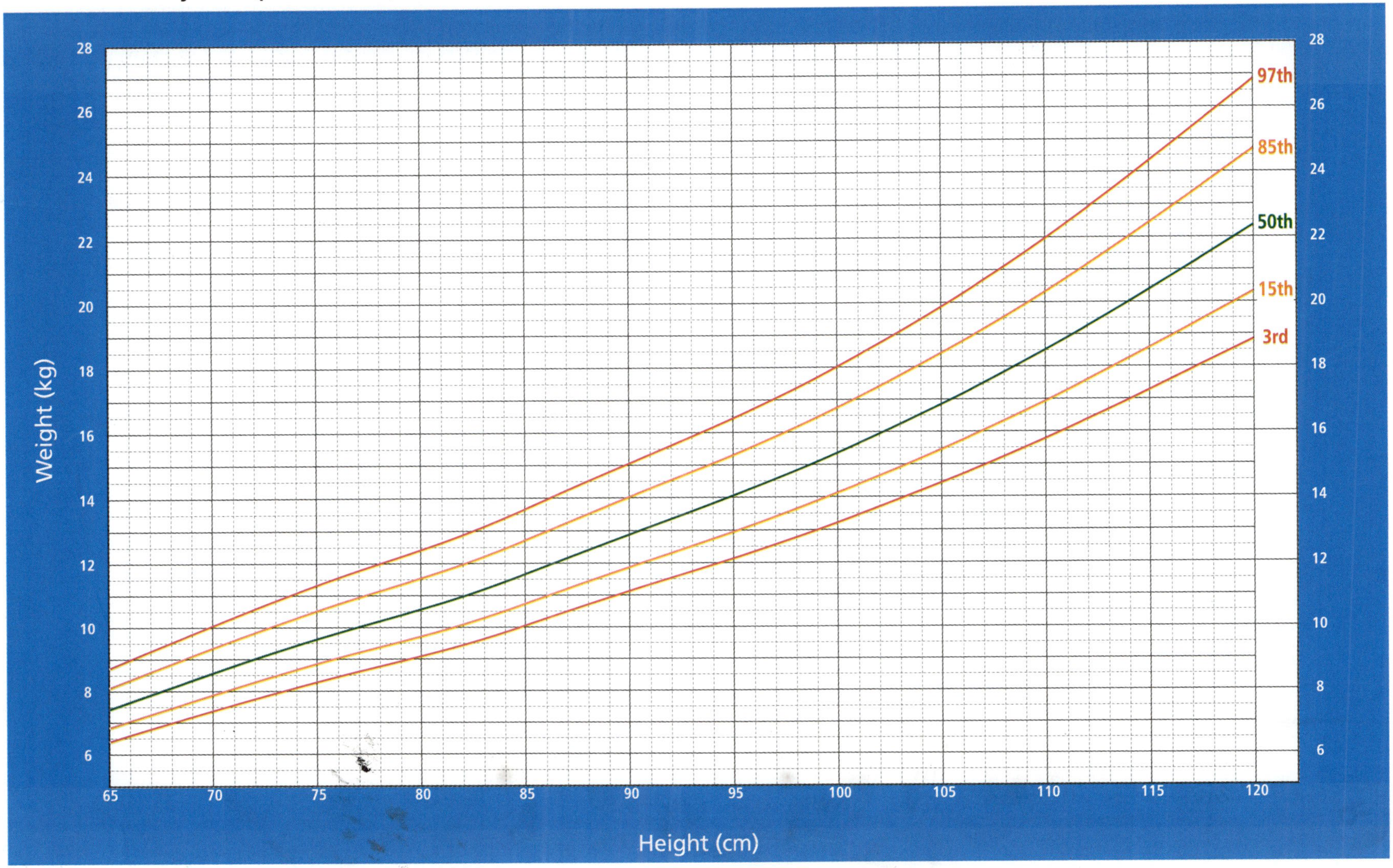

WHO Child Growth Standards

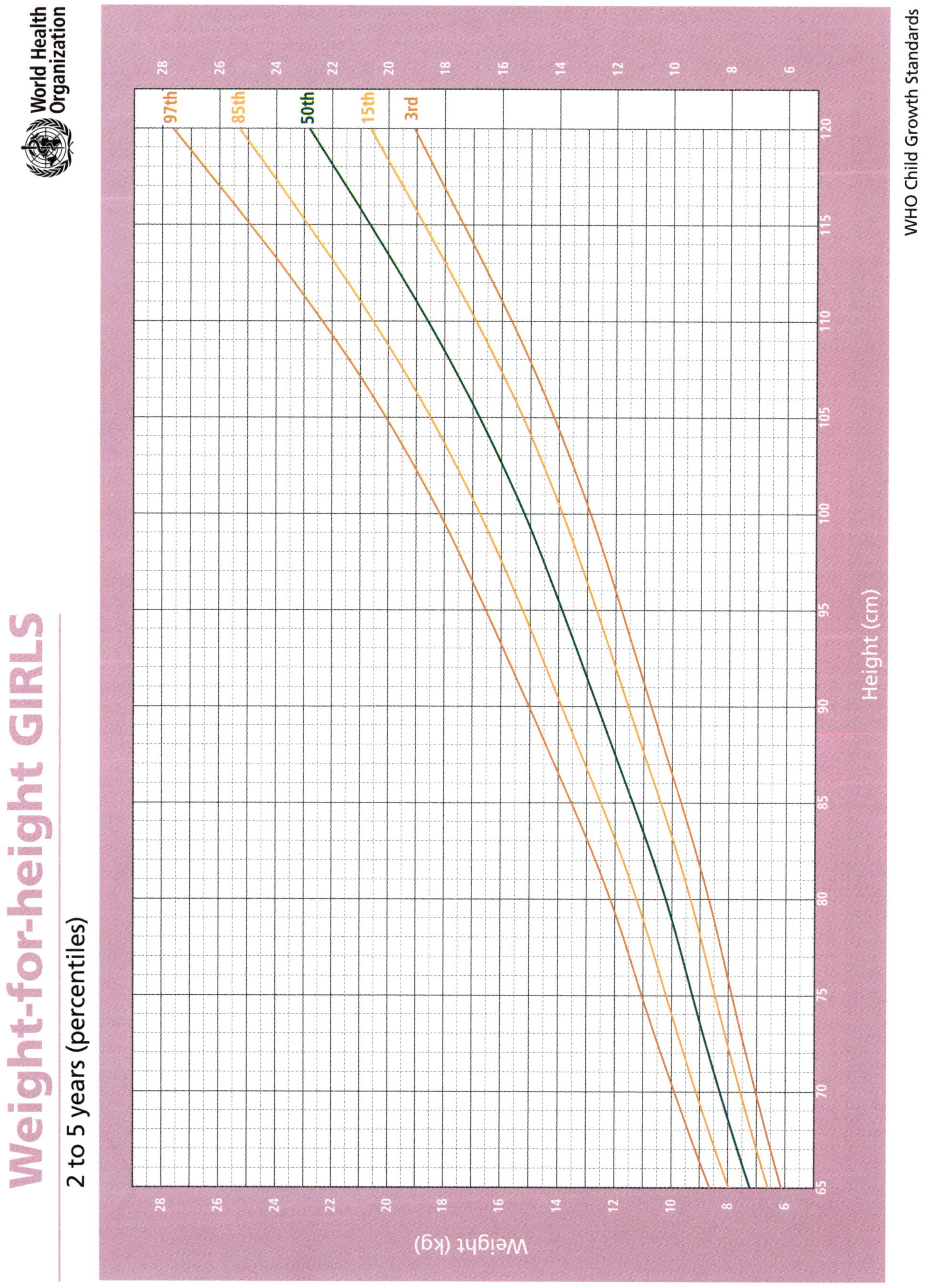
Weight-for-height GIRLS
2 to 5 years (percentiles)
World Health Organization
WHO Child Growth Standards
97th
85th
50th
15th
3rd
Height (cm)
65 70 75 80 85 90 95 100 105 110 115 120
Weight (kg)
6 8 10 12 14 16 18 20 22 24 26 28

Weight-for-length BOYS

World Health Organization

Birth to 2 years (percentiles)

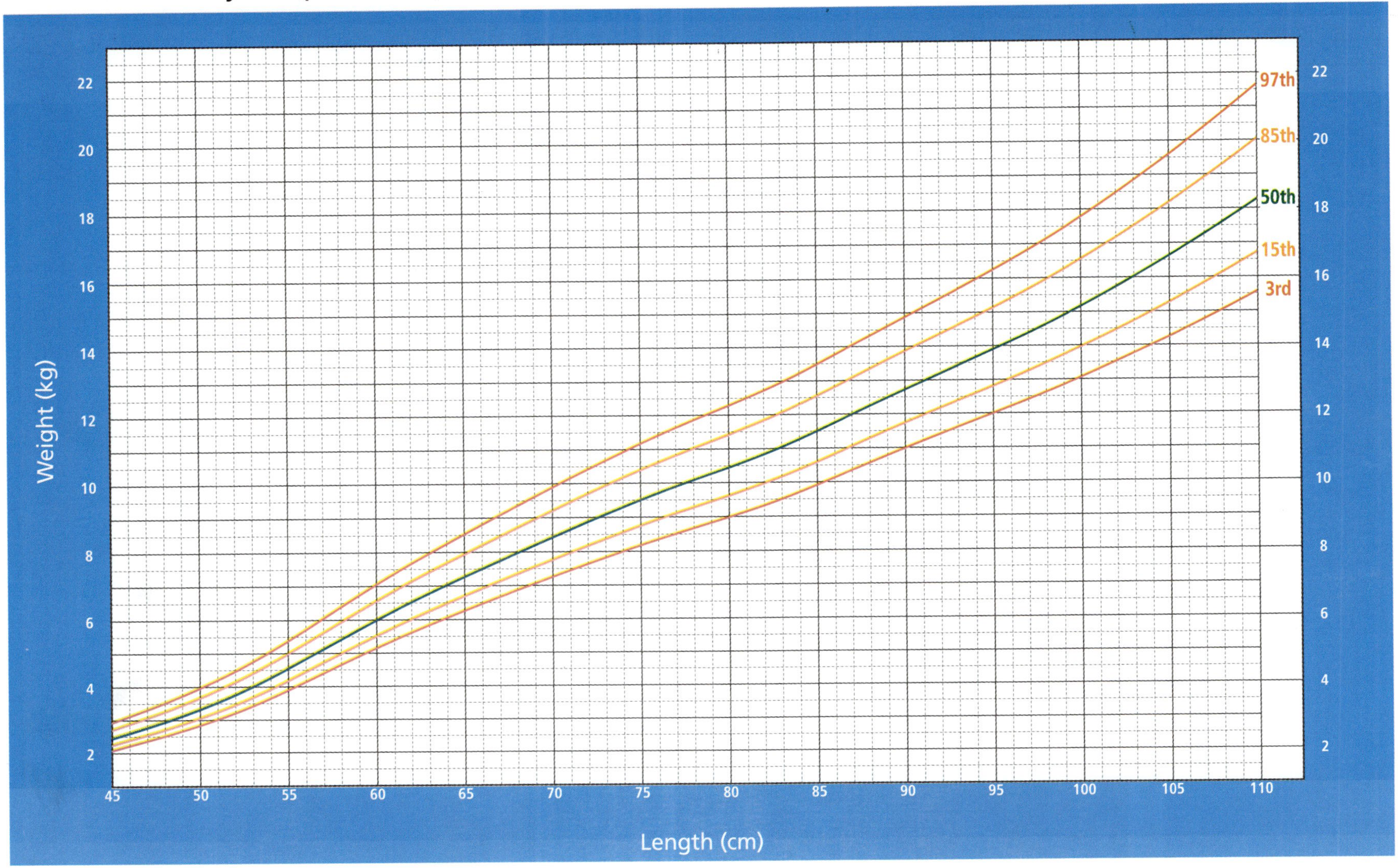

WHO Child Growth Standards

Windows of achievement for six gross motor milestones

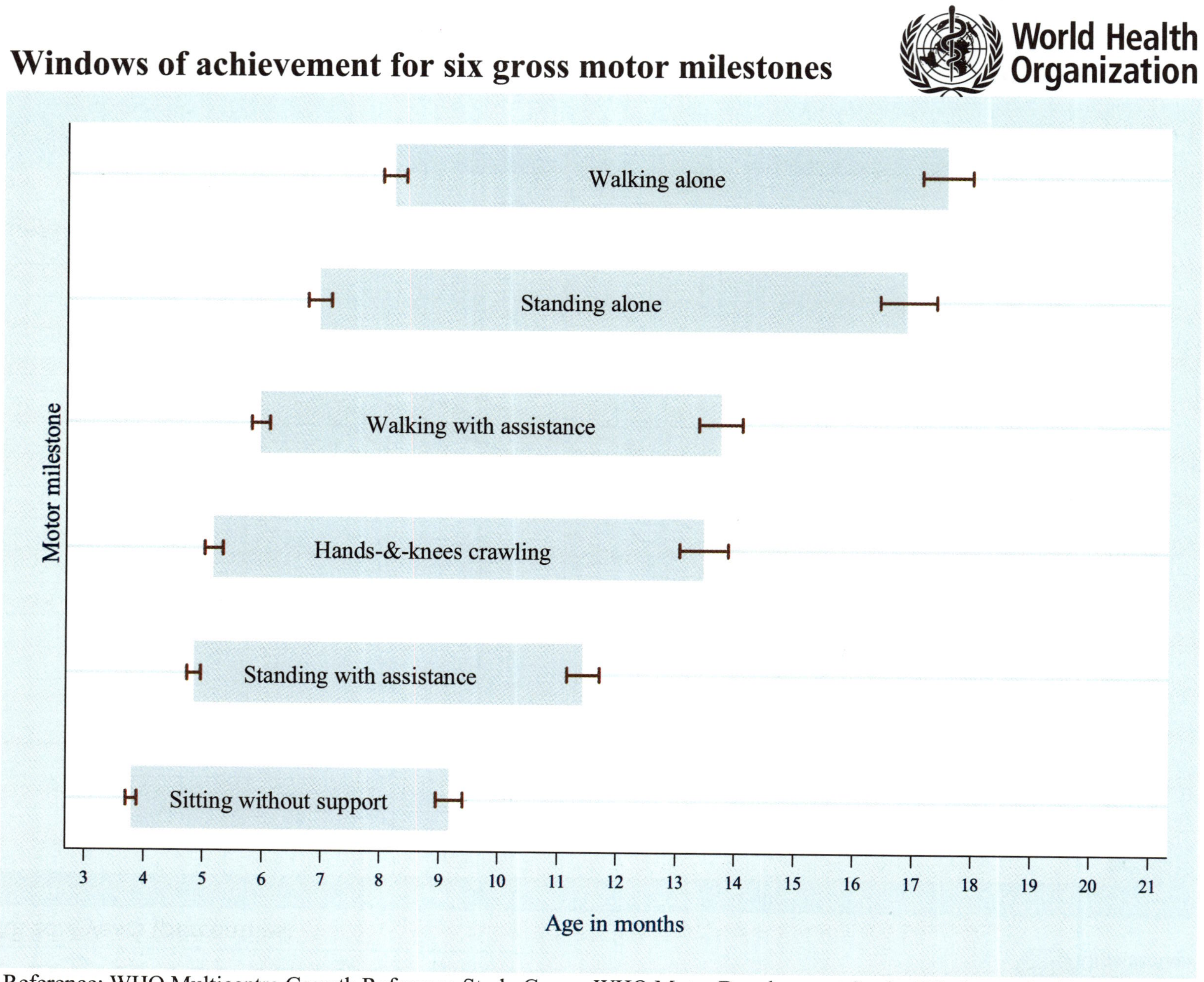

Reference: WHO Multicentre Growth Reference Study Group. WHO Motor Development Study: Windows of achievement for six gross motor development milestones. Acta Paediatrica Supplement 2006;450:86-95.

Index